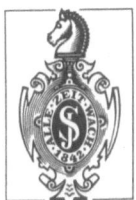

ATHERO-SCLEROSIS III

Proceedings of the
Third International Symposium

Edited by G. SCHETTLER and A. WEIZEL

With 349 Figures and 222 Tables

Springer-Verlag
Berlin Heidelberg New York 1974

Proceedings of the Third International Symposium on Atherosclerosis

Held in West-Berlin, October 24–28th, 1973

Sponsored by the

Bundesministerium für Jugend, Familie und Gesundheit
Senat der Stadt Berlin
American Heart Association
British Atherosclerosis Discussion Group
European Atherosclerosis Group
International Society of Cardiology
National Institutes of Health, Bethesda, MD/USA
Ontario Heart Foundation

ISBN-13: 978-3-642-65956-0   e-ISBN-13: 978-3-642-65954-6
DOI: 10.1007/978-3-642-65954-6

Library of Congress Cataloging in Publication Data. International Symposium on Atherosclerosis, 3d, Berlin, 1973. Atherosclerosis. Bibliography: p. 1. Arteriosclerosis-- Congresses. I. Schettler, Friedrich Gotthard, ed. II. Weizel, A., 1940- ed. [DNLM: 1. Arteriosclerosis--Congresses. W3 IN916AG 1973a/WG550 162 1973a] RC692.Is 1973   616.1'36   74–14636

Softcover reprint of the hardcover 1st edition 1974

ACKNOWLEDGEMENTS

We wish to express our gratitude to the Minister, Mrs. Focke, and to the "Bundesministerium für Jugend, Familie und Gesundheit" and the "Senat der Stadt Berlin" for their generous financial support which enabled the organization of this symposium and the publication of its proceedings.

This Symposium would not have been possible without the generous financial support of the following foundations, individuals and companies:

Bundesministerium für Jugend, Familie und
  Gesundheit
Senat der Stadt Berlin
American Heart Association
British Atherosclerosis Discussion Group
European Atherosclerosis Group
International Society of Cardiology
National Institutes of Health
Ontario Heart Foundation

and by the following:

Asta-Werke AG, Brackwede
Astra Läkemedel, AB, Södertälje, Sweden
Baxter Laboratories, Morton Grove,
  Illinois, USA
Bayer, Leverkusen-Bayerwerk
Behringwerke AG, Frankfurt/Main
Best Foods, Union, N.J., USA
Boehringer Mannheim GmbH, Mannheim
C. H. Boehringer Sohn, Ingelheim
Bofors Nobel Pharma, Mölndal, Sweden
Byk-Gulden Lomberg, Chem. Fabrik GmbH
Cassella-Riedel Pharma GmbH,
  Frankfurt/Main
Chemiewerk Homburg, Frankfurt/Main
Ciba-Geigy AG, Wehr/Baden
Cilag-Chemie GmbH, Alsbach a. d. Bergstr.
The Dow Chemical Company, USA
Deutsche Kabi GmbH, München
Eternit AG, Berlin
Farbwerke Hoechst AG, Frankfurt/Main
Fisons Corporation, Bedford, MA, USA
Gödecke AG, Freiburg
Hoffmann-La Roche AG, Grenzach/Baden
Hoffmann-La Roche, Nutley, N. J., USA
Immuno GmbH, Heidelberg
Janssen GmbH, Düsseldorf
Kali-Chemie AG, Hannover

Adolf Klinge & Co., München
Knoll AG, Ludwigshafen
Eli Lilly GmbH, Gießen
Lilly Research Laboratories, Indianapolis,
USA
Live Stock & Meat Board, USA
Luitpold-Werk, München
Dr. Madaus & Co., Köln
Maizena Gesellschaft mbH, Hamburg
E. Merck, Darmstadt
Merck, Institute for experim. research,
Rahway, N.J., USA
L. Merckle KG, Blaubeuren
A. Nattermann & Cie GmbH, Köln
Nestle, Vevey, Schweiz
Nordmark-Werke GmbH, Hamburg
Pharma Stern GmbH, Wedel
Pharmacia AB, Uppsala, Sweden
Pfizer GmbH, Karlsruhe
Pfizer AB, Täby, Sweden
Pfizer, Kent, England
Procter & Gamble Company, Cincinnati,
Ohio, USA
Rhein-Pharma Arzneimittelwerk, Plankstadt
Albert Roussel Pharma GmbH, Wiesbaden
Sandoz AG, Nürnberg,
Sandoz AB, Täby, Sweden
Sandoz-Wander Inc., East Hanover,
N.J., USA
Sanol Arzneimittel Dr. Schwarz GmbH,
  Monheim
Scanmeda, Göteborg, Sweden
Schering AG, Berlin
Schering Corp., Bloomfield, N.J., USA
Sharp & Dohme GmbH, München
Siegfried GmbH, Säckingen
Smith Kline & French Laboratories,
  Philadelphia, USA

Solco GmbH, Wyhlen, Schweiz
Svenska-Hoechst AB, Stockholm, Sweden
Syntex Laboratories Inc., Palo Alto,
  California, USA
Dr. Karl Thomae GmbH, Biberach a. d. Riß
Troponwerke Dinklage & Co., Köln
Union Deutscher Lebensmittelwerke
  (Deutsche Unilever) GmbH, Hamburg
The Upjohn Company, Kalamazoo,
  Michigan, USA

Wander GmbH, Frankfurt/Main
Hans Weist, Heppenheim a. d. Bergstraße
Wellcome Research Laboratories, N.C., USA
Wirtschaftsverband Asbest E.V.,
  Frankfurt/Main
Johann A. Wülfing-Bauer & Cie., Neuss
Wyeth Laboratories Inc., Philadelphia, USA

CONTENTS

X

VIII. Animal Models of Atherosclerosis

IX. Liproprotein and Lipid Metabolism in Experimental Animals

X. Hyperlipoproteinemia and Lipoprotein Disorders – Genetics and Epidemiology

XI. Plasma Lipids

Cholesterol and Triglyceride Metabolism

Fatty Acids

XIV. Plasma Lipoproteins

XV. Risk Factors

XVI. Prevention

XVII. Dietary Management of Hyperlipoproteinemias

XVIII. Drug Therapy of Hyperlipoproteinemia

Experience with Absorbable Drugs

Adamson, J. L. *(235*)*, see Bell, F. P.**

Alaupovic, Petar, Lipoprotein Laboratory, Oklahoma Medical Research Foundation, Oklahoma City, OK 73104/USA *(629, 676)*

Albers, J. J., The Northwest Lipid Research Clinic, Dept. of Medicine, Univ. of Washington, Seattle, WA 98104/USA *(469)*

Alexander, C. *(672)*, see Day, Ch. E.

Alexander, M. *(389)*, see Portman, O. W.

Alfin-Slater, R. B. *(339)*, see Morrison, L. M.

Altschuler, Stanley L., Medical College of Pennsylvania, Pulmonary Disease Section, Veteran's Administration Hospital, Philadelphia, PA/USA *(803)*

Armstrong, Mark L., Dept. of Internal Medicine, Univ. of Iowa Hospitals, Iowa City, IA 52240/USA *(300, 336)*

Assmann, Gerd, Molecular Disease Branch, NHLI, National Inst. of Health, Bethesda, MD 20014/USA *(569, 641)*

Atsumi, T. *(806)*, see Shimamoto, T.

Bajwa, G. S. *(339)*, see Morrison, L. M.

Bankovskaya, E. B. *(85)*, see Klimov, A. N.

Barndt, R. *(481)*, see Blankenhorn, D. H.

Barrett, A. M., Dept. of Pharmacology, School of Medicine, Leeds/England *(608)*

Bastenie, P. A., Dept. of Medicine, Hopital Universitaire Saint-Pierre, Brussels/Belgium *(608)*

Beaumont, J. L., Unité de Recherches à l'Institut National de la Santé et de la Recherche Médicale (I.N.S.E.R.M.), Hôpital Henri-Mondor, Créteil/France *(579)*

Beaumont, V., *(579)*, see Beaumont, J. L.

Beckenbach, E. S. *(484)*, see Blankenhorn, D. H.

Becker, C. D., Dept. of Pathology, The New York Hospital, Cornell Medical Center, New York, NY 10021/USA *(166)*

Becker, C. *(476)*, see Krishan, J.

Bell, F. P., Dept. of Pathology, McMaster Univ., Hamilton/Canada *(235)*

Berenson, G. S., Louisiana State Univ. Medical Center, New Orleans, LA 70112/USA *(6)*

Berg, Kare, Inst. of Medical Genetics, Univ. of Oslo, Oslo/Norway *(481)*

Berger, H. *(488)*, see Vogelberg, K. H.

Berjon, J. J. *(353)*, see Larrue, J.

Berkowitz, D. *(803)*, see Altschuler, St. D.

Bersohn, J. *(478)*, see Stein, E. A.

Bierman, E. L., *(464, 543, 547)*, see Hazzard, W. R.

Bihari-Varga, M. *(591)*, see Gerö, S.

Bing, R. J. *(118)*, see Tillmanns, H.

Biss, Kurt, DeKalb Clinic, DeKalb, I.L. 60115/USA *(512)*

Björkerud, Sören, Dept. of Histology, Göteborg/Sweden *(14, 110, 245)*

---

* The number in parenthesis indicates the beginning of a contribution.
** Only the complete address of the first author of a contribution is given.

Gilbert, C. H., Diabetes Research Laboratory, St. Bartholomew's Hospital, London/England *(140)*

Glomset, J. A. Dept. of Medicine, Univ. of Washington, Seattle, WA/USA *(499, 543, 548)*

Goldstein, J. L., *(413, 422, 464)*, see Hazzard, W. R.

Ghosh, P., Dept. of Biochemistry, Univ. of Cambridge, Cambridge/England *(529)*

Goto, Y., Dept. of Medicine, Keio Univ. School of Medicine, Tokyo/Japan *(761)*

Gotto, A. M., Jr., Dept. of Medicine and Biochemistry. Baylar College of Medicine and Methodist Hospital, Houston, TX/USA *(629)*

Greene, D. G., *(376)*, see Lofland, H. B.

Gresham, G. A., Dept. of Pathology, Cambridge/England *(297, 348)*

Greten, H., Medizinische Universitätsklinik, Heidelberg/BRD *(543, 557)*

Gries, F. A., Diabetes Forschungsinst., Univ. Düsseldorf, Düsseldorf/BRD *(488/816)*

Groleas, A. *(191)*, see Picard, J.

Gross, Richard C., Dept. of Medicine, Univ. of California, San Diego, La Jolla, CA 92037/USA *(155)*

Grundy, S., Dept. of Medicine, School of Medicine, La Jolla, CA/USA *(761, 816)*

Gutstein, W. H. *(299)*, see Pearl, F.

Hahn, K. J., Medizinische Universitätsklinik, Heidelberg/BRD *(816)*

Hales, C. N. *(529)*, see Gosh, P.

Hames, C. G. *(476)*, see Krishan, J.

Hamilton, Robert M. G., Dept. of Biochemistry, Univ. of Western Ontario, London/Canada *(406)*

Hartmann, G., Medizinische Klinik der Univ. Inselspital, Bern/Switzerland *(761)*

Hauss, W. H., Medizinische Klinik und Poliklinik der Westfälischen Wilhelms-Univ., Münster/BRD *(210)*

Haust, M. D. *(205, 366)*, see Trillo, A.

Havel, R., Univ. of California. San Francisco, School of Medicine, Cardiovascular Research Inst., San Francisco, CA/USA *(499)*

Havenstein, N., *(788)*, see Nestel, P.

Hazzard, William, R., Northwest Lipid Research Clinic, Harborview Medical Center, Seattle, WA 98104/USA *(464, 469)*

Heiberg, Arvid, Inst. of Medical Genetics, Univ. of Oslo, Oslo/Norway *(455)*

Hellström, Kjell, Medicinska Kliniken, Serafimerlasarettet, Stockholm/Sweden *(532)*

Hermelin, B. *(191)*, see Picard, J.

Hernell, O. *(543)*, see Olivecrona, Th.

Herrlinger, H. *(242)*, see Zöllner, N.

Hess, Hans, Medizinische Poliklinik, München/BRD *(358)*

Heyrovsky, A. *(429)*, see Sobra, J.

Ho, K.-J. *(512)*, see Biss, K.

Hollander, William, Boston University, School of Medicine, Boston, MA 02118/USA *(604)*

Holmes, W. L., Division of Research, Lankenau Hospital Philadelphia, PA/USA *(413)*

Honohan, Th. *(822)*, see Parkinson, Th. M.

Hood, B., Dept. of Internal Medicine, Malmö General Hospital, Malmö/Sweden *(604)*

Hornstra, G., Unilever Research Vlaardingen, Vlaardingen/The Netherlands *(279)*

Horsch, A. K., Medizinische Universitätsklinik, Heidelberg/BRD *(103)*

Houtsmuller, A. J., Erasmus Univ., Oogziekkenhuis, Rotterdam/The Netherlands *(782)*

Howard, Alan, N., Dept. of Investigative Medicine, Downing Site, Cambridge/England *(308, 816)*

Ilebekk, A., Inst. for Experimental Medical Research, Univ. of Oslo, Ulleval Hospital, Oslo/Norway *(233)*

Imai, H. *(344)*, see Lee, K. T.

Atherosclerosis and its complications have become a major problem in industrialized nations. More than half of all deaths result from circulatory diseases, and within this category degenerative cardiovascular disease is leading by far. Forty per cent of all cases of death occur between age 35 and 64, and that means in the working population. The main causes are occlusive diseases of the cerebrovascular system, and of the coronary, renal and peripheral arteries.

It is a specific trend of atherosclerotic lesions that they start in early childhood and progress at different rates in different individuals. It is rarely possible to make long term predictions as to the time when the atherosclerosis manifests itself as a disease with clinical symptoms. Results of epidemiologic studies have revealed the factors which tend to accelerate the atherosclerotic process and which lead to earlier and mor severe complications in comparison with subjects lacking such factors. In 80 per cent of all patients dying from atherosclerosis, one or more risk factors can be determined catamnestically.

Thus, certain prognostic indices have been developed. It is an important task for the epidemiologist to recognize conditions of risk in the population and in the individual, to try to eliminate these risk factors and to evaluate the results of these measures.

An important but rather neglected task is my opinion the study of so-called negative risk conditions such as the occurrence of idiopathic hypotension in conjunction with underweight and low lipoprotein levels. In the 1930s, it was claimed in this country that patients with chronic anemia, particularly pernicious anemia, developed only mild forms of atherosclerosis, and never suffered atherosclerotic occlusions. Negative risk conditions occurred when the times seemed biologically unfavorable, as during the semi-starvation of the war and post-war periods. They were the result of a deplorable worldwide experiment, but have stimulated in an important way research in atherosclerosis and particularly in preventive medicine. The results of comparative geopathology and clinical epidemiology indicate that the search for the "simple" life should be the best preventive measure against degenerative cardiovascular desease. We should thoroughly study the life habits of the "have nots", to use a term of Ian Prior, and look for the narrow road between luxury and starvation in order to prevent the rapid increase of death from atherosclerosis. A solution for this number one health problem can come only from a world-wide effort and particularly from world-wide education. If we succeed in eliminating the factors which produce or which favor the development of disease, the benefit to all mankind would be invaluable. Available results in the area of degenerative cardiovascular diseases are far more promising than those in the fight against cancer, the number two killer among human beings.

This symposium is not to be a meeting on cardiac infarction although coronary atherosclerosis and myocardial infarction are the most deadly complications of atherosclerosis. It is also not supposed to deal extensively with sudden death, with cerebrovascular disease, with aortic or renal artery stenosis, or with peripheral vascular occlusions. As the preceding meetings in Athens and Chicago, this symposium will center around problems of pathogenesis and etiology which are the prerequisites for an understanding of clinical manifestations and their complications. The main purpose of each conference on atherosclerosis will then be prevention and therapy. There have been many new findings during of many small pieces as is the case for any meeting. Even the experienced scientist often encounters difficulties in finding his way through the many results and in recognizing their significance. This meeting thus reflects the research in atherosclerosis which is going on in thousands of laboratories and hospitals all over the world. It is an urgent challenge of our time to centralize and organize these world-wide efforts.

As I see it, there are various possibilities for cooperation. If we should be successful in suggesting or even planning one or the other common project, this meeting would have achieved a worthwhile objective.

It is necessary to intensify basic research even though it has frequently been overestimated in this country in comparison with clinical medicine. On the other hand, Europeans scientists have contributed important concepts and hypotheses in the area of atherosclerosis. Rudolf *Virchow* has done research and teaching in another part of this city. His pupils and successors *Aschoff, Verse, Marchand,* who coined the term "Atherosclerosis", have had a close cooperation with the Russian pathologists *Ignatowski, Chalatow,* and *Anitschkow* as well as with Austrian and Swiss pathologists such as *Rokitansky* and *Erdheim;* they investigated problems of common interest and exchanged their coworkers. Several apparently new concepts of our time are based on their old theories, and it is interesting that improved and more specialized methods tend to confirm the ideas of these great men. It is particularly in this area of basic research where it would seem relatively easy to plan and investigate projects on a cooperative basis.

Other points of emphasis in atherosclerosis research include: Classification of lesions and their epidemiology in different geographical areas, as started by the pathologist *Folke-Henschen;* establishment of clinical criteria of atherosclerosis by direct and indirect methods. The importance of using reliable methods for measurement of circulatory parameters cannot be overemphasized since inadequate techniques are frequently applied to obtain these data. These procedures should be critically reviewed and recommendations should be made for coordinated studies. This applies also for the direct methods of angiography. Too few clinical studies are available that deal with arteriosclerosis as a generalized disease. Pathologists, internists, cardiologists, neurologists, ophthalmologists, and psychiatrists should supplement the findings of the clinical angiologists. Biochemists, physiologists and coagulation specialists should contribute to the elucidation of various clinical courses of atherosclerosis ("Gangarten" according to *Rühl* and *Doerr*).

Individual cases should be observed on a long term basis over decades. In this country, Max *Bürger* has used the term "Biorheutik" and has assigned a central position to atherosclerosis research. Within certain limitations, it is still true today that a man is as old as his vascular system.

Epidemiological studies should center on recognition and evaluation of risk factors; the actual goals should be prevention and therapy. National programs should be established and co-ordinated internationally. Efforts have already been made to set up national centers, including hospitals, for the prevention of cardiovascular, cerebrovascular and peripheral-vascular disease. I refer to the achievements of our American and Russian friends, and may also mention the contributions from this country. Cooperative research projects should be developed such as the WHO study on the occurence of myocardial infarction in young adults. Risk factors such as cigarette smoking, hypertension, hyperuricemia, hyperlipoproteinemia and chronic alcoholism are easily recognized, but their elimination requires highly specialized knowledge and extraordinary effort.

An important problem is the continued investigation of the relationships between nutrition and atherosclerosis or degenerative cardiovascular disease. It seems to me that we have today several well controlled long-term studies which justify the recommendation of certain diets for patients with atherosclerosis and for high-risk subjects. It is a different question whether recommendations should be generalized for the nutrition of the population as a whole. In my opinion, it is more promising to pursue well controllable objectives of limited duration, instead of conducting, with hundreds of thousands of people, mass experiments, that are difficult to control in many essential details. Again, projects on an international scale would be particularly important here.

The significance for the atherosclerosis process of socioeconomic and psychological stress, in my opinion, is still controversial, as is the role of physical exercise in prevention. Interesting projects are going on in this area and I think they should be coordinated by critical teams. Careful planning and supervision is necessary, particularly with regard to the methods applied. Documentation and processing of data should be available on an international basis; they would be of special value for long-term studies on the role of medication for prevention and therapy. The controversies surrounding long-term anticoagulation therapy and measures to influence platelet aggregation are additional problems that should be investigated.

Of particular significance is the rehabilitation of patients suffering from atherosclerotic sequelae. A number of important and promising projects are under way here. The solution of problems resulting from atherosclerosis can come only from common efforts. Support by the government is essential. If we turn to society, this society must be defined. Are we to depend on the government and on the official health agencies, on political groups, on doctors, sociologists, and psychologists, or on behavioral scientists if we want to see progress? I think we should establish efficient research teams as well as sufficiently funded research institutes and hospitals. Financial support by the taxpayers will have to be so great that a system of scrupulous control of funds becomes a prime necessity. A true engagement of the individual is needed. Many people today consider good health their right, and too many forget that health is also a responsibility and obligation of the individual. Too many people have become used to living at the expense of others and when problems arise they call on the government for help. There seems to be very little willingness to become personally involved and to undergo personal sacrifice, and one has the impression that this willingness decreases with increasing wealth. The solution of world-wide problems is possible only if the individual is ready for personal sacrifice. He is the one to benefit from it, by elimination of risk factors or by a change of unhealthy habits. In addition, the example of the individual is of educational value. We should turn to the young people and familiarize them with practical problems of atherosclerosis research through the curricula of high schools and universities.

This is an ambitious program. It can only be accomplished one step at a time. But a great goal is worth such world-wide efforts. International co-operation in medical science is needed *now*. Doctors and scientists everywhere in the world stand ready.

G. SCHETTLER

I

The Arterial Wall
in the Pathogenesis of Atherosclerosis

Chairmen: E. B. Smith, Great Britain
          S. Björkerud, Sweden

Participants: R. H. More, Canada
             D. Sinapius, BRD
             G. S. Berenson, USA
             W. Insull, USA
             S. Dayton, USA

DEFINITION OF EARLY HUMAN LESIONS - MORPHOLOGY AND HISTOCHEMISTRY

R. H. More

There is considerable controversy on what actually constitutes the 'early lesion', on whether all lesions begin in the same way and whether all develop into fibro-fatty plaques. This introduction outlines the morphology and histo-chemistry of lesions regarded as 'early' in terms of chronology and the general pathology of atherosclerosis (Movat et al., 1959; Haust, 1971a; Geer and Haust, 1972).

Fatty Dots and Streaks

The first of these presents itself on gross examination as a yellow (fatty) dot or streak; microscopically the changes vary from a stage considered to be early to somewhat more advanced. In the early yellow dot, fat droplets are present in the native smooth muscle cells (Geer et al., 1961; Haust et al., 1961; More et al., 1963) of a focal area. As the lesion grows in size, the number of fat droplets in a given smooth muscle cell as well as the number of these cells involved in the change increases. When much of the cytoplasm is occupied by fat, the cell acquires the appearance of a foam cell. By electron microscopy it is often possible to recognize the foam cell derived from the smooth muscle cell ("myogenic" foam cell) (Balis et al., 1964) and distinguish it from that which appears only in advanced fatty streaks and is of histiocytic origin (Balis et al., 1964). In the advanced fatty streaks there is also extracellular fat. Much of it resembles by light microscopy the finely distributed fat "dust" present in small amounts along the elastic lamellae of normal intima. By electron microscopy, in addition to these small osmiophilic bodies, fat may present itself in the form of myelin figures and droplets resembling those of intracellular fat (Haust et al., 1967). Cellular necrosis progresses with advancement of the lesion, but possibly these 'developed' fatty streaks should no longer be regarded as early lesions. Using the fluorescent and ferritin antibody techniques, in small fatty dots there appears to be no definite increase in albumin or in α- or β-lipoproteins, and fibrin appears to be absent, but in the larger raised fatty streaks there appears to be an increase in all the plasma proteins, and fibrin can be demonstrated (Wyllie et al., 1964; Cho et al., 1966; Haust, 1968).

'Normal' Diffuse Intimal Thickening. In all human subjects there is a progressive age-related thickening of the intima in both the aorta and the coronary arteries (Movat et al., 1958; More and Haust, 1968) which probably should not be regarded as part of the atherosclerotic process, but which must be used as the baseline for assessing the changes in 'early lesions' in any age group.

'Gelatinous Elevations'. These translucent thickenings are not very conspicuous
on gross inspection, particularly in young subjects, but become larger and more
prominent in the 4th - 6th decades. They appear as focal swellings of the intima
reminiscent of a blister, or a gelatinous elevation (Movat et al., 1959; Haust,
1971). Microscopically, it shows an intimal area in which the extracellularly
formed connective tissue components are either "wiped" out, or distorted,
fragmented, separated and swollen. There is a decrease or absence of metachromasia indicating either a change in the physico-chemical state, or "disappearance" of the acid mucopolysaccharides of the ground substance. The picture
is that of serous insudation, but often, fibrin may be found in the insudate.
The presence of fibrin in such areas may be easily confirmed on electron microscopic examination. Often, fibrin concentrates around the smooth cells — a
feature noticed long ago but not explored in depth. The cellular elements of the
lesion may be entirely free of change (Haust, 1971a; Haust, 1971b) but there
may be some extracellular fat. Occasionally, particularly when on gross examination there is a slight yellow tint to the lesions, the smooth muscle cells
contain fat droplets (not unlike those in fatty streaks), so that the lesion
has features both of the fatty streak and gelatinous elevation (Haust, 1971a).
With fluorescent antibody techniques (Haust et al., 1964; Wyllie et al., 1964;
Cho et al., 1966; Haust, 1968) one may demonstrate the presence of fibrin and
low-density lipoproteins, and increased amounts of albumin and high density
lipoproteins.

Mural Microthrombi

The third early lesion is seldom, if ever, seen by naked eye and is often found
on microscopic examination by chance. It represents a microthrombus which may be
observed in various stages. Most often it is composed largely of fibrin, but
microthrombi with a considerable core of platelets or predominantly consisting
of platelets may be also found. Some of such microthrombi are covered by endothelium and may be in various stages of "contraction" of their fibrin mass and
organization. Microthrombi may extend over somewhat larger area of the intima,
but most commonly are focal. They may be found at all ages, even in small children, and over microscopically unaltered intima (Haust and More, 1960). Microthrombi consisting predominantly of platelets resemble closely those produced
experimentally by various means.

It has been reasonably well established that the above three lesions occur in
man. However, even investigators who consider these to be the "forerunners" of
the atherosclerotic plaques and thus to represent early atherosclerotic lesions,
do admit that at present it is not known how often each of the three occurs in
relation to the other two, and how often each progresses to the atherosclerotic
plaque, becomes arrested or regresses. Moreover, it is not known whether there
is an interdependence of the three lesions in their steps of evolution to the
atherosclerotic lesion. All these problems are not easily solved in man and must
be approached through the co-ordinating and collaborative efforts of many investigators.

MODIFICATION OF LESIONS BY LOCATIONAL FACTORS

D. Sinapius

In *cerebral* arteries fatty streaks occur as well as in the aorta and in the
coronaries. But I suppose that they are less common in this region. On the contrary mural thrombi seem to play an important role in cerebral arteries, microthrombi as well as thicker ones. I have never seen typical intime edema in cerebral arteries such as is well known in the aorta.

In the *coronaries* fatty streaks are a very frequent condition. Also microthrombi and thicker mural thrombi occur frequently. Microthrombi very often include foam cells or extracellular lipids adsorbed from the bloodstream, probably lipoproteins.

Also in the *femoral* artery fatty streaks occur very often, with or without microthrombi. Not rarely cushions of microthrombi rich in erythrocytes and including many large foam cells are to be seen, not yet overgrown by a new endothelium. Thick mural thrombi as early lesions play an important role in the beginning and in the progression of femoral atherosclerosis.

In addition I would like to point out 2 early lesions which are not yet described by others: 1. elevations of thrombotic material mixed with crystals of cholesterol, but without endothelium at the surface, and 2. lipids, probably lipoproteins, adsorbed to the surface of the coronary artery intima which are phagocytized by endothelial cells, smooth muscle cells or monocytes and then overgrown (and thus incorporated) by a new endothelium.

Discussion

Dr. Adams: The question of edema, intimal swelling, serous inflammation, and what Lendrum has called fibrinous vasculosis is somewhat confusing. Is it an inflammatory lesion? Actually, it has only got *one* component of the inflammatory lesion, *viz.* the actual leakage, *i.e.* the exsudation of a liquid through the endothelium. It neither has the cellular, polymorphonuclear component of the general inflammatory response, nor the vascular changes connected to this general process. I would like to make a plea: let us give the early arterial change I am referring to a concrete finite name, so that we do not talk about different things for semantic reasons.

Dr. Haust: Professor More was mentioning for years the information we have today on the subject that we call gelatinous lesion. Originally, Dr. Elspeth Smith was responsible for coining the term "gelatinous lesion". At least with regard to certain aspects, it is a serous inflammation. However, it is often overlooked that sometimes such lesions may contain fibrin, and, consequently, are no longer exclusively serous in nature. The term "gelatinous lesion" was termed with respect to its gross appearance. By gross criteria it is, indeed, a gelatinous elevation. Microscopically it represents the topical reaction to injury with an insudation of plasma protein into the intimal tissue. The word *insudation* is used to convey that it is *not*, in a general sense, an exsudation, *i.e.* the material does not leave the vessel wall, as exsudates do by definition. I like to suggest that we should agree on calling this type of lesion "gelatinous lesion or elevation". It represents an inflammatory reaction that is devoid of the presence of inflammatory cells, and comprises an exsudation which we call insudation *only* to denote that material is being arrested *within* rather than outside the vessel wall.

Dr. Adams: I think that Daria Haust's point about plasmatic insudation is a very good one. We should realize that edema is a low-protein transsudate. What Daria Haust mentioned is actually an exsudate. I suggest we drop the term edema and use her term insudation.

PLASMA AND SYNTHESIZED LIPID CONSTITUENTS IN INTIMA AND THEIR COMPARTMENTALIZATION

E. B. Smith

The concepts which have developed from our analytical studies are summarized in the diagram where two lipid indices – the percentage of the cholesterol which is free (unesterified) and the ratio of linoleic acid to oleic (18:2/18:1) in the cholesterol esters – are related to the morphological characteristics of the intimal lipid and to the amount of intact LD-lipoprotein in the tissue (Fig.1).

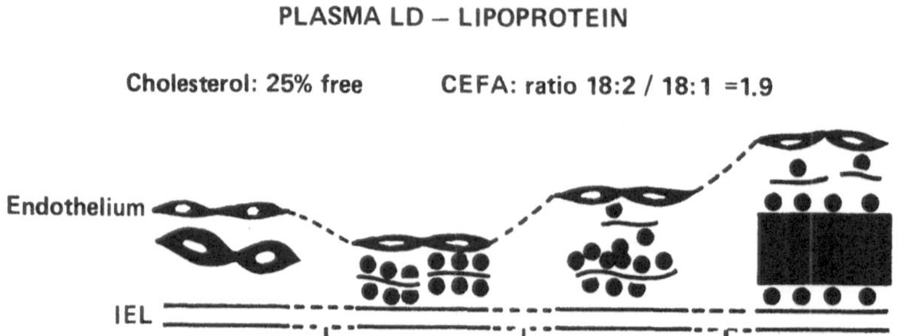

PLASMA LD – LIPOPROTEIN

Cholesterol: 25% free   CEFA: ratio 18:2 / 18:1 =1.9

	Fatty streak	Adult normal	'Gelatinous'	Amorphous lipid
LP concentration % of normal level	22%	100%	200 - 400 %	100 - 200 %
Cholesterol % free	22%	27%	24 %	40 - 50 %
CEFA Ratio 18:2 / 18:1	0.2 - 0.3	1.4 - 1.5	1.8	1.4

Figure 1. Relation of unesterified cholesterol and ratio of linoleic acid to oleic acid to morphological characteristics of the intimal lipid and amount of intact LD-lipoprotein in the tissue.

The endothelial surface is bathed with LD-lipoprotein in which about 25% of the cholesterol is free and linoleic acid is the major component in the cholesterol esters. In 'normal' aortic intima of the fourth decade and upwards there is diffuse intimal thickening and accumulation of fine perifibrous lipid droplets along collagen and fragmentary elastic fibres in the deep layers. The overall lipid pattern resembles LD-lipoprotein and linoleic is the major cholesterol ester fatty acid (CEFA) although its proportion is slightly lower. On a crude volumetric basis the concentration of intact LD-lipoprotein in the intima is approximately the same as in the plasma.

In the juvenile type fatty streak described by Dr. More, and by Dr. McGill in his plenary lecture, the lipid indices are totally different and most of the lipid is within fat-filled cells. *Oleic* acid is the major component of the CEFAs and there is extensive evidence for local esterification (see Dr. Dayton's contribution). There is no evidence of differential hydrolysis which could convert this pattern of cholesterol ester into the pattern found beneath large fibrous plaques (Smith & Slater, 1972) and the chemical evidence supports the epidemiological evidence presented by Dr. McGill that these lesions are on a different pathway to adult fibrous plaques (Smith and Slater, 1973a,b).

The 'gelatinous' or 'insudation' lesions were fully described by Dr. More (see also review by Haust, 1971); morphologically the lipid occurs as fine perifibrous droplets and/or 'diffuse sudanophilia'. The lesion contains greatly increased concentrations of intact LD-lipoprotein which may account for 75% of the total cholesterol; the lipid indices are virtually identical with LD-lipoprotein.

I postulate that this is the precursor of the large fibrous plaque, but the amorphous lipid in the core shows some changes. There is a slight decrease in the proportion of linoleic acid and a marked increase in the proportion of free cholesterol, which could indicate cholesterol esterase activity with a slight preference for cholesterol linoleate.

Three major questions arise from these observations.
1. What factors make fat-filled cells fill themselves with fat? Are they actively destroying LD-lipoprotein?
2. Is the great increase in the concentration of plasma constituents in 'gelatinous' lesions primarily the result of increased endothelial 'permeability' or of changes in the intracellular matrix causing increased retention?
3. What happens when the lipid of the soluble lipoprotein in the intima is 'deposited?

Discussion

Dr. Adams: Could I ask about the question concerning the change from soluble lipoprotein to stainable deposited cholesterol. Why could not the answer be very simple: that the cholesterol becomes dissociated from the apoprotein vehicle?

Chairman Smith: I think that the cholesterol really must come from a dissociated apoprotein vehicle, but the question is: what causes it to become dissociated? It may be that in a gelatinous lesion the lipoprotein can re-equilibrate with the plasma lipoprotein; if the lipoproteins remain soluble, the lesions may perhaps disappear again. But I feel that once something has initiated the dissociation of the lipid from the apoprotein, then it might be retained in the tissue. Why this happens may be one of the most important questions facing us in this field. Furthermore, why does deposition seem to occur at certain stages in the development of atherosclerosis? We find quite large, fairly early looking fibrous plaques which contain very little lipid.

Dr. Adams: I have the impression that low-density lipoprotein is a very unstable molecule. Rather than "why should it split up?", why should it *not* split up, if it is an unstable molecule? What happens if, for example, you inject lipoprotein under the skin – does it stay intact or does it rapidly shed its lipid? I have the feeling it's something that is rather unstable.

Dr. Hoff: I would like to add some information on lipoprotein retention in human atherosclerotic lesions. We have studied the presence of lipoprotein, actually the apoprotein of LDL, in different sites of the arterial wall. The apo-LDL was present in the elastic membranes in the thickened intima. The apo-LDL was confined quite specifically as judged from the immunofluorescence to the elastic membranes or to fragments of elastic membranes. It is possible that these fragments could also represent newly formed elastin material. We also found specific zones in large accumulations of collagen that contained apo-LDL distributed rather diffusely, whereas other areas of collagen, such as in atheromatous plaques, were mostly negative.

Dr. Caro: Looking at Dr. Smith's slide on the fatty streak, how about this suggestion: the lipoprotein is entering to pick up lipid from the wall. We have argued, and I think shown, that the wall permeability tends to be low in certain regions exposed to low shear. Under low wall shear I would expect less lipoprotein to enter and then, if my suggestion is right, one would find a lower lipo-

protein protein content and a higher lipid content in such specific areas which
could correspond to fatty streaks.

Chairman Smith: We have, in fact, got some rather crude measurements on the lipid
content of the lipoprotein that we get out of the wall by electrophoretic migration. It appears to be identical with the patients own circulating lipoprotein.

ARTERIAL CONNECTIVE TISSUE AND POSSIBLE ROLE OF MATRIX
FOR PERMEABILITY AND RETENTION*

G. S. Berenson with collaboration of S. R. Srinivasan,
B. Radhakrishnamurthy, and E. R. Dalferes, Jr.

Numerous investigators have observed response by the arterial wall to a variety
of injuries, in an effort to simulate and study mechanisms for development of
atherosclerosis. The primary role of the connective tissue matrix is to maintain
integrity of the arterial wall (Berenson et al., 1971) and in a general sense,
connective tissue of cardiovascular structures responds by a repair and remodeling to any type of inflammatory reaction–stress, blood pressure changes, hypoxia,
viruses, or infiltration of lipids. In this response two or more cell types,
endothelial and the multi-potential myofiber cell, play a key role in the synthesis of the complex connective tissue macromolecules. Interestingly, the recent work using tissue culture by Roos and Glomset, 1973, and Fischer-Dzoga et al.,
1973, suggests that proliferation of cells and metabolic activity can be enhanced
by lipoproteins. The changes of carbohydrate protein macromolecules of the matrix
and fibrous structures composing the arterial wall are obviously governed by
metabolic activity of these cells.

The connective tissue interstitial matrix is composed of a variety of carbohydrate-protein macromolecules; of these, acid mucopolysaccharides (MPS) and glycoproteins are both quite heterogeneous. Actually, little is known about the
sialic acid-containing glycoproteins in the development of atherosclerosis. From
studies in our laboratory we know that they are genetically determined, show differences from one individual to another, have enzymatic activity, and are immunologically active (Berenson et al., 1966; Srinivasan et al., 1971; Dugan et al.,
1967). In addition, serum glycoproteins have also been shown to complex with
collagen fibers (Franzblan et al., 1973). The studies of Buddecke 1960 and Robert
1970 have demonstrated glycoprotein increases during atherosclerosis, but their
role in atherosclerosis is not clear.

Considerably more work has concerned MPS, in part due to the observation by
numerous histochemical studies that they increase in atherosclerosis. The MPS
exist both as free and protein-bound; they are quite heterogeneous, vary in
composition (e.g., sulfation), and are even polydisperse in molecular weight.

Although the precise role of the MPS in the development of the atherosclerotic
lesion remains unclear, certain observations of MPS as a group indicate a relationship to permeability and retention of lipids by the arterial wall matrix.
These are:

1. MPS are highly charged, reactive macromolecules capable of trapping water,
binding electrolytes and ions, such as Ca^{++}.
2. MPS have an inter-relationship with the fibrous structures--collagen, elastin.
3. The amount and composition of MPS vary in different sites in the aorta. For

---

*Supported by funds from USPHS and NHLI (HL15103-HL02942) and the American Heart
Association.

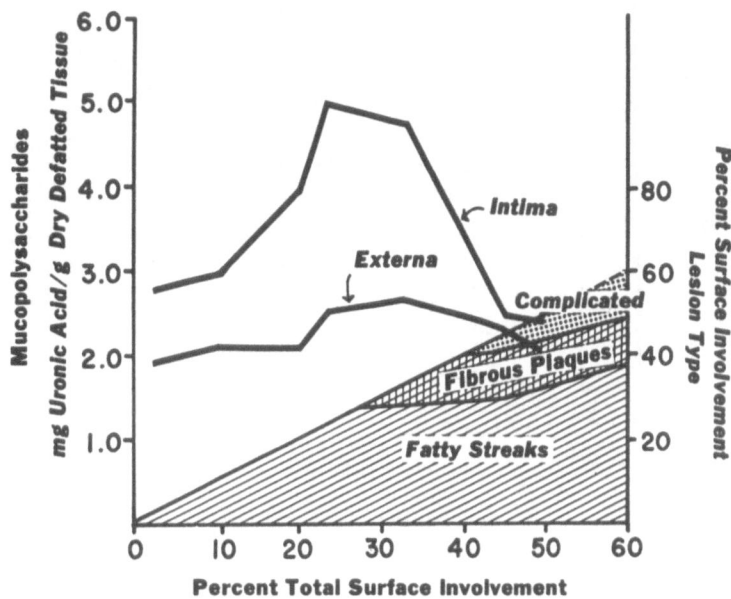

AORTIC MPS VARIATIONS WITH EXTENT OF ATHEROSCLEROSIS AND TYPE OF LESION

Figure 1. Concentration of acid MPS in the inner and outer layers of aorta with increasing degrees of atherosclerosis. The relationship of the MPS content to the lesion type suggests that with increasing formation of fatty streaks there is a significant increase of the MPS content. With progressive atherosclerosis a decrease of the concentration of MPS occurs

example, the intima contains a high content of sulfated MPS and a much greater concentration occurs in the abdominal aorta than in the thoracic. Sites predisposed to the development of atherosclerosis have higher concentrations of MPS. 4. MPS are functional in initiating processes related to atherosclerosis, e.g., lipoprotein lipase, anticoagulation, platelet activity.
5. MPS vary with aging; cardiovascular connective tissue might be considered a target organ for hormonal changes.

Studies from our laboratory have shown that an increase of MPS in the intima parallels the extensiveness of the early atherosclerotic lesion (Kuinar et al., 1967a,b). Fig. 1 illustrates changes of the total MPS with the degree and varying types of atherosclerotic lesions and indicates a progressive increase with the extensiveness of fatty streaks and perhaps fibrous plaques. However, with more advanced disease and complicated lesions there is an actual decrease in the MPS content. In young males between the age of 12-25 years the total amount of MPS correlates closely with the degree of atherosclerosis in both thoracic and abdominal aorta tissue (Dalferes et al., 1971). Studies of the specific changes of MPS indicate alterations occur primarily with chondroitin sulfates and heparin sulfate.

Fig. 2 shows the general direction of changes of MPS with Ca^{++}, collagen and lipids. Elastin should also be included, since it has been shown to predispose to deposition of lipoproteins and Ca^{++} and likely has a close relationship with MPS.

From these observations, one concept for the role of connective tissue matrix can be inferred. The matrix is a highly charged gel-sieve capable of expanding and contracting with various states of hydration. As a charged gel-sieve it is

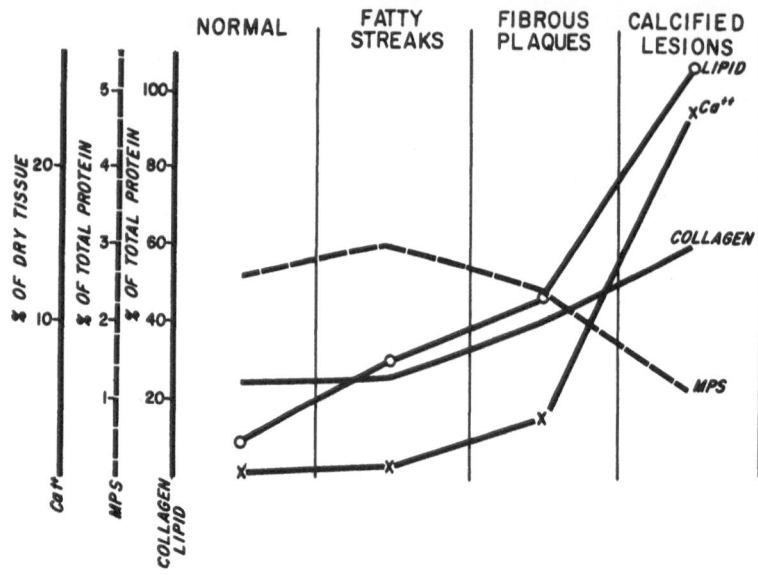

Figure 2. A composite illustration of the changes of total MPS, collagen, lipids, and calcium in the normal aorta and in various types of atherosclerotic lesions

capable of influencing not only permeability but also the influx and egress of ions, proteins, and nutrients transported in plasma.

Is there any evidence for a role of retention of lipids by the matrix in pathogenesis of atherosclerosis?

SCHEMATIC REACTION MECHANISM OF β-LIPOPROTEIN-HEPARIN COMPLEXES

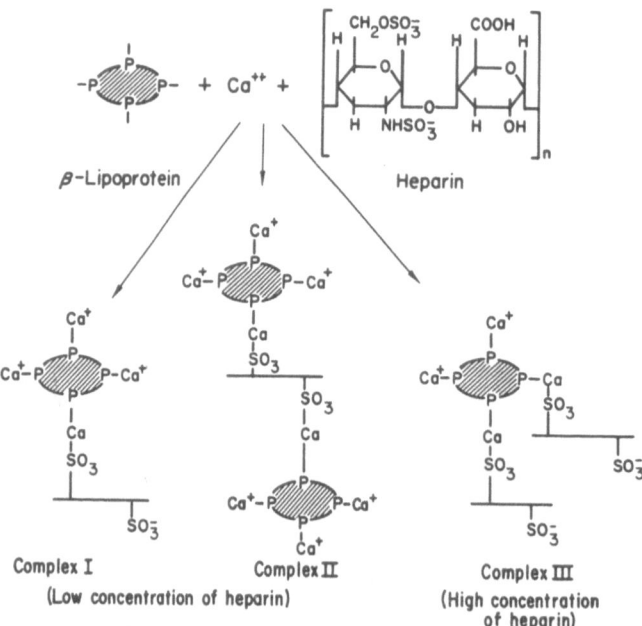

Figure 3. A schematic representation of a proposed mechanism of complexing of MPS (heparin) with serum lipoproteins and Ca^{++} (courtesy of Srinivasan et al., Atheroscler. 12:321, 1970)

A number of studies, presented at this symposium indicate an active movement of protein from plasma into the arterial wall. Also, it has been known for some time that highly charged polysaccharides, i.e. MPS and specifically heparin, form complexes in vitro with serum low density lipoproteins (LDL). A model of this complexing was developed with the use of serum lipoproteins, heparin and calcium (Srinivasan et al., 1970). The complexing as it occurs in vitro has been studied in detail, and a schematic representation of the complexes is shown in Fig. 3. These studies indicate a rather selective ability of sulfated MPS to complex with serum ß- and pre-ß-lipoproteins in the presence of divalent cations. Ca^{++} and Mg^{++} appear to be more specific in this regard, although heparin is much more reactive than the other MPS found in higher concentration in blood vessels.

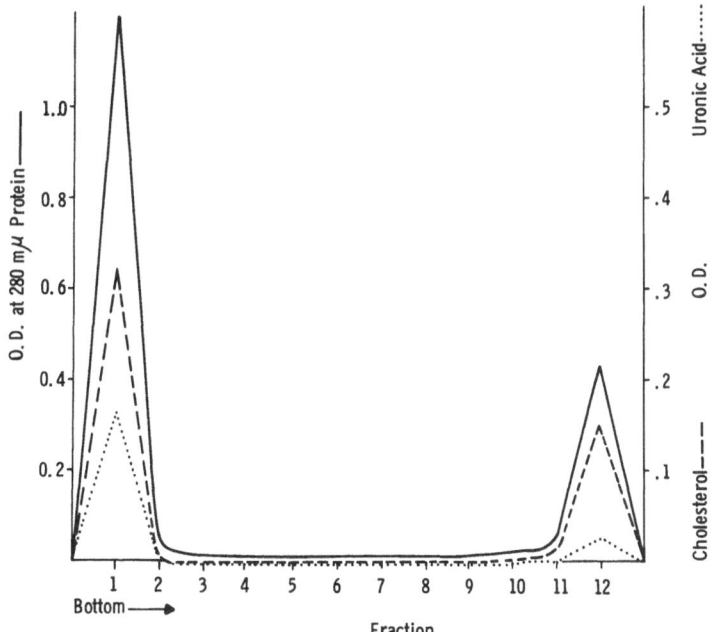

Figure 4. Ultracentrifugal profile of lipoprotein-MPS complexes obtained by the fractionation of fibrous plaque extracts on Bio-Gel P-300 columns. Ultracentrifugation of the complexes was carried out in the solvent density 1.006 (with NaCl) at 114,000 g. These studies indicate the presence of very low density lipoprotein-MPS complexes present in the top fraction. Recentrifugation of the bottom fraction at 1.065 D using D_2O yielded low density lipoprotein-MPS complexes in the top layer

In order to study similar complexing as might exist in the arterial wall, a method of extraction of lipoprotein-MPS complexes from fatty streaks and fibrous plaques was developed (Srinivasan et al., 1972). Extracts were obtained which were composed of lipoprotein and the amount extractable from the arterial wall can be reduced by the addition of Ca^{++} in the extracting medium. Ca^{++} presumably stabilizes the complex. The lipoprotein-MPS complexes after partial purification by gel chromatography were then further studied by ultracentrifugation. Fig. 4 illustrates the presence of VLDL and LDL material complexed to MPS.

Further studies were conducted on complexes from fatty streak and fibrous plaques to determine the nature of MPS present. MPS materials were isolated from the complexes and studied by electrophoresis. Chondroitin sulfates (CS-C/A) and hyaluronic acid were found in the complexes of fatty streaks and plaques. The major MPS, CS-C, was indicated by both electrophoretic and enzymatic studies. Heparin was also detected in material from fibrous plaques.

9

The ability of charged MPS to complex with lipoproteins thus introduces the second possible role of the matrix in development of the early atherosclerotic lesion. MPS are capable of complexing, trapping, and ultimately sequestering serum lipoproteins which can diffuse or be transported into the arterial wall. Although this movement of lipoproteins appears to occur even in a normal state, it is evident that with an additional load or movement of lipoproteins the egress or clearance may be altered by forming complexes with the MPS. Ultimately, material may be sequestered in the form of an extra cellular lesion.

The arterial wall matrix and the connective tissue carbohydrate-protein macro-molecules play an important role in the pathogenesis of atherosclerosis.

Discussion

Dr. Hoff: I think most of us detected a certain discrepancy between your data, that of Dr. Berenson and that of Dr. Smith concerning the amount of LDL or lipo-protein in general that is found in the fatty streak lesion. You showed quite a bit more than the normal tissue, and she showed quite a bit less. I wonder, in brief time, if we could reconcile this discrepancy?

Chairman Smith: Dr. Berenson and I have talked about this problem. We really have not come up with any good answer to it. One possibility is that we are de-fining our "fatty streaks" differently. *My* fatty streaks are specifically fat-filled cell early lesions and his may, I think, include the fatty infiltrations which were described in Dr. McGill's plenary lecture. Another possibility is that the lipoprotein is irreversibly bound to the mucopolysaccharide, and is not mobile in my electrophoretic system. This seems rather unlikely, because we found the same thing when we did extraction experiments, and then we had condi-tions of salt concentration and pH under which one would imagine they should dissociate. But this is a problem that we have discussed between ourselves and really come up with no solution.

Dr. Berenson: I think I can add one more reason. In these studies the main pur-pose was to try to demonstrate that complexing actually occurred in the arterial wall. These are large aggregates, perhaps in excess of 50 million, and, strangely enough, we found hyaluronic acid there which does not bind *in vitro*. Therefore, it is suggestive of real aggregation of large macromolecules. We did *not* make an assay to try to quantitate these and the whole variety of lipids that is present, but merely to get the complexes.

Dr. Wissler: Dr. Tracy, about ten years ago, extracted lipoproteins from the artery wall and in lesions very much like the ones I think Dr. Berenson is speak-ing of, and found that they did still retain their immunological reactivity at least on gel-diffusion test. When he tested them on electrophoretic mobility, however, they had a different mobility. He found that this was the mobility that he would get if he mixed some of the acid mucopolysaccharides with lipoproteins. Therefore, the bound lipoproteins probably still will react immunologically. If you try to test the electrophoretic mobility, it will be different. It seems pertinent in this discussion, which I have listened to with a great deal of interest so far, to raise the question, how much what we have been calling in-sudation really is an accumulation of new acid mucopolysaccharides produced by the cells of the artery wall. The increase of mucopolysaccharides may in turn make the lesions look edematous. One interesting feature of the mucopolysacchar-ides is that you can't see them in ordinary microscopy. They are there, and un-less you stain for them very specifically, you are not very aware that they are there.

Dr. Finlayson: Dr. Berenson, may I ask you, have you examined mucopolysaccharides in tendons. If you have, what do they share in common with mucopolysaccharides of the aorta? The thing they share in common, I think will help us to elucidate why lipoproteins are sticky.

Dr. Berenson: I am aware of this peculiar site of predilection of the xanthomatous material. We have not analysed tendons.

Dr. Hodara: I would like to make some comments on Dr. Berenson's work. I have been hearing about complex formation between mucopolysaccharides of this complex, although it has been shown that they occur *in vitro*. I have sampled tangential sections of bovine and human aortas. There is no relationship between the lipid content, also with regard to lipid subfractions, and the mucopolysaccharides, especially the sulphated ones. I don't see any physiological significance for this complex formation.

Dr. Berenson: You would not deny that they are present, though? The difference, I think, resides in methodology.

PHYSIOCHEMICAL ASPECTS OF LIPIDS IN THE PATHOGENESIS AND COMPOSITION OF EARLY LESIONS OF HUMAN ATHEROSCLEROSIS

W. Insull

The accumulation of lipid is one of the early manifestations of the occurrence of atherosclerosis and is commonly accepted as strong evidence for a developing lesion. Lipids accumulate in lesions in the form of aggregates visible with the microscope. Recent studies have been describing in detail these lipid aggregates in man. The physical and chemical properties of the aggregates are unusual and appear likely to have a significant influence on the metabolism of the lipids in the lesions. To use the study of metabolism of these lipids as a tool to explain the pathogenesis of atherosclerosis it is essential that we understand the effects of the physicochemical properties on the lipids' metabolism.

Three types of lipid aggregates have been observed: 1. perifibrous lipid droplets seen in grossly normal intima in the extracellular spaces, 2. lipid inclusions in gross fatty-streak lesions, seen in stellate cells, in ovoid cells, as well as in extracellular spaces, 3. and lipid inclusions in gross fibrous-plaque lesions, also seen in the two types of cells as well as extracellularly. The physicochemical properties of all these fall into three categories, morphology, chemical composition, and structure. For each of the lipid aggregates some of these properties have been determined, but others are yet unknown. No aggregate has been completely described.

At present, some major concepts about these lipid aggregates appear established, while others are developing. The concepts that appear established are that cholesterol esters are the dominant lipid in the mixtures occurring in the aggregates, that cholesterol oleate and linoleate are the dominant esters, that cholesterol, triglyceride and phospholipid are also present but in smaller proportions, that the lipid composition varies significantly with each kind of lesion and the composition of its aggregate is characteristic of the lesion. Developing concepts are that lipids may exist in the aggregates as liquids and as liquid crystals, and that inclusions are physically discrete compartments of specific composition. Examples are drawn from studies with my coworkers Drs. Yoshiya Hata, John Hower and Dieter Lang.

The inclusions can be isolated from the tissues of the gross fatty streak and fibrous plaque of human aorta. They appear as spheres with diameters of about 2 micra. With the polarizing microscope and 1/4 wavelength plate they appear as mixtures of two forms. The anisotropic forms have the characteristic image of a circle with a black Formée cross with quadrants of yellow and blue. Isotropic forms true liquids, are grey (Lang and Insull, 1970). In fatty streaks the proportion of anisotropic forms is higher than in fibrous plaques.

Chemical analyses of the lipids show that cholesterol ester is the dominant lipid, 81% of total lipids in fatty streaks, and 59% of total lipid in fibrous plaques. The proportions of ester and other lipids are distinctly different for the fatty streak and fibrous plaque inclusions (Table 1)(Insull, 1972). The cholesterol ester fatty acids are predominantly oleic and linoleic acids. The proportions of these and other acids are significantly different for the inclusions from fatty streaks and fibrous plaques (Table 2).

The optical characteristics of the anisotropic forms, their Formée cross image, interference colors, and high refractive index, and their high content of cholesterol esters indicate that these are probably liquid crystals of cholesterol esters. We propose that their basic internal structure is a solid sphere of many concentric lamellae of ester molecules in a smectic mesophase. The major axis of each ester molecule is perpendicular to the plane of its lamella and is aligned along a radius of the sphere.

Table 1. Proportions of lipid classes in lipid of inclusions from human aortic fatty streaks and fibrous plaques

	Cholesterol esters	free	Phos-lipid	Triglycerides
		% of total lipids		
Fatty streaks	81.2	5.2	9.5	4.1
Fibrous plaques	59.6	12.9	17.6	9.9

All differences between lesions are significant at P<0.001.

Table 2. Proportions of major fatty acids in the cholesterol ester fatty acids of inclusions from human aortic fatty streaks and fibrous plaques

Fatty acid		Fatty streak		Fibrous Plaques
		%		%
Palmitic	16:0	8.9	*	11.0
Palmitoleic	16:1	5.3		5.4
Stearic	18:0	1.6		1.5
Oleic	18:1	46.9	*	38.7
Linoleic	18:2	17.6	*	28.2
Arachidonic	20:4	5.4	*	6.8

*Difference is significant at P<0.02.

Scanning electron microscopy confirms that the isolated inclusions have a spherical shape, and shows the presence of a variety of surface defects, pits, holes and conical depressions, of a wide range of size. Mixtures of inclusion from fibrous-plaque lesions have significantly more forms with defects than do mixtures from fatty streaks, 15% vs. 3% respectively (Insull et al., 1971).

These studies show that the variety of physical and chemical properties of the inclusions occur in specific patterns related to the types of lesion. This supports the concept that the inclusions are physically discrete compartments of lipid of specific composition, and are unique products of lipid metabolism in the atherosclerotic process.

Considering the significance of these observations for the metabolism of lipids in the artery raises several questions. Do the physical properties of lipids control the selection of lipids for segregation in the inclusions? What is the role of self-assembly in the formation of lipid aggregates and inclusions from individual lipid molecules? Does the physical state of the lipids in inclusions influence the lipids' availability to metabolic mechanisms for further synthesis and for catabolism?

Future studies must evaluate these possibilities.

Discussion

Question: I am very interested in the phospholipid part of the lipid structures you have described, Dr. Insull. The phospholipids influence, as we all know, the physical state of lipid liquid crystals. However, Dr. Insull, you have focused your presentation to a very great extent on cholesterol and the esterification of cholesterol. We know that the composition of the phospholipids changes in several situations. My point is that the physical state of your lipid aggregates is very much dependent on such surfactant components as the phospholipids. If you assume that these phospholipids are constant both with regard to quantity and quality in your lipid crystals, then the physical state would perhaps be entirely dependent upon the cholesterol and the cholesterol esters. However, the phospholipids do change, and if you do not take this fact into consideration, I think you do injustice to the scientific method.

Dr. Insull: I could not go into the details in the time I had. There are two points that bear directly on that. First point is: we have analyzed the phospholipids in detail in these studies and do know the proportions of lecithin, sphingomyelin etc. We have demonstrated that there is a predominance of lecithin in the fatty streaks. In the fibrous plaques there is more sphingomyelin. We have, furthermore, performed analyses correlating the proportions of these with the fatty acids etc., looking for relationships. We have not found these. The only relationship that we found in the fatty streaks, for example, was in lysolecithin in work that Dr. Lang did several years ago. When we repeated it on a more recent group of fatty streak preparations, we could not confirm this correlation. Therefore, I feel that this relationship may just have been a factitious observation. One other observation in the same general area is that one can make models of these inclusions and can do this with pure cholesterol esters in which we have no phospholipid. There is a tendency to form liquid crystals by the cholesterol esters without the presence of phospholipid. The phospholipid is not necessarily essential. This does emphasize the significance of the physical properties of cholesterol esters alone.

Dr. Adams: I think my former co-worker Dr. Roy Weller and I did a lot of work on liquid crystals and I think he was finding quite a lot of phospholipid and cholesterol in them; it also suggested *in situ* transformation of cholesterol into cholesterol ester. If I understand you correctly, your isolated liquid crystals were just pure cholesterol esters; is that right?

Dr. Insull: The data we presented here indicated that the inclusions were predominantly cholesterol esters: in the fatty streaks there was 80% and in the fibrous plaques 59%. They did have phospholipid in them, but it was only a minor part of them. We are very much aware of Dr. Weller's work. Dr. Weller actually helped us to get started on some of the techniques, and we realize there is a discrepancy between his observations and ours. However, I feel this can probably be explained on methodological grounds. He had a rather limited number of observations. We now have fatty streak preparations from ca. forty different individuals and fibrous plaque preparations from ca. twenty. I believe that the pattern of composition that was seen, is rather firmly established. I don't understand how he got a predominance of phospholipid. This does not fit in with analysis of whole tissue or with Dr. Smith's observations on specific regions that were isolated by microdissection.

ENDOTHELIAL PERMEABILITY; INTERPRETATIONS FROM EXPERIMENTAL LESIONS

S. Björkerud

We all know that extrapolation from experimental to human biology may be hazardous. However, experimental information may be needed to supplement that which can be obtained from man. It may also provide information on the dynamics and the time sequence of events. This kind of information may be difficult or impossible to obtain from man.

This introduction will be focused on the role of the endothelium. It will be performed in two steps - which can be defined as two questions:
Step one: Are the basal arterial tissue reactions or responses, as known from experimental studies, applicable to man?
Step two: Can some of the properties of human early lesions be understood in terms of certain basal arterial tissue reactions?

The arterial endothelium is a monolayer of cells with a limited life-span. The rate of cell turnover varies in different regions of the artery. A larger proportion of newly formed (Wright, 1970; Schwartz and Benditt, 1973) and of injured or dead endothelial cells (Björkerud and Bondjers, 1972; Gutstein et al., 1973) is present in relation to branching points. This suggests hemodynamic strain as one of many possible factors which could influence the rate of the endothelial cell turnover. The basal physiological concepts related to arterial endothelium are summarized in Fig. 1.

Material may be carried through intact endothelium by pinocytotic vesicles (Stein and Stein, 1972) and through intercellular clefts (Schwartz and Benditt, 1972; Hüttner et al., 1973). The latter pathway seems to be restricted for small and medium-sized particles (Stein and Stein, 1972). Both pathways are probably subject to control both quantitatively and qualitatively (Fig. 2). In certain regions where increased hemodynamic strain may be expected to occur, the endothelial layer is discontinuous (Fig. 2) due to abundance of injured or dead cells even in the normolipidemic animal (Björkerud and Bondjers, 1972; Gutstein et al., 1973). Such regions are also characterized by more or less unregulated passage of *e.g.* lipoprotein (Bondjers and Björkerud, 1973a). Active contraction of arterial endothelial cells (Fig. 2) has also been proposed as a mechanism for unregulated passage (Shimamoto and Sunaga, 1972; Robertson and Khairallah, 1973), but definite evidence for this mechanism is still lacking (for review see Björkerud, 1974).

The effect of the presence or absence of endothelium can be studied conveniently in an experimental system where the degree of experimental endothelial desquamation can be controlled (Björkerud, 1969a and b). Fig. 3 depicts schematically the principles for and consequences of graded endothelial removal. Three different response patterns follow (Fig. 3). The induction of a denudation with small area is followed by rapid overgrowth of endothelium and a transient thickening of the intima - if combined with a low degree of medial injury; or calcification, encapsulation and capillarization - if combined with marked medial injury

MONOLAYER

WITH

SELECTIVE PERMEABILITY AND ANTITHROMBOTIC

PROPERTIES

- - - - - - - - - - - - - - - - - -

CELLS TURN OVER

DUE TO

CELL DEATH   CELL RENEWAL
(CELL AGE; INJURY)   (MITOTIC)

BALANCED BY

- - - - - - - - - - - - - - - - - -

ENDOTHELIAL PERMEABILITY MODIFIES OR

CONTROLS (?) LIFE OF SMOOTH MUSCLE IN

ARTERY (THROUGH FEEDBACK MECHANISM ?)

Figure 1. Scheme depicting some basal physiological concepts related to arterial endothelium

(necrosis). These conditions probably represent the experimental analogues to progressive fibro-elastic intimal thickening and medial (Mönckeberg) sclerosis in man.

The right side of Fig. 3 illustrates the sequential changes which follow a very large endothelial desquamation. This is new information, recently published (Björkerud and Bondjers, 1973a) and may require a somewhat more detailed description. After desquamation of the endothelium, intimal proliferation follows as for a small desquamation with a low degree of medial injury. The aortic branches are sources of new endothelium (Fig. 3, II A, B). Regions near enough to sources of endothelium to be reendothelialized within ca. 3 weeks heal (Fig. 3, II C) as for the small injury with low degree of medial damage (Fig. 3, I 1). In areas remote enough not to be covered within ca. 3 weeks, endothelial overgrowth is retarded, in some lesions for more than a year, and the thickening of the intima proceeds (Fig. 3, II C, "pond" is a designation for the non-reendothelialized central, slightly depressed part and "bank" of the surrounding, more elevated part of the plaque; "land" is healed or uninjured regions). Histologically, lipid is present as a faint diffuse extracellular stain in the non-reendo-thelialized regions, *i.e.* the ponds (Björkerud and Bondjers, 1973a). We know from chemical studies that the cholesterol content is increased about fourfold, and the increase of cholesterol ester is about 12-fold in normolipidemic rabbits in the pond region of this type of lesion (Bondjers and Björkerud, 1973b). It should be emphasized that we here are dealing with a tissue containing *masked* lipids and one cannot really trust the impression obtained from tissue sections treated with traditional lipid stains concerning the absolute amounts of lipids present. It is very probable that we face the same problem in human arterial lesions.

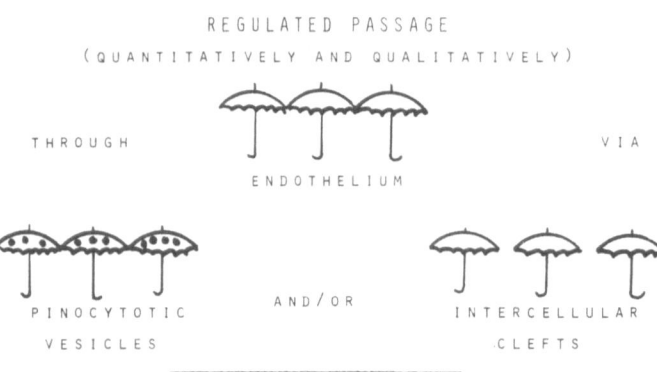

Figure 2.   Illustration of some functional and pathophysiological concepts
related to arterial endothelium

This type of lesion will eventually be reendothelialized in the normo-lipidemic
rabbit (Fig. 3, II D). Late reendothelialization is connected with the appearance of masses of intracellular lipid in granular form, *i.e.* foam cells occur.
From general tissue biological criteria, this tissue is more or less necrotic
(Fig. 3, II D, black area). In contrast to the abundance of lipids as seen in
sections, the actual cholesterol *content* its considerably lower and the proportion of cholesterol ester is also lower than in the preceding stage (Bondjers
and Björkerud, 1973b; Björkerud and Bondjers, 1973b). Here again the histological picture deceives us.

We interpret these findings as follows: A prolonged exposure to serum due to the
absence of an endothelial barrier changes the tissue beyond the point of return.
When the endothelial permeability barrier is reestablished the tissue dies, probably because of insufficient (relative) influx of nutriments or oxygen.

Connected to the necrosis is a demasking of the histologically masked lipids.

At this point it is possible to make the following generalizations, at least for
this model system.

1. The presence of *intact endothelium* seems to be related to either *no* histo
logically stainable lipid *or* the presence of masses of intracellular lipid.
2. The *absence of endothelium* or the presence of *injured* endothelium is related
to low amounts of histologically stainable lipid, if any. In contrast, we know
from other studies that the content of both free and esterified cholesterol is
high. These statements may seem somewhat untraditional and paradoxical. However,
it can be tested if they apply to human arterial tissue. If they do, it would
be a strong indication that the basal arterial tissue reactions, as just described, do not only occur experimentally, but also spontaneously, in man.

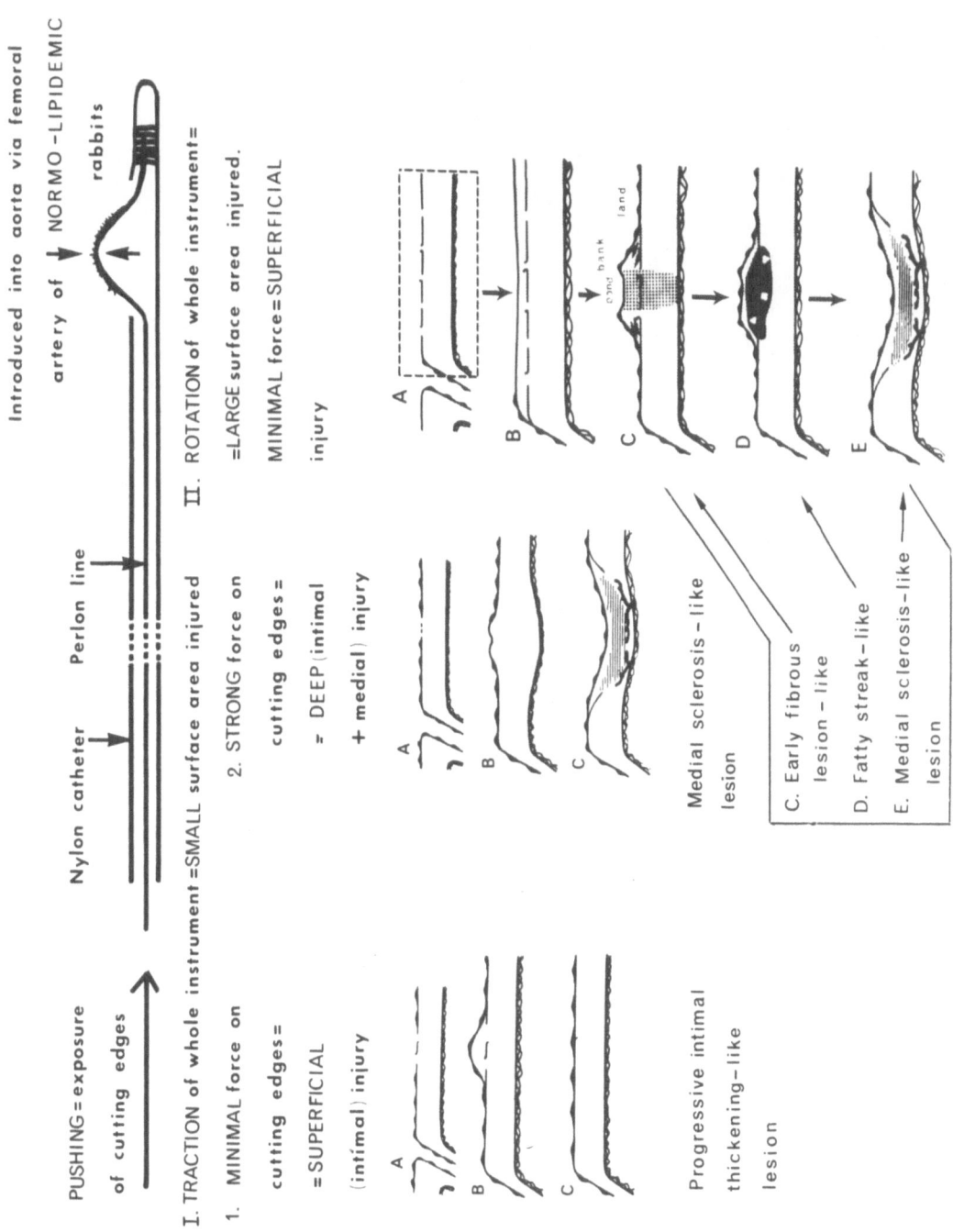

Figure 3. Schematic illustration of the principles for and consequences of the induction of different types of mechanical injury in the rabbit aorta. By means of a microsurgical instrument equipped with microscopic diamonds as cutting edges it is possible to induce injuries the extent of which is defined both with regard to surface area and depth (Björkerud, 1969a,b; Björkerud and Bondjers, 1971, 1973a). For explanation of designations see text

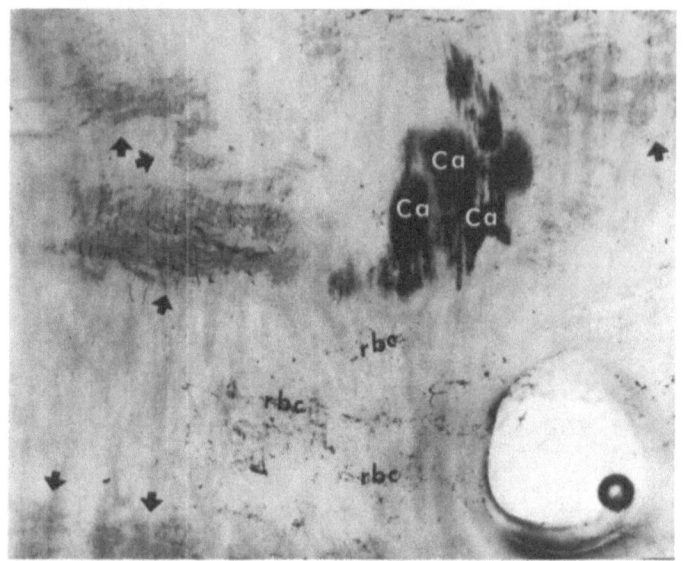

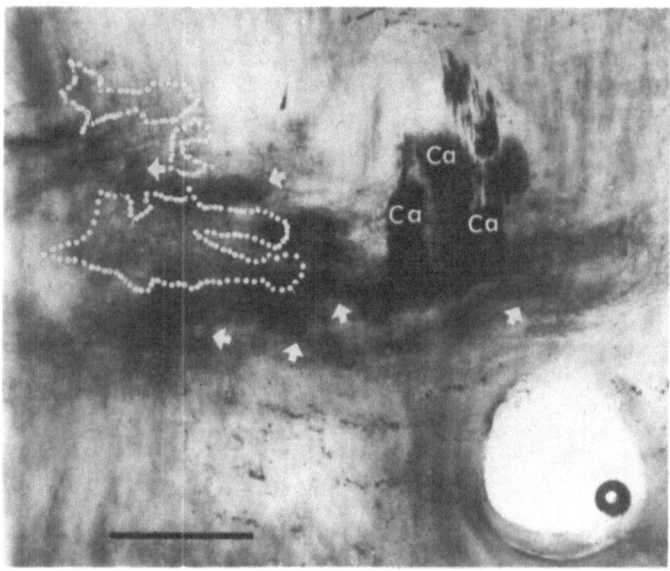

Figure 4. Semimicrograph of a part of the femoral artery of a 36 year old man
as seen from the luminal surface. Amputation of the leg was performed for therapeutic reasons. The living artery was stained for endothelial injury with uncomplexed Evans blue (Björkerud and Bondjers, 1972). After fixation it was cut
open, mounted flat, stained for lipids with oil red O, for peroxidase, and embedded in starch hydrolysate to render the tissue transparent (Björkerud, 1972).
To enable illustration in black-and-white the blue colour (cellular injury; a)
was separated from red (stainable lipid; b) by photography in red and blue light,
respectively
a) Stainability with uncomplexed Evans blue indicates the presence and the
distribution of areas with injured endothelium (black arrows). Ca=calcified
tissue. rbc=red blood cells. In the lower right corner of the picture is the
opening of a branch (the small sphere is an air bubble in the embedding medium).
b) Same as a, but photographed in blue light to visualize the distribution of oil
red O-stained lipid (white arrows). Note that stainable lipid predominantly
occurs in regions with intact endothelium. The white dots indicate the extension
of areas with injured endothelium (cf.a). Line corresponds to 1 mm

In Fig. 4 is shown a surface view of an about 5 mm long segment from the femoral artery of a 36 year old man. The artery was excised surgically for clinical reasons – small malignant pelvic tumour and hemipelvectomy.

The degree of endothelial injury was visualized in the living artery by dye exclusion test for endothelial injury with uncomplexed Evans blue (Björkerud and Bondjers, 1972). Stained regions indicate endothelium with a high degree of injury (Fig. 4a). Unstained regions have uninjured endothelium. Oil red 0 was used as stain for lipids. As can be seen in Fig. 4b, most of the stained lipid is not confined to areas with injured endothelium, but occurs in unstained, intact regions. A large proportion of regions with intact endothelium do not stain for lipid at all.

Furthermore, the calcified region present (Fig. 4) is covered with intact endothelium, as is the case for mechanically induced experimental calcified lesions (Fig. 3, I 2; Björkerud and Bondjers, 1971).

The human lesion shown in Fig. 4 would probably be classified as a fatty streak in traditional pathological terms. However, it is possible to discriminate different characteristic parts of this lesion which are similar to those present in the experimental lesion following a superficial injury with large area (Fig. 3, II). The central region with discontinuous injured endothelium would correspond to the "pond" region and the surrounding oil red 0-stained area to a broad, reendothelialized bank (Fig. 3, II C).

In conclusion, as an answer to the first question raised initially: the basal arterial tissue reactions as seen in this experimental model seem to be applicable to man. With this as a basis I think it is reasonable to propose some possible analogies between human and experimental lesions.

In Fig. 5 is shown, schematically, the possible development of uncomplicated human lesions as deduced from the experimental information referred to above. The lesions conventionally classified as "early" are encompassed in the scheme.

The most likely analogue to the early fibrous lesions is the lesion following superficial injury with large area at the specific stage of its development which is characterized by retarded reendothelialization (Fig. 3, II C). If induced in hyperlipidemic animals, the last-mentioned lesion acquires properties very similar to uncomplicated human atheromata (Björkerud and Bondjers, in preparation). This may reflect a similar mechanism for the formation of atheromata in man. It should be emphasized that the term hyperlipidemia as used in this context is not equivalent to the traditional clinical term. It may comprise, in terms of serum cholesterol, concentrations exceeding a threshold value of ca. 145 mg per 100 ml or even less (Constantinides, 1965).

We propose that there are at least two etiologically different types of fatty streaks. One type (Fig. 5, fatty streak 1) may not be as early as generally presumed for fatty streaks; rather we comprehend it as related to rapid regression of arterial tissue. The fact that fatty streak-like lesions follow the induction of superficial injuries with small areas in hyperlipidemic animals suggest that fatty streaks may simply also represent a proliferating intima combined with hyperlipidemia (see above) (Fig. 5; Björkerud and Bondjers, in preparation).

However, it must be stressed that the situation is much more complex in man. Many lesions may represent synchronous mixtures of different response patterns or sequential pattern of responses which may, in addition, partially overlap each other.

In conclusion, as an answer to the second question raised initially: It seems possible to understand some of the properties of, and maybe also certain relationships between, human early lesions in terms of different characteristic basal arterial tissue reactions which can be elicited experimentally under defined conditions.

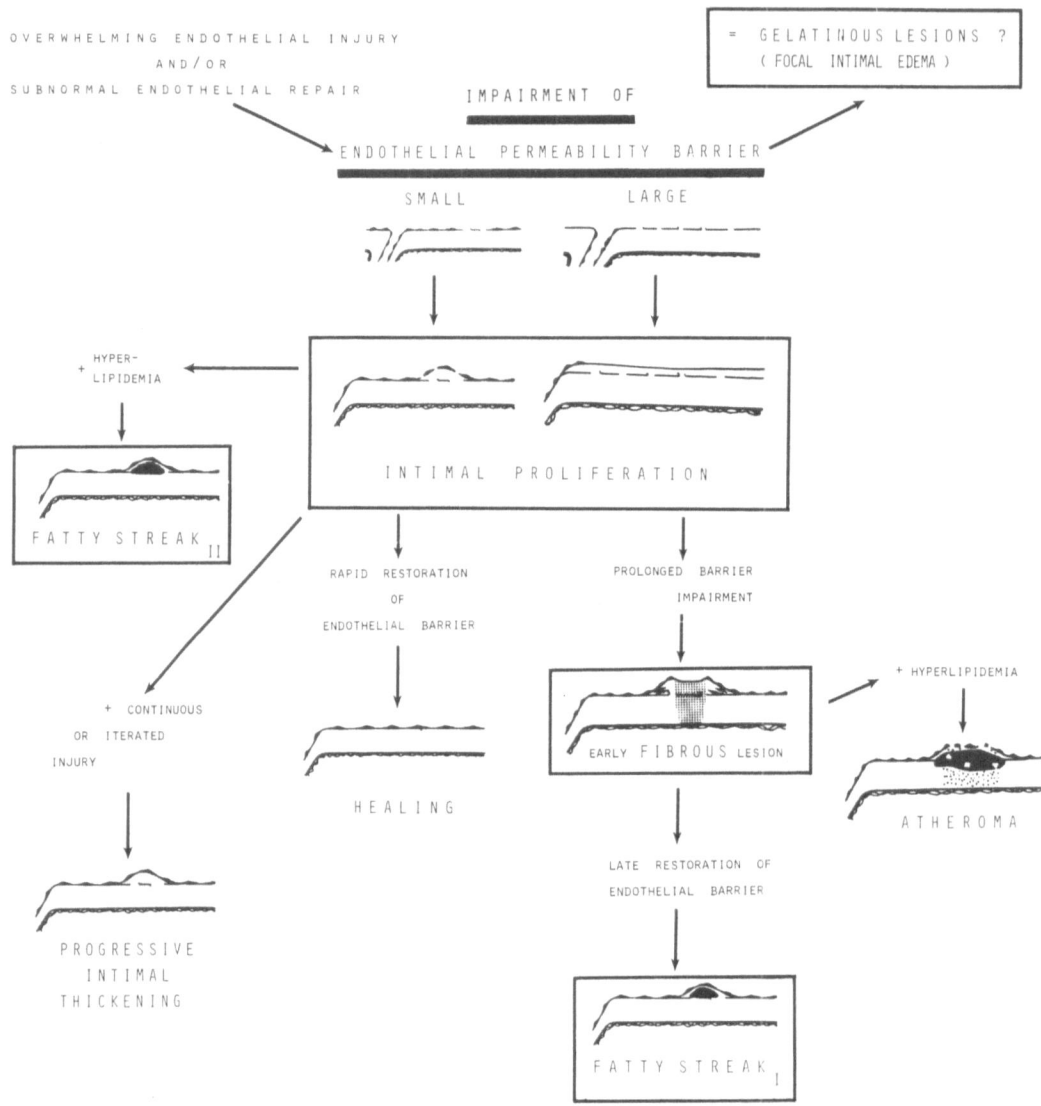

Figure 5. Scheme depicting hypothetically the development and possible interrelationships between early human atherosclerotic lesions. The term hyperlipidemia as used in this context is not equivalent to the traditional clinical term. It may comprise, in terms of serum cholesterol, concentrations exceeding 145 mg per 100 ml or even less (Constantinides, 1965)

DYNAMIC ASPECTS OF FREE AND ESTERIFIED CHOLESTEROL ACCUMULATION

S. Dayton

On the question of cholesterol influx we can probably agree on the following points :- There is some influx of intact plasma lipoprotein. There is also some influx of free cholesterol independent of peptide. This independent influx is much faster than lipoprotein influx, but mainly represents physico-chemical exchange rather than a biological process.

This leaves a number of unanswered questions: 1. Does cholesterol oleate – the dominant lipid of experimental atheroma – get there by influx of plasma cholesterol oleate, or by esterification of free cholesterol *in situ* ? The answer appears to be that both contribute. We have shown in the experimental rabbit lesion that 20% or more of the cholesterol oleate arose by local synthesis (Dayton and Hashimoto, 1968, 1970). Dr. Smith (1972), studying large human lesions by entirely different techniques, concluded that 80% of the cholesterol ester came from plasma and 20% from local synthesis. I consider it safe to say that local synthesis of cholesterol ester within the incipient and growing atheroma is a quantitatively significant process.

Question number 2 follows logically: what factors influence local cholesterol ester synthesis? What enzyme pathway is involved? Abdulla et al. (1968) reported evidence for LCAT activity in the atheroma, and Proudlock & Day (1972) have identified another enzyme active at low pH. In common with St. Clair et al.(1970) we have centered our attention on a third enzyme having acyl CoA: cholesterol acyl-transferase activity. Homogenates of rabbit atheroma were incubated with palmityl CoA, labeled in the fatty acyl group. The ß-fatty acid of lecithin achieved much higher specific activity than did cholesteryl ester; furthermore, the specific activity of the cholesteryl ester stopped rising as soon as the substrate was exhausted, suggesting that lecithin was not acting as an intermediate (Fig. 1).

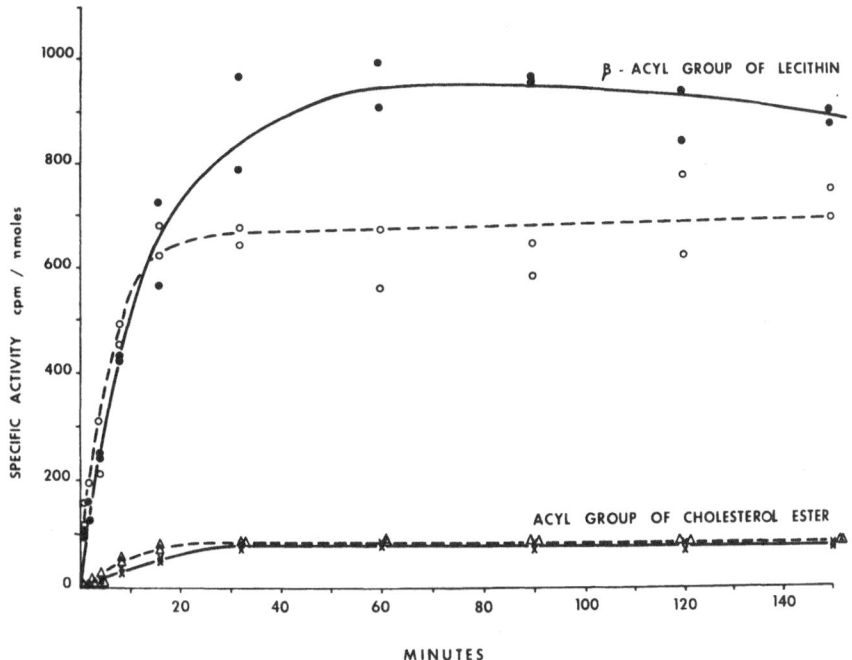

Figure 1. Atherosclerotic cell – free homogenate

Most of the activity was in the microsomes. In a typical experiment (Fig. 2) enzymatic activity of atherosclerotic microsomes was about 40-fold greater than activity of normal microsomes. It is difficult to avoid the inference that the massive acceleration of cholesterol ester formation through this pathway is associated with their accumulation. Available evidence suggests that there may be

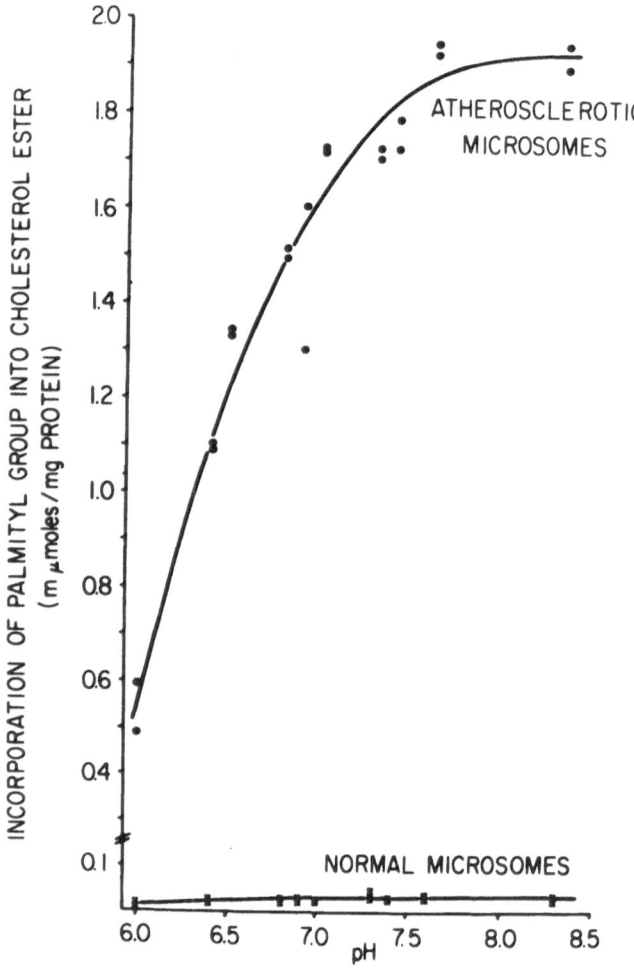

Figure 2

more enzyme in atherosclerotic microsomes, but this requires further studies. Another factor which might influence the rate of cholesterol ester synthesis is increased availability of free cholesterol; we find its concentration tripled in microsomes of cholesterol-fed rabbits.

Recently, Dr. Hashimoto has shown that mitochondria from atheromas display consistent depression of their ability to oxidize palmityl CoA to CO_2 (Fig. 3). The mitochondria are, however, responsive to carnitine. The possible relevance of this observation to cholesterol ester accumulation is shown in Fig. 4. Normally, mitochondria oxidize roughly half the fatty acyl CoA available to the cell, so that suppression of mitochondrial oxidation could result in significant increase in the amount of acyl CoA available to the major microsomal pathways, including cholesterol ester synthesis.

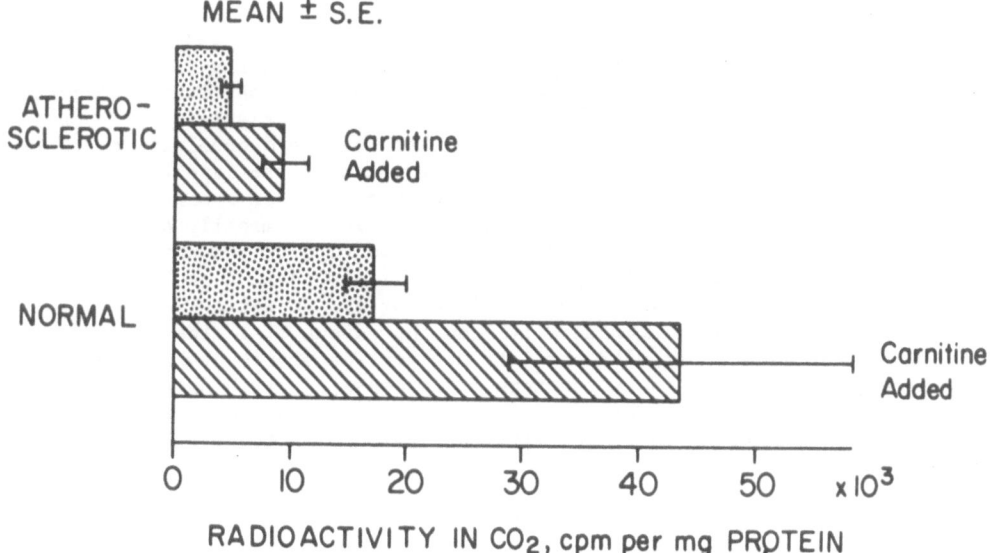

Figure 3. $(1 - ^{14}C)$ Palmityl - CoA $\longrightarrow$ $^{14}CO_2$ in aortic mitochondria

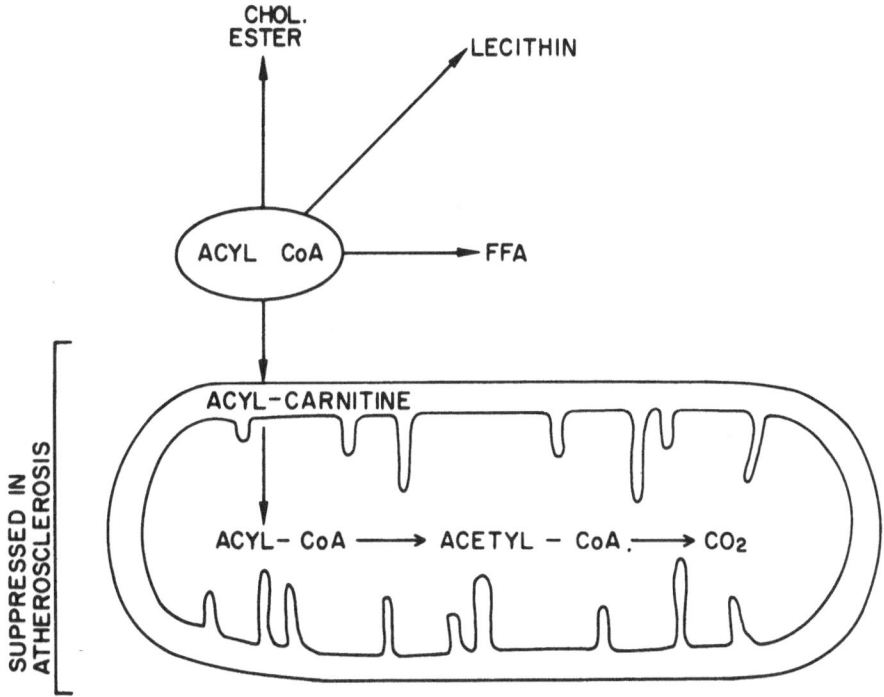

Figure 4

To recapitulate - three different local factors might augment cholesterol ester formation in the arterial microsomes of the cholesterol-fed rabbit. First, their microsomes contain more free cholesterol. Second, their mitochondria provide less competition for acyl CoA. Third, but not yet conclusively demonstrated, their microsomes may contain more cholesterol-esterifying enzyme.

Discussion

Dr. Smit Sibinga: May I demonstrate some information relating to the scheme Dr. Björkerud showed on possible relationships between different atherosclerotic lesions? I have been using an experimental model where arterial injury caused by experimental irradiation has been combined with feeding of cholesterol to rabbits. With this system it is possible to gain information on the importance of permeability changes in the vessel wall for the deposition of cholesterol in normolipidemic as well as hyperlipidemic animals. No histochemically demonstrable accumulation of lipids occurs after irradiation damage in the normolipidemic animal. On the other hand, if hyperlipidemia is induced in a rabbit with arteries injured with X-rays, a very marked deposition of lipids follows. However, if the carotid artery is injured mechanically from the adventitial side, a strikingly different picture follows, with complete destruction of the media and the formation of mural thrombi. This latter type of response is strikingly different from the one following the destruction of the endothelium and the intima which follows X-rays, which I referred to in the first part of this presentation (Smit Sibinga, 1972).

Chairman Björkerud: The combined effects of the induction of a proliferation of the intima and hyperlipidemia has been studied by many workers. I think it is a general consensus that a fatty streak-line lesion is produced. The lesion which follows cholesterol-feeding exclusively, is rather different from the human atherosclerotic lesions, a fact which also has been pointed out by a number of workers. However, the combination of injury and hyperlipidemia produces lesions which are more similar to the lesions occurring in man. This subject has been treated in detail in Constantinides' monograph "Experimental Atherosclerosis".

Dr. Caro: Is there a missing link between endothelial injury and presence of lipids in the underlying tissue?

Chairman Björkerud: The point you are referring to is the paradoxical distribution of histochemically demonstrable lipids and the presence of endothelial injury. One would believe that where the endothelium is injured, more lipid would be seen in the underlying tissue. However, this is not the case. One of the points in my presentation was, that due to the fact that lipids be histochemically masked, we might have been misled for years regarding the actual chemical content of lipids in the tissue. As a consequence of this, we may also have misinterpreted the true nature of the different types of human lesions and the true sequential development of the different stages of the atherosclerotic lesion. If I may add one further comment on the hypothetical scheme of possible relationships between the different kinds of lesions shown in my presentation. Due to lack of time it was only possible to touch upon some of the evidence underlying this scheme. I would like to add here briefly the further evidence provided by the findings by Dr. Elspeth Smith. I proposed that at least one type of fatty streak in man followed late reendothelialization and actually represents regression of a tissue which before the reendothelialization was characterized by marked intimal proliferation and imbibition of serum constituents. The presence of a continuous, "tight", endothelium covering the fatty streak would prevent the influx of serum lipids. This is consistent with the low content of intact lipoprotein in human fatty streaks, as found by Dr. Smith. Furthermore, the absence of extracellular lipids conforms with *removal* of lipids, in other words, regression. The abundance of foam cells which, no doubt, show many signs of cellular injury would also be consistent with regression of tissue, *i.e.* tissue death.

Dr. Caro: One might see, perhaps, a correlation between arterial injury and a low lipid content? Could it be that hemodynamic events, as an increased flow velocity could increase the egress of lipids?

Chairman Björkerud: I must disappoint you on this point, because the actual cholesterol and cholesterol ester content, as determined by chemical methods, is high in the tissue underlying injured endothelium, at least in the rabbit. If this also is valid for man is uncertain, because studies involving chemical analyses of human arterial samples with defined endothelial integrity have not been carried out as yet, to my knowledge. Our dye-exclusion technique would be suitable for this purpose, if it is applied to living arterial segments that have not been damaged during the excision.

Chairman Smith: Perhaps I can make a comment here, that in the gelatinous lesions intact lipoprotein can account for up to 75% of the total cholesterol present in the lesion. If you electrophorese the lipoprotein out of the tissue and then measure the cholesterol that has not moved out of the tissue by electrophoresis, this may be very much less than the cholesterol accounted for by intact lipoprotein. This could well fit in with some of your findings, Dr. Björkerud, because I don't think that lipoprotein will stain with the ordinary Sudan stains. I think one requires a "lipid droplet" of a certain minimum size to get the proper staining. It is possible that this is where the apparent discrepancy may arise, that we have got intact lipoprotein present in really quite large amount. If the cholesterol is measured chemically, one will find quite a lot, and a large part of this is in intact lipoprotein.

Dr. Wissler: In our very early studies, frequently we could find lipoprotein by fluorescence microscopy before we could see it with Sudan staining. We also ran into a paradox in a sense similar to Dr. Björkerud's. In the Rhesus monkey, where we admittedly were dealing with rather high cholesterol or lipoprotein levels, we expected a correlation between the *in vivo* staining with albumin-complexed Evans blue, and where first lesions occurred. Neither grossly nor microscopically, did we find a very good correlation. The blue areas frequently did not have any lesion, and lesions were frequently where there were no blue areas. These observations were obtained in acute experiments. Of course, one needs better observations with time, to be able to draw more firm conclusions on this question in the model system we used. Finally, I would like to ask Dr. Insull whether he would put on a left handside of his relatively established observations that there are lipoproteins in the arterial wall which might be different from the kinds of bodies you are observing? I would like to point out that there seem to be at least three rather widely divergent analyses even for fatty streaks, either in terms of the fatty acids in them, or the proportion of the cholesterol ester. It may be so that we call different lesions fatty streaks. We may not even be observing the same kinds of lesions in different parts of the world.

Chairman Smith: They first appeared in either Canada or Germany.

Dr. Adams: Could I just comment on the staining of the lipoprotein. I would agree with you absolutely that the Sudan type of dyes, as oil red O, Sudan black, and Fett Rot would stain cholesterol ester and triglycerides. When you have lipids dispersed by protein, they become hydrophilic, and a physical dye of this sort should not stain them. I agree entirely what you are saying, and what Dr. Wissler said, but Kenneth Walton tells me he used oil red O to stain lipoprotein lipid on paper. I remember we did this at one time and it stains lipoprotein on paper. Why this difference?

Chairman Smith: One usually denatures it. It is fixed in some way before you stain.

Dr. Adams: So that would be the explanation?

Chairman Smith: Yes, It's either heated or denatured in some other way before it is stained.

Dr. Walton: We have recently been studying lesions in the iris and in the iridial vessels sequentially in the cholesterol-fed rabbit (Walton, 1973). There is a stage at which one gets lipoprotein fluorescence in the endothelium of the small iridial vessels, but lipids cannot be demonstrated with conventional lipid stains. On the electronmicroscopic level the same lesions show endothelial cells with marked pinocytosis of small lipid particles. So this is one instance where there is a discrepancy in the sensitivity of the tool. I agree that you really have to have some change in the lipoprotein, in order to be able to stain it. Furthermore, I want to underline the last point raised by Robert Wissler: The last time there was an international conference on nomenclature, the lesion that we have been talking about today, the gelatinous lesions, mucoid elevation, insudation spot, or whatever we are going to call it, was dismissed as entirely physiological. I think most of us would agree on now that it probably is not. It seems to me that if this conference does nothing else than to reverse that opinion, it will be really quite useful.

Question: I came here to learn: what is the initial factor, regardless of the anatomy of the fatty streak, gelatinous lesion etc. What ideas do you have? Is it diet, is it catecholamines, genetic factors, a virus, an enzyme? What are your ideas? I take anything right now.

Chairman Smith: If I knew I would have got the Nobel prize by now.

THE LESION

Henry C. McGill, Jr.

Introduction

The etiology and pathogenesis of mural atherosclerotic lesions remain central issues in the problem of the atherosclerotic diseases. Primary prevention, now accepted as the long-range goal for control of atherosclerotic disease, depends on knowing what stage in pathogenesis is amenable to intervention. The mural atherosclerotic lesions have been thoroughly described and illustrated in several reviews and symposia (Geer and Haust, 1972; Wissler and Geer, 1972; McMillan, 1973). Therefore, the purpose of this article is to review information accumulated since the Second International Symposium on Atherosclerosis (Jones, 1970), and to examine the implications of these finding for our concepts of pathogenesis and for preventive intervention. Emphasis is placed on reports that have appeared since 1969, and on selected reports from previous years that are pertinent to current issues.

Unsolved Problems of Pathogenesis

The conventional concept of pathogenesis is indicated in Fig. 1. The earliest distinctive lesion of atherosclerosis is seen as intimal lipid deposition (the fatty streak), which is converted into an elevated lesion with a lipid core and a fibromuscular cap (the fibrous plaque). The fibrous plaque undergoes a variety of changes, some of which (particularly thrombosis) result in arterial occlusion. Ischemia of vital organs results in various clinical disease syndromes depending on the organ affected.

Although the general framework of the scheme described above remains the most widely accepted concept of pathogenesis, conclusive proofs of some steps are still lacking and new information suggests that some concepts of pathogenetic sequences should be altered. The major problem areas are the following:

1. Intimal thickening that precedes lipid deposition. Does this represent the earliest stage of atherosclerosis? Is it a "lesion" in the sense of being a reaction to injury? If so, what causes it, and is it preventable?
2. The origin of the fatty streak, and the conditions responsible for it. Is there more than one kind of fatty streak?
3. The relationship of the fatty streak to the fibrous plaque. Do fibrous plaques arise from fatty streaks, or do they arise independently?
4. The role of smooth muscle proliferation in the pathogenesis of lesions. To what degree is smooth muscle proliferation a normal growth phenomenon, and to what degree is it a reaction to injury?
5. The mechanism of action of the risk factors on mural arterial lesions. Do all the risk factors increase lipid deposition, or do they act on different stages in the pathogenetic sequence?

These, of course, are not the only unsolved questions. For example, the role of thrombosis as the terminal occlusive event in the coronary arteries has been questioned repeatedly, particularly in cases of sudden death. However, in this discussion, we will concentrate on problems related to the earlier stages of atherogenesis.

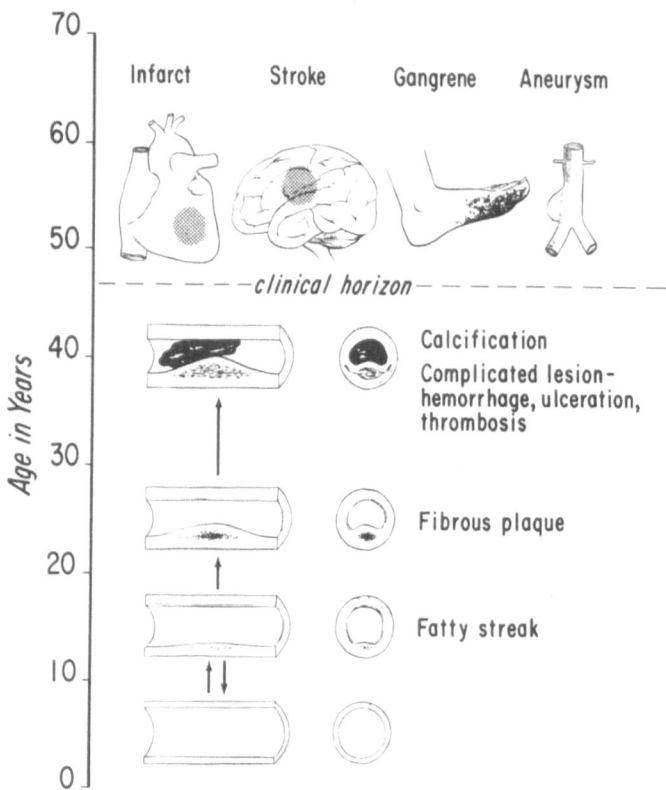

Figure 1. Diagrammatic description of the natural history of human atherosclerotic lesions and their clinical manifestations. (From McGill, H.C., Geer, J.C.,
and Strong, J.P., in Atherosclerosis and Its Origin, edited by Sandler, M. and
Bourne, G.H., Ch. 2, New York, Academic Press, Inc. 1963)

Fibromuscular Intimal Thickening

The Problem. Fibromuscular intimal thickening without abnormal lipid deposition
is a characteristic feature of the coronary arteries of young humans. By the end
of the second decade of life, the intima of the main coronary arteries equals the
media in thickness. This thickened intima is made up of longitudinally oriented
smooth muscle cells, collagen, and elastic fibers. Intimal thickening appears at
about the same age in the abdominal aorta, and at a later age in the thoracic
aorta. In neither aortic segment does it become as prominent as in the coronary
arteries. In almost all persons after young adulthood, the thickened intima of
the coronary arteries and aorta becomes inextricably mixed with focal lipid
deposition and associated chronic inflammatory and proliferative reactions
typical of atherosclerosis. Thus, the existence of fibromuscular intimal
thickening independently of atherosclerosis is obscured, and divergent views
of their relationship to one another have developed. The issue is limited, for
the most part, to lesions of the coronary arteries because intimal thickening
is more prominent in them than in other arteries.

Coronary Intimal Thickening as a Developmental Phenomenon. Geer and Haust (1972)
have thoroughly reviewed observations on the development of the thickened coronary artery intima, which was recognized long ago as an essentially normal structure. Gross (1934) described its formation from birth to old age in meticulous
detail, but avoided a distinction between the process of proliferation in childhood and the process of atherosclerosis. Dock (1946) found coronary artery intimal muscular proliferation more extensive in male newborn infants than in fe-

male infants, and attributed the predilection of males for coronary atherosclerosis to this structure. He interpreted the intimal muscular thickening itself,
however, as an inherited characteristic rather than as a response to a
specific injury. Moon (1957) found the same process at birth and interpreted
it as a response to injury and a precursor of atherosclerosis. Neufeld (1962)
found muscular intimal thickening beginning at or shortly after birth, and found
the total artery wall thickness and the external diameter of the artery wall to
be greater in males than in females from birth. However, the ratio of intimal
thickness to total thickness of the arterial wall was equal in males and females
until 20 years of age.

Population Comparison of Childhood Intimal Thickening. Data on the extent of
fibromuscular intimal thickening among children of different population are also
conflicting. Vlodaver (1969) found differences that corresponded with the severity of adult atherosclerosis, but other studies have found no significant differences among young persons (Robertson, JH, 1960; Robertson, WB et al., 1963;
Scott et al., 1966; Geer et al., 1968). On the basis of comparison of coronary
arteries with other arteries (Glagov, 1972), and on the basis of hemodynamic
studies (Fry, 1973), others have concluded that the fibromuscular intimal thickening occurring before 20 years of age represents a physiological remodeling of
the arterial wall, an adaptation to organ growth and increased flow.

Coronary Intimal Thickening as Atherosclerosis. The alternative view, that fibromuscular intimal thickening results from a specific injury and is the initial
lesion of atherosclerosis, is supported in part by the experimental induction of
intimal muscular proliferation without lipid deposition by a variety of methods.
This phenomenon has been reported in several species of animals after feeding
certain oils, particularly peanut oil, which contain long-chain fatty acids
(Kritchevsky, 1970; Kritchevsky et al., 1971). Increased proliferative activity
in arterial smooth muscle cells is caused by feeding cholesterol to experimental
animals (McMillan and Duff, 1948; McMillan and Stary, 1968). Proliferation begins
even before serum cholesterol is significantly elevated (Florentin and Nam, 1968;
Thomas et al., 1968; Florentin et al., 1969; Thomas et al., 1971). A fibromuscular intimal layer may also be produced by injuring the artery with a suture
(Poole et al., 1971) or denuding the endothelium with an intravascular balloon
catheter (Stemmerman and Ross, 1972; Ross and Glomset, 1973b). Ross and Glomset
(1973a) recently amplified this view by proposing that plasma proteins penetrate
endothelium of increased permeability to stimulate intimal smooth muscle cell
proliferation and thereby initiate atherosclerosis. Although smooth muscle proliferation undoubtedly contributes to the pathogenesis of atherosclerosis, it
does not seem likely that the fibromuscular intimal thickening of coronary arteries in childhood is the result of a specific environmental agent. Smooth
muscle proliferation and connective tissue accumulation after age 20 years are
very likely the result of environmental agents and are unquestionably involved
in the process of atherosclerosis.

In summary, we conclude that fibromuscular intimal thickening in the coronary
arteries of persons under 20 years of age is an essentially normal anatomic structure. Atherosclerosis proper develops only when other changes take place within
this structure.

Fibromuscular Intimal Thickening in Animals. Focal intimal plaques of smooth
muscle and variable proportions of connective tissue are common findings in the
large arteries of most animals, even without experimental manipulation. They
occur both at the orifices of branching vessels and in straight segments. An impression exists that both diffuse and focal fibromuscular intimal thickening are
greater in larger animals, but this impression has not been subjected to systematic controlled analysis. Stary and Strong (1973) have shown that fibromuscular
intimal plaques consistently occur in the main segments of the extramayocardial
coronary arteries of rhesus monkeys. These muscular plaques become foci of predilection for lipid deposition when the animals are fed cholesterol (Stary 1974).

The fibromuscular cushions that occur at points of branching have been recognized
in animals as well as in man and have been interpreted as responses to hemodynamic stress (Fry, 1973). Although these cushions are also sites of predilection
for lipid deposition in cholesterol-fed animals, they do not seem to predispose
to occlusive lesions in humans.

The distribution of focal fibromuscular cushions in the arteries of experimental
animals needs more thorough investigation in order to assess their relevance to
experimental atherosclerosis and their relationship to intimal thickening in man.

The Fatty Streak

"Fatty streak" is widely used as a descriptive term for flat or slightly raised
intimal lesions in which the predominant abnormality is an accumulation of intracellular or extracellular lipid. These accumulations occur frequently in the
large muscular and elastic arteries of humans from infancy to old age, alone and
in association with other types of atherosclerotic lesions. We have an enormous
body of information about the structure, chemical composition, metabolism, and
other characteristics of fatty streaks, both occurring naturally in the human and
experimentally induced in experimental animals. Nevertheless, controversy abounds
regarding the significance and fate of the fatty streak, particularly regarding
its relationship to the fibrous plaque and other advanced lesions.

Histology and Ultrastructure. The light and electron microscopic characteristics
of human fatty streaks recently have been reviewed and illustrated comprehensively
(Haust, 1971; Geer and Haust, 1972). The fatty streak in young humans characteristically is made up of smooth muscle cells that contain varying amounts of lipid;
other lipid-filled cells resembling phagocytic mononuclear cells (macrophages);
and extracellular lipid. Both intracellular and extracellular lipid particles
appear in a variety of structural forms under the electron microscope due either
to differing chemical composition, or to variations in fixation and processing,
or to both. Experimentally induced fatty streaks are similar to fatty streaks
of young humans in structure and composition (Scott et al., 1967a; Geer et al.,
1968; Tucker et al., 1971).

Fatty streaks can be subclassified into many types according to location of the
lipid, amount of lipid, relative proportion of connective tissue elements, and
other morphologic characteristics. However, such classifications are of little
value unless they are related to a pathogenetic sequence. We will return to this
problem in discussing the relationship of the fatty streak to the fibrous plaque.

Lipid Composition. Most investigators agree that the lipid in fatty streaks from
young persons is predominantly cholesterol and its esters, with lesser proportions
of triglycerides and phospholipids (reviewed by Cornwell et al., 1973). The distinctive characteristic of the cholesterol ester in human fatty streaks is the
high proportion of cholesterol oleate. This feature distinguishes it from normal
artery, from advanced atherosclerotic lesions, and from plasma cholesterol esters. Experimentally induced fatty streaks also have a high proportion of cholesterol oleate (St. Clair et al., 1968; Peterson et al., 1971).

Connective Tissue Composition. Fatty streaks also contain all the connective tissue elements of normal artery -- collagen, elastic fibers, microfibrils, and
glycosaminoglycans. However, less is known about alterations of these components
than about alterations in lipids, and it has not been possible to describe a
simple, consistent relationship between connective tissue elements and lipid
(Smith, 1973). Furthermore, it has not been possible to identify any distinctive
alterations in connective tissue that precede lipid deposition.

Permeability and Fatty Streaks. Many recent investigations have been directed
toward increased intimal permeability as a possible precursor of the fatty streak.

In humans, these efforts are limited to searching for variations in the concentration of normal plasma constituents in different segments of the intima. Plasma components demonstrated in fatty streaks include lipoproteins (Kao and Wissler, 1965; Woolf and Pilkington, 1965; Smith and Slater, 1968, 1970, 1973) and fibrinogen or fibrin (Woolf and Crawford, 1960; Haust et al., 1967; and Walton and Williamson, 1968).

In experimental animals, focal areas of increased intimal permeability have been demonstrated *in vivo* with plasma proteins labelled with I-131 (Packham et al., 1967) and with Evans Blue (McGill et al., 1957; Friedman and Byers, 1963; Somer and Schwartz, 1971, 1972; Fry, 1973. This observation is cited as evidence that focally increased endothelial permeability could be responsible for focal intimal lipid deposition, particularly when the plasma is rich in low-density lipoprotein as Page suggested many years ago (1954). It has not been possible to test this hypothetical mechanism of the origin of intimal lipid deposition in humans, nor is it likely to be possible to do so in the near future. Any altered endothelial permeability associated with an established human fatty streak could be secondary to the underlying abnormal lipid deposition. Thus, the presence of excess plasma constituents in human fatty streaks does not demonstrate that these substances initiate the fatty streak. Their presence however, does provide a mechanism for explaining progression of fatty streaks to more advanced lesions.

Metabolism. The metabolism of human and experimental arterial fatty streaks has been investigated extensively with regard to lipid influx and efflux, lipid biosynthesis, and energy metabolism (St. Clair et al., 1968, 1969; Dayton and Hashimoto, 1970; Lofland and Clarkson, 1970; Day et al., 1970; Geer et al., 1972; Scott et al., 1972; Chobanian and Manzur, 1972; Adams, 1973; Zilversmit and Hughes, 1973; Stein and Stein, 1973; Peters et al., 1973). These data, together with knowledge of the complex structure and composition of fatty streaks, indicate that arterial lipid deposition is a more complex process than simple passive infiltration of lipid-rich plasma and physical trapping of excess lipid. Developments in this area are reviewed elsewhere in this symposium.

The Natural History and Distribution of Fatty Streaks. Many years ago, pathologists observed fatty streaks in the aortas of children and speculated on their origin and significance (Klotz and Manning, 1911; Zinserling, 1925). They begin to appear within a few months after birth and are present in almost all children after the age of three years (Holman et al., 1958; McGill, 1968; Strong and McGill, 1969). In the second decade of life, the mean extent of aortic intimal surface involved by fatty streaks increases rapidly in succeeding age groups, with wide individual variability from less than 5% involvement of the intimal surface to nearly 100% involvement. There is a progressive increase in the extent of aortic fatty streaks until about the fourth decade, after which the extent remains constant or declines slightly. Since fibrous plaques and other advanced lesions begin to involve the aorta to an appreciable degree in the fourth decade, it is difficult to measure fatty streaks in any meaningful way after age 40.

Coronary artery fatty streaks begin to appear in the middle of the second decade of life, and increase in extent rapidly in the third decade (Strong and McGill, 1962; McGill, 1968; Eggen and Solberg, 1968; Strong and McGill, 1969). Thus, the pattern of development of coronary artery fatty streaks follows that of the aorta by about 10 years. The increase in extent with age is less rapid than for aortic fatty streaks, but coronary artery fatty streaks tend to involve increasing proportions of surface area at older ages, rather than to reach a plateau as do aortic fatty streaks. As in the aorta, they become mixed with and replaced by fibrous plaques in the fourth and subsequent decades.

In the carotid and intracranial arteries, fatty streaks begin in the third and fourth decades of life and increase in prevalence and extent slowly in subsequent years (Solberg et al., 1968; Solberg and Eggen, 1971; Solberg and McGarry, 1972).

"Spontaneous" Fatty Streaks in Animals. Although fatty streaks have been the focus of attention as endpoints in experimental atherosclerosis, usually as a result of cholesterol feeding, fatty streaks also occur "spontaneously" in some species without serum lipid elevation and without cholesterol feeding. For example, baboons (*Papio* sp.) examined in their natural habitat show a high prevalence of aortic fatty streaks (McGill et al., 1960; Van der Watt et al., 1973). So also do squirrel monkeys (*Saimiri sciureus*), and to a lesser degree, cebus monkeys (*Cebus apella* and *Cebus albifrons*) (Middleton et al., 1967; Eggen et al., 1969). Some strains of swine develop fatty streaks (French and Jennings, 1965). The newly hatched chick has aortic and coronary artery fatty streaks (Nichols et al., 1961). These spontaneous lesions are considered by some investigators a curse, requiring more numerous control animals in experiments; and by others a blessing, simulating more closely the human situation. At the very least, their existence demonstrates that hyperlipidemia and the other conditions associated with severe human atherosclerosis are not absolute requirements for arterial intimal lipid deposition.

The Fate of Fatty Streaks. The prevailing concept holds that continued lipid accumulation, smooth muscle and connective tissue proliferation, necrosis, and possibly fibrin and platelet deposition cause fatty streaks to progress in subsequent decades to fibrous plaques and other more advanced atherosclerotic lesions, which in turn produce stenosis, thrombosis, occlusion, and ischemic necrosis of vital organs. The fatty streak therefore is seen as the initial lesion of atherosclerosis, or at least at the earliest lesion recognizable as distinctive to the process of atherosclerosis. Whether fatty streaks can, and in fact do, progress under certain conditions to fibrous plaques was mentioned initially as a controversial problem regarding the fate of the fatty streak. We will return to this problem after a consideration of the fibrous plaque itself.

Regression of Fatty Streaks. There seems little doubt that simple fatty streaks may undergo regression, particularly in experimental animals, after the stimulus for hypercholesterolemia is withdrawn (Armstrong et al., 1970; Tucker et al., 1971). The histologic and ultrastructural characteristics of human fatty streaks suggest that they, too, are capable of regression with minimal residual stigmata, but there is no direct evidence for such regression. Regressed experimental fatty streaks initially leave an intima which contains somewhat more connective tissue than the normal intima, a phenomenon that may explain in part the diffuse fibrous intimal thickening seen in the arteries of adults and elderly persons. This connective tissue component eventually returns to approximately normal levels, but decreases much more slowly than the lipid content (Armstrong and Megan, 1973).

The Fibrous Plaque

The typical fibrous plaque is made up of a core of extracellular lipid-rich material surrounded by a capsule of smooth muscle and connective tissue. Like the term "fatty streak", "fibrous plaque" is a gross descriptive term. Common changes in fibrous plaques include vascularization, hemorrhage, calcification, ulceration, and mural thrombosis. The fibrous plaque and its sequelae are unquestionably the precursors of arterial occlusion (Tejada et al., 1968; Strong et al., 1968; Deupree et al., 1973), and are associated with the risk factors for clinical disease (Robertson and Strong, 1968; Scott et al., 1966; Strong et al., 1969; Strong et al., 1972).

Lipid Composition. The lipid of fibrous plaques, like that of fatty streaks, is predominantly cholesterol and its esters, but the fatty acids esterified to cholesterol contain a higher portion of linoleate (Cornwell at al., 1973; Smith and Slater, 1973). Thus, fibrous plaque lipid resembles plasma lipid. This finding supports the idea that the lipid core of the fibrous plaque is likely to be derived from infiltration of plasma lipid. Although lipid is a constant component of the fibrous plaque, the amount relative to the size of the entire lesion varies greatly. Lipid may be the principal component, or it may be so small as to appear insignificant in comparison with the smooth muscle and connective tissue.

Role of Smooth Muscle. Since fibroblasts are either nonexistent or rare in the arterial intima and in fibrous plaques, and since arterial smooth muscle in tissue culture has been shown to be capable of producing collagen and elastin (Ross, 1971; Ross and Klebanoff, 1971; Ross and Glomset, 1973b), it is now presumed likely that the connective tissue in fibrous plaques is produced by smooth muscle. Emphasis on the smooth muscle and connective tissue has led to consideration of the fibrous plaque as a proliferative reaction rather than as a degenerative lesion. Evidence that fibrous plaques may have a monoclonal origin (Benditt and Benditt, 1973) further supports this view and introduces the concept of cellular transformation as a mechanism.

Natural History and Distribution of Fibrous Plaques. Fibrous plaques begin to appear in the abdominal aorta and the coronary arteries in the third decade of life, and in the thoracic aorta and cerebral arteries in the fourth decade. Thereafter, they increase progressively in all arterial systems in succeeding age groups from all populations examined (Eggen and Solberg, 1968; Solberg and McGarry, 1972). Thus, in their appearance they lag behind fatty streaks by 5 to 10 years. Although fibrous plaques are present to some degree in all populations, their prevalence and extent parallel closely the incidence of clinical disease due to atherosclerosis in the corresponding population.

Experimental Production of Fibrous Plaques. While fatty streaks have been the usual lesions of experimental atherosclerosis, fibrous plaques have been relatively rare. Consequently, less is known about conditions that favor their development in experimental animals. Pigeons (Clarkson and Lofland, 1961) and swine (Scott et al., 1972) which have sites of predilection for lesions under experimental regimens, develop human-like fibrous plaques after 6 months of cholesterol feeding. In rabbits, intermittent periods of cholesterol feeding tend to produce lesions resembling fibrous plaques (Constantinides, 1965), perhaps because rabbits do not tolerate a continuous high cholesterol diet for long periods. In nonhuman primates, cholesterol feeding must be continued for several years before lesions like human fibrous plaques appear. A recent report indicates that one non-human primate species, the vervet monkey (*Cercopithecus aethiops*), is more likely to develop fibrous plaques on atherogenic regimens than are other species (Bullock et al., 1972). Generalizing about the experimental production of fibrous plaques is hazardous, but it seems that animals with moderate elevations of serum cholesterol concentration (200 - 300 mg/dl) for several years are more likely to develop human-like fibrous plaques than are those with extremely high elevation of serum cholesterol for shorter periods.

Relationship of Fatty Streaks to Fibrous Plaques

Evidence Against a Sequential Relationship. Some investigators have challenged the conventional concept that fatty streaks progress to fibrous plaques. In both the aorta and the coronary arteries, the extent and localization of fatty streaks in younger persons do not correlate well with the extent and localization of fibrous plaques in older persons. Aortic fatty streaks appear first in the proximal portion of the arch and later in the thoracic and abdominal aorta, while severe advanced atherosclerosis typically affects the abdominal aorta (Holman et al., 1958; Mitchell and Schwartz, 1965). Negro children have more extensive aortic fatty streaks than do white children, while Negro adults have less extensive fibrous plaques than do white adults (McGill, 1968). Young females of all ethnic groups in all parts of the world have more extensive aortic fatty streaks than do young males of the corresponding populations, but older females have less extensive fibrous plaques and less frequent clinical disease (Tejada et al., 1968; McGill, 1968). There is no consistent association in young persons between extent of aortic fatty streaks and diet, serum lipids, obesity, geographic residence, terminal or complicating illness, or other conditions or characteristics commonly associated with severe adult atherosclerosis and clinically manifest disease due to atherosclerosis. Aortic fatty streaks typical of present-day children were present in children many years ago (Klotz and Manning, 1911; Zinserling, 1925). Aortic fatty streaking appears to be a universal phenomenon in young humans, unaffected by environment, and in particular unaffected by environmental conditions associated with advanced lesions and clinical disease.

The coronary arteries also show discrepancies between fatty streaks and fibrous plaques. Negroes have more extensive coronary artery fatty streaks than whites or other ethnic groups, and females have more extensive coronary artery fatty streaks than males (McGill, 1968). In contrast, it is well known that Negroes and females are less likely to develop coronary artery fibrous plaques and advanced coronary atherosclerosis than are whites and males in the corresponding populations.

With these discrepancies between fatty streaks in young persons and fibrous plaques in older persons, it is reasonable to question the relationship of fatty streaks to fibrous plaques and clinically significant atherosclerosis. It is also reasonable to suggest that fibrous plaques arise by a process more or less independent of fatty streaks.

Evidence Supporting a Sequential Relationship. Other observations indicate that the hypothesized relationship between fatty streaks and fibrous plaques cannot be dismissed easily. The average extent of coronary artery fatty streaks in young individuals among white populations parallels the extent of severe atherosclerosis in older persons from the same groups (McGill, 1968). The most convincing evidence, however, is the presence of lesions in young adults that have the gross and microscopic characteristics of both fatty streaks and fibrous plaques. Such lesions that appear "transitional" are relatively common in the coronary arteries of North American males between 20 and 40 years of age. They have not been studied extensively because 20 to 40-year-old males have low mortality rates, and their most common cause of death is accidental. Tissues from this age group, therefore, are not readily available in autopsy material collected from conventional hospital autopsy services. Consequently, transitional lesions are not frequent in material usually collected for histologic study or chemical analyses, and their occurrence is minimized or their existence denied. More intensive study of lesions from 20 to 40-year-old persons from populations subject to a high incidence and extent of severe atherosclerosis would provide valuable information on this point.

Although there are discrepancies in the localization of aortic fatty streaks and aortic fibrous plaques, the axial localization of fatty streaks in younger persons corresponds to that of fibrous plaques and other advanced lesions in the coronary arteries (Montenegro and Eggen, 1968) and in the carotid and vertebral arteries (Solberg and McGarry, 1971).

Factors Determining the Fate of the Fatty Streak. Factors that determine the fate of the fatty streak have been sought within the structure and composition of the fatty streak itself. For example, at one time it was hypothesized that fatty streaks in high risk populations such as North Americans might contain an abnormal lipid, for example, a distinctive fatty acid esterified to cholesterol, that would incite a more intense chronic inflammatory reaction than other lipids (Robertson, 1963). No such lipid has been found. Analyses of coronary arteries from different populations have shown that they contain similar lipids (Scott et al., 1966). The possibility remains that more lipid is deposited in the coronary arteries of high risk populations than in the coronary arteries of other populations, but the differences found so far do not seem great enough to account for the differences in fibrous plaques and their sequelae. More investigation is needed on this point.

Proliferation as a Link Between the Fatty Streak and the Fibrous Plaque.
McMillan and Duff (1948) first demonstrated mitotic figures in intimal cells of
cholesterol-induced lesions in rabbits. Later, electron microscopy showed that
these intimal cells were smooth muscle cells. Tritiated thymidine radioautography
demonstrated labeling of such cells in several animal species (McMillan and
Stary, 1968; Thomas et al., 1968; Stary, 1969; Stary and McMillan, 1970; Cavallero et al., 1971). This topic has been thoroughly reviewed by Stary (1973a).
Since the fibrous plaque, at least in its formative stage, may essentially be a
proliferative reaction, smooth muscle proliferation may be the link between the
fatty streak and the fibrous plaque. However, the data on proliferation are
based exclusively on cholesterol-fed animal models, and there is no similar
direct evidence indicating proliferative activity in human fatty streaks.

Different Types of Fatty Streaks. Part of the difficulty in resolving the relationship between fatty streaks and fibrous plaques may be due to the wide
variety of lesions that are included in the descriptive and generic term "fatty
streak". Differentiation among fatty streaks may assist in reconciling the conflicting data.

At least one type of fatty streak, that occurring in childhood and adolescence,
is universal in humans regardless of environment. The lipid in the juvenile fatty
streak is predominantly intracellular in smooth muscle cells and foam cells.
There is minimal connective tissue, and there are no large pools of extracellular
lipid. We do not know whether smooth muscle proliferation is involved in the
juvenile fatty streak. Juvenile fatty streaks increase rapidly in the aorta during adolescence; they are more extensive in females than in males; and they are
more extensive in Negroes than in whites.

A second type of fatty streak occurs in young adults, particularly in young
adults from populations with high levels of advanced atherosclerosis and high
frequencies of clinical disease. This fatty streak contains more extracellular
lipid, particularly as aggregates of extracellular lipid in areas devoid of
intact cells. In other portions the lesion contains many cells, including smooth
muscle cells, foam cells of both smooth muscle and mononuclear origin, and mononuclear cells similar to those of chronic inflammation. Lipid-containing cells
often appear to be undergoing necrosis. The lesion often shows increased connective tissue elements, particularly about the pool of extracellular lipid. Although no data on proliferative activity in any human lesions are available, the
numerous nuclei in sections of such lesions suggest that there may be proliferation as well as cellular infiltration. This type of fatty streak appears to be
"progressing"; it has some of the characteristics of the fibrous plaque; and it
is identical to the transitional lesion between fatty streaks and fibrous
plaques previously mentioned.

It is possible to distinguish still another type of fatty streak in which there
is diffuse infiltration into a thickened intima of fine extracellular lipid
particles, often clustered around elastic tissue fibers. There are few lipid-
filled mononuclear or smooth muscle cells, and there are no pools of extracellular lipid. These fatty streaks occur principally in middle aged and elderly
persons, and occur both with and without other advanced atherosclerotic lesions.

Significance of Different Types of Fatty Streaks. The juvenile fatty streak has
the appearance of a localized intracellular lipid storage phenomenon. It is fairly certain that its distribution cannot be accounted for by hyperlipidemia, hypertension, cigarette smoking, diabetes mellitus, or other conditions associated
with severe atherosclerosis and clinical disease. The juvenile fatty streak may
be a genetically programmed process that, at some point in the evolutionary
process, had survival value. Dock (1946) suggested a similar evolutionary origin
for coronary intimal thickening in childhood. McKusick (1963) has pointed out
that obesity, diabetes mellitus and hypercholesterolemia, systemic disorders
associated with increased risk of several diseases in modern times, may have developed originally through natural selection as mechanisms for coping with famine.

The juvenile fatty streak may have a similar origin in our evolutionary history.

The characteristics and associations of what we have called the advanced fatty streak suggest that it is the precursor of the fibrous plaque. Its cellular appearance suggests active proliferation, infiltration, and chronic inflammation. Pools of extracellular lipid presage the gruel that forms the core of the fibrous plaque. Increased connective tissue elements suggest the beginning of the fibromuscular cap of the fibrous plaque. Its frequency in young adults from high risk populations suggests that it is associated with the conditions predisposing to severe atherosclerosis.

The third type of fatty streak, described as diffuse fatty infiltration, does not seem to be associated consistently with other atherosclerotic lesions and appears to come closest to passive lipid infiltration into the intima. It may represent partial regression of the juvenile fatty streak. It does not seem to progress to lesions that produce clinical disease.

Mechanism of Action of Risk Factors. It is possible that some or all of the risk factors now identified so closely with coronary heart disease may exert their influence on the frequency of disease not by initiating the juvenile fatty streak, but by selectively altering the balance of lipid exchange and cellular replication in the juvenile fatty streak. Proliferation, excessive lipid accumulation, and necrosis may then lead to the advanced fatty streak and eventually to the fibrous plaque.

Current investigative work on arterial smooth muscle metabolism and proliferation suggests many mechanisms of action of the risk factors on lesions. For example, the previously mentioned finding that cholesterol feeding increases mitoses in arterial smooth muscle cells within a few days after initiation indicates that dietary cholesterol may affect arterial smooth muscle before it induces hyperlipidemia (Thomas et al., 1971). Hyperlipidemic serum also has been reported to stimulate arterial smooth muscle cells in tissue culture (Myasnikov and Block, 1965). It would be paradoxical indeed if hyperlipidemia, the strongest and most consistent risk factor for coronary heart disease, were not responsible for the initial human fatty streak (the juvenile form), but were responsible for the smooth muscle proliferative response typical of the fibrous plaque. Hyperlipidemia may also contribute to the further accumulation of lipid in an established focus of extracellular lipid through passive infiltration.

The increase in atherosclerotic lesions associated with hypertension and cigarette smoking, two other well-documented risk factors for clinical disease, is predominantly an increase in fibrous plaques and a minimal increase in fatty streaks (Robertson and Strong, 1968; Strong et al., 1969). It has not been possible to determine whether these risk factors lead first to an increase in or an alteration of fatty streaks, which later become converted into fibrous plaques. Their effect on clinical disease is independent of an effect on serum lipids (Stamler et al., 1972). Experiments have shown that hypertension, when combined with cholesterol feeding, increases arterial lipid influx and lipid deposition in experimental animals (Campbell et al., 1973). Pick (1972) has noted that hypertension increases the connective tissue component of cholesterol-induced lesions in stump-tailed macaque monkeys. More experiments should be directed toward determining the effect of hypertension on the proliferation of vascular smooth muscle and the generation of connective tissue in experimental lesions.

Except for experiments that have shown enhancement of fatty streaks by carbon monoxide in cholesterol-fed animals, we have no information regarding the mechanism of the cigarette smoking effect.

The effect of maleness is principally on coronary atherosclerosis, and involves an increase in fibrous plaques rather than fatty streaks. Intimal muscular proliferation in childhood has been suggested as a predisposing mechanism (Dock, 1946), but, as mentioned previously, the observation of increased intimal muscular proliferation in the coronary arteries of males has not been consistently confirmed.

Whatever the mechanism of their effect, the common risk factors do not appear to be responsible for the initiation of the juvenile fatty streaks. They may alter the character of juvenile fatty streaks by stimulating proliferation of smooth muscle and by increasing the amount of lipid diffusion into an already established lesion. It is possible that they also lead to the formation of fibrous plaques without any relationship to pre-existing fatty streaks. The two possibilities are not mutually exclusive.

Selective Effects of Risk Factors. The effects of the various risk factors on advanced atherosclerotic lesions are often selective for specific arterial segments. Hypertension, for example, leads to a greater increase in coronary atherosclerosis than in aortic atherosclerosis, and to an even greater increase in cerebral atherosclerosis (Solberg, 1972). There is a suggestive trend that cigarette smoking affects the abdominal aorta more than other arterial segments (Strong et al., 1969). Although specific data are not available, it is possible that cigarette smoking and diabetes mellitus may exert a selective effect in accelerating atherosclerosis of the arteries of the extremities, and thereby account for the well-known strong association of these two risk factors with peripheral vascular disease. A closer look at the effect of risk factors on specific arterial segments, particularly in experimental animals, is needed.

Implications of This Pathogenetic Relationship. If the juvenile fatty streak is an essentially normal phenomenon which, under certain conditions, is converted to an advanced fatty streak and eventually to a fibrous plaque, it appears that it would be impossible or at least impractical to prevent the juvenile fatty streak. The most likely point of intervention would be to prevent the formation of the fibrous plaque.

Since fibrous plaques begin to appear with appreciable frequency and extent in the third decade of life, and since significant differences in extent of fibrous plaques develop among populations in the third decade, it appears that it would be reasonable to begin such intervention at least in the latter part of the second decade and possibly earlier. The objective of such intervention, however, should be recognized explicitly as being to retard the progression of the process to advanced lesions, and not to prevent initial lipid deposition, the juvenile fatty streak.

Summary

The modifications in our concept of the natural history of human atherosclerotic lesions are shown in Fig. 2. The major change is the introduction of fibromuscular intimal thickening as an essentially normal process of growth and adaptation, and division of fatty streaks into two major types. The sequence implies that when one or more of the risk factors for clinical disease are present, some juvenile fatty streaks undergo changes that eventually result in the formation of fibrous plaques. The effects of the risk factors are selective for different arterial segments. Prevention of the juvenile fatty streak, which is not related to hyperlipidemia or the other risk factors, does not appear practical. Prevention should be aimed at the advanced fatty streak and the fibrous plaque, which begin to develop at about the beginning of the third decade of life. The search for mechanisms should be directed toward how the risk factors cause progression of selected fatty streaks to fibrous plaques.

Lesion	Age in years	Process	Cause
Fibromuscular intimal thickening	0-15	Physiological adaptation	Growth
Juvenile fatty streak	5-15	Lipid storage in intimal smooth muscle cells	Genetically programmed
Advanced fatty streak	15-30	Proliferation, necrosis, chronic inflammation, infiltration	Hyperlipidemia Hypertension Cigarette smoking Maleness
Fibrous plaque	30+	Continued proliferation, necrosis, chronic inflammation, infiltration	Continued effect of risk factors
Complicated lesion	40+	Vascularization, ulceration, hemorrhage, thrombosis	Maturation of fibrous plaque

Figure 2. Modified description of the natural history of human atherosclerotic lesions and their relationship to the risk factors for clinical disease

METABOLISM OF THE ARTERIAL WALL[*]

David Kritchevsky and Himanshu V. Kothari

The enzymes of lipid, carbohydrate, protein and nucleic acid metabolism in normal and arteriosclerotic aorta have been studied (Kirk, 1963). In a survey of enzyme activities, Kirk (1969) pointed out that aortic enzymic activity could not be directly correlated with the severity or type of arteriosclerotic involvement, some activities rising and some falling (Table 1). Since it is not possible to deal with all enzymic activities in the aorta, we shall deal with those relating to that particular component which showed the greatest degree of change, namely, lipid. Smith (1965) has shown that the mucopolysaccharide content of the fatty streak was 115% of that in the normal aorta but in the fibrous and calcified plaque, the mucopolysaccharide content was 96% and 46% of normal. Collagen content was 106%, 166% and 285% that of normal in the fatty streak, fibrous plaque and calcified plaque, respectively. Lipid content rose most strikingly with progression of the lesion in the fatty streak being 312% or normal, 483% in the fibrous plaque and 1112% in the calcified plaque. Among the lipid classes, the most marked increase was that observed in the aortic cholesterol ester. This increase was observed by Windaus (1910) and was further quantitated by Böttcher (1961) and Smith (1965). The phospholipid content of the artery did not vary sharply with age and atherosclerosis, but the sphingomyelin content of human arteries showed a sharp rise in atherosclerotic lesions (Böttcher, 1961). Thus lecithin comprises 43% of the phospholipids of normal aorta, and sphingomyelin, 35%. In early atherosclerosis, these percentages become 32 and 53 for lecithin and sphingomyelin, and in late atherosclerosis, lecithin accounts for 23% of the total phospholipid and sphingomyelin 63%. The significant increase of aortic sphingomyelin with age has been confirmed by Eisenberg et al. (1969).

Table 1. Effect of arteriosclerosis on vascular enzymes (compared to normal tissue) (Kirk, 1969)

Sample	No.	Significantly lower	Significantly higher	No change
Aorta, lipid arteriosclerotic	37	11	8	18
Aorta, fibrous arteriosclerotic	29	18	3	8
Aorta, mixed arteriosclerosis	23	9	2	12
Coronary artery, arteriosclerotic	42	11	5	26

This discussion will deal with ester cholesterol and sphingomyelin metabolism under two conditions, aging and atherosclerosis. Although atherosclerosis is not a necessary concomitant of aging, much of the data on the two conditions are parallel and consideration of both may provide better insight into aortic metabolism.

---

[*]This work was supported in part by Research Grants HL-03299, HL-13722 and a Research Career Award (HL-00734) from the National Heart and Lung Institute and by a grant from the John A. Hartford Foundation, Inc.

The spectrum of cholesterol ester fatty acids in serum differs from that in plaques primarily in the ratio of oleic to linoleic acids. Based on a compilation of data from various sources the ratio of 18:1/18:2 in serum was 0.64 and in plaques it was 0.95 (Kritchevsky, 1967). Nelson et al. (1961) compared the oleic,palmitic and "unsaturated" fatty acids in normal and abnormal intimal tissue of five accident victims and found the percentage of oleic acid went from 21.1 to 42.2 (p <0.001), palmitic acid dropped from 20.3 to 12.6% (p <0.05) and total unsaturated fatty acids rose from 57.8 to 78.6% (p <0.001). Examination of aortas of children has, in one study at least, shown no aortic cholesterol ester (Scott et al., 1966). Newman and Zilversmit (1964) fed rabbits cholesterol for 120 days and observed that the aortic free/esterified cholesterol ratio went from 40 on Day 0 to 2 on Day 20 and reached a level of 1 by Day 40. It did not change much thereafter. This change in free/esterified cholesterol ratio is also observed in aortas of rabbits fed atherogenic, cholesterol-free diets (Kritchevsky and Tepper, 1968).

We undertook the study of cholesterol esterase activity in acetone powder preparations of aorta. The details of the preparation of these powders have been published (Kothari et al., 1973). The acetone powder preparations have both cholesterol ester synthesizing and hydrolyzing activity depending upon substrate preparation and pH. For synthesis, an emulsion (pH 6.1) containing 2.05 µmoles of cholesterol, 6.22 µmoles of oleic acid and 4.10 µmoles of sodium taurocholate was used. The addition of coenzyme A or of ATP singly or together did not affect ester formation (Table 2). Using this system the specificity for a number of fatty acids was investigated. It is evident (Table 3) that with either rat or rabbit aorta preparations oleic acid is the preferred substrate.

Table 2. Effect of cofactors on the synthesis of cholesteryl oleate by rat and rabbit aorta enzyme

Incubation system		nmoles cholesterol esterified	
		Rat	Rabbit
Control		52	24
"	plus 2 µmoles CoA	55	21
"	plus 10 µmoles ATP	52	22
"	plus (2 µmoles CoA and 10 µmoles ATP)	56	22

Esterification was measured with the usual emulsified substrate with or without the indicated amounts of CoA and ATP. The table is a composite of two experiments.

The esterification of a number of sterols with oleic acid has also been studied. It can be seen from Fig. 1 that cholesterol and cholestanol are the preferred substrates for oleate formation.

Hydrolysis of cholesterol esters was studied using a micellar substrate (pH 6.6) containing 1.30 µmoles cholesterol ester, 2.58 µmoles sodium taurocholate and 3.0 mg lecithin. A study of the hydrolysis of a number of cholesterol esters (Table 4) showed preferential hydrolysis of linoleate. The synthesis and hydrolysis of different cholesterol esters bears directly on aortic metabolism in the course of atherogenesis. The atherosclerotic rabbit aorta shows an enormous increase in fatty acid synthesis (Whereat, 1964). The fatty acids synthesized are probably palmitic and oleic. Dayton and Hashimoto (1970) have estimated that about half of the aortic cholesterol esters may be attributable to local synthesis. When Portman (1970) fed squirrel monkeys an atherogenic diet, the 18:1/18:2 ratio in the aortic cholesterol esters was 0.8 in the control animals and remained at or near that level through the eight-month experiments. After three months, the monkeys fed the experimental diet exhibited an 18:1/18:2 ratio of 4.25. At this time some monkeys were returned to normal monkey chow and after five months on this regimen their 18:1/18:2 ratio was 1.00; in monkeys maintained on the atherogenic regimen it was 3.20 at eight months.

Table 3. Fatty acid specificity for synthesis of cholesterol esters by acetone dry powder extract of rat and rabbit aorta (nmoles of cholesterol esterified)

Fatty acid used (15 μmoles)	Rat aorta		Rabbit aorta	
	Expt. 1	Expt. 2	Expt. 1	Expt. 2
Oleic acid	49	56	38	35
Linoleic acid	41	44	29	26
Linolenic acid	26	20	24	19
Palmitoleic acid	22	24	18	15
Palmitic acid	19	16	13	10
Stearic acid	13	13	7	7
Arachidonic acid	23	21	21	24
Butyric acid	-	6	4.5	5

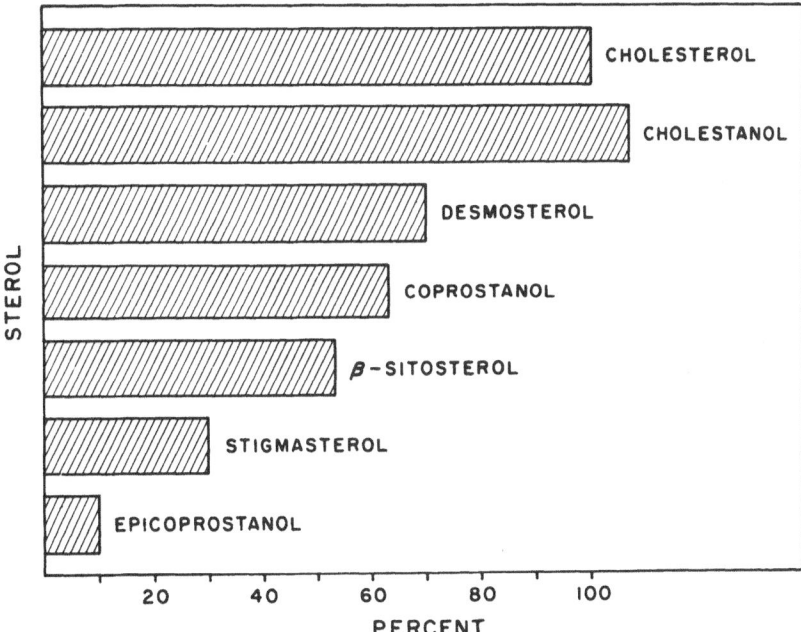

Figure 1. Esterification of $[1-^{14}C]$-oleic acid with different sterols using rat aorta acetone powder (cholesterol=100)

Table 4. Hydrolysis of various fatty acid esters of cholesterol by acetone dry powder extract of rat and rabbit aorta (nmoles of cholesterol released)

Ester used	Rat		Rabbit	
	Expt. 1	Expt. 2	Expt. 1	Expt. 2
Oleate	93	84	37	31
Linoleate	105	91	44	39
Laurate	55	47	24	19
Myristate	44	44	16	18
Palmitate	68	52	25	32
Stearate	38	28	17	16
Acetate	82	87	31	30

Table 5. Serum cholesterol, aortic atherosclerosis and aortic cholesterol esterase activity of rabbits fed 2% cholesterol in 6% corn oil[a]

Day	Serum Cholesterol (mg/dl)	Atheromata Arch	Atheromata Thoracic	Synthetase (S) nm/mg protein/hr	Hydrolase (H) nm/mg protein/hr	S/H
0	84 ± 8[b]	0	0	3.60 ± 0.74	4.98 ± 1.27	0.72
7	685 ± 147	0	0	13.65 ± 6.75	7.85 ± 2.93	1.74
11	506 ± 140	0	0	8.85 ± 2.33	3.23 ± 0.92	2.74

[a]Four rabbits taken at each time period.
[b]Standard Error.

Table 6. Serum and liver lipids, atherosclerosis and aortic cholesterol esterase activity in rabbits fed 2% cholesterol in 6% corn oil[a]

Day	Cholesterol Serum (mg/dl)	Cholesterol Liver (g/100g)	Atheromata Arch	Atheromata Thoracic	Synthetase (S) nm/mg protein/hr	Hydrolase (H) nm/mg protein/hr	S/H
0	49±6[b]	0.52±0.05	0	0	3.13±0.43	2.67±0.33	1.17
5	173±29	1.01±0.12	0	0	5.58±0.52	3.33±0.61	1.68
12	495±230	2.04±0.96	0.5	0	9.31±0.29	5.15±0.75	1.81
20	1874±316	4.16±0.77	1.0	1.0	7.83±1.35	4.83±1.69	1.62
30	925±107	3.73±0.47	1.1	0.5	8.03±1.27	4.65±0.90	1.73

[a]Four rabbits taken at each time period.
[b]Standard Error.

Table 7. Sphingomyelin accumulation with age (Stein and Stein, 1972)

Species	Age	Sphingomyelin µg P/mg DNA	Sphingomyelin hydrolyzed
Rat	1 mo.	4.3	0.32
	18-24 mo.	13.1	0.41
Rabbit	1 mo.	8.9	0.09
	18-24 mo.	26.9	0.15

Rabbits maintained on an atherogenic regimen (Table 5) for only 7 days (Kritchevsky et al., 1974b) showed a 279% increase in cholesterol ester synthesizing capacity and a 58% in ester hydrolyzing activity. A second experiment (Table 6) yielded similar results. St. Clair et al. (1970) found that the cholesterol ester synthetase activity of pigeon artery increased significantly after only a few days of cholesterol feeding.

The sphingomyelin of human aorta has been shown to increase with age (Böttcher, 1961). Portman (1970) in a study of the phospholipids of normal and atherosclerotic squirrel monkey aorta reported a 28% increase in lecithin, a 425% increase in lysolecithin but no change in sphingomyelin with atherosclerosis. Stein and Stein (1972), on the other hand, reported a 204% increase in rat aorta sphingomyelin with age and a 202% increase in rabbit aorta (Table 7). Cholesterol uptake by tissue culture cells is enhanced by lysolecithin and inhibited by sphingomyelin (Rothblat et al., 1968). Zilversmit et al. (1954) demonstrated an increased phospholipid synthesis in atheromata with the principal increase being in the sphingomyelin fraction (McCandless and Zilversmit, 1956). Possibly sphingomyelin accumulation is a defense against cholesterol infiltration. Patelski et al. (1970) reported increased phospholipase A activity in rabbits fed an atherogenic diet.

Studies of rat aortic metabolism with age have shown that lipolytic activity in aortas of seven-month rats is almost double that in two-three month old rats (Zemplenyi and Grafnetter, 1959). Our own studies with aortic cholesterol ester hydrolase in rats (Table 8) have shown that both synthesis and hydrolysis of cholesterol oleate rose with age, but whereas synthetic activity at twelve months was 1.4 times higher than that at two months, hydrolytic activity had risen 3.5 times (Kritchevsky et al., 1974a). Stein and Stein (1972) have measured aorta phospholipases in aging rats (Table 9) and found a huge increase in lecithinase but no change in sphingomyelinase.

Table 8. Influence of age on synthesis and hydrolysis of cholesterol oleate by rat aorta preparations

Age (mo)	No. pools	Avg.protein (mg/ml)	Synthesis[a] (S)	Hydrolysis[a] (H)	S/H
2	4	2.04	3.9 ± 0.17a[b]	2.0 ± 0.62a	1.95
12	3	1.49	5.5 ± 1.62	6.9 ± 2.36b	0.80
24	4	0.90	7.0 ± 0.41a	23.2 ± 2.46ab	0.31

[a] nm/mg protein/hr.

[b] standard error.

Values with same subscript are significantly different.

Table 9. Rat aorta phospholipases, effect of age (from Stein and Stein, 1972)

| Age (mo) | % Change from 1 month | | | |
	PC	PE	Sph	LL
1.5	325	140	17	14
3	650	280	17	50
6-12	2025	1200	17	54
18-24	2150	1150	17	96

Table 10. Sphingomyelin choline-phosphohydrolase activity (Rechmilewitz et al., 1967)

| Species | Sphingomyelin hydrolized (mcg P/hr) | |
	per mg DNA	per g wet wt.
Rat	8.60	13.88
Dog	4.67	6.92
Guinea Pig	4.42	8.61
Rabbit	2.53	4.56

Table 11. Cholesterol ester synthesizing (S) and hydrolyzing (H) activities of acetone dry powder preparation of aortas of various species[a]

| Species | Experiment 1 | | | Experiment 2 | | |
	S	H	S/H	S	H	S/H
Susceptible						
Human	6.5	8.3	0.78	6.6	6.9	0.96
Baboon	6.2	7.5	0.83	5.4	6.2	0.87
Swine	5.5	4.8	1.15	6.7	7.0	0.96
Rabbit	6.5	7.0	0.93	5.8	6.0	0.97
Chicken	8.0	8.1	0.99	6.3	6.5	0.97
Resistant						
Rat	10.0	16.0	0.63	10.6	19.6	0.54
Mouse	9.2	14.0	0.66	7.3	12.7	0.57
Dog	4.0	14.5	0.28	6.5	18.0	0.36

[a]Synthesis and hydrolysis of cholesterol ester is described as nmoles of substrate converted per mg of protein per hour.

Finally, we should examine species differences in aortic metabolism to see how they correlate with known suspectibility to atherosclerosis. Zemplenyi et al. (1963) showed that rat aorta displayed greater lipolytic or esterolytic activity than aortas of rabbit, guinea pig or cockerel. Rachmilewitz et al. (1967) reported that rat aorta had greater sphingomyelinase activity than did aortas of dog, guinea pig and rabbit (Table 10). Our determinations of the ratio of aortic cholesterol ester synthesis to hydrolysis (S/H) indicated that the so-called resistant species have a lower S/H ratio (about 0.94) than do the susceptible species (about 0.51) (Table 11). Experiments to determine possible intraspecies differences were performed using aortas from White Carneau (susceptible) and Show Racer (resistant pigeons) (Lofland and Clarkson, 1959). The ratio of aortic cholesterol ester synthetase to hydrolase (S/H) was 1.21 in the White Carneau pigeon and 0.73 for the Show Racer. Since the spontaneous atherosclerosis which occurs in White Carneau pigeons was found almost exclusively in the distal portion of the artery (Clarkson, et al., 1959) we determined the S/H ratios in proximal and distal portions of arteries from White Carneau and Show Racer pigeons. The results (Table 12) suggest that an aberration in cholesterol ester metabolism may be among the elements of aortic metabolism which predispose to atherosclerosis.

Table 12. Cholesterol ester synthetase (S) and hydrolase (H) activity in proximal and distal portions of aortas of White Carneau and Show Racer pigeons

Aorta portion	No. pools	S/H ratio $\pm$ S.E.M.	
		White carneau	Show racer
Proximal	5	0.65 ± 0.08[a]	0.48 ± 0.03[b]
Distal	5	0.95 ± 0.10	0.52 ± 0.05[b]

[a] vs WC distal, $p < 0.05$.
[b] vs WC distal, $p < 0.01$.

This discussion has covered only one aspect of the constellation of events which lead to atherosclerosis. The focal nature of the disease suggests that measurements of any parameter in arterial tissue can identify only one underlying metabolic factor. Precisely how and to what extent the various metabolic factors interact remains to be elucidated.

BIOPHYSICAL FACTORS IN VASCULAR STRUCTURE AND CALIBER

Simon Rodbard

Each segment of every blood vessel in the body continuously adapts its strength
to the stretching and compressive forces that it must bear, and adjusts its
caliber to the size and metabolic activity of the tissue that it serves. These
adaptations proceed without the appearance of unnecessary overgrowths of wall
thickness, even as the structural properties of the entire vascular system
undergo continuous change. The metamorphoses transform the small thin-walled
gelatinous vessels of the embryo into the large firm vessels of the adult. They
also contribute to the production of arteriosclerosis and arterial occlusions.

The mechanism of such striking adaptations of structure to function requires
analysis. Some view these changes as evidence for the operation of a remarkably extensive memory and computer network, whose programs continuously adjust
the quantities and distributions of the many elements of the vessel walls, or
for the operation of a growth hormone. No such network has been found. The
continuing adaptation of blood vessels in the parts of the body distal to hemi-
section of the cord, indicates that the nervous system does not make these
adjustments. The localized uterine vascular enlargements of pregnancy have been
attributed to hormonal changes, but hormones circulate throughout the body
without producing comparable vascular changes at other sites.

Adaptation of the strength of the wall of each vessel segment and of its caliber
must be operative from the beginning of the embryonic circulation, with appropriate modifications as the life of the individual unfolds its great variations in
activity and pressures. Specific stresses such as birth, pregnancy, illness, the
training of particular muscle groups of the body and other situations must be
met by appropriate strengthening or enlargement or closure of vessels. Since
these remarkable adaptations ordinarily give rise to no specific disorders they
have received only passing interest and the processes are therefore considered
to be normal.

Rarely, the strength of a given vessel segment is inadequate to meet the forces
that act against it, and the vessel ruptures. Vessel segments sometimes appear
to enlarge excessively, as in aneurysms, post-stenotic enlargements and in
fistulae. Much more commonly, the caliber of a segment of a blood vessel or even
an entire length may so decline in caliber that delivery of blood to its peripheral vascular bed is limited. The search for the cause and prevention of these
narrowings, usually classified as disease states, receives nearly the entire
effort of the research establishment devoted to the study of arteriosclerosis.
Much less study is directed to the many vascular occlusions that are welcomed as
"normal" processes. Such accepted and wished-for stenoses include closures of
some of the gill arches, the atrial, ventricular and arterial septal openings,
the ductus arteriosus and venosus, and the disappearance of vessels whose
function has apparently been completed as in the large uterine arteries and
veins after parturition. These closures are usually viewed as beneficial.

Occasionally, in transposition of the great arteries, spontaneous closure of an
atrial or ventricular defect isolates the circulation of the right heart from
that of the left heart. Such closures are viewed with alarm and the defect must
be surgically re-opened to facilitate mixing of the blood of the two separate
circulations. By contrast, closures of the coronary or cerebral arteries generate
disabling or even mortal disease. These well-documented vascular changes require

analysis in terms of the potential for changes in vascular structure and of the search for those forces that may contribute to their development.

Since each vascular segment apparently adapts satisfactorily to a wide spectrum of local conditions, local factors must be operative in each segment in the determination of vascular structure. The present study is based on the thesis that mechanical stresses at each site are the inducers of the local changes that adapt vascular thickness and caliber to the forces in operation. The mesenchymal cells that form the blood vessels are considered to be sensitive to these stresses, and capable of responding to the forces with counteracting mechanisms.

Stresses. Engineering science classifies mechanical stresses as 1. tensile (stretching), 2. compressive, or 3. shearing (sliding) forces. The directions and magnitudes of these forces can vary greatly from point to point in each structure. Thus, the blood pressure compresses the intimal lining of the blood vessels as it stretches the circumferential elements of the wall, and causes the layers of the wall to slide on each other. At the boundary between the stream and the vessel lining, shear forces tend to drag the endothelial cells downstream. The pulsations of pressure waves produce continuous rates of change in the strength of each of these forces. The resulting complex dynamics of the stress in the vessel wall are countered by information in the DNA memory banks accumulated in the course of evolution.

Evolutionary selection appears to have favored those organisms whose mesenchymal cells can manufacture specific, adequate materials which can remove the stress from the cells (Fig. 1). Data that examine this general thesis are reviewed in a recent report (Rodbard, 1970). Each mesenchymal cell responds to the specific forces that impinge on it, thereby providing local adjustments to the forces in operation. These responses are modified to some extent by hormonal and other general effects, but the major adjustment is of local origin.

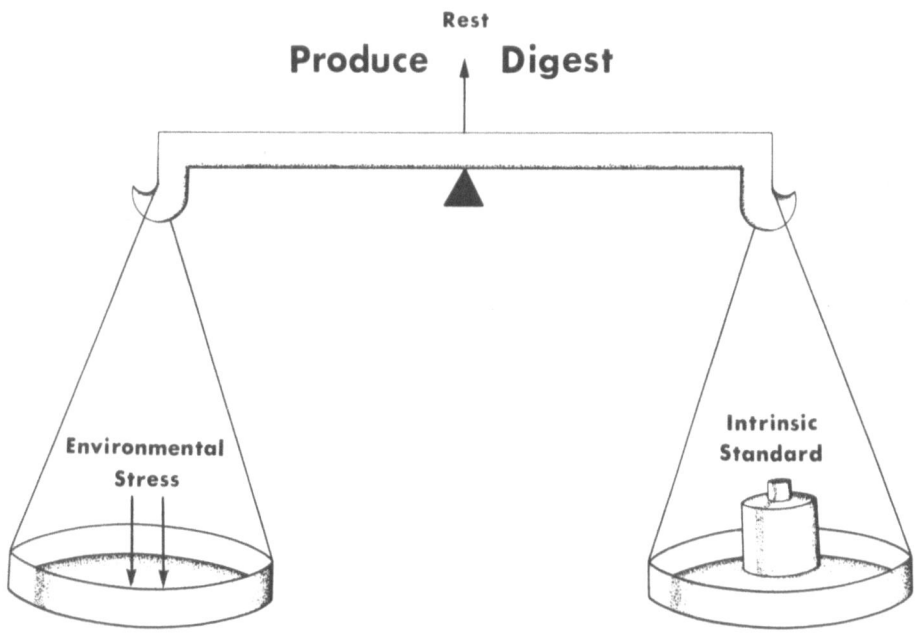

Figure 1. Negative feedback mechanism illustrated as a balance. Since the intrinsic setpoint standard (weight in the right pan) is balanced by an applied mechanical force (2 arrows) on the left pan, the system is at rest

The present brief survey of this approach will be captioned in a manner that gives the mechanical force acting on a mesenchymal cell, and the induction and manufacture (arrow) by the cell of a specific material that removes the stressing force from the cell. This negative feedback mechanism provides for local adaptations in strength and caliber (Fig. 2).

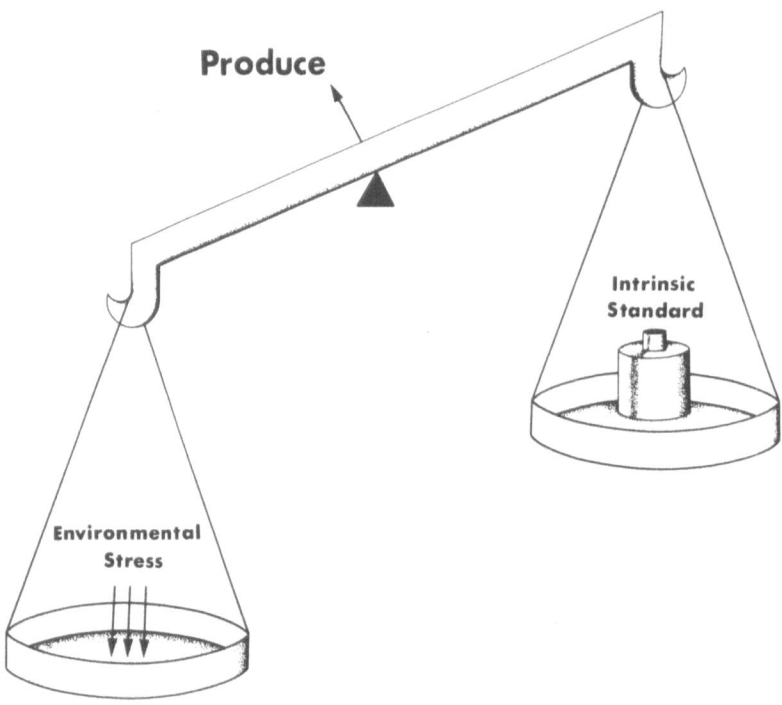

Figure 2. When mechanical stress (three arrows) exceeds the intrinsic set-point, the cell is induced to produce materials which counteract and balance the stress

Tension → Collagen. Tensile forces that stretch mesenchymal cells induce these cells to manufacture collagenous ropes. The cells attach these fibers to the sites of origin of the stretching forces (Fig. 3). Manufacture and alignment of collagen continues until the number and strength of the collagenous fibers are sufficient to relieve the cell of the pulling forces. In this way, the quantity of collagen at each locus is sufficient to meet the accustomed applied stresses, with sufficient reserve to withstand extraordinary, but still limited, stresses. The tension on the cells of the vessel wall increases when the blood pressure rises, or the vessel enlarges. The number of collagenous fibers in the wall increases in proportion to the tension, thereby protecting the vessel wall against rupture. Studies of tendons and bones following the application of tensile stresses illustrate such adaptations. Adjustments in the strength of tendinous structures also follow when the stretching forces are chronically reduced. The cells then operate as fibroblasts which dissolve collagen at those sites where the collagen is excessive relative to the magnitude of the stretching forces. The cells of the vessel wall and of the connective tissues of the body appear to use such negative-feedback mechanisms to adjust the strength of each segment of the wall to local changes in the stretching forces produced by the tension (pressure x radius)(Fig. 4).

Rate of Change of Tension → Elastin. In addition to the relatively steady stretching force that the mean arterial pressure applies against the vessel wall, pulsations generate an oscillating force or a rate of change of tension, i.e., the first derivative of the tensile forces. Connective tissue cells that sense

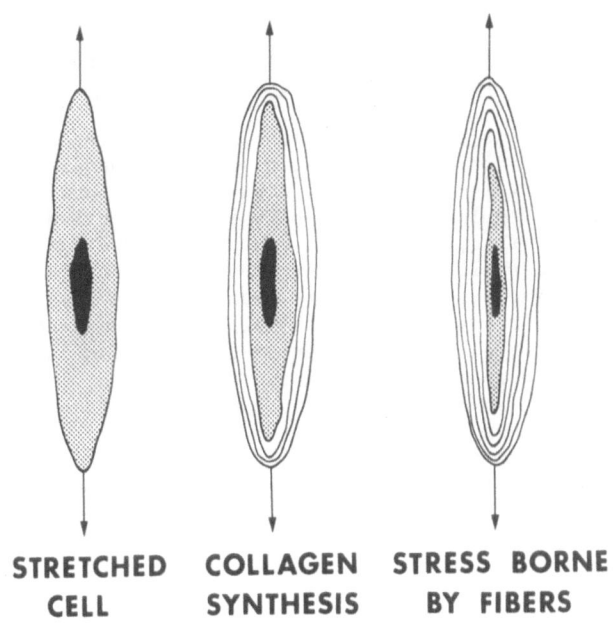

STRETCHED CELL **COLLAGEN SYNTHESIS** **STRESS BORNE BY FIBERS**

Figure 3. A fibroblast at left is stretched, inducing collagen synthesis (middle) until the number of fibers is sufficient to relieve the cell of the pulling force (right). The cell then appears as a resting fibrocyte, enclosed in its collagenous sheath

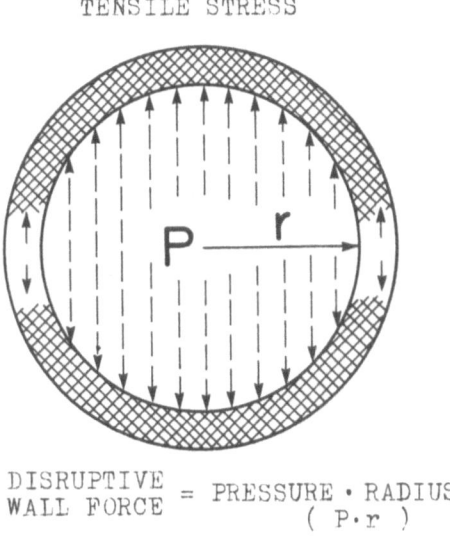

TENSILE STRESS

$$\frac{\text{DISRUPTIVE WALL FORCE}}{} = \text{PRESSURE} \cdot \text{RADIUS} \ (\text{P} \cdot \text{r})$$

Figure 4. The stretching forces on the cross section of the wall of a blood vessel (divergent arrows inside the wall) vary with the product of the pressure (arrows inside lumen) and radius of the vessel (number of such arrows) divided by the thickness of the wall

this rate of change of tension appear to be induced to produce elastin. This rubbery material is manufactured and aligned in positions that relieve the cell of the oscillating forces.

Elastin is present only in sites that are exposed to rates of change of tension (Hass, 1939). Thus, elastin does not appear in the embryo until the heart begins to beat. The quantity of elastin in various tissues varies with the local amplitude of pulsation, most of which is supplied by the arterial pulse wave. The aortic root, which is markedly distended during each ventricular ejection and decreases in volume during the following diastole, has the greatest amounts of elastin. Vessels that are expanded to a lesser extent by each pulse, such as the thoracic aorta, the abdominal aorta, the arteries and the arterioles, have progressively smaller concentrations of elastin. The capillaries and venules are not exposed to significant rates of change of tension, and they have no elastin. Fig. 5 shows that rigidity induced by placement of a suture is associated with the disappearance of elastin. The elastic components of the vessel wall are well developed in the carotid arteries prior to their entry into the foramina of the cranium. The elastin in the wall of the artery decreases as the artery passes through the carotid foramen into the cranial cavity. Inside the cranium, the cerebrospinal fluid applies a counter-pressure to each pulse wave, and only an internal elastic membrane is present.

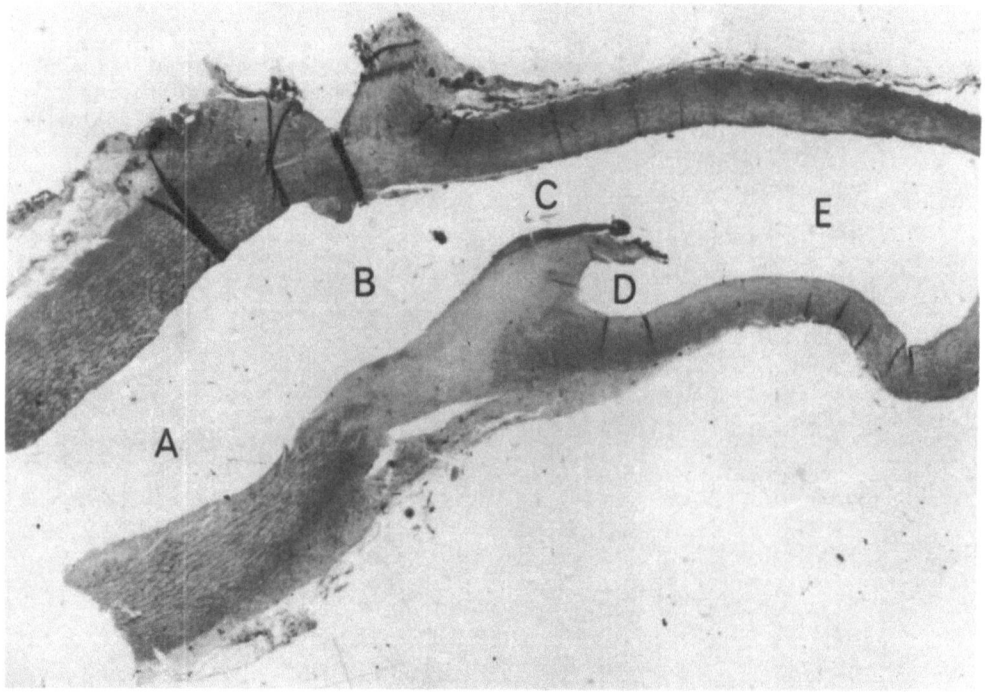

Figure 5. Adjustments in the quantities and arrangements of components of the wall to applied stresses. Placement of a tuck suture at B, partially narrowed the aorta, as in a coarctation. Ingrowths resembling a narrowing are present at B and a "valve" is seen at C with a sinus at D. Elastin disappeared in the region of fixation (B) and was replaced by collagen. The wall above the valve-like narrowing (A) is thickened in accord with the higher pressure in this segment. The wall downstream to the narrowing is much thinner, in accord with the reduced pressure. The downstream segment (E) exhibits a post-stenotic dilatation

We have enclosed the common carotid artery in plastic sheaths (Rodbard et al., 1962) which prevent distension of the vessel by the pulse wave; the elastin in these vessels quickly disappears. The quantities of elastin are essentially equal in the embryonic pulmonary artery and in the aorta. Following birth, the elastin in the aorta increases markedly with the rise in the systemic pulse pressure, while the quantity in the pulmonary artery declines. These and other data are consistent with the thesis that the quantity and alignment of elastin in tissues vary with the time rate of change of tension that acts locally on the mesenchymal cells. The formation of elastin appears to be associated with a relatively uniform rate of change of tension. When the rate of change oscillates more abruptly, the acceleration of the tensile forces produces a strikingly different effect on the mesenchymal cells.

Acceleration of Tension → *Muscle*. Muscle is a specialized connective tissue in which the sudden application (acceleration) of tension triggers an equally sudden active shortening or counter-acceleration. Muscle may therefore be viewed as consisting of cells that respond to a sudden application of tension by transferring the applied abrupt pull to specialized contractile elements. The number of contractile elements in each muscle fiber varies with the magnitude of the accelerative tensions that the muscle fiber must bear. This adjustment of strength to load is achieved by the manufacture of contractile elements in parallel, under the stimulus of the acceleration (rate of change of rate of change of tension). While collagenous and elastic fibers are deposited outside the cell, the contractile fibers whose formation is induced by the second derivative of tension are deposited in orderly arrays in parallel with similar fibers already present *inside* the cell.

In the arterial wall the smooth muscle cells are attached to adjacent sleeves of elastin in positions where they can respond to rapid accelerations of tension and thereby achieve a reduction of excessive movements of the wall. The amount of smooth muscle appears to vary with the acceleration of tension in the vessel wall. This is well appreciated in the differences between the aorta and the pulmonary artery. Increased steepness in the rate of rise of pressure and therefore in the acceleration of tension may determine the thickness (hypertrophy) of the layers of muscle in the arterial wall. When the load is chronically diminished, the number of muscle elements per unit cross-sectional area decreases (atrophy)(Fig.5).

The arterial wall is therefore a composite multiphase structure in which an acceleration of tension triggers a counter-contraction of its smooth muscle, a rate of change of tension that is absorbed by the elastin,and steady tensile forces which are met by the stretching of collagen. When the muscle, elastin or collagen in the wall are inadequate to counteract the specific derivative of tension, the connective tissue cells affected by the force are induced to produce more of the specific material.

Tensile forces at one site in a structure are invariably associated with nearby compressive forces. The mesenchymal cells respond by specific negative feedback mechanisms with materials that reduce the forces of compression that act on them.

Compression → *Osteoid*. Mesenchymal cells in a region subjected to steady compression are induced to secrete a firm organic matrix (osteoid) which can protect the cell against a limited compressive force. Since compressive and tensile forces are invariably associated, collagenous fibers are also deposited in the matrix. Marked compression is followed by mineral deposition along the collagen fibers, with the result that the cell may be enclosed in a mineralized field. This appears to be the case in the aorta in which cells may be partially enclosed by tiny calcific crystals. In some of these sites the cell may then resemble an osteoblast or an osteocyte.

Bone forms normally in only a few sites of the cardiovascular system. Boney spurs are found in sclerotic plaques where the aortic pressure steadily compresses components of the wall against adjacent unyielding vertebral structures. Steady compression as occurs at the root of the great arteries is associated with the formation of bone, as in the *os cordis* of cattle.

Rate of Change of Compression Cartilage. Cartilage, a dense tissue with the consistency of hard rubber, is found at sites at which oscillating compression induces cells to secrete chondroitin sulphates. The cell organizes this material into a set of concentric shells in which it envelopes itself. The firm rubbery material acts as a shock absorber that relieves the affected cell of the rate of change of compression that initiated the change.

We have performed several types of experiments in which the application of rates of change of compression induces cartilage. The insertion of a stainless steel wire into an arterial segment is followed within days by the appearance of a colony of hyaline cartilage cells immediately adjacent to the wire (Fig. 6) (Rodbard, 1958). The cartilage appears to be induced by the recurrent hammering blows of the pulse wave on mesenchymal cells that lie against the anvil-like wire.

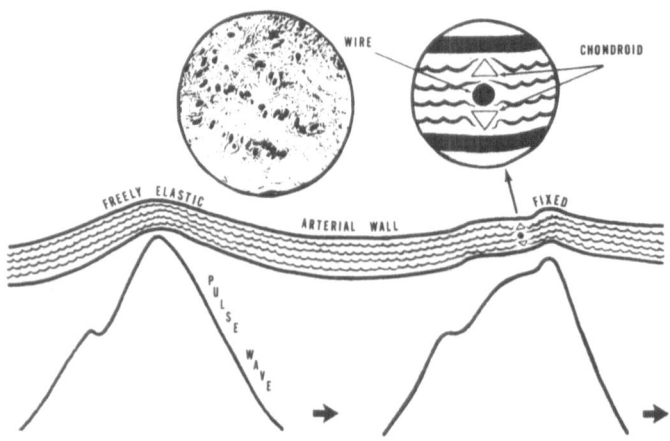

Figure 6. Hammering effects of pulse wave on arterial wall. At left, the pulse wave distends the freely elastic vessel wall. At right, the artery is fixed by a stainless steel wire (black dot). Chondroid (left insert) develops adjacent to wire (right insert)

In other experiments we have injected a bleb of gelatinous carrageenin into the arterial media. The molecular structure of carrageenin, a mucopolysaccharide obtained from seaweed, resembles that of the hyaluronic acids of the ground substances. The bleb is quickly invaded by mesenchymal cells which are thereby exposed to recurrent arterial pulsations that apply high rates of change of compression. This oscillating compression appears to trigger the affected cells to synthesize chondroitin sulfates (Fig. 7). These mucopolysaccharides become organized into chondroid shells that damp the oscillations on the cell in the manner of a shock absorber (vibration isolator) (McCandless et al., 1963).

Analysis of the vascular bed involved in the formation of the cartilage of the skeleton suggests that cartilage production in these sites is dependent on the application of rates of change of compression. This is clearly seen in the healing fracture callus (Mindell et al., 1971). In embryonic amphibia, removal of the heart and thus of the source of recurrent compressive forces results in cessation of cartilage formation, even though many other structures continue to develop (Kemp and Quinn, 1954). Each chondrocyte provides a unit of damping. The number of chondrocytes in each location appears to be dependent upon the magnitude of the applied rate of change of compression.

In addition to the tensile and compressive forces and the specific cellular responses presented above, all structures are subjected to forces that act to cause their parts to slide on each other. These shearing forces may be illustrated by applying a force to the back of the spine of a book, thereby causing the pages of the book to slide on each other. As such materials tend to move with respect to each other, friction is generated.

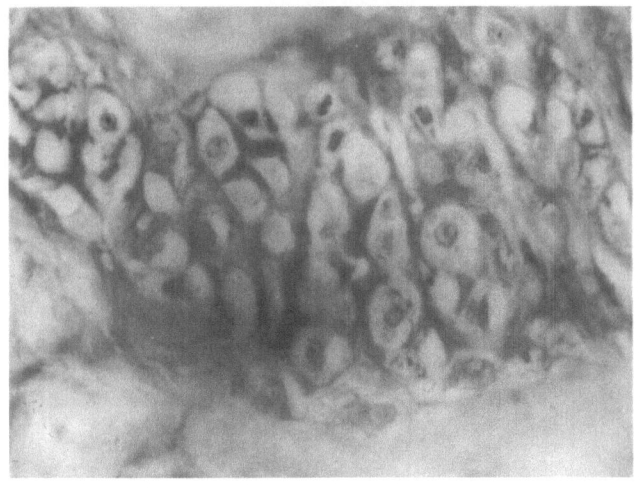

Figure 7. Cartilage in a carrageenin bleb injected into the aortic wall of the chick

Friction → *Papilliferous Growths.* We have induced endocardial papillomas by arranging that adjacent endocardial surfaces rub against each other (Rodbard et al., 1964). The atrial appendage of dogs was invaginated to form an epicardial sheath. A silastic ball was placed into this sheath which was then closed by sutures. This introduced an undamaged endocardium-lined mass into the atrium (Fig. 8). Grossly visible, round, slightly raised cauliflower-like growths appeared on the endocardium of the intra-atrial mass, and on the endocardium of the adjacent atrium and valve (Fig. 9). Each growth on the intra-atrial mass was matched by a similar growth on the opposing parietal endocardium or on the inlet valve. The growths were richly vascularized, endothelium-lined excrescences of numerous branched papillae. The motion of the heart produced a frictional to-and-fro contact of the mass against adjacent atrial and valvular surfaces. The appearance of papillary growths at such sites suggests that shearing, sliding forces induce growths which resemble pedunculated friction-reducing ball bearings. Similar papillomata occur on the surface of inflamed valves during rheumatic fever. They may also appear on the arterial wall. The appearance of papillomata on skin and on other surfaces where friction takes place (Rodbard and Epstein, 1965) support this thesis.

We have previously analyzed factors that may participate in the regulation of vascular caliber (Rodbard et al., 1967).

As noted above, the caliber of most blood vessels usually matches the size and metabolic activity of the vascular bed it serves. In accord with this general rule, the huge calibers of the aorta, pulmonary artery and of the venae cavae appear to be adjusted to the flow of the total cardiac output, while the lumen of each smaller vessel reflects that portion of the output that flows through it. In general, the diameter of each segment of a blood vessel varies with the cube

root of the volume of flow that passes through it. The drag generated by a
laminar stream also varies with the cube root of the rate of flow.

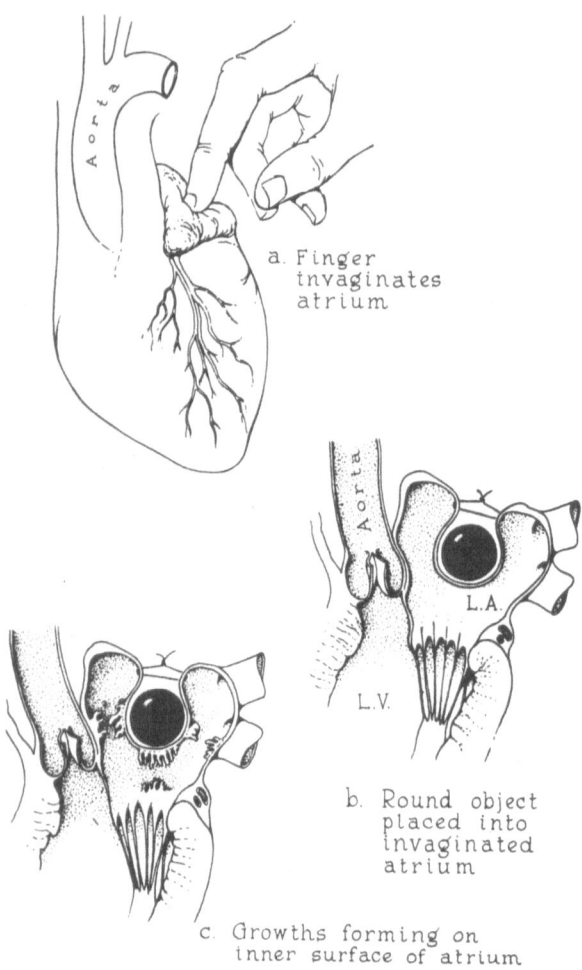

a. Finger
   invaginates
   atrium

b. Round object
   placed into
   invaginated
   atrium

c. Growths forming on
   inner surface of atrium

Figure 8. Method of induction of intra-arterial papillomas

An increase in the activity of a tissue, as occurs in growth, or during the
training of a specific set of muscles, is soon followed by an increase in blood
flow to the tissue and then by a comparable enlargement of its blood vessels.
Specialized vascular segments, such as the heart chambers, their orifices and
valves, also grow with the individual(Rowlatt et al., 1973; Lueker et al., 1970).
Even the growth of tumors is associated with the rapid appearance of arteries and
veins in numbers and calibers sufficient to supply such growths (Wright, 1938;
Cudkowicz and Armstrong, 1953). Decreases in activity, as in invalidism or sen-
escence, are followed by caliber reductions. These important adjustments are
accepted by physiologists and pathologists with hardly a comment, even though
fundamental aspects of vascular modifications are evident.

Segments of vessels sometimes enlarge excessively and without apparent relationship to the rate of flow, as in post-stenotic dilatations, aneurysms and
varicosities. At other sites, vascular segments exhibit progressive narrowing,

as at coarctations, at stenotic plaques or at heart valves. A vessel that has been adequate for a given stream may impede flow by narrowing partially or even by closing. These and other exceptions, which are the special interest of workers in arteriosclerosis, challenge the *general rule* that vascular caliber varies with the blood flow through its vascular bed.

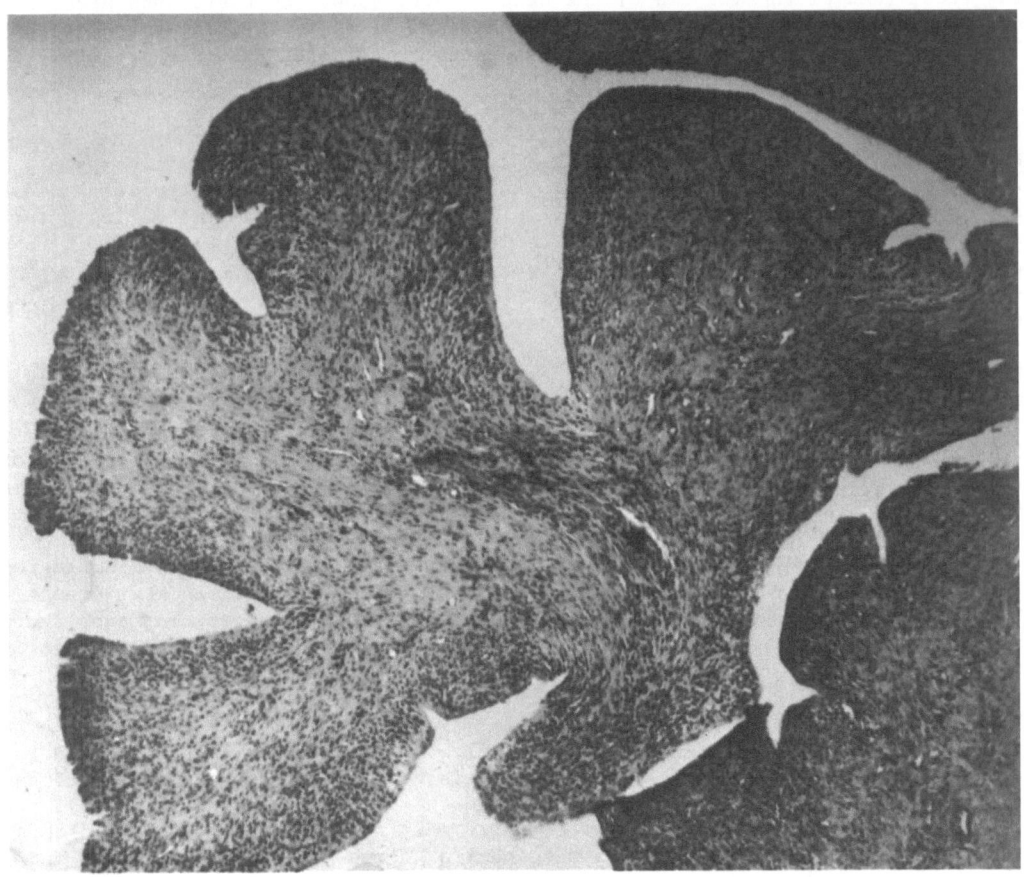

Figure 9. Papilloma on the atrial wall, induced by method in Figure 8

The general rule, together with many of its exceptions, as well as of the complexities of congenital and acquired heart diseases can be accounted for almost entirely on the basis of endothelial responses to the magnitude of the force of hydrodynamic drag. The few circumstances in which pressure may affect caliber will be discussed first.

The blood stream generates mechanical forces that operate perpendicular to the vessel lining, or parallel to the lining. Pressure, the force perpendicular to the wall, is usually positive, but at highly localized sites it may be negative with respect to the ambient pressure.

Pressure. Vascular caliber is independent of the positive pressure in the vessel. Thus, the pressure at the origin of each intercostal artery is identical with that in the immediately adjacent, vastly larger thoracic aorta. Further, the calibers of the aorta and of the pulmonary artery in normal subjects are approximately equal even though the pressures in these vessels may differ by an order of magnitude.

Ligation of an artery usually is followed by a decline in its caliber, even though the arterial pressure remains unaffected.

Changes in pressure and therefore in mechanical tension (Schaper, 1971) induce changes in wall thickness and strength, as noted above. This is evident in the characteristically much greater thickness of the dependent arteries and veins of the feet, than of the vessels of the head (Short, 1954). However, such pressure differences have no significant effects on vascular caliber. Compression of the layers of the wall can similarly be discounted as a factor that significantly affects vascular cross-sectional area.

Lift. A local increase in stream velocity will lower the pressure against the adjacent segment of the vessel lining (Bernoulli, 1938). Thus the velocity of the stream that passes through a narrowing may be so marked that the local pressure against the lining of the artery will fall below the pressure on its outer wall. This negative pressure or *lift* can deform the lining of the vessel, especially when its tissues are gelatinous as they are in the embryo. The dynamic effects of lift have been demonstrated in channels that have been lined with deformable materials (Rodbard et al., 1967).

Lift generated by local high velocities can form cushions and valves. It can also metamorphose these structures into severe stenoses or dissections (Rodbard, 1971). Such lifting forces can be operative only at a relatively restricted segment of the arterial wall. If excessive lift pulls the inner wall of an artery away from its outer media and adventitia, damage to the arterial vasa vasorum may facilitate a local hemorrhage into the media. The blood accumulated in the medial laceration will in turn push the vessel lining into the lumen, generate a still higher velocity and augment the lift forces. The intramural hemorrhage can then progressively dissect the vessel wall and obstruct the lumen. This effect may account for dissections in the aorta and in the coronary arteries. Except for such acute local effects, lift is probably not a general or chronic determinant of vascular caliber.

Hydrodynamic Drag — Vascular Caliber. All streams exert drag, a force that acts parallel to the wall, in the direction of flow. Many of the changes observed in vascular caliber can be explained on the basis of the hydrodynamic drag that the viscous blood stream applies against the endothelial lining (Rodbard, 1956), and by the responses of the endothelial cells to this force. This hypothesis offers a general experimental approach to the study of normal growth and decline, and also to many of the pathological modifications observed in blood vessels.

A laminar stream resembles a set of concentric sleeves of fluid (Fig. 10). The fluid layer immediately adjacent to the wall moves very slowly because of the viscosity of the fluid. The adjacent sleeve of fluid moves with the layer in contact with the wall, but the perfusion pressure impels it to a higher velocity. Each succeeding concentric sleeve moves with the velocity of its adjacent mural sleeve, plus an increment imposed by the more central sleeve. Velocities therefore increase from sleeve to sleeve, with the highest velocity in the axial core.

The vessel lining can receive no *direct* information concerning either the maximal velocity, or the volume flowing through the vessel. Such information can be transmitted to the wall only indirectly through the fluid layer in contact with the endothelium. The force generated by this outermost lamina of the stream tends to pull the lining cells downstream. Being firmly fixed to the vessel wall, the endothelial cells remain in place. However, the stream generates a shear stress in the lining cells.

Each endothelial cell appears to be equipped with receptors (Fig. 11) that can respond to the magnitude of the drag force that impinges on it. The system is in equilibrium as long as the stream deforms endothelial receptors to a certain set point value. Deviations of the drag force from this set point stimulate the cell to initiate negative feedback mechanisms that can return the magnitude of the

DRAG DETERMINES VASCULAR CALIBER

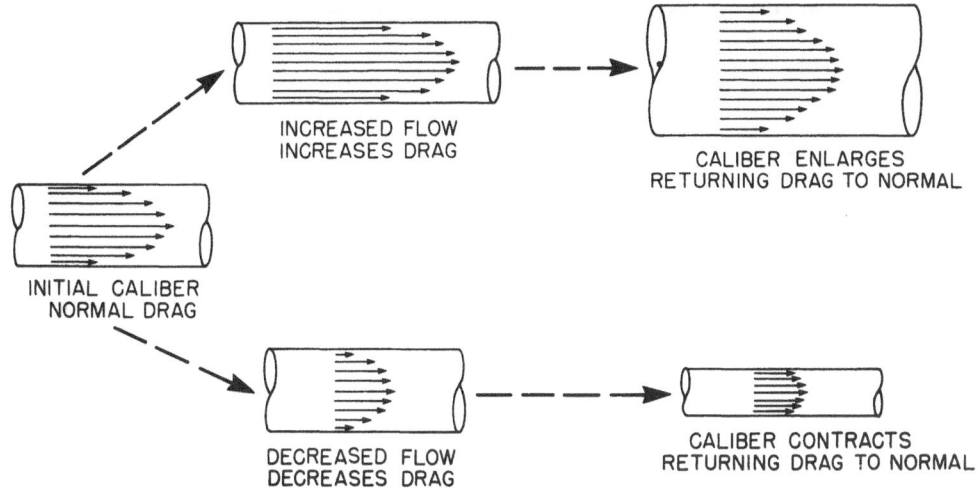

INCREASED FLOW
INCREASES DRAG

CALIBER ENLARGES
RETURNING DRAG TO NORMAL

INITIAL CALIBER
NORMAL DRAG

DECREASED FLOW
DECREASES DRAG

CALIBER CONTRACTS
RETURNING DRAG TO NORMAL

Figure 10. At left, initial distribution of velocities in laminar flow. Arrows adjacent to the wall exert a drag on the vessel lining. Above, an increased flow increases velocity and drag, inducing enlargement of caliber (at right above). Below, a decreased flow decreases drag, and the caliber of the vessel declines (right, below)

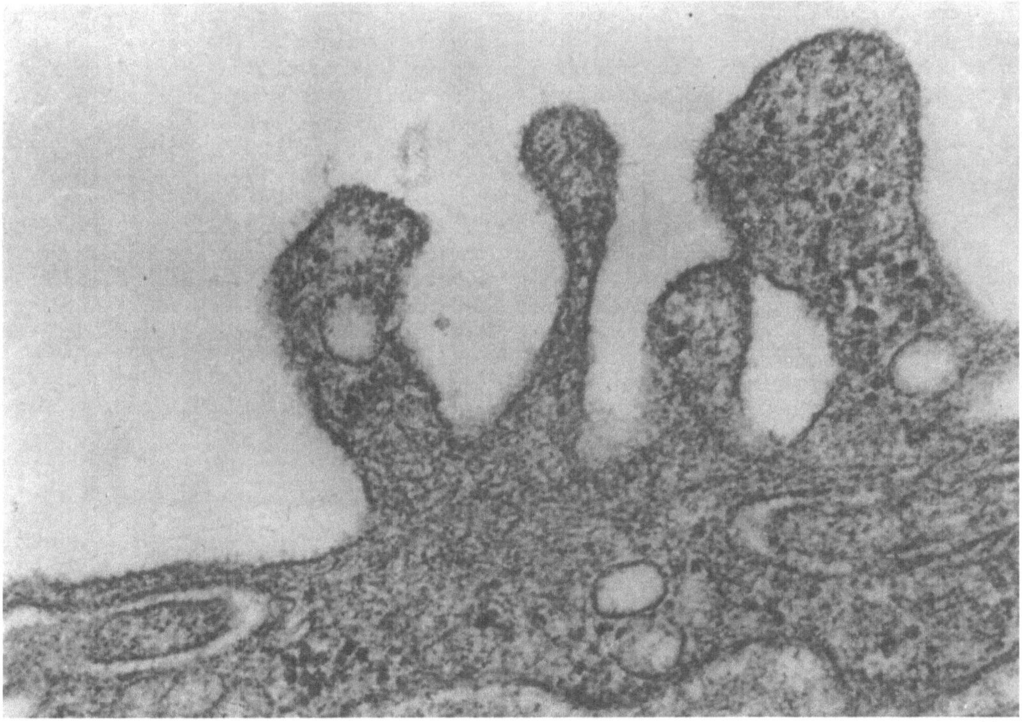

Figure 11. Endothelial projections. Electron microscopy. Courtesy U. Smith, *Science*

drag to its set point. These effects appear to operate through two sequentially
related mechanisms: a) the change in flow rate and the associated change in drag
induce an immediate physiological adjustment in the tension of the smooth muscle
of the wall. If the changed flow rate persists, b) an anatomical change of the
vessel follows (Fig. 12).

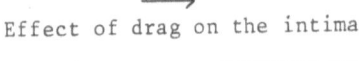

Effect of drag on the intima

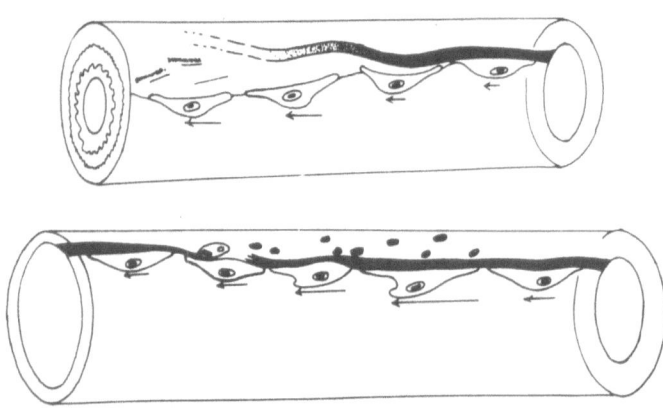

Figure 12. The potential role of hydrodynamic drag in the determination of
vascular caliber. In the upper drawing the first arrow indicates a normal
(set-point) drag acting on an endothelial cell. An increased flow applies an
augmented shear stress (second arrow) to the endothelial cell. Acute dilatation
widens the lumen, reducing velocity and drag (third arrow) to normal values. If
the increased drag is persistent the lumen is reorganized (at fourth cell) around
a larger lumen in which the drag returns to normal values (fifth arrow). In the
lower drawing, a reduced rate of flow results in a subnormal drag force (short
arrow at left). The vessel lumen decreases, thereby increasing the velocity and
drag (third arrow) to normal values. The vessel is then reorganized around the
reduced lumen (at right)

a) Physiological Adjustments. Contraction of a muscle is immediately followed by
a local marked increase in blood flow (exercise hyperemia). The smooth muscle of
the wall of the supplying artery relaxes almost immediately (Schretzenmayr, 1935).
Dilatation reduces the energy losses involved in flow and thereby facilitates the
increase in flow. When the flow returns to its resting rate, the artery contracts
to its previous caliber. These acute changes in association with sudden flow
changes have been demonstrated in femoral (Schretzenmayr, 1935), cerebral, and
other arteries. The veins that receive the increased volume of returning blood
exhibit similar changes in caliber.

The foregoing forms the basis for our hypothesis that *hydrodynamic drag* is the
specific stimulus for the determination of vascular caliber. An increase in the
flow and in the velocity of a laminar stream through a vessel produces a proportional increase in the hydrodynamic drag on its lining, and imposes an added
shear stress on each endothelial unit of surface area that faces the stream. Our
hypothesis holds that endothelial cells perceive the magnitude of this force,
perhaps by means of surface receptors, and that the endothelial cells transmit
this information to the arterial smooth muscle.

Endothelial cells extend filaments through fenestrations in the internal elastic
membranes to the medial smooth muscle cells. Let us assume that an increase in
the shear stress on receptors of an endothelial cell induces the cell to transmit
an impulse directly to subjacent medial smooth muscle cells, and that these cells
respond by relaxation. The resulting vascular enlargement will diminish the

velocity of the stream and return the drag on the endothelial cells toward control values.

If the increase in flow is brief and non-repetitive, the subsequent return of flow to basal rates will reduce the drag. Perception of the reduced shear stress by the endothelial cell then stimulates the subjacent smooth muscle cells to increase their tone. The resulting decrease of vessel caliber to its resting value returns the endothelial drag to its set point. The sensitivity of the vascular lining to drag can also account for normal vascular growth, as indicated below.

b) Anatomical Changes in Caliber. Numerous instances in which anatomical vascular calibers are adapted to the volume flow may be cited. Thus, hydrostatic forces perfuse more of the pulmonary blood flow through the basal vessels of the normal lung than through the apical vessels (Rodbard, 1956). In accord with this, basal (dependent) pulmonary vessels are larger than apical (elevated) vessels. When more of the stream is deviated to the pulmonary apices as occurs in mitral stenosis, the apical vessels enlarge while the basal vessels decline in caliber. Radiological assessment of such patterns of enlargement or decline often facilitates the diagnosis of associated congenital and acquired cardiovascular disorders.

General Enlargement

Long persistence or frequent recurrence of an increased flow and a consequent prolonged vascular dilatation, is known to be followed by anatomical enlargement of the vessel. Thus, animals that are exercised daily exhibit enlargement of the heart; cessation of the exercise is followed by regression of heart weight (Tepperman and Pearlman, 1961). Swimming or running on a treadmill is followed by an increase in the weights of the heart and of casts of the coronary arterial tree. These vascular growths take place even though body weight gain of the exercised animals is abnormally slow. Extracoronary collateral and coronary arteries also increase significantly over control values. The number of capillaries per muscle fiber also increases. Vascular growth is therefore related to blood flow, but not necessarily to general body growth. In cyanotic congenital heart disease in which the cardiac output increases even though the oxygen transported per unit volume of blood may decline, the blood vessels including the coronary arteries may be remarkably enlarged.

Vascular growth depends on the response of individual cells to the local stresses that operate on them. The number of endothelial cells increases with the surface area of a growing vessel (Hughes, 1937), perhaps because these cells are exposed to increased surface tension which induce them to proliferate until the surface tension is returned to its set point. The enlarged radius applies increased tensile forces and their derivates to the media, inducing the formation of more elastin, muscle and collagen, and these materials are organized into structural patterns that prevent vascular rupture. The foregoing chain of events can account for general vascular growth during embryogenesis and in the post-natal period.

Regional Enlargement

Vascular growth sometimes affects only a portion of the cardiovascular system. Regional enlargement of caliber is usually associated with a local increase in flow; vascular segments that do not share in the added flow do not enlarge. Thus, congenital or acquired arteriovenous fistulae are associated with enlargement not only of the communicating arterial and venous segments, but also with the growth of the entire pathway that carries the increased flow (Holman, 1968). In such fistulae, enlargement is also present in the vena cava, all the chambers of the heart, their valve rings, leaflets and orifices; and the pulmonary artery and aorta up to the abnormal connection. The vessels in the remainder of the body remain unaffected. This differential growth shows that vascular modification is not due to general or circulatory hormones or other materials.

Turbulence. A number of workers have held that stream turbulence triggers vascular widening. Turbulence develops when the inertial forces of the stream exceed the viscous forces that tend to maintain laminar (streamline) flow. The phenomenon of turbulence encompasses many processes including mixing of the stream, heating effects, and increased drag (Rodbard and Johnson, 1968).

As noted, drag varies with velocity in a laminar stream. However, in a turbulent stream, drag varies with the square of the velocity. The increased drag in a turbulent post-stenotic segment can therefore account for the local enlargement, even though the flow volume is the same as that in the arterial segment upstream to the narrowing where flow is laminar (Fig. 5). Enlargement of the post-stenotic segment reduces the local velocity and thereby returns the endothelial drag or shear stress to its set point value. The dilated segment is subsequently anatomically reorganized around the enlarged lumen. The magnitude of the dilatation therefore offers information regarding the magnitude of the turbulence and through this, of the severity of the stenosis, and of the pressure drop across the stenosis

General Decline

Generalized decline of vascular caliber is ordinarily relatively gradual and undramatic; as a result, these changes have attracted little study. Vessels decline in caliber when the cardiac index is chronically subnormal as in the hypometabolic states of myxedema, chronic debility, or paralysis. Output also declines when a stenosis at a critical site impedes blood flow. For example, when severe mitral stenosis limits the volume of blood that can be delivered into the left ventricle, physical activity is restricted and hyperemic responses are limited or even absent. In accord with this reduction in activity, patients with severe mitral stenosis tend to have arteries and veins of subnormal caliber. Similar declines in general vascular caliber are observed in other conditions with reduced cardiac index, as in severe aortic stenosis, chronic coronary artery disease, and congestive failure.

A reduced flow diminishes the drag on the endothelial cells and may thereby lead to a reduction in caliber. The immediate response to a decreased drag is considered to be an increase in the tone of vascular smooth muscle. The resulting reduction in caliber increases the stream velocity and the drag force on each endothelial cell, until the set point is again achieved. If the flow persists at the reduced rate, the vessel remains at its reduced caliber, and subendothelial proliferation then diminishes the lumen. This process is clearly seen after ligation of an artery (Buck, 1961; Williams, 1965). Proliferation of the subendothelial connective tissues reduces the arterial caliber to a slit within a week.

Similar subendothelial ingrowths are observed in the post-natal progressive closure of the ductus arteriosus. When pulmonary conductance (flow rate/pressure) increases at the onset of breathing, the foramen ovale closes. The resulting precipitous reduction in flow and drag through the ductus is associated with an immediate contraction of its smooth muscle, further reducing the flow through this potential bypass. A persistent reduction in flow permits progressive subendothelial proliferation. Similar processes probably close the ductus venosus and many other embryonic vessels.

When the function of a given tissue declines, blood flow through the tissue is reduced, and its vessels become smaller. Conditions that lead to reduced physical activity and cardiac output also appear to induce subendothelial proliferation, followed by progressive vascular closure. Vascular changes of this type have been viewed as due to specific components of the disease that produced the invalidism. Some of these subendothelial proliferations may be facilitated by the reduced

flow associated with inactivity, operating through a reduced drag on the
endothelium. In the vascular narrowings of thromboangiitis obliterans, the
primary disturbances may be sympathetic stimulation and arteriolar constriction.
When blood flow remains persistently reduced, the resulting arterial narrowing
may produce those pathological changes in the larger vessels that limit the blood
flow to the limbs. Indeed, a localized stenosis in an artery may, by reducing
flow to the segment beyond the stenosis, lead to subendothelial proliferation in
downstream segments of the vessel. Similarly, coarctation of the aorta can, by
reducing flow beyond the narrowing, result in a markedly atrophic distal aorta.
A local stenosis can therefore lead to the reduction of vascular caliber beyond
the narrowing, even though the tissues served by these vessels become ischemic.

Streamline Separation. Ligaments (Carter, 1972), spurs, plaques and sites of
injury in the lumen of an artery will deviate the streamlines and may thereby
lead to smoothing of the vessel (Fig. 13). Streamlines are accelerated as they
flow around the longer path introduced by an irregularity in the vessel wall. The
increased velocity separates the streamlines from the wall, thereby generating a
local region of reduced drag at the downstream end of the irregularity. Endothelial perception of this decreased drag can induce local subendothelial
proliferation that will smooth out the irregularity and restore the drag on the
local endothelium to its set point. Under slightly different conditions, this
process can lead to a progressive stenosis.

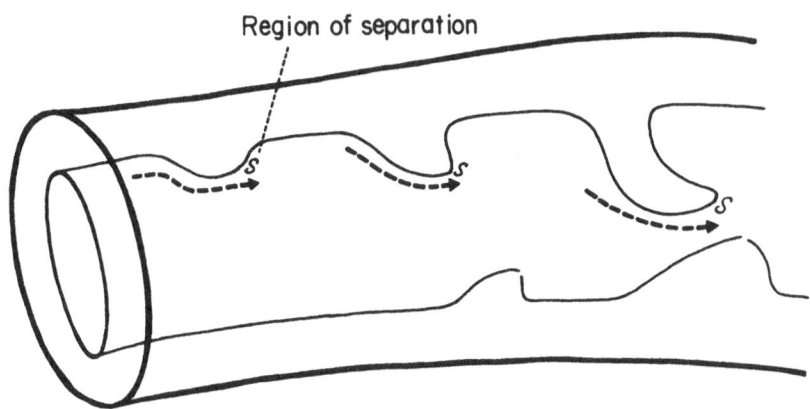

Region of separation

Figure 13. Deviation of streamlines at downstream end of a plaque (at left)
produces a region of separation (S) and locally reduced drag. Ingrowth in the
region of separation leads to progressive downstream subendothelial growth,
enlarging the plaque, and providing a new region of separation. As the process
continues, a growth on the opposing wall may be induced

Progression of Stenosis. When the velocity of the stream passing around the
downstream end of a plaque is very rapid, the streamlines separate from this
segment of the wall, thereby exposing the endothelial cells at this site to a
markedly reduced drag. Local subendothelial proliferation will then cause the
downstream tip of the new growth on the plaque to become the site of most severe
narrowing. The locally enhanced velocity separates the streamlines from
this new segment of the wall. Ingrowth in this new region of separation
narrows the lumen further. When the narrowed arterial segment becomes the
limiting conductance of the vascular bed, ischemia and even infarction of the
affected tissues will follow.

The foregoing suggests that a delicate balance of increased flow sufficient to
hold vessels open, but not great enough to produce a region of high velocity

and separation may facilitate a desired enlargement of the cross-sectional area of a stenotic arterial lesion. On the other hand, when the configuration of the vessel and the velocity of the stream operate to produce separation of the streamlines from the wall, progressive closure is facilitated. This can occur particularly at critical flow velocities in regions of roughness of the wall where slight disturbances in a lamina can amplify oscillations and accelerate these processes.

General Considerations

The present study has focused on the potential role of hydrodynamic forces in the adjustments of wall strength and caliber of blood vessels. Specialized vascular segments such as valves and heart chambers apparently also respond to the same tensile, compressive and shear stresses. Similar principles may be operative in determining the structure and caliber of other vital tubes, including the lymphatic vessels, the airways, the gastro-intestinal, biliary, and genito-urinary tracts, and other passages. The wall thickness, the distribution of its fibrous and other components, and the caliber of each segment of these tubes tend to vary with the mechanical forces that operate on it (Table 1). Proper applica-tion of the mechanical principles outlined in this study may make it possible to control the calibers of these channels in accord with the wishes of the physician and his patient.

Of primary importance is the fact that each of the mechanical forces operating on the vessel wall can be experimentally evaluated and modified. The subsequent changes in the wall or lumen can be measured. The present hypothesis is therefore subject to testing as an approach to the analysis of biophysical factors in vascular structure and caliber. The approach appears to hold promise in the analysis of vascular structure and in the directed modification of the vascular lumen.

Table 1

Stress	Derivative of stress		
	0	1	2
tension	collagen	elastin	muscle
compression	osteoid	cartilage	enamel
shear	caliber	papillomata	synovia

Table 1 is a matrix that shows stresses and their derivatives (column at left). These stresses induce mesenchymal cells to produce specific materials which can relieve the cell of the specific stress. Stresses less than the set point value of the cell induce it to generate processes that dissolve excess materials.

Summary

Primary features of the structure and caliber of blood vessels are determined by the mechanical forces that operate on the cells of the vascular system. The mechanical forces include tension, compression, and shear, which operate on all structures. Tensile forces stretch the materials of the wall, compressive forces push the components of the wall together, and shearing forces cause contiguous tissues to slide on each other along their contact plane.

Stretching of a connective tissue cell induces it to produce collagen fibers which it attaches to the source of the tensile forces; sufficient collagen is generated to relieve the cell of the stretching force. On the other hand, a diminution in the tensile forces induces the cell to digest some of the collagen, thereby adjusting the strength of the fibers to the load. Similar negative feedback mechanisms appear to account for other components of the vessel wall. Oscillating tensile forces induce each affected mesenchymal cell to produce elastin, and to attach this material to sites where it can damp the rate of change of tension acting on the cell. Mesenchymal cells respond to a sudden pull, i.e., an acceleration (rate of change of rate of change) of tension, by the manufacture and alignment of contractile elements within the cell. A sudden pull on the cell thereby activates its contractile machinery so that the muscle pulls back with an equal force and neutralizes the effect on the cell.

Mesenchymal cells appear to respond to compression by secreting relatively firm gels (osteoid) which remove the compressive force from the cell parenchyma. Calcification can then cause the vessel wall to become rigid, thereby relieving the fibrous connective tissue cells of the compressing force. An oscillation of compression (rate of change of compression) induces the mesenchymal cell to secrete sulfated mucopolysaccharides which it organizes into relatively firm concentric shells that enclose the cell, thereby relieving it of the oscillating force.

Similar negative feedback mechanisms have been shown to be in operation in the production of papilliferous growths on the heart valves and in other sites. Friction, a shearing force that causes contiguous planes of tissues to slide relative to each other, induces the formation of the cauliflower-like profusion of pedunculated "ball-bearings" (papillomata) that reduce the friction.

The velocity of the stream generates a drag force on the endothelial cells. When drag is at the set point value of the lining cells, these cells are at rest. An increase in flow rate through the vessel increases the drag force on its lining, and the affected endothelial cell induces relaxation of the subjacent smooth muscle of the wall. This results in a functional local enlargement of the vessel with a reduction in stream velocity and local drag. If the increased flow rate and functional enlargement persist, tensile and compressive forces will then induce an anatomical reorganization of the components of the vessel wall around the larger lumen, i.e., the vessel grows with the increased vascular conductance of the tissues it supplies. This can account for ordinary vascular growth, as well as for abnormal growth as in arteriovenous fistulae. Wherever turbulence occurs, drag increases with the square of the velocity of the stream, and the augmented drag induces a post-stenotic dilatation. Drag generated by a jet increases with the cube of the volume of the stream and such forces can induce aneurysms and related marked enlargement.

A reduction in flow rate and in the drag on the endothelium is followed by the contraction of the smooth muscle of the vessel wall, a reduced caliber and a return of the endothelial drag to its set point. Persistence of the reduced flow permits subendothelial proliferation, reducing the anatomical caliber of the vessel in accord with the flow through it. This occurs in the uterine vessels when flow diminishes, as after parturition. Streamlines tend to separate from the wall at the downstream end of an irregularity in the vessel lining, as occurs at a plaque. The region of separation is a region of reduced drag. This induces a highly localized subendothelial proliferation which further reduces caliber and flow rate. Such a process appears to be operative in vascular closures, as in the ductus arteriosus and ductus venosus at the time of birth. Similar processes may be in operation in occlusions of coronary, cerebral and other arteries.

The study indicates that negative feedback mechanisms operating through each connective tissue cell of the vessel wall may account for the structure and caliber of blood vessels. Similar mechanisms may account for the structure of the other connective tissues of the body.

CONTRACTION OF ENDOTHELIAL CELLS AS A KEY MECHANISM IN ATHEROGENESIS AND TREATMENT OF ATHEROSCLEROSIS WITH ENDOTHELIAL CELL RELAXANTS

T. Shimamoto

Sixty years have passed since Anitschkow (1913) succeeded in producing an atheroma in his experiment by "cholesterol loading" in rabbits. To this date, however, the mechanism of atherogenesis remains unresolved. It appears, though, that new findings obtained in our laboratory may contribute to some extent in unraveling this long-standing enigma.

It has been found by us (Shimamoto and Sunaga, 1972; Shimamoto and Sunaga, 1973; Shimamoto, 1972; Shimamoto and Numano, 1972) that the endothelial cells of internal lining of arteries exhibit contractile reaction immediately following Anitschkow's one-shot treatment with cholesterol in rabbits. We have named this phenomenon "endothelial cell contraction". The contraction (contracting activity) of the endothelial cells results in enlargement of the intercellular space, thus allowing penetration of relatively large particles of serum components such as ß-lipoprotein (150-250 Å in diameter) into the subendothelial layer via the widened intercellular space channel and activating at the same time the membrane flow of the large particles by the contraction (Bennet, 1956).

That the migration and subsequent deposition of ß-lipoprotein and pre-ß-lipoprotein into the subendothelial layer lead to the formation of atheroma is today textbook knowledge, but the "how" of this infiltrative mechanism had been an unanswered question (Haust and More, 1972). Here it is noteworthy, as shown by us (Shimamoto and Sunaga, 1972; Shimamoto and Sunaga, 1973; Shimamoto, 1972; Shimamoto and Numano, 1972) and also Robertson and Khaivallah (1972), that the endothelial cell contraction can also be caused by the hitherto well-known substances that can induce the so-called edematous arterial reaction (Stamler et al., 1972).

Based on the new findings aforementioned (activation of the contracting and swallowing activity of the endothelial cell - penetration of lipid particles into the subendothelial layer), we have been able to formulate a new concept of prevention and treatment of atherosclerosis (Shimamoto, 1972; Shimamoto and Numano, 1973).

Epidemiologic Studies of Atherosclerosis - Facts and Achievements

Internationally controlled epidemiologic studies revealed several important aspects of atherosclerosis. There is no doubt at this time that a clear-cut correlation exists between the severity of atherosclerosis and the incidence of heart attack as well as stroke. Stamler et al. (1972) have pointed out that the progression of atherosclerosis is significantly related to 3 major risk factors. These are 1. hypercholesterolemia, 2. hypertension, and 3. cigarette smoking. As far as atherosclerotic coronary artery disease goes, the risk factors were found to contribute, alone or in combination, to morbidity and mortality of myocardial infarction. Similar facts were confirmed in postmortem studies of the severity of atherosclerosis as related to these three risk factors. The progress of cerebral atherosclerosis in Japanese has been shown to be faster than that of Americans by Resch et al. (1967) despite the lower serum cholesterol level in Japanese than in Americans. However, the incidence of hypertension is actually quite high among Japanese due to their habitual high salt intake in the diet.

What Questions Are to Be Answered?

Why do the 3 major risk factors play important roles in the etiology of atherosclerosis? Our investigation must start at this point. The result of the epidemiologic study (Stamler et al., 1972) also tells us that, among the risk factors, hypercholesterolemia alone demonstrated no specific relation to atherosclerosis. Each of the 3 factors bears equivalent weight in pathogenesis, and when two or three factors were combined, a synergistic relationship was found in terms of progression of atherosclerosis and in particular, of incidence of myocardial infarction. Why? This question must be answered first.

Laragh (1971) and Kaneko (1972) reported that among hypertensive diseases, those associated with a low blood level of renin have a good prognosis and least incidence of heart attack or stroke. These findings are important enough to require further investigation to elucidate the linkage between the renin-angiotensin system and progression of atherosclerosis.

It has been suspected until recently that neutral fats together with cholesterol shared in the production of atherosclerosis, but current lines of investigations have revealed facts contrary to this assumption (Insull, 1972). Epidemiological studies (Kuo, 1972) show that it is rather hyperlipidemia with ß-lipoprotein and pre-ß-lipoprotein (Types II,III, IV, V after Fredrickson) that accounts for atherosclerosis. Why is just this type of hyperlipidemia associated with the progression of atherosclerosis?

One exceptional case gives us a clue. It is of extreme interest to note that again the epidemiological study (Kuo, 1972) revealed that in families with Type I hyperlipoproteinemia there are few atherosclerotic cases, and practically no progression of atherosclerotic lesions were detected among these families (Kuo, 1972).

It is almost incredible that patients who suffer from Type I hyperlipoprotein-emia, who have an extremely high level of lipids, quite often including cholesterol, whose condition is lifelong because of a genetic trait, can be minimally attacked by an atherosclerotic process. One would have to give an answer that accounts for this striking phenomenon. All in all, we can only start atherosclerosis research by thinking much about the aforementioned mysterious facts and by trying hard to give answers to the questions raised above.

Brief Summary of Our Findings

The beginning of our atherosclerosis research dates back many years when we had confirmed a peculiar edematous reaction occurring on the internal lining of the arterial wall of rabbits and rhesus monkeys whenever the animals had been treated with atherogenic substances. We termed this phenomenon "edematous arterial reaction" (Shimamoto, 1963). Among atherogenic substances, those definitely producing atheroma, as in the case of repeated administration of cholesterol, have been categorized into one group, while others including epinephrine and angiotensin II have been placed into another category which was deemed to be responsible for the progression of atherosclerosis. Needless to say angiotensin II is also an active agent in renal hypertension and epinephrine is also an active agent in cigarette smoking. In either case, rabbits and rhesus monkeys treated with these substances all showed "edematous arterial reaction" (Shimamoto, 1963), while rats, not susceptible to atherosclerosis, showed almost no such or a minimal reaction. We now recognize that the edematous arterial reaction is nothing but part of a complex and integral chain reaction involving both the arterial wall and the blood component, especially platelets, in terms of changes in morphology as well as physicochemical properties, and the reaction is always accompanied by a thrombogenic tendency (Shimamoto, 1963). The fact that acid mucopolysaccharides appear in the edematous portion of the arterial wall (Shimamoto, 1963) and that it is highly similar to the pathologically defined

pattern of early-stage atherosclerosis has motivated us to delve deeper into
this topic.

As will be described in detail later, we have been fortunate in discovering
substances that can prevent or offset the said edematous arterial reaction
(Shimamoto, 1963) at a relatively early stage of our investigation. Pyridinolcarbamate (PDC) was found to be one of the above "preventive substances" (Kuo,
1972). This agent (PDC) has been shown to be effective in the prevention of the
following experimentally induced atherosclerotic conditions: a) atheroma in the
rabbit produced by cholesterol loading (Shimamoto et al., 1966; Wu et al., 1969),
b) arteriosclerosis induced by calciferol loading (Grafnetter et al., 1969),
c) arteriosclerosis due to experimental lathyrism (Zamura, 1969), and d) diabetic
angiopathy and nephropathy of K.K. mice (Camerini-Davalos et al., 1973). It is
also the first so-called platelet drug in the history of medicine. Bearing all
the above findings in mind, we reached the conclusion that, whatever may be the
cause, the key portion of atherogenesis lies in the edematous arterial reaction
(Shimamoto, 1963) in which the triggering mechanism that leads to full-blown
atherosclerosis is concealed.

In 1971, we were able to demonstrate the presence of serum ß-lipoprotein in the
edematous parts of the aortic wall showing edematous arterial reaction (Shimamoto
and Sunaga, 1973; Shimamoto, 1972, Shimamoto et al., 1972). Within a very short
time of cholesterol loading, i.e. just a few hours after a single-dose treatment
of animals with cholesterol, particles like ß-lipoprotein with dimensions between
150-250 Å infiltrated into the intima and further down to the media. The mode of
infiltration was such that the particles entered the subendothelial space first,
then the muscular layers via pores in the internal elastic lamina, and eventually
were carried away, possibly by the lymphatics (Shimamoto and Sunaga, 1973;
Shimamoto, 1972; Shimamoto et al., 1972). PDC itself proved to
reduce or prevent this infiltrative process (Shimamoto and Sunaga, 1973;
Shimamoto, 1972). At this juncture, we were faced with the underlying mechanism
that can possibly provide an explanation as to why large particles such as
ß-lipoprotein could be transported into the subendothelial layer so rapidly that
it is almost instantaneous. We were inclined to believe that the rapid infiltration does occur not only via the vesicular system, but rather mainly by a
transient enlargement (widening) of the interendothelial cellular space, which
may well provide enough room and accessibility for the large lipid particles to
enter. Furthermore, in order for the intercellular space to enlarge, the possibility of endothelial cell contraction was considered as the step preceding
enlargement of the intercellular space.

Studies on the Contracting and Swallowing Activity of the Endothelial Cells

In our laboratory, investigations dealing with the problem of endothelial cell
contraction were initiated in 1971. A catheter is introduced into the left
ventricle of the rabbit under anesthesia, through which the fixative solution is
perfused under constant pressure (110 mmHg) in order to achieve in situ fixation
of the aortic endothelial cells. The fixative consists of isotonic glutaraldehyde
with phospate buffer pH 7.4. It is warmed to room temperature before perfusion.
The temperature is then gradually lowered to ice-cold during the procedure. The
specimen obtained in this fashion is finally subjected to electron microscopic
study.

The presence of contractile protein in the endothelial cells has been known since
Becker and Murphy's description (1969). Among various contractile proteins, the
presence of thin filaments (40-90 Å) with dense bodies, thick filaments (130-160
Å), and intermediate filaments (70-120 Å) are easily recognized in the endothelial cells of rabbit and monkey (Fig. 1). As a result of contraction, the nucleus
shrinks, forming hollows at its periphery. When actomyosin contracts vigorously,
hollow formation becomes extreme to such a degree that both poles at the ceiling
of the hollow can be seen in conjunction. Majno et al. (1969) referred to this

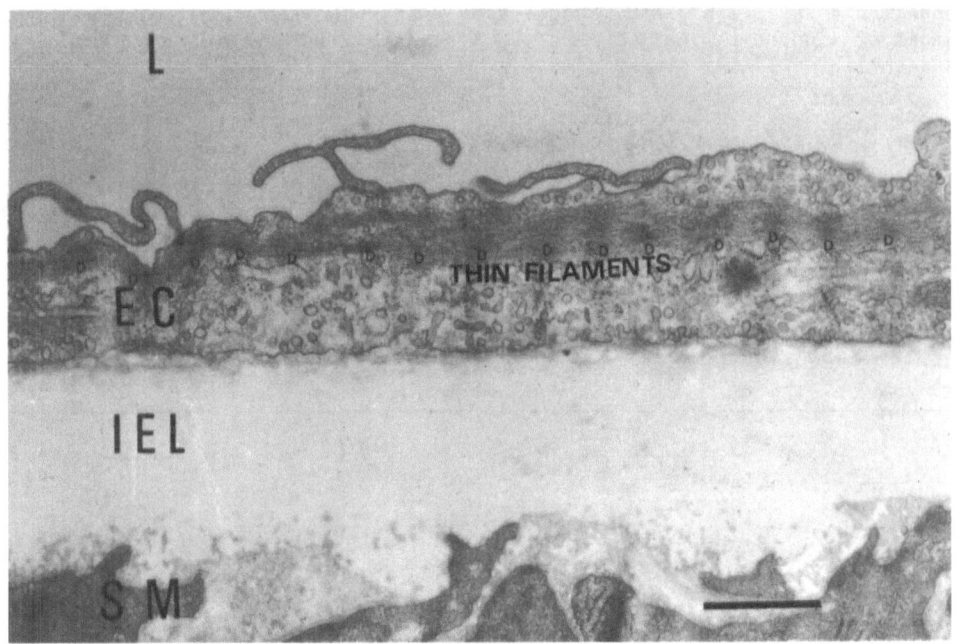

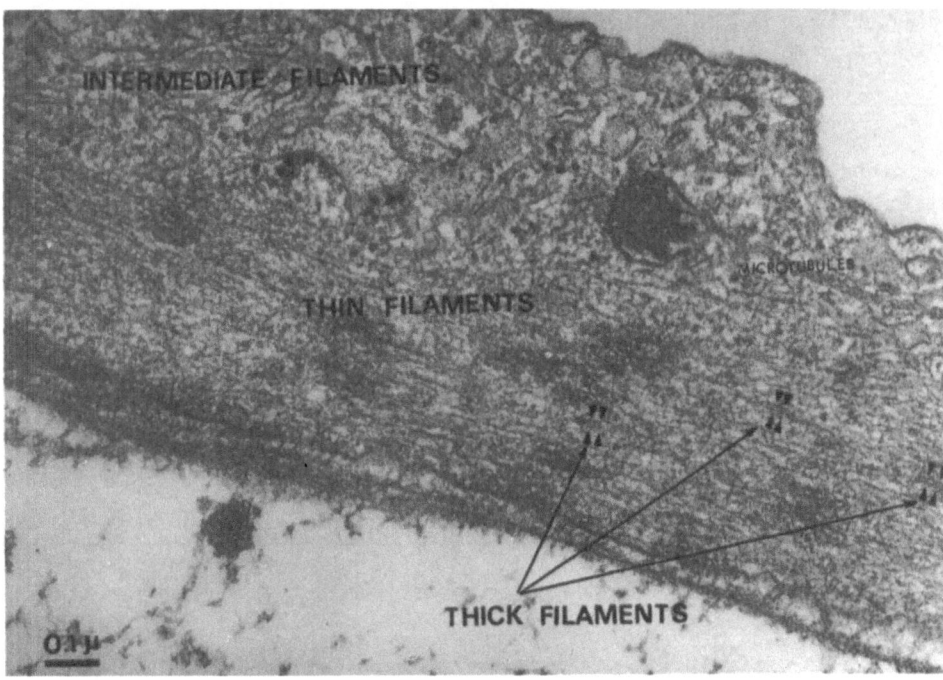

Figure 1. Longitudinal transection of endothelial cell of rabbit aorta.
(1) *Note:* Longitudinally running thin filaments with dense bodies (D) are seen.
The dense bodies correspond well with the concave parts of the endothelial
surface.
(2) *Note:* Thick filaments are seen among thin filaments resembling those of smooth
muscle cells. Intermediate filaments are also present, apart from thin
filaments.

L: Lumen   D: Dense body   EC: Endothelial cell
IEL: Internal elastic lamina   SM: Smooth muscle

phenomenon as "pinch", and we have used appearance and number of pinches as an index of endothelial cell contraction. We have also measured the size of inter-endothelial cellular space.

Table 1. Contraction of Endothelial Cells

Challenge	Pretreatment	T E M			Immunofluorescent antibody technique	
		No. of Anim.	No. of EC Counted	Pinches	No. of Anim.	Infiltration of ß-lipoprotein
no	no	10	934	0	7	- ~ +
Cholesterol 1g/kg p.o.	no	10	972	6.2 ± 1.1[a]	7	+++[b]
	Premarin 5mg/kg i.v.	5	526	0	3	- ~ +
	Pyridinol-carbamate 10mg/kg p.o.	5	548	0	5	- ~ +
Epinephrine 1µg/kg i.v.	Placebo	5	536	4.1 ± 1.2[c]	5	+++
	Pyridinol-carbamate 10mg/kg p.o.	5	529	0	5	- ~ +
Angiotensin II 1µg/kg i.v.	Placebo	7	453	4.3 ± 1.2[c]	5	+++[b]
	Pyridinol-carbamate 10mg/kg p.o.	6	510	0	5	- ~ +
Bradykinin 10µg/kg i.v.	Placebo	6	520	2.7 ± 1.0[c]	5	+++
	Pyridinol-carbamate 10mg/kg p.o.	6	515	0	5	- ~ +
Serotonin 10µg/kg i.v.	Placebo	5	486	5.4 ± 1.8[a]	5	+++
	Pyridinol-carbamate 10mg/kg p.o.	5	503	0	5	- ~ +

Control vs Challenged.

[a] $p < 0.001$.　　[b] $p < 0.5$.　　[c] $p < 0.01$.

This table summarizes the results obtained by electron microscopic observation (75 rabbits) and by immunofluorescent observation (62 rabbits).
The contraction of endothelial cells with nuclear pinch was observed in the endothelial cells of the thoracic aorta at the level of 1st and 2nd inter costal arteries between their orifices and at its dorsal aspect. The immunofluorescent observation was made on thoracic and abdominal aorta.
Note: The contraction of endothelial cells with pinch was induced by single dose treatment of the animal with cholesterol, epinephrine, angiotensin II, bradykinin, and serotonin. Migration of ß-lipoprotein into the arterial wall was achieved at the same time by the same challenge. Pyridinolcarbamate and Premarin exhibited a preventive effect against both contraction of endothelial cells and migration of ß-lipoprotein to the subendothelial space.

Results (Table 1)

In a group of rabbits used for control we were unable to observe any "pinch" phenomenon nor an enlargement of the intercellular space. The same was true with another group fed with placebo. To further demonstrate that no enlargement of the intercellular space had taken place, we gave ferritin by i.v. bolus, but no ferritin was observed in the intercellular space and little was seen in the subendothelial layer.

On the contrary, in a group of 10 rabbits which were given cholesterol (1g/kg p.o.) and killed one to two hours later, about 6.2% of their aortic endothelial cells exhibited "pinch" of the nucleus indicating strong endothelial cell contraction (Fig. 2).

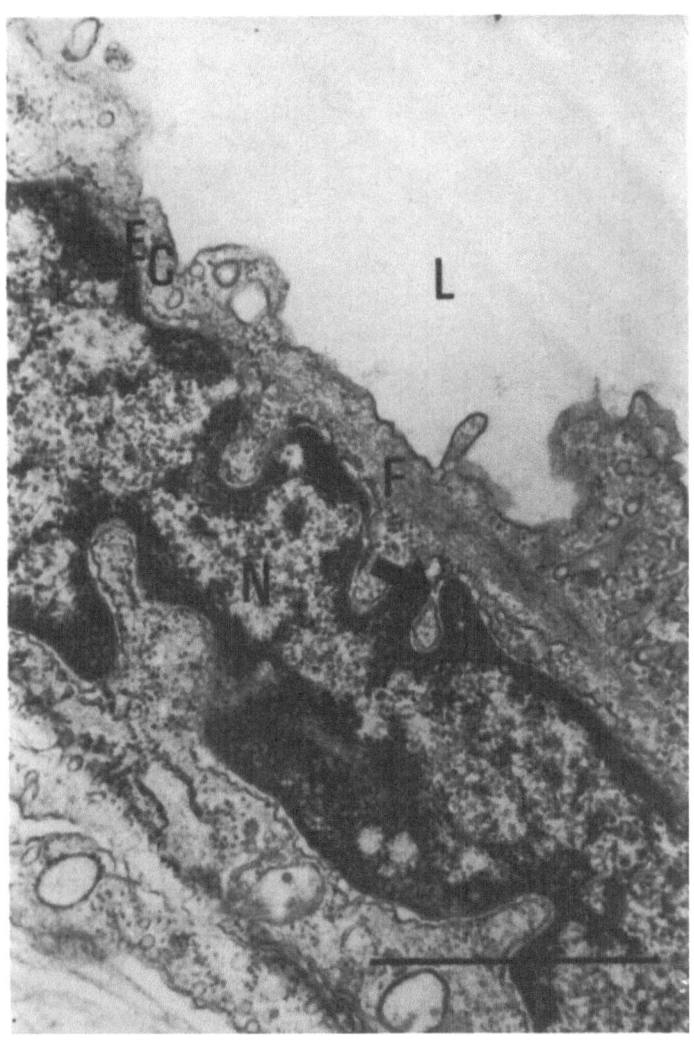

Figure 2. Endothelial cells of thoracic aorta of rabbit sacrificed 2 hours after cholesterol challenge (1g/kg p.o.)
Note: The nucleus shows marked indentations and pinch (↑) formation. In the neighboring cytoplasm of the pinch, many thin filaments are seen running longitudinally and are considered to be the contracting actomyosin responsible for the formation of pinch

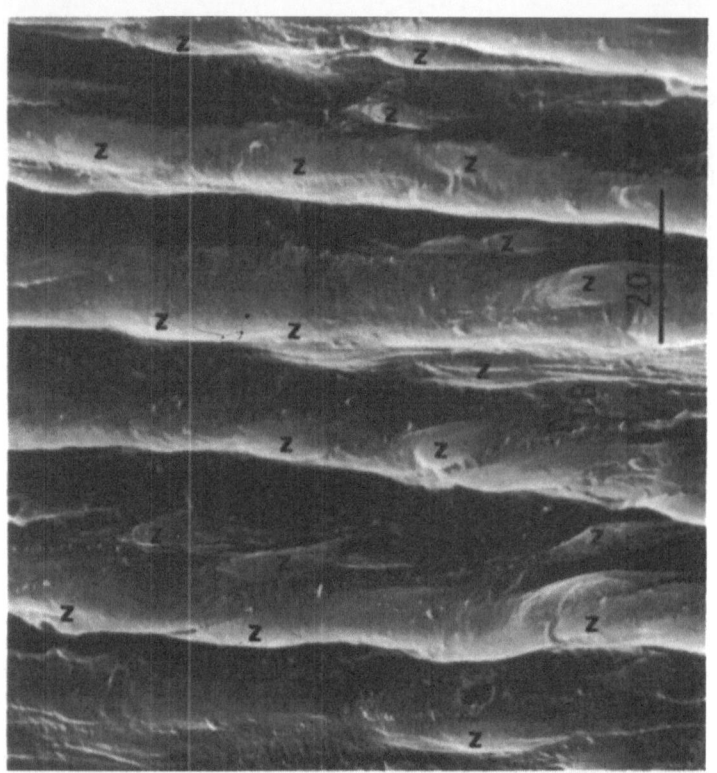
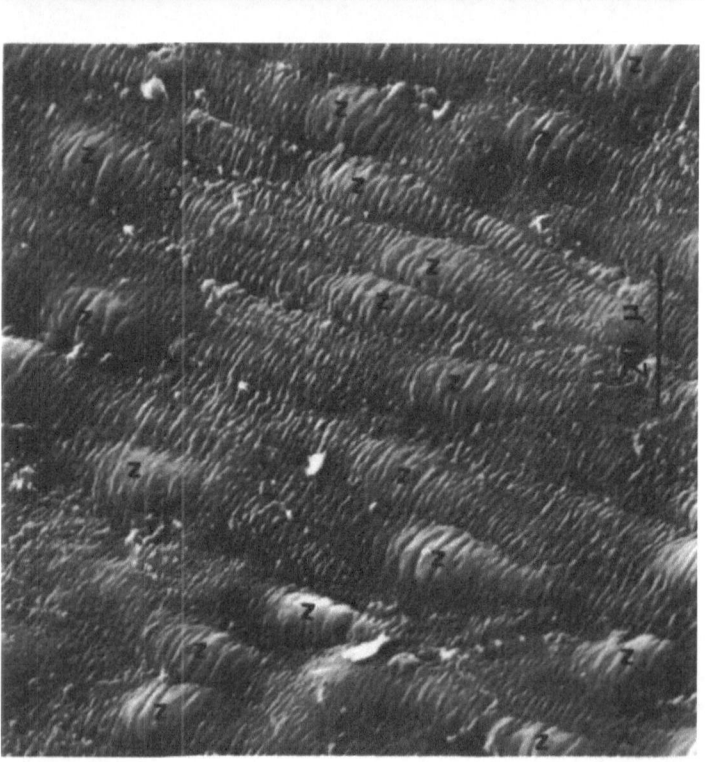

Figure 3. Scanning electron microscopic demonstration of endothelial cell contraction
Left (1). Angiotensin II side and right (2): Saline side.
Both common carotid arteries were temporarily clamped and saline or 10 ng/ml angiotensin II were separately injected into the lumen of the right and left carotid artery respectively at the peripheral part of the clamp; immediately after removing the clamps, the endothelial surface of (1) the left and (2) the right carotid artery was simultaneously fixed by 2.5% glutar-aldehyde by the catheter placed in the left ventricle
CB: Cell boundary

Note: (1) The angiotensin II side was fixed at moderate vasodilation. The boundaries of endothelial cells are relatively clear and the vertical wrinkles of endothelial cells were produced by their contraction due to angiotensin II. They look like a washing board ("the washing board phenomenon"). They are considered to contribute to the increase in thrombogenic activity of platelets because the wrinkles are just vertical to the direction of the blood flow. (2) The saline side: The surface of each endothelial cell is smooth, despite the moderate vasoconstrictive state with deep folds due to the contraction of arterial smooth muscles

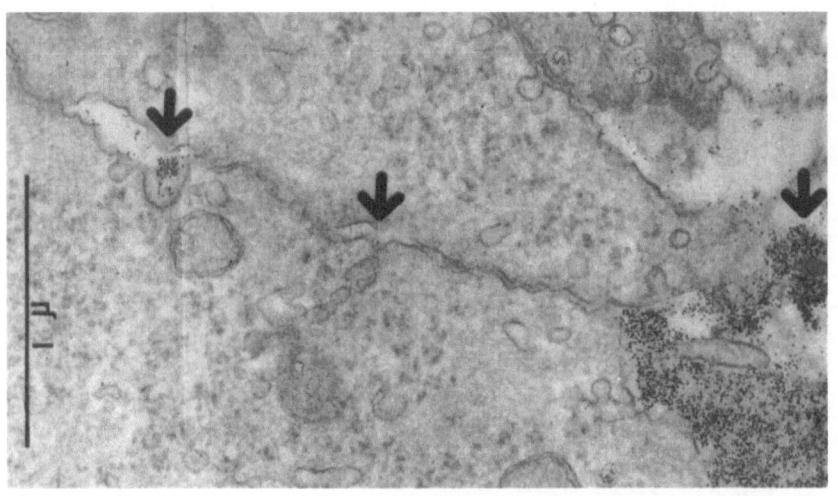

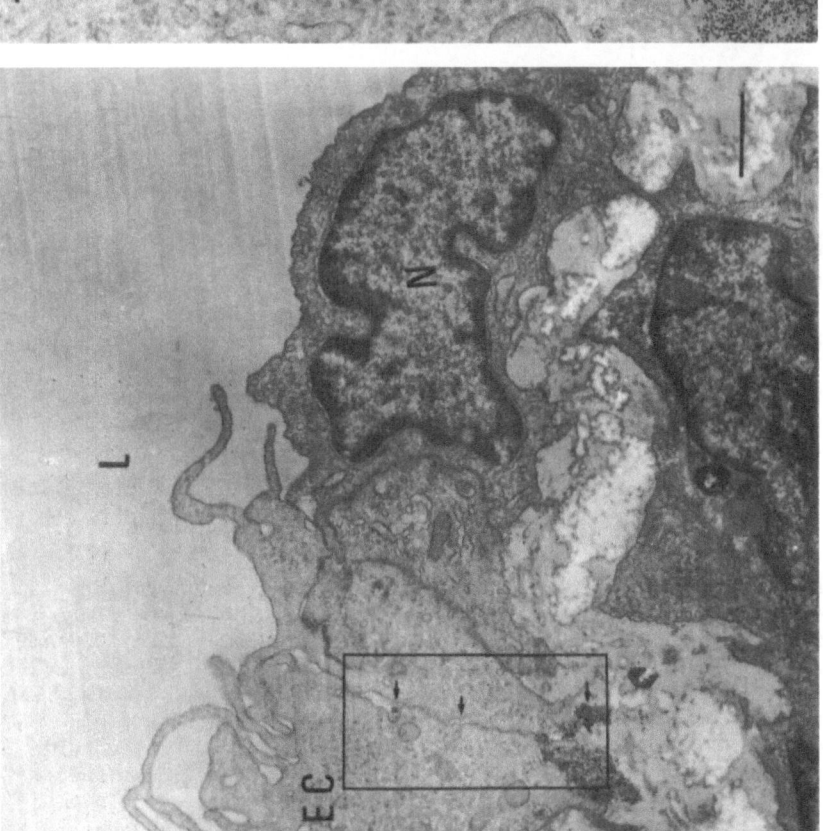

Figure 4. Transection of the intima of thoracic aorta of a rabbit receiving angiotensin II. 1 μg/kh, i.v. and ferritin, 700 mg, i.v. as a marker, 10 minutes later. This specimen was sampled following vital fixation of the aorta, performed 10 minutes after intravenous injection of ferritin.

Note: Ferritin particles are passing into the intercellular space from the aortic lumen to the subendothelial space. They are seen as widened area (↑) in the intercellular space at its orifice (↑) in the subendothelial space. L: aortic lumen. EC: endothelial cell. N: nucleus; ← Ferritin

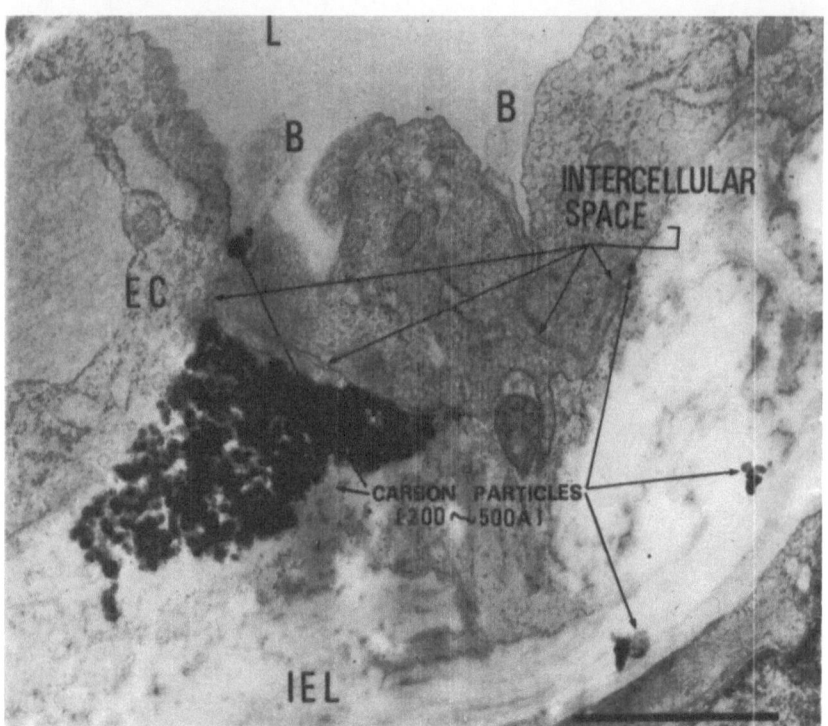

Figure 5. Transection of intima of thoracic aorta of a rabbit receiving cholesterol, 1 g/kg p.o., and carbon particles i.v. 2 hours later.
Note: Carbon particles (↑) are deposited in the subendothelial space after
passing through the intercellular space. Three carbon particles (↑) are seen
in the widened area of the intercellular space of endothelial cells, whereas
one carbon particle (↑) is already seen in the orifice of the subendothelial
space. L: aortic lumen. E.C.: endothelial cell

Similar findings were obtained with rabbits treated with epinephrine, angiotension
II, bradykinin, serotonin, and prostaglandin E-1 (Fig. 3). The degree of
enlargement of the interendothelial cellular space can sometimes reach 300 Å in
diameter, although the enlargement was usually seen as localized widening
scattered interruptedly along the cellular junction. Occasionally, we could see
a localized enlargement measuring up to 900 Å in diameter. When ferritin or
carbon particles (200-500 Å) were given in addition to cholesterol or other
above-named substances, they appeared as clusters in the intercellular space.
As shown in Fig. 4, ferritin can be seen as scattered small clusters along the
course of the intercellular space, and at its opening into the subendothelial
layer there appears a large aggregate of ferritin despite of scantiness of
ferritin particles in vesicles at this stage. As shown in Fig. 5, carbon particles
also passed the course of the intercellular space into the subendothelial layer.
The membrane flow (Bennett, 1956) through cytoplasm was also activated in the
later stage in the case of carbon transportation by the above-mentioned challenge,
when the contraction of the endothelial cell was extremely strongly induced,
and the enhancement of membrane flow seemed to be induced also by contracting
activity of the endothelial cells.

Interrelationship Between the Size of Lipoprotein, Endothelial Cell Contraction with Subsequent Enlargement of the Intercellular Space, and Transportation of the Lipid Particles

Speaking of the enlargement of the intercellular space again, we have observed that the greatest enlargement can be obtained after injection of angiotensin II (Fig. 6). In the case of cholesterol, a considerable enlargement is usually elicited, with upper limit of the range at 300–360 Å. The enlargement of the intercellular space can reach 700 A, although rarely[*]. Naturally, with this degree of enlargement, one can easily deduce that small particles up to ß-lipoprotein (150–250 A) could enter into the subendothelial layer with

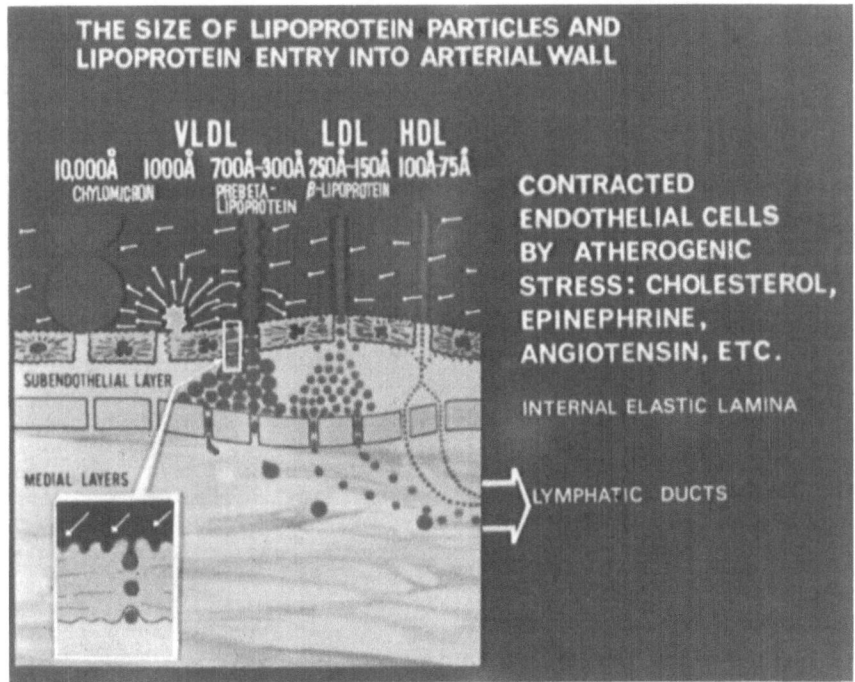

Figure 6. Contraction of endothelial cells widens the intercellular space resulting in increased entry of ß-lipoprotein and possibly pre-ß-lipoprotein passing through it into the subendothelial space. The wrinkles, which are induced by the contraction of endothelial cells and are vertical to the blood flow ("the washing board phenomenon (Shimamoto)"), contribute to the sticking of platelets and especially of large plasma particles like pre-ß-lipoproteins, accelerating the membrane flow (Bennett 1956) and vesicle activity; this results in increased entry of lipoproteins including pre-ß-lipoprotein into the subendothelial space. However, chylomicrons are too large to enter the intercellular space or endothelial cell itself by membrane flow

---

[*] In our experiment, ferritin particles entered the subendothelial space with ease. The carbon particles (500–700 A) enter the subendothelial space with relative difficulty when cholesterol alone is given. It is easier, however, when combined challenge with cholesterol and epinephrine is attempted. Angiotensin II is quite potent: it enlarges the intercellular space and enhances significantly the transportation of carbon particles by the intercellular space and also by the membrane flow.

relative ease, and the intercellular route seems to be the main route for smaller particles, although the vesicle system and membrane flow for ferritin transportation were also activated by the above-mentioned challenges. It is not impossible, although not always, for the larger particles of pre-ß-lipoprotein (300-700 Å) to enter through the enlarged intercellular space, and the entry by membrane flow may be possible for pre-ß-lipoprotein, as in the case of carbon particles, when endothelial cells are strongly activated as for carbon entry. As far as the chylomicron is concerned, its passage through the enlarged intercellular space is considered difficult, since the maximum enlargement we have ever observed was in the range of 900 A in diameter, and this only exceptionally, even its passage through cytoplasm by membrane flow is also considered difficult because of its large size.

Haust and More have stated in their recent book (1972): "It is nowadays widely accepted that once invasion of ß-lipoprotein and pre-ß-lipoprotein into the subendothelial layer occurs, atherosclerosis can be eventually formulated through chain reactions. The mechanism of this invasion is not clear." In this context, it is probably not an overstatement when we say that our findings have shown a clue to the solution of the enigma for all those who have been engaged in the research into atherosclerosis.

Studies Using the Immunofluorescence Method

As stated previously, the ß-lipoprotein invades the arterial wall immediately following a single dose treatment of test animals with cholesterol, epinephrine, or angiotensin II (Shimamoto and Sunaga, 1973; Shimamoto, 1972; Shimamoto et al., 1972). This finding was obtained by the immunofluorescence method. Of extreme interest at this juncture is our finding with the rhesus monkey. In monkeys, for the ß-lipoprotein to further penetrate into the muscular zone after passing through the subendothelial layer as well as the pores of internal elastic lamina, it takes relatively longer as compared with that of immunoglobulin G (IgG). There is a 30-minute to one-hour delay in the case of ß-lipoprotein. This implies, at least as one possibility, that particles the size of ß-lipoprotein could hardly penetrate through the internal elastic lamina which, therefore, tend to stagnate in the subendothelial layer. Even in the case of the ferritin particle, transportation through the holes in the internal elastic lamina took place just one by one. For carbon particles the size of pre-ß-lipoprotein, the passage through internal elastic lamina is quite difficult and their stagnation in the subendothelial space is marked (lasting at least over one to several hours or more) when carbon particles once penetrate the endothelial lining due to angiotensin II or other agents. With the increase of particle size such as in the case of pre-ß-lipoprotein, the situation is deemed to become more realistic, although, at this time, we do not have any experimental data yet. Here, the reason why men with high blood levels of ß- and pre-ß-lipoprotein are more prone to atherosclerosis, could well be explained on the basis of the above findings. The toxicity of Lp(a) may also be related to the larger size of Lp(a) than ß-lipoprotein.

While the fact that the cholesterol content of ß-lipoprotein is as high as 40% is in itself significant, the cause of atheroma formation lies in the stagnation of lipoproteins in the subendothelial layer, particularly due to the difficulty for ß-lipoprotein to further penetrate downwards through the internal elastic lamina.

In the case of Type I hyperlipoproteinemia, in which chylomicrons constitute the major carrier of cholesterol in the blood, we would assume that atherosclerosis could rarely occur merely because of the large size of chylomicron particles (1,000-10,000 Å). This is because, as stated before, the widening of the intercellular space secondary to the contraction of endothelial cells can, at the most, reach only 900 Å and it is almost impossible for the membrane flow to carry such large particles.

Endothelial Cells Covering Atheromatous Lesions - Their Contraction and Relaxation

When we studied the endothelial cells covering the atheroma in experimentally induced atheromatous rabbits, we were able to confirm that the "pinch" indicative of cell contraction appeared in 6.2% of all endothelial cells observed. There was concomitant enlargement of the interendothelial cellular space and enhancement of the membrane flow (Bennett, 1956 . Furthermore ferritin and carbon particles were easily detectable on the electron micrograph in the fashion already mentioned. These facts fit the finding of Lofland and Clarkson (1970), who demonstrated increased influx of labeled cholesterol in atheromatous lesions as compared with the unaffected area. Administration of PDC or EG467 or Premarin by mouth to such animals in a sufficient dose showed a statistically significant decrease of the percentage appearance of pinch (Fig. 7) and the pharmacological study of the same data revealed a statistically significant therapeutic effect of PDC on atherosclerotic lesions. When the PDC dose was increased to 30 mg/kg, or the animals were given EG467 1 mg/kg p.o. or Premarin 5 mg/kg i.v., cells showing the pinch had completely disappeared. In other words, the above three substances exhibited a strong relaxing action on the contracting and swallowing activity of endothelial cells.

What we then have considered was the possibility that, as the widened inter-cellular space is narrowed, membrane flow limited, and infusion of lipoprotein blocked, only physiologic particles together with water is infused into the atheromatous lesion. Could it conceivably be the case that physiologic perfusion would help washing out the diseased focus? Thus, cholesterol could be removed; edema would subside; and eventually, the atheroma could well be absorbed leading to plain sailing toward recovery. There is another reason for us to state that the above hypothetical thinking is not unsound. In fact, the ongoing pharmacological study (Shimamoto, 1969) in our laboratory dealing with the effect of long-term administration of PDC, EG467, or Premarin to atheromatous rabbits has already indicated healing of the atheroma which is statistically significant in terms of acceleration rate of the healing process. For the sake of simplicity, we give the general term of "endothelial cell relaxants" to substances such as PDC, EG467, and Premarin. The criterion of

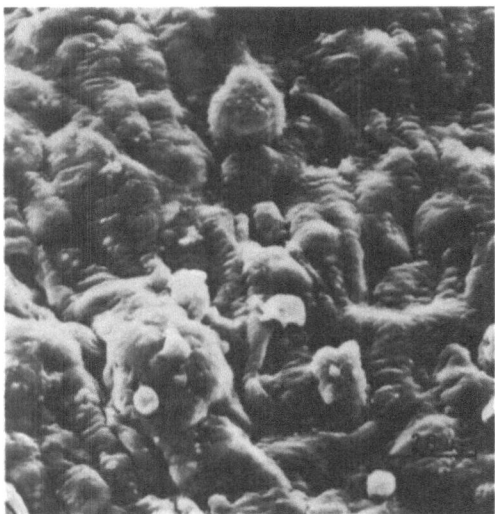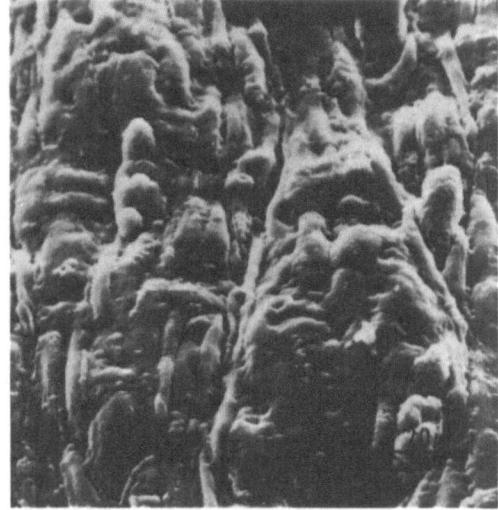

Figure 7. Endothelial cells covering atheroma - in cholesterol-fed rabbits. Left: Untreated; many horizontal lines represent the contraction of endothelial cells. Right: Treated by endothelial cell relaxant; horizontal lines have been markedly reduced by pyridinolcarbamate (10 mg/kg p.o. given 2 hours before sacrifice)

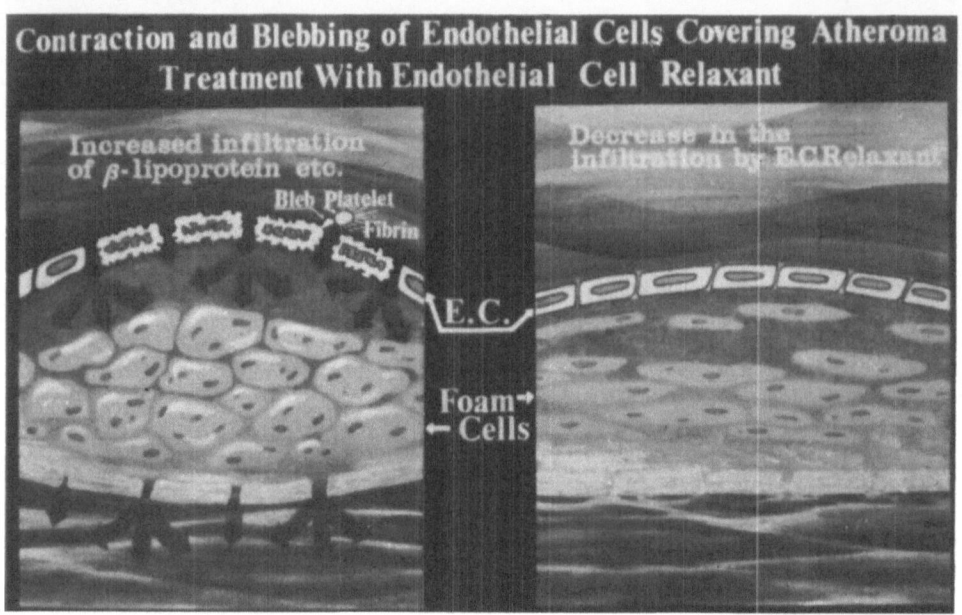

Figure 8. The left picture shows that contraction of endothelial cells enlarges
the intercellular space, inducing penetration of cholesterol-bearing large
lipoproteins from the bloodstream into the subendothelial space. This results in
stagnation of cholesterol-bearing lipoproteins, leading to formation of
atheromatous lesions in the subendothelial space (left). The right picture shows
that relaxation of endothelial cells reduces the size of the intercellular space,
which in turn, inhibits or reduces the infiltration of large plasma particles
through the intercellular into the subendothelial space, thus exhibiting the
curative effect of endothelial cell relaxant

the therapeutic effect of endothelial cell relaxants may well be based on
the following: it relaxes the endothelial cells; it can decrease or block the
contraction of endothelial cells as well as subsequent enlargement of the intercellular space and enhancement of the membrane flow (this chain reaction is
usually caused by the active substances of 3 major risk factors such as
cholesterol, epinephrine, angiotensin, bradykinin, serotonin, histamine, prostaglandin E-1, and some causative agents of inflammation); finally, it
displays the vital effect of preventing infusion of ß-lipoprotein and pre-ß-
lipoprotein into the subendothelial space. It appears that, based on the
above-mentioned preventive as well as therapeutic effect of the endothelial cell
relaxants, prevention of atherosclerosis is not unfeasible, and that treatment
of established atheroma could, if not always, be facilitated (Fig. 8). At this
juncture, it is noteworthy that recent enzymatic studies covering these areas
have proven positive biochemical aspects of PDC in favor of its preventive and
therapeutic effect on atherosclerosis. Numano et al. (1971) and Yamazawa et al.
(1973) reported that PDC activated enzymes relevant to the repair process of
atheroma, while Kritchevsky and Tepper (1971) demonstrated enhancement of
cholesterol oxidation by PDC. These new biochemical aspects of endothelial
relaxants will, of course, play supplemental and complemental roles in our understanding of the mechanism of atherogenesis and its treatment.

Interrelationship Between Endothelial Cell Contraction and Thrombus Formation

The linkage between endothelial cell contraction and thrombus formation is an important problem. When the endothelial cell goes into extreme contraction from whatever cause - cholesterol, epinephrine, angiotensin II, etc., etc. - its ultrastructural appearance on electron microscopy is characterized by the formation of vertical wrinkles due to contraction of the longitudinally running actomyosin. We call this phenomenon "the washing board phenomenon", because of its similarity. These wrinkles may undoubtedly induce turbulence of peripheral blood flow and tend to accelerate the morphological and functional changes of platelets responsible for the increase in platelet aggregation. In addition,

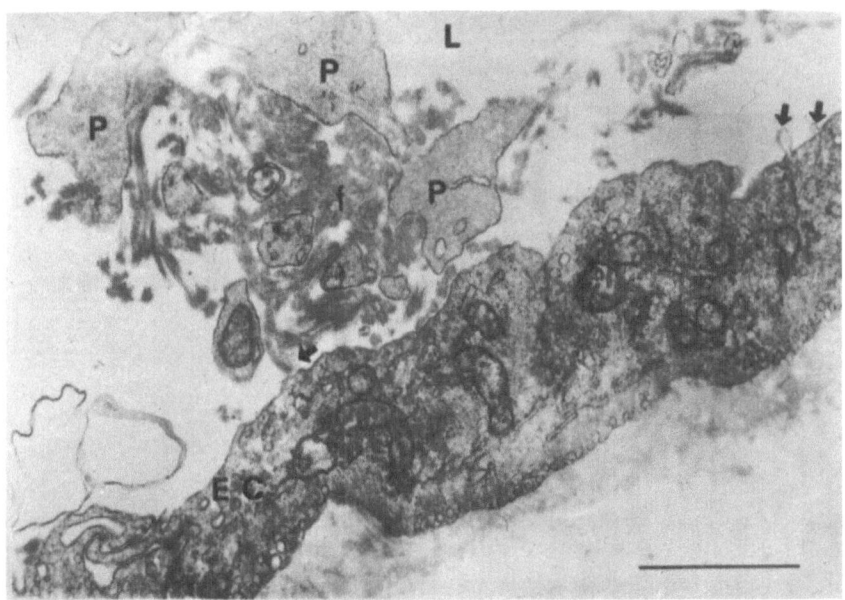

Figure 9. Endothelial cell (EC) with bleb (↑) stuck to platelet (P) and the formation of fibrin (f)

the strong contraction of the endothelial cells frequently accompanies formation of blebs (Shimamoto and Sunaga, 1973; Shimamoto, 1972; Shimamoto and Numano, 1972).[*] In addition to this basic change, one frequently sees sticking of the platelets to the blebs, and there is usually fibrin deposition (Fig. 9). It seems to me that the part of the cell membrane beneath which the bleb is formed is actually injured in such a way that the repelling ability against the platelet has been lost. Losing the physiologic platelet-repelling activity, the normal cell membrane tends to play a part in the aggregation of platelets, thus leading to fibrin formation. We have observed in rabbits that whenever they were treated with a single dose of epinephrine, angiotensin II, and/or cholesterol, there has been a transient increase of coagulability of the blood. Among the mechanisms of this phenomenon, a serial reaction consisting of: injury of the platelet - its sticking and releasing serotonin, a potent endothelial cell contractor; platelet factors - segregation of platelets stuck to and from the part of a

---

[*]Controversy exists regarding the nature and significance of the bleb. The author feels that parts of the blebs are exhibited in close association with injury of, or in a stimulated state of endothelial cells, such as in the case of increased apocrine secretion. It should be emphasized, however, that blebs are always seen in company with contraction of endothelial cells with nuclear pinch.

qualitatively altered cell membrane - recirculation of such segregated platelet aggregate into the blood stream (platelet aggregation is now enhanced) and final increase of coagulability of the blood was suggested. This type of chain reaction will probably be repeated progressively, resulting in formation as well as structural reinforcement of the atheromatous lesions.

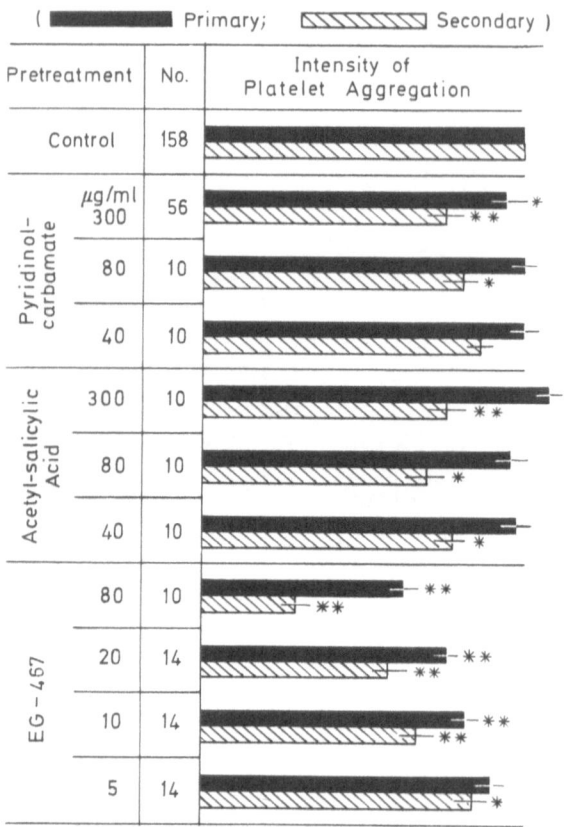

Effect of Pretreatment on Intensity of Platelet Aggregation Induced by 3×10^{-6} M of ADP

Figure 10. Human platelets, suspended in citrated platelet-rich plasma, were incubated with saline solution at different concentrations of PDC or aspirin or EG467, and as a control, with saline for 5 minutes at 37°C, and the ADP-induced platelet aggregation was then measured by the optical density method. (Didisheim, P., Sturm, R.E. and Owen, Jr., C.A.: Experiments on Thrombosis and its Prevention. Current Concepts of Coagulation and Hemostasis. pp. 177-185, 1971, F.K. Schattauer Verlag, Stuttgart-New York).
Note: The primary aggregation of platelets is significantly inhibited by PDC and EG467, but not by acetylsalicylic acid, while the secondary aggregation is inhibited by all these substances. Highly potent inhibitory effect of EG467 is noted.

PDC (Shimamoto, 1972, Sano et al.) and EG467 (Yamazaki et al., 1972) showed a direct effect on platelets in both, humans and rabbits. By in vitro studies we were able to demonstrate a strong inhibitory action of these agents against primary and secondary aggregation of platelets which had been induced by ADP, epinephrine, or collagen. In this regard, the strength of PDC in terms of aggregation-inhibition was equivalent to aspirin, whereas EG467 was more potent than aspirin (Fig. 10).

In the meantime, we looked into the preventive effect of PDC (Shimamoto, 1972; Sano et al.) and EG467 (Yamazaki et al., 1972) against the thrombogenic trend as well as the increase of blood coagulability in rabbits who had been given cholesterol, epinephrine, and/or angiotensin II by the one-shot method. These two agents showed a striking preventive effect against the ehhancement of coagulability and related thrombus formation. The effective dose with PDC was 10 mg/kg, and 1 mg/kg with EG467 (Yamazaki et at., 1972). To our surprise, however, the effective blood levels of these agents were much lower than had been anticipated. In other words, it was lower than in the case of in vitro studies in which, as was mentioned before, investigations on platelet aggregation and its inhibition by PDC and EG467 were made. Our finding is compatible with that of Cotton et al. (1972), who observed the normalizing effect of PDC treatment on elevated platelet aggregation of patients suffering from severe arteriosclerosis obliterans whose PDC blood level was not sufficiently high to lower directly the platelet-aggregation on in vitro testing. At any rate, the fact that thrombosis contributes as a factor in the pathogenesis of atherosclerosis (Duguid, 1948) has been well known to us now for more than two decades. When the pathologic section of atheromatous lesions is carefully examined one can often see the characteristic picture that symbolizes the formative process of atheroma. This includes sticking of the platelets to the arterial intima and formation of thrombi which are frequently encapsulated by newly generated endothelial cells. Here, one may argue about the possible role of collagen as a factor giving rise to thrombus formation, for endothelial cell contraction can also expose intercellular collagen tissue to the circulating blood by widening the intercellular space. Of course, it may be important in the case of injured endothelial cells, but we feel that "the washing board phenomenon" by endothelial cell contraction, the loss of platelet-repelling activity by the cell membrane due to injury, or the blebbing caused by vigorous contraction may possibly be significant, as in the case of exposed collagen tissue.

Use of Endothelial Cell Relaxants as Therapeutic Agent for Atherosclerotic Diseases

We first used PDC for treatment of atherosclerosis in 1963 (Shimamoto and Yamazaki, 1964; Shimamoto et al., 1970). Cerebral, coronary, and peripheral atherosclerosis had been chosen as major targets, and to date, there are considerable numbers of reports of clinical trials on PDC from many countries all over the world (Shimamoto, 1972) including U.S.S.R. (Shkhvatsabaya, 1973; Kyusov et al., 1972; Januskevichius and Blouyhas, 1973).

As regards prevention of cerebrovascular accident and/or myocardial infarction (MI), I feel, on the basis of dialectics, that the use of endothelial cell relaxants as drugs deserves certain merit. Needless to say, intentional removal or avoidance of various risk factors on the part of patients, combined with establishment of sound ecology is of primary importance but it sometimes takes too much time and is often impossible, so that endothelial cell relaxants are required.

Especially in the prevention of arterial thrombosis, in which platelets and the endothelial surface play an essential role, PDC and EG467 exhibited a highly potent preventive effect in our experimental model of arterial thrombosis in rabbits (Fig. 11). In man, Fukui tried PDC on as many as 4,083 patients who had survived strokes with resultant hemiplegias (Fukui, 1969). These patients were divided into two groups for the purpose of studying the frequency of recurrence of stroke or development of MI. One group was treated with PDC, and the other, which formed the control group was treated differently. The PDC group showed a lower incidence of both recurrent stroke and MI than did the other group, which was statistically significant. Atsumi et al. (1971) also carried out a similar study, but dealt with advanced cases of occlusive peripheral arterial desease. All these patients had presented either severe intermittent claudication or

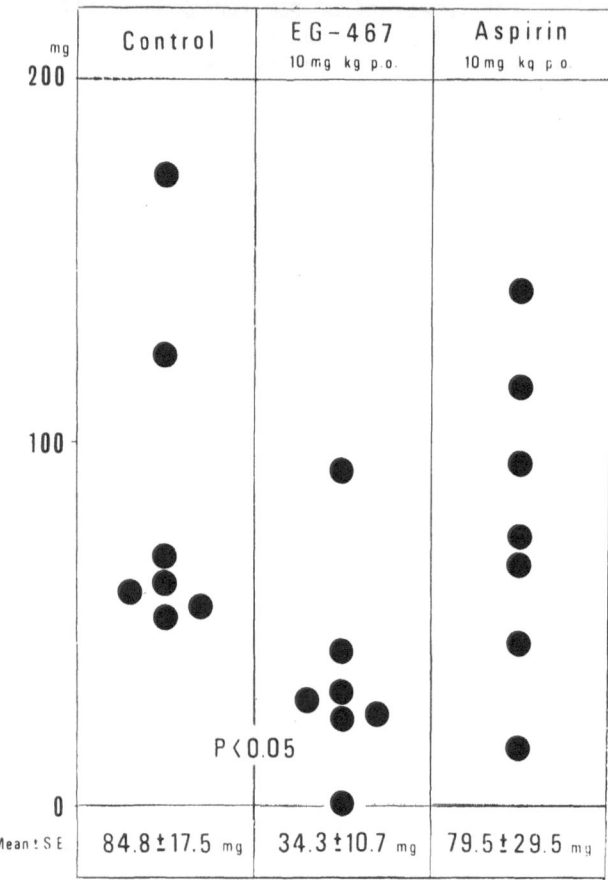

Figure 11. Weight of thrombus in experimental model of rabbit.
Note: Experimental arterial type of thrombus was produced in rabbits by our technique (Ochanomizu Med. J. 13:189, 1965) and EG467 was shown to have a definite antithrombotic effect, while aspirin remained without a statistically significant effect in this experimental model

cyanosis of the lower extremities with or without ischemic ulcers. Forty-five cases were given PDC and 60 cases were given other treatment, and all were followed up for a period of 4 years. In the PDC group, none developed MI and only one had a stroke, which he survived (zero mortality rate, P<0.05). Among the control group, however, six had MI and two had a stroke, and all succumbed (Table 2).

Future Perspective

Up to now, atherosclerosis research has accumulated a vast amount of new knowledge regarding the relationship between atherogenesis and lipid metabolism as well as enzymatic processes involved therein. This new knowledge is of inestimable value in our understanding of atherogenesis and the repair processes of the arterial wall. Needless to say, further development in these fields is essential, ways and means to correct or modify abnormal lipid metabolism and to expedite the repairing process of the injured arterial wall.

However, at the present moment, it seems not unreasonable to emphasize the importance of efforts to further elucidate the nature of contractile protein within the endothelial cells of the arterial intima, because we know so little about it. The current studies on the effects of endothelial cell relaxants on

Table 2. Follow up study on patients suffering from arteriosclerosis obliterans under pyridinolcarbamate treatment and other treatment (Atsumi, T., Honda, Y., and Matsuda, M.: J. Jap. Coll. Angiol. In press)

	Pyridinolcarbamate Group	Non-Pyridinolcarbamate Group
Total Number of Patients	45	60
Age (years)	50.7 ± 2.4	53.0 ± 1.5
The History of Disease (months)	50.0 ± 10.9	48.9 ± 6.8
The Severity of Disease (types) II	39	57
IV	6	3
Blood Cholesterol Level (mg/dl)	198.8 ± 8.7	187.2 ± 5.2
Blood Pressure (mmHg) Systolic	149.4 ± 5.0	152.9 ± 5.1
Diastolic	83.5 ± 2.7	90.4 ± 2.4
Complications Diabetes Mellitus	6	4
Myocardial Infarction	2	2
Observation Period (weeks)	211.5 ± 17.4	165.4 ± 13.0
Number of Deaths by Apoplectic and Heart Attacks	0	8 [*]
Apoplectic Attacks	(1)survived	2
Heart Attacks	0	6

($p < 0.05$)

various vascular injuries must be expanded and appraised carefully by continued, well-controlled methods. At this point, it is worthwhile to refer to the work of Camerini et al. (1973) who used a large dose of PDC in K.K. mice in order to evaluate its preventive as well as therapeutic effects on diabetic angiopathy and/or nephropathy. The result was encouraging although the working mechanism of PDC is not fully understood. Nevertheless, it seems to me that the current lines of study on the pathophysiology of arterial endothelial cells, especially the investigation of actomyosin, will soon become a new and important field in cardiovascular research. In a way, the current status of atherosclerosis research is as specific and extensive as that which we experienced in the past years with topics like "hypertension versus actomyosin of arterial smooth muscle".

Conclusion

The contraction of endothelial cells, which induce the entry of large particles such as ß-lipoprotein (and presumably pre-ß-lipoprotein) into the subendothelial space and, at the same time, the enhancement of thrombogenic activity of the blood, especially of platelets, seems to be the key mechanism in atherogenesis and thrombogenesis. For the prevention and treatment of atherosclerosis, the above-mentioned findings may suggest the importance of two active procedures besides the removal of risk factors. The lowering and normalizing of ß-lipoprotein and pre-ß-lipoprotein of the blood, instead of simple hypocholesterolemic procedures, in cases with elevated ß- and pre-ß-lipoprotein. The inhibition and reduction of the entry of ß-lipoprotein and pre-ß-lipoprotein into the subendothelial space in all atherosclerotic conditions with or without hyperlipoproteinemia by the endothelial cell relaxant, which inhibits at the same time the sticking and aggregating activity of platelets.

II

Lipoproteins and Proteins
of the Arterial Wall

UPTAKE OF INTACT PLASMA LIPOPROTEINS INTO THE ARTERIAL WALL OF THE RABBIT

A.N. Klimov, T.N. Loviagina, A.V. Popov, and E.B. Ban'kovskaya

It appears that accumulation of lipoproteins in the arterial wall should be regarded as a first stage in the development of atherosclerotic injury of vessels. Therefore it is of primary importance to study the mechanism of penetration of plasma lipoproteins into the arterial wall and their destiny therein.

We investigated the uptake of rabbit plasma lipoproteins into the aortic wall in healthy animals and animals with experimental atherosclerosis. For this purpose we used ß- and pre-ß-lipoproteins, radioactively labeling the lipid or protein part of the lipoproteins or both simultaneously (lipoproteins with a double label). The labeled lipoproteins were injected intravenously into animals or employed for perfusion of the isolated rabbit aorta.

Methods

Radioactive lipoproteins were isolated from the serum of rabbits with experimental hypercholesterolemia. The latter was induced by feeding animals cholesterol according to Anichkov. Radioactive precursors of lipoproteins were introduced in the following way: $4-^{14}C$-cholesterol was given either through the feeding tube in alcohol solution in a dose of $1-1.9 \cdot 10^8$ cpm or intravenously by the method of Whereat and Staple (1960) in a dose of $7-16 \cdot 10^8$ cpm 24 h before blood-taking. $Na_2H^{32}PO_4$, ^{35}S-methionine and ^{14}C-hydrolysate of protein were injected intramuscularly in the following doses: $1.7-4.2 \cdot 10^8$, $1.1-2.0 \cdot 10^8$, and $7-15 \cdot 10^9$ cpm 24 h, 3 h and 9 h before blood-taking respectively.

In some experiments the total fraction of radioactive ß- and pre-ß-lipoproteins was separated by heparin precipitation in the presence of calcium ions. In other experiments the same fraction (LDL+VLDL) was isolated by ultracentrifugation. In all the cases isolated lipoproteins were dialysed against physiological saline for two days at $4^{o}C$, while lipoproteins intended for aortic perfusion were subjected to dialysis against the Eagle medium during 12 h. The techniques of lipoprotein isolation from aorta and determination of radioactivity were described previously (Klimov et at., 1972, Popov and Gerchikova, 1973).

Results and Discussion

The data presented in Table 1 show that after intravenous injection of the ß- and pre-ß-lipoprotein fractions, which were radioactively labeled at different sites of the lipoprotein particle, radioactivity was revealed in all cases both in the aorta and in the analogous lipoprotein fraction isolated from the aorta of the recipient rabbits.

Table 2 contains data obtained after the injection of double-labeled lipoproteins. As one can clearly see the ratio between the radioactivity of isotopes in lipoproteins administered to animals and lipoproteins extracted from their aortas remains close. This is an indication that lipoproteins penetrate the aortic wall rather as intact particles.

The results obtained from perfusion of the isolated rabbit aorta with a perfusate containing double-labeled lipoproteins support our conclusion on the whole (Table 3). It is of interest that lipoproteins penetrate the atherosclerotic aorta much more rapidly than the normal one.

Table 1. Penetration of radioactive LDL+VLDL into the arterial wall of rabbits 48 hours after intravenous injection

No	Site of the radioactivity in LDL+VLDL	Dose of radioactivity administered, cpm	Total radioactivity in the aorta, cpm/g of tissue	Radioactivity in LDL+VLDL isolated from the aorta	
				cpm	% of dose administered
1	^{14}C-cholesterol	$1.8 \cdot 10^5$	140	75	0.04
2	^{35}S-protein	$4.4 \cdot 10^5$	329	91	0.02
3	^{32}P-phospholipid	$1.4 \cdot 10^5$	369	222	0.16

If by the end of perfusion the ratio $\dfrac{^{14}C\text{-lipid}}{^{14}C\text{-protein}}$ in the lipoproteins of the perfusate is assumed to be 1.00, it will be 1.02 ± 0.10 in the lipoproteins of the perfused normal aorta and 1.35 ± 0.14 in the lipoproteins of the perfused atherosclerotic aorta (p 0.05). The increased ratio in lipoproteins of the atherosclerotic aorta after perfusion, although not statistically significant, does not rule out the possibility that part of the label may be carried to the aortic lipoproteins from perfusate lipoproteins by exchange, as Dayton and Hashimoto (1970) suggest for non-esterified cholesterol.

Thus, the results of experiments with intravenous injection of radioactive lipoproteins with single or double labels, and experiments with perfusion of the isolated rabbit aorta with a perfusate containing double-labeled lipoproteins show that plasma lipoproteins penetrate the arterial wall on the whole as intact particles. This mechanism probably is the most important in lipid transport from blood plasma into vessel.

Table 2. Penetration of double-labeled lipoproteins of rabbits 48 hours after intravenous injection

No	Fraction of LP	Total radio-activity adminis-tered, cpm	Site of radioactivity	Ratio of radioactivity	Serum Total activ-ity of ß+pre-ß-LP, cpm/ml of serum	Serum Ratio of radioactivity	Aorta Total activity of ß+pre-ß-LP, cpm/g of tissue	Aorta Ratio of radioactivity
1	ß+pre-ß	$19 \cdot 10^5$	^{32}P-PL; ^{35}S-Pr	$\dfrac{^{32}P}{^{35}S} = 1.5$	1042	$\dfrac{^{32}P}{^{35}S} = 1.5$	284	$\dfrac{^{32}P}{^{35}S} = 1.4$
2	"	$8 \cdot 10^5$	"	" 2.3	888	" 2.3	120	" 2.5
3	"	$13 \cdot 10^5$	^{32}P-PL; ^{14}C-Ch	$\dfrac{^{32}P}{^{14}C} = 2.4$	1104	$\dfrac{^{32}P}{^{14}C} = 2.8$	368	$\dfrac{^{32}P}{^{14}C} = 3.3$
4	"	$9 \cdot 10^5$	"	" 2.6	354	" 3.3	148	" 3.3
5	ß	$28 \cdot 10^5$	^{14}C-Ch; ^{14}C-Pr	$\dfrac{^{14}C\text{-}Ch}{^{14}C\text{-}Pr} = 12.0$	8395	$\dfrac{^{14}C\text{-}Ch}{^{14}C\text{-}Pr} = 12.3$	164	$\dfrac{^{14}C\text{-}Ch}{^{14}C\text{-}Pr} = 15.4$
6	"	$17 \cdot 10^5$	"	" 1.4	3025	" 2.3	305	" 1.8

In experiments 1 and 2 the lipoproteins for intravenous injection were isolated by the precipitation method, in experiments 3 to 6 by the ultracentrifugation method.

LP - lipoproteins; PL - phospholipids; Ch - cholesterol; Pr - protein

Table 3. Perfusion of the isolated rabbit aorta by solutions containing lipoproteins labeled in the lipid and protein moieties

No	Aorta	LP used for perfusion	Time of perfusion min	Content of LP, mg%	Perfusate, 20 ml Total radioactivity, cpm	S.A. of LP cpm/mg	$\dfrac{^{14}C\text{-lipid}}{^{14}C\text{-protein}}$	Radioactivity in LDL+VLDL isolated from the aorta Total activity of LP, cpm	LP penetrated into aorta, µg/mg of tissue	$\dfrac{^{14}C\text{-lipid}}{^{14}C\text{-protein}}$
1	Normal	LDL+VLDL	360	2075	8 790 000	21 180	1.53	2090	$32 \cdot 10^{-2}$	1.99
2	Atherosclerotic	"	"	3050	14 873 000	21 200	1.62	4672	$55 \cdot 10^{-2}$	2.25
3	Normal	"	"	835	3 546 000	21 500	1.84	167	$2 \cdot 10^{-2}$	2.34
4	Atherosclerotic	"	"	1825	7 723 000	21 159	1.45	779	$13 \cdot 10^{-2}$	2.57
5	Normal	VLDL	240	536	3 365 680	32 455	2.1	360	$5 \cdot 10^{-2}$	1.7
6	Atherosclerotic	"	"	"	"	"	"	1277	$15 \cdot 10^{-2}$	3.4
7	Normal	"	"	270	1 374 000	25 444	2.2	580	$9 \cdot 10^{-2}$	2.8
8	Atherosclerotic	"	"	"	"	"	"	735	$12 \cdot 10^{-2}$	2.8
9	Normal	LDL	"	405	3 892 260	48 052	2.1	873	$6 \cdot 10^{-2}$	2.1
10	Atherosclerotic	"	"	"	"	"	"	1869	$17 \cdot 10^{-2}$	3.6
11	Normal	"	"	250	2 509 720	41 828	2.8	422	$3 \cdot 10^{-2}$	2.4
12	Atherosclerotic	"	"	"	"	"	"	550	$4 \cdot 10^{-2}$	2.8
13	Normal	"	"	379	2 109 675	27 781	11.9	105	$6 \cdot 10^{-2}$	7.7
14	Atherosclerotic	"	"	"	"	"	"	878	$8 \cdot 10^{-2}$	8.5
15	Normal	"	2	250	2 509 720	41 828	2.8	0	0	–
16	"	"	2	379	2 109 675	27 781	11.9	0	0	–

BETA-LIPOPROTEIN ENTRY INTO THE ARTERIAL WALL AND ITS PREVENTION

Takio Shimamoto and Fujio Numano

The authors (Shimamoto et al., 1972; Shimamoto and Sunaga, 1972a; Shimamoto and Sunaga, 1972b; Shimamoto and Numano, 1972c; Shimamoto, 1972; Shimamoto, 1973) previously found that the acute entry of ß-lipoprotein, fibrinogen and r-globulin is induced into subendothelial and medial layers of the artery directly after a single-dose treatment of rabbits with cholesterol, epinephrine and angiotensin II and it is induced by stimulation of arterial endothelial cells by these challenges. The stimulated endothelial cells show strong contracting and swallowing activities, resulting in entry of relatively large particles with the size up to pre-ß-lipoprotein in the subendothelial space, although it is not yet known what active agent is involved in the effect of cholesterol given orally. In this experiment the authors used rhesus monkeys to see whether such a phenomenon exists in this species.

Materials and Methods

Thirty-three rhesus monkeys weighing 2.1 ± 0.3 kg (1.8 to 2.3 kg) were anesthetized by Sernylan (1.5 mg/kg i.m.), then the oral or intravenous adminis-tration of placebo or test drugs was performed. As a placebo, potato starch was given by gastric tube or saline was given by intravenous injection and as a test drug, angiotensin II (1 µg/kg i.v.), epinephrine (1 µg/kg i.v.), norepinephrine (10 µg/kg i.v.) or cholesterol (1 g/kg p.o.) was given as a single-dose treatment and thereafter, the animals were serially sacrificed at 30 minutes, 1, 2, 4, 6, 12 and 24 hours after the challenge and aortic specimens were sampled and examined for the presence of IgG and ß-lipoprotein by immunofluorescent antibody technique.

The specimens were obtained from thoracic and upper abdominal aortas at the ventral parts remote from orificium of aortic branches. Each of 5 animals also received pretreatment with pyridinolcarbamate (10 mg/kg p.o.) or EG 467 (1 mg/kg p.o.) or Premarin (5 mg/kg i.v.) 2 hours before each challenge, in order to ascertain the preventive effect of these substances against the combined chal-lenge with cholesterol and epinephrine or the angiotensin II challenge. Rabbit immunoglobulin against rhesus monkey serum IgG and ß-lipoprotein and their conjugations with F.I.T.C. (F/P molar ratio; 1.0 and 1.0 resp.) were used. They were produced by Prof. T. Matuhasi using the modified Marshall's method (Kawamura, 1969). The specificity of each antiserum had been confirmed by gel diffusion and by immunoelectrophoresis. The presence of IgG and ß-lipoprotein was observed by immunofluorescence and interference filter techniques (Rygaard and Olsen, 1971).

Results

The fluorescence due to ß-lipoprotein or IgG was green and the aortic tissue including elastic fibres was red, so that the presence of these plasma proteins was clearly identified. In thoracic and abdominal aortas of untreated and placebo control monkeys, a weak immunofluorescence due to ß-lipoprotein was found in highly limited areas of the subendothelial space (Fig. 1), but it was absent in media, while a definite but weak fluorescence due to IgG was found in limited areas of the subendothelial space and often in limited areas of the innermost layers of media.

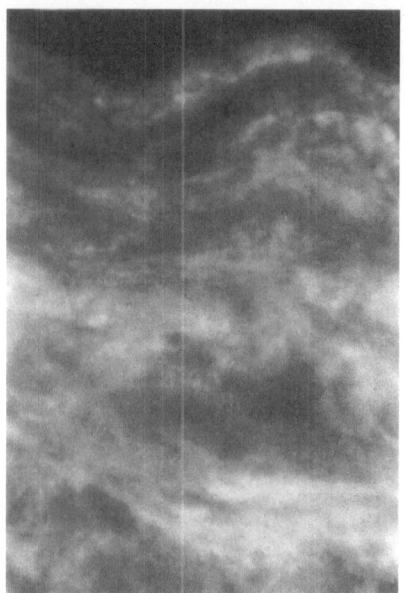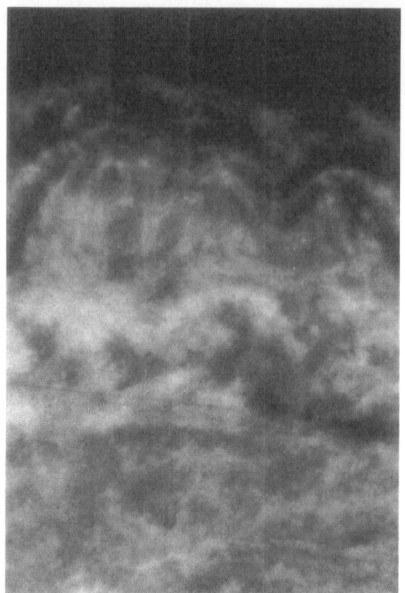

Figure 1. (A) Transection of abdominal aorta of monkey treated by placebo (saline)
and stained by anti-monkey ß-lipoprotein antibody conjugated with F.I.T.C.
Note: Fluorescence due to ß-lipoprotein is absent in the intima and media, except
for adhered blood
(B) Transection of abdominal aorta of untreated monkey and stained by anti-monkey
ß-lipoprotein antibody conjugated with F.I.T.C.
Note: Some spotty fluorescence due to ß-lipoprotein is seen in the subendothelial
space but not in the medial layers

In animals challenged with cholesterol (1 g/kg p.o.) or epinephrine (1 g/kg i.v.)
or norepinephrine (10 g/kg i.v.) or angiotensin II (1 g/kg i.v.), a definite
and strong fluorescence showing the acute entry of ß-lipoprotein and IgG from the
vessel lumen into the subendothelial space and then into the medial layers of the
arterial wall was clearly shown by serial sacrificing of animals after each
challenge (Fig. 2, Fig. 3). The fluoresence was strong in the innermost layers,
but in the course of 5 to 6 hours after the cholesterol challenge or 2 to 3 hours
after the epinephrine, norepinephrine or angiotensin II challenge, a definite but
spotty fluorescence due to both proteins was also found in the middle of the
media and sometimes even in the outer part of the media. The passage of ß-
lipoprotein through the internal elastic lamina into the medial layer was
characteristically delayed approximately 30 minutes to one hour as compared with
that of IgG. Fluorescence due to the infiltration of IgG and ß-lipoprotein had
disappeared almost completely in animals sacrificed at 7 to 12 hours after each
challenge. In animals pretreated with pyridinolcarbamate (10 mg/kg p.o.) or EG 467
(1 mg/kg p.o.) or Premarin (5 mg/kg i.v.), the acute entry of these plasma
proteins was statistically significantly inhibited.

Discussion

The acute entry of ß-lipoprotein and presumably pre-ß-lipoprotein into the subendothelial space was induced by a relatively small dose of physiological substances and it may be a trigger mechanism in atherogenesis, because ß-lipoprotein
tends to stagnate in the subendothelial space dammed by the internal elastic
lamina. Another experiment of the authors even showed that the passage through
the lamina is impossible for particles with the size of pre-ß-lipoprotein. The
preventive effect of pyridinolcarbamate, Premarin, and EG 467 is considered to be
the essential mechanism involved in their antiatherosclerotic effect.

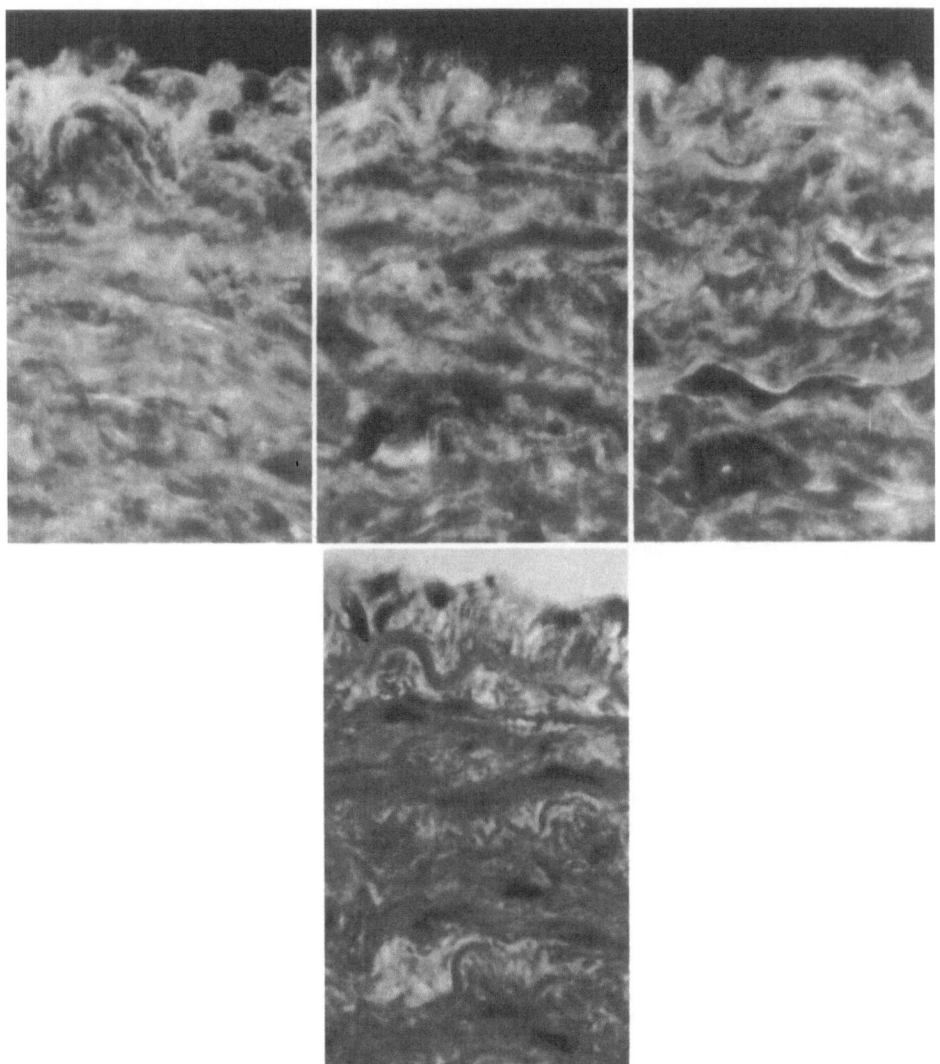

Figure 2. Transection of abdominal aorta of the monkey sacrificed at 3 hours (A),
6 hours (B) and 12 hours (C) respectively after cholesterol challenge (1 g/kg p.
o.) and stained by anti-monkey ß-lipoprotein antibody conjugated with F.I.T.C.
Note: (A) Fluorescence due to ß-lipoprotein is seen in the subendothelial space
but is barely discernible in the limited areas of the innermost medial layers.
(B) Fluorescence due to ß-lipoprotein is seen in the subendothelial and medial
layers. The fluorescence was often kept inside the elastic laminae of medial
layers showing the relative barrier function of elastic laminae.
(C) Some spotty fluorescence due to ß-lipoprotein remains in the subendothelial
space.
(D) The same specimen of (B) was stained by hematoxylin-eosin and photographed by
ordinary methods.
Note: The areas with the positive fluorescence due to ß-lipoprotein in (B) fit
exactly to the areas with a definite extracellular edema showing the presence of
the plasma protein in the edematous parts

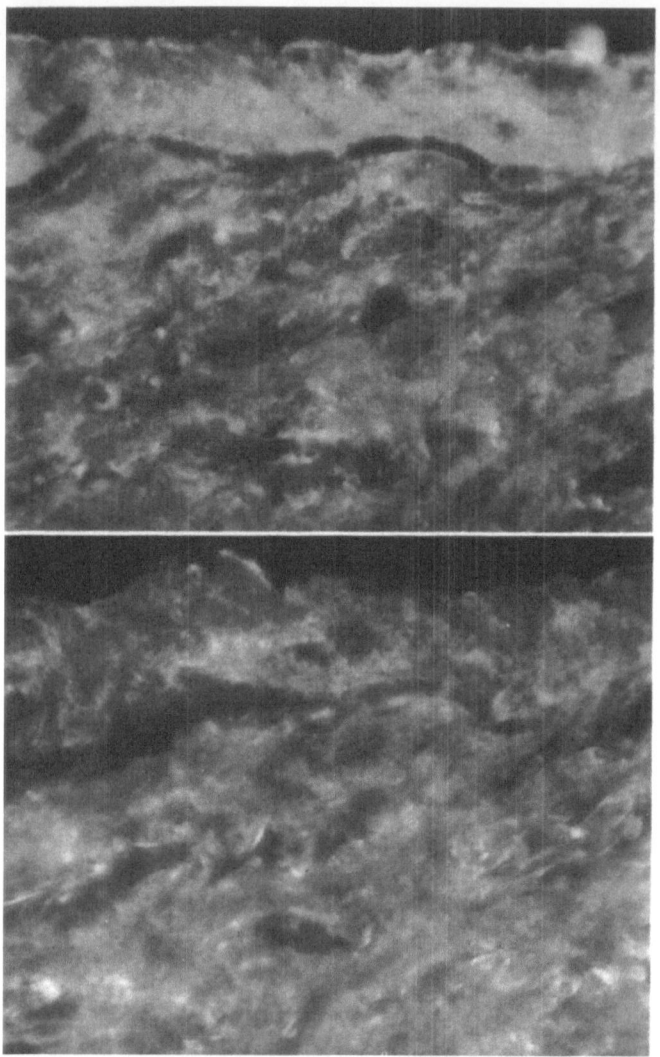

Figure 3. Transection of abdominal aorta of the same monkey sampled 30 minutes
after epinephrine challenge (1 μg/kg i.v.).
(A) Stained by anti-monkey IgG antibody conjugated with F.I.T.C.
Note: Fluorescence due to IgG is present not only in the subendothelial space,
but also in the innermost layers of the media beyond the internal elastic lamina.
(B) The next specimen of the specimen (a) transected serially and stained by anti-
monkey ß-lipoprotein antibody conjugated with F.I.T.C.
Note: Fluorescence due to ß-lipoprotein is seen in the subendothelial space clearly limited by internal elastic lamina, but not seen beyond internal elastic
lamina in the media

Summary

A single-dose treatment of a rhesus monkey with cholesterol (1 k/kg p.o.),
epinephrine (1 μg/kg i.v.), norepinephrine (10 μg/kg i.v.) and angiotensin II
(1 μg/kg i.v.) has been shown to induce an acute infiltration of ß-lipoprotein
and IgG first into the subendothelial space of the aorta and then into internal
parts of its medial layers. ß-lipoprotein is characteristically delayed in its
passage through internal elastic lamina as compared with IgG. The acute entry of
ß-lipoprotein and IgG was inhibited by pretreatment of animals with Premarin
(5 mg/kg i.v.), and cyclic AMP phosphodiesterase-inhibiting substances such as
pyridinolcarbamate (10 mg/kg p.o.) and EG 467 (1 mg/kg p.o.).

IDENTIFICATION OF LIPOPROTEINS INVOLVED IN HUMAN ATHEROSCLEROSIS

Kenneth W. Walton

It has been shown previously, using immunofluorescence, that a close topographic relationship is demonstrable between the extracellular lipid revealed by conventional lipid 'stains' (such as oil red O) and that of specific fluorescence due to LDL or VLDL at all stages of the development of atherosclerotic arterial lesions. But no similar relationship could be shown for HDL (Walton and Williamson, 1968). In this previous work: a) comparisons were made by photographing corresponding fields of consecutive sections of the same material; and b) the antisera used were raised to intact native lipoproteins derived from pooled plasma.

It is now reported that even more precise results can be obtained by applying immunofluorescence and conventional lipid 'staining' sequentially to the *same* section. The technique used has been previously detailed (Walton et al., 1970). Experiments have also been carried out employing antisera directed against other (minor) antigenic components of lipoproteins.

1. Genetic Markers in Lipoproteins

Berg (1963) showed that some rabbit antisera, raised to crude LDL fractions from *individual* human donors and cross-absorbed, contained residual antibodies reacting with the sera of some individuals and not others. The antigen thus detected was called the Lp(a) lipoprotein. Population and family studies (Berg, 1966) suggested that Lp(a) reactivity is genetically determined (*i.e.*, is an allotypic characteristic) and is present in about 20 per cent of random Caucasian populations as determined by gel-diffusion.

Antisera detecting Lp(a)[+] reactors have been raised in the rabbit and sheep. Using more sensitive immunological methods, in our hands a much higher proportion of a British population shows some degree of Lp(a)[+] reactivity but the sera from other individuals, even after concentration, do not react (Walton et al., 1973a). These antisera have been used to type, retrospectively, the blood of subjects coming to autopsy. Examination of arterial lesions from the same subjects has been carried out using fluorescein-labelled anti-Lp(a).

It has been found that, in the lesions of Lp(a)[+] subjects, not only is there precise correspondence between material reacting with oil red O and with anti-LDL (Fig. 1) but that a similar distribution is given with the labelled antiserum to Lp(a) (Fig.2). On the other hand, in the arterial lesions of Lp(a)-negative subjects while specific fluorescence is obtained with anti-LDL, no material reacting with anti-Lp(a) is detectable.

The significance of this observation is that, in appropriate subjects, it is possible not merely to demonstrate that a low-density lipoprotein is present, but that a molecule with a genetic marker peculiar to a given individual occurs, in his atherosclerotic lesions.

2. Possible Role of VLDL in Atherogenesis

When antisera are raised to intact LDL and VLDL respectively, the antisera do not distinguish between these lipoprotein classes (Walton and Darke, 1964)

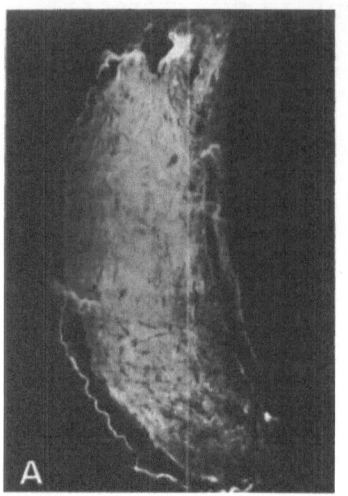
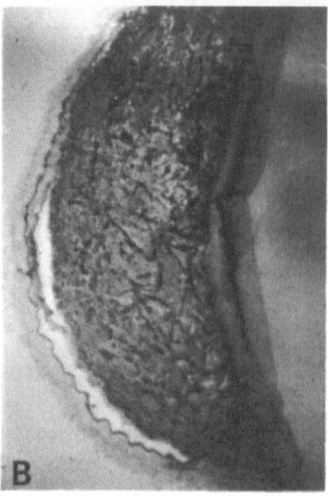

Figure 1. Frozen section of plaque in cerebral artery from Lp(a)[+] subject:
(A) treated with fluorescein-labelled anti-LDL; (B) 'stained' with oil red O,
light green and haematoxylin. Note close correspondence in distribution of
specific fluorescence in A (white in picture, bright green in original) with
that of lipid in B (dark grey in picture, bright red in original)

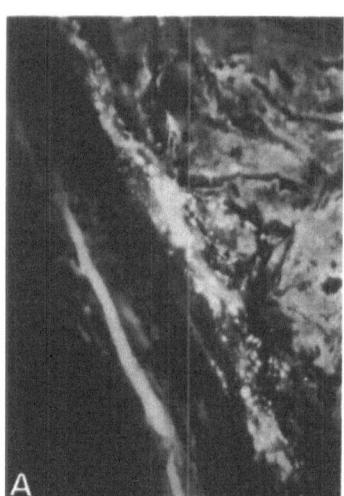
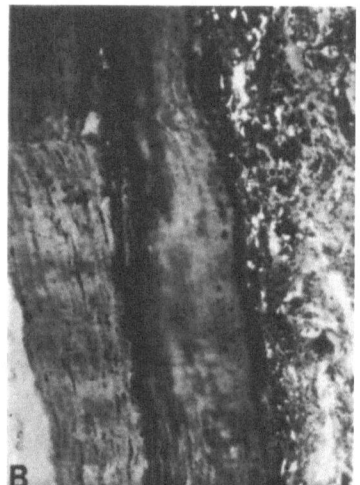

Figure 2. Higher magnification of portion of same material as shown in Fig. 1.
(A) treated with labelled anti-Lp(a); (B) stained for lipid and examined in
polarized light. Note similar correspondence between specific fluorescence in
A and that of extracellular lipid 'staining' with oil red O in B. But note black
streaks (negative reaction) in A corresponding to position of cholesterol crystals
in B

being directed against the protein part of the molecule which is common to both
LDL and VLDL (apolipoprotein B). But when antisera are prepared to delipidated
VLDL, antibodies can be obtained to an additional component (apolipoprotein C)
not present in LDL (see Alaupovic, 1971). Using an antiserum kindly provided by
Professor Alaupovic, in our hands apolipoprotein C has been found to be present
in both 'intermediate' (S_f10-20) lipoproteins and in VLDL (S_f20-400) lipoproteins.
The demonstration by immunofluorescence of apolipoprotein C in the atherosclerotic
lesion of both hyperlipidaemic (Fig. 3) and normolipidaemic individuals therefore

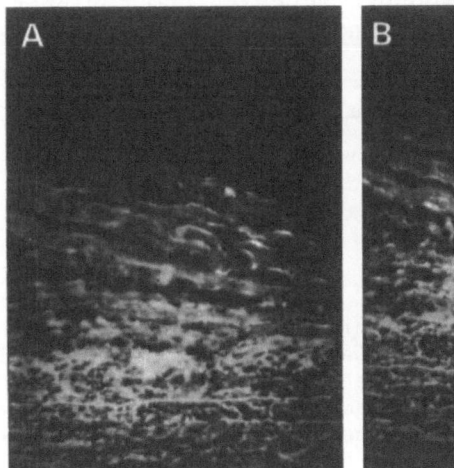

Figure 3. Consecutive frozen sections of fibro-fatty aortic plaque: (A) treated
with fluorescein-labelled anti-apolipoprotein B; (B) treated with fluorescein-
labelled anti-apolipoprotein C. Note similarity of distribution of specific
fluorescence in intima

does not define precisely the upper limit of molecular size of lipoproteins
exhibiting atherogenic potential. However, it does suggest that lipoproteins
of even larger molecular size than LDL are involved in the process (see below).

Conclusions

The sequential application of immunofluorescence and of conventional lipid
'stains' to the *same* section provides even more precise correlation between these
two techniques. It has been pointed out previously (Walton et al., 1970; 1973b)
that antibodies to lipoproteins are directed mainly or exclusively against the
protein portion of the molecule, while dyes such as oil red O are selectively
soluble in the lipid moiety but are unreactive with the protein portion. The
identity of distribution found by the two techniques thus makes it reasonable to
infer that material thus reacting is in the form of intact lipoprotein.

The work of Ehnholm et al. (1971; 1972) suggests that, immunologically, the
protein moiety of Lp(a) lipoprotein consists essentially of the apolipoprotein B
of LDL to which is attached an additional peptide (apolipoprotein Lp(a)). The
close similarity of distribution found in Lp(a)-positive subjects using antisera
directed against these two different apolipoproteins is thus consistent with the
presence of intact Lp(a) lipoprotein in their lesions. By the same token, since
the distribution found in a given lesion for apolipoproteins B and C is again
similar, this suggests that both apolipoproteins are very closely associated, as
they would be expected to be in intact 'intermediate' lipoproteins and in VLDL.

QUANTITATIVE INTERRELATIONSHIPS BETWEEN PLASMA CONSTITUENTS AND NORMAL AND ATHEROSCLEROTIC HUMAN INTIMAL TISSUE

Elspeth B. Smith, Rosalind S. Slater, and D.C. Crothers

Introduction

Most of the cholesterol which accumulates in arterial intima appears to be derived from plasma (reviewed by Dayton and Hashimoto, 1970; Portman, 1970). The cholesterol esters which accumulate in extracellular locations also appear to be derived directly from plasma, but those which accumulate inside fat-filled cells are probably formed by esterification *in situ* (Smith et al., 1967; Smith and Slater, 1972a). Using the technique of immunofluorescent microscopy numerous investigators have demonstrated LD-lipoprotein in normal intima (with the exception of the youngest age groups, Kao and Wissler, 1965) and in lesions of all types (reviewed by Smith and Slater, 1970). There is less agreement on the presence of other plasma constituents, but albumin, HDL and fibrinogen or fibrin have also been demonstrated (Haust et al., 1965; Wyllie et al., 1964; Haust, 1968). It seems probable that all plasma proteins are present in the intima with the possible exception of intact VLDL.

Smith and Slater (1971, 1972b) developed a method for the quantitative assay of LD-lipoprotein in small samples of intima by electrophoresis directly from the minced tissue into an antibody-containing gel. Surprisingly large amounts of LD-lipoprotein have been found; in 'normal' intima from the fourth decade upwards the concentration per unit volume of intima is approximately the same as the plasma concentration and is highly correlated with it. In the 'gelatinous' lesions (reviewed by Haust, 1971 and Geer and Haust, 1972) which we believe are the precursors of fibrous lesions (Smith and Slater, 1973a) the overall concentration is increased up to fourfold compared with normal intima, with very much greater increases in the deep layers of the lesion (Smith and Slater, 1973a,b). The method can be adapted for measurement of other plasma antigens including albumin (Smith and Slater, 1972b), fibrinogen and fibrinogen/fibrin-reactive antigens (FRA) (Smith et al., 1973) and HDL. In the study reported here we have attempted to obtain information on factors such as permeability or specific binding which may influence intimal lipoprotein concentration by comparing the relative concentrations of LD-lipoprotein, albumin and FRA in normal intima and lesions.

Results

Plasma Antigens in Normal Intima. In 24 subjects aged 35-69, with no history of hypertension, from whom blood samples were obtained during the week before death a very high correlation ($r = 0.971$; $p \ll 0.001$) has been found between the concentration of LD-lipoprotein in normal intima and the serum cholesterol level (Smith and Slater 1972b, 1973a). In the assay by electrophoresis in an antibody-containing gel the samples of intima are run on the same plate as a standard LD lipoprotein preparation and 10 μl of the patient's own serum or plasma. This means that the intimal lipoprotein can be expressed as absolute amount, and also in terms of the volume of the patients plasma from which it has been derived. On this basis the correlation with serum cholesterol level is much lower, suggesting the concept that a relatively constant volume of 'plasma' may enter the intima; if the plasma LD-lipoprotein is high this volume of plasma will carry a large amount of LD-lipoprotein into the intima, but if the LD-lipoprotein is low the amount carried into the intima will be small. In 6 known hypertensives the 'volume of plasma' in the intima was significantly higher than in normotensive subjects ($p < 0.001$).

Using the same technique albumin and fibrinogen/fibrin reactive antigens (FRA) have also been measured. In normal intima, the ratio LD-lipoprotein/albumin in terms of volumes of the patients plasma is approximately 7, and the ratio LD-lipoprotein/FRA is approximately 3 (Smith et al., 1973). Thus, surprisingly, the largest molecule is present in relatively the largest amount and the smallest molecule is present in the smallest amount. The actual concentrations of LD-lipoprotein and albumin in normal intima are approximately equal although in plasma there is 7-10 times more albumin than lipoprotein. These findings are compatible with the idea that 'whole plasma' enters the intima, and the relative amount of any constituent found depends on its relative rate of egress.

Changes in LD-lipoprotein, FRA and Albumin Concentrations in Early Lesions. Because of the very high correlation between the concentration of the antigen in the intima, and blood pressure and plasma concentration, the absolute amount found in early lesions may be misleading, therefore in Table 1 the concentration is expressed as a percentage of the concentration in normal intima from the same aorta. In typical fatty streaks containing numerous fat-filled cells all three plasma components are *reduced;* for LD-lipoprotein and FRA the reduction is highly significant (p = or <0.001) but for albumin the reduction is probably not significantly greater than the reduction in FRA or albumin (p <0.001 for both). By contrast, in gelatinous thickenings and the gelatinous peripheries of plaques, all components show significant *increases* (p = or <0.01). LD-lipoprotein and FRA increase in parallel, and in the peripheries of the plaques their increase is significantly greater than the increase in albumin.

Table 1. Changes in plasma constituents in early lesions; the concentrations are expressed as percentage of the level in normal intima from the same aorta

	Number of pairs	Percentage of level in normal intima		
		LD-lipoprotein	FRA	Albumin
Fatty streaks	11	23%	62%	69%[a]
		←------p = 0.001----→		
		←------------p = 0.001-------→		
Gelatinous thickenings	16	225%	255%	177%
		←------N.S.------------N.S.---		
Gelatinous peripheries of plaques	16	360%	425%	220%
		←------N.S.----------→		
		←------------P = 0.015------→		

[a]Not significantly different from normal (p = 0.05); all other values are significantly different from normal (p = 0.01 or less).

The Relationship Between the Plasma Constituents in Different Layers of Lesions. In normal intima dissected into two layers the concentration of lipoprotein in the lower layer is only 16% of the concentration in the upper layer (Smith and Slater, 1973a), but in gelatinous lesions and early fibrous plaques there is a great increase in the proportion of LD-lipoprotein in the lower layers (Table 2). The ratio LD-lipoprotein/FRA shows no significant change either between the upper and lower layers, or between normal intima and lesions. This seems to suggest that LD-lipoprotein and fibrinogen enter the intima together, and their relative retention is unchanged in the gelatinous lesions. By contrast, there is a highly significant increase in the ratio LD-lipoprotein/albumin in the lower layers (Table 2) and this is even more marked in larger lesions dissected into three layers (Table 3).

Table 2. The ratios of LD-lipoprotein to FRA and albumin, expressed as equivalent volumes of the patients plasma, in the upper and lower layers of normal intima and early lesions

| | No. | Concentration of LP in lower as % of upper | RATIOS | | | |
| | | | $\frac{\text{LD-lipoprotein}}{\text{FRA}}$ | | $\frac{\text{LD-lipoprotein}}{\text{albumin}}$ | |
			Upper	Lower	Upper	Lower
Normal	9	14.5%	2.5+0.3[a]	3.9+1.4	7.4+0.7	4.3+0.5
Gelatinous thickenings	6	37.7%	2.0+0.8	3.1+1.6	10.8+2.7	8.4+2.5
Gelatinous peripheries of plaques	6	64.6%	2.5+0.7	3.6+1.8	10.4+4.0	18.5+9.8
"White" fibrous plaques	6	142.0%	1.7+0.7	1.6+0.8	9.0+1.8	16.9+6.3

[a] S.E.M.

Table 3. The ratios of LD-lipoprotein to FRA and albumin, expressed as equivalent volumes of the patients plasma, in 9 large plaques dissected into three layers

| | Relative concentration of lipoprotein | RATIOS | |
		$\frac{\text{LD-lipoprotein}}{\text{FRA}}$	$\frac{\text{LD-lipoprotein}}{\text{albumin}}$
Upper cap	1.0	3.2 ± 0.6	10.5 ± 0.7
Lower cap and cap/lipid junction	2.1	3.8 ± 1.2	21.0 ± 5.5
Deep layers	1.6	3.9 ± 0.4	19.2 ± 5.5

α-Lipoproteins (HDL) in Intima. Between 10% and 30% of the plasma cholesterol is carried by the α-lipoproteins (HDL 2 and 3) which could theoretically contribute to cholesterol accumulation in the intima. In preliminary experiments with the immunoelectrophoresis system whole plasma and an ultracentrifuge fraction of plasma isolated between densities 1.063 and 1.21 both gave compact peaks which stained very faintly for lipid (oil red O) and strongly for protein (amido-black). An S_f0-20 lipoprotein fraction gave no reaction, and an S_f>20 fraction gave an irregular band, not a peak, which stained strongly for lipid but gave no detectable staining for protein; this probably represents large molecules from the lightest part of the fraction which were retarded in the 1% agarose gel. Four samples of intima gave large peaks which stained very faintly for lipid and strongly for protein; the ratio LD-lipoprotein/α-lipoprotein in terms of volumes of plasma was about 5, thus the relative retention of α-lipoprotein is slightly greater than albumin. This means that it will only contribute about 5% of the lipoprotein-bound cholesterol in the intima.

Summary and Conclusions

In capillary transudates the relative concentrations of the plasma proteins are inversely proportional to their molecular weights so that the proportion of albumin is larger and of α_2 globulin and LD-lipoprotein much smaller than in plasma. In the adult human aortic intima the reverse is found; relative to plasma, LD-lipoprotein is the largest component and albumin the smallest. This suggests the concept that 'whole plasma' enters the intima and the small molecules then pass through into the media or back into the intima at a faster rate than the large molecules; LD-lipoprotein might be subject to nonspecific retardation or specific binding to glycosaminoglycans. Recent studies support the idea that large molecules cross intact aortic endothelium in pinocytotic vesicles (Schwartz and Benditt, 1972; Stein and Stein, 1973) and the latter authors showed that apo-HDL passed rapidly into the media. However, there seems to be no information on the condition of the endothelium in the middle-aged human; it is possible that it is not intact and that 'whole plasma' can leak into the sub-endothelial tissue through defects.

If the concentration of LD-lipoprotein in a lesion differs from the concentration in normal intima this could be the result of change in permeability, change in retardation or specific reversible binding, or change in destruction or irreversible binding. In fatty streaks containing numerous fat-filled cells LD-lipoprotein is reduced to a quarter of the level in normal intima, and the reduction is significantly greater than the reduction in fibrinogen or albumin, suggesting specific destruction of the lipoprotein by the fat-filled cells. The moderately reduced levels of fibrinogen and albumin are surprising; it is difficult to believe that intimal permeability is *decreased* in fatty streaks.

In the gelatinous lesions all components increase, suggesting a general increase in permeability. There is a significantly greater increase in LD-lipoprotein than in albumin, particularly in the deep layers of the lesions. However, the relationship between fibrinogen and LD-lipoprotein remains constant, so if it is postulated that there is an increase in specific binding of lipoprotein there must be an equal increase in the binding of fibrinogen.

Acknowledgments

This work has been supported by grants from the British Heart Foundation and the Medical Research Council. We wish to thank A. Singer for technical assistance and the Department of Pathology, University of Aberdeen, for help in obtaining autopsy material.

III
Lipids of the Arterial Wall

LIPID METABOLIC POOL IN SUBCELLULAR FRACTIONS OF RABBIT AND HUMAN ATHEROSCLEROTIC LESIONS[*]

A.J. Day, A.K. Horsch, and J.W. Proudlock

The intracellular accumulation of lipids is an early feature of atherogenesis and the active involvement of the arterial wall in this process is well established (Day and Wahlqvist, 1968, Wahlqvist et al. 1969). The intracellular lipid is present as lipid droplets, which differ in composition from the extracellular lipid (Smith et al., 1967). Two types of lipid droplets have been demonstrated in human atherosclerotic lesions, one isotropic, the other anisotropic (Lang and Insull, 1970). On the basis of electronmicroscopic studies it has been suggested, that the anisotropic droplets are formed from the cell membrane and are subsequently transformed into isotropic droplets and that these changes are associated with the esterification of free cholesterol (Weller et al., 1968).

In order to obtain further information regarding the metabolic activity of morphologically different fractions from the atherosclerotic intima, studies were carried out using I^{14}-C-labelled oleic acid and the incorporation of this precursor into lipids of different subcellular fractions in the arterial wall was investigated for both rabbit aortic intima and for human femoral artery intima.

Atherosclerotic aortas were obtained from male New Zealand white rabbits fed daily 1 g cholesterol and 3 ml peanut oil in 100 g rabbit chow for 19 - 22 weeks. Human femoral arteries were obtained post mortem from patients aged 23 - 82 years.

The procedure was essentially the same for all arteries: Following removal the artery was dissected free of adventitial connective tissue and a segment incubated in vitro for 4 hrs at $37^{\circ}C$ in an incubation medium containing equal volumes of serum (rabbit or human respectively) and TCM 199 or Hanks solution to which was added a known amount of I^{14}-C-oleic acid. For human arteries incubation was commenced within 1 hr of clinical death. At the end of the incubation period, the artery segment was removed, thoroughly washed in 0.9% sodium chloride solution and the intima stripped at the cleavage plane formed by the internal elastic lamina. Media and adventitia were discarded. The intima was homogenized and spun for 5 min at 1 000 g to remove cellular debris. This low speed supernatant was then recentrifuged at 1 00 000 g for 1 hr and three fractions separated: a floating lipid skin, a clear supernatant and a particulate fraction. These were individually extracted with chloroform-methanol (2 : 1, v/v) and the resulting extracts washed by the method of Folch (1957). Aliquots from all fractions were separated by thin layer chromatography and gas liquid chromatography and assayed for radioactivity. Quantitative recovery of label was obtained. Detailed descriptions of the procedures involved have been published elsewhere (Proudlock et al., 1973).[**]

Table 1 gives the percentage distribution of cholesterol ester, free cholesterol and phospholipid between the three subcellular fractions for the rabbit. Most of the cholesterol ester is present in the lipid skin fraction whereas the free cholesterol and phospholipid are mainly associated with the particulate fraction.

---

[*]These studies were in part supported by the Deutsche Forschungsgemeinschaft within the SFB 90 Cardiovasculäres System.

[**]Details of the rabbit aorta studies will be reported more fully elsewhere (Proudlock et al., Exp. Molec. Pathol., 19, 389-401 (1973)).

Table 1. Percentage distribution of lipid in subcellular fractions of atheromatous thoracic intimas of cholesterol fed rabbits[a]

	Cholesterol ester	Free cholesterol	Phospholipid
P 104	25.8 ± 1.5	50.4 ± 5.3	73.3 ± 2.6
SN	15.7 ± 5.8	34.3 ± 4.7	21.2 ± 2.4
L.S.	58.5 ± 9.5	15.3 ± 3.4	5.5 ± 1.3
Total amount present	137. ± 62.	73. ± 23.	75. ± 28.
(μg / mg dry wgt.)			

[a]Mean of 4 rabbits with S.E.M.
P 104   -   104 000 g deposit,
SN   -   104 000 g supernatent,
LS   -   lipid skin.

The fatty acid composition of the cholesterol esters of the various subcellular fractions for the rabbit thoracic intima is given in the Table 2. The fatty acid composition of the serum cholesterol ester from similar cholesterol fed rabbits is also given and it will be noted that the serum cholesterol ester is almost identical to that in the aortic supernatant fraction.

The lipid skin fraction shows a significantly higher cholesterol oleate content ($p < 0.02$) and a significantly lower cholesterol linoleate content ($p < 0.01$) than either the serum or supernatant fraction. The particulate fraction shows an enrichment in cholesterol oleate and a depletion in cholesterol linoleate compared to the supernatant.

Table 2. Percentage distribution of cholesterol ester fatty acids in subcellular fractions of atheromatous thoracic intimas of cholesterol fed rabbits[a]

	16:0	16:1	18:1	18:2[c]
P 104	12.2 ± 0.29	4.8 ± 0.54	57.6 ± 0.90	19.2 ± 0.74
SN	13.4 ± 0.75	5.5 ± 0.72	51.6 ± 1.00	23.2 ± 0.80
L.S.	12.3 ± 0.81	4.1 ± 0.37	61.4 ± 0.52	16.2 ± 0.65
Serum[b]	13.9 ± 0.5	6.7 ± 0.5	51.3 ± 1.1	21.0 ± 0.9

[a]Mean of 4 rabbits with S.E.M.   [b]Mean of 13 rabbits with S.E.M.   [c]$p < 0.01$.

The fatty acid composition of the phospholipid fatty acids shows no significant differences between the three subcellular fractions but each differs from the serum phospholipid fatty acid pattern.

The incorporation of I [14]-C-oleic acid into phospholipid and cholesterol ester by the rabbit aortic intima is shown in Table 3 together with the percentage distribution of the label between the different subcellular fractions. The cpm incorporated into phospholipid and cholesterol ester are similar.Most of the label incorporated into phospholipid, however, is associated with the particulate fraction,while that incorporated into cholesterol ester is largely in the lipid skin. Further series of incubations were carried out for various time intervals (5 min - 4 hrs) in order to determine whether redistribution of labelled oleic acid occurred during the incubation period. Distribution of the labelled fatty acid was similar at all incubation times.

Table 3. Percentage distribution of ^{14}C-oleic acid in subcellular fractions of atheromatous thoracic intimas of cholesterol fed rabbits[a]

	Cholesterol ester	Phospholipid
P 104	28.5 + 7.4	76.0 + 3.0
SN	1.2 + 0.26	10.9 + 0.5
L.S.	70.3 + 7.6	13.1 + 2.9
Total cpm (x 10^{-3})	66.9 + 2.1	65.6 + 11.8

[a]Mean of 4 rabbits with S.E.M.
P 104 - 104 000 g deposit,   SN - 104 000 g supernatent, L.S. - lipid skin.

The distribution of the labeled phospholipid,triglyceride and cholesterol ester between the three subcellular fractions for the human femoral artery is given in Table 4. In the normal intima, little incorporation of I^{14}-C-oleic acid into cholesterol ester occurred; in the atherosclerotic intima considerably more uptake and incorporation of I^{14}-C-labelled oleic acid into cholesterol ester took place.

Table 4. Percentage distribution of labelled phospholipid, triglyceride and cholesterol ester between subcellular fractions of human femoral arterial intimas

	Normal intima[a]		
	Phospholipid	Triglyceride	Cholesterol ester
P 100	78.8 + 18.8	63.4 + 8.2	58.6 + 2.5
SN	20.8 + 19.1	9.8 + 5.7	21.0 + 12.7
L.S.	0.4 + 0.64	26.6 + 6.1	20.4 + 11.9
	Atherosclerotic intima[b]		
	Phospholipid	Triglyceride	Cholesterol ester
P 100	77.0 + 14.4	36.5 + 15.3	37.9 + 20.0
SN	18.2 + 10.6	10.9 + 4.5	10.4 + 6.7
L.S.	4.7 + 6.4	52.6 + 18.3	51.7 + 20.2

[a]Mean of 3 human arteries with S.E.M.   [b]Mean of 11 human arteries with S.E.M.
P 100 - 100 000 g deposit,   SN - 100 000 g supernatent, L.S. - lipid skin.

In the normal artery more than 50% of the oleic acid incorporated into cholesterol ester is associated with the particular fraction with a relatively low proportion associated with the lipid skin. In contrast the cholesterol ester labelled in the atherosclerotic intima is found predominantly in the lipid skin fraction.

The distribution of triglyceride between the subcellular fractions follows closely that of the cholesterol ester. The labelled phospholipid on the other hand in both normal and atherosclerotic vessels is primarily in the particulate fraction. These findings suggest the separation of phospholipid and cholesterol ester synthesis into separate metabolic pools in the atherosclerotic lesions.

GLUCOSE AND LIPID METABOLISM IN THE HUMAN ARTERIOSCLEROTIC AORTA

I. Filipovic, K. von Figura, and E. Buddecke

The chemical composition and the origin of human arteriosclerotic lesions have been extensively studied, but information on the metabolism of human arterial tissue and its changes in arteriosclerosis is limited. Though the ability of mammalian arterial tissue to synthesize fatty acids has been the subject of several reports (Whereat et al., 1967; Howard Jr., 1968; Filipovic and Buddecke, 1971; Filipovic et al., 1973), the lipid accumulation in human arteriosclerosis is thought to be the result of infiltration of plasma lipids into the arterial wall. In this study it will be shown that ^{14}C-fatty acid and triglyceride synthesis, respectively, in arteriosclerotic parts is much greater than that in nonarteriosclerotic parts of the same aorta.

Results

^{14}C-glucose uptake and ^{14}C-lactate formation in nonarteriosclerotic and arteriosclerotic parts of the same aorta shows a linear rate over a period of 6 h, thus indicating the adaption of the human aorta to a steady state of in vitro metabolism. Measurements of metabolic events in glucose at the end of the incubation period (Table 1) revealed that about 60% of the glucose present in the incubation medium was utilized, but that nearly 90% of this was converted to ^{14}C-lactate. The incorporation of ^{14}C-radioactivity into CO_2 and lipids and glucosaminoglycans (Table 1) reflects oxidative and biosynthetic processes under in vitro conditions.

Table 1. [U-^{14}C] glucose uptake, lactate formation and percentage of total radioactivity incorporated into the metabolites and products of synthesis. 60% of the added [U-^{14}C] glucose were utilized during an incubation period of 6 h

		Glucose uptake	Lactate formation	cpm/µmol Lactate	Percent of total radioactivity incorporated into			
		umol/g wet weight			Lactate	CO_2	Lipids	GAG
[U-^{14}C] Glucose [a]	non arteriosclerotic tissue	7.4	26.3	10900	89.6	0.69	0.64	0.38
	arteriosclerotic tissue	7.5	33.3	8600	91.3	0.31	0.56	0.32

[a]Specific radioactivity 68100/µmol.

In order to obtain more information about lipid synthesis and its changes in arteriosclerosis, the arterial lipids were labelled with ^{14}C-acetate, its radioactivity being nearly quantitatively incorporated into the fatty acid moiety of arterial lipids. Table 2 summarizes the results of ^{14}C-acetate experiments. As is known and to be expected, the total lipid content of arteriosclerotic parts of arterial tissue is two to three times higher than that of nonarteriosclerotic areas, consequently the specific radioactivity of total lipids is lower in arteriosclerosis. However, when the total radioactivity incorporated into lipids is calculated per gram wet weight of tissue or per μmol DNA (Table 2), a higher rate of fatty acid synthesis in arteriosclerotic parts of the arterial wall is evident. Moreover, fractionation of total lipids into their subfractions revealed a higher specific radioactivity of the triglyceride fraction in arteriosclerosis, thus indicating that the increased fatty acid synthesis refers mainly to the triglyceride fatty acids.

Table 2. Total lipids, lipid subfractions and their radioactivities isolated from nonarteriosclerotic and arteriosclerotic parts of human aortae after in vitro incubation in the presence of $[1-^{14}C]$ acetate (means of 3 incubation experiments). Labelling of lipids by ^{14}C-glucose revealed 6400 cpm (nonarteriosclerotic) and 4000 cpm/mg total lipids (arteriosclerotic), the bulk of the ^{14}C-radioactivity being incorporated into the glycerol moiety

| Part of aorta | mg total Lipids/ g wet weight | Specific radioact. (cpm) | | | | Radioact. (cpm)incorp. into total Lipids/ | |
		Total Lipids	Tri- glyc.	Phospho Lipids	Total Cholest.	g wetweight	μMol DNA
Nonarterio- sclerotic	14,2	2000	1900	4700	800	28400	389000
Arterio- sclerotic	34,4	1200	2300	4300	280	41500	629000

A more detailed analysis of the radioactivity of the fatty acids revealed a remarkable difference in the radioactivity distribution within the palmitic and palmitoleic acid fraction (Table 3). Both fatty acids account for 20 - 30% of the total fatty acids. After decarboxylation and determination of that proportion of radioactivity which is present in the carboxyl group, the bulk of the radioactivity was found in the carboxyl group in arteriosclerosis, while in the nonarteriosclerotic parts only 65% of fatty acid radioactivity was present in the carboxyl carbon. The ratio of the radioactivity present in the carboxyl group and the acyl residue is highly consistent with the concept that chain elongation of preformed fatty acids is the predominant mechanism of fatty acid synthesis in arteriosclerosis, while in nonarteriosclerotic parts of arterial tissue at least part of the fatty acids is synthesized by a de novo mechanism, as far as the synthesis of C_{16} and $C_{16:1}$ fatty acids is concerned.

Table 3. Radioactivity of C_{16} and $C_{16:1}$ fatty acids present in the carboxylic group as determined by decarboxylation. The C_{16} and $C_{16:1}$ fatty acids were prepared from the total lipids following in vitro incubation of nonarteriosclerotic and arteriosclerotic parts of human aortae in the presence of ^{14}C-acetate (means of 3 incubation experiments)

| Part of aorta | % of total fatty acids | % Radioactivity Incorporated into | |
		carboxylic group	acyl residue
Nonarteriosclerotic	23,6	66	34
Arteriosclerotic	31,9	94	6

Conclusions

The results of the ^{14}C-glucose metabolism experiments suggest a reduction of oxidation metabolism in arteriosclerotic parts of human aortae as judged by diminished $^{14}CO_2$ production and increased ^{14}C-lactate formation. This metabolic state closely resembles hypoxic incubation conditions which are characterized by a decreased ATP/ADP and a rise of the NADH/NAD ratio. The accelerated fatty acid synthesis in arteriosclerotic segments - as indicated by increased synthesis of triglyceride fatty acids after ^{14}C-acetate incorporation (Table 2 and 3) - represents a regulating mechanism in which the accumulating NADH can be reoxidized by storing acyl units. Under these conditions the chain elongation mechanism in the course of the fatty acid synthesis is favored (Table 3) as being an ATP-saving process. From our results, the capacity of arterial tissue to synthesize fatty acids, and the apparent stimulation of this process in arteriosclerosis, must be considered an important pathogenetic factor.

CHOLESTEROL TRANSFER IN VITRO BETWEEN THE RABBIT AORTA AND SERUM LIPOPROTEINS[*]

Göran Bondjers and Sören Björkerud

The question, whether atherosclerotic lesions are reversible or not, has for a long time been controversial. However, recent studies on the development of experimental atherosclerosis induced by mechanical trauma in the aorta of normo-lipidemic rabbits, have established that such atherosclerotic lesions may revert entirely, or develop into lesions reminiscent of media sclerosis (Björkerud and Bondjers, 1973). During the formation of this type of athero-sclerotic lesion, cholesterol is accumulating in the aortic tissue, but during restoration of the normal arterial wall structure cholesterol is rapidly eliminated (Bondjers and Björkerud, 1973). It seems reasonable to assume that the mechanisms underlying cholesterol removal may be of significance for the reversion of atherosclerotic lesions, and perhaps also for the maintenance of a normal cholesterol content in non-atherosclerotic arterial tissue. The purpose of the present study was to investigate the relative significance of local arterial tissue factors and different blood-borne factors for cholesterol elimination *in vitro*.

Materials and Methods

Male, albino rabbits of the Danish country strain were obtained from the same breeder. They were fed 125 gms daily of low-calorie, high fiber-contents rabbit pellets ("maintenance food", Astra-Ewos AB, Södertälje, Sweden). Experimental atherosclerosis was induced in the aorta of normo-lipidemic rabbits with a micro-surgical instrument as described previously (Björkerud, 1969). The rabbits were killed four weeks after the operation.

Six days before the animals were killed they were injected intravenously with 1 mCi per kg body weight of ^{3}H-cholesterol incorporated into serum lipoproteins *in vitro*. Unoperated rabbits, and rabbits with experimental atherosclerosis were anaesthesized with Nemumal, and killed by bleeding during continuous aortic perfusion with Ringer's glucose solution. The aorta was cut in 1 mm segments with a McIlvain tissue chopper. The adventitia was carefully dissected away under a dissecting microscope, and normal (from unoperated animals) and atherosclerotic segments incubated 4 hours in different incubation media (see below).

Unlabelled serum was collected from normo-lipidemic rabbits after intra-cardial punction. Different serum lipoprotein fractions (VLDL, LDL, and HDL) and a serum infranatant at d>1.21 (i.e. including VHDL) were isolated with ultracentrifugation (Hatch and Lees 1968). The different fractions were dialysed for 24 hours against physiological saline at $4°C$. During the entire preparation procedure sterile material and solutions were used.

Serum lipoproteins in different combinations (VLDL, LDL, HDL single or all three combined) were mixed with serum infranatant and Krebs Ringer Bicarbonate buffer, pH 7.4. After removing an aliquot for lipid analysis, normal and atherosclerotic arterial segments were added and the samples transferred to a water bath main-tained at $37°C$. After 4 hours incubation with continuous shaking, the samples were cooled in ice water and the arterial segments removed.

[*]This investigation was supported by grants from the Swedish National Association against Heart and Chest Diseases, the University of Göteborg, Tore Nilsson's foundation and the Swedish Medical Research Council (Project No. 19X-2589).

Tissue lipids were extracted and washed as described by Folch et al. (1957). The lipids of the incubation medium were extracted and washed as described by Svennerholm (1968). Free and esterified cholesterol were determined as described by us (Bondjers and Björkerud, 1971). Radioactivity was determined with liquid scintillation counting in a Packard 3380 liquid scintillation spectrometer.

Results and Discussion

After incubation of normal arterial tissue with reconstituted serum (*i.e.* containing VLDL+LDL+HDL) we observed an increased cholesterol content in the incubation medium (Table 1). This increase was balanced by a decrease in the cholesterol content of the incubated tissue samples compared to unincubated controls (Table 1). Comparable observations in whole serum have been published by Murphy (1962, 1965) after incubation with erythrocytes, and by Rutenberg and Soloff (1971) after incubation with arterial tissue obtained at autopsy. However, in the present study, cholesterol transfer from the tissue to the incubation medium was observed also in control samples heated to $80^{\circ}C$ for 5 minutes and in control samples incubated in only KRB buffer (Table 1). Therefore, we do not feel that the present results allow the suggestion that these observations indicate biologically meaningful elimination of cholesterol from the arterial tissue. Other possible explanations to these observations, as *e.g.* desintegration of the arterial tissue with release of tissue debris into the incubation medium should be taken into consideration.

Table 1. Cholesterol concentration in incubation media (µg/ml) before and after incubation with normal and atherosclerotic arterial tissue, and cholesterol concentration (µg/mg dry weight) in incubated tissue samples and unincubated control tissue. Means ± S.E.M.

	Incubates with normal tissue			Incubates with atherosclerotic tissue		
	Incubation medium		Arterial tissue	Incubation medium		Arterial tissue
	Before	After		Before	After	
VLDL+LDL+HDL	91.8±5.3	115.6±6.2	4.6±0.1	146.3±5.4	127.4±1.1	6.1±0.2
VLDL+LDL+HDL (heated)	95.9±1.8	107.3±5.3	4.5±0.1	-	-	-
KRB buffer	-	7.9±2.4	4.4±0.1	-	5.2±2.2	7.0±0.3
VLDL	14.3±0.7	11.0±1.6	7.0±0.2	14.5±1.8	8.4±0.2	7.0±0.5
LDL	67.3±4.5	65.6±3.4	7.3±0.1	70.7±3.6	58.8±1.4	7.2±0.2
HDL	86.7±6.8	68.6±4.5	7.2±0.1	154.9±3.8	150.0±1.0	6.6±0.3
(unincubated control tissue)			5.6±0.1			7.5±0.1

Abbreviations

LDL = low density lipoproteins, ß-lipoproteins. HDL = high density lipoproteins, α-lipoproteins. VLDL = very low density lipoproteins, pre-ß-lipoproteins. LCAT = lecithin cholesteryl acyl transferase.

Incubation of normal arterial tissue with one isolated lipoprotein fraction, either of VLDL, LDL, or HDL, resulted in a decreased cholesterol content in the incubation medium, balanced by an increased cholesterol content in the incubated arterial tissue samples (Table 1). This net transfer of cholesterol into the arterial tissue was not simply due to contamination of the tissue with serum lipoproteins, as the percentage of esterified cholesterol actually decreased in the incubated arterial tissue (Table 2). Therefore, these results suggest actual net transfer of cholesterol into the arterial tissue, perhaps to cell membrane lipoproteins. This observation is qualitatively different from observations made after *in vitro* incubations with whole serum (see above), but does, on the other hand, correlate well with observations made on hereditary lipoprotein abnormalities. Thus, in hereditary as well as in experimental abetalipoproteinemia, the cholesterol content of erythrocytes appears to be increased (McBride and Jacobs, 1970). It has been suggested that this increase may be due to decreased efflux of cholesterol to a serum containing only HDL (McBride and Jacobs, 1970). In Tangier's disease, where normal HDL is absent, deposition of cholesteryl ester in retriculo-endothelial tissue is characteristic (Fredrickson et al., 1972). Furthermore, in one of the twelve patients with this rare disease frequent fatty streaks in the pulmonary artery were observed (Fredrickson et al., 1972), suggesting that lipid deposition might also involve the arterial tissue. Taken together with these observations, those of the present study suggest that a marked dysbalance in the lipoprotein pattern *per se* might promote transfer of cholesterol into arterial tissue, also when the dysbalance involves a decrease of specific lipoprotein fractions.

Table 2. Esterified cholesterol as per cent of total cholesterol in incubation media, before and after incubation with normal and atherosclerotic arterial tissue, and in incubated and unincubated arterial tissue samples. Means ± S.E.M.

Components of incubation medium	Incubates with normal tissue			Incubates with atherosclerotic tissue		
	Incubation medium		Arterial tissue	Incubation medium		Arterial tissue
	Before	After		Before	After	
VLDL+LDL+HDL	62.4±0.8	73.0±1.2	12.3±5.8	79.6±1.9	92.2±0.6	8.6±1.6
VLDL	60.3	65.0±2.8	8.2±0.8	58.3±2.5	66.4±2.5	13.0±4.2
LDL	53.9 55.3	68.1±2.1	4.3±0.5	72.0±2.9	83.6±2.5	5.0±0.7
HDL	60.2 68.8	76.0±2.4	6.3±1.7	85.4±2.2	95.1±1.2	11.6±2.6
(unincubated control tissue)			11.8±1.1			5.6±0.9

After incubation of atherosclerotic tissue in various media, we observed a decreased cholesterol content in all media except that one containing HDL (Table 1). However, this decrease was not balanced by an increased cholesterol content of the tissue samples (Table 1). Thus, the recovery of cholesterol was below 100% in these incubates. Whether this depicts actual decomposition of cholesterol, transfer of cholesterol to a form giving decreased recovery with our analytical methods, or other processes cannot be assessed at present.

The cholesterol content of atherosclerotic tissue samples incubated in incubation media containing HDL was lower than that of unincubated controls or controls incubated in KRB buffer solution (Table 1). This suggests that the presence of HDL is an important factor in the removal of cholesterol from atherosclerotic tissue. Such a mechanism may explain results from clinical studies, indicating that patients with myocardial infarction or intermittent claudication have a decreased concentration of HDL-bound cholesterol in comparision with healthy men (Eriksson and Carlson, 1973).

Correlated with observations on net transfer of cholesterol, studies on the transfer of radioactive cholesterol may give pertinent information. Thus, in incubates with HDL and atherosclerotic arterial tissue, net removal of cholesterol from the tissue was parallelled with specific radioactivies far higher in free cholesterol than in cholesteryl ester (Table 3). This suggests that primarily free cholesterol was transferred from the atherosclerotic tissue to the incubation medium, a mechanism which would be in agreement with our previous suggestion from *in vivo* studies that cholesterol is mobilised from atherosclerotic tissue in its free form (Bondjers and Björkerud, 1972). However, elimination of free cholesterol from the atherosclerotic tissue was parallelled by esterification of cholesterol in the incubation medium (Table 2). The low specific radioactivity in the cholesteryl ester fraction (Table 3) does clearly indicate that free cholesterol in the incubation medium is the substrate for this esterification activity.

Cholesterol esterification was observed in all incubation media (Table 2), presumably reflecting the presence of LCAT and VHDL, which may serve as a primary substrate for LCAT (Fielding and Fielding, 1971), in the infranatant. However, our results indicate that the direction of cholesterol transfer is totally independent of LCAT activity. Thus, net transfer of cholesterol to the arterial tissue, as well as out of the arterial tissue, were observed in incubates with roughly the same esterification activity (Tables 1 and 2). Our results suggest that the main prerequisite for net cholesterol transfer out of arterial tissue *in vitro*, is that the tissue is atherosclerotic. If this is the case, the presence of HDL appears to be obligate for net transfer of cholesterol out of the tissue. However, it is possible that when these prerequisites are fulfilled, LCAT activity may be an important component in the cholesterol elimination process.

Table 3. Specific activity (DPM/μg) of free and esterified cholesterol in incubation media after 4 hours incubation with atherosclerotic arterial tissue labelled with ^{3}H-cholesterol. Means ± S.E.M.

Components of incubation medium	Free cholesterol	Cholesteryl ester
VLDL+LDL+HDL	25.3 ± 3.8	1.0 ± 0.1
VLDL	40.8 ± 4.0	11.7 ± 1.3
LDL	16.5 ± 4.5	1.1 ± 0.1
HDL	53.4 ± 9.2	1.4 ± 0.2

The fact that cholesterol is deposited in normal arterial tissue when incubated with HDL, but eliminated from atherosclerotic arterial tissue under similar experimental conditions, could conceivably reflect that the direction of cholesterol transfer is determined by the cholesterol concentration of the tissue. Such a mechanism has been proposed by Sardet et al. (1972) for the transfer of cholesterol between erythrocytes and serum lipoproteins. However, when normal arterial tissue is incubated with HDL, the cholesterol concentration increases to values above those for atherosclerotic tissue incubated with HDL. Therefore, it appears more probable that the capacity for cholesterol elimination is a property which is specific for atherosclerotic arterial tissue. This property may perhaps develop in response to the drastical changes in permeability for serum constituents into the arterial tissue, which appears to be involved in atherogenesis (*e.g.* Björkerud and Bondjers, 1971; Bondjers and Björkerud, 1973).

ARTERIAL LIPID METABOLISM IN DIABETIC ANIMAL MODELS WITH REDUCED OR ELEVATED PLASMA INSULIN LEVELS*

A.V. Chobanian, G.C. Gerritsen, L. McCombs, and P.I. Brecher

Introduction

Hyperlipidemia, hyperinsulinemia, and abnormal arterial metabolism all have been proposed as causes of the accelerated atherogenesis observed in diabetic patients. The incidence of atherosclerotic disease is increased in hyperlipidemic diabetic populations but is relatively low with normal serum lipids (Rudnick and Anderson, 1962). Abnormal carbohydrate metabolism (Wahlberg, 1966) and hyperinsulinemia (Stout and Vallance-Owen, 1967) are common in patients with ischemic heart disease. Increases in insulin concentration could stimulate arterial lipid synthesis (Stout, 1967), although any increase may be confined to the adventitial adipose tissue (Vost and Hollenberg, 1969). Hyperglycemia is an independent risk factor for ischemic heart disease (Epstein, 1971). An adverse effect of hyperglycemia could possibly be mediated via the polyol pathway; increase in glucose levels in vitro induces arterial accumulation of polyol derivatives, increases arterial water content, and reduces arterial oxygen uptake (Morrison et al., 1972).

The present investigation has examined the relationship between diabetes, hyperlipidemia, and arterial lipid metabolism in 2 contrasting diabetic animal models with either reduced (Chinese hamster) or elevated (obese KK mouse) plasma insulin. Both dia betic strains may have microvascular involvement and other features resembling the human disease (Gerritsen and Dulin, 1967; Felderman and Gerritsen, 1970; Dulin and Wyse, 1970; and Camerini et al., 1970).

Materials and Methods

The diabetic animals, obtained from the Upjohn Co. Colony, had persistent hyperglycemia and glycosuria. The control hamsters were non-diabetic siblings of similar age, sex, and weight. The controls for the KK mice were of the C57 strain and were of similar age and sex but of lighter weight to correct for differences in body fat. All animals were maintained on Purina Mouse Breeder Chow.

Fasting plasma glucose and immunoreactive insulin were assayed as described (Gerritsen and Dulin, 1967). Plasma cholesterol was determined by a micro-modification of the method of Abell. Following sacrifice, the total aorta was removed and the adventitia carefully teased away. The intima-media segments were incubated for 2 hrs in KRB buffer containing $[2\text{-}^{14}C]$ acetate or $[U\text{-}^{14}C]$ glucose (5mM). Arterial cholesterol and DNA content and lipid radioactivity were determined as described (Chobanian, 1968; Chobanian and Manzur, 1972). Light and electron microscopic studies were performed using fixation and staining methods previously reported (McCombs et al., 1969).

Results

The diabetic hamsters demonstrated marked increases in fasting plasma glucose and mild decreases in plasma insulin; the KK mice exhibited moderate increases in

*Supported by USPHS Grants HL 12869 and HL 07299 and the U.A. Whitaker Fund.

glucose but massive elevations in plasma insulin (Table 1). Plasma cholesterol was elevated above 200 mg% in 14 of 30 diabetic hamsters studied with levels as high as 450 mg% being observed. The degree of hypercholesterolemia did not correlate significantly with levels of plasma glucose or insulin. Hypercholesterolemia was not observed in the KK mice.

Arterial cholesterol content was significantly elevated in the hypercholesterolemic diabetic hamsters but not in the normocholesterolemic diabetic hamsters or mice (Table 1). The results were similar whether related to tissue wet weight or DNA content.

Table 1. Plasma and Arterial Cholesterol Content in the Diabetic Hamster and KK Mouse

Group	Blood Glucose (mg%)	Plasma Insulin (uU/ml)	Plasma Cholesterol (mg%)	Arterial Cholesterol (mg/mg DNA)
Diabetic Hamsters (hypercholesterolemic)	354 ± 29	52 ± 8	251 ± 14	3.09 ± 0.21
Control Hamsters	102 ± 12	65 ± 7	139 ± 4	1.58 ± 0.19
Diabetic Hamsters (normocholesterolemic)	331 ± 26	55 ± 6	133 ± 8	1.64 ± 0.23
Control Hamsters	97 ± 10	64 ± 7	124 ± 6	1.73 ± 0.23
Diabetic KK Mice	224 ± 15	1275 ± 125	104 ± 5	1.40 ± 0.15
Controls (C57)	124 ± 12	78 ± 13	110 ± 5	1.14 ± 0.07

Incorporation of acetate into total arterial lipids or into any major lipid fraction was not significantly different in the diabetic or control hamsters (Table 2). Glucose conversion to lipid was reduced significantly in the diabetic hamsters; the degree of reduction was greater in the ketotic than the non-ketotic diabetics.

Table 2. Influence of Diabetes on the Aortic Incorporation of $[U-^{14}C]$ Glucose and $[2-^{14}C]$ Acetate into Lipid

Group	Incorporation into Lipid	
	$U-^{14}C$ Glucose	$2-^{14}C$ Acetate
	(dpm/mg DNA)	
Diabetic Hamsters	35,500 ± 5600	74,200 ± 7800
Control Hamsters	66,300 ± 6100	69,600 ± 9300
Diabetic KK Mice	37,900 ± 5100	-
Control (C57)	44,700 ± 4300	-

No significant abnormality in glucose incorporation into lipid was apparent in the KK mice.

No grossly visible lesions were apparent in diabetic hamster aortas, but light microscopy revealed occasional lesions with mild intimal thickening and fragmentation of the internal elastic lamina. EM studies of these lesions demonstrated prominent lipid droplets and intracytoplasmic vesicles in endothelial cells, lipid micelles, and increased ground substance (Fig. 1). Increased numbers of lipid droplets were also seen in the smooth muscle cells.

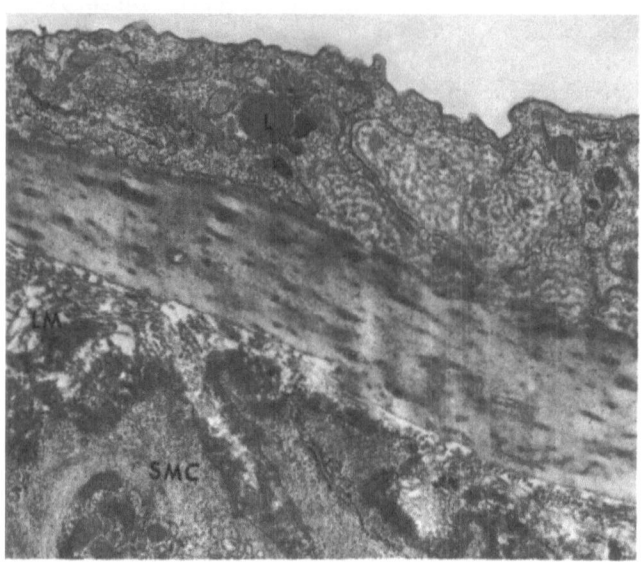

Figure 1. Transverse section of descending thoracic aorta of a male diabetic hamster. Note the lipid droplet (L) in an endothelial cell with very prominent organelles and large numbers of intracytoplasmic vesicles. Lipid micelles (LM) are present in the extracellular space surrounded by collagen strands and abundant ground substance. Smooth muscle cells (SMC) of the media have large numbers of mitochondria. Uranyl acetate and lead citrate stain. X 11.400

Discussion and Conclusion

Spontaneous hypercholesterolemia is a relatively frequent occurrence in the diabetic Chinese hamster. The hypercholesterolemia has been shown previously to be associated with increased serum triglycerides, reduced fractional turnover rate of plasma cholesterol, expansion of the rapidly exchanging cholesterol compartment (Chobanian and Gerritsen, 1971) and increased VLDL (C. Day, personal communication). Hypercholesterolemia and decreased fractional turnover of plasma cholesterol have also been observed in cholesterol-fed squirrel monkeys with insulin deficient diabetes induced by alloxan (Lehner et al., 1972). In contrast, hypercholesterolemia was not observed in the hyperinsulinemic obese diabetic mice. Nevertheless, adipose tissue appears to be an important storage site for cholesterol (Angel and Farkas, 1970) and one might expect total body cholesterol content to be elevated in these animals.

Elevations in aortic cholesterol were confined to the hypercholesterolemic hamsters. These findings coupled with studies which failed to demonstrate elevations in arterial lipid synthesis in the diabetic animals suggest that hyperlipidemia is a major factor contributing to the increased arterial lipid deposition. The relatively low incidence of vascular disease in diabetic populations with normal serum lipids (Rudnick and Anderson, 1962) lends indirect support to this hypothesis

The reduced incorporation of glucose to lipid in the diabetic hamster was part of a generalized decrease in aortic glucose utilization previously reported by us (Chobanian and Gerritsen, 1971) and similarly observed in the alloxan-diabetic rabbit (Winegrad et al., 1965). While this abnormality could be secondary to a decrease in plasma insulin, a reduced sensitivity to insulin could also be a factor since supraphysiological doses of insulin have been necessary to normalize aortic glucose utilization in the diabetic hamster. The lack of increase in aortic glucose utilization in the KK mouse despite markedly elevated plasma insulin could also be consistent with relative insulin insensitivity. These findings cast doubt on the hypothesis that hyperinsulinemia may induce atherogenesis by stimulating arterial lipogenesis. Other detrimental arterial effects of insulin cannot be excluded, however. Recently, insulin stimulation of smooth muscle cell proliferation has been observed in arterial tissue cultures (Stout et al., 1973).

The arterial lesions and the mild increases in arterial cholesterol content in the diabetic hamster may reflect early atherosclerotic changes, but further studies will be needed to clarify the significance of these findings. An increased tendency of diabetic animals to develop atherosclerotic lesions has been observed in cholesterol fed alloxan-diabetic rats and squirrel monkeys (Martin and Hartroft, 1965; Lehner et al., 1971).

LIPID METABOLISM IN PERFUSED HUMAN CORONARY ARTERIES AND SAPHENOUS VEINS[*]

H. Tillmanns, I.S.M. Sarma, K. Seeler, and R.I. Bing

Our paper deals with lipid metabolism in perfused human coronary arteries and saphenous veins. Some of these studies have been reported before (Hashimoto et al., 1974). This paper, therefore, represents a summary of our data on this subject. Experiments will also be reported which deal with the effect of carbon monoxide on these mechanisms.

Materials and Methods

Our techniques consist in principle, in perfusion of human coronary arteries obtained from autopsy material up to 5 hours after death. Sterile techniques were used during the preparation and perfusion. Coronary arteries were removed at autopsy from patients who ranged in age from 2 to 22 years. Saphenous veins were removed from patients prior to performing aortic-coronary saphenous grafts. The length of the veins and arteries used in the perfusion experiments ranged from 2 to 3 cm. The vessels were dissected free of fat and connective tissue. Perfusion was carried out for a period of 4 hours at $37^\circ C$ with a perfusion pressure of 130/100 mmHg at a pulsatile rate of 80. Veins were perfused at two pressure ranges, one from 45/33 mmHg, the other at arterial pressure of 130/100 mmHg. Pressures less than 30 mmHg could not be obtained in our perfusion system. A modified Carrel-Lindbergh pump was used in all experiments, as described previously (Carrel and Lindberg, 1938). The basic perfusion fluid consisted of sterile human plasma collected within 10 days prior to the experiment. A mixture of 75% nitrogen, 20% oxygen, and 5% carbon dioxide was employed to drive the fluid through the artery. Purity of $2-^{14}C$-sodium acetate ($^{14}-C$-acetate, 2 Ci/mole) and cholesterol-1, $2-^3H$ (^3H-cholesterol, 55 Ci/mmole) was tested as previously described. ^3H-cholesterol (100-200 µCi) was added to about .01 ml of concentrated lipid extract from human serum which contained 118.4 µmoles/ml of total cholesterol, 15.2 umoles/ml of free cholesterol, and 32.6 µmoles/ml of phosphorus of phospholipids. The mixture was evaporated in vacuo to a small volume. Final evaporation was carried out under a stream of nitrogen. After addition of about 5 ml of human plasma, the mixture was sonicated in an ice-water bath 3 times for 1 minute each, at intervals of about 1 minute, using a Biosonik III (20 KHz) with a microtip. The sonicated mixture was then made up to a volume of about 60 ml with plasma and shaken again for two hours at $37^\circ C$. Cellulose acetate membrane electrophoresis of the incubated plasma mixture was carried out according to the method of Chin and Blankenhorn (1968). It could be shown that the tritium radioactivity was located mainly in the alpha-2-lipoprotein and beta-lipoprotein fractions. The incubated mixture was then combined with a basic perfusion fluid to which 250 µCi of ^{14}C-acetate had been previously added. The total perfusion mixture was made up to 250 ml. In every instance the perfusion fluid was tested for sterility at the onset and at the termination of the experiment. In addition, pieces of arteries were histologically examined. No histological changes were noticed following the period of perfusion.

Lipids were analyzed in the perfusion fluid prior to and following perfusion. Extraction was carried out according to the method of Folch et al. (1957).

[*]Supported by grants from the Kenneth T. and Eileen L. Norris Foundation and The Council for Tobacco Research--U.S.A., Inc.

Analyses were carried out on the whole blood vessel with the exception of the adventitia. After weighing the tissue and freezing it in liquid nitrogen, it was crushed in a mortar. The crushed tissue was then collected in an Erlenmeyer joint flask with the Folch mixture of chloroform and methanol (2:1 v/v) and kept under nitrogen gas for 20 hours at $5^{\circ}C$. The mixture was then refluxed for 30 minutes and filtered using analytical filter paper. The residue on the filter paper and in the Erlenmeyer flask was refluxed again with the Folch mixture for 30 minutes.

Separation of lipids was accomplished by means of thin-layer chromatography on silica gel (silica gel F-254) according to the method of Freeman and West (1966). Location of spots on the plates was detected by ultraviolet light or by exposure to iodine vapors. The separate fractions were eluted from thin-layer plates with elution solvents appropriate for the corresponding fraction. Recovery of the fraction was tested by counting the radioactivity of the eluate and comparing it with the radioactivity of the residue gel.

Radioactivity of the extracts was counted in a Tri-Carb liquid scintillation spectrometer in the presence of a toluene-dioxane scintillator.

The method of Zlatkis et al. (1953), or the method of Zak et al. (1956), was used for determination of cholesterol in plasma extract and in the eluate. Phosphorus of phospholipids was analyzed according to Lowry et al. (1954), modified by Wagner et al. (1963). When the amount of cholesterol esters taken up was calculated, the mean value of the specific activity of ^3H-cholesterol esters into plasma before and after perfusion was used.

The following technique was carried out when the effect of carbon monoxide was investigated:

In the first 5 experiments, where high concentrations of HbCO were maintained, a gas mixture containing CO, CO_2, O_2 and N_2 in the ratios 5:5:20:70 by volume, was bubbled through the whole blood until the HbCO level rose above 80%; this blood was then added to the remaining part of the radioactive plasma to form the perfusate for the experimental specimen. For the tests in which lower levels of HbCO (< 15%) were used, the blood which usually contained less than 5% HbCO was directly mixed with labelled plasma, with no pretreatment. The Hb, HbCO and HbO_2 levels of the final perfusate were measured before and after the perfusion.

During the perfusion the system is closed to the outer atmosphere and gas mixture can be introduced into the system at a controlled pressure to form the local atmosphere. This gas mixture is referred to as perfusion gas. In the control experiments this consisted of O_2, N_2 and CO_2 in the ratios 20:75:5. In the experiments where high level CO was used, the perfusion gas contained CO, CO_2, O_2 and N_2 in the ratios 0.5:5:20:74.5; for the low level CO experiments the corresponding ratios were 0.05:5:20:74.95.

Results

Although there is considerable incorporation of ^{14}C radioactivity into phospholipids, free fatty acids, and diglycerides and triglycerides, no synthesis of cholesterol from ^{14}C-acetate could be demonstrated (Table 1). No incorporation of ^{14}C radioactivity into cholesterol esters could be shown. Distribution of ^{14}C radioactivity was greater in triglycerides than in phospholipids (2p < 0.001).

Saphenous veins perfused at a pressure of 45/35 mmHg were unable to synthesize significant amounts of free cholesterol (Table 1); small amounts of cholesterol esters were synthesized. The largest amount of ^{14}C radioactivity was again found in the triglycerides. Similar to nonatherosclerotic coronary arteries, incorporation into phospholipids was greater than that into free fatty acids or diglycerides. No statistical difference was found between incorporation of ^{14}C-acetate

Table 1. Incorporation of acetate-2-^{14}C into lipids of human coronary arteries and saphenous veins, as % of ^{14}C radioactivity of total lipids.

	Atherosclerotic coronary arteries (n = 8)	Nonatherosclerotic coronary arteries (n = 6)	Saphenous veins perf. press. 45/35mmHg (n = 9)	Saphenous veins perf. press. 130/100mmHg (n = 9)	Saphenous veins with nict. perf. press. 45/35mmHg (n = 6)	Statistical Analysis A vs B	A vs C	C vs B
FC	0.3±0.2	0.2	0.8±0.2	0.2±0.1	0.9±0.3	ND	ND	ND
CE	2.1±1.1	1.4±0.9	3.0±0.6	3.2±0.7	2.5±1.0	NS	NS	NS
PL	35.0±1.7	23.8±3.1	27.5±1.8	29.1±1.4	23.4±2.0	p<0.005	p<.01	NS
FFA	8.7±1.7	8.3±1.4	7.7±0.8	8.4±1.0	7.5±0.4	NS	NS	NS
DG	2.0±1.3	8.2±3.8	3.9±0.7	6.7±0.6	3.7±0.7	NS	NS	NS
TG	49.1±2.4	45.9±4.5	48.1±1.6	44.5±1.1	46.4±3.6	NS	NS	NS
TC[a]	10.1±2.8[b]	20.3±8.1	35.5±7.8	36.1±6.4	23.1±7.6	ND	ND	NS

The figures represent mean values ± standard error.

FC = free cholesterol,
CE = cholesterol esters,
PL = phospholipids,
FFA = free fatty acids,
DG = diglycerides,
TG = triglycerides

a = radioactivity in total lipids,
b = concentration of ^{14}C acetate in perfusion fluid; 150 uCi/250ml,
ND = not determined,
NS = no significant difference.

into any of the lipid fractions of these veins as compared to nonatherosclerotic cornonary arteries (Table 1).

Distribution of ^{14}C radioactivity did not differ in saphenous veins perfused at high pressure as compared to veins perfused at a pressure of 45/35 mmHg or to perfused coronary arteries (Table 1). The distribution of ^{14}C radioactivity was greatest in triglycerides, followed by phospholipids, free fatty acids, and diglycerides. The percent of ^{14}C radioactivity incorporated into free cholesterol was insignificant. There was slight synthesis of cholesterol esters from ^{14}C-acetate.

Cholesterol and Cholesterol Ester Content in Coronary Arteries and Saphenous Veins

The contents of cholesterol and cholesterol esters are represented in Table 2. The very high lipid content in atherosclerotic arteries as contrasted to that in saphenous veins and nonatherosclerotic arteries is seen. In saphenous veins, the content of cholesterol esters was lower than that of free cholesterol.

Uptake of Free Cholesterol and Cholesterol Esters from the Perfusion Fluid by Nonatherosclerotic Coronary Arteries and Saphenous Veins

Table 2 illustrates that considerable amounts of free cholesterol were taken up by the arteries from the perfusion fluid. The mean uptake was 45.0 ± 10.7 mμmoles/gm of tissue. The uptake of cholesterol esters by these tissues was considerably higher than that of free cholesterol.

In contrast to normal coronary arteries, saphenous veins perfused at low pressure incorporated considerably smaller amounts of cholesterol from the perfusion fluid (Table 2). Only 7.5 ± 1.1 mumoles/gm of tissue were incorporated. Uptake of cholesterol esters was small but varied, possibly because of the low specific activity of cholesterol esters in the perfusion fluid.

Saphenous veins perfused at arterial pressure of 130/100 mmHg took up considerable amounts of free cholesterol from the perfusion fluid (Table 2). The average uptake was 34.4 ± 9.9 mμmoles/gm tissue. Table 2 illustrates that the uptake of ^{3}H-cholesterol in saphenous veins perfused at high pressure was greater than in veins perfused at low pressure ($p < .01$). Equally significant was the difference in cholesterol uptake between saphenous veins perfused at low pressure and nonatherosclerotic arteries ($p < .01$). This illustrates that perfusion pressure plays a considerable role in determining the uptake of cholesterol.

As in the case of lipid synthesis, nicotine failed to influence uptake of ^{3}H-cholesterol into saphenous veins perfused at low pressure (Table 2).

As previously described in our publications, lipid synthesis and cholesterol uptake did not differ in atherosclerotic coronary arteries from those of normal vessels.

Effect of Carbon Monoxide

These results are now in print in a separate publication (Sarma et al., in prev.). No significant changes in the lipid synthesis (^{14}C incorporation) were observed in arteries exposed to carbon monoxide (Table 3). Apparently, at either high or low levels of CO in the perfusate, cholesterol uptake by the arteries is increased to the same extent (Tables 3 and 4). Large variations in the cholesterol uptake were found. This could be due to variations in the inner geometry of the arterial specimens leading to different turbulent flow patterns which could influence cholesterol transport. It is unlikely that differences in the degree of atherosclerosis of the arterial specimens could have affected the cholesterol uptake,

Table 2. Lipid content and ^{3}H-cholesterol uptake in human coronary arteries and saphenous veins

	A Athero-sclerotic coronary arteries	B Nonathero-sclerotic coronary arteries	C Saphenous veins perf. press. 45/35mmHg	D Saphenous veins perf. press. 130/100mmHg	E Saphenous veins with nict. perf. press. 45/35mmHg	Statistical Analysis				
						A vs B	B vs C	C vs D	A vs C	C vs E
Tissue lipid content cholesterol (μmoles/g tis.)	3.67±0.92 (n = 8)	1.33±0.40 (n = 5)	0.85±0.24 (n = 6)	ND	ND	p<0.05	NS	ND	p<0.025	ND
Tissue lipid content cholesterol ester (μmoles/g tis.)	10.40±2.37 (n = 8)	4.54±1.61 (n = 4)	0.53±0.08 (n = 6)	ND	ND	p<0.05	p<0.025	ND	p<0.005	ND
Cholesterol uptake (mμmoles/g tis.)	33.0±11.7 (n = 8)	46.0±10.7 (n = 3)	7.5±1.1 (n = 7)	34.4±9.9 (n = 9)	11.8±2.3 (n = 5)	NS	p<0.01	p<0.01	p<0.05	NS

The figures represent mean values ± standard error.

ND = not determined,
NS = no significant difference.

since it was reported earlier (Hashimoto et al., 1974) that arterial cholesterol uptake is not influenced by the presence of atherosclerosis.

It is likely that the increased uptake of cholesterol by arteries perfused with CO is the result of tissue hypoxia as shown by Goldsmith (1969) and Ayres et al. (1973). Carbon monoxide may also directly interfere with tissue metabolism because of its higher affinity to myoglobin as compared to hemoglobin (Oburn, 1970; Astrup, 1972). The myoglobin takes part in the transport of oxygen from blood hemoglobin to tissue mitochondria while also accomplishing oxygen storage to a limited degree (Ayres et al., 1973; Wittenberg, 1965). Astrup and coworkers (Astrup et al., 1967; Kjeldsen et al., 1968; Wanstrup et al., 1969; Astrup et al., 1970) demonstrated that hypoxia as well as exposure to carbon monoxide significantly increase the permeability of the endothelial membranes. They found that rabbits when exposed to carbon monoxide develop arterial lesions resulting in a considerable accumulation of lipids. Siggaard-Andersen et al. (1968) found that exposure to CO results in a greater increase in the permeability of the vascular walls than hypoxia alone. Parving (1972) and Parving et al. (1972) also studied the transvascular protein flux during CO exposure and confirmed that the disappearance rate from blood of albumin ^{131}I increased about 50% after 3 hours of exposure to 20-25% carboxyhemoglobin levels in blood.

No difference in cholesterol uptake was found using 2 different levels of CO in the perfusion fluid. This suggests that the rate of cholesterol uptake under these experimental conditions is an all or none process. No influence of CO on lipid synthesis in the arterial wall could be demonstrated (Tables 3 and 4) in this study.

Summary

Lipid synthesis and cholesterol uptake was measured in vitro in perfused human coronary arteries and saphenous veins obtained at autopsy. The results reveal:

1. Cholesterol is not synthesized by normal or atherosclerotic human coronary arteries or saphenous veins.
2. Saphenous veins take up cholesterol, the amount of uptake depending on the perfusion pressure.
3. Nicotine failed to influence cholesterol uptake or lipid synthesis.
4. Carbon monoxide leads to a marked increase in cholesterol uptake of human coronary arteries, regardless of the concentration of CO in the perfusion fluid. Carbon monoxide does not interfere with lipid synthesis in the arterial wall.

Table 3. Cholesterol uptake and lipid synthesis with and without carbon monoxide.

Experiment No.	Age - Sex	COHb % in perfusate	Chol. perfusate μmoles/ml	Chol. content tissue μmoles/gm t.	Chol. uptake by the tissue μmoles/gm t.	Lipid Synthesis[a]					
						Chol.	CE	PL	FFA	DG	TG
4-C	62 F	0	1.04	2.57	20.5	1.3	4.1	14.1	7.0	6.1	46.2
5-E		97	0.90	5.35	26.7	0.9	4.2	14.0	4.0	2.6	49.2
6-C	61 M	0	1.27	29.0	32.1	2.8	1.8	50.6	12.9	5.2	13.9
7-E		97	1.25	25.5	37.6	5.4	2.4	32.1	33.6	1.0	22.5
8-C	69 M	0	1.02	36.5	9.4	1.4	4.8	35.0	9.6	19.5	29.4
9-E		76.7	1.04	21.1	24.8	3.3	5.4	26.1	12.0	26.1	27.2
10-C	70 F	0	1.11	2.64	78.8	6.0	2.6	14.6	11.8	15.5	49.5
11-E		89	1.12	23.62	90.9	1.6	2.4	26.5	12.4	21.3	35.9
12-C	60 F	0	1.29	25.0	105.6	2.5	8.0	31.8	9.3	25.5	23.0
13-E		92.4	1.27	63.1	108.7	4.0	4.0	35.4	10.2	36.5	10.0
14-C	86 F	0	0.85	8.5	92.4	9.2	7.9	33.5	9.2	9.4	30.9
15-E		26	0.85	3.0	130.8	2.5	0	31.9	14.2	5.6	45.7
16-C	49 F	0	1.03	18.2	38.9	0	0	7.0	0	37.9	56.1
17-E		6.6	1.05	31.4	59.2	0	0	4.6	0	39.2	56.2
18-C	48 M	0	0.97	12.8	70.5	5.6	6.0	24.6	3.8	12.8	47.2
19-E		5.8	0.87	5.2	188.4	8.5	2.3	21.4	5.4	15.4	47.1
20-C	8 M	0	0.89	43.3	297.0	31.0	3.0	17.5	7.3	7.6	33.3
21-E		14.2	0.91	3.4	398.0	38.8	3.3	14.4	8.5	5.3	29.7
22-C	54 F	0	0.78	2.4	187.3	0.5	1.2	18.0	0.4	4.7	75.0
23-E		14.0	0.80	3.0	138.7	2.3	0	13.0	2.8	8.7	73.0

C = control, E = experimental, Chol. = cholesterol, CE = cholesterol ester, PL = phospholipid, COHb = carboxyhemoglobin, FFA = free fatty acid, DG = diglyceride, TG = triglyceride, t = tissue.

a = % of ^{14}C radioactivity of total lipids.

Table 4. Statistical Analysis

Data Compared	Statistical Parameter	P Value	Significance
Cholesterol uptake by arteries (control vs. experiment)	x = 66.2	p < 0.001	S
Cholesterol uptake by arteries (low concentrations vs. high concentrations of CO)	t = 2.1	p > 0.05	NS
Lipid synthesis by arteries (control vs. experiment)			
C	t = 0.2	p > 0.05	NS
CE	t = 1.1	p > 0.05	NS
PL	t = 0.5	p > 0.05	NS
FFA	t = 0.9	p > 0.05	NS
DG	t = 0.3	p > 0.05	NS
TG	t = 0.1	p > 0.05	NS

S = significant, NS = not significant.

IV

Enzymes of the Arterial Wall

Chairmen: A.J. Day, Australia
          J. Patelski, Poland

Participants: S. Eisenberg, Israel
              Y. Stein, Israel
              A. Vost, Canada
              D.E. Bowyer, England
              J.D. Pearson, England
              R. St. Clair, USA

Studies carried out on the lipid composition of the normal arterial wall and of the atherosclerotic lesion in both man and experimental animals indicate that both the content and composition of arterial wall phospholipids and cholesteryl esters alter as a result of aging and of atherosclerosis. These observations have been supplemented by studies on the synthesis and metabolism of phospholipids and cholesteryl esters and it is now well-recognized that both the synthesis and hydrolysis of these two lipid fractions occurs in the arterial wall and that changes in the enzymes responsible for these effects are involved in the atherogenetic process. It is the purpose of this Workshop to discuss arterial wall enzymes with particular emphasis on the synthesis and degradation of phospholipid and of cholesteryl ester.

PHOSPHOLIPID SYNTHESIS AND DEGRADATION IN THE ARTERIAL WALL

S. Eisenberg and Y. Stein

Several studies have demonstrated that the content of phospholipids--mainly sphingomyelin--in arteries increases during aging and atherogenesis (Buck and Rossiter, 1951; Smith, 1960; Böttcher and Van Gent, 1961; Eisenberg et al., 1969b). The pioneering work of Chernick et al. (1949) demonstrated that lipids are synthesized by arterial tissue and called attention to the possible role of *in situ* metabolism to account for phospholipid accumulation in arteries. The following precursors have been used for aortic phospholipid synthesis in arteries: fatty acids, acetate, glucose, alphaglycero-phosphate, lysolecithin, phosphate and choline (Zilversmit et al., 1954; Newman et al., 1961; Stein and Stein, 1962; Stein et al., 1963a,b; Parker et al., 1964, 1966; Newman et al., 1966; Day and Wahlqvist, 1968, 1969). Studies by Zilversmit and his associates have conclusively proved that in both the normal and atherosclerotic arteries the contribution of *in situ* synthesis to the arterial phospholipid pool exceeds that of phospholipid transported from the blood stream (Zilversmit and McCandless, 1959; Zilversmit et al., 1954, 1961).

Several years ago we investigated the role of catabolism in phospholipid accumulation in arteries. The following enzymic activities were characterized: sphingomyelin choline phosphohydrolase, phosphatide-2-acyl hydrolase (phospholipase A2) and lysophosphatide acyl hydrolase (lysolecithinase) (Rachmilewitz et al., 1967; Eisenberg et al., 1968; Eisenberg et al., 1969a,b; Eisenberg et al., 1971). The rate of hydrolysis of various phospholipids by aortic homogenates derived from rats, rabbits or humans varied both with respect to age and with respect to the phospholipid substrate. With increasing age, the rate of hydrolysis of lecithin and phosphatidyl ethanolamine increased 5 to 10 times and that of lysolecithin 2 to 3 times. In contrast, sphingomyelin hydrolysis was either unaffected or decreased with age. Since no effect on the rate of phospholipid synthesis was present, it was concluded that the phospholipid content in arteries may be regulated by the observed change in pattern of hydrolysis of the individual phospholipid. This hypothesis is compatible with further observations on the effect of thyroid and sex hormones on aortic phospholipid content and metabolism (Blatt et al., 1971).

The following questions are pertinent for discussion.

1. What are the sites of phospholipid accumulation and the location of the enzymes involved?
2. Is phospholipid accumulation a physiological or pathological process?
3. What regulation mechanisms exist for phospholipid synthesis and catabolism?

Discussion

Dr. Smith observed that in the human artery, the proportion of sphingomyelin increased with age in the media but not in the intima and the question of the location of the phospholipases responsible for the progressive accumulation of sphingomyelin was raised. Dr. Stein indicated that although their data related to combined intima-media preparations most of the sphingomyelin was, in fact, present in association with the smooth muscle cells of the media. Dr. Smith suggested that since the amount of lipoprotein which entered the artery wall contained considerable amounts of phospholipid including sphingomyelin that the major substrate for sphingomyelin hydrolase may come from the plasma. Dr. Stein considered that although whole lipoprotein may filter into the arterial wall there was appreciable metabolic capacity to take care of its various components with the exception of cholesterol which was relatively inert and tended to accumulate.

The question of location of the phospholipid which accumulated in the arterial wall and of its relationship to membrane turnover was raised. Dr. Smith pointed out that in the normal intima the phospholipid:free cholesterol ratio remained constant over a wide age range from 6 months to 60 years of age. Dr. Bowyer indicated that there appeared to be two pools of phospholipid in the arterial wall; an extracellular pool which arises from the plasma and another pool which represents cell membrane phospholipid. The question was raised, therefore, as to whether the sphingomyelinase activity associated normally with the plasma membrane is associated with the catabolism of plasma lipoprotein phospholipid.

Dr. Olga Stein presented some electron microscopic data relevant to the question of the location of sphingomyelin in the smooth muscle cell of the normal rat aorta. This data supported the conclusion that the plasma membrane differed in composition from the intracellular membrane in that it was richer in sphingomyelin relative to cholesterol. The increase in sphingomyelin could, therefore, be accounted in part by this increase in plasma membrane. Sphingomyelinase activity was lysosomal, however, not in the plasma membrane, although lecithinase activity may be present in the plasma membrane.

The question of relative rather than absolute increases in phospholipids were raised by Dr. Hodara and he suggested that the high levels of accumulated phospholipid may be associated not only with their reduced degradation but with increased synthesis. Dr. Stein indicated, however, that the synthesis of phospholipid was similar in all portions of the media.

Dr. Day raised the question of the role of phosphatidyl inositol in the normal arterial wall. It has been demonstrated by P^{32}-incorporation studies that the turnover of phosphatidyl inositol is faster than any other of the phospholipids in the normal intima and further that a reduction in its turnover occurs as atherosclerosis proceeds (Newman *et al.*, 1966). Dr. Stein suggested that although phosphatidyl inositol turnover has been linked with transport phenomena (Hokin and Hokin, 1955) the role of phosphatidyl inositol in the arterial wall has not been determined.

ARTERIAL WALL TRIGLYCERIDE HYDROLASES

A. Vost

Despite the early observation of Korn (1955) that acetone powders of aortas released glycerol or monoglyceride from chylomicrons, the investigation of arterial lipases has been sparse. Progress in this area has been hampered by studies in which substrates have been inappropriate or without adequate specificity. However, the two major groups of lipases, storage glyceride lipases (Patelski et al., 1967) and lipoprotein triglyceride lipase (Vost and Pocock, 1973) have been demonstrated in mammalian aorta. Storage glyceride lipases in the human aorta have two pH optima, one at 5.4 and the other at 8.8, and it is possible that earlier findings of a single alkaline pH optimum in other mammals reflect inactivation of acid lipase by distiled water extraction (Hayase and Miller, 1970). The acid lipase, by analogy with liver and other tissues may be lysosomal. As in adipose tissue, aortic storage lipase activity exhibits hormonal control and is stimulated by epinephrine, norepinephrine, glucagon and ACTH; however, insulin, in contrast to its effect in adipose tissue, also stimulates lipolysis according to Chmelar and Chmelarova (1968).

Lipoprotein lipase-like activity had been observed in aortas but the inhibition characteristics of the crude enzyme activity with protamine and saline had not been those of classical lipoprotein lipase. These difficulties may have been due to lack of substrate specificity and recent studies with ^{14}C-labeled triolein preincubated in serum have shown that the aortic enzyme has the same inhibition characteristics as the classical adipose tissue enzyme (Vost and Pocock, 1973). From the limited data available, chylomicron triglycerides in perfused aorta are hydrolyzed to a small extent but this is after arterial uptake (Vost, 1972). Consequently, a major unresolved problem is the position of lipoprotein lipase in the arterial wall and the transport pathway of its large diameter substrates-- chylomicrons and VLDL, from serum to the site of enzyme action.

As an adenyl cyclase system is present in arterial wall (Schonhofer et al., 1971) and there is hormonal stimulation of storage lipase activity, it is possible that co-ordinated regulation of lipoprotein lipase and storage lipase exists as in adipose tissue and is mediated by nucleotides.

Discussion

Dr. Patelski considered that the differences in pH optima reported for lipase activity could be explained by the different methods of extraction used. Distilled water has been successfully used for lipase extraction. It is possible that other extractants may give better results. He also pointed out that chylomicrons present a more physiological substrate to lipase than hydrosols, though they contain substrates for other esterases as well. When glycerol trioleate hydrosol is used, the enzyme activity measured is lipase though other esterases are present in the crude enzyme preparation. Dr. Day raised the question of a connection between lipase activity and neutral fat accumulation in the arterial wall. Triglycerides do not markedly increase in the atherosclerotic artery. Comment was invited on the role of lipase with respect to triglyceride turnover in regard to the atherosclerotic lesion. Dr. Vost indicated that very little information was available regarding glyceride turnover in relation to the atherosclerotic lesion or of the quantitative contribution of chylomicron triglyceride fatty acids compared with

free fatty acids as substrates for cellular triglyceride synthesis in arterial
wall. Dr. Vost speculated that a lipoprotein lipase enzyme in arterial wall might
partially degrade chylomicrons removing triglycerides but allowing chylomicron
remnants, with higher concentrations of cholesteryl esters and other lipids, to
remain. No data on the formation or uptake of chylomicron remnants by the arterial
wall is available. Dr. Olga Stein indicated that it was unlikely that chylomicrons
could contribute significantly to the arterial wall lipid in view of their size
relative to low density lipoprotein. Dr. Vost concurred that, in quantitative
terms, this was true but that transport of other large diameter particles (such
as high M.W. dextrans) across continuous endothelium was well established; his
data demonstrated that some chylomicron triglyceride uptake did occur in normal
arterial wall.

STEROL-ESTER HYDROLASE (EC3.1.1.13)

D.E. Bowyer and J.D. Pearson

Sterol-ester hydrolase is the systematic name given to the enzymes which are responsible for the reaction:

Sterol-ester $\rightleftharpoons$ Sterol and fatty acid.

These enzymes are often referred to as cholesteryl ester hydrolase or cholesterol
esterase, implying.that cholesteryl esters are preferred substrates. Sterol-ester
hydrolase could bring about the synthesis of sterol-esters under some conditions
by the reversal of the hydrolytic cleavage, but there is no evidence to show that
such conditions pertain *in vivo* and thus bring about cholesteryl ester accumulation in tissues.

Enzymatic cholesteryl ester hydrolysis was first demonstrated by Klein (1938,
1939) in extracts of pancreas and other organs (see the review of cholesteryl
ester metabolism by Goodman, 1965). Subsequently the pancreatic enzyme was extensively studied, especially by Swell and Treadwell (1955). This enzyme has an
absolute requirement for taurocholate and a pH optimum of 6.6. Other enzymes catalysing sterol-ester hydrolysis, not requiring bile salts, and with a broad pH
optimum between 7 and 8 are present in tissues which have a high turnover of cholesterol esters such as liver, adrenal, testes, ovaries and developing brain. An
arterial sterol-ester hydrolase was first demonstrated by Patelski (1964) but the
earliest reference commonly cited for the demonstration of sterol-ester hydrolysis
by aortic tissue is Day and Gould-Hurst (1966).

Our particular interest in the arterial enzymes centers on the fact that cholesteryl esters accumulate in all forms of atherosclerotic lesion. It is clear that
these may be derived either from the plasma lipoproteins or from local synthesis.
Extracellular cholesteryl esters have the same composition as the plasma lipoprotein cholesteryl esters, which in man are rich in linoleic acid, whilst intracellular cholesteryl esters are mainly cholesteryl oleate (Smith et al., 1967). Thus
sterol-ester hydrolase could be important in controlling the fatty acid composition of the intracellular cholesteryl ester pool. Furthermore, tissue culture
studies from Werb and Cohn (1972) and Rothblat and Kritchevsky (1968) indicate
that only free cholesterol and not cholesteryl esters can leave cells and this
suggests that sterol-ester hydrolase activity could control the intra-cellular
concentrations of cholesteryl esters. By analogy with cholesteryl ester storage
disease and Wolmans disease (Sloan and Fredrickson, 1972) and other lipidoses
(Brady, 1972), an enzyme deficiency would lead to cholesteryl ester accumulation.
In contrast to studies of lipidoses, however, in which estimation of enzymeactiv-
ity *in vitro* has lead to the unequivocal realisation that an enzyme deficiency
exists *in vivo*, measurements of arterial cholesteryl ester hydrolase has not
produced such obvious conclusions. Difficulties exist partly because of the low

Table 1. Sterol-ester hydrolase activity in aortic tissue: Summary of published results which can be referred to aortic tissue weights.

Author	Species	Enzyme preparation	Assay method	Substrate concentration	pH	Notes[a]	Rate[b]
Patelski et al., 1967; Patelski et al., 1968b	Pig	Extracts from AcBu powders	pH-Stat	1mM	8.6	U U,TC U,TC,GSH	20 50 400
Patelski et al., 1968a	Rat	Extracts from wet tissue	pH-Stat	1mM	8.6	U,TC,GSH D,TC,GSH	500 45
Patelski et al., 1968a	Rabbit	Extracts from wet tissue	pH-Stat	1mM	8.6	U,TC,GSH D,TC,GSH	210 40
Patelski et al., 1970	Rabbit	Extracts from AcBu powders	pH-Stat	1mM	8.6	U,TC,GSH D,TC,GSH	45 14
Patelski and Tipton, 1971	Pig	Subcellular fractions	pH-Stat	1mM	8.6	U,TC,GSH	30-60
Howard et al., 1971	Baboon	Extracts from AcBu powders	pH-Stat	1mM	8.6	U,TC,GSH D,TC,GSH	40 34
Howard and Portman, 1966	Rat	Subcellular fractions	radio-activity	5-40μM	7.4	U,GSH	0.01
Howard and Portman, 1966	Monkey	Subcellular fractions	radio-activity	5-40μM	7.4	U,GSH	0.01
Felt and Benes, 1969	Rat	Tissue slices	radio-activity	?	7.4	U	0.1
St. Clair et al., 1970	Pigeon	Subcellular fractions	radio-activity	10uM-1mM	7.5	U D,3 mths D,8 mths	<0.1 5.0 <0.5
Kothari et al., 1970	Human	Subcellular fractions	colori-metric	2.6mM	6.6 and 7.5	U,TC ±GSH	0.7
Kothari et al., 1973	Rat	Extracts from Ac ether powders	radio-activity	0.6-1.3mM	6.6 and 7.5	U,TC	1.0 0.4
Kothari et al., 1973	Rabbit	Extracts from Ac ether powders	radio-activity	0.6-1.3mM	6.6 and 7.5	U,TC	1.0 0.4

[a]Notes - U = undiseased tissue, D = diseased tissue, TC = sodium taurocholate present, GSH = reduced glutathione present.

[b]All rates expressed as nmol/mg dry tissue/h.

activity of the enzyme in aorta, and also because the conditions of the *in vitro* assay affect the apparent enzyme activity.

The following considerations, pertinent to measurement of enzyme activity, emerge from a survey of previous studies.

1. Method of Measurement

These have included:

a) the chemical assay of released fatty acid or cholesterol (e.g. Kothari et ál., (1970);
b) continous titration of released fatty acid at constant pH in the pH-stat (e.g. Patelski et al., 1967);
c) radiochemical assay of the released product from a labelled substrate (e.g. Howard and Portman, 1966).

The first two techniques are barely sensitive enough. As shown in Table 1, the results obtained with the pH-stat show a large discrepancy from those obtained by the radiochemical technique.

2. Method of Enzyme Preparation

In order to measure enzyme specific activity, it is necessary to purify the enzyme protein from other tissue proteins. This is particularly important for the arterial wall, because the amounts of collagen, elastin and connective tissue are very variable, depending in part upon age and atherosclerosis. The methods have included:

a) preparation of a subcellular fraction by centrifugation after homogenization. Homogenization of whole tissue is difficult and sub-cellular localization of of enzyme activity may be lost. Studies directed at sub-cellular distribution are best done on isolated cell preparations (Peters et al., 1973);
b) extraction of wet tissue slices with water or salt solutions or glycerol-water (Patelski et al., 1967);
c) preparation of an acetone or acetone-butanol powder from homogenate or sub-cellular fraction followed by drying of the powder and extraction of the enzyme protein as in (b) above. This approach is also important because it removes endogenous substrate. Acetone-butanol powders are apparently stable if kept at low temperature although the enzyme extract is inactivated by heating and also by -SH inhibitors; the latter is prevented by reduced glutathione (see Patelski et al., 1968a).

3. Method of Substrate Presentation

In studies of enzymes of lipid metabolism, the method of presentation of the substrate may markedly affect the apparent activity of the enzyme. Essentially three methods have been used in studies of cholesteryl ester hydrolase.

a) Dispersion of the cholesteryl ester as a hydrosol by injection of a solution of the ester in acetone or ethanol into water or directly into the reaction mixture (Patelski et al., 1967, Howard and Portman, 1966). The particle size of the dispersion varies depending upon the temperature of the preparation, extent of mixing, and upon the particular cholesteryl ester and its final concentration. The homogeneity of particle size may be improved by sonication. The volume of acetone used should be less than 1% of the final reaction volume, because it may inhibit the enzyme (see Brecher et al., 1973).
b) Preparation of a micellar substrate containing surfactants such as lecithin, free fatty acids or bile salts which are then sonicated (Kothari et al., 1970).

Care should be exercised in adding free fatty acids because they may act as product inhibitors (Brecher et al., 1973).

c) The substrates may be stabilized as an emulsion with protein such as albumin, although a more physiological stabilizer such as apolipoprotein might be desirable (Kothari et al., 1970).

The form of the substrate presentation may influence the pH optimum of the enzyme, possibly because of an effect on the charge distribution or zeta potential of the lipid-water interface at which the enzyme acts. Thus, Kothari et al. (1970) have shown in acetone dry powder of normal rat and rabbit aorta and in homogenate fractions of human aorta that a micellar substrate had a pH optimum of 6.6 and was better hydrolyzed by the same preparation than an albumin emulsified substrate which had a pH optimum in the range pH 7.4 to 7.8. A further consideration is that detergent molecules such as taurocholate may affect activity by:

a) improving the emulsification;

b) being a specific cofactor for the enzyme or stabilizing a polymeric form of the enzyme in an active configuration and preventing its breakdown. This has been demonstrated for the pancreatic enzyme (Vahouny et al., 1967), although it seems unlikely to be the case in the arterial wall;

c) causing the release of enzyme from sub-cellular fractions such as lysosomes into the reaction mixture. Latency of the lysosomal enzymes studied by Peters et al. (1973) and Kothari et al. (1970) was observed by addition of Triton.

4. Role of Enzyme Inhibitors

The enzyme has been shown to be inhibited *in vitro* by excess substrate (Patelski, 1964 and Johnson and Moskowitz, 1968). Product inhibition has also been demonstrated by free fatty acid even in the presence of albumin, but was not found with cholesterol (Brecher et al., 1973). Enzyme inhibitors which have also been described include 1 mM-para-chloro-mercuri-benzoate (which is reversed by reduced glutathione) and 1mM concentration of salts of Hg^{++}, Zn^{++}, Cu^{++} (Kothari et al., 1970, Ca^{++}, Na^+, and K^+ (Patelski et al., 1968b).

Some Conclusions Concerning the Role of Cholesteryl Ester Hydrolase in Atherogenesis

Early studies (Patelski et al., 1968a) had suggested that the activity of arterial cholesteryl ester hydrolase is higher in species resistant to atherosclerosis, such as rat, than in susceptible ones such as rabbit. This idea now receives support from the work of Bonner et al. (1972) and Kritchevsky (1974), although the absolute rates of ester hydrolysis found in the studies of Patelski et al., using pH-stat, are unaccountably high. This may be because the pH-stat has a low specificity, measuring only released acidity, and that a non-specific esterase was also being assayed. The pH optimum (pH 8.6) was also higher than has been found in other studies (Kothari et al., 1970, pH 6.6 - 7.8 depending on substrate presentation and Peters et al., 1973, pH 4.25 for a lysosomal enzyme). The work of Patelski (Patelski et al., 1968a, Patelski et al., 1970) had also suggested that within one species there is a decreased activity of the enzyme in aorta during the induction of the experimental fatty streak. More recent studies have failed to substantiate this (Brecher et al., 1973; Peters et al., 1973), although St. Clair et al. (1970) have pointed out that interpretation of such a study depends upon whether it is assumed that the exogenous substrate equilibrates with the endogenous cholesteryl esters or not. In the study of St. Clair, only if it was assumed that no equilibration had occurred, was there a fall in apparent activity.

It is becoming clear that a major part of sterol-ester hydrolase activity is lysosomal and the activity increases together with the activities of other lysosomal enzymes during fatty streak formation (Peters et al., 1973; Bonner et al., 1972; Kothari et al., 1970; Kothari et al., 1972). Nonetheless, the lysosomal activity may be inadequate to prevent cholesteryl ester accumulation in the cell especially

in susceptible species which have a relatively low activity of the enzyme. This
is made more likely by the discovery (Peters et al., 1973) of a class of low density lysosomes in smooth muscle cells from aortic fatty streaks in rabbits, which
have a high concentration of cholesterol, but a cholesteryl ester hydrolase activity which is relatively lower than that in high density lysosomes. The possibility
of increasing the effective action of cholesteryl ester hydrolase by lysosomal
activation, or by enzyme activation, as occurs in some tissues under hormonal control, for example in ovary (Behrman et al., 1971) remains speculative.

Discussion

Dr. Patelski described some of the problems relating to the quantitation of cholesteryl ester hydrolases, which depended on some of the different methods used.
Changes of substrate concentration, incubation times etc. give a marked difference
in the amount of enzyme activity determined. The ratio of synthesis to hydrolysis
reported by Kritchevsky may also be subject to some question. Comparison on this
basis may not necessarily be valid.

Dr. St. Clair raised the question of the function of cholesteryl ester hydrolysis
within cells in regard to removal of cholesterol from cells, and some discussion
with respect to the role of cholesteryl ester hydrolase in the removal of cholesteryl ester from the atherosclerotic wall and in the regression of lesions
ensued. The paper reported by Howard and Patelski (1973) in which accentuation of
cholesteryl esterase activity by lipostabil was described, but in which no regression occurred as evidenced by loss of lipid might be interpreted to suggest that
sterol-ester hydrolase does not play a role in the removal of lipid from the
atherosclerotic arterial wall. However, the stage at which stimulation of cholesteryl ester hydrolase activity is present may be important so that the above conclusion may not necessarily be valid.

Dr. Smith pointed out that extracellular free cholesterol accumulation is a characteristic of older lesions and that the removal of cholesteryl ester was not
associated with a reduced level of total cholesterol. Thus the hydrolysis of
cholesteryl esters and the accumulation of free cholesterol may take place in the
evolution of the older lesions, and not be associated with regression but with the
accumulation of more extracellular free cholesterol in the plaque.

CHOLESTEROL ESTERIFYING ENZYMES OF ARTERIAL TISSUE

R. St. Clair

The increase in the cholesteryl ester content of arterial tissue is a hallmark of
atherosclerosis in man and virtually all experimental animals that have been studied. The origin, however, of this accumulated cholesteryl ester is not clear.
Some appears to come from esterification of cholesterol within cells of the arterial wall while some cholesteryl esters also come from the plasma (Dayton and
Hashimoto, 1968; Smith et al., 1967).

Several investigators have shown in a number of animal species that cholesterol
esterification is enhanced in atherosclerotic compared with normal arterial tissue
(Dayton and Hashimoto, 1968; St. Clair et al., 1970; Day and Wahlqvist, 1968).

The rate of esterification of fatty acids to cholesterol is positively correlated
with the extent of atherosclerosis (Fig. 1). In the experiments described in this
figure, squirrel monkey aortic tissue was maintained in organ culture for four
days with radioactive oleic acid as substrate. There is a positive and significant
correlation of stimulation of cholesterol esterification with the extent of

atherosclerosis as measured by the cholesterol content of the arterial tissue.
Increased cholesterol esterification can be demonstrated early in the progression
of the disease and suggests a role in the early events in the development of the
atherosclerotic lesion (St. Clair et al., 1970).

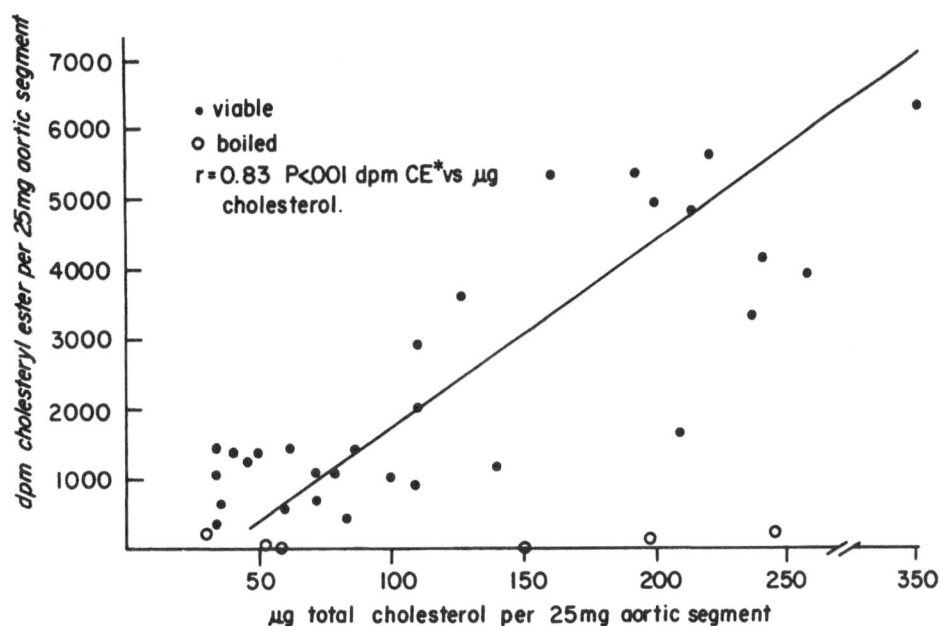

Figure 1. Effect of arterial cholesterol content on esterification of exogenously-
derived cholesterol by organ cultures of squirrel monkey aorta. The culture
medium contained 29% bovine serum and squirrel monkey LDL with $(1,2-^3H)$ cholesterol; *cholesterol ester

We have recently been able to demonstrate stimulation of cholesterol esterification *in vitro* using either fatty acid or cholesterol as substrate, with organ
cultures of normal pigeon aorta incubated for relatively short periods of time
with hypercholesterolaemic pigeon serum (Table 1). This provides further evidence
that stimulation of cholesterol esterification is one of the earliest changes in
atherogenesis. Most evidence suggests that the increased cholesterol esterification is taking place within the foam cells of the lesions (Day and Tume, 1970).
In our studies with pigeons, an increase in cholesterol esterification parallels
the appearance of fat-filled cells within the arterial wall. When cholesterol is
removed from the diet of these birds, the foam cells gradually disappear (Wagner
and Clarkson, 1973) along with a rapid decline in cholesterol esterification
(St. Clair et al., 1972). Indirect evidence obtained from studies on chemical
composition of human lesions also suggests that the fat-filled cells are a site
of active cholesterol esterification (Smith et al., 1967).

There are now several reports indicating at least three mechanisms for cholesterol
esterification in arterial tissue.

1. Lecithin cholesterol fatty acyl transferase (cholesterol + lecithin - cholesteryl ester + lyso-lecithin).
2. Fatty acyl-CoA-cholesterol acyl transferase (cholesterol + fatty acyl-CoA -
   cholesteryl ester + CoASH).
3. Cholesterol ester synthetase (cholesterol esterase) (cholesterol + fatty acid
   - cholesterol ester + H_2O).

Table 1. Stimulation of cholesterol esterification in organ cultures of pigeon aorta: effect of hypercholesterolemic pigeon serum[a]

	Substrate	N	Medium Cholesterol Content	Cholesterol Ester Synthesis	Arterial Cholesterol	
					FC	CE
			mg/ml	µg/25 mg segment	µg/25 mg segment	
50% NCS[b]	Chol.-1,2-^{3}H	3	1.65	6.1	-	-
50% HCS[c]	Chol.-1,2-^{3}H	3	6.92	11.8	-	-
5% NCS	Oleate-1-^{14}C	3	0.17	0.08	51.9	5.3
50% NCS	Oleate-1-^{14}C	6	1.69	0.64	57.6	5.1
50% HCS	Oleate-1-^{14}C	6	7.33	4.26	71.6	20.7

[a]All cultures were maintained for nine days. [b]NCS = normocholesterolemic pigeon serum. [c]HCS = hypercholesterolemic pigeon serum.

Abdulla and coworkers (1968) have reported the presence of lecithin cholesterol fatty acyl transferase in arterial tissue from man and rabbit. Evidence from several other laboratories, however, suggests that if present this enzyme is in low concentration in arterial wall tissue.

Most evidence suggests that the primary stimulation of cholesterol esterification in atherosclerotic arteries is by the enzyme fatty acyl-CoA-cholesterol acyl transferase (St. Clair et al., 1970; Felt and Benes, 1969; Proudlock and Day, 1972; Hashimoto et al., 1973; Brecher et al., 1973). This enzyme requires ATP and Coenzyme A, has a pH optimum of 7.0-7.5, and is localized primarily in the microsomal fraction. Increases of greater than 50 fold in the activity of this enzyme have been reported for atherosclerotic pigeon and rabbit aorta (St. Clair et al., 1970; Brecher et al., 1973).

More recent evidence suggests that in atherosclerotic tissue there is an increase in the activity of an acid pH active cholesterol ester synthetase (Proudlock and Day, 1972; Brecher et al., 1973; Kothari et al., 1970). Whether this is a lysosomal enzyme remains to be determined. Whether all or only certain of these enzymes are increased in atherosclerotic lesions of different morphological types from different animal species under different sets of experimental conditions is not known. The relative contribution of each of these enzyme systems to the total newly synthesized cholesteryl ester is unknown.

Although considerable information is available on the mechanisms and changes in cholesterol esterification in atherosclerotic arterial tissue, there are still major questions that remain unanswered. Some of the questions include:

1. What actually stimulates cholesterol esterification and by what mechanism?
2. Is cholesterol esterification important only in the fatty streak and not in fibrous lesions?
3. Is cholesterol esterification involved in the etiology of the development of the lesion or is its stimulation simply a result of the disease?
4. What is the role of the lysosome in the accumulation of cholesterol esters?
5. What is the relative importance of cholesterol esterification, cholesteryl ester hydrolysis and influx of cholesteryl esters from the plasma on the accumulation of cholesteryl esters in the arterial wall?

Discussion

The presence of lecithin cholesterol acyl transferase in arterial wall was considered. Dr. Adams pointed out that although their finding of LCAT activity in
the arterial wall had been confirmed (Patelski et al., private communication),
other laboratories had failed to demonstrate such activity. Dr. Day indicated the
possibility of induction of cholesterol esterifying enzymes by mechanisms apart
from increased cholesterol entry into the arterial wall. For example, there is
data suggesting that hypertension in the absence of cholesterol feeding (Bretherton, Day and Skinner, unpublished data) and also platelet thrombi (Day et al.,
1973) may both result in increased esterification of cholesterol in the arterial
wall.

A COMPARISON OF THE RATES OF LIPOLYSIS AND LIPOGENESIS IN THE RAT AORTA

C.H. Gilbert and D.J. Galton

Many external factors such as hypertriglyceridaemia and hypercholesterolaemia may be involved in the deposition of subintimal lipid in the arteries of susceptible animals. But the aorta wall can synthesise neutral and phospholipids de novo; and the pathways for synthesis of neutral lipid in rat aorta are similar to liver and adipose tissue (Stein et al., 1963). The contribution that de novo lipogenesis makes to the atheromatous plaque is not clear. However, one local tissue factor that may be of importance for the accumulation of subintimal lipid is the relative rates of lipid synthesis and mobilisation of lipids by lipolysis. We have, therefore, compared the rates of lipogenesis from glucose in the rat aorta to the maximal rates of lipolysis of glycerolipids produced by stimulation with catecholamines.

Methods

Measurements were performed with intact pieces of aorta from Wistar rats (150-180 g) which had been fed ad libitum on laboratory chow. The rats were transferred to the laboratory and allowed to acclimatise for at least 1 hour to reduce stress before sacrifice. Aortas were removed quickly and dissected in 0.9% saline. All visible surrounding fat and connective tissue were dissected away and histological examination showed that nearly all adventitial adipose tissue had been removed.

Lipolysis

Aorta pieces (15-40 mg) were pre-incubated for 30 min at 37° in 5 ml of Earle's bicarbonate buffer (pH 7.4) containing 1% crystalline bovine serum albumin. The aorta pieces were then transferred to fresh buffer containing appropriate agents and incubated for 5 min for assay of cyclic-AMP and for 2 hrs to measure release of glycerol according to the methods of Gilbert and Galton (1973).

Lipogenesis

Aorta pieces (15-40 mg) were incubated in 0.5 ml of Earle's bicarbonate buffer (pH 7.4) containing 1% crystalline serum albumin and ^{14}C-U-glucose (8 mM, 1 μCi/ml). At the end of incubation, aorta pieces were washed, blotted and then weighed. Tissue lipids were extracted and radioactivity measured in 10 ml of a toluene PPO scintillator as described by Galton et al. (1971).

Results

Evidence for the presence of a hormone-sensitive cyclase system in rat aorta is presented in Fig. 1 and 2. Fluoride (10^{-2} M), an agent which activates adenyl cyclase, was found to elevate levels of cyclic-AMP in aorta wall; and theophylline, which inhibits the phosphodiesterase, had a similar effect. Adrenergic stimulation by isoprenaline (10^{-6} M) and noradrenaline (10^{-4} M) also raised the levels of cyclic-AMP in aorta walls. A dose response curve for isoprenaline is shown in Fig. 2 and maximal stimulation of cyclic-AMP was observed at 10^{-6} M (p <0.01, verus controls). This was followed by release of glycerol 50 minutes after the peak

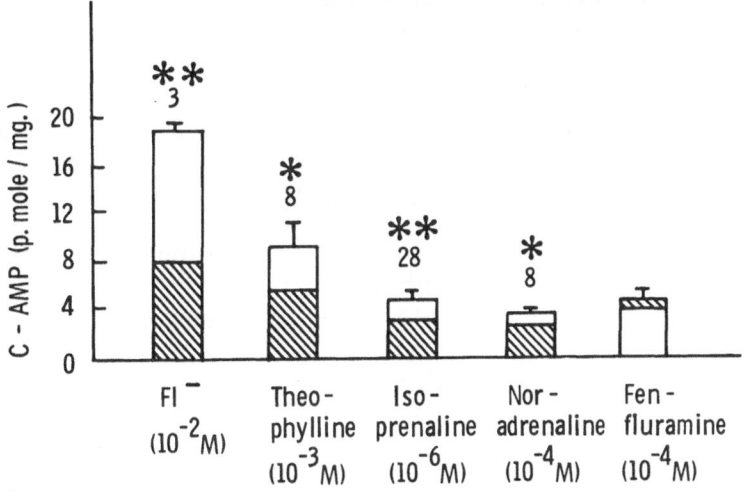

Figure 1. The effect of lipolytic agents on the level of cyclic-AMP in rat aorta. Small pieces of rat aorta (15-40 mg) were incubated for 5 min in 0.6 ml of albumin-bicarbonate buffer. Additions to the medium were made as listed above and the tissue was extracted and assayed for cyclic-AMP. Results are means of the number of observations in the absence (hatched colums) and presence (open columns) of the respective agent. Significance of differences were tested by Students t; $p^{**} < .01$, $p^{*} < .05$

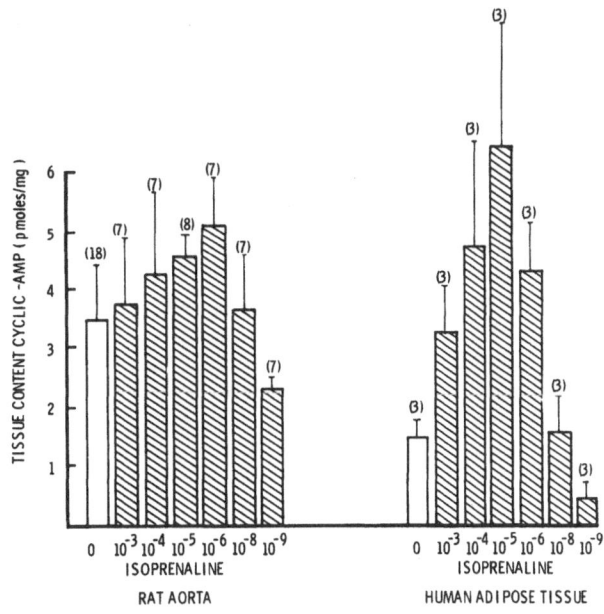

Figure 2. A dose response curve for action of isoprenaline on rat aorta and human adipose tissue. Small pieces of rat aorta (15-40 mg) or human adipose tissue (50-120 mg) were incubated for 5 min in 0.6 ml of albumin-bicarbonate buffer with increasing amounts of isoprenaline. Results are means of the number of observations indicated and bars enclose S.E.M.

response in cyclic-AMP. However, the maximal rate of release of glycerol from aorta walls stimulated by isoprenaline was a quarter that of the rate of conversion of glucose into lipids (Table 1). The corresponding values for adipose tissue are also shown in Table 1, the lipolytic activity of this tissue being approximately tenfold greater than the lipogenic capacity.

Table 1. A comparison of lipolysis and lipogenesis in aorta and adipose tissue

Tissue	Lipolysis μmoles/g/hr		Lipogenesis from glucose μmoles/g/hr
	basal	+ adrenaline	
Aorta	0.62 ± 0.09 (35)	0.95 ± 0.14 (35)	4.2 ± 2.6 (4)
Adipose tissue	0.47 ± 0.08 (5)	3.4 ± 0.9 (5)	0.35 ± 0.17 (7)

Representative values for adipose tissue are taken from previously published data using similar methods (Galton and Bray, 1967; Galton, 1969).

Discussion

The lipolytic sequence of ß-receptor, adenyl cyclase and lipase is demonstrated in rat aorta, and we confirm observations of Mahler (1966) and Chmelar and Chmelarova (1968) that this tissue contains a hormone-sensitive lipase. However, maximal release of glycerol from aorta was small and many replicates were required to observe statistically significant increases. This may partly reflect the low content of glycerolipids in aorta walls, but it also suggests a low lipolytic activity of the tissue. This is supported by the small increments in levels of cyclic-AMP in rat aorta after stimulation with catecholamines. In the rabbit, a species more susceptible to atheroma, Schonhaffer et al. (1971) were unable to observe any effects of isoprenaline on the accumulation of cyclic-AMP in strips of aorta.

By contrast, the lipogenic activity of rat aorta is readily demonstrated, and there is active incopropration of glucose (and palmitate) into neutral lipids of the aorta wall. It is possible that the discrepancy between lipolytic and lipogenic activities of aorta wall makes this tissue a particularly susceptible site for ectopic lipid deposition. The lipolytic activity of the aorta may be insufficient to mobilise lipids without consideration of the exogenous lipid derived from the blood stream.

PROPERTIES AND POSITIONAL SPECIFICITY OF LIPASES IN THE HUMAN AORTA

Akio Noma, Hiroaki Okabe, Toyozo Sakurada, Hajime Orimo, and
Mototaka Murakami

The presence of lipase in the human aortic wall was demonstrated by Adams et al.
(Adams et al., 1969). A detailed study on the properties of the enzyme was
reported by Hayase and Miller (Hayase et al., 1970). However, they used the whole
aortic tissue for preparing the enzyme sources. In this paper studies on the properties of lipases in the human aortic intima and media and on the role of these
enzymes in the development of atherosclerosis are presented.

Materials and Method

Aortas of human male adults were obtained at autopsy within 6-10 h of death. They
were separated into intima and media under a stereomicroscope. Intima and media
were homogenized separately in 8 volumes of ice-cold 0.01 M phosphate buffer,
pH 7.0, and centrifuged at 20,000 g for 15 min in a refrigerated centrifuge. The
supernatant was filtered through a layer of glasswool in order to remove the fatty
material floating on top of the tube. The filtrate was used as the enzyme source.

Lipolytic activity of the aorta was determined using ^{3}H-glyceryl trioleate as substrate. The incubation mixture consisted of 4 μmoles of substrate, 0.5 ml of 1%
of gum arabic in buffer, and 0.5 ml of enzyme solution. Final volume was 1 ml.
After 1 h of incubation at 37°C, the reaction was stopped by the addition of 3 ml
of a mixture of hexane-diethyl ether-ethanol (1:1:1, v/v/v). The extracted lipids
were applied on either silica gel G thin-layer plate or boric acid-impregnated
silica gel H plate. The silica gel plate was developed with a mixture of haxane-
diethylether-methanol-acetic acid (90:20:3:2, v/v/v/v) and the boric acid-impregnated plate with a mixture of chloroform-acetone (96:4, v/v). The spots on the
thin-layer plate were scraped off into counting vials and the radioactivity was
determined using an automatic scintillation spectrometer. Free ^{3}H-glycerol was
determined by taking an aliquot of the lower phase after extraction of the lipids
from the incubation.

Results and Discussion

Fig. 1 shows the effect of pH on the final composition of the glycerides obtained
when glyceryl trioleate was hydrolyzed by aortic intimal and medial lipases. Two
pH optima of 5.0-5.5 and 8.8 were observed in both intima and media. Increases of
diglyceride content were observed with increasing lipolytic activities, and monoglyceride contents were not significantly changed at any pH values.

The products of hydrolysis of glyceryl trioleate by aortic lipases were separated
by thin-layer chromatography using the boric acid-impregnated silica gel H plate.
This plate was used for the isolation of 1- and 2-monoglycerides and 1,2- and
1,3-diglycerides. As shown in Table 1, about 90% of the diglyceride fraction was
of 1,2-configuration and 70-80% of the monoglyceride fraction was of 2-configura-
tion in both intimal and medial acid lipases at all incubation periods. On the
other hand, gradual decreases in their percentages were observed in the alkaline
condition with increasing time of incubation. This might be due to the isomerization which took place in alkaline conditions (Noma et al., 1971) during incubation. In both intima and media, 2-monoglyceride occupied more than 73% of the
total monoglyceride and 1,2-diglyceride occupied more than 97% of the total diglyceride at 15-min-incubation. These results demonstrate that both acid and alkaline

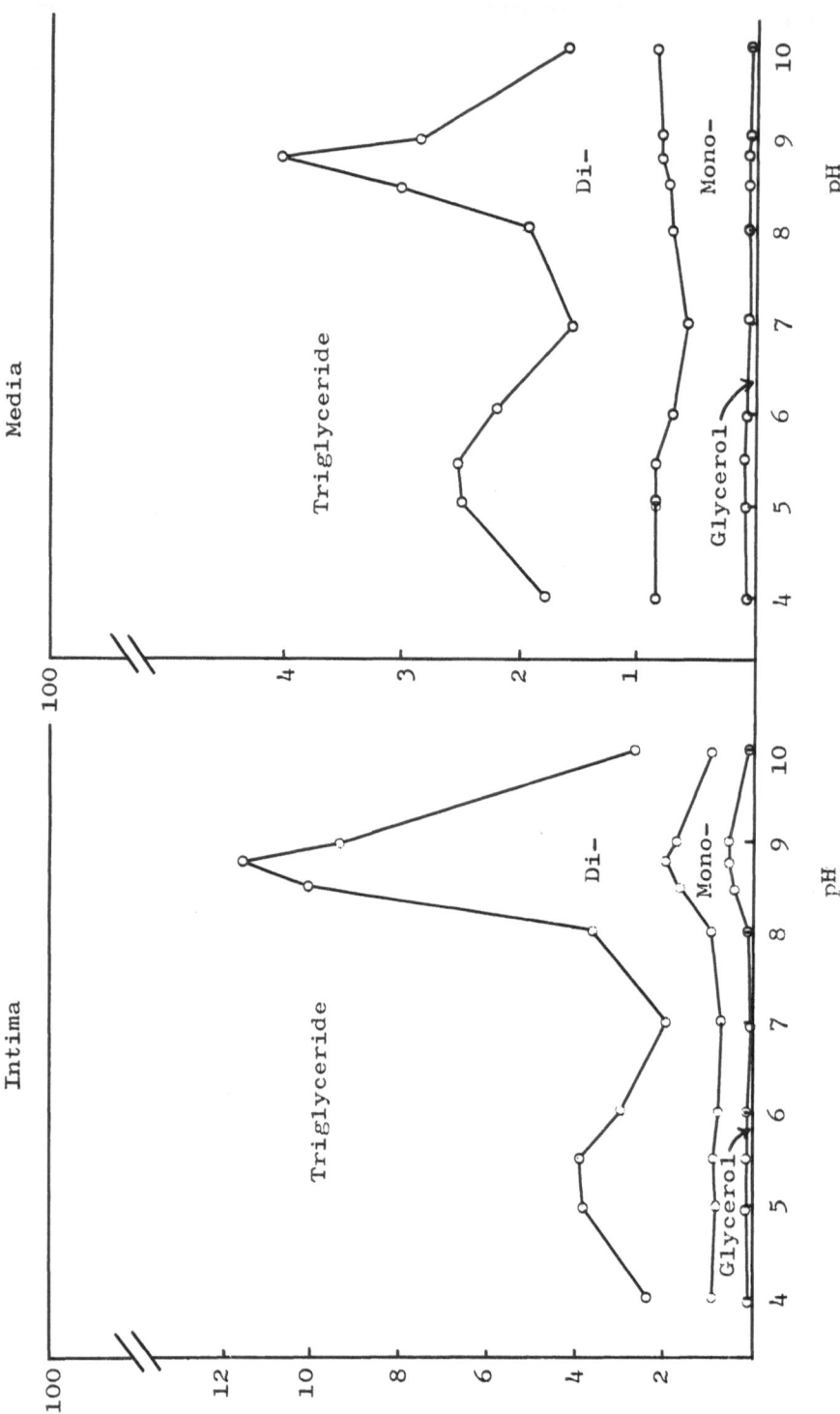

Figure 1. Molar percentage composition of glyceride products formed during lipolysis at different pH values by human aortic intimal and medial lipases. Substrate 4 μmoles of ^{3}H-glyceryl trioleate. Final volume 1 ml, incubation 1 h at 37°C

lipases of the intima and media act on the primary ester bonds of triglyceride. Furthermore, the specificities of alkaline lipases were stronger than those of acid ones.

Table 1. Percentages of 2-monoglyceride in total monoglyceride and 1,2-diglyceride in total diglyceride at various incubation periods

	Incubation Time min.	pH 5.0		pH 8.8	
		2-MG %	1,2-DG %	2-MG %	1,2-DG %
Intima	15	80.8	91.1	75.2	97.2
	30	76.1	90.8	72.0	96.3
	60	75.4	90.9	70.7	95.0
	90	79.7	91.2	70.2	93.3
	120	78.3	90.7	68.0	91.1
Media	15	71.4	89.3	73.0	97.1
	30	68.1	90.4	71.0	96.2
	60	72.6	91.0	67.4	96.0
	90	70.7	90.7	66.0	95.0
	120	70.8	91.5	65.6	92.3

Table 2 summarizes the results of the effect of various compounds on the hydrolysis of glyceryl trioleate by the intimal and medial alkaline lipases. Calcium ions had no effect on the activities of both alkaline lipases. Sodium deoxycholate activated both alkaline lipases, but the magnitude of the activation of the medial lipase was more marked than that of the intimal. 1 M of sodium chloride and 200 µg/ml of protamine sulphate significantly inhibited the activity (up to 70%) of the intimal alkaline lipase, but had no effect on the medial lipase. 2.5 ug/ml heparin slightly increased the activities of both lipases, but that of the intimal lipase was inhibited by 10 µg/ml of heparin.

These observations lead us to speculate that the main part of the intimal lipase might be lipoprotein lipase acting on lipoprotein triglyceride permeated from serum, and the medial lipase might be true lipase acting on triglyceride molecules.

Table 2. Effect of various compounds on lipolysis by aortic intimal and medial alkaline lipases

Addition	Intima	Media
Calcium chloride	no effect	no effect
Sodium deoxycholate	slightly activated	markedly activated
Sodium chloride (1 M)	markedly inhibited	no effect
Protamine sulphate	markedly inhibited	no effect
Heparin (Low concentration)	slightly activated	slightly activated
" (High concentration)	inhibited	no effect
Lecithin	slightly inhibited	no effect

THE INFLUENCE OF ATHEROSCLEROSIS ON CHOLESTEROL ESTERIFYING ACTIVITY OF RABBIT AND MONKEY AORTA[*]

P.I. Brecher, A. Tercyak, and A.V. Chobanian

Introduction

Cholesterol ester accumulation within the arterial wall appears to result from both intracellular synthesis and infiltration of plasma lipoproteins (Dayton and Hashimoto 1968; Chobanian and Manzur, 1972; Newman and Zilversmit, 1962; Smith et al., 1968). Recently there have been several reports demonstrating increased activity of arterial cholesterol esterifying enzymes in response to cholesterol feeding in While Carneau pigeons (St. Clair et al., 1970) and rabbits (Hashimoto et al., 1973). Two different enzyme systems in intimal homogenates from atherosclerotic rabbit aorta were recently described (Proudlock and Day, 1972). One system had a pH optimum of 5.0 and was independent of ATP and CoA while the second had a pH optimum of 7.5 and required ATP and CoA. We have studied some properties of these enzyme systems in both the rabbit and the Rhesus monkey and have investigated the effect of chlorophenoxyisobutyrate (clofibrate, CPIB) on these enzymes in rabbit aorta.

Methods

Female rabbits were maintained on an atherogenic diet containing 1% cholesterol for 2-36 weeks. The entire aorta was removed, stripped free of adventitia and homogenized in 10 volumes of sucrose buffer. The homogenates were centrifuged at 9000g for 20 min and the resulting supernatant spun at 161,000g to obtain the microsomal pellet and high speed supernatant.

Rhesus monkeys were maintained on a 1% cholesterol-0.5% cholic acid diet for 3 years. Extensive lesions in both thoracic and abdominal regions were observed. Details concerning the characteristics of these animals and the methodology are reported elsewhere (Brecher et al., 1973a).

The standard incubation mix used to assay for fatty acyl CoA:cholesterol acyltransferase contained 70 umoles tris (pH 7.4), 0.8 μmoles $MgSO_4$, 1 μmole dithiothreitol, 2 μmoles ATP, 0.25 μmoles CoA, 0.6 nmoles labeled oleic acid and 50 μg microsomal protein. Total incubation volume was 0.25 ml. Control incubations without ATP and CoA were routinely included. Following incubation at 37°C for 90 min, the reaction was terminated with chloroform:methanol (2:1). The lipids were extracted (Folch et al., 1957), the lipid classes were separated by TLC, and the radioactivity in the cholesterol ester fraction was determined as described (Brecher et al., 1973b).

Activity at pH 5.2 was measured by adding 0.5 volume of sodium acetate buffer (pH 5.2) to 1.0 volume of aortic high speed supernatant. The reaction was performed in a total volume of 0.2 ml and initiated by the addition of 4 μl of an acetone solution containing labeled oleic acid (0.25 mM). Incubations were routinely performed at 37°C for 60 min, and radioactive incorporation into cholesteryl ester determined as described above. Protein was measured by the method of Lowry et al. (1951) and cholesterol determined by gas chromatography (Brecher et al., 1973b).

---

[*]Supported by USPHS Grants HL 12869 and HL 13262 and the U.A. Whitaker Fund.

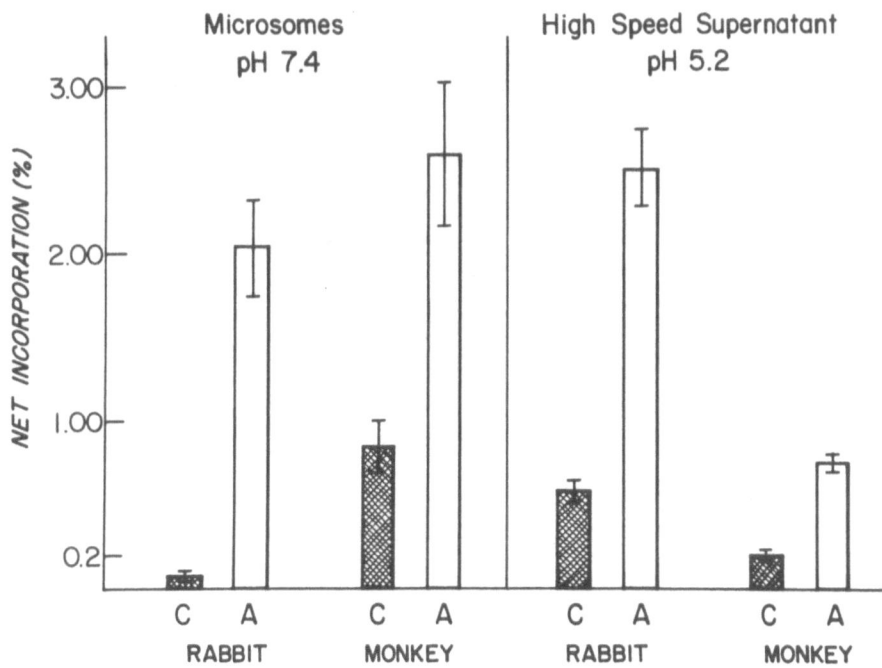

Figure 1. Incorporation of 1-^{14}C-oleic acid into cholesteryl esters in subcellular fractions of rabbit and Rhesus monkey aortas. The number of animals per group was 6 and 4 for rabbit and Rhesus monkey, respectively. C = control; A = atherosclerotic

Results and Discussion

The incorporation of labeled oleic acid into cholesteryl ester was much greater in subcellular fractions from atherosclerotic tissue of both rabbit and monkey than in the non-atherosclerotic controls (Fig. 1). Preliminary studies showed that the ATP and CoA dependent system was localized in the microsomal fraction, whereas the activity at pH 5.2 was mainly in the supernatant fraction. The most dramatic increase occurred in the microsomal fraction of rabbit atherosclerotic aorta, although significant increases were seen in both species for both enzyme systems. Studies of the characteristics of these systems indicated that the microsomal enzyme was a fatty acyl CoA:cholesterol acyltransferase, as suggested by other workers (St. Clair et al., 1970; Hashimoto et al., 1973), whereas the activity at pH 5.2 was not clearly defined.

Microsomal enzyme activity was determined in rabbit aortic tissue with varying degrees of atherosclerosis. The correlation between total aortic cholesterol content and activity is shown by Fig. 2. This data was obtained from thoracic and abdominal segments from 15 rabbits fed an atherogenic diet for 2-16 weeks. The high correlation coefficient (r=0.93) emphasizes the relationship between activity and the degree of atherosclerosis. It is possible that the increased enzymatic activity seen in atherosclerotic preparations could be a result of greater free cholesterol content since the exogenously added labeled oleic acid is esterified to endogenous microsomal cholesterol. When the free cholesterol content of microsomal preparations was compared with enzymatic activity, a less significant correlation (r=0.51) was obtained, suggesting that endogenous cholesterol does not fully account for the increased activity. The increased activity seen in atherosclerotic tissue could be related to the proliferation of endoplasmic reticulum previously demonstrated in rabbits as a result of cholesterol feeding (Parker et al., 1966).

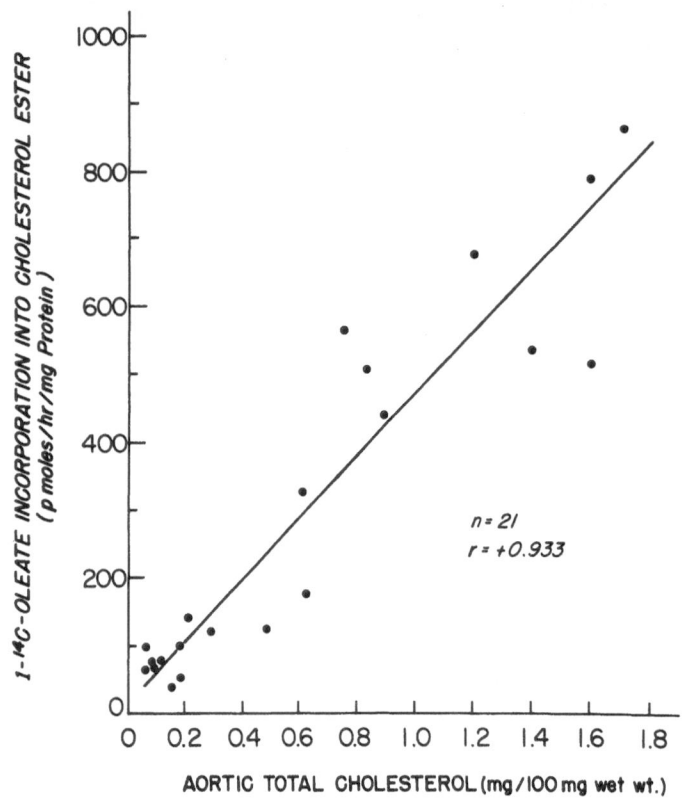

Figure 2. Correlation between fatty acyl CoA cholesterol acyltransferase activity and total aortic cholesterol content of thoracic and abdominal sections from normal and cholesterol fed rabbits

The increased incorporation of oleic acid into the high speed supernatant fraction at pH 5.2 in both monkey and rabbit aorta has not been previously reported. Although significant increases in oleic acid incorporation were observed in atherosclerotic supernatant fractions, increases in the cholesterol content of these fractions were also seen. Thus, in comparing the pH 5.2 activity in the high speed supernatant fraction of 6 control and 6 cholesterol-fed rabbits (8-12 weeks), we found an 8 fold increase both in oleic acid incorporation and in free cholesterol content. One therefore cannot exclude the possibility that increased substrate was responsible for the greater activity seen in the atherosclerotic preparations. The significance of this activity is not clear since exchange mechanisms, free cholesterol content, or other factors may play a role within the in vitro system. The acidic pH of this activity may indicate a lysosomal origin, the aortic lysosomes being disrupted and solubilized during homogenization.

The effect of clofibrate on both enzyme systems in shown in Fig. 3. Inhibition was observed in both cases but the microsomal enzyme was clearly more sensitive to the drug. A 50% reduction in microsomal activity was seen at a clofibrate concentration of about 5 mM, whereas much greater amounts of the drug were required to obtain a comparable inhibition of the activity at pH 5.2. Clofibrate has been shown to inhibit other microsomal enzymes involved in lipid metabolism (Avoy et al., 1965; Lamb and Fallon, 1972; Lamb et al., 1973), but no effects of clofibrate on aortic cholesterol metabolism have been reported previously.

Our data adds to the evidence that intracellular synthesis contributes to the accumulation of cholesteryl ester seen in atherosclerotic lesions. We have shown that two arterial enzyme systems exhibited increased activity as a result of

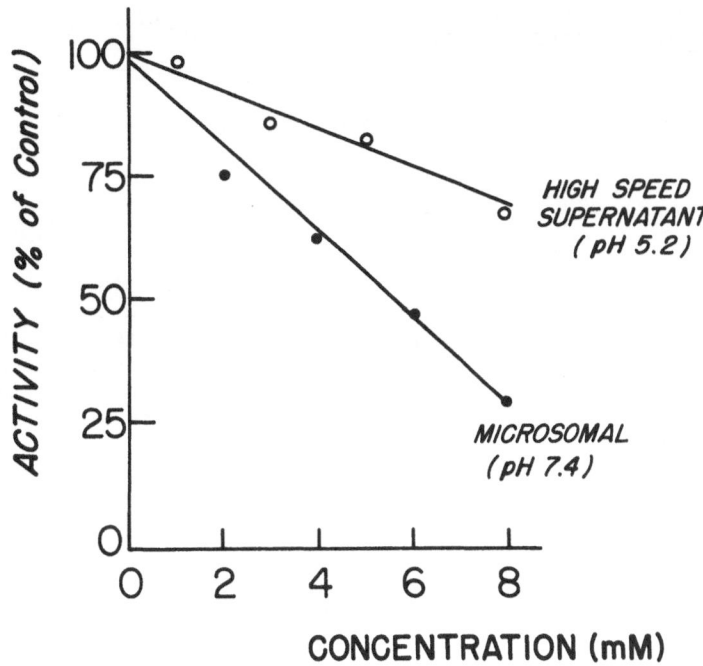

Figure 3. The effect of clofibrate on the microsomal (pH 7.4) and high speed supernatant (pH 5.2) activities in atherosclerotic rabbit aorta

cholesterol feeding in both the rabbit and a primate species, the Rhesus monkey. Furthermore, the hypolipemic agent clofibrate can inhibit both enzyme systems under in vitro conditions.

AORTIC UPTAKE OF CHYLOMICRON TRIGLYCERIDE IN VIVO AND AORTIC LIPO-PROTEIN TRIGLYCERIDE LIPASE IN RAT[*]

Alan Vost and Dorothy M-E. Pocock

In humans, high dietary fat intake is associated with high fasting serum cholesterol and a high incidence of ischemic heart disease. It is generally assumed that this effect of exogenous lipid on the arterial wall is mediated by its effect on serum cholesterol. However it remains possible that dietary fat may have an independent effect on the arterial wall. The possible uptake of the major lipid of chylomicrons, triglyceride, by rat aorta *in vivo* was examined for this reason.

Chylomicron triglyceride fatty acid uptake (TGFA) by adipose tissue is dependent on hydrolysis to partial glycerides and FFA during uptake (Scow et al., 1972). A Previous study of rabbit aorta perfused in situ indicated that triglyceride hydrolysis was not required for aortic uptake of TGFA (Vost, 1972).

Chylomicrons labeled in the fatty acid moiety of triglycerides (^{3}H-triglyceride >90% of chylomicron ^{3}H lipid) were prepared by feeding glyceryl tri[^{3}H] 9; 10 palmitate to rats and collecting thoracic lymph. Chylomicrons were purified by flotation twice through 0.9% saline and their estimated minumum diameter was 90 mµ. Under light ether anesthesia rats were injected intravenously with 40 - 70 mg chylomicron triglyceride per kg body weight and returned to their cage. Ten minutes later rats were exsanguinated and plasma and tissue lipids extracted. Major lipid classes were separated on glass fiber paper impregnated with silica gel (Pocock et al., 1972).

In these experiments ^{3}H-triglyceride in aorta could have been derived either by direct uptake of plasma ^{3}H-triglyceride or by aortic esterification of ^{3}H-FFA released by hydrolysis of chylomicron triglyceride in aorta or other tissues. In addition a small quantity of ^{3}H-FFA (3% of ^{3}H-lipid) was present in the injected chylomicrons. To distinguish the two processes of direct triglyceride uptake and of esterification, ^{14}C palmitate bound to serum albumin was injected with ^{3}H-chylomicrons. As initial experiments had shown that injected albumin-bound ^{14}C-palmitate and ^{3}H-palmitate were incorporated into aortic lipid esters in identical fashion in ten minutes, the following equation was derived

$$^3\text{H-TG d.p.m.} = \frac{^{14}\text{C-TG d.p.m.}}{^{14}\text{C-PHL d.p.m.}} \times {}^3\text{H-PHL d.p.m.} \qquad (1)$$

where TG and PHL are newly synthesised triglyceride and phospholipid respectively. Consequently the esterification pattern of ^{14}C-palmitic acid could be used to estimate the esterification pattern of ^{3}H-palmitic acid.

In experiments in which ^{3}H-chylomicrons and ^{14}C-FFA were injected analysis of aortic lipids is shown in Table 1. ^{14}C-phospholipid was the major labeled ester lipid derived from ^{14}C-FFA. In contrast 60% of the ^{3}H-ester lipid was ^{3}H-triglyceride. By applying Eq (1), the fraction of labeled aortic TG derived by esterification was 40 ± 3%. The assumption in using the equation is that aortic ^{3}H-phospholipid is derived only by esterification of ^{3}H-FFA. As it remains possible that some aortic ^{3}H-phospholipid was derived from the small fraction of plasma ^{3}H-phospholipid the calculated esterification value is a maximum value. These results indicate that 10 minutes after injection of chylomicron ^{3}H-triglyceride, a

[*]This study was supported by grants from the Medical Research Council of Canada and the Quebec Heart Foundation and a Research Scholarship (A.V.) and Fellowship (D.P.) of the Canadian Heart Foundation.

Table 1. Aortic ester lipid radioactivity % distribution after intravenous injection of chylomicrons containing ^{3}H-palmitate-triglyceride and ^{14}C-palmitate (FFA)

	^{14}C	^{3}H
Triglyceride	36 ± 3.3	57 ± 2.6
Phospholipid	51 ± 2.3	32 ± 2.2
Diglyceride	13 ± 2.1	11 ± 0.7
Cholesteryl Ester	<1	0

Mean values ± S.E. (n = 8).

minimum of 60 ± 3% of labeled aorta TG was derived directly from plasma triglyceride without hydrolysis. To confirm this, the generation of ^{3}H-FFA from ^{3}H-TG was blocked in similar experiments by pretreating animals with the lipoprotein lipase inhibitors cyclohexamide (Wing et al., 1967) 6 mg/kg injected i.p. 4 hr before labeled lipid injection (n=3) or cyclohexamide plus protamine sulfate 10 mg/kg i.v. 1 hr before lipid injection (n=3). In the inhibitor treated groups (n=6) 81.7 ± 2% of aortic ^{3}H-triglyceride was derived by direct uptake of plasma unhydrolysed TG, a value greater than that in the 6 controls (P<0.001).

The specific radioactivity of injected chylomicron and terminal plasma triglyceride and the half life of ^{3}H-triglyceride in serial plasma samples from rats of similar weight injected with similar loads of chylomicron triglycerides, were measured. From these results the specific permeability co-efficients for chylomicron triglyceride passing from blood to aorta in these experiments was approximately 0.25 x 10^{-7} M cm^{-2} sec^{-1} M^{-1} ml^{-1}. This value is similar to the co-efficient for chylomicrons in perfused rabbit aorta calculated from previous data as 0.49 x 10^{-7} (Vost, 1972) and is several orders of magnitude less than co-efficients calculated for albumin in other tissues (Landis et al., 1963).

The possibility that aortic ^{3}H-TG represented contamination from blood or periaortic brown fat was explored. Three rats were injected with ^{51}Cr-tagged red cells and after equilibration, aortas were removed and processed in the usual manner. No significant radioactivity was detected in aortas although the sensitivity was sufficient to detect 18 nl of blood in the presence of aortas. From this result and the triglyceride radioactivity in the terminal blood samples it was calculated that <12.8 ± 1.5% of aortic ^{3}H-triglyceride could have been derived from contaminating plasma. Although brown fat contained 130 times more ^{3}H in lipid per g wet weight than aorta it did not apparently contaminate aortas since both fasting and lipoprotein lipase inhibitors reduced brown fat ^{3}H lipid to 19% and 15% of control values without associated falls in aortic ^{3}H lipid.

These experiments show that chylomicron triglyceride is taken up unhydrolysed by rat aorta *in vivo* and that the apparent permeability rates of chylomicrons are very low consistent with their large particle radius.

In view of the above results the presence of an aortic lipoprotein triglyceride lipase was investigated using a specific assay with ^{14}C-triolein substrate. Groups of aortic acetone-ether powders from 6 male rats were incubated for 60 min in 0.4 ml TRIS buffer (0.2M), 1.5 mls 15% bovine serum albumen, 0.1 ml heparin (0.125 µ), 0.8 ml dog serum, 0.2 ml 10% Ediol (coconut oil emulsion) with ^{14}C-triolein (1µc) and 1.0 ml NH3:NH4 Cl buffer (0.025M). The reaction was terminated by acidification and lipids were extracted in heptane-isopropanol and ^{14}C-fatty acids extracted in an alkaline wash. The incubation conditions were optimal for substrate concentration and pH (8.1) and ^{14}C-FFA release was linear for 60 min. Blank tubes without tissue and control tubes with boiled aortic powders were included. Aortic lipoprotein lipase activity was 75 ± 2 nmoles FFA released/g wet weight/hr. Using the same assay with similar weights of brown and white adipose tissue, aortic

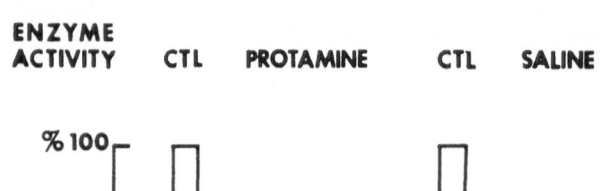

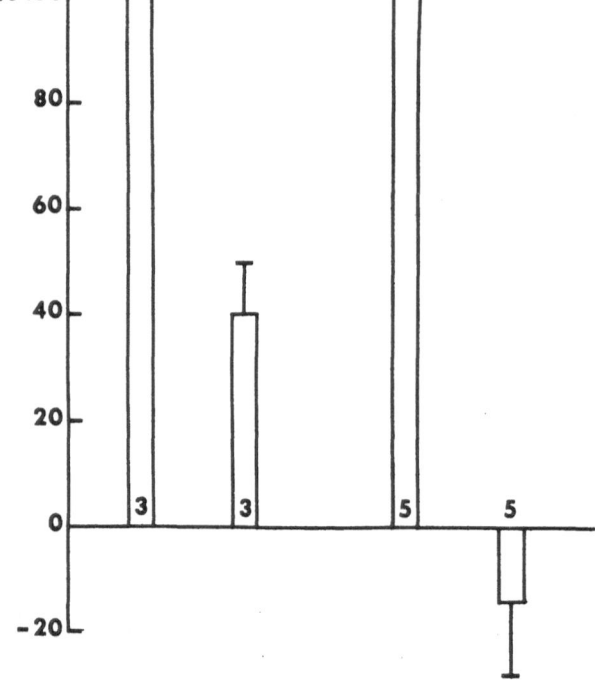

Figure 1. Aortic lipoprotein lipase activity in groups of 6 rat aortas. Effects of lipase inhibitors, 0.5 M NaCl and protamine sulfate 0.8 mg/ml assay medium

activity was only 8% and 2% respectively of that in these tissues. Protamine and 0.5 M saline produced major inhibition of aortic lipolytic activity (Fig. 1). These results with a specific assay demonstrate that lipoprotein triglyceride lipase is present in aorta and its inhibition characteristics are similar to adipose tissue enzyme. Previous difficulties in assaying this enzyme in aorta (Zemplenyi, 1968) may have been due to lack of specificity of the assay systems.

The combined results of these studies indicate that chylomicron triglyceride is taken up rapidly by aorta in vivo and triglyceride hydrolysis is not required for uptake. From the previous (Vost, 1972) and present studies it is concluded that the uptake rates of chylomicron triglyceride are quantitively small. The enzyme lipoprotein triglyceride lipase is present in aorta. Consequently the pathways for physiological uptake and metabolism of chylomicron triglyceride are present in mammalian aortas.

V
Metabolic Functions of the Arterial Cell

WORKSHOP: Metabolism and Function of Arterial Cells in Culture

Chairmen: A.L. Robertson, Jr., USA
O.J. Pollak, USA

Participants: R.C. Gross, USA
S.C. Smith, USA
E.C. Smith, USA
C. Becker, USA
A.S. Daoud, USA
Katti Fischer-Dzoga, USA

The potential value of cell, tissue and organ culture techniques in studies of the vascular wall and its role in the pathogenesis of the multifactorial disease we call atherosclerosis is receiving increasing attention.

As part of the studies on viability of arterial transplants by tissue culture over 20 years ago, an exhaustive literature search only yielded a few references (Lazzarini-Robertson, 1953).

A number of fundamental questions are to be answered before interpretation of data from different laboratories can be compared with the behavior of arterial cells *in vivo*. Questions range from stabilization of vascular cells in culture by provision of standardized and well-defined environmental conditions, to the evaluation of culture requirements by arterial cells from susceptible or atheroma-prone primates and other animals in comparison to those from more resistant species.

METABOLISM OF PLASMA LIPOPROTEINS BY CULTURED HUMAN FIBROBLASTS AND RAT HEART CELLS

R.C. Gross

Introduction

Cultured cells may provide useful models for study of mechanisms involved in hyperlipoproteinemia and atherosclerosis. During the past few years we have studied the uptake and utilization of plasma lipoproteins by several types of isolated and cultured mammalian cells.

Human skin fibroblasts are a particularly attractive model. They are easily grown*. They are readily obtained from patients with familial hyperlipoproteinemia as well as normal subjects, the hope being that metabolic errors present in patients will be reflected in the handling of lipoproteins by these cells. Cardiac muscle is known to utilize lipids avidly. It has abundant lipoprotein lipase (Korn, 1955). Harary and associates (1967) have shown that primary cultures of heart cells from newborn require fatty acids for beating and maintenance of certain enzyme levels. Thus these cells might provide means of investigating regulation of lipoprotein metabolism by non-adipose, lipoprotein lipase-rich tissues.

---

*Goldstein and Brown (1973) have recently demonstrated that skin fibroblasts from patients homozygous for familial hypercholesterolemia have elevated 3-hydroxy-3-methylglutaryl coenzyme A reductase activity. This appears to be due to failure of suppression by low density lipoproteins, and results in overproduction of cholesterol.

Methods

Skin biopsies were obtained from normal subjects and a number of patients with familial hyperlipoproteinemia. They were grown in monolayers in Eagle's Minimum Essential Medium (Gibco) with 10% fetal calf serum. The cells grew to confluence in 7-10 days, and had the typical appearance of fibroblasts (Fig. 1). Most experiments were carried out with confluent cultures. Hearts were excised from 5-7 day old rats and were treated with minor modifications of the method described by Harary and Farley (1967) to isolate heart cells. These were grown in MEM with 10% fetal calf serum in small petri dishes. They became confluent in 5-7 days, and were noted to beat spontaneously between 3 and 5 days of growth (Fig. 2). LDH activity from these cultures was 60% suppressible by pyruvate, compared with 37.7% suppressibility of fibroblast LDH activity, indicating that the heart cell culture was composed largely of myocardial cells (Cahn et al., 1962).

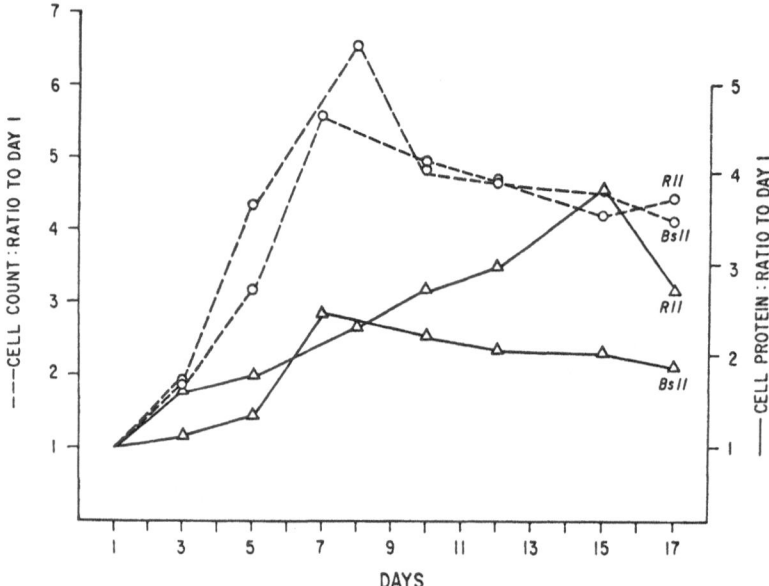

Figure 1. Human fibroblast growth curves

Uptake and utilization of triglycerides of human very low density lipoproteins was the main object of study with both culture systems. Labeled VLDL was prepared by incubating human serum with glyceryl trioleate-1-^{14}C or ^{3}H dispersed on Celite. Lipoproteins were then isolated by preparative ultracentrifugation.

Triglyceride-labeled lipoproteins were washed once with fatty acid-free serum albumin to remove labeled free fatty acids. After this treatment, 96-98% of lipoprotein radioactivity was associated with triglycerides. A typical VLDL preparation contained 100,000-200,000 dpm and 500-1500 nmole triglyceride. The average specific activity was 187 dpm/nmole triglyceride. Lipoproteins prepared in this manner were similar to native unlabeled lipoproteins from the same plasma pool in lipid composition, and electrophoretic mobility. Their triglycerides were readily hydrolyzed by lipoprotein lipase prepared from cow's milk.

For *in vitro* experiments, growth medium was removed from the cells, and media containing MEM, 1% fatty acid-free serum albumin, and the labeled lipoprotein were added. Incubations were carried out up to 24 hours. Incorporation of radioactivity into cell lipids and CO_2, and changes in distribution of radioactivity in medium

lipids were determined using thin-layer chromatography and liquid scintillation
spectrometry.

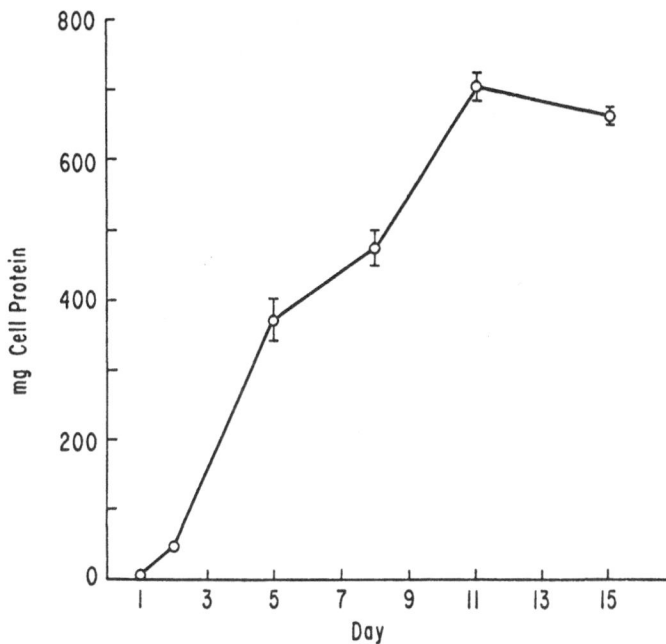

Figure 2. Rat heart cell growth curve

Results

Experiments with Cultured Human Skin Fibroblasts. After 24 hours incubation with
triglyceride-labeled VLDL, these cells had usually incorporated from 1-5% of medium radioactivity into their lipids. In Table 1, results are seen from 13 recent
experiments under basal conditions. The mean uptake was 2.39% ± 0.60 (S.E.M.) percent of added radioactivity, or 0.90 ± 0.13 percent/mg cell protein. Incorporation
into CO_2 was approximately 10% of the amount of radioactivity in cell lipids in
those studies in which it was measured. 67.0 ± 4.29% of cell lipid radioactivity
was in phospholipids (PL) and 20.7 ± 3.20% was in triglycerides (TG). As total
incorporation of radioactivity into cell lipids increased, relatively more of this
tended to appear in PL (Gross, 1972). The remainder of cell lipid radioactivity
was in fatty acids (FA) and diglycerides (DG), with only small amounts seen in
monoglycerides, and insignificant amounts in free and esterified cholesterol. This
distribution is similar to that seen after incubation with small amounts of
albumin-bound labeled free fatty acids (Table 2). Changes in medium radioactivity
were small, with three times more radioactivity and mass in unesterified fatty
acids when cells were present. No differences were noted between cells from normals and patients with hyperlipoproteinemia.

Though these findings all indicated active uptake and utilization of VLDL triglycerides by fibroblasts, rather than merely passive adherence of lipoprotein to
cells, this uptake was too low to allow study of inhibitors, or to detect impairment of uptake or metabolism of lipoprotein triglycerides by patients' cells
because it did not result in marked changes in the medium. Therefore, conditions
were sought which might enhance this uptake. Cells were studied during the log
phase of growth (5-7 days, Fig. 1). Incorporation did not differ significantly
from that observed in confluent cultures (Table 1). Suspensions of fibroblasts
which had been scraped from their culture bottles were also studied allowing

higher concentrations of both lipoproteins and cells to interact (Table 1). Uptake was somewhat higher than with monolayers in spite of shorter incubation times. When cells were trypsinized to facilitate removal from culture bottles, a further increase in uptake may have been produced. However, in all experiments done with cell suspensions, incorporation of radioactivity into cell PL was considerably lower than it was with monolayers. This suggested to us that the greater uptake might be due to increased adherence of lipoproteins to cells without subsequent utilization.

Table 1. Effects of culture conditions on incorporation of radioactivity from triglyceride-labeled VLDL by human fibroblasts

Condition	Uptake by cells		Distribution in cell lipids	
	Percent	Percent/mg	Percent in PL	Percent in TG
1. Monolayers[a]				
A. Confluent (n=13)	2.39±0.60[c]	0.90±0.13	67.0±14.2	20.7±10.6
B. Log phase	1.41	1.18	43.5	21.9
Log phase	1.71	1.05	61.2	23.1
2. Suspension[b]	2.32	0.89	7.5	83.4
Suspension	1.46	0.39	8.0	82.8
Suspension	2.77±0.09	2.90±0.36	7.1±0.56	80.2±0.66
"Trypsinized	5.32±0.31	3.32±0.26	12.8±1.21	69.8±0.92

[a]Incubated 20 or 24 hr.　　[b]Incubated 6 or 8 hr.　　[c]S.E.M.

Table 2. Incorporation of radioactivity from triglyceride-labeled VLDL and fatty acid-labeled albumin by cultured human fibroblasts

	Uptake by cells			
	Percent	Percent/mg	nmoles	nmoles/mg
Triglyceride fatty acid	1.80	1.55	21.34	18.37
Albumin- fatty acid	32.3	30.70	3.88	3.69

	Distribution in cell lipids			
	% in PL	% in DG	% in FFA	% in TG
Triglyceride fatty acid	74.92±1.91[a]	3.12±0.24	11.20±0.74	10.75±1.05
Albumin- fatty acid	82.93±1.01[b]	2.53±0.18	8.07±0.23[b]	6.40±0.91[c]

[a]S.E.M.　　[b]$p < 0.01$.　　[c]$p < 0.05$.

Factors which are known to influence cell growth also appeared to be without significant effect on incorporation of VLDL radioactivity into fibroblasts (Table 3). Neither insulin nor putrescine (Pohjanpalto and Raina, 1972) consistently influenced any of the parameters followed. Fetal calf serum decreased the uptake of radioactivity; this is probably due to lowering of specific activity of the VLDL by lipids in the serum.

Table 3. Effects of additions to medium on incorporation of radioactivity from triglyceride-labeled VLDL by cultured human fibroblasts

Addition	Uptake by cells		Distribution in cell lipids	
	Percent	Percent/mg	Percent in PL	Percent in TG
Insulin 0	0.49±0.08[a]	1.55±0.41	52.7	30.8
" 100uU/ml	0.81±0.34	1.58±0.04	53.4	19.2
" 1000uU/ml	1.22±0.39	2.08±0.53	64.0	16.5
Insulin 0	0.62	0.37		
" 200uU/ml	0.44	0.33		
" 500uU/ml	0.39	0.35		
" 1000uU/ml	0.35	0.33		
Putrescine 0	0.68±0.08	0.38±0.03	48.2±4.6	31.0±3.9
" 1x10^{-7} M	0.57±0.02	0.39±0.05	60.3±1.7	23.1±1.2
Putrescine 0	1.88	1.26		
" 1x10^{-7} M	1.20	1.40		
Fetal calf serum				
" 0,1% Alb	2.14	1.00		
" 0,2% Alb	1.52	0.88		
10% 0 Alb	1.62	0.66		

[a] S.E.M.

Because there was some evidence of hydrolysis of VLDL triglycerides by fibroblasts, stimulators of lipoprotein lipase activity were tried (though we had previously been unable to demonstrate any lipase activity with the characteristics of LPL in homogenates of these cells). Heparin was without effect (Table 4). Addition of apolipoprotein glu, the polypeptide activator of LPL which is normally present in VLDL, did increase uptake significantly, and also may have enhanced incorporation of radioactivity into cell PL (Table 4). These results suggest that if PLP has a role in lipid metabolism by fibroblasts, it is not releasable by heparin.

Table 4. Effects of stimulators of lipoprotein lipase activity on incorporation of radioactivity from triglyceride-labeled VLDL by cultured human fibroblasts

Stimulator	Uptake by cells		Distribution in cell lipids	
	Percent	Percent/mg	Percent in PL	Percent in TG
Heparin 0	0.66±0.05[a]	0.78±0.06		
" 5u/ml	0.53±0.02	0.74±0.04		
Apolipoprotein				
Glu 0	1.35±0.03	1.30±0.07	70.4±4.69	16.8±4.02
" " 20 μg	1.98±0.04	2.34±0.15[b]	76.1±3.15	10.1±1.72
" " 40 μg	2.34±0.17	2.36±0.17[b]	77.4±1.19	9.1±0.67

[a] S.E.M.   [b] $p < 0.01$.

Incorporation of parts of the lipoprotein molecule other than triglyceride were also examined. Nearly 15% of labeled cholesterol was taken up from VLDL (Table 5). Uptake of the protein moiety of LDL was quite small, with ten times more of the extremely small amount of $I125$ labeled lipid present in the lipoprotein being taken up (Table 6).

Table 5. Uptake of radioactivity from triglyceride and cholesterol-labeled VLDL by cultured human fibroblasts

	Percent	Percent/mg	nmoles	nmoles/mg	TG/Chol. Molar ratio
Triglyceride	0.68	0.21	10.8	3.3	
					0.07
Cholesterol	14.6	4.50	144.5	44.3	
			Medium VLDL		1.60

Table 6. Uptake of radioactivity from $I125$-labeled LDL by cultured human fibroblasts

Time	Incorporation into cell protein			Incorporation into cell lipids	
	Percent[a]	Percent/mg	ug LDL protein/mg	Percent[b]	Percent/mg
6 hr	0.041	0.0099	6.80	0.41	0.099
16 hr	0.040	0.0124	8.43	0.44	0.137
24 hr	0.044	0.0132	8.80	0.58	0.174

[a]3,073,330 DPM in LDL protein.   [b]62,700 DPM in LDL lipid.

In spite of the difficulties owing to low uptake of VLDL TG by fibroblasts, a few preliminary studies of the effects of lipid-lowering drugs have been done. Table 7 shows results of experiments with CPIB and another agent which lowers triglycerides in man, Tibric Acid (2-chloro-5(3,5-dimethylipiperidinosulfonyl) benzoic acid; CP-18,574). Cells were grown in the presence of these compounds for 4 days prior to incubation with labeled VLDL. CPIB inhibited incorporation of radioactivity at the highest concentration used, 1000 µg/ml. It had no effect on cell protein levels. Tibric acid, on the other hand, tended to promote uptake of radioactivity, just missing statistical significance in this and other experiments. Treatment with this compound was also associated with somewhat higher cell protein levels.

Experiments with Cultured Rat Heart Cells. Knowing that myocardium is a rich source of lipoprotein lipase, it was expected that heart cells would be more active than fibroblasts in metabolizing VLDL triglycerides. Initial results have borne this out. After 24 hours of incubation, heart cells under basal conditions incorporated from 10 to 30 percent of total medium radioactivity into cell lipids (30-45%/mg cell protein) (Table 8). Usually over 60% of this was in cell TG at 24 hours, with less than 25% in PL. Around 10% was in cell FA and the remaining 5% in DG. Radioactivity in medium lipids changed greatly during the 14 hour incubation, with radioactivity increasing in FA as it fell in TG (Table 9). There was an increase in radioactivity in medium TG between 6 and 24 hours which may be due to release of radioactive TG into the medium from cells. The role of lipoprotein lipase in producing these changes was assessed by adding heparin, apolipoprotein glu, and a lipase inhibitor polypeptide also associated with VLDL, apolipoprotein ala. Heparin appeared to increase incorporation of radioactivity into cells, with

Table 7. Effects of hypolipidemic drugs on incorporation of radioactivity from triglyceride-labeled VLDL by cultured human fibroblasts

| Drug | Uptake by cells | | Distribution in cell lipids | |
	Percent	Percent/mg	Percent in PL	Percent in TG
CPIB 0	1.47 ± 0.10^a	1.26 ± 0.18	52.1 ± 3.96	33.4 ± 2.19
" 200ug/ml	0.97 ± 0.05	1.21 ± 0.08	-	-
" 500ug/ml	1.20 ± 0.16	0.94 ± 0.11	-	-
" 1000ug/ml	1.15 ± 0.12	0.75 ± 0.07^b	47.4 ± 6.47	43.1 ± 5.48
CPIB 0	3.14 ± 0.67	1.14 ± 0.15	73.4 ± 1.15	13.2 ± 0.25
" 1000ug/ml	1.44 ± 0.30	0.70 ± 0.12	62.9 ± 3.46^b	23.1 ± 2.54^b
Control	2.00 ± 0.21	0.78 ± 0.06	50.8 ± 3.26	32.3 ± 1.72
CPIB 400ug/ml	1.54 ± 0.26	0.59 ± 0.05^b	49.5 ± 2.62	31.6 ± 2.60
Tibric Acid 4ug/ml	3.06 ± 0.68	0.99 ± 0.07	56.2 ± 1.34	27.6 ± 0.81^b

[a] S.E.M.   [b] $p<0.05$.

Table 8. Effects of heparin on incorporation of radioactivity from triglyceride-labeled VLDL by cultured rat heart cells

| Time | Heparin | Uptake by cells | | Distribution in cell lipids | | | |
		Percent	Percent/mg	% in PL	% in DG	% in FA	% in TG
2 hr	0	1.25 ± 0.05^a	3.86 ± 0.12	24.9	17.2	14.5	43.4
	5U/ml	1.30 ± 0.0	3.88 ± 0.12	14.6	16.7	17.4	51.6
6 hr	0	3.65 ± 0.35^a	13.98 ± 2.65	19.8	9.7	14.0	56.5
	5U/ml	3.08 ± 0.51	18.80 ± 0.28	22.3	15.5	11.5	50.8
24 hr	0	11.20 ± 0.17^b	46.20 ± 6.55	18.4	6.1	9.8	65.7
	5U/ml	13.20 ± 0.83	73.50 ± 5.46^c	23.9	18.7	9.4	48.0

[a] $\frac{Range.}{2}$ [b] S.E.M.   [c] $p<0.05$.

slightly more appearing in PL and DG and less in TG compared with non-treated cells (Table 8). It also caused more loss of radioactivity from medium TG, and a greater increase in medium FA radioactivity (Table 9). In the absence of cells, heparin had no effect on medium radioactivity. Apolipoprotein glu did not appear to stimulate the uptake of VLDL TG by cells significantly, but did significantly increase the hydrolysis of medium VLDL TG in the presence of cells, as evidenced by the increased radioactivity in medium FFA (Table 10). Stimulation of hydrolysis of VLDL TG by apolipoprotein glu with no increase of cell uptake of TGFA has also been seen with isolated rat adipocytes. Apolipoprotein ala may inhibit both cell uptake and hydrolysis of VLDL (Table 11). The results just missed statistical significance. In spite of decreased uptake, the percent (and absolute amount) of radioactivity incorporated into cell PL was increased by apolipoprotein ala. These results suggest that lipoprotein lipase plays an important part in metabolism of VLDL by heart cells.

Table 9. Effects of heparin and cultured heart cells on distribution of radio-activity in incubation medium

	Percent in PL	Percent in DG	Percent in FA	Percent in TG
With cells				
_2 h_				
Heparin 0	3.2	2.1	20.7	74.0
Heparin 5u/ml	2.2	1.6	57.4	38.8
_6 h_				
Heparin 0	2.8	1.8	48.1	47.3
Heparin 5u/ml	1.2	3.4	73.2	22.2
_24 h_				
Heparin 0	0.4	2.8	38.0	58.7
Heparin 5u/ml	0.4	1.7	59.9	38.0
No cells				
_0 h_				
Heparin 0	0.4	2.7	1.7	95.4
Heparin 5u/ml	0.2	1.8	1.0	96.9
_24 h_				
Heparin 0	0.2	2.0	0.7	97.1
Heparin 5u/ml	0.3	1.9	0.8	97.0

Table 10. Effects of apolipoprotein glu on incorporation of radioactivity from triglyceride-labeled VLDL by cultured rat heart cells

Apolipoprotein glu added	Uptake by cells		Distribution of radioactivity			
			Cell lipids		Medium lipids	
	Percent	Percent/mg	% in PL	% in TG	% in FA	% in TG
0	31.6±3.5[a]	38.1±3.0	24.8	54.7	32.1	62.0
68 ug	33.3±1.2	55.1±6.2	32.4	46.3	44.7	49.5
136 ug	29.3±1.7	37.7±3.7	39.3	39.7	47.3	47.1

[a]S.E.M.

Table 11. Effects of apolipoprotein ala on incorporation of radioactivity from triglyceride-labeled VLDL by cultured rat heart cells

Apolipoprotein ala added	Uptake by cells		Distribution of radioactivity			
			Cell lipids		Medium lipids	
	Percent	Percent/mg	% in PL	% in TG	% in FA	% in TG
0	26.4±1.2[a]	32.9±3.1	12.7	55.4	31.7	63.5
73 ug	21.3±3.4	27.6±1.36	20.6	45.9	26.0	69.4
146 ug	18.2±2.6[b]	24.7±4.2	27.3	39.6	22.1	73.1

[a]S.E.M.   [b]p<0.05.

Comparison of Results from Study of Two Cell Types

Comparing results obtained from study of fibroblasts with those from heart cells, a number of basic differences must be kept in mind which could profoundly influence results obtained. 1. One obvious difference is that between species. As a control, we are doing studies with fibroblasts from rats. 2. Fibroblasts are studied after numerous passages, whereas heart cells are primary explants. Harary and associates have propagated heart cell lines through many passages, and they appear to lose many of their characteristics (1967). We have not yet studied metabolism of lipoproteins in established cultures of heart cells. 3. The heart cells are from newborn animals, whereas most of our fibroblast lines are from middle-aged adults. However, we have noted no difference in lipoprotein metabolism due to age of skin donors. 4. Heart cells are cultured in smaller vessels and are thus exposed to a more concentrated solution of lipoprotein. However, the experiments with suspensions of fibroblasts were done with similarly concentrated solutions and the uptake and further metabolism of lipoproteins still differed from that seen with heart cells.

That triglyceride which was incorporated into fibroblasts was probably hydrolyzed prior to or at the time of uptake. It appeared mainly in cell phospholipids. No lipase activity resembling lipoprotein lipase has been demonstrable in fibroblasts, and heparin has no effect on uptake of triglycerides from VLDL. Inconsistently, apolipoprotein glu did produce a small but significant increase in incorporation of triglyceride — an effect which has not been observed with other cell types studied. In contrast, heart cells from newborn rats appear to hydrolyze and incorporate triglyceride fatty acids from human VLDL quite avidly. Results of experiments with stimulators and inhibitors of lipoprotein lipase activity suggest that this enzyme plays an important role in the metabolism of VLDL, a not unexpected finding.

Uptake of VLDL cholesterol by fibroblasts may be more active than triglyceride uptake. The work of Maca and Connor (1971) with LDL and mouse fibroblasts suggested net uptake of cholesterol. It remains to be seen whether the uptake we have observed is a net change. The very low uptake of labeled protein from LDL is similar to that observed by Robertson (1965) with cultured human aortic intimal cells. Similar studies have not yet been done with heart cells.

Additional studies are clearly needed to elucidate the reasons for the observed differences in lipoprotein metabolism by these two kinds of cells; however, one explanation may lie in the different lipoprotein lipase activity. If this is so, it would seem that cells lacking lipoprotein lipase cannot have an important role in metabolism of lipoprotein triglycerides.

CELLULAR ASPECTS OF ATHEROGENESIS IN PIGEONS

S.C. Smith and E.C. Smith

Some years ago, Robertson (1963) postulated that the underlying cause of atherosclerosis is a metabolic defect in arterial intimal cells of susceptible individuals. Atherosclerosis-susceptible White Carneau (WC) and atherosclerosis-resistant Show Racer (SR) pigeons offered a unique animal system in which to search for such a defect since Clarkson, Lofland, Prichard, and co-workers (Lofland and Clarkson, 1959; Prichard, 1965) failed to demonstrate differences between the intact birds which would explain susceptibility and resistance to spontaneous atherosclerosis. Development of spontaneous atherosclerosis in WC aortas is highly predictable in terms of site specificity, lesion severity, and disease progression (Santerre et al., 1972). The celiac bifurcation of the aorta is a site of severe lesions in all WC over four years of age, and by one to two years of age foam cells are common within the muscular foci at this site. In SR, few foam cells are observed within the celiac foci, and severe lesions are uncommon.

In order to isolate the experimental system from blood factors which affect lesion development in the intact animal, we chose what was then a relatively new technique for studying genetic defects, the use of primary cell culture. Genetic diseases or metabolic defects are often accentuated in cell culture, and for this reason the use of cultures in diagnosis of various inherited lipidoses and mucopolysaccharidoses has become routine (Brady, 1971; Danes, 1969). Primary cell cultures were established from the inner medial layers of the thoracic aorta from embryonic pigeons of both breeds (Smith et al., 1965). In all subsequent experiments, WC and SR cultures were studied in parallel to compare the susceptible with the resistant control. These comparisons also permit us to compensate for artifacts of the cell culture technique in our interpretations since differences between WC and SR cells indicate a difference in cell response or cell capabilities.

Similar to cells in the celiac muscular focus *in vivo*, pigeon aorta cells in culture are predominatly (>90%) smooth muscle cells as evidenced ultrastructurally by numerous, 60-90Å diameter myofilaments with dense bodies, micropinocytotic vessicles, and a thickened glycocalyx. Histochemically, many myosin-ATPase positive bundles of filaments are also evident. These cells *in vitro* undergo a sequence of maturation (SR) or degeneration (WC) similar to that seen *in vivo* except for the accelerated age scale *in vitro* (Fig. 1) (Cooke and Smith, 1968; Wight, 1972). Furthermore, the degenerative sequence in WC cells resembles that described in early stages of human atherogenesis, the key process being the transformation of modified smooth muscle cells into lipid-containing foam cells (Wissler and Vesselinovitch, 1968).

Comparisons of the lipid composition between celiac foci in 4-6 month WC (preatherosclerotic) and SR showed similar differences (underlined in Table 1), as did comparisons between 16-day WC (early degeneration) and SR cultures (Nicolosi et al., 1972). Much of the lipid accumulating in WC cells *in vivo* and *in vitro* is squalene and cholesteryl ester. This difference in culture strongly suggests a metabolic defect in WC cells as originally hypothesized. Correlation of the data in Table 1 with the morphological features outlined in Fig. 1 further suggests that the presence of excess lipid interrupts the process of normal maturation and initially involves the granular endoplasmic reticulum (GER).

Table 1. Lipid composition of celiac foci (4-6 month pigeons) and cell cultures (16 day) from pigeon aortas

Lipid class	Celiac Foci			Cell cultures		
	WC	SR	WC/SR	WC	SR	WC/SR
Hydrocarbon	90.1[a,b]	33.5[a,b]	2.7	12.3[a,c]	7.1[a,c]	1.7
Cholesteryl ester	17.3[b]	8.2[b]	2.1	12.2[c]	7.0[c]	1.7
Triglyceride	10.9	8.7	1.3	11.3[c]	7.3[c]	1.5
Nonesterified fatty acid	3.7[b]	1.7[b]	2.2	2.8	2.1	1.3
Sterol	10.1	9.4	1.1	3.9	3.3	1.2
Phospholipid	22.9	34.1	0.7	5.8	5.0	1.2
Total	155.0[b]	95.6[b]	1.6	48.3[c]	31.8[c]	1.5

a   ug Lipid/ug DNA.
b,c   Difference between breeds significant, $P < 0.05$.

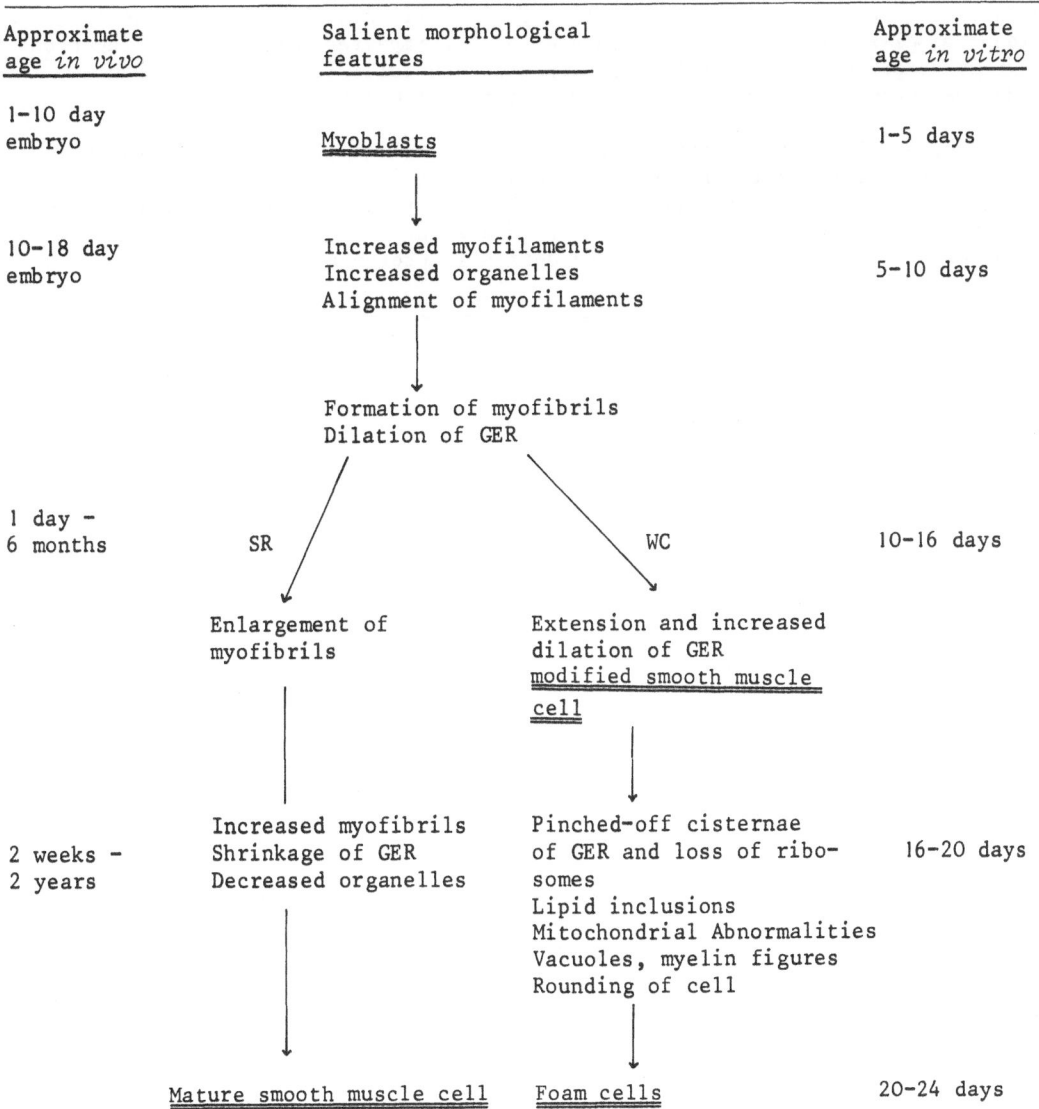

Approximate age *in vivo*	Salient morphological features	Approximate age *in vitro*
1-10 day embryo	<u>Myoblasts</u>	1-5 days
10-18 day embryo	Increased myofilaments Increased organelles Alignment of myofilaments	5-10 days
	Formation of myofibrils Dilation of GER	
1 day - 6 months	SR WC	10-16 days
	Enlargement of myofibrils	Extension and increased dilation of GER <u>modified smooth muscle cell</u>
2 weeks - 2 years	Increased myofibrils Shrinkage of GER Decreased organelles	Pinched-off cisternae of GER and loss of ribosomes Lipid inclusions Mitochondrial Abnormalities Vacuoles, myelin figures Rounding of cell	16-20 days
	<u>Mature smooth muscle cell</u> <u>Foam cells</u>	20-24 days

Note: GER = Granular Endoplasmic Reticulum.

Figure 1. Maturation and degeneration of pigeon aorta cells

We are now studying metabolic processes responsible for intracellular squalene and cholesteryl ester accumulation which may lead to foam cell formation. Our current effort is to distinguish *in vitro* between processes responsible for this lipid accumulation by either: 1. greater lipid incorporation, 2. greater lipid synthesis, 3. reduced lipid catabolism, or 4. reduced lipid excretion by aortic WC cells.

Interpretation of our earlier findings of little mitochondrial phosphorylating ATPase in vacuolated WC cells *in vitro* (Smith et al., 1966) and decreased respiratory control in celiac foci of 4-6 month (pre-atherosclerotic) WC *in vivo* (Santerre,

1971) as indicative of lesser catabolism in WC cells must be reserved until the chronological sequence of lipid accumulation vs. impaired mitochondrial function has been determined. Accumulation of lipid within cells is known to uncouple oxidative phosphorylation (Vasquez-Colon et al., 1966).

Pigeon aorta cell cultures offer a useful and pathologically relevant system in which to study intracellular aspects of atherogenesis. Differences found between WC and SR cells in this simplified, controlled culture model can be examined subsequently in the celiac foci of these pigeons to determine the significance in the atherogenic process. This research design is presented in Fig. 2.

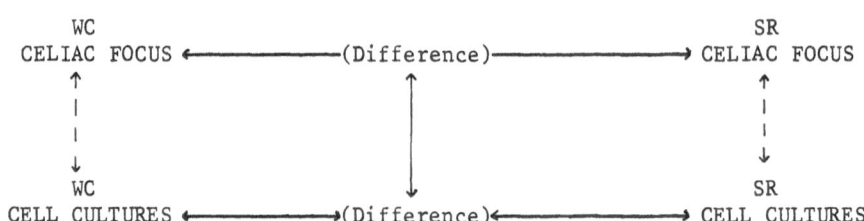

Note: Solid arrows represent primary comparisons in the research design. Broken arrows represent secondary comparisons.

Figure 2. Design to maintain pathological reference of findings in pigeon aorta cell cultures

CHARACTERISTICS OF ENDOTHELIAL CELLS CULTURED FROM HUMAN UMBILICAL CORD

C.D. Becker, E.A. Jaffe, R.L. Nachman, and R. Minick

Endothelial cells were cultured from human umbilical veins. In order to identify the cultured cells as endothelial cells and to study their functional characteristics, the cells were examined by a variety of techniques including light and immunofluoresence microscopy, scanning and transmission electron microscopy, mixed cell agglutination reactions, and tissue typing. In the course of these experiments it was observed that the cultured cells grew as monolayers of closely opposed, polygonal, flattened cells (Fig. 1). In contrast, smooth muscle cells and fibroblasts grew as slender, spindle-shaped cells which tended to form parallel arrays or whorls. Ultrastructurally, cultured endothelial cells possessed bundles of myofilaments (Fig. 2) and attachment bodies. By immunofluorescence microscopy, it was observed that cultured endothelial cells contained actomyosin of smooth muscle type (Fig. 3) (Jaffe et al., 1973b) and tropomyosin (Becker, manuscript in preparation). It was also observed that they contained material which was reactive with antisera against blood clotting Factor VIII (Jaffe et al., in press). By mixed cell agglutination reaction it was observed that cultured endothelial cells, unlike cultured fibroblasts or smooth muscle cells contained ABH blood group antigens appropriate to the tissue donor's blood type (Jaffe et al., 1973b). Cultured endothelial cells were also observed by microcytotoxicity tests to contain HL-A antigens appropriate to the tissue type of the tissue donor (Gibofsky et al., manuscript in preparation).

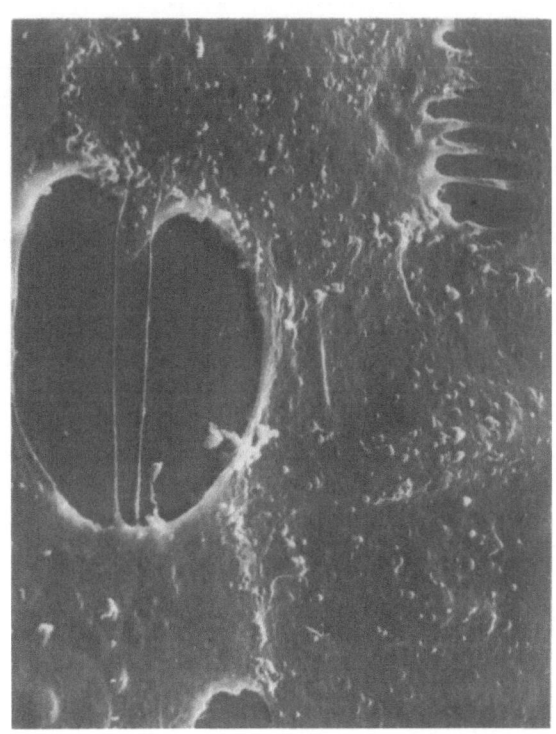

Figure 1. Scanning electron photomicrograph of cultured umbilical vein endothelial cells. The cells form a monolayer, and are large, flat, and polygonal. Intercellular interdigitations are present. X 0.927

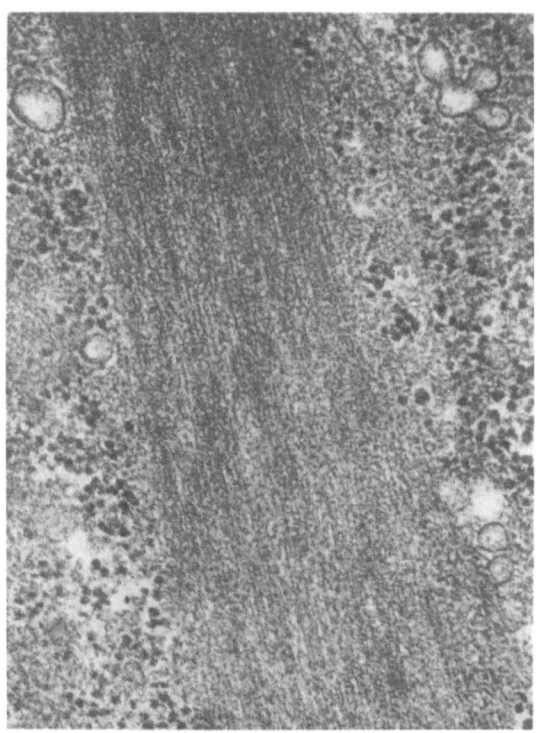

Figure 2. Myofilaments and vesicles in cytoplasm of cultured endothelial cell. X 57.170

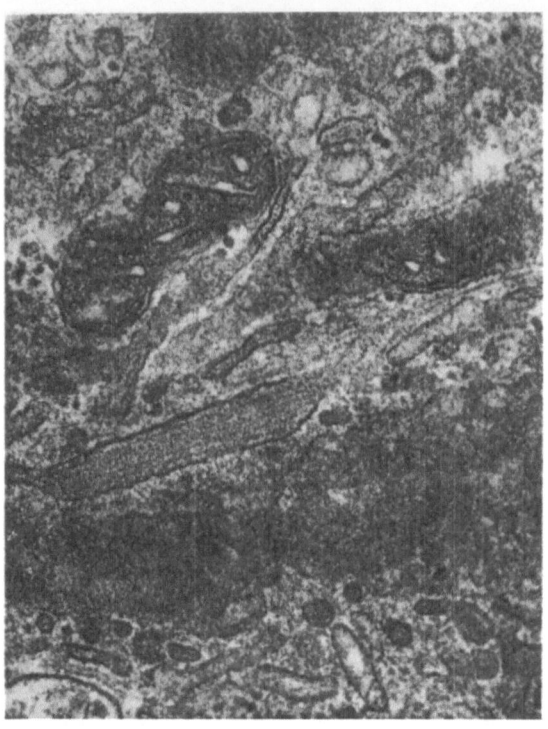

Figure 3. Weibel-Palade body in cytoplasm of cultured endothelial cell. X 61.50

Methods

Culture and Isolation of Endothelial Cells. Endothelial cells were isolated from human umbilical cord veins according to methods described previously (Jaffe et al., 1973b). In brief, segments of umbilical cord were obtained at delivery. The umbilical vein was rinsed with buffer (0.14M NaCl, .004M KCl, 1.001M phosphate buffer containing .011M glucose, pH 7.4), cannulated, filled with 10 ml of 0.2% collagenase solution, clamped and incubated at 37°C for 15 minutes. The vein was then perfused with buffer. Cells were sedimented, washed and cultured in plastic petri dishes containing Medium 199 with 20% fetal calf serum. The yield of cells was 0.5 to 1.5 x 10^6 per cord specimen and plating efficiency was 50-75%. The isolation and culture of smooth muscle cells and dermal fibroblasts for purposes of comparison are described previously (Jaffe et al., 1973b).

Scanning and Transmission Electron Microscopy. Umbilical cord tissue and cultured cells were prepared for examination by SEM and TEM by methods previously described (Jaffe et al., 1973b).

Immunofluorescence Microscopy. Preparation of umbilical cord tissue and cultured cells for immunohistologic studies, and the preparation and specificity of anti-sera to human uterine actomyosin and to human platelet actomyosin (thrombosthenin) are described previously (Becker and Murphy, 1969; Becker and Nachman, 1973). Antisera to purified human uterine tropomyosin was prepared in rabbits. Immunodif-fusion and absorption studies confirm the specificity of this antisera for tropo-myosin (Becker, manuscript in preparation). Unlike antisera to uterine or platelet actomyosins which react only with smooth muscle or smooth muscle-like structures, antisera to uterine tropomyosin reacts with both smooth and striated muscle.

Antisera to human blood coagulation factor VIII prepared in rabbits and in goats were obtained, respectively, from Dr. Leon Hoyer of the University of Connecticut School of Medicine and Dr. Harvey Grolnick of the National Institutes of Health.

Mixed Cell Hemagglutination Reactions. MCAR was performed with commercial anti-A and anti-B sera and anti-H lectin extracted from Ulex europaeus according to the method of Coombs et al. (1965).

Histocompatibility Typing. This was performed according to a modification of the method of Mittal et al. (1972).

Results. The results of these experiments are summarized in Table 1.

Table 1.

	Endothelial cells	Vascular smooth muscle cells	Fibroblasts
Cell morphology	polygonal	spindle	spindle
Growth pattern	monolayer	multilayered parallel arrays whorled	multilayered parallel arrays whorled
Myofilaments	+	+	+ or - variable
Immunofluorescent staining with anti-sera to smooth muscle actomyosin	+	+	+ or - variable
Immunofluorescent staining with anti-sera to smooth muscle tropomyosin	+	+	+ or - variable
Presence of major blood group antigens	+	-	-
Presence of histo-compatibility antigens	+	not tested	not tested
Immunofluorescent staining with anti-sera to Factor VIII	+	-	-

EFFECTS OF HOMOLOGOUS AND HETEROLOGOUS SERA ON EXPLANTS OF SWINE AORTIC MEDIA

A.S. Daoud

The assessment of the role of individual factors in the pathogenesis of atherosclerosis by means of *in vivo* studies is extremely difficult because of the complexity of the disease. In the last decade *in vitro* systems have been used advantageously (Jarmolych et al., 1968; Daoud et al., 1970; Robertson, 1967; Ross, 1971; and Wissler, 1973) in the study of various aspects of atherogenesis. The system which we have devised and characterized consists of aortic medial explants which, under our culture conditions, develop a peripheral growth having many features resembling those found in the early atherosclerotic plaque (Fig. 1). Both cell proliferation and cell necrosis, which are two important components of the lesions, are observed early in the culture period and continue throughout the life of the explants. The cells in the peripheral growth are identical to those

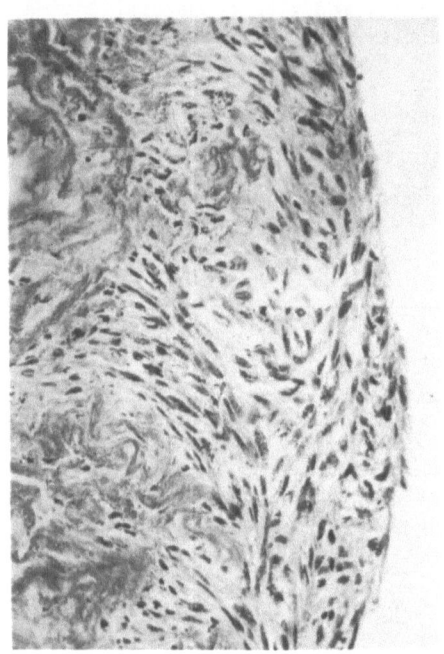

Figure 1. Photomicrograph of 21-day culture. The growth is composed of multiple cell layers arranged in various orientations. The deeper layers show some pyknosis and karyolysis of cell nuclei. The viable cells are elongated and fusiform,resembling medial cells. "Modified cells" are present mostly in the outer layers. Histochemical study shows the presence of mucopolysaccharide, elastic tissue, and collagen in the extracellular substance. The included portion of the explant proper is almost completely acellular. X 280

described in the early atherosclerotic lesions and secrete collagen, mucopolysaccharides and elastic tissue, which are the major extracellular substances in the lesion and normal arterial wall (Fig. 2) (Jarmolych et al., 1968).

For the development of peripheral growth, the explants require the presence of serum or serum derivative. Explants grown in semisynthetic medium (M199) only, develop no peripheral growth and show little DNA and protein synthetic activity. However, if parallel explants are cultured in medium containing, in addition to M199, 20% serum (normal or hyperlipemic),a peripheral growth occurs together with increase in both cell proliferation and cell death. Hence it is only logical to assume that serum contains factors which cause cell death, cell proliferation and formation of peripheral growth. Work in this laboratory has confirmed the presence of these factors (Fritz et al., 1972).

We have carried out investigations designed to compare the effects of human and swine sera on the swine explant system. We sought answers to the questions: 1. does inclusion of human serum in the growth medium result in a type of swine explant growth similar to that resulting from swine serum? and 2. if so, how do the various reactions influenced by serum compare quantitatively?

The growth pattern of explants grown in the presence of human serum seems to be analogous to that seen with swine serum. By light and electron microscopy, the peripheral growth resulting from culture in the presence of human serum was qualitatively indistinguishable from that resulting from culture with swine serum in the medium (Daoud et al., 1973). There were similar areas of acellularity within the explant proper in both culture types and autoradiography showed varying numbers of similarly labeled nuclei in each. Collagen, elastic tissue and mucopoly-

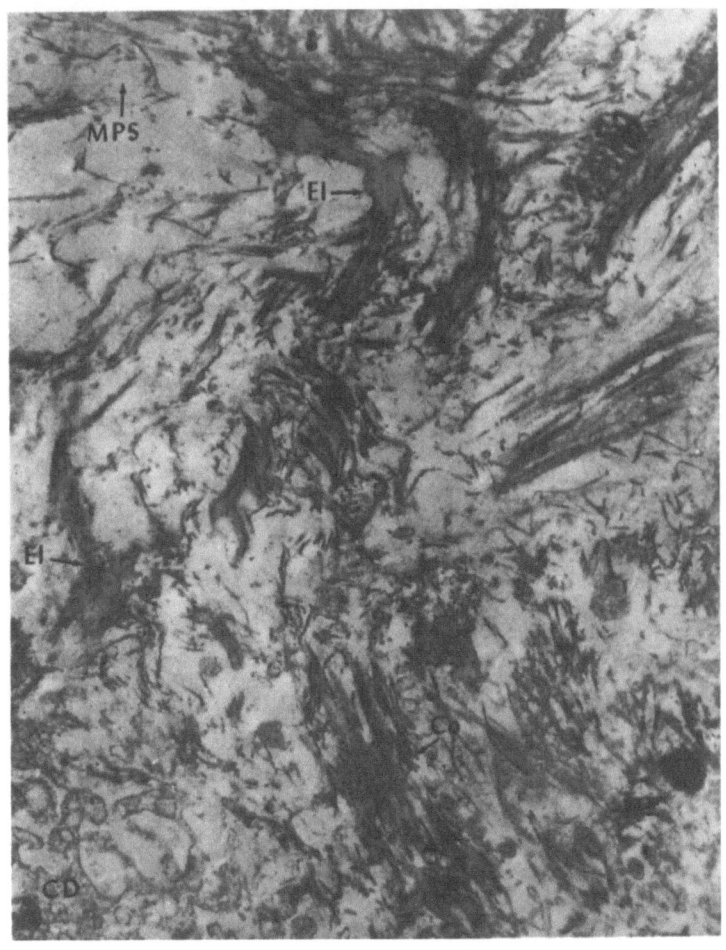

Figure 2. Electromicrograph of intercellular substance from the peripheral new growth of a 21-day culture. Large numbers of collagen fibers (Co) and elastic fibers (El), together with mucopolysaccharides (MPS), are present. Cell debris (CD) suggesing cell degeneration is also present. X 8.938

saccharides were demonstrated microscopically in the peripheral growth of each type of culture (Daoud et al., in press).

Quantitatively, several interesting findings, summarized in Table 1, emerged from these experiments. In many instances human sera resulted in a more copious peripheral growth than the normal swine serum. But there was a marked variation among human sera in their capacity to elicit the peripheral growth. There was no difference between human sera and swine sera in their capacities to cause DNA degradation. However, when all human sera tested were compared to the reference normal swine sera, a significantly greater terminal rate of synthesis of DNA resulted from the human sera (Daoud et al., 1973). Another interesting point was that the range of synthetic activities among the human sera was much greater than that among normal swine sera, showing in several instances as much as a ten fold difference. There was also a significantly greater terminal rate of total protein synthesis resulting from human sera than from swine sera. The range of differences among the human sera in this respect was commonly three fold, more rarely five fold. In quantitative studies of collagen synthesis overall, the percentage of total protein synthesis represented by collagen synthesis or the actual amounts of collagen synthesized were not different in human serum cultures than they were in swine serum cultures. However, again the range of percentages of collagen synthesis was much greater among the human serum cultures, both the highest and lowest percentages being in human cultures.

The wide differences in DNA, protein and collagen synthesis observed among human sera suggest that the explant system may prove to be a sensitive bioassay for the prediction of individual susceptibility to atherosclerosis. Studies aimed at confirmation of this potential application are now in progress.

Table 1.

Culture medium	Peripheral growth	Terminal DNA synthesis	Terminal protein synthesis	Collagen synthesis (as % of total protein synthesis)
M199	0	$\pm$	$\pm$	$\pm$
Normal swine serum	+ — ++	+ — ++	+ — ++	++
HC swine serum	+ — +++	+ — +++	+ — +++	—[a]
Human serum	+ — ++++[b]	+ — ++++[b]	+ — ++++[b]	+ — +++[c]

[a] Not investigated.
[b] Among individual sera there was good correlation between DNA and protein synthesis but not between amount of peripheral growth and terminal DNA synthesis.
[c] There is good correlation between the percent of total protein synthesis involved in collagen synthesis and the amount of peripheral growth.

RESPONSE OF AORTIC MEDIAL CELLS TO HYPERLIPEMIC SERUM *IN VITRO*

Katti Fischer-Dzoga

The aortic smooth muscle cell has been implicated in mammalian atherogenesis. In order to document this further and to develop more quantitative measurements of the response of these cells to selected atherogenic stimuli we developed an *in vitro* system using the outgrowth of small explants of thoracic media. Cultures of smooth muscle cells, as judged by morphological (EM) and immunohistochemical criteria, were obtained in this manner. They readily take up lipids and by means of special stains they could be shown to produce collagen and acid mucopolysaccharides. Mostly thoracic aortas of Rhesus monkeys and of rabbits were used. Our main concern, once a reproducible system was established, (Fischer-Dzoga et al., 1973) has been to investigate the response of these cells to exposure to hyperlipemic serum (induced in homologous donor animals by a high lipid and cholesterol diet) as compared to their behavior in normal serum. It is within this framework that our experiments were set up.

We concentrated our efforts on two problems: the effects of the presence of hyperlipemic serum on the proliferation of and lipid uptake by these cells. One important finding was that these primary cultures, which in normal serum reach a stationary growth phase after about six weeks can be stimulated to a second phase of growth by the addition of 5% of hypercholesteremic serum to the culture medium. This proliferative effect can be measured as increase in surface area or it can be visualized by radioautography after a pulse label with ^{3}H thymidine. The fraction found to be responsible for this second spur of growth was the low density lipoprotein (Sf 0-20). LDL of normal serum has no such effect on these cells even when given in higher concentrations so as to approach concentrations of cholesterol

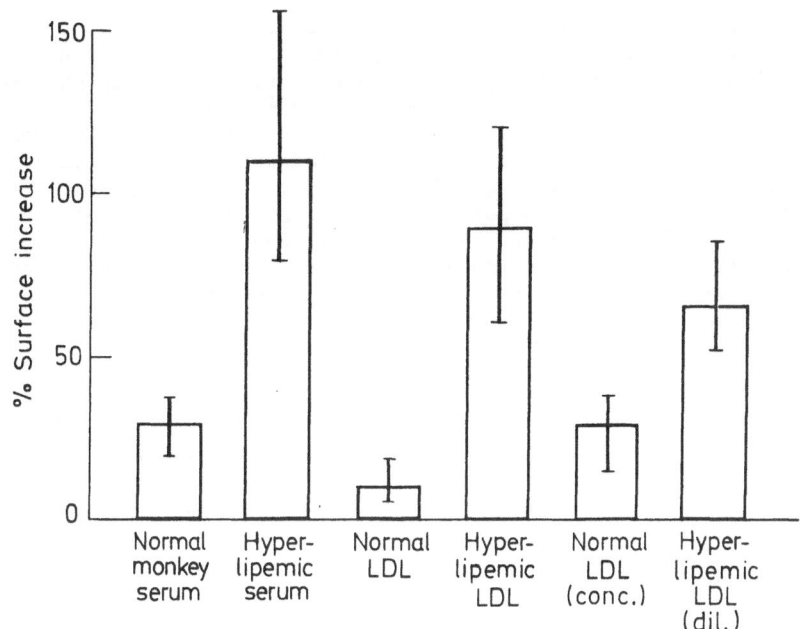

Figure 1. Effect of normal and hyperlipemic serum lipoprotein fractions on the growth of primary cultures of aortic smooth muscle cells: % increase in surface area during a 10-day period (summary of 5 experiments)

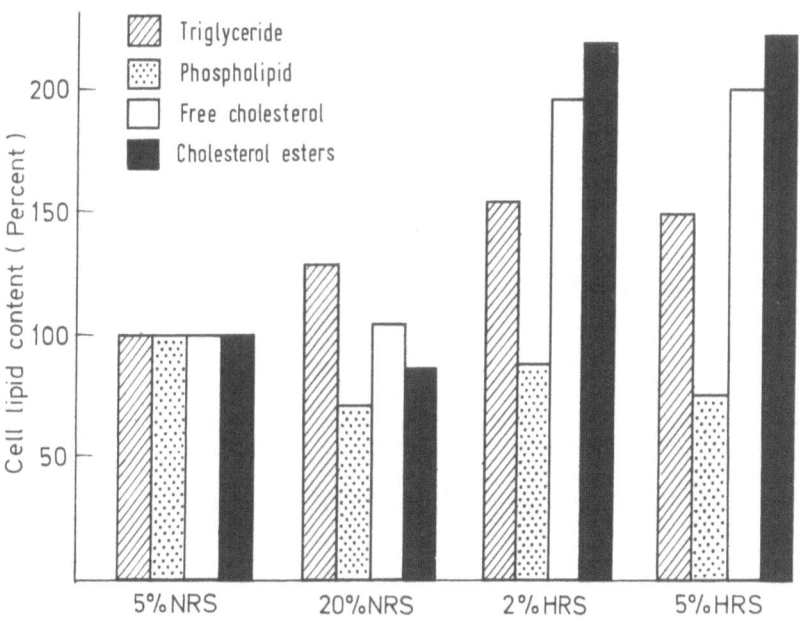

Figure 2. Lipid distribution in rabbit aortic medial cells incubated in media containing different concentrations of normal and hyperlipemic serum

comparable to the values in hypercholesteremic LDL (Fig. 1). It thus appears that the type of serum is much more important than the amount of lipoprotein added. An increase in uptake of lipids by these cultures was also observed and by immuno-histochemical methods the major apoprotein of LDL could be demonstrated within these cells. No positive reaction could be obtained with labeled antibodies to HDL. Extraction of the lipid accumulated within these cells and subsequent thin layer chromatography revealed an increase in total lipids. After exposure of these cell lipids to hyperlipemic serum or LDL from hyperlipemic serum, there was also a striking increase in cholesterol and cholesterol esters, compared to the amounts found in cells incubated in normal serum. Again the type of serum seemed to determine the pattern of lipid uptake, not the lipid lipoprotein concentration in the medium (Fig. 2). Some increase in triglycerides was also observed.

Table 1. Response of aortic medial cells to hyperlipemic serum in vitro

Animals used	Monkey and rabbit	Rabbit
Type of culture	Primary	Subcultures
Characteristics of cells EM Immunochemical staining	1. Morphology of smooth muscle cells 2. React positively with anti-smooth muscle acto-myosin	Morphology of smooth muscle cells
Growth Measurement of colony size H^3 thymidine incorporation Protein determination Cell count	1. Increased proliferation after 24-36 hours 2. Responsible fraction: hyperlipemic LDL 3. No linear dose-response relationship	Increased prolifera-tion *and* increased degeneration
Lipid accumulation ORO Stain Immunochemical staining Lipid extraction, follow-ed by TLC	1. Accumulation of lipids, generally reversible 2. Positive reaction with anti-LDL, no reaction with anti-HDL 3. Increase in cholesterol and cholesterol esters	1. 2-4 fold increase in cholesterol ester and free cholesterol 2. Some increase in triglycerides 3. Time dependent, generally reversible

Most of these biochemical studies were done with trypsinized subcultures of rab-bit aorta, but preliminary experiments with primary cultures of monkey aorta gave comparable results. A summary of these findings is shown in Table 1.

Effect of hyperlipemic serum on lipid content of rabbit aortic medial cells. Cells grown in 5% of normal serum served as the control group, and the lipid per mg of cell protein of control was used as one unit. The other groups were compared to this control unit. Cells exposed to 2-5% of hyperlipemic serum showed striking increase of cholesterol ester and free cholesterol.

FUNCTIONAL CHARACTERIZATION OF ARTERIAL CELLS INVOLVED IN SPONTANEOUS ATHEROMA

A.L. Robertson, Jr.

Since 1954, we have been interested in identifying the metabolic characteristics of human cells involved in the initial stages of spontaneous atheroma. What follows is a short review of some of the findings as well as a summary of current studies aimed at the eventual development of therapeutic measures to slow progression or induce regression of atheroma in man.

The long-term goals of these investigations are: 1. to obtain short-term cultures of homogenous monoclonal diploid arterial cells for repetitive quantitative analyses; 2. stabiliation of both karyotype and metabolic requirements of such cells *in vitro;* and 3. identification of specific biochemical abnormalities, susceptible to therapy, in cells from atheromatous vessels.

Using isolation of arterial layers by cell culture methods described several years ago (Lazzarini Robertson, 1959), we have been able to study arterial intimal, medial and adventitial cells and identify some of their cytological characteristics.

In the adult human arterial intima, two major cell populations have been identified by cell culture (Lazzarini Robertson, 1959). Based on their functional response to the incorporation of extracellular lipids *in vitro,* the terms "atherophils" and "fibrophils" were suggested, since morphological identification of such cells in mixed cultures have proved to be inadequate for the evaluation of large cell numbers (Robertson, 1967). Atherophils fulfill many of the cytochemical, immunofluorescent and ultrastructural characteristics of vascular smooth muscle and are by far the most common cell type both in normal intima and early atheroma. Fibrophils, on the other hand, are much less numerous and usually are overgrown by rapidly dividing atherophils in primary cultures. The third component of the arterial intima, the endothelial cells, share some functional and metabolic characteristics with atherophils and medial smooth muscle cells *in vitro.* They respond to stimulation with nanogram concentrations of some vasoactive agents and rapidly incorporate colloidal electron markers and extracellular lipoproteins (Robertson and Khairallah, 1973b). These findings have been interpreted as an indication that large arteries, endothelium, atherophils, and medial smooth muscle cells may share a common ancestry and represent specialized transitional stages of metabolically and functionally similar cell populations in the adult vessel (Robertson, 1973). Average cell composition of atherophils *in vitro* have been compared with those of rapidly dividing adult human tumor cells shown to be within the same range as other diploid mesenchymal cells.

	Diploid Human Atherophil	Polyploid Human Hepatoma
DNA	7×10^{-12} g/cell	2×10^{-11} g/cell
RNA	2.2×10^{-12}	2.5×10^{-11}
Total cell protein	2×10^{-10}	1×10^{-9}

Fig. 1-1 and 1-2 show that, in contrast to similarities in culture of intimal and medial cells, striking differences in morphology and growth characteristics may be found when such cells are compared to those of the adventitial layer of the same arterial segment. Arterial adventitial cells are similar in culture to connective tissue cells from other organs.

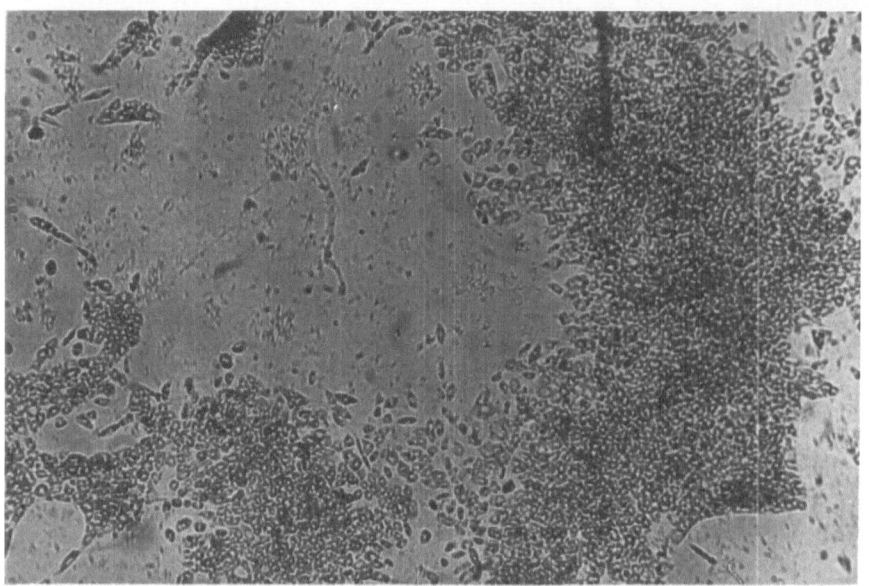

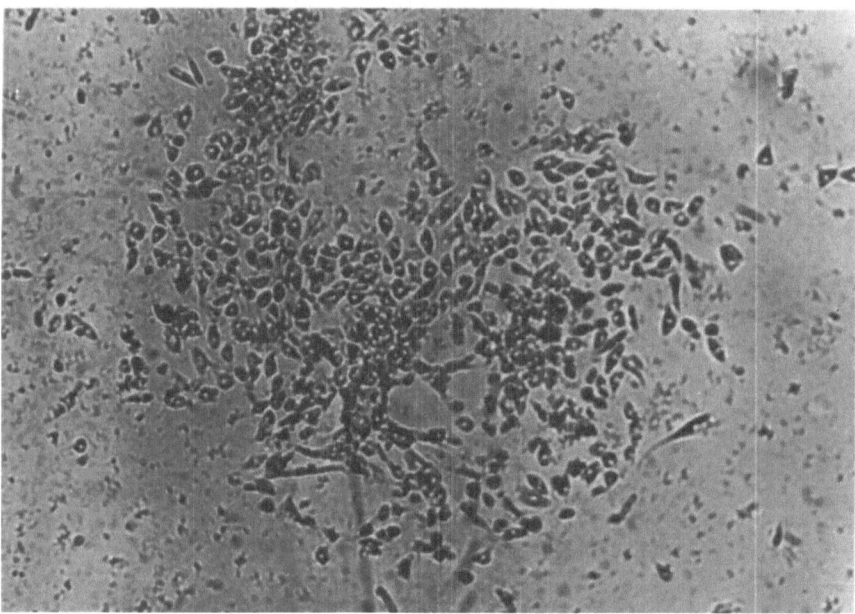

Figure 1. Morphological differences and growth characteristics of mixed cultures of atherophils and fibrophils (1) and adventitial cells (2) from the same arterial segment. Human coronary artery. Phase contrast microscopy. Unstained preparations

Sensitivity to the incorporation of lipoprotein lipids was found to be an important phenotypic characteristic useful in the identification of atherophils in culture (Robertson, 1965). As shown in Fig. 2, cells obtained from disease-free areas of aortas with severe atheroma elsewhere showed increased uptake rates of labeled cholesterol from low density lipoprotein fractions when compared with those of atheroma-free aortas. In contrast, Table 1 shows results of similar studies done with arterial cells from species considered less susceptible or more resistant to spontaneous atherosclerosis than primates. Chick, rat or rabbit arterial cells showed consistently lower incorporation rates of labeled cholesterol

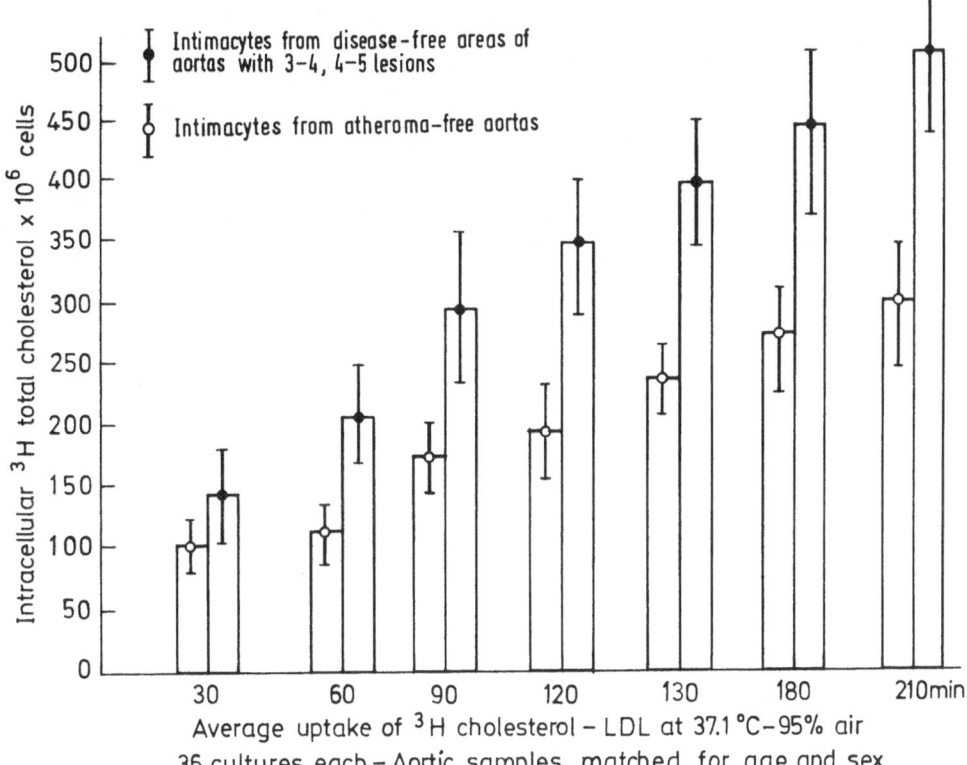

Figure 2. Differences in rates of cholesterol uptake of human aortic cells
(intimacytes) *in vitro*

after incubation in tissue culture medium containing homologous sera of matching
cholesterol concentrations from arterial cells of swine, monkey, or man.

Table 1. Species differences in intracellular sterol accumulation arterial cells
from atheroma-free donors. Individually challenged with media containing *homologous* sera of matching cholesterol concentrations

| | Incubation time in minutes | | | |
	30	60	120	240
Chick	0.16/4.2	0.21/4.0	0.31/3.8	0.49/3.6
Rat	0.24/3.9	0.36/3.8	0.48/3.6	0.39/3.8
Rabbit	0.42/4.0	0.59/4.2	0.84/3.9	1.2/3.3
Swine	1.26/4.3	2.43/4.1	4.94/3.2	16.3/2.7
Monkey	3.4/3.8	16.7/3.2	87.2/2.7	183/2.6
Human	98/3.21	246/0.84	548/0.39	847/0.21

Average μg of total cholesterol per mg cell protein/FC/CE ratio 28 cultures for
each value

An unusual metabolic characteristic of matching cultures of diploid human coronary intimal cells is shown in Table 2 following incubation in pooled normolipemic or hyperlipemic sera. Intracellular cholesterol ester concentrations were significantly higher than those of any of the other lipid fractions after incubation in hyperlipemic serum. In contrast to cultures of human skin fibroblasts, skeletal muscle cells, or adipocytes also tested, this intracellular ester accumulation did not decrease simultaneous *de novo* synthesis of cholesterol from ^{14}C labeled acetate or tritiated mevalonate. The absence of this important regulatory feedback mechanism for sterol synthesis in the atheromatous artery may be responsible, at least in part, for the development of typical "foam" cells during atherogenesis.

In agreement with the very interesting observations with monkey medial cells reported at this meeting by Dr. Fisher-Dzoga, we have found that in both human adult and fetal arterial cells, mitotic activity and tritiated thymidine incorporation were stimulated by LDL fractions from hyperlipemic sera (Robertson, 1971). Other powerful inducers of arterial cell proliferation have been found to be suppressor concentrations of vasoactive agents such as the actapeptide angiotension II, 5-hydroxytriptamine (serotonin) and prostaglandin $F_2\alpha$ (Robertson and Khairallah, 1973a). In contrast, catecholamines seem to inhibit mitotic activity and thymidine uptake under similar experimental conditions.

Table 2. Monoclonal diploid human coronary intimal cells in culture. Average intracellular lipid concentrations[a] after incubation

Uptake of Extracellular Lipids	in 10% NS[b]	in 10% HS[c]
Triglycerides	52	142 µg L/mg cell protein
Free cholesterol	84	194
Cholesterol esters	32	520
C/CE ratio	2.62	0.37

Same cells "*De Novo*" synthesis from ^{14}C acetate or ^{3}H mevalonate

	in 10% NS[b]		in 10% HS[c]	
	% Total lipids	Average dpm/µg L	% Total lipids	Average dpm/µg L
Free cholesterol	96	620	8	28
Cholesterol esters	12	94	81	146

[a] 32 cultures each incubated for 120 minutes at 37°C in 5% CO_2-Air.

[b] Pooled normolipemic human serum: TC 220 mg%   TG 89 mg%,
CE 184 mg%   PH 292 mg%.

[c] Pooled hyperlipemic human serum: TC 396 mg%   TG 104 mg%,
CE 294 mg%   PH 290 mg%.

Time lapse cinematography has been used to follow morphological changes occurring during early stages of intracellular lipid deposition. Fig. 3 shows selected single frames from such a study demonstrating the appearance of large perinuclear vacuoles after incubation for 60 minutes or longer in tissue culture medium containing 20% type II hyperlipoproteinemic sera.

At ultrastructural level, the storage of intracellular lipids is initiated by localized dilatations of the cisternae of rough endoplasmic reticulum shown in Fig. 4. They are followed by formation of single unit membrane limited vacuoles of different electron density (L_1 and L_2), some of which are eventually released to the extracellular space after cell lysis. We have recently found that LDL fractions from hyperlipemic donors also induce rapid secretion of amorphous extracellular material by these arterial cells (Fig. 5). These phenomena are followed by appearance of poorly differentiated extracellular fibrilar components resembling elastin as well as by more electron dense and well defined fibrils with the periodicity of collagen (Fig. 6).

In summary, the above findings suggest that some lipoprotein fractions, particularly LDL isolated from hyperlipemic sera, may induce three major changes in human arterial cells from atheromatous arteries:

1. accelerated intracellular lipid storage, particularly of cholesterol esters;
2. increased mitotic activity resulting in larger cell populations; and
3. *de novo* synthesis of extracellular components.

While these *in vitro* alterations in arterial cell function are also shared by arterial cells *in vivo* during the initial stages of spontaneous atheroma, more research is needed to fully assess their significance in both the development and progression of atherosclerosis in man.

Discussion

Dr. R. St. Clair asked Dr. Smith if he had cross-tested sera from White Carneau and Show Racer pigeons to determine if the variations found in susceptibility to spontaneous arterial lesions were related to genetic changes in arterial cells or to unknown serum factors. Dr. Smith replied that while the suggested test was difficult to perform, since sera from embryos would be needed, the reported differences in his studies were found with cells from both types of pigeons incubated in heterologous culture medium containing normolipemic horse serum. Dr. St. Clair concurred with these comments and mentioned that preliminary studies in his own laboratory also suggested that the observed increased susceptibility was due to some biochemical component in the arterial wall rather than in the serum. Dr. Daoud commented that sera from less atheroma-prone species, such as the dog, induced slower growth rates of swine medial arterial explants than human serum under similar laboratory conditions. Dr. Pollak stressed the need to standardize both the sources of sera and tissues for such comparative studies.

Dr. G. Rothblat asked Dr. Robertson to clarify whether the absence he described of a feedback mechanism in adult human intimal cells to regulate sterol synthesis in the presence of increased extracellular cholesterol uptake, was also found in other cell types. Dr. Robertson answered that this was true also for fetal vascular smooth muscle cells but not for human skin fibroblasts or for several established human cell lines. These findings suggested to him that a potentially important metabolic inability to handle excessive sterol loads may be present in human arterial cells.

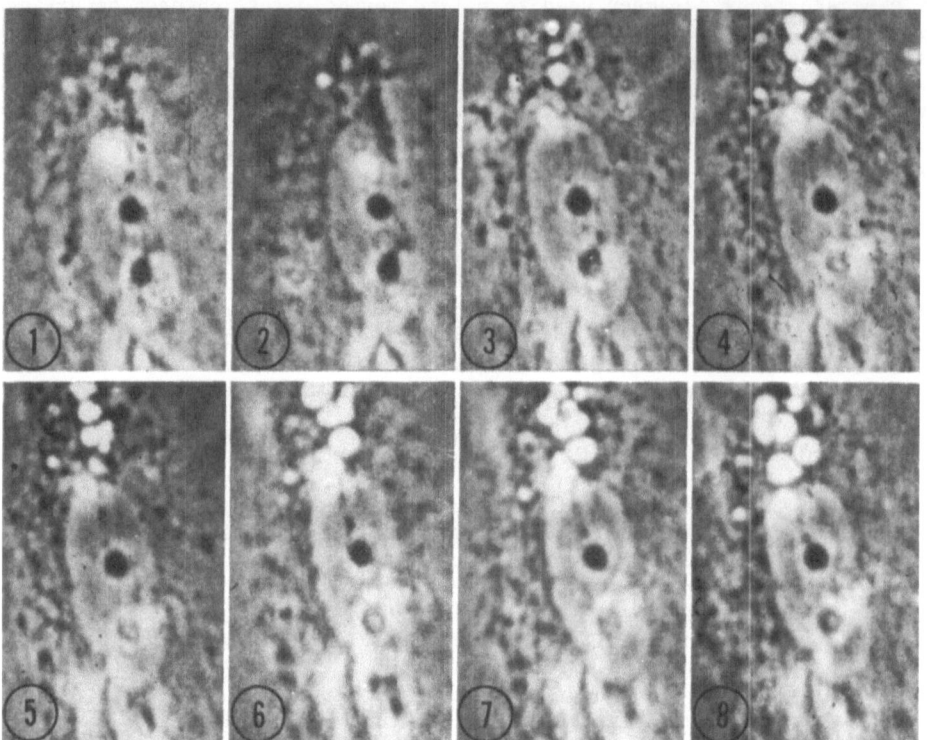

Figure 3. Selected frames from time lapse cinematography showing intracellular
lipid incorporation during incubation of an atherophil from human coronary artery
in media containing 20% pooled homologous sera from Type II hyperlipoproteinemic
patients. Frame 1 after 60 minutes incubation; each subsequent frame was taken at
10 minute intervals. Phase contrast microscopy. X 787

Dr. Rothblat also questioned Dr. Gross regarding differences in incorporation of
labeled triglycerides between heart cells and skin fibroblasts and suggested that
this may be due to the presence of lipases since Dr. Gross's data suggested that
triglyceride uptake occurred as free fatty acids. Dr. Gross answered that this
indeed could be possible and that this lipase release may be heparin dependent.
Dr. Rothblat then asked Dr. Fischer-Dzoga if, when lipoproteins were added to
induce increased proliferation of smooth muscle cells in her experiments, the
presence of such lipoprotein was necessary throughout the experiment or if only a
short exposure was required. Dr. Fischer-Dzoga's reply was that experiments are in
progress to study this interaction in her tissue culture system. Dr. Rothblat
then asked how long can vascular smooth muscle be maintained as differentiated
cells *in vitro*. Dr. Fischer-Dzoga mentioned that after 8-9 passages in her experiment, cells showed morphological changes consistent with neoplastic transformation.
Several other participants agreed with this view. Dr. W. Thomas mentioned that in
their studies with medial swine cells in culture, prolonged cultivation induced
irreversible cytological alterations with profound morphological changes. Dr.
Robertson then mentioned that in human arterial cultures, polyploidy is a common
finding after 6-10 passages. In contrast with short-term cultures, after 10 passages *in vitro*, cells from atheromatous arteries lose their metabolic characteristics, including incorporation of labeled lipids at a faster rate than cells from
atheroma free arteries. Dr. Rothblat asked the group if these changes could be
considered examples of cytological "dedifferentiation" *in vitro*. There was general

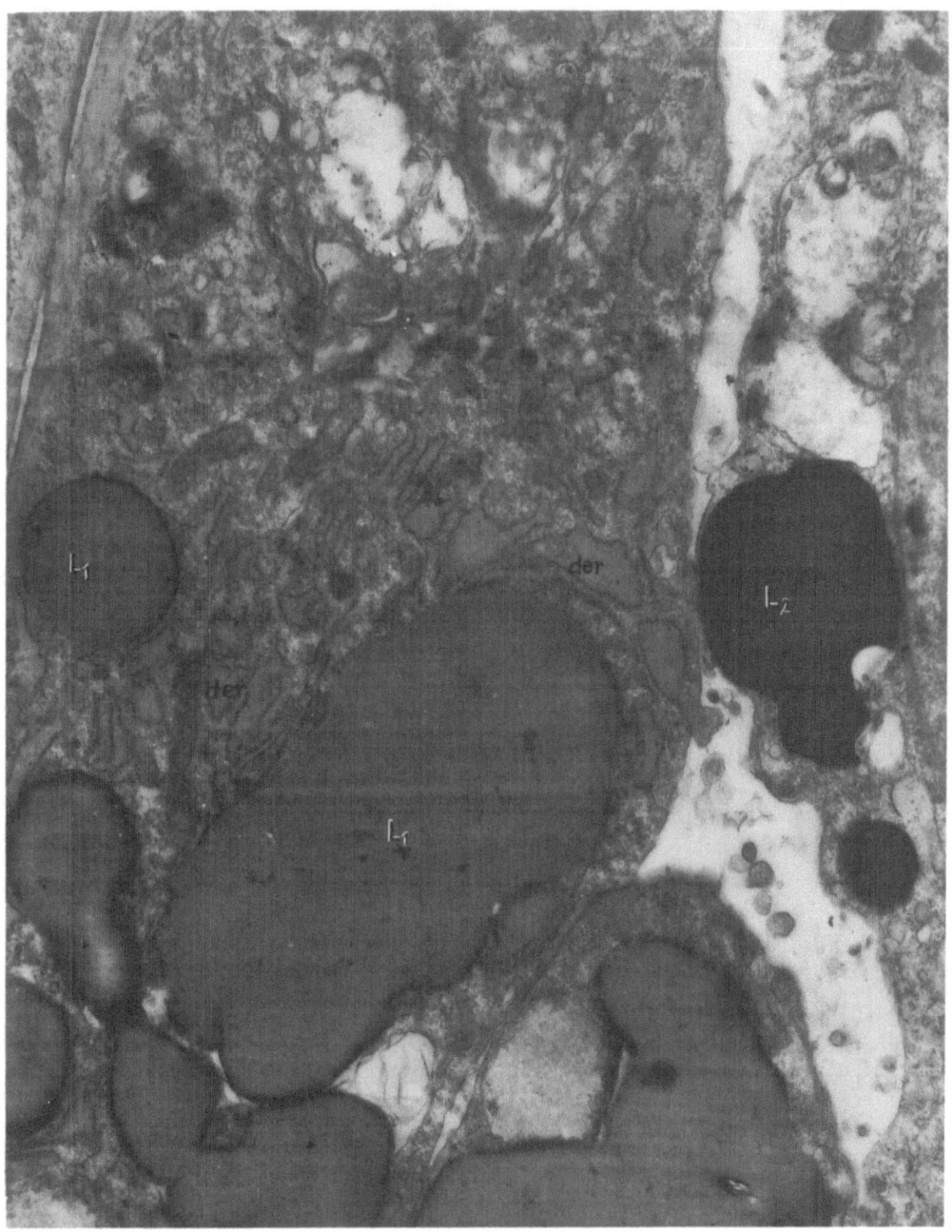

Figure 4. Ultrastructural changes found during initial storage of intracellular lipids (dilated cisternae of rough endoplasmic reticulum) (der) are surrounded by membrane bound lipid droplets of different electron density related to concentration of triglycerides and FFA. Water embedding technique, followed by uranyl acetate-lead citrate staining. X 13.020

agreement that this was the case but that the term "dedifferentiation" has a number of confusing connotations and should be avoided. In answer to Dr. Rothblat's question as to whether an outgrowth of preexisting fibroblasts could explain such behavioral changes, Dr. T. Wight did not believe so. In studies done in collaboration with Dr. R. Ross, they have noted such changes using what may be considered a pure population of medial smooth muscle cells only occasionally contaminated with endothelial elements.

Dr. W. Hauss asked Dr. Fischer-Dzoga if the low density lipoprotein fraction used in her study was a specific stimulant for vascular smooth muscle proliferation or if other substances also may have such properties. Dr. Fischer-Dzoga answered that LDL seems to be specific for vascular smooth muscle since it has no effect on uterine smooth muscle, subcutaneous fibroblasts, or in primary cultures from other tissues. Dr. Hauss then asked if sera from hypertensive animals was used by Dr. Fischer-Dzoga and to that she replied that it had not been tested.

Dr. W. Thomas then commented that the sudden transformation observed in swine arterial and medial cell cultures after several passages favors the idea of a cytological alteration occurring in preexisting cells rather than an overgrowth of preexisting fibroblasts. With regard to Dr. Fischer-Dzoga's presentation, he then mentioned that the experimental design of her dilution studies with hyperlipemic sera could not exclude the possibility that other cell factors may also be diluted besides lipoproteins.

Dr. St. Clair then asked if information was available as to whether or not all smooth muscle cells in a culture are simultaneously stimulated or whether individual clones or cells respond to such stimuli. Dr. Daoud answered that their autoradiographic studies were inconclusive, while Dr. Fischer-Dzoga believed that in primary primate cultures the stimulation is indeed spotty and varies considerably from explant to explant. Dr. Robertson then asked Dr. Becker if endothelial cells from umbilical veins do not aggregate or superimpose on one another, as is the case with arterial endothelium, or if they show basement membrane or "tight" intercellular junctions. Dr. Becker referred this question to Dr. R. Minnick who replied that in their ultrastructural studies, they would occasionally find basement membranes and "tight" junctions.

Dr. Rothblat then asked the Workshop if cell culture studies would be a good system for the screening of anti-atherogenic agents. Dr. Gross referred to examples of the evaluation of cytological effects of clofibrate in such systems and there was general agreement that, indeed, this is an important contribution that tissue culture techniques can make to the field of atherosclerosis research.

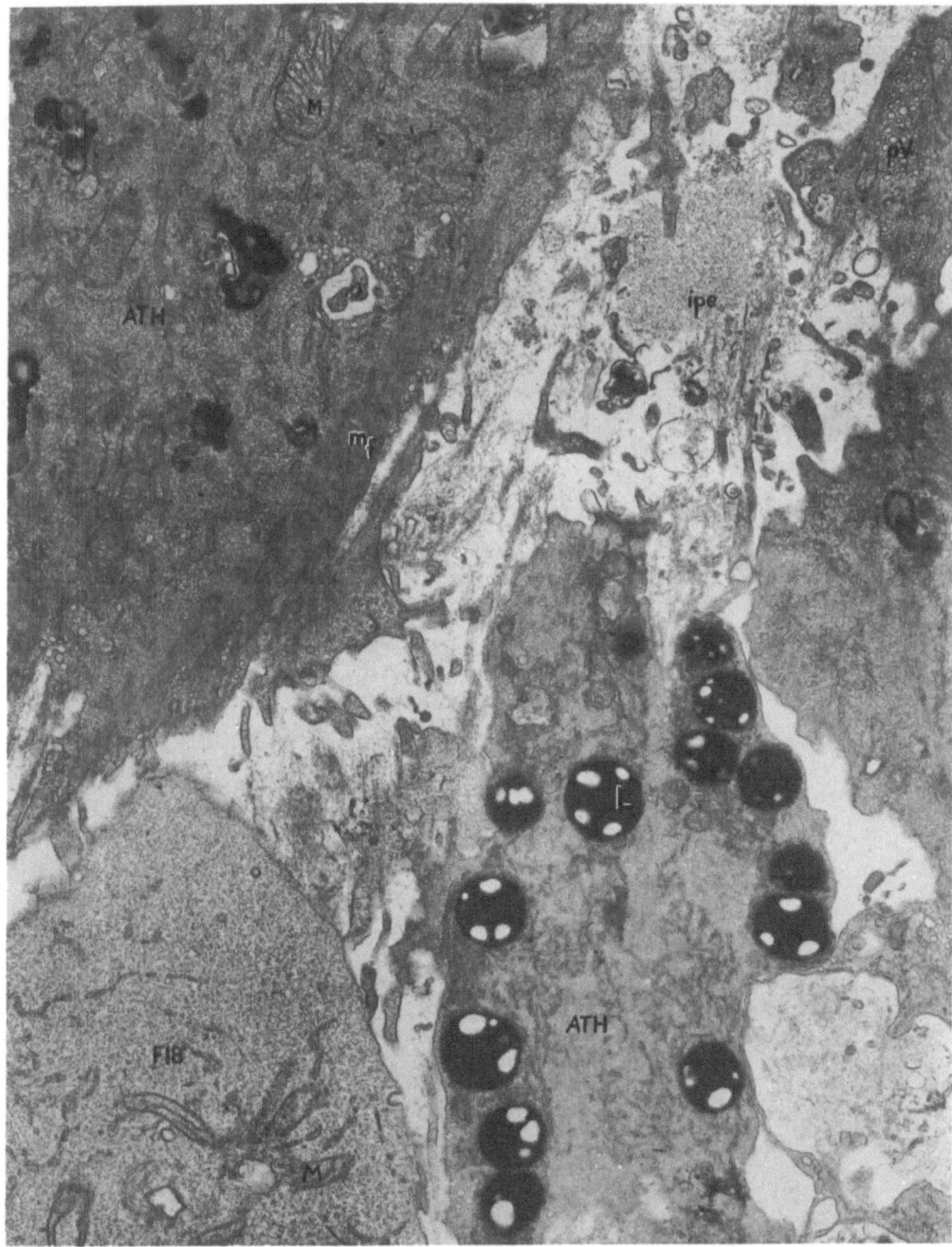

Figure 5. Ultrastructural differences between atherophils (ATH) and fibrophils (FIB) during incorporation of extracellular lipids. Note amorphous extracellular elements (lpe) and abundance of pinocytotic vesicles in ATH cells (pV). Uranyl acetate-lead citrate staining. X 16.728

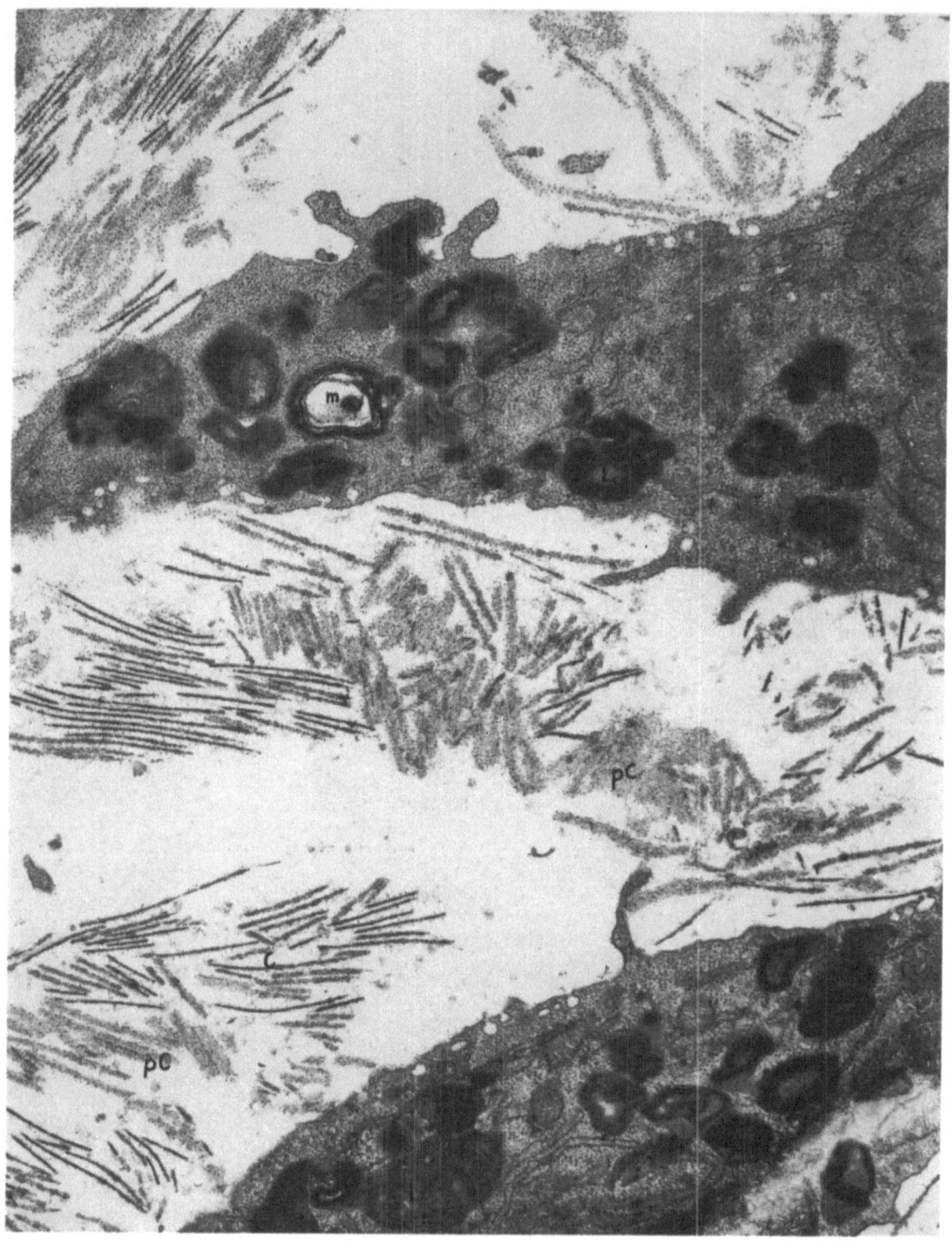

Figure 6. Increased extracellular fibrillar material found after incubation in LDL fraction from hyperlipemic donors. Note amorphous or poorly differentiated fibers (pC) as well as defined fibrils (C). Uranyl acetate, lead citrate staining. X 22.168

SUMMARY OF WORKSHOP ON TISSUE CULTURES

O.J. Pollak

As background for my remarks I selected one facet of the problem faced by tissue culture workers in the field of atherosclerosis.

Let us consider the "appearance of intracellular lipids". There are various possible *modes* which may operate singly, in sequence, or in combination: phagocytosis, pinocytosis, trans-membrane transport with or without physicochemical change to the lipids, synthesis regulated (according to Dr. Robertson) by cellular homeostasis, phanerosis (referring to Dr. Simms' lipfanogens), aging or degeneration. There are even more numerous *factors*, operative again in sequence or in combinations. The origin of the explant ... the species differences which were mentioned here by all speakers, the donor's age ...also mentioned, the donor's health ... not mentioned, the quality of the explant ... with obvious differences between intact and altered tissues, then, the culture method ... CO_2 percentage, to mention only one aspect, the composition of the nutrient and the availability of lipids, the purity of the cell line, and the age of the cell population ... stressed by the participants at this workshop. Only after we have solved all of this can there be progress in the attempts to influence the modes and the factors.

Attention has been paid to the lipid metabolism on the cellular level. But, very little attention has been given to glycoaminoglucans, carbohydrates, proteins, amino acids, etc. Whatever happened to the differences in arachidonic acid found by Dr. Smith in cell cultures from two breeds of pigeons? This line of research must be pursued. Study of enzymes by histochemical and chemical methods could yield interesting information. I found differences in the results of enzyme stains applied to arteries and veins. And I am glad to learn that Dr. Becker is working with veins. Comparison of my results proved difficult because of the differences in growth rates between arterial and venous cells and the qualitative and quantitative shifts of enzymes during aging of the cells.

This brings me to the problem of standardization of methodology. It may be that complete standardization - which would result in stagnation - is not essential. It seems to me essential, however, that everybody reports his work in greatest detail to facilitate reconciliation of seemingly incompatible results. One important observation agreed upon here in answer to a query by Dr. Rothblat was that smooth muscle cells lose their morphologic and metabolic characteristics after 6 to 8 passages. Here then may be a real need for standardization: Investigators should agree to study cells between F_2 and F_4. Hopefully, similar criteria will be established for other vascular cell types.

Drs. Daoud, Dzoga, and Smith discussed smooth muscle cells, Dr. Becker spoke about endothelial cells, and Dr. Gross about fibroblasts. Nobody mentioned the fourth type of cell cultured regularly from arterial lesions - the metabolically active, light reflecting, highly mobile, burr-shaped macrophage. Dr. Robertson suggested that this may be a modified, fat-laden smooth muscle cell. I have my doubts since these cells appear very early in culture and much earlier than smooth muscle cells. They also differ in many ways from fat-bearing cells from blood vessels - the three types referred to before.

Dr. Gross studied myocardial cells. This is good. There were difficulties in obtaining myocardial cell cultures free of fibroblasts. Much can be learned from comparison of myocardial cells with vascular smooth muscle cells.

The question of drug screening was asked by Rothblat and was commented on by Dr. Smith. This - hopefully profitable - application of tissue culture work is still in its infancy. As I pointed out in a chapter on cytopharmacology in my monograph on tissue cultures in atherosclerosis, it is regrettable that fibroblasts only have been used for this line of investigation. Certainly, our concern is with smooth muscle cells and endothelial cells which are involved in the fat metabolism.

Two more fascinating observations were reported today by Dr. Dzoga and confirmed by others in response to a question by Dr. Hauss:
one, that increased cholesterol uptake by smooth muscle cells is nearly specifically caused by low-density lipoproteins (LDL); the second, that within a given time span (5 hours) a saturation point (of 20%) of cholesterol uptake is reached by these cells. Hopefully, criteria along these lines will be established for other vascular cell types.

As the cell *in vitro* and the whole body *in vivo* reach a saturation point so does the audience at this workshop. And thus I am closing my summation with a "Thank you!" to all the participants.

CELL PROLIFERATION AND ULTRASTRUCTURAL CHANGES IN REGRESSING ATHEROSCLEROTIC LESIONS AFTER REDUCTION OF SERUM CHOLESTEROL

H.C. Stary

Dietary cholesterol causes cell proliferation in the intimal atherosclerotic lesions of arteries (Stary, 1967; McMillan and Stary, 1968; Stary and McMillan, 1970). This paper reports an experiment designed to study whether cell prolifera- tion will return to normal levels when cholesterol is removed from the diet and hypercholesterolemia is reduced. Changes in cell proliferation are compared with the rate of lipid removal, and with alterations in cellular fine structure during lesion regression.

Methods

The design of this study is described elsewhere in detail (Stary, 1972). Briefly, rhesus monkeys received normal commercial primate food (NF), or atherogenic food (NF supplemented with a saturated fat and cholesterol) for 12 weeks. At the end of the 12-week period of lesion induction, monkeys receiving atherogenic food (AF) were ranked according to serum cholesterol elevation, divided into three groups with similar mean serum cholesterols, and returned to NF. One group was killed 3 weeks after return to NF at which time the serum cholesterol had just returned to normal levels. These animals provided a measure of the extent of lesions induced. Other groups were killed 16 and 40 weeks following return to NF. Two i.v. injec- tions of thymidine-^{3}H were given to each monkey, 8 hours and 1 hour before kill- ing. Radioautographs were prepared from the entire length of the aorta by a technique described previously (Stary and McMillan, 1970). Tissue for electron microscopy was taken from four standard locations in the aorta, fixed with buffer- ed osmium tetroxide, embedded in Maraglas, fine sectioned, and stained with lead citrate and uranyl acetate.

Results

The mean total serum cholesterol level was 120 mg/100 ml in animals given NF only. It was 435 mg/100 ml in animals on AF during the 12-week lesion induction period. These elevated values returned to normal within one to three weeks after return to NF (Stary, 1972).

NF Only. Most segments of aortic intima had one or several strata of smooth mus- cle cells (SMC). Intracellular lipid was rare, and there was no extracellular lipid in the intima. Tritiated thymidine radioautography showed infrequent label- ing of the nuclei of endothelial cells, and intimal and medial SMC.

12 Weeks AF Followed by 3 Weeks NF. There were many intimal lesions, more numer- ous and extensive in the thoracic than in the abdominal aorta. Just beneath the endothelial lining of lesions there were interdigitating mats of foam cells (FC), that is cells with lipid inclusions lacking features of smooth muscle. FC lipid was in the form of clear vacuoles, cholesterol clefts, phagolysosomes, and resi- dual bodies. The SMC in intimal lesions were of varying differentiation and many contained homogeneous lipid inclusions of moderate electron density. Some SMC showed degenerative changes. Necrotic FC and SMC appeared to be the source of extracellular lipid visible with the electron microscope. Tritiated thymidine labeling of SMC and FC in intimal lesions was frequent, and endothelial cells on the surface of lesions also showed more frequent labeling than endothelial cells in animals given NF only. The lesions were indistinguishable from those of

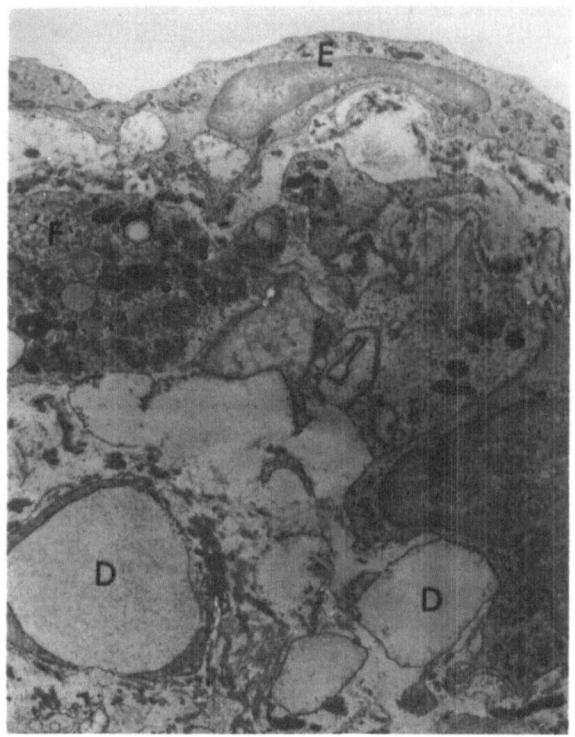

Figure 1. Intimal lesions in the distal part of the descending thoracic aorta of a monkey given atherogenic food for 12 weeks followed by normal food for 16 weeks. A foam cell (F) in the upper intima shows lipid inclusions and phagolysosomes. Necrotic cells and portions of cells with degenerative changes (D) are seen in the lower intima. Endothelial cell (E). (Rhesus No. 61; X 7200)

monkeys killed immediately after a 12-week period of AF in another experiment (Stary, 1970, 1972). Thus, the 3-week period of NF in the present group appeared to have caused no visible lesion regression.

12 Weeks AF Followed by 16 Weeks NF. Compared with the preceding group, intimal lesions were less cellular and contained less lipid. This was mainly due to a marked decrease in the number of FC. The morphology of the small number of FC seen in the intimal lesions of this group differed from that of FC in the preceding group. FC lipid was mainly in the form of phagolysosomes (Fig. 1 and 2), while clear lipid vacuoles and residual bodies were less frequent. Most of the residual lipid in these lesions was in the form of extracellular lipid, and lipid in well differentiated intimal SMC. The appearance of the lipid inclusions had not changed in the intimal SMC. Necrotic cell fragments and degenerative changes in cells (Fig. 1) were similar to those seen in the preceding time period. There was a marked reduction in tritiated thymidine labeling of all types of cells in the intimal lesions.

12 Weeks AF Followed by 40 Weeks NF. The number and extent of aortic intimal lesions had decreased markedly. Remaining lesions had only an occasional, rare FC and less extracellular lipid than lesions in the preceding group. Residual lipid now was in the deep parts of the intima, as extracellular lipid on the intimal side of the internal elastic lamina, and in the form of homogeneous lipid inclusions in well differentiated intimal SMC (Fig. 3). The nature of the lipid inclusions in intimal SMC remained the same, unchanged since the preceding time period.

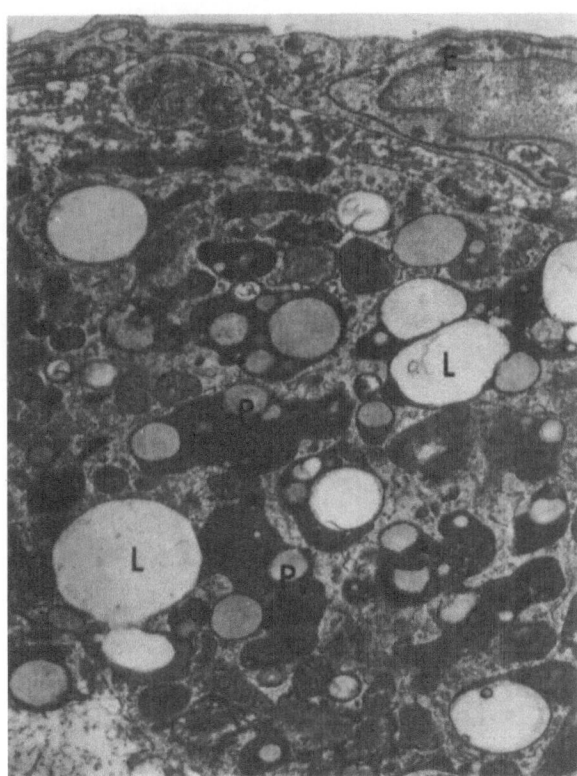

Figure 2. Intimal lesion in the proximal part of the descending thoracic aorta of a monkey given atherogenic food for 12 weeks followed by normal food for 16 weeks. A portion of a foam cell is seen beneath an endothelial cell (E). Almost all the intracytoplasmic lipid inclusions (L) in the foam cell are in association with laminated bodies to form phagolysosomes (P). (Rhesus No. 61; X 12900)

Necrotic cell fragments were infrequent. The rare residual FC did not label with tritiated thymidine. Labeling of intimal SMC and of endothelial cells was at the level of monkeys given NF only.

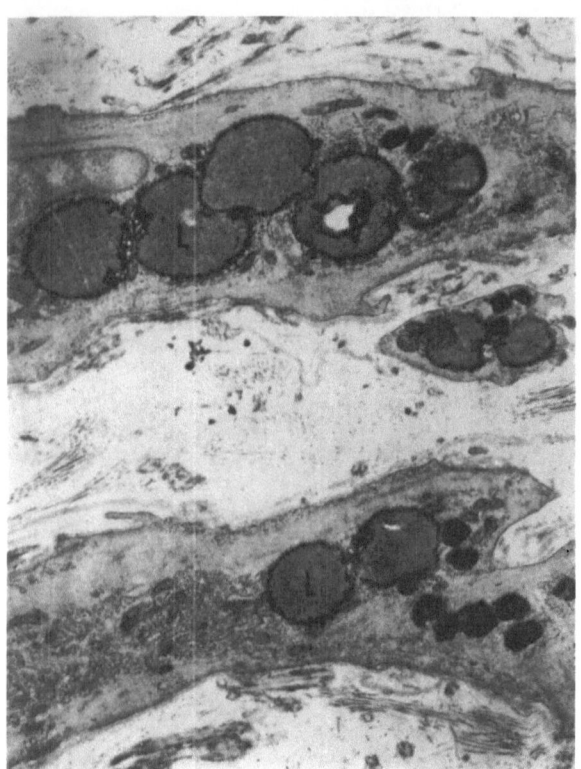

Figure 3. Intimal lesion in the abdominal aorta of a monkey given atherogenic food for 12 weeks followed by normal food for 40 weeks. Several well differentiated smooth muscle cells in the deep part of the intima are characterized by numerous myofilaments. They contain homogeneous lipid inclusions (L), predominantly of the moderately electron-dense type. (Rhesus No. 57; X 10125)

GLUCOSAMINEGLYCANS IN CELL MEMBRANES AND THE EXTRACELLULAR COMPARTMENT OF THE ARTERIAL WALL

J. Picard, P. Levy, B. Hermelin, M. Douillon-Breton, A. Groleas, and E. Deudon

Variations in the structure and distribution of arterial glucosamineglycans have been observed with aging and in experimental atherosclerosis (Picard and Gardais 1962; Gardais et al., 1973).

Accumulation of glucosamineglycans (mucopolysaccharides) in the arterial wall during early lesions of atherosclerosis is well-known. For this reason we attempted to elucidate in vitro the pathway of biosynthesis of proteoglycans in the arterial wall and to demonstrate the incorporation of labeled sugars from uridine nucleotide precursors by membrane enzymes (Picard and Levy, 1973).

The results indicate that for N-acetyl hexosaminyl-transferase and glucuronyl-transferase the optimum pH is approximately 6.8. These activities are present in both the submicrosomal fractions isolated according to the method of Dallner. As noted in Table 1, the yield of incorporation is 13.4% for UDP Glc NAc ^{14}C and 7.6% for UDP Glc UA [14]C.[*] These yields are approximately equal in rough and smooth membranes.

Table 1. Incorporation of carbohydrate in membrane proteins

	A	B
Unfractionated membranes	950	690
Rough membranes	13 400	7 600
Smooth membranes	12 600	7 300

The incubation mixture is described in previous studies (Picard and Levy, 1973). It contained sugar nucleotides UDP Glc NAc [14]C : 0.05 µC (A) or UDP Glc UA [14]C 0.05 µC (B). Results are given in specific activity : CPM / mg protein.

For the two enzymic activities the yield of incorporation is clearly lower in the nonfractionated membranes. The higher activity for hexosamine incorporation in the submicrosomal fractions results from its utilization in the biosynthesis of glycoproteins, while the glucuronate incorporation concerns only the biosynthesis of glucuronoglucosamineglycan proteins. The small amount of incorporation observed with ^{14}C-glucosamine involved utilization of labeled sugars from essentially uridine nucleotide precursors. In this case, the yield of incorporation is one-sixth the yield of incorporation with the correspondent nucleotide sugar. In previous studies we established that the incorporation of N-acetylhexosamine and glucuronate into proteoglycans of membranes concern all glucuronoglucosamineglycans that suggest efficient polymerases in the arterial wall. Chondroitin sulfate and heparin sulfate are labeled in these experiments. The incorporated radioactivity is higher in hyaluronic acid and heparan sulfate than in chondroitin sulfate.

---

[*]Abbreviations: UDP glucuronate : UDP Glc UA; UDP-N-acetylhexosamine : UDP Glc NAc.

Thus, it has been reported that the turnover of the chondroitin sulfate was 5 or 10 times slower than the turnover of heparin sulfate (Hermelin et al., 1973, in press). The glucosamineglycans are efficiently synthesized in the arterial wall as in embryonic cartilage.

Glucosamineglycans were also degraded by pig aortic enzymes. N-acetylhexosaminidase and ß-glucuronidase showed a high activity in the postnuclear supernatant from medial homogenates. Chondroitinase activity was detected in lysosomes, after density-gradient sucrose centrifugation (Table 2).

Table 2. Enzymic activities of isolated aortic smooth muscle cells

Enzyme	Specific activity[a]		pH optimum
	HT[d]	PNS[d]	
Acid phosphatase[b]	98.0	–	5.0
ß-glucuronidase[b]	2.3	4.1	5.6
N-acetyl-ß-glucosaminidase[c]	11.4	20.0	4.7 .

[a] Expressed as 10^{-9} mole of substrate / mg protein / hour.
[b] 0,1 M Acetate buffer.
[c] 0,0t M Citrate Phosphate buffer.
[d] HT : Homogenate ; PNS : Postnuclear supernatant.

These results indicate that the glucosamineglycan metabolism depends on cellular enzymes. Proteoglycans were isolated from matrix and medial and intimal cells.

These data agree with the existence of different pools of glucosamineglycans in the arterial wall. Glucosamineglycans were detected in rough and smooth membranes, and also in plasma and basement membranes. In the last, a small quantity of glucosamineglycans, hydrolyzable by chondroitinase AC, was separated from sialoglycoproteins by electrophoresis (Picard et al., 1973) (Table 3).

These macromolecules are implicated in tissue permeability and autoimmunization which could concern the atherosclerotic process.

Table 3. Components of intimal plasma membranes

Components	/ mg Protein
Hexosamines	19 ug
Sialic acid	4.2 ug
Glucosamineglycans	10 ug
5' Mononucleotidase	21 u Moles Pi per h

(Protein content of membranes : 50 ug / g $(W_{/W})$

INCREASED MITOTIC ACTIVITY IN PRIMARY CULTURES OF AORTIC MEDIAL SMOOTH MUSCLE CELLS AFTER EXPOSURE TO HYPERLIPEMIC SERUM

Katti Fischer-Dzoga, Rose M. Jones, Dragoslava Vesselinovitch, and Robert W. Wissler

The vascular smooth muscle cell has been demonstrated to play an active part in the pathogenesis of mammalian atherosclerosis. For several years now, we have been using primary cultures of aortic medial cells in order to study their response to an isolated atherogenic stimulus, namely, diet induced hypercholesteremia. Morphological and immunohistochemical evidence suggest that these cultures consist almost exclusively of smooth muscle cells. Our method of culturing is to place small explants of aortic media in tissue culture flasks with an appropriate medium, let them attach to the bottom of the flask and after a 5-10 day period, the first cells can be observed growing from this explant. Within 5-6 weeks, this outgrowth reaches a diameter of about 15-18 mm. These cell colonies can be maintained in culture for another 2 months or longer. However, they increase very little during that period, not more than 1-2 mm, and only few mitotic figures can be observed. This plateau is quite characteristic for these cells and it is at this stage that we use the cells for our experiments. The cells are elongated, mostly arranged in parallel fashion, often forming characteristic patterns of multilayered growth. Electron microscopical examination and special stains indicate that there is no loss of contact-inhibition in these areas, but rather that the layers are separated by elastin, collagen, or mucopolysaccharides.

Overnight labeling with H^3-Thymidine reveals that very few of these cells are synthesizing DNA, an expression of mitotic activity. Usually less than 10% of the nuclei are labelled by the isotope.

Presence of lipids can be visualized by staining with a fat stain, e.g., Oil Red Oil or Sudan black, and lipid distribution shows a wide variation at this stage, but mostly there is little lipid present within these cells. When the normal serum in the medium is replaced by diet induced hypercholestemic serum two things happen: first, the cells take up lipids in large amounts and second, the labeling index goes up to over 30% within 24 hours, indicating that these cells were stimulated into DNA synthesis by the presence of the hyperlipemic serum. This is illustrated in Table 1, which summarizes the results of 5 different experiments.

Table 1. Effect of hyperlipemic serum on mitosis of medial cells in vitro

Duration of incubation	% Labeled nuclei
2 hours	10.6 ± 6.6
4 hours	5.9 ± 4.6
6 hours	8.0 ± 8.2
18 hours	35.0 ± 12.5
24 hours	31.6 ± 20.7
2 days	29.5 ± 11.5
3 days	53.8 ± 12.0
4-5 days	43.6 ± 17.9
7-10 days	49.0 ± 21.7

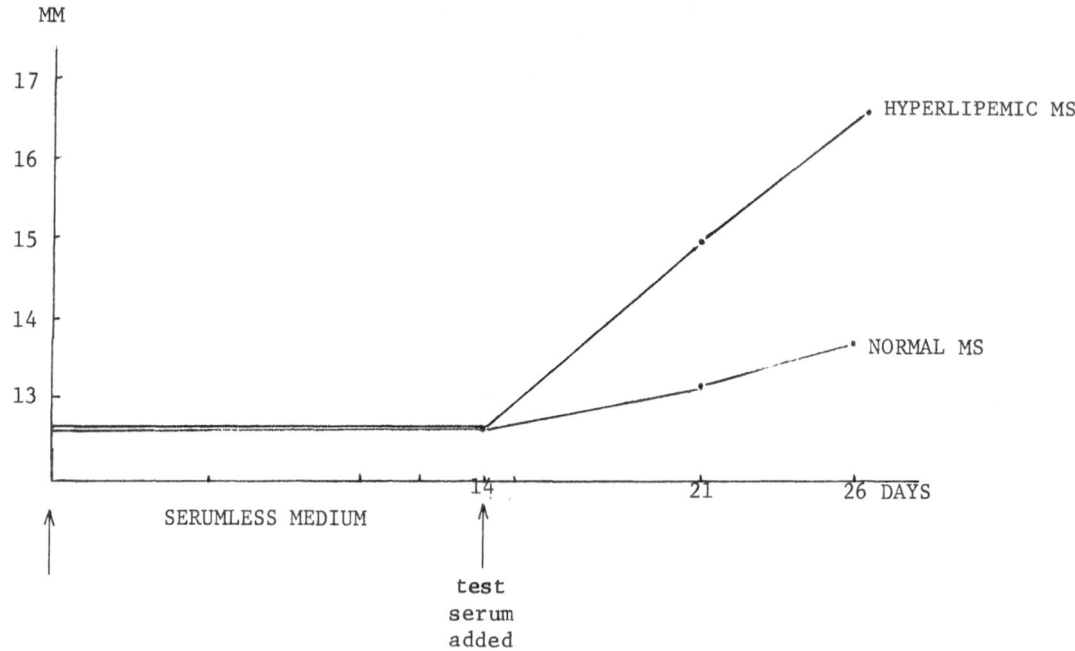

Figure 1. Effect of hyperlipemic and normal monkey serum on the growth of primary aortic smooth muscle cell cultures after exposure to serumless medium for 2 weeks (12 cultures/group)

At least 15 cultures were counted for each time point. While the mitotic index increased rapidly and consistently within 24 hours and stayed high, no clear pattern emerged as to lipid uptake. The amount of lipid within these cells showed a wide variation and we still do not know if there is any relationship between increased lipid uptake and increased proliferation or if these are two unrelated phenomena in response to hyperlipemia. We have reported previously that it is mainly the low density lipoprotein (LDL) of the hyperlipemic serum that induces proliferation, high density lipoprotein has no such effect. Chylomicrons or the very low density lipoprotein usually result in considerable lipid uptake, but generally little proliferation. We also found that the proliferative effect is not dose dependent; diluted LDL to near normal cholesterol levels is still active. In contrast to the high lipid diet induced hypercholesteremic serum, postprandial serum has no effect on proliferation of these cells, although lipid uptake may be increased.

We like to think that lipid uptake and proliferation are in some way related, but so far we could not establish any clear relationship. In another series of experiments we withdrew all serum for 2 weeks or overloaded the cells with lipid by adding post prandial serum for 10 days, in order to test what effect the subsequent addition of either normal or hyperlipemic serum would have. The idea was, that lipid overload might block the proliferative effect of hyperlipemic serum, and on the other hand, that the cells might start to proliferate even with normal serum after a 2 week no-serum withdrawal period. However, this was not the case. Fig. 1 shows one of the withdrawal experiments: as before, the cultures were in the stationary phase, e.g., 6 weeks old when the experiments were started. As can be seen, serum withdrawal had no effect on the subsequent proliferation pattern of these cells. The addition of hyperlipemic serum results in an appreciable increase in cell colony surface, while normal serum has no effect. When the cells were exposed to chylomicrons or postprandial serum, which resulted in a massive lipid deposition within the cells, the hyperlipemic serum still stimulated these cultures (Fig. 2).

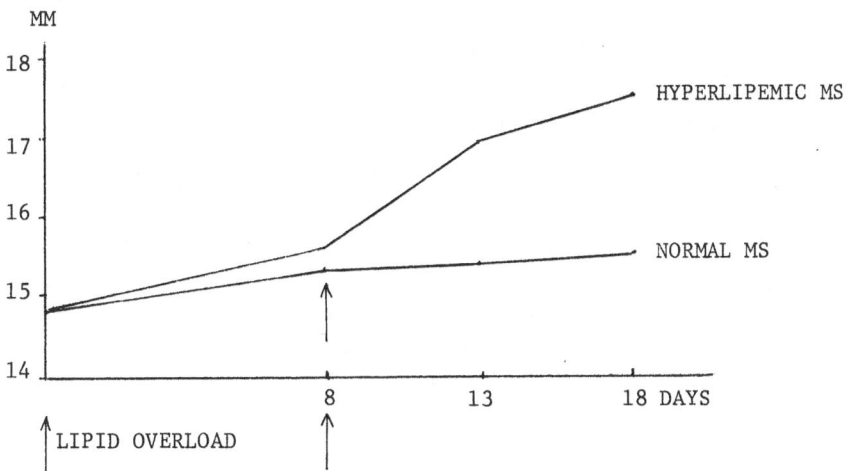

Figure 2. Effect of hyperlipemic and normal monkey serum on the growth of primary aortic cultures after 8-day exposure to post prandial serum (10 cultures/group)

Primary cultures of nonvascular origin, including uterine smooth muscle cells, were tested in the same manner. Hyperlipemic serum generally did not have any effect on the growth of these cells as compared to normal serum. However, quite often it proved to be toxic.

To summarize, increased DNA synthesis starts within 24 hours after the addition of hyperlipemic serum. Increase in surface area can be measured after about 5 days and it lasts for 2-3 weeks. It then levels off. The relatively prompt onset and the limited duration of this proliferative phenomena and the relative absence of a dose dependence on effect of cholesterol content suggests a direct action of one as yet unidentified factor in the hyperlipemic LDL on the mechanism of cellular DNA synthesis.

THE SYNTHESIS AND SECRETION OF SULFATED GLYCOSAMINOGLYCANS BY VASCULAR SMOOTH MUSCLE CELLS IN VITRO

Thomas Wight and Russell Ross

Although it is now well established that the arterial smooth muscle cell is the major cell type involved in atherosclerosis, knowledge of the metabolic capabilities of this cell is still very limited. Recent *in vivo* and *in vitro* experiments in our laboratory (Ross and Klebanoff, 1971; Ross, 1971) have demonstated that arterial smooth muscle cells are capable of synthesizing and secreting collagen and elastic fiber proteins, two of the three major connective tissue matrix components present in blood vessel walls. Based on these observations, it has been suggested that this cell should be considered a functioning connective tissue synthetic cell. We would like to reaffirm this role for arterial smooth muscle by demonstrating that these cells are also capable of synthesizing and secreting glycosaminoglycans, the third major component of the extracellular matrix. Since changes in glycosaminoglycan content have been demonstrated in blood vessels involved in atherosclerosis (Berenson et al., 1971), knowledge of their cellular source, distribution and metabolic control is essential if we are to delineate the role of glycosaminoglycans in atherogenesis.

This paper is addressed to the following 3 questions:

1. Do arterial smooth muscle cells synthesize and secrete glycosaminoglycans *in vitro?*
2. If so, what types are made and in what amounts?
3. At what stage in their growth phase do these cells engage in the synthesis of these macromolecules?

Arterial smooth muscle cells were isolated from the thoracic aorta of the nonhuman primate pig tail monkey, *Macaca nemestrina,* and grown in cell culture (Ross and Alomset, 1973).

Since the medial layer of primate blood vessels consists solely of smooth muscle cells, this tissue offers a convenient source for growing pure populations of smooth muscle cells in culture. Segments of intimal-medial tissue were explanted in Dulbecco-Vogt modification of Eagle's medium supplemented with 5% monkey serum from the same species. Cells were allowed to grow in monolayer to confluency at which time they were trypsinized and passed. Confluent cultures from the second to sixth passage were used for all experiments. Ultrastructural studies of these cultures demonstrated that all of the cells possess ultrastructural features that are characteristic of smooth muscle (Ross and Alomset, 1973).

To examine glycosaminoglycan synthesis, cells were grown to confluency in 250ml Falcon flasks in 10ml of medium and either single labelled with 20uCi ^{35}S-sulfate or double labelled with 20uCi ^{35}S-sulfate and 20uCi ^{3}H-acetate per flask for 24 hours. Eight flasks comprised one experiment which yielded 12-25x10^6 cells. Sulfur is a common precursor to all sulfated glycosaminoglycans while ^{3}H-acetate is a common precursor to all glycosaminoglycans, in addition to other macromolecules, and is used in these experiments to measure the synthesis of hyaluronic acid, a non-sulfated glycosaminoglycan.

Following labelling, glycosaminoglycans were extracted from the medium and cell layer according to the procedure of Nameroff and Holtzer (1967). Briefly, this procedure consists of boiling the samples, followed by digestion with pronase for 18 hrs at 60°C. Proteins and nucleic acids were precipitated with trichloracetic acid at 4°C at a final concentration of 10%, removed by centrifugation, and the supernatants dialyzed initially against 0.01M Na$_2$SO$_4$ and then against distilled H$_2$O for 4 days. The samples were concentrated by contact dessication and aliquots were taken for liquid scintillation counting, enzyme digestion assays and electrophoresis.

Results indicate that mass cultures of arterial smooth muscle cells incorporate ^{35}S-sulfate as well as ^{3}H-acetate into TCA soluble material (Table 1). The majority of the activity is present in the medium (90%) with less activity (10%) associated with the cell layer.

Table 1. Incorporation of ^{35}S-sulfate and ^{3}H-acetate into non-dialyzable, TCA soluble material by primate arterial smooth muscle cells *in vitro*

| ^{35}S | | ^{3}H | |
Medium	Cell layer	Medium	Cell layer
117,412[a]	3,843	36,597	4,511
89,349	5,698	37,210	11,139
86,267	4,303	237,181	29,188

[a]All values are specific activities DPM/10^6 cells.

Within the past few years, success has been achieved in isolating and purifying enzymes that specifically degrade individual types of glycosaminoglycans. Subsequently, these enzymes have been used as assays to determine small quantities of glycosaminoglycans (Saitu et al., 1968). The assay system that we have used was developed by Toole and Gross (1971) with recent modifications by Dorfman (personal communication). It consists of incubating isotopically labelled glycosaminoglycans with each of the following enzymes: a) leech hyaluronidase; b) testicular hyaluronidase and c) chondroitinase ABC for a maximum period of 96 hours followed by separating the digestion products by gel filtration on Sephadex G-25 columns. Controls consisted of sample plus buffer without enzyme. By determining the percentage of the sample degraded in each enzyme digest, it is possible to obtain an estimate of the types of glycosaminoglycans present in the sample. Leech hyaluronidase specifically degrades hyaluronic acid; testicular hyaluronidase specifically degrades chondroitin sulfate A and chondroitin sulfate C in addition to hyaluronic acid; chondroitinase ABC specifically degrades dermatan sulfate in addition to chondroitin sulfates A and C. Chromatographic analysis of ^{3}H-acetate labelled glycosaminoglycans from the medium after digestion with leech hyaluronidase demonstrated that all but a very small fraction of the activity eluted in the same position as the control. Chromatographic analysis of ^{35}S-sulfate labelled glycosaminoglycans from the medium after treatment with testicular hyaluronidase showed slight retardation (10-12%) of activity, indicating partial digestion of the sample. In contrast, the elution profile of ^{35}S-sulfate labelled glycosaminoglycans from the medium after digestion with chondroitinase ABC showed that the majority of the activity (80-90%) was retarded and eluted as a distinct second peak, indicating extensive degradation of the sample. Enzymatic digests of the cell layer gave essentially the same elution profiles.

By calculating the percentage of activity retarded on Sephadex G-25 columns in each digest as a function of total activity applied to the column, we are able to make the following estimates of the types of glycosaminoglycans synthesized and secreted by these cells: hyaluronic acid (0-5%); chondroitin sulfate A and C (10-20%); dermatan sulfate (60-80%); other sulfated glycosaminoglycans (10% or less).

To verify the enzyme assays, parallel aliquots of labelled glycosaminoglycans were characterized by cellulose acetate electrophoresis against known glycosaminoglycan standards. The major peak of activity corresponded to the dermatan sulfate standard with lesser peaks associated with the chondroitin sulfate C standard and a fraction which migrated behind dermatan sulfate.

In order to determine at what stage in the growth phase these cells are most active in the synthesis of glycosaminoglycans, cells were grown in various concentrations of serum and labelled with ^{35}S-sulfate during log and stationary phases of growth. Subsequently, the glycosaminoglycans were extracted from the cell layer and medium as previously described. Cultures maintained in 1% serum remained stationary and did not increase in cell number over a 16 day period. On the other hand, cultures maintained in the presence of 5% serum grew logarithmically until saturation density. The specific activity of isotopically labelled glycosaminoglycans present in the medium of stationary phase cultures at 9, 13 and 16 days was consistently higher than the specific activities of comparable cultures in logarithmic growth.

In conclusion, primate arterial smooth muscle cells synthesize and secrete glycosaminoglycans *in vitro*. Under our conditions of culture, these cells synthesize and secrete primarily dermatan sulfate with smaller amounts of chondroitin sulfate A and C and trace amounts of hyaluronic acid. Both cell layer and medium gave similar results. Dividing and non-dividing smooth muscle cells are capable of synthesizing sulfated glycosaminoglycans although non-dividing cells are more active in the synthesis of these macromolecules.

This research was supported in part by a grant from the USPHS HL-14823 and by a fellowship from the USPHS HL-53109.

The authors would like to thank Ms. Beverly Kariya and Ms. Lynne Phillips for their excellent technical assistance.

ETIOLOGY OF MYOINTIMAL CELL PROLIFERATION[*]

Clarke Stout

Although many investigators feel that fatty streaks are the primary precursors of myointimal cell plaques, several extensive studies of atherosclerosis in humans suggest that this is not the case (Mitchell and Schwartz, 1965; McGill et al., 1969). Our studies indicate that fatty streaks and myointimal cell plaques also have a different pathogenesis in the aortas of captive wild animals. For example, myointimal cell plaques were found in the aortas of 11 out of 12 seals and sea lions. These plaques were located around branch orifices, particularly in the abdominal segments, and occupied up to 11% of the total intimal surface, but no appreciable lipid could be demonstrated by Sudan IV or Oil Red O staining. About half of these animals were juveniles or adolescents and the remainder were young adults or adults. The extent of myointimal cell plaques was positively related to age (Stout, 1969).

The hoofed mammals were another group in which fatty streaks and myointimal cell plaques appeared to be unrelated. Myointimal cell plaques were found in 57 out of 121 hoofed mammals, being most common at the aortic trifurcation. Fatty streaks were present in 61 of 121 hoofed mammals. In 14 of 35 newborn and juvenile hoofed mammals these fatty streaks were confined to the thoracic aortas. In older animals, fatty streaks were usually associated with myointimal cell plaques, being located primarily around the periphery of the lesions. Fatty streaks were not seen at the aortic trifurcation in the absence of myointimal cell plaques (Stout and Bohorquez, 1969; Stout and Bohorquez, 1973).

Sudan positive material was found at the periphery of many myointimal cell plaques in multiple species. Although this finding could be interpreted to indicate that lipid insudation caused myointimal cell proliferation, the appearance of the lesions suggested that the reverse was true. Examination of serial step sections revealed that the lipid tended to be located in the "shoulders" of the plaques or within a slightly thickened intima immediately adjacent to the plaques (Fig. 1).

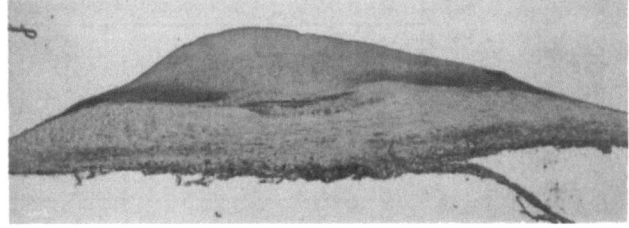

Figure 1. Myointimal cell plaque from an ostrich showing lipid deposits primarily in the shoulders of the lesion. Oil Red O stain (lipid appears black)

Sometimes the lipid extended along the outermost layer of the intima beneath the entire plaque; at other times the center of the lesion contained little or no lipid. In plaques with a double hump due to the central exit of a branch vessel,

[*]Supported by Grants HE 08725 and HE 11044 from the National Heart Institute, United States Public Health Service.

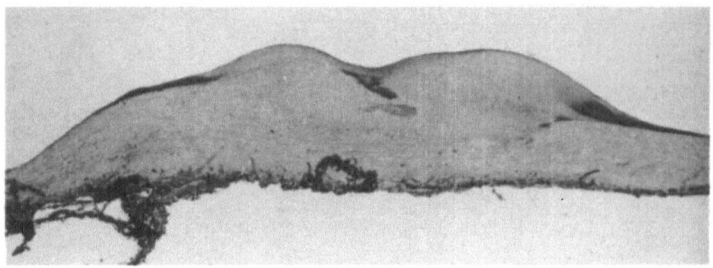

Figure 2. Myointimal cell plaque with a double hump from an ostrich showing lipid deposits at both shoulders and in the central depression. Oil Red O stain (lipid appears black)

the lipid was sometimes seen at both shoulders and in the central depression (Fig. 2). Most of the above described lipid was in fine droplets layered along collagen and elastic fibers. The appearance and distribution of this lipid suggests that the lipid entered the plaque after its formation, possibly because of changes in blood flow characteristics engendered by the plaque itself. This interpretation is supported by the fact that lipid was also found at the periphery of raised plaques caused by medial degeneration with only minimal associated intimal thickening.

Focal areas were found in the shoulders of some of the plaques in which the myointimal cells were randomly aligned and contained many large cytoplasmic lipid droplets. One such area was found in the center of a plaque, but step serial sections revealed that the process had apparently originated at a shoulder caused by the exit of a branch vessel. Histologically, these areas resembled those described by Fry (1973) in which the intima was exposed to unstable stress patterns or endothelial erosion. The findings in the above described plaque suggest that this mechanism could lead to the accumulation of excessive lipid in the center of a myointimal cell plaque, thereby converting it into an atheroma.

Table 1. Aortic intimal lesions in shocked and control pigs

| | Number of elevated lesions | | | | | | | | |
	1	2	3	4	5	6	7	Totals	Means
Shocked pigs	31	14	7	18	12	11	15	108	15.4
Control pigs	6	2	7	5	9	1	3	33	4.7
	Percent elevated lesions								
	1	2	3	4	5	6	7	Totals	Means
Shocked pigs	7.9	7.8	1.3	3.1	1.5	2.3	0.9	24.8	3.5
Control pigs	0.2	0.1	1.6	1.7	1.7	0.8	1.6	7.7	1.1
	Percent fatty streaks								
	1	2	3	4	5	6	7	Totals	Means
Shocked pigs	1.3	0.9	0.3	3.3	1.3	0.4	1.4	8.9	1.3
Control pigs	1.8	1.5	6.2	5.9	4.1	0.3	3.2	23.0	3.3

Because of the above findings, we attempted to see if chronic stress would induce myointimal cell proliferation without a high fat diet. Seven miniature pigs were given low intensity electric shock for 3 seconds each hour for 6 months. Seven control pigs were housed on the shocking device but did not receive shock. Serum cholesterol, phospholipid and triglyceride concentrations remained the same before, during and at the end of the experiment (mean serum cholesterol concentrations were 110 mgs% for shocked pigs, 120 mgs% for control pigs). At sacrifice, the experimental pigs had 2 to 3 times as many myointimal cell plaques as the controls (Table 1). Surprisingly, the controls had more fatty streaks, consisting of fine lipid droplets within a normal or slightly thickened intima.

VI
Permeability of the Arterial Wall and Connective Tissue Reactions

: Factors Affecting Permeability and Connective Tissue
Reactions in Atherosclerosis

Chairmen: M.D. Haust, Canada
L. Robert, France

Participants: H. Jellinek, Hungary
B. Jacotot, France
W.H. Hauss, West Germany
K.W. Walton, Great Britain
J.P. Lindner, West Germany

WHAT INDICATIONS ARE THERE THAT PERMEABILITY IS ALTERED AND WHICH FACTORS AFFECT IT IN ATHEROSCLEROSIS?

H. Jellinek

Colloidal iron was employed as a marker of vascular permeability under six different experimental conditions: hypertension, hypoxia, sensitization with horse serum, adrenalin administration and repeated injections of inflammatory and vasodilatory drugs. Under all of the above conditions the transmural transport of colloidal iron was increased as compared with controls.

Colloidal iron entered the intima through the widened endothelial junctions and reached the intercellular matrix of the subendothelial region. It could be demonstrated even in the smooth muscle cells of the media and in the fibroblasts of the adventitia. In animals on cholesterol rich diets the presence of colloidal iron could be demonstrated in the arterial wall even earlier than that of lipids, thus indicating that an increased permeability preceded the appearance of lipids.

The transport phenomenon through the arterial wall may be considered at three levels: the permeability of the intima, the permeability of the media, and the removal of substances by drainage in the adventitia. Concerning this last point we have examined the lymphatic channels in hypoxia and have observed the presence of macrophages containing colloidal iron particles in the dilated channels. Following cholesterol feeding the same phenomenon was seen, but in addition, lipids were observed both in the macrophages and in the endothelial cells.

That permeability changes do occur under the above experimental conditions, may be shown by ruthenium red staining of the glycocalix on the endothelial surface. After a two months diet containing cholesterol, the staining property is diminished.

The reaction of alkaline phosphatases at the interface of media-adventitia is increased by hypertension, and completely abolished by anoxia. The last enzyme-reaction coupled with colloidal iron demonstrates the same location for the enzyme reaction, showing again disturbances in the flow of transmural circulation.

Accumulation of plasma proteins in the arterial wall results in hyaline formation in the subendothelial zone, while in the media, it causes the destruction of smooth muscle cells (demonstrable by electron-microscopy), as well as the deposition of fibrin. Smooth muscle cells which escape this destruction, do proliferate and elastic fibers of a "remodeled" structure make an appearance. In this process the smooth muscle cells play an important role.

Discussion

Dr. Pollak: In our work we have used graphite instead of colloidal iron to show an increased permeability with results similar to those shown by Dr. Jellinek. Have you observed regional permeability differences? These differences exist as was shown by Haimovici et al. by exchanging aortic and pulmonary artery segments. This resulted in the formation of the same type (and extent) of lesions in spite of relocation. I wonder whether the increased permeability "happens" through an intact or injured (swollen) endothelial cell, through the gaps between cells (as suggested by Shimamoto's work on contracting endothelial cells), or both.

Dr. Jellinek: Our work suggested that the endothelial cells are not normal in increased permeability, and that indeed, there were regional differences particularly in experimental hypertension. The substances from the lumen entered the intima under conditions of increased permeability either through the cell or the widened cell junctions, but there remain many problems regarding these routes.

Dr. Adams: I believe that the selective (normal) permeability is abolished once and for all when the endothelium is damaged, as shown by the experiments that thorium does enter atherosclerotic lesions but not the normal arterial intima. We have some evidence from our own work that albumin enters much faster into plaques when the atheroma is already formed. I would like to ask how long does the endothelium remain normal in the atherosclerotic process?

Dr. Jellinek: In our experimental models the endothelium appears to remain normal, even on electron microscopic examination, up to two or three weeks.

Dr. Holvig: How did you assess the values for thickness of the ruthenium red stained layer and what were the variations in the width of that layer?

Dr. Jellinek: We have based the assessment of the width of the ruthenium red stained layer on morphometric studies; only aorta was examined.

Dr. Rona: I wish to comment on problems related to Dr. Pollak's and Dr. Adams' questions. The existing regional differences in permeability, even within the same vessel, may relate to the regional variations in the structure of incomplete tight junctions of endothelial cells as demonstrated by us to exist in the aorta. In short model experiments one can demonstrate increased permeability even through normal endothelium, this being a physiological adaptation mechanism. The increased transport takes place through the normal pathways, i.e. via the endothelial junctions and the pinocytotic vesicles. I would like to ask how does Dr. Jellinek relate the processes in his experimental models to the process of atherosclerosis.

Dr. Jellinek: Basically the process of increased permeability is probably similar or identical in many disease states including atherosclerosis, but the difficulty is to be able to confirm this in man, for the increased permeability is an early step and impossible to follow at the stage of already visible human lesions.

Dr. Scott stated that work initially undertaken with his colleague, Dr. P.J. Hurley, in men, had recently been extended by Dr. G.D. Calvert working in adolescent pigs. The studies strongly supported the concept that some low-density lipoprotein molecules (LDL), of mean molecular weight about 2×10^6, did move into arterial intima, subintima, and towards the adventitia. The evidence had been obtained with ^{125}I-LDL, direct counting and autoradiography of pigs killed hours to 5 weeks after injecting the ^{125}I-LDL. Light-microscopic autoradiographs suggested, but did not prove, that the bulk of the isotope demonstrated by direct counting of aortic tissue, was present extracellularly. Simple washing procedure and salt extraction removed the isotope bearing molecules from aortic tissues. The isotope thus recovered was not present as radio-iodide, iodotyrosine or on lipid. 85 to 90% was regularly found to be TCA precipitable. Immunodiffusion and density studies suggested that much of the isotope was still present on lipoprotein molecules bearing porcine "B" antigen. These pigs possess two LDL species approximating 220 A$^\circ$ and 185 A$^\circ$ (Sf 5 and Sf 3). Both molecular classes appear to enter intima and subintima in small amounts relatively rapidly, with maximal entry in anterior aortic arch. After 24 hours the isotope moves progressively outwards towards outer media. Isotope is also found around adventitial vessels, but this appears to represent a small area or pool of local LDL exchange. (G.D. Calvert and P.J. Scott; unpublished observations).

INTERCELLULAR MACROMOLECULES OF THE ARTERIAL WALL AND PLASMA LIPIDS[*]

B. Jacotot

Qualitative and quantitative changes in the intercellular matrix macromolecules of the arterial wall were described recently in aging individuals and in atherosclerosis. The isolation and purification of these connective tissue macromolecules in recent years enabled the study of their interaction with lipids and lipoproteins. Interaction between proteoglycans and lipoproteins has been reported first in vitro by Gero and coworkers (1967). Recently, Robert et al. (1972), Moczar and Robert (1970), and Kramsch and Hollander (1973) described binding between elastin and lipids. Collagen was shown to have also some affinity for lipids (Nikkari and Heikkinen, 1968).

The four main classes of the extracellular macromolecules of the arterial connective tissues are:

Collagen: It was shown by Nikkari and Haikkinen (1968) that collagen shows some affinity for lipids.

Proteoglycans may interact with lipoproteins, largely through their glycosaminoglycan chains. Complexes between these macromolecules may facilitate the degradation of lipoproteins and the local deposition of lipids (Bihari-Varga et al., 1968; Srinivasan et al., 1972). As proteoglycans (heparan-sulphate or dermatansulphate) are present in the arterial wall (for review see Robert, 1970), this mechanism may be of importance in the initiation of lipid deposition in the intima, and later in the media.

Structural glycoproteins (SGP) isolated from a variety of connective tissues (Robert et al., 1973) may play an important role in the formation of the atherosclerotic lesions. They have a microfibrillar structure with a 100 Å diameter (Kadar et al., 1973). The SGP fraction extracted from aorta contains a certain amount of lipid which is not removed by organic solvents before the "chemical dissection" of the arterial wall. Pig aortas used for this study were delipidated and then submitted to a sequential extraction (Moczar and Robert, 1970). The fraction containing SGP was rich in lipids (20-40% of total dry weight). In rats maintained in isotopic equilibrium by a diet containing ^{14}C-cholesterol, we found high specific radioactivity in SGP extracts of aorta and skin, confirming the great turnover of lipids bound to SGP (Szigeti et al., 1972).

Elastin: elastic laminae result from the interaction of "microfibrils" which were shown to be composed of SGP, surrounding the (elementary) elastic core or proelastin ("elastic unit" of Haust et al., 1967). Proelastin is probably secreted as a globular molecule of about 74,000 molecular weight (Sandberg et al., 1970) and associated with this microfibrillar array probably through Coulombic forces.

---

[*]In collaboration with M. Claire and L. Robert. The experiments reported were carried out under contract with the DGRST (71-7-2809) INSERM (714 54) and the CNRS (ER No 53).

Globular proelastin subunits are held together by lysino-norleucine, desmosine and isodesmosine bridges (Partridge, 1969). Elastin is rich in aliphatic and non-polar amino-acids, its tertiary and quaternary structure are mainly stabilised by hydrophobic interactions (Jacotot et al., 1973). Many hydrophobic regions are present on the surface of these macromolecules explaining thus their ability to bind lipids. Binding of lipids to elastin results in stable complexes (Szigeti et al., 1972; Jacotot et al., 1973; Robert et al., 1972). Kramsch and Hollander (1973) observed binding between elastin and LDL and VLDL but not between elastin and chylomicrons or HDL.

Lipids bound to elastin can be eluted after filtration on DEAE Sephadex columns (Robert et al., 1969; Robert and Robert, 1970). The composition of this lipid fraction is being presently investigated.

Several authors, particularly Kramsch and Hollander (1973) have found differences between the amount of lipids bound to the elastin of normal and atheromateous aorta ("plaque elastin"). We think that "plaque elastin" is formed from elastin and structural glycoproteins, and that the presence of this last macromolecule influences the amount of lipids bound. It appears that SGP are capable of binding significant amounts of lipids.

Binding of ^{14}C-cholesterol by arterial elastin was demonstrated in men by Kramsch and coworkers (1971), and in rats by Jacotot et al. (1971); and Szigeti et al. (1972). It was shown that: stable complexes were formed in vivo and it was possible to determine, for every differentiated form of connective tissue (aorta, dermis, sponge-tissue), an extraction diagram the slope of which reflected the tissue's affinity for cholesterol. The rate of delipidation of aorta was the fastest, that of skin and sponge tissue were significantly slower. The slope of the plots for tissues of rats maintained on normal and those on a cholesterol rich diet was approximately the same.

In another experiment, we studied the intima and media of human aorta with minimal to moderate and severe atherosclerosis. These tissues were submitted to a sequential chemical extraction (Table 1).

In the first lipidic extract are the lipids easily extracted in aortic homogenate; in the second extract are lipids fixed by elastin and obtained before elastase digestion; lipids extracted with urea and associated with polymeric collagen, proteoglycans and structural glycoproteins are present in the third extract; the fourth extract contains lipids associated with elastin and obtained after elastase digestion.

Thin layer chromatography of the lipids extracted from elastin before and after elastase digestion showed the presence of many spots, representing probably monoglycerides and carotenoids. In the fourth extract (elastin-associated lipids) a significant difference exists between the two types of lesions:

- In the aortas with stage I (minimal) lesions, there are more cholesteryl-esters and triglycerides than in the aortas with predominatly stage II-III (severe) lesions.
- In the aortas with more advanced lesions there are much more free fatty acids than in the aortas with the first degree lesions.

These data suggest that there may be a defect of fatty acid esterification (or an increased rate of hydrolysis) in aortas with more severe atherosclerosis.

Discussion

Dr. Smith: I think that all plasma proteins enter the intima. We have certainly found all the plasma proteins that we have looked for and that includes low-density lipoprotein, high-density lipoprotein, albumin, fibrinogen, thrombin and

Table 1

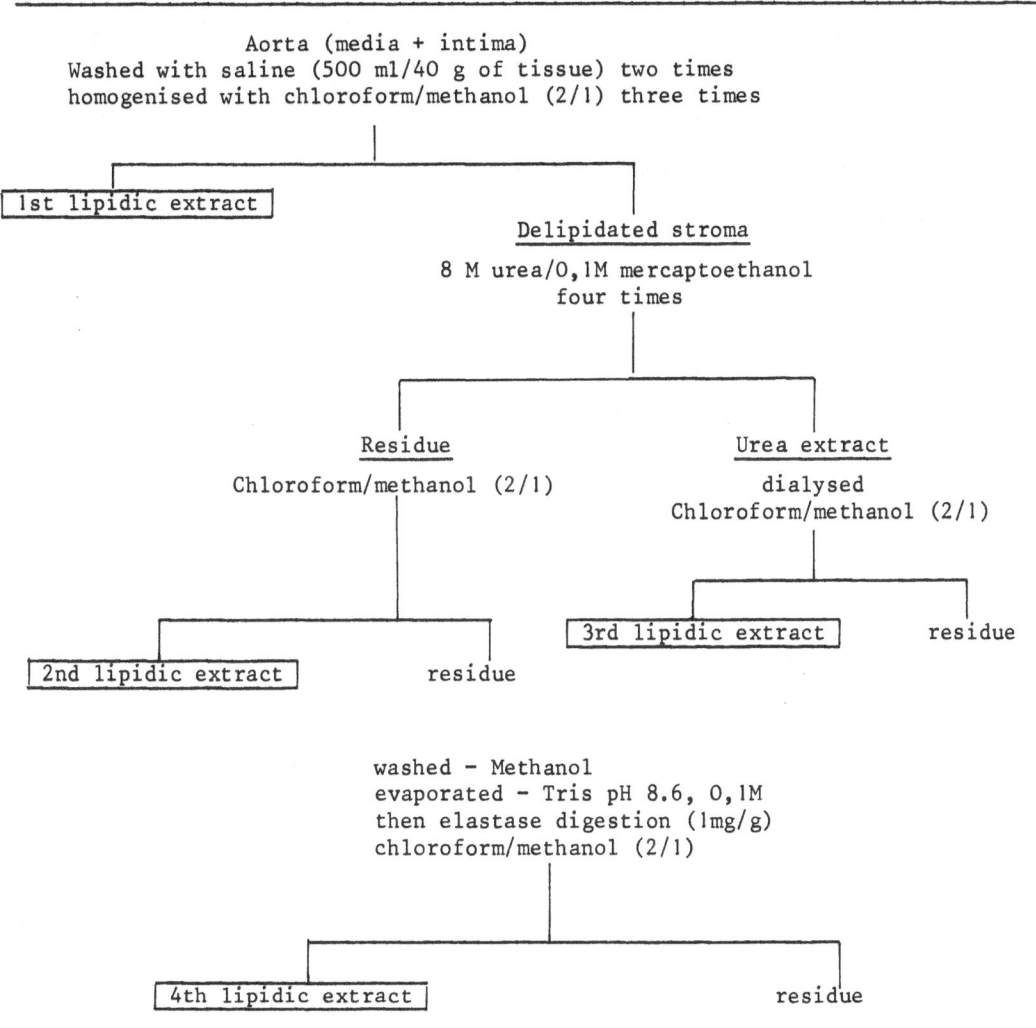

Aorta (media + intima)
Washed with saline (500 ml/40 g of tissue) two times
homogenised with chloroform/methanol (2/1) three times

1st lipidic extract

Delipidated stroma
8 M urea/0,1M mercaptoethanol
four times

Residue
Chloroform/methanol (2/1)

Urea extract
dialysed
Chloroform/methanol (2/1)

3rd lipidic extract   residue

2nd lipidic extract   residue

washed - Methanol
evaporated - Tris pH 8.6, 0,1M
then elastase digestion (1mg/g)
chloroform/methanol (2/1)

4th lipidic extract   residue

plasmin, and there is no doubt that when we have found suitable antibodies and suitable systems for measuring them we will find that all plasma proteins are present. I particularly mention HDL because you suggested that it was not, in fact, present. Two points were of great interest in your presentation. One is the interaction of lipid with elastin. I am sure that this is a major factor in the breakdown of elastic laminae, and I believe that the breakdown and erosion of elastic laminae is probably an important factor in diffuse intimal thickening. Do you think that the intact lipoprotein itself is interacting with the elastin, or do you think that the lipid must already have been detached from the lipoprotein before it *can* interact with the elastin?

Dr. Jacotot: I think lipoproteins are more-or-less degraded during their transfer across the arterial wall and we see the lipids fixed with elastin but I don't know what happens to intact lipoproteins and particularly to apoproteins.

Dr. Adams: I just wanted to comment that there is very good histological evidence for the binding of lipids to elastic tissue. About 12 years ago we showed that in some very early lesions (they were hardly lesions), particularly in the cerebral vessels, there was a peculiar localization of stainable cholesterol along the elastic tissue.

Chairman Robert: Thank you for this comment. I think Dr. Adams was one of the first to show that elastin can be stained as a lipoprotein. Perhaps this might not be even a pathological finding but merely an expression of normal aging. It was shown recently that elastin picks up also calcium.

Dr. Werthesson: I would like to ask whether Dr. Jacotot compared tissues with different stages of atherosclerotic lesions that also included normal tissue from the same artery?

Dr. Jacotot: There was no normal tissue. It was tissue with atherosclerotic lesions. They were not derived from the same artery, but from two different kinds of arteries.

Dr. Werthesson: The point I wish to make is that had you chosen an artery where there was sufficient *normal* tissue to do the same analysis, I have a very strong suspicion that you would have found a great deal of similarity between the normal and the presumed abnormal. I think it would be an excellent idea to add this to your comparison.

Dr. Hauss: I wonder how strong is the evidence that the lipids destruct the elastic tissue directly? I am not able to decide what is the evidence for, and the mode of the possible destruction of the elastin directly by the lipoproteins. I have always suggested that the lipoproteins were "irritating" to the cell and that as a result the mesenchymal cell begins to produce altered elastin which is subject to damage and disintegration. This idea is just as attractive as the direct damage to the elastic tissue by lipoproteins.

MESENCHYMAL CELLULAR REACTIONS AND CONSEQUENCES

W.H. Hauss

More than ·ten years ago, we showed that in human atherosclerosis the mesenchymal metabolism in the arterial wall is accelerated as could be demonstrated by the accelerated ^{35}S-sulphate incorporation into the proteoglycans of the aorta. Studying the effect of atherogenic factors we learned that they regularly and instantly induce a reaction of mesenchymal metabolism. Thus, hypertension induces in less than one hour an impressive increase of ^{35}S-sulphate incorporation into the proteoglycans of aortic mesenchyme. Hypertension likewise induces acceleration of fatty acid and cholesterol synthesis in the cells of the aortic wall (Fig. 1).

Acceleration of ^{14}C acetate incorporation into lipid acids and cholesterol induced by chronic renal hypertension (tissue slides of rats' aortas)

	Normotensive rats	Chronic renal hypertensive rats
Lipid acids mumoles acetate/g/day	240.00	422.50
Cholesterol mumoles acetate/g/day	8.03	15.43

Matthes, K.J., G. Junge-Hülsing, G. Schmitt, H. Wagner, W. Oberwittler and W.H. Hauss: J. Atheroscler. Res. 9, 305-318 (1969)

Figure 1

Moreover, atherogenic factors induce regularly and immediately a proliferation of the arterial wall cells. While cell reduplication is slow in aortas of normotensive rats, mitotic activity is increased by hypertension and by other atherogenic factors, for example, the emotional stress.

Direct consequences of this mesenchymal reaction in the arterial wall are well demonstrated by electron microscopy. In the coronary artery wall of a normotensive rabbit (Fig. 2a) the subendothelial space is narrow (Fig. 2b). After some weeks of arterial hypertension this subendothelial space is widened (Fig. 2c). Moreover, the endothelial cells are filled with vacuoles (Fig. 2d). And finally, cells with

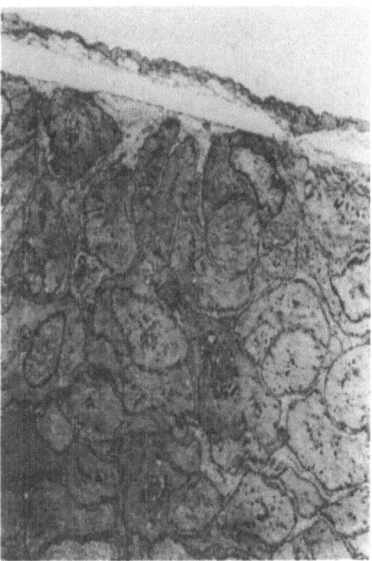

Figure 2a

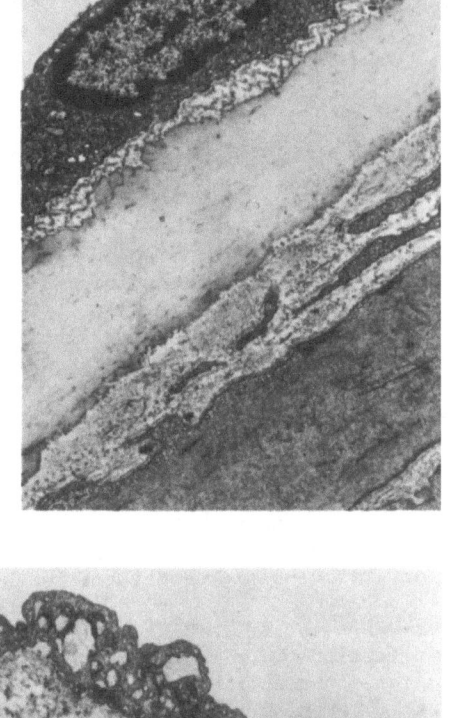

Figure 2b

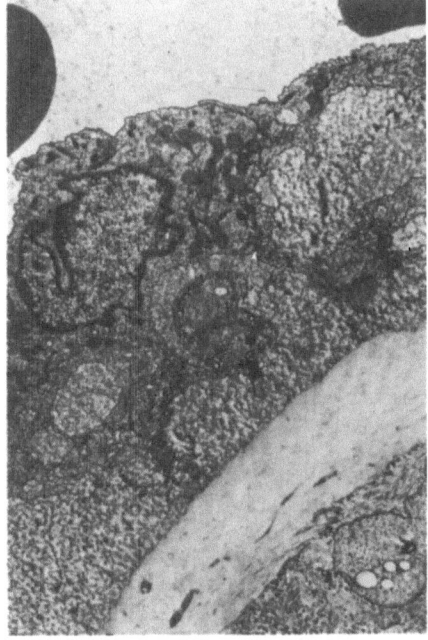

Figure 2c

Figure 2d

211

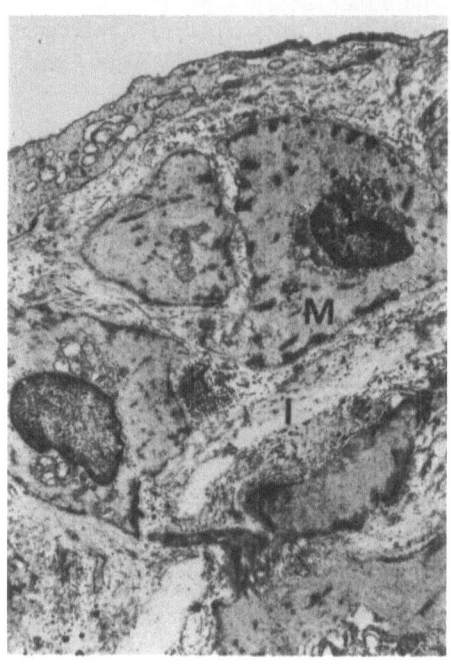

Figure 2e

the characteristics of smooth muscle cells "encroach" upon the endothelial zone and produce ground substance and fibres (Fig. 2e).

As mentioned above (Fig. 1) arterial wall cells synthesise lipids, and arterial hypertension and other sclerogenic factors induce increased synthesis of fatty acids and cholesterol in the arterial wall. Nevertheless, the increased lipid synthesis in these cases is too small to explain the increase of lipid deposition in the wall, found in our short term experiments. Incorporation of acetate into cholesterol after shock had been 0.26 mμ moles of acetate incorporation/g aorta/ hour. The increase of cholesterol deposition in this time was 440 mμ moles, an amount too high to have been induced only by an increased synthesis. However, in chronic hypertension the increased synthesis of lipids may play a more important role for the lipid deposition in the arterial wall.

Using an albumin complex of ^{14}C-labelled palmitate Matthes, Schmitt and I studied penetration velocity of this complex from the aortic lumen into the aortic wall of rats by measuring the diminution of ^{14}C-palmitate activity in a sac of the aortic lumen tied on both sides; the branching arteries were also tied tightly. The pressure in the sac could be varied (Fig. 3). We speak of penetration half life, these parameters following an e-function.

The penetration half life into the aortic wall of normotensive **and of** hypertensive rats depends on perfusion pressure (Fig. 3). It means that at higher blood pressure lipids penetrate quicker into the wall. Moreover, the penetration half life into the aortic walls of chronic renal hypertensive rats under pressure conditions is longer than in normotensives (Fig. 3). It means that the lipids enter quicker into the wall of normotensive than of hypertensive rats.

Using the same method with albumin complex of the ^{14}C-labelled palmitate we studied the elimination velocity of this complex leaving the aortic wall. The lipid elimination half life of the aortic walls depends on the perfusion pressure being shorter at higher pressures (Fig. 4). Beyond this the experiment showed that the elimination half life from the aortas of the chronic renal hypertensive rats was considerably higher than from the aortas of normotensive rats. It means that in the aortas of hypertensive rats the lipids are piled up by the hypertension induced, transformed aortic wall structure.

Penetration half lifes of a ^{14}C palmitate albumin complex in the aortic wall of normotensive resp. hypertensive rats by different aortic pressures

	Normotensive rats		Chronic renal hypertensive rats	
Perfusion pressure:	80 mm Hg	160 mm Hg	80 mm Hg	160 mm Hg
Penetration half life:	6,25 min.	4,0 min.	7,6 min.	5,6 min.

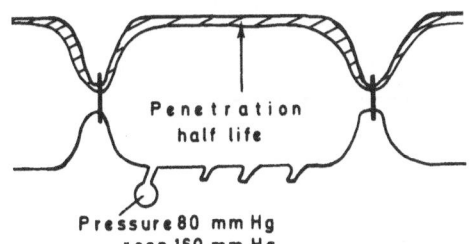

Figure 3

Penetration half life

Pressure 80 mm Hg resp.160 mm Hg

Elimination half lifes of a ^{14}C palmitate albumin complex out of the aortic wall of normotensive resp. hypertensive rats by different aortic pressures

	Normotensive rats		Chronic renal hypertensive rats	
Perfusion pressure:	80 mm Hg	160 mm Hg	80 mm Hg	160 mm Hg
Elimination half life:	6,0 min.	3,2 min.	15,6 min.	8,0 min.

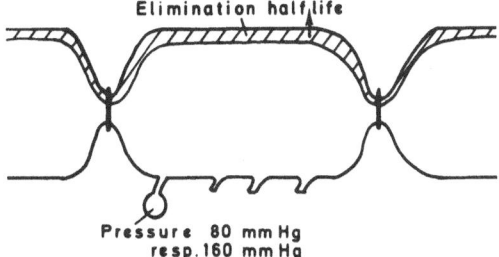

Elimination half life

Figure 4

Pressure 80 mm Hg resp.160 mm Hg

We have showed previously that the accumulation of cholesterol and lipids does not begin immediately after the onset of pressure elevation. Thus, lipid concentration can be observed only after prior pronounced changes in mesenchymal metabolism have taken place (Fig. 5). In experiments with an acute hypertension only 24 hours after the beginning of the pressure elevation, lipid concentration is increased at the time even when arterial pressure elevation still has returned to normal.

Our experiments indicate that:

1. the mesenchymal reaction is regularly and immediately induced by all atherogenic factors studied by us;
2. the mesenchymal reaction induces oedema, hyalinosis, and fibrosis of the arterial wall;
3. the reactively induced structural alterations block partially the transit ways in the wall and they are responsible for lipidosis; and
4. stronger blocked transit ways may cause necrosis of cells in the wall, alterations of endothelial cell and facilitate contacts between tissue elements (procollagen and thrombocinase for instance) thus inducing thrombosis.

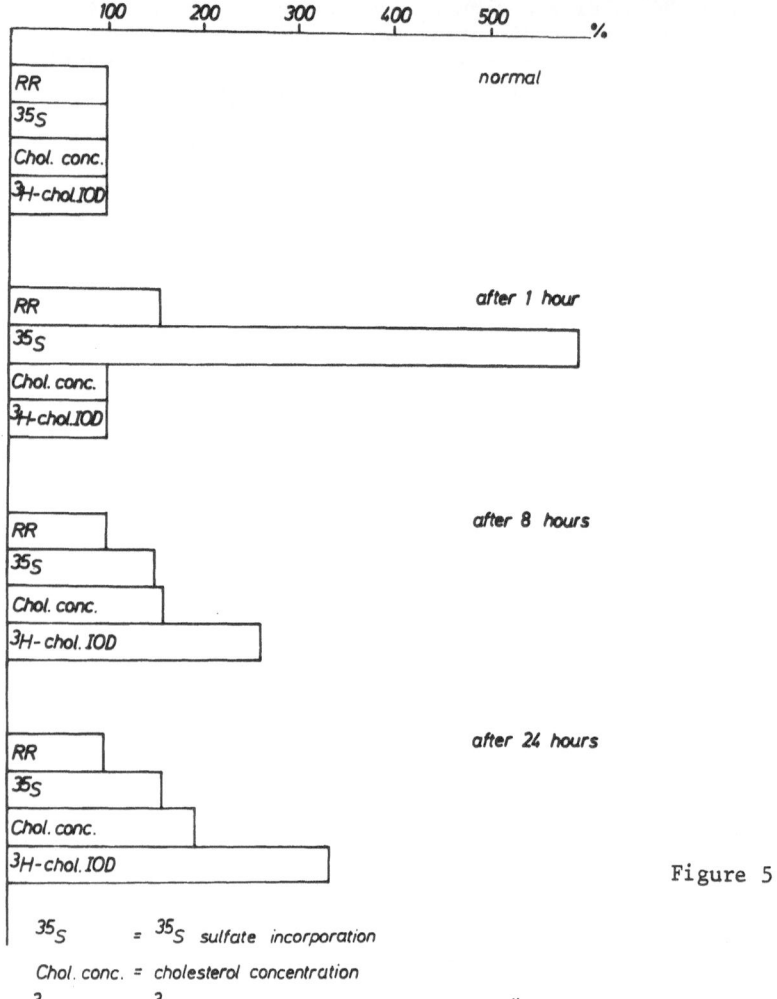

Figure 5

35$_S$ = 35$_S$ sulfate incorporation

Chol. conc. = cholesterol concentration

3H-chol. IOD = 3H-cholesterol "inflow-outflow-difference"

Discussion

Chairman Haust: Thank you Dr. Hauss. It is of interest that the inception of the process of atherosclerosis is looked upon either as entirely dominated by lipid deposition, and we have heard this view presented this morning in the Plenary Session by Dr. McGill, or as being the result of an initial mesenchymal reaction, a concept supported by the data presented to us by Dr. Hauss.

Dr. Caro: Dr. Hauss would you give us briefly some detail about your elimination experiments. I gather this was a prefusion experiment on isolated arteries?

Dr. Hauss: The aortae were left in the body. The abdomen was opened and the arteries remained on the vena cava so that the outflow could take place; all the branches of the aortae had been tied.

Dr. Caro: Duncan, Buck and Lynch about 10 years ago showed that the permeability of the wall is affected in a peculiar way by stretch; presumably, by using a higher pressure one stretches the artery more but the flux per unit area is constant, so that although one would expect to eliminate more material from a dilated artery I would still assume that the flux per unit area of the artery would not be changed in such studies. It is a very peculiar feature that we don't understand.

Dr. Thomas: Dr. Haust just posed the question whether (the initial stage of) atherosclerosis must be an either or phenomenon (lipid only or mesenchymal reaction only). It does not have to be that way. We are dealing with a complex disease and it seems there can be multiple phases. For example, in Albany we have demonstrated quite clearly that within a very short time, i.e. two or three days after feeding cholesterol to swine there is an increase in mitosis, DNA-synthesis, and so on, in the aorta, before we can see any lipid by electron microscopy or demonstrate any excess lipid chemically. This process progresses slowly and in approximately one month when lesions appear there are lots of lipids and at that stage the DNA-synthesis and mitosis rate are increased about tenfold as compared to the twofold increase present earlier. We have come to think of this as a two-phase phenomanon and perhaps even more phases are operational as the lesions progress.

Dr. Hauss: I think that there are several possibilities (or phases ?) depending upon timing. What I showed was an acute experiment with hypertension. In less than half an hour there is the reaction of the cells one may follow by the incorporation of a precursor and in less than half an hour the mitotic rate is high, 5-6 times higher than before. Was this true also in your experiments Dr. Thomas? When one experiments with diets it takes longer to produce this effect perhaps as long as 14 days. The mitotic rate remains high for two months and decreases thereafter but not to normal levels.

Dr. Thomas: In our experience with cholesterol feeding in the pigs this early response of the mesenchyme has continued for as long as at least a year in the areas of the artery where no lesions were present.

Chairman Haust: Perhaps the difference observed by you gentlemen relates at least in part to different species employed (pigs versus rats).

Dr. Gerö: There is only a small variation in the reactivity of connective tissues in response to different injuries, namely, changes in the mucopolysaccharides and composition of the ground substance. In our review, and in agreement with the concept of Dr. Hauss, this non-specific reaction of the vascular connective tissue is a common link in the long chain of events culminating in atheroma formation. The mucopolysaccharides of the vascular wall have many functions and are involved in permeability, anticoagulation, fibrillogenesis, ion exchange, clearing activity, and others. Moreover, they may form complexes with beta-lipoprotein and with fibrinogen, inhibit the lipolytic activity in the vessel wall, and influence the beta-glucuronidase activity. All these possible biochemical changes may be favourable or unfavourable to the formation, or evolution of the atheroma.

Dr. Hauss: I agree that this is an unspecific reaction.

LIPOPROTEINS - CONNECTIVE TISSUE INTERACTIONS

K.W. Walton

There is now wide agreement that the lipids in *early* atherosclerotic lesions originate from the plasma, although in later lesions they may be modified, or supplemented, by metabolic processes in the arterial wall itself (for reviews, see Walton, 1969; 1973a). However, there is still divergence of opinion about the mechanism underlying the initial stages of the process in relation to the retention of lipids (lipoproteins) in the arterial wall. For example, selective retention of plasma lipids in the connective tissues of the arterial intima has been postulated to be due to:

a) Mechanical arrest of lipid in the intima secondary to changes in the tunica media such as 1. blockage of fenestrations in the internal elastic lamina (Gofman and Young, 1963; Lendrum, 1964); 2. intimal thickening and fibrosis of the muscular media (Wilens and McCluskey, 1954); 3. enzymic medial defects due to anoxia (Adams et al., 1962); or
b) A 'molecular sieving' effect of the intimal connective tissue gel (ground substance) resulting in failure of lipids (lipoproteins) to permeate through the intima (Adams, 1967); or
c) Interaction of low- and very low-density lipoproteins (LDL and VLDL) with the sulphated glycosaminoglycans (S-GAG) of the intimal connective tissues (Amenta and Waters, 1960; Gero et al., 1960; Walton and Williamson, 1968).

Studies using radioisotopically-labelled plasma proteins (Walton et al., 1963; Scott and Hurley, 1970); immunofluorescence (Watts, 1959; Haust et al., 1964; Kao and Wissler, 1965; Walton and Williamson, 1968); or immunochemical analysis of arterial extracts (Ott et al., 1958; Tracy et al., 1961; Smith and Slater, 1970, 1972) have established that: 1. Some plasma proteins *normally* permeate the arterial wall; 2. In atherosclerotic vessels, LDL, VLDL and fibrinogen are selectively *localized in lesions* while other plasma proteins are not; 3. In particular, although LDL, VLDL and high-density lipoproteins (HDL) all act as carriers for the same lipids (cholesterol, phospholipids and triglycerides) these studies confirm the clinical evidence (derived from measurement of serum lipoprotein levels) suggesting that LDL and VLDL, but *not* HDL, are involved in atherogenesis.

These studies suggest that it is the *nature of the vehicle for lipids* (i.e. possibly some aspect of the physico-chemical characteristics of intact LDL and VLDL), rather than the nature of the lipids being carried, that determines initial localization. As far as the postulates discussed above are concerned they suggest that:

a) Initial sub-endothelial lipid accumulation cannot be due to a mechanical barrier 'damming-back' plasma in the intima since this would be expected to cause accumulation of *all* rather than selective plasma proteins, and also because LDL is demonstrable in very early lesions ('fatty streaks') *before* changes in the elastic lamina or media are demonstrable (Walton, 1973b), and in heart valves where no muscular barrier exists (Walton et al., 1970);

b) When antisera deliberately chosen to cover a range of molecular sizes are used, no evidence of specific localization of other macroglobulin components of plasma, such as α2M- of IgM globulins, is found (Walton and Williamson, 1968; Walton et al., 1970) indicating that molecular size alone does not determine the selectivity of localization of plasma proteins in the intima.

c) On the other hand, direct and indirect evidence supporting the postulate that selective interaction occurs between LDL, VLDL or fibrinogen and the S-GAG's of the intima can be summarised as follows: 1. VLDL, LDL and fibrinogen selectively form precipitates (co-acervates) with charged acidic polysaccharides such as heparin, dextran sulphate etc. *in vitro* and these co-acervates are stabilized by an optimum concentration of calcium ions (Walton, 1952; Walton and Scott, 1964). Similar interactions occur with S-GAG's and proteoglycans extracted from the aorta and other connective tissues. 2. Studies using histochemical methods or techniques based upon radiosulphate uptake (Curran and Crane, 1962; Gero et al., 1967) have shown a significant correlation between the topographic distributions of calcium, S-GAG's and lipid (lipoprotein). Of these components, conventional histological methods are probably least sensitive for calcium but it has been shown by electron probe analysis that calcium is bound to the GAG's of the arterial wall from an early age (Hale et al., 1967), while many authors have noted, from chemical analyses, that an increase of the calcium content of arteries occurs with age and atherosclerosis, the rate of accumulation being roughly parallel with the incidence of atherosclerosis in a given population (see Walton, 1969).

Experimental studies with radioactive sulphate (Buck, 1955) suggest a correlation between turnover-rate (rather than absolute amount) of S-GAG's and the rate of lipid deposition. There is some evidence to suggest that these changes in the ground substance of the arterial wall may *precede* and thereby determine the sites of entrapment of lipoproteins. Many pathologists have noted tiny mucoid elevations of the intima at sites where atherosclerotic lesions develop subsequently. Such sites show oedema (suggesting altered endothelial permeability) and increase of histochemical reactions for GAG's. At sites of altered arterial permeability experimentally induced by catecholamines, hypoxia and other manipulations, a 'mesenchymal reaction' is induced associated with increased local synthesis of S-GAG's and other evidence of activity of mesenchymal cells (Hauss et al., 1969).

If the stimuli giving rise to localized alteration of permeability thus also pro- mote synthesis of those components of the intimal gel which are reactive with LDL, VLDL and fibrinogen, one can begin to see why these proteins are selectively en- trapped. It is possible that the extent of calcium-binding might determine the stability or reversibility of the co-acervates formed, thus accounting for the tendency of some early lesions to regress. On the other hand stable complexes can be envisaged as providing a stimulus to further mesenchymal cell reaction to give rise to fibrogenesis and other features of the more fully-developed lesion.

Discussion

Dr. Klimov: To determine the concentration of lipoproteins in the arterial wall we use the following method to obtain lipid from vascular tissues: a segment (disc) of human or pig aorta is placed inside a special syringe. Under pressure one can squeeze out a small volume of tissue fluid and with a glass capillary this fluid is collected. From one disc of the aorta containing intima and media and having a diameter of 2 cm., one may collect 0.2 - 0.3 ml. of tissue fluid. To obtain more tissue fluid it is necessary to process several discs. This tissue fluid is very convenient for the study of the concentration of lipoproteins. The electrophoresis of serum and aortic tissue fluid of man and pig shows the same spectrum of lipoproteins in serum and in the aortic tissue fluid. Immunological investigations confirm the identity of the aortic and the serum lipoproteins. We have investigated within 24 hours many aortas from men who died or were killed in accidents. The tissue fluid was prepared and the precipitation method was used to determine the fractions of beta- and pre-beta-lipoproteins. Tissue fluid prepared from the aorta without atherosclerotic changes contained approximately 160 mg.%. The content of lipoproteins in tissue fluids prepared from aortae with fatty streaks was significantly higher and that from aortae with plaques and atheroma was several times higher than in the tissue fluid obtained from aortae without atherosclerotic lesions. It is very interesting to note that the content of lipo- proteins in the inferior vena cava was not increased even when the atherosclerotic process was very severe in the arteries.

Dr. Walton: It is very nice to have this evidence from yet another quarter in sup- port of the view that the lipoproteins are actively involved in the lesion. In relation to Dr. Klimov's closing comment that he finds beta-lipoprotein in the artery but not in the vein, this again reflects the fact that one gets athero- sclerotic lesions in arteries but not in veins. However, there are circumstances in which one can produce atherosclerotic lesions in veins and that is where a vein has been made to behave like an artery. We have looked at autologous venous grafts replacing atherosclerotic arteries and in these it is possible to demon- strate with the passage of time the deposition of beta-lipoproteins just as in the original artery. One could say that in relation to the artery the material is moving from the lumen outward whereas the main purpose of a vein is to act as a collector in the other direction, mostly collecting material from the tissues. Presumably, the large molecules are screened out in the tissue, so the vein is acting as a drain rather than a pressure vessel.

Dr. Bihari-Varga: Following the publications of Gero et al., and Amenta and Waters on the possible role of attractive forces between serum lipids and vascular mucoid substances in atherogenesis, in vitro studies were performed in our laboratory on glycosaminoglycan-beta-lipoprotein complexes, with the aim to analyse their physico-chemical and biochemical properties and testing the specificity of the reaction. Glycosaminoglycans, and their individual fractions, prepared from human aorta, were precipitated with lipemic serum or with isolated low-density lipoproteins in the presence of bivalent metal ions at various pH. In the physiologically presumably relevant calcium complexes the degree of complex formation and the amount of calcium bound in the complex, showed a parallel change with the amount of acidic groups present in the glycosaminoglycan molecules. The solubility of the complexes was affected by the increase in pH and in the presence of sodium, potassium and ammonium ions.

When calcium was replaced by other bivalent metal ions, the degree of complex formation was found to be proportional to the ratio of the second power of charge to the ionic radius of the ion. These findings support the presumption that in the complexing process the uronic acid and sulfate groups of the glycosaminoglycans are linked through bivalent cations to the phosphate groups of beta-lipoprotein and that the bond is, at least partly, maintained by electrostatic forces.

We have also demonstrated that the glycosaminoglycans bind only the beta-lipoproteins of the serum protein fraction to form a complex. When the complexes precipitated from hyperlipemic human sera by the calcium salt of aortic glycosaminoglycans were removed from the system and the supernatant was subjected to immunoelectrophoresis, the immunoelectrophoretic pattern showed virtually complete and isolated removal of beta-lipoproteins. There was a significant correlation between the concentration of beta-lipoprotein in serum and the amount of complex formed. Furthermore, the lipid composition of the isolated complexes corresponded to that of the Sf 0-20 beta-lipoprotein fraction. Titration of glycosaminoglycans with beta-lipoprotein and that of beta-lipoprotein with glycosaminoglycans yielded complexes in which the ratio of the components remained the same.

Tracy et al. succeeded in extracting glycosaminoglycan-beta-lipoprotein complexes from the aorta, which had the same electrophoretic mobility as the in vitro complexes previously demonstrated by us. Furthermore, glycosaminoglycan-beta-lipoprotein complexes were demonstrated in our laboratories in the atherosclerotic intimal tissue by means of a thermoanalytical method. The thermal decomposition of glycosaminoglycans takes place at about 240°, as indicated by a peak on the differential thermal gradient curves. We found that the thermostability of glycosaminoglycans characteristically increased when they were bound specifically in the form of glycosaminoglycan-beta-lipoprotein complex. A similar increase in the thermostability was observed in the atherosclerotic human vessel wall, as well as in the aortas of cholesterol-fed rabbits.

WHAT IS THE MORPHOLOGICAL AND (PHYSICO-) CHEMICAL EVIDENCE THAT CONNECTIVE TISSUE IN LESIONS ARE INDEED ALTERED?

J.P. Lindner

The vascular oedema is the first nonspecific reaction of disturbed vascular connective tissue metabolism after most injuries caused by a variety of factors, and follows a disturbed permeability. The main morphological evidence of disturbed permeability is the increased intensity of histochemical staining for acid mucopolysaccharides (MPS).

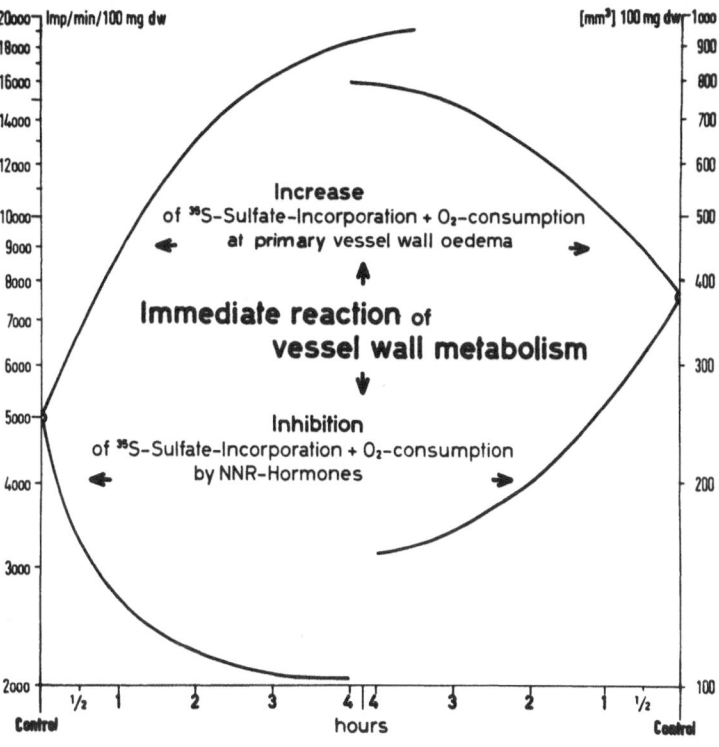

Figure 1

This increased metachromasia may depend upon the degradation of proteoglycans, changes of polymerisation, or decreased binding of MPS to proteins with enchanced liberation of anionic groups of MPS (glycosaminoglycans) for bindings with cationic stains, and on an absolute quantitative increase of the total content of the MPS after enhanced synthesis. Therefore, for true assessment the biochemical evidence is needed.

Most often, the enhanced S^{35}-sulfate incorporation is found as the first changed metabolic parameter (Fig. 1). A half an hour to four hours following an injection of low or high molecular solutions, an increased oxygen consumption is observed as an unspecific manifestation of an increased metabolism in rat aorta as well as in vascular tissues of other species, including men. The S^{35}-sulfate incorporation as in indicator method for the proteoglycan synthesis is increased as well as the activities of the involved enzymes, mostly in early lesions. The same is true for collagen synthesis.

The increased catabolism of proteoglycans and collagen is measured by the indicator enzymes, morphohistochemically, for localization, for example for beta-glucuronidase.

Biochemical quantification for collagen peptidase, even normally with highest activity in aorta of rabbit in comparison with other tissues, shows an increase in disturbed permeability and in early lesions (Fig. 2).

The increased catabolism and enhanced synthesis indicate an increased turnover of intercellular substances. Quantitative immunological estimations of serum proteins in arterial tissue sections, carried out with the so-called ring-test-dilution-method show (Fig. 3), that the serum albumin content is higher in the intima than the media, and is higher than the globulin content at every stage of

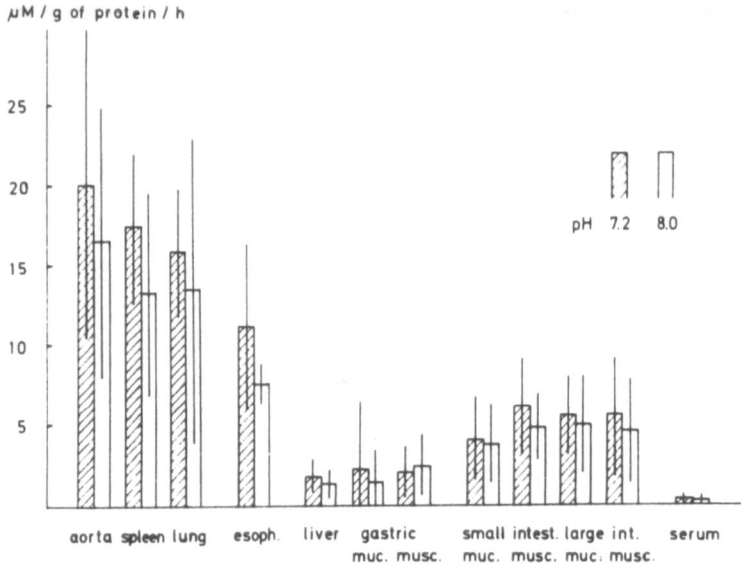

Figure 2. Collagenase activity of several rabbit organs compared with that of serum

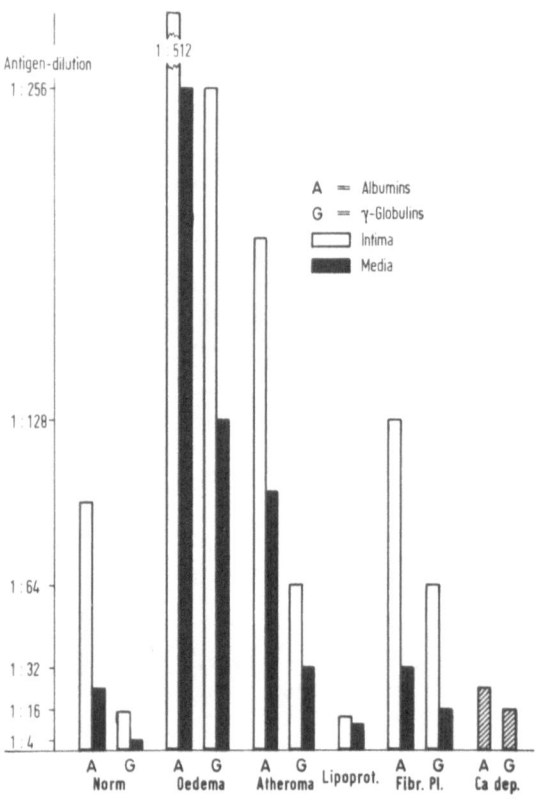

Figure 3. Quantitative serumprotein content of intima and media different art.-stages of the same aorta

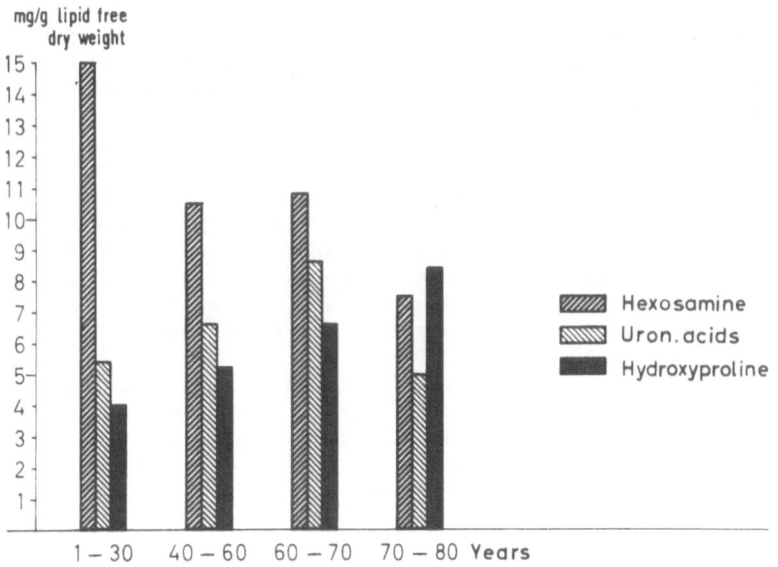

Figure 4. Changes of collagen- and MPS-content in oedema-plaques of aorta in several age groups

atherosclerosis. The highest content of both serum proteins is in the oedematous plaques, in accordance with the biochemical results.

The aminosugar content is highest in oedema in the first 30 years of life and lowest in the oldest age group. Aminosugars indicate the MPS - and glycoproteid-content; since the uronic acid content (only for acid MPS) is lower than the hexosamine content, it becomes evident, that the increase of hexosamines depends on an enhancement of neutral, especially serum, glycoproteids in oedematous plaques. The age dependent increase of MPS- is accompanied by an increase in collagen content as evident (Fig. 4) by the increase in hydroxyproline content.

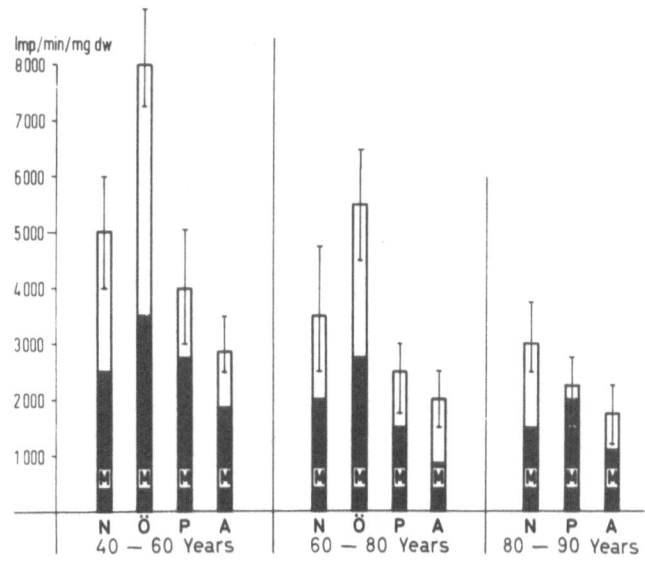

Figure 5. Comparison of MPS-syntheses of intima ▭▭▭ and media ▬▬▬ on 4 stages in 3 age groups

The S^{35}-incorporation as an indicator method for ground substance synthesis in human material decreases with age at all atherosclerotic stages, is higher in the intima than in the media, and most importantly, it is highest in oedematous plaques at every age and in comparison with unchanged parts of the same vessels (Fig. 5). The oxygen consumption runs parallel.

The total content of the ground substance and collagen depends at any given time upon the balance of synthesis = influx and breakdown = output (Fig. 6). Immediately following injury, and before there is morphological evidence for early lesions, there will be breakdown of ground substance and collagen before the synthesis increases. This results in a decreased total content (as is also seen in the first stage of inflammation). Alternatively, the synthesis may increase earlier than the breakdown is at its peak and thus the total content increases.

Both ana- and catabolism are increased in the following second stage resulting in an enhanced turnover, but the same total content. Turnover decreases in the later stages with the catabolism decreasing more markedly and earlier than the anabolism. This results in an increased total content, by morphologic and biochemical findings, or metachromatic ground substance, and later of collagen content, with disorganization and destruction, and lipid and calcium deposition.

Summarizing these observations one may state that the synthesis and the degradation of MPS - and collagen - fractions increase, and so does the total content of vascular MPS and collagen and their turnover rates, whereas their half live times are shortened (Fig. 7).

In progressing atherosclerosis there is a decrease of anabolic and catabolic processes and therefore a decrease in the turnover rates and the total content of the MPS and the soluble collagen fractions. The total content of the insoluble

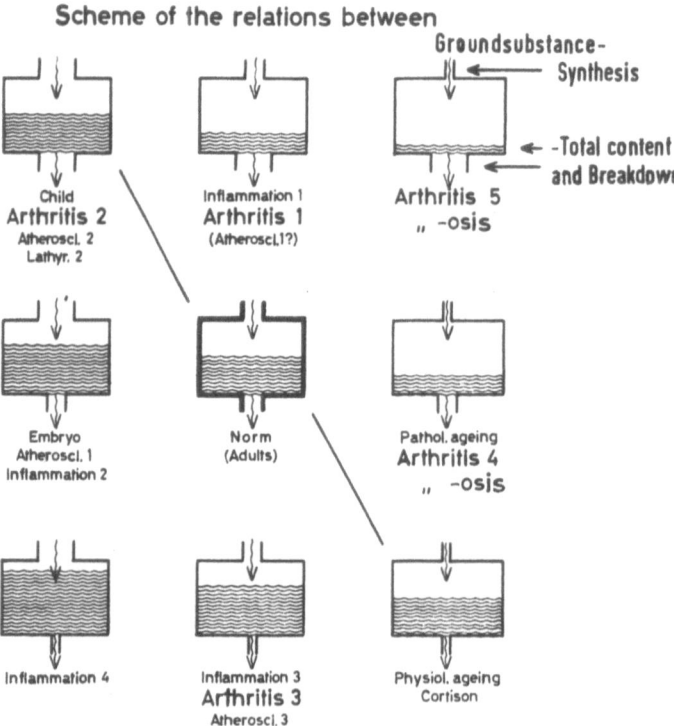

Figure 6

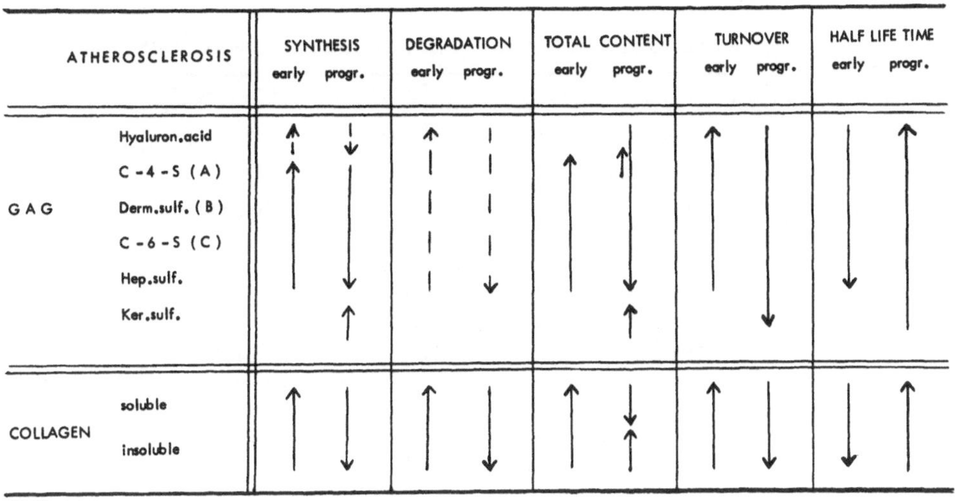

Figure 7

ATHEROSCLEROSIS		SYNTHESIS early progr.		DEGRADATION early progr.		TOTAL CONTENT early progr.		TURNOVER early progr.		HALF LIFE TIME early progr.	
GAG	Hyaluron.acid	↑↓	↓	↑	↓	↑	↑	↑	↓		↑
	C-4-S (A)	↑		↓	↓						
	Derm.sulf. (B)	↑	↓	↓	↓	↑	↓	↑	↓		↓
	C-6-S (C)			↓	↓						
	Hep.sulf.			↓	↓						
	Ker.sulf.		↑				↑				
COLLAGEN	soluble	↑	↓	↑	↓	↑	↓	↑	↓	↑	↑
	insoluble		↓		↓		↑		↓		↓

collagen fraction increases, as does also half life time of the vascular connective tissue components.

The consequences of the disturbed metabolism of the vascular connective tissues
are hypertrophy and hyperplasia of cellular and extracellular components as shown
also by Hauss, culminating in the disturbance of the transit across the artery
and morphologically in advanced and complicated lesions (Fig. 8).

In closing, one may state (Fig. 9) that there is clear evidence of connective
tissue alterations in the development of atherosclerotic lesions on the basis of
combined morphological and biochemical data. There is an enhanced metabolism,
which is higher also in the morphologically unchanged parts of the involved arteries.

Among the unresolved problems remains the question whether the disturbance in
metabolism of ground substance begins prior to, or following the disturbance of
permeability.

Discussion

Chairman Haust: Thank you Dr. Lindner for the summary on our state of knowledge
regarding the connective tissues in the lesions. I would like to call now upon
Dr. Poole, who some years ago with Dr. Charles Levine produced a paper showing
that there is an increase in collagen in arteriosclerotic versus non-arteriroscler-
otic aorta and stating that this was a preliminary report only. Hopefully, you
had followed up this work by further qualitative studies. Dr. Poole, would you
care to comment?

Dr. Poole: There were no further studies apart from that paper that you have mentioned and the facts are extremely simple: with increasing age there is increasing collagen content in normal intima, but there is an even greater increase of
collagen in atherosclerotic lesions. No qualitative studies followed.

Dr. McCullagh: I would like to come back to the questions posed by Dr. Walton,
and his statement that some of the plasma proteins normally "percolate" through
the intima. It is clear from some data presented this afternoon that the transfer
rate for fibrinogen was much slower than it was for albumin. Extrapolating from
the above in terms of molecular size, the amount of low-density lipoprotein that

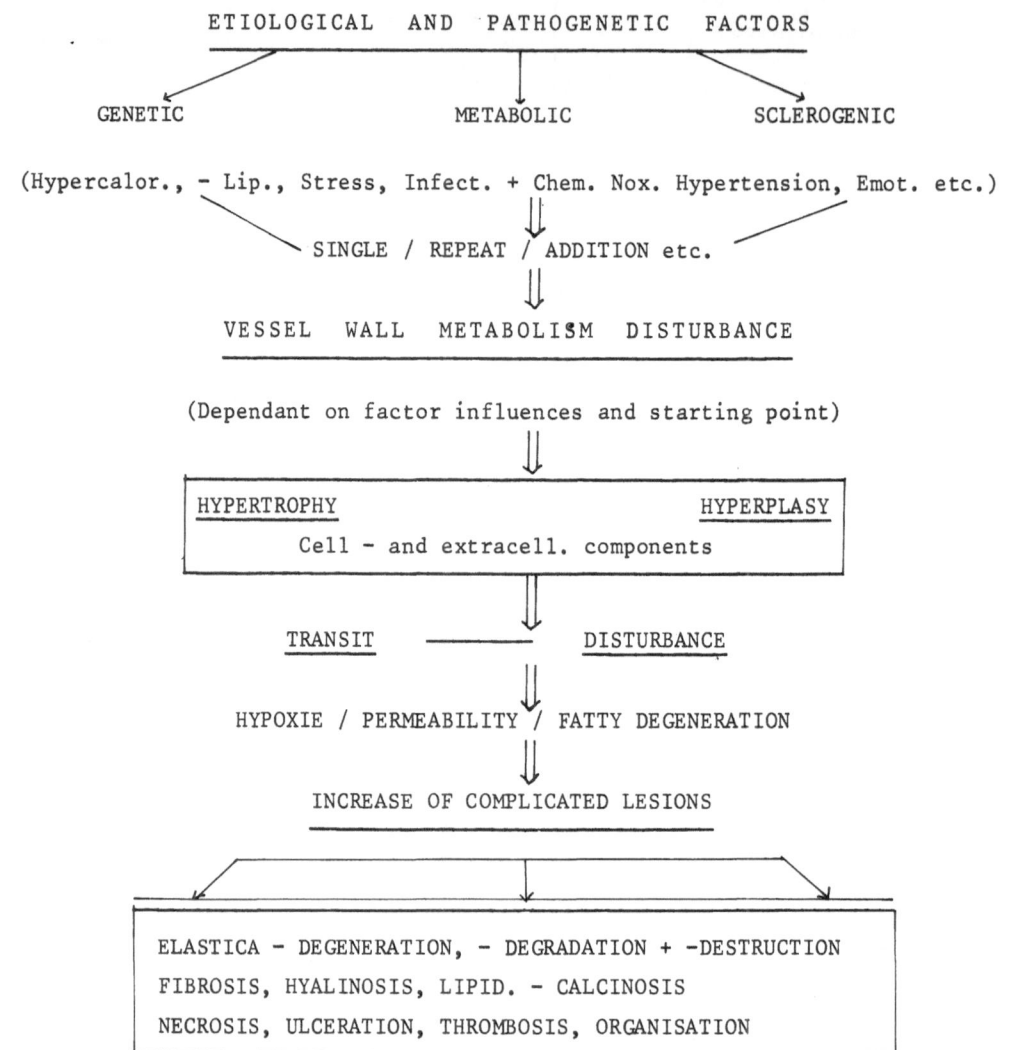

ETIOLOGICAL AND PATHOGENETIC FACTORS

GENETIC   METABOLIC   SCLEROGENIC

(Hypercalor., - Lip., Stress, Infect. + Chem. Nox. Hypertension, Emot. etc.)

SINGLE / REPEAT / ADDITION etc.

VESSEL WALL METABOLISM DISTURBANCE

(Dependant on factor influences and starting point)

HYPERTROPHY   HYPERPLASY
Cell - and extracell. components

TRANSIT ———— DISTURBANCE

HYPOXIE / PERMEABILITY / FATTY DEGENERATION

INCREASE OF COMPLICATED LESIONS

ELASTICA - DEGENERATION, - DEGRADATION + -DESTRUCTION
FIBROSIS, HYALINOSIS, LIPID. - CALCINOSIS
NECROSIS, ULCERATION, THROMBOSIS, ORGANISATION

Figure 8

can be expected to be transported directly through the normal intima is very small, indeed, and our studies in perfusion with rabbit show that in a normal intact artery the amount of low-density lipoprotein that is measurably going into the arterial wall is very small. And so I think we have to be very careful when stating that low-density lipoprotein is normally diffusing into the intima. It may be that only when the intima and the endothelial cells are damaged does that molecule enter the intima. Therefore, the accumulation of the low-density lipoprotein within the artery is obviously a function of permeability.

Dr. Smith: In a very few early lesions representing intimal edema, one may find collagen budles faintly perfused by lipids, but often lipid appears to be "plastered" on to the collagen fibers. Characteristically, these collagen bundles are rather thick.

EVIDENCE

1. for CONNECTIVE TISSUE ALTERATIONS in lesions by biochemical and
   morphological methods

2. for ORDER of 1. biochemical, 2. morphological findings (= on
   alterations) in EARLY LESIONS

3. for RESULT: as earlier as more unspecific REACTIONS of CONNECTIVE
   TISSUE COMPONENTS (esp. in the EXTRACELLULAR SUBSTANCES)

NOT enough EVIDENCE

1. for CAUSAL and TEMPORAL RELATIONSHIP between DISTURBANCES of
   PERMEABILITY and of VASCULAR CONNECTIVE TISSUE METABOLISM

2. for ELASTIN METABOLISM in EARLY LESIONS

3. for RELATIONSHIPS between DENATUR! COLLAGEN? NO - COLLAGEN -
   PROTEINS and AMYLOID in PROGRESSED LESIONS in arterial AGEING.

Figure 9

Dr. Lindner: The vessel walls *are* connective tissues and when the artery is diseased the connective tissues are altered. Naturally it is possible that lipids
derived from whatever source may come to lie between collagen fibers, but this
doesn't mean that these are specifically associated with the collagen or other
connective tissues, or that there are affinities. This is only a morphological
picture.

Chairman Haust: I think that at issue is the question whether or not the mesenchymal, or smooth muscle cells, when called upon to proliferate in the sense as
indicated by Dr. Hauss, are in these lesions producing normal connective tissues.
I think this is the key issue but we are almost attempting to avoid discussing it
directly, because there are no hard data other than those suggested by Dr. Lindner
here, i.e., that the solubility of the collagen is altered in atherosclerosis.
However, we can not continue to overlook the status of connective tissues in
atherosclerotic lesions very much longer; I was hoping that someone in the audience will contribute newly compiled or accumulating data regarding this matter,
but this does not seem to be the case.

Dr. Buddecke: There were many reports on the glycoproteins and glycosaminoglycans
in the course of this Symposium and I really wonder why nobody mentioned in effect
that there are four different glycosaminoglycans in the arterial wall, namely
hyaluronate, chondroitin sulfate, dermatan sulfate and heparin sulphate. And it
is a matter of fact that these four glycosaminoglycans do not react uniformly in
response to the hypertension, and they are not evenly distributed in the arterial
wall. It has been shown ten years ago that about 70% of chondroitin sulphate is
present in the subintimal layer, while the rest is distributed throughout the
media. And I should like to give two examples of the different metabolic reaction
of the individual glycosaminoglycans. The first example concerns the age-dependant
changes in the specific radioactivity of the glycosaminoglycans in bovine arterial
wall. When the sulphated glycosaminoglycans are examined one can see an exponential decrease in the specific radioactivity of all sulphated glycosaminoglycans,
in contrast to the hyaluronate; the specific activity of the hyaluronate increases
with increasing age reaching a plateau in the 5th or 6th decade. The other example for different metabolic reactions of glycosaminoglycans concerns hypertension.
We can confirm the results of the Hauss-group as we found an increase in the

specific activity of the sulphated glycosaminoglycans in spontaneous hypertension of rats. Moreover, we found that not all sulphated glycosaminoglycans participate in this increased specific radioactivity. This specific radioactivity increase does not apply, however, to the chondroitin sulphate; only the dermatan sulphate and the heparan sulphate increase in the course of hypertension.

GENERAL DISCUSSION

Dr. Adams: I wouldn't at all disagree with Dr. Walton about the mucopolysaccharides, but I wonder if he is not being a little bit too unitary and not looking at the likelihood of multiple factors being involved. We have heard, for example, of collagen binding of cholesterol, of elastin binding of lipids and lipoprotein. That was one comment I wish to make. The second relates to the barrier role of certain components in the arterial wall. The elastic laminae certainly do act as a barrier as one can judge by cholesterol radiography work. One does find an accumulation of autoradiograph granules on the inside of elastic laminae and then one can also show them "flowing" through the fenestrations of the elastic laminae, so there is some holding up of the flow at that point. The third comment concerns the question of hypoxia of the media, particularly in larger human arteries. It has been recently reported in studies on oxygen consumption that there is in animals a defect of oxygen utilization in the inner part of the media. Whereas hypoxia per se would not influence the outflow of proteins and lipoproteins, it would interfere with the local handling, i.e., the dispersion and phagocytosis of cholesterol that has already been deposited in the tissue. If you damage smooth muscle fibers by hypoxia and they lose their enzymes, then they are not going to work so well in their dispersing phagocytic action against cholesterol deposits.

Dr. Björkerud: I should like to address myself to the issue whether the connective tissues in atherosclerotic lesions are different from those of other lesions or normal artery. There may be at least one, almost qualitative, difference in some experimental lesions. In lesions which proliferate and which are covered with endothelium there are formed fine elastic laminae which bridge over the experimental injury. However, if one induces a proliferative lesion where the re-endotheliazation is retarded there is no formation of such oriented elastic laminae. There is elastin but under the light microscope the small fibrillae appear without any definite orientation, and in the electron microscope one only sees small lumps of pro-elastin. This could be one very important difference between a non-atherosclerotic lesion (oriented elastic laminae) and the atherosclerotic type of lesion lacking endothelium (disoriented elastic laminae).

Dr. Shimamoto: Of the various factors implicated in changing the permeability of the arterial wall the contracting substance of the endothelial cell plays an important role. If one injects animals with Angiotensin II that produces endothelial contraction, and administers either ferritin or carbon particles intravenously at the same time, one may observe under the electron microscope that the endothelial cells by contracting provide avenues between them for the passage of the above particles. On the other hand, if one administers an endothelial cell relaxant (i.e., estrogen proved in our hands to have this property), then there will be no passing of either ferritin or carbon particles between the endothelial cells into the intima. Such endothelial "relaxants" will also prevent the development of atherosclerotic lesions in hypercholesterolemic animals. We are in the process of testing several substances with the endothelial cell relaxing property.

Dr. Schmit: If one exposes the vessels in rabbits to an ionizing radiation injury alone lesions develop that have few features of atherosclerosis. However, when similar injury is applied to animals on a hypercholesterolemic diet, the developing lesions are similar in many ways to atherosclerotic lesions; the outcome is a thickened intima with sclerosis and atheromatosis. Some arteries that do not develop atherosclerosis on diet alone (e.g., carotid arteries) will become the site of fat infiltration when simultaneously, these arteries will be irradiated. Many drugs, commonly used in medicine, have been tested in our laboratories for their effect upon the arteries in experimental animals, and to our surprise quite a few promoted infiltration of fat into the intima. Among these were several anti-inflammatory drugs presently in use, and a Vitamin B-derivative.

Dr. Wight: Relevant to the question as to why collagen and lipid may interact, are perhaps the following observations. If one takes precautions in preserving glycosaminoglycans in experimental lesions, a very convenient way of doing this is to fix the tissue in the presence of ruthenium red. This seems to keep glyco-saminoglycans within the tissue. If one then looks at the collagen fibers in so treated experimental lesions, one sees large granules deposited on the major interbands along the collagen fibrils indicating one of two things: either that the glycosaminoglycans are deposited along the collagen molecule representing a negative charge site, or that the collagen molecule is strongly anionic at that point. If there be any credence to the idea that beta-lipoproteins and glyco-saminoglycans interact electrostatically, then this might be a way in which the beta-lipoprotein complexes with the collagen molecule. It is of interest that in addition to the basement lamina the plasma membrane of the smooth muscle cell also stains with ruthenium red indicating that there is a possible anionic charac-ter of that plasma membrane. This might suggest selective uptake of beta-lipopro-tein by the smooth muscle cell provided that beta-lipoprotein remains intact and keeps its positive charge.

Chairman Haust: I should like to call now upon my Co-Chairman, Dr. Robert, to deliver his Summary remarks.

Chairman Robert: The vascular wall may be considered as a differentiated form of connective tissue. As such, it contains a relatively abundant intercellular matrix. This matrix comprises all four types of macromolecules which are also present in other differentiated connective tissues, i.e., collagen, elastin, proteoglycans and structural glycoproteins. There is evidence accumulating in favour of the local synthesis of all these macromolecules by the smooth muscle cells of the mam-malian aorta, whereas the endothelial cells and fibroblasts of the adventitia may be concerned with the synthesis of some types only.

The major problem that remains to be answered concerns the "program" of the syn-thesis of these macromolecules in well defined ratios, i.e., the regularity mechanisms enabling the cells to synthesise the aforementioned macromolecules of the intercellular matrix, as well as those retained within the cells such as ac-tin, myosin, and so on.

The problem of the permeability of the vessel wall was discussed by several speakers at this Workshop (Dr. Jellinek, Dr. Jacotot, Dr. Walton). The penetra-tion of macromolecules from the blood stream into the vessel wall appears to be limited by two factors: uptake by cells, largely by the endothelium, and the dif-fusion through the elastic laminae. The selective penetration of lipoproteins appears to be well documented and Dr. Walton's presentation was informative re-garding this topic. The selective uptake of LDL and VLDL in the atherosclerotic vessel wall and the exclusion of HDL points to the importance of the peptide por-tion of lipoproteins. In addition, physicochemical factors such as the size, com-position and surface properties of particles play a role in their interaction with the vessel wall elements. None of these factors alone seems to be determin-ing.

An important aspect, discussed by Prof. Jacotot, concerns the interaction of lipids vehicled by the penetrating serum lipoproteins, with the individual macro-molecules of the intercellular matrix. Although most of these macromolecules appear to be able to interact with lipids, elastin seems to play an important role in the fixation of lipids in the intercellular matrix. A mechanism involving "hydrophobic stacking" of lipid molecules, mainly cholesterol, in the peptide folds of elastin was proposed to account for lipid accumulation, loss of elasticity and gradual breakdown of elastic laminae with age and arteriosclerosis. Recent studies show that the composition of lipids associated with the individual macromolecular extracts of the arterial wall changes with the degree of arteriosclerosis. These studies together with those on the molecular mechanism of calcium fixation in elastin may throw new light on the detailed molecular mechanism leading from lipoprotein penetration to the pathological alteration of the vessel wall in atherosclerosis.

The metabolic studies reported by Dr. Hauss here stress the importance of the altered reactivity of the mesenchymal cells as demonstrated by the increase of ^{35}S-incorporation into the aortic glycosaminoglycans. This "non-specific mesenchymal reaction" is induced by several factors such as hypertension, toxin, emotional stress, etc. The altered synthesizing activity of the mesenchymal cells results in the modified composition of the connective tissue of arterial wall in atherosclerosis. These modifications were expertly summarised by Dr. Lindner.

Dr. Jellinek drew attention to the patho-physiological aspects of the permeability of the arterial intima, studied by original histochemical methodology. His presentation exemplified the present-day attempts at approaching the problem of atherosclerosis by combined efforts at molecular, morphological, patho-physiological and hemodynamic levels.

It became also obvious in the course of this Workshop that many questions remain unanswered with respect to the role of permeability and mural connective tissues in the process of atherosclerosis, and these problems need to be pursued.

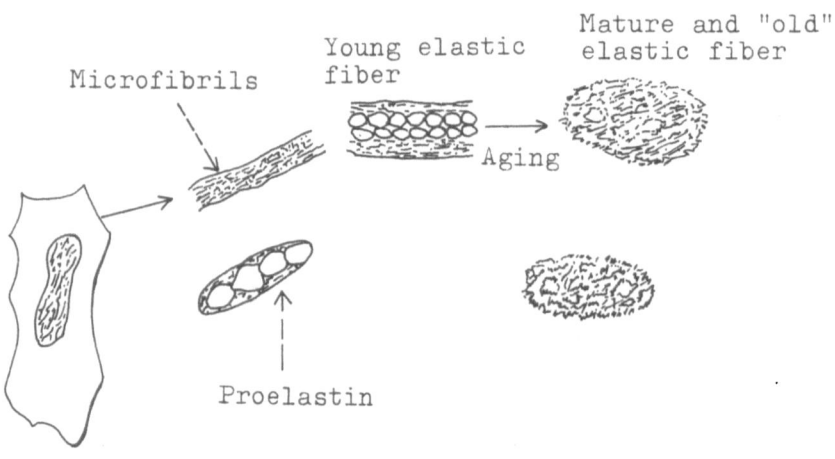

Figure 1. Schematic representation of elastogenesis. The smooth muscle cell produces "microfibrillar" structural glycoproteins. Proelastin monomers associate with the microfibrillar scaffolding through electrostatic interactions and are then crosslinked through the action of lysine oxydase and formation of lysinonorleucine and desmosine. The ratio elastin / glycoprotein increases with age, but "microfibrils" are present also in mature elastic lamellae. In "plaque-elastin" this ratio decreases again and elastin becomes fragmented through the action of elastases

ASSOCIATION OF CORONARY ARTERY ENDOTHELIAL INJURY WITH ELEVATION OF SERUM BILE ACIDS IN THE RAT

Fritz Parl and William H. Gutstein

Emotional factors have been implicated in atherogenesis. Employing electric stimulation of the lateral hypothalamus we previously found functional biliary obstruction associated with hypercholesterolemia in the rat (Gutstein et al., 1969). Using ligation induced biliary tract obstruction, ultrastructural evidence of coronary artery endothelial injury was encountered in the same species (Gutstein and Parl, 1973).

In the present investigation, serum total cholesterol, alkaline phosphatase and bile acids were measured and correlated with morphologic changes of coronary artery endothelium 24 hr after bile duct ligation.

Male and female rats of the Sprague - Dawley strain weighing 200 to 250 gm were divided into experimental and control groups. Experimentals were subjected to bile duct ligation for a 24 hr period and controls were sham operated with manipulative exposure of the bile duct, omitting ligation. Both groups received ad libitum cream feeding post-operatively to stimulate bile flow. At the conclusion of the experimental period, the hearts were removed while the animals were under anesthesia. The hearts were fixed by immersion in full strength Karnovsky's medium after which small transverse sections of coronary artery were selected with the aid of a dissecting microscope and processed for electron microscopic examination. Baseline venous blood samples were obtained prior to ligation or manipulation of the bile duct and at the end of the experimental period. Samples were analyzed for serum total cholesterol and alkaline phosphatase activity. Serum bile acids were hydrolyzed enzymatically, extracted, and separated by thin-layer chromatography from phospholipids, triglycerides and fatty acids. Following methylation and trifluoroacetylation, the bile acids were identified and quantitatively determined by gas-liquid chromatography.

Table 1 presents means of total and individual serum bile acids, cholesterol and alkaline phosphatase for ligated and sham operated animals. In experimental animals serum total bile acids, chenodeoxycholic acid, cholic acid, cholesterol, and alkaline phosphatase increased significantly ($p<0.01$) within 24 hr, whereas in controls there was either no change or a decrease in these parameters. The disappearance of secondary bile acids (deoxy- and hyodeoxycholic acid) from the blood of obstructed animals is a consequence of the interruption of the enterohepatic circulation.

Electron microscopic changes of coronary artery endothelium disclosed cytologic degenerative changes in the majority of ligated animals similar to those reported previously (Gutstein and Parl, 1973). These generally consisted of intracellular edema with cytoplasmic vacuole formation often associated with attenuation and disruption of the plasma membrane on the luminal side. Intercellular junctions, however, appeared to be intact (Fig. 1, 2).

The serum bile acid levels in the general circulation of untreated rats were found to be exceedingly low, in accordance with observations by Okishio and Nair (1966). After 24 hr bile duct ligation, however, they increased approximately 200 times and were associated with the morphologic changes described. In rats, total bile acid levels of portal blood under physiologic conditions have been determined to be approximately 55 times those normally present in the systemic circulation. Ultrastructural examination of the portal vasculature by other investigators, however, did not reveal any morphologic changes comparable to those described here

Table 1. Means ± S.D. of total bile acid, deoxycholic acid, chenodeoxycholic acid, hyodeoxycholic acid, cholic acid, total cholesterol and alkaline phosphatase concentrations in serum of experimental and control animals before and after treatment

Serum parameter	Experimental		Control	
	Pre-ligation	Post-ligation	Before	After sham-operated
Total bile acids (µg/ml)	3.12 ± 1.08 (11)[a]	251 ± 112 (11)	1.79 ± 0.69 (6)	1.88 ± 0.89 (6)
Deoxycholic acid (µg/ml)	0.45 ± 0.23 (11)	0.00[b] (11)	0.20 ± 0.18 (6)	0.30 ± 0.30 (6)
Chenodeoxycholic acid (µg/ml)	0.42 ± 0.40 (11)	19.4 ± 8.1 (11)	0.19 ± 0.17 (6)	0.21 ± 0.18 (6)
Hyodeoxycholic acid (µg/ml)	0.92 ± 0.29 (11)	0.00 (11)	0.58 ± 0.24 (6)	0.54 ± 0.35 (6)
Cholic acid (µg/ml)	1.33 ± 0.64 (11)	232 ± 102 (11)	0.85 ± 0.55 (6)	0.66 ± 0.43 (6)
Total cholesterol (mg/100 ml)	72 ± 11 (10)	183 ± 81 (9)	77 ± 12 (5)	52 ± 8 (6)
Alkaline Phosphatase (mU/ml)	101 ± 31 (10)	208 ± 67 (10)	123 ± 31 (6)	67 ± 14 (6)

[a] The number of animals "n" is indicated as (n).

[b] Values of 0.00 µg/ml indicate that the respective bile acids were not detected at these concentrations.

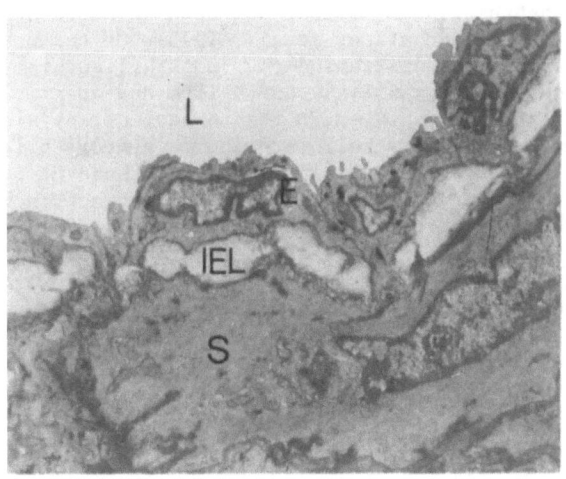

Figure 1. Coronary artery of sham operated (control) rat sacrificed 24 hours after surgery. Nucleus and cytoplasm of endothelial cells (E) are intact. L = lumen, IEL = internal elastic lamina, S = smooth muscle cell (Original magnification X 2280)

in the coronary artery (Rouiller and Jezequel, 1963). It is therefore possible that the observed endothelial injury is related to the surfactant effect of the bile acids above certain threshold concentrations. This possibility is further supported by the demonstration that direct injection of deoxycholate into the rat femoral artery resulted in extensive degenerative endothelial damage (Constantinides and Robinson, 1969). The concentration of deoxycholate employed was several times higher than that of total bile acids found in this study.

The role of dihydroxy bile acids as injurious agents compared with trihydroxy bile acids is somewhat more difficult to assess. For example, an increased intrahepatic concentration of chenodeoxycholic acid following ligation induced biliary

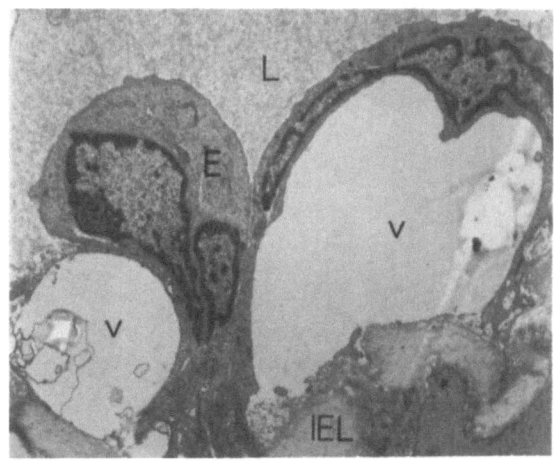

Figure 2. Coronary artery of rat 24 hours after bile duct ligation. Two large vacuoles (V) are present within endothelial cells. One vacuole appears almost empty while the other contains membrane like material (Original magnification X 3000)

obstruction in the rat has been shown to be associated with toxic changes in hepatocytes (Schaffner et al., 1973). On the other hand, in rats rendered cholestatic by the administration of α-naphthylisothiocyanate (ANIT), degenerative changes of hepatocytes, biliary epithelium and arteriolar endothelium of the portal tract have been observed in the absence of any significant concentrations of intrahepatic chenodeoxycholic or other dihydroxy bile acids. This raises the possibility that our observations as well as those of other investigators concerning cell injury associated with biliary obstruction may be due to other factors in association with increased bile acid concentrations operating either locally in hepatocytes, distantly in various target organs or in the circulation itself.

Whatever the ultimate mechanism involved, it appears clear that biliary obstruction sustained for even a relative short time is capable of injuring not only endothelial cells of various target organs, but of the coronary artery itself. As such, it may be viewed as a potentially atherogenic factor.

EFFECT OF NICOTINE ON SEVERITY OF ACUTE MYOCARDIAL ISCHEMIC INJURY

Arnfinn Ilebekk and Ole D. Mjøs

According to the combined studies of Albany and Framingham, the incidence of myocardial infarction in heavy smokers is three times as great as in non-smokers (Doyle et al., 1962). Mortality from coronary heart disease is also substantially higher in cigarette smokers than in non-smokers. It is believed that the deleterious effects of cigarette smoking are partly due to nicotine (Aronow et al., 1971), but mechanisms involved remain in doubt.

The actions of nicotine are primarily mediated through stimulation of the sympathetic nervous system and release of catecholamines from the adrenal medulla, with a consequent rise of arterial blood pressure, mechanical activity of the heart and myocardial oxygen consumption ($M\dot{V}O_2$). Moreover, Kershbaum et al. (1961) have shown that nicotine intravenously (or through cigarette smoking) raises plasma concentration of free fatty acids (FFA). Since recent studies (Mjøs, 1971 a,b) indicated that increased delivery of FFA to the heart may increase $M\dot{V}O_2$ through a metabolic stimulation - independent of changes in mechanical activity of the heart - the first purpose of the present study was to determine if the rise in $M\dot{V}O_2$ caused by nicotine was to any degree related to increased myocardial consumption of FFA. This could be studied by inhibition of nicotine-induced lipolysis by nicotinic acid or its derivative ß-pyridyl-carbinol (Ronicol, F. Hoffman-La Roche & Co. A.G. Basel, Switzerland), without altering the nicotine-mediated rise in mechanical activity of the heart (Mjøs and Ilebekk, 1973). The effect of intravenous (I.V.) infusion of nicotine (15 µg per min. kg) on $M\dot{V}O_2$ was studied before and during inhibition of lipolysis by continuous I.V. infusion of Ronicol (5–10 mg. per min), in intact, sodium pentobarbital anesthetized dogs (Mjøs and Ilebekk, 1973). Although mechanical responses to nicotine were similar in both settings, $M\dot{V}O_2$ increased by 4.1 ± 0.9 ml per min · 100g before and 2.1 ± 0.6 ml per min · 100g ($p<0.005$) during inhibition of lipolysis. Thus with intact lipolysis about 50 per cent of the nicotine-induced rise in $M\dot{V}O_2$ was related to enhanced mechanical activity of the heart, the remainder being attributable to a metabolic stimulation of high concentrations of FFA.

Various agents which augment myocardial oxygen requirements have recently been shown to increase the extent and magnitude of an experimental myocardial injury in dogs, and agents lowering the oxygen requirements of the heart have been shown to decrease the size (Maroko et al. 1970; Kjekshus and Mjøs, 1973). Since nicotine intravenously in normal dogs increased $M\dot{V}O_2$ - partly due to an "uncoupling" effect of FFA and partly due to increased cardiac work -, the next step was to study if nicotine I.V. would also increase the severity of an ischemic myocardial injury following acute coronary occlusion in open-chest dogs, and furthermore to study if the nicotine-induced ischemic injury was reduced during inhibition of lipolysis with Ronicol. Myocardial ischemic injury was assessed quantitatively by the S-T segment elevations in epicardial ECG at easily recognizable sites on the epicardial surface surrounding the occluded artery. Recordings were performed with a cotton wick electrode. Previous studies (Maroko et al., 1970) showed that this technique provides rapid and reproducible determinations of the ischemic injury at repeated coronary occlusions in the same animal, provided recovery periods of 30 minutes are allowed. According to Jennings et al. (1969), irreversible myocardial cellular injury does not occur during the first 20 minutes of coronary occlusion. In the present study the sum of S-T segment elevation (ΣST) at 10 minutes occlusion was used as an index of ischemic injury. The results showed that ΣST during coronary occlusion alone averaged 25.6 ± 4.6 mV. During I.V. infusion of nicotine (15 µg per min · kg) ΣST increased to 29.2 ± 4.3 mV ($p<0.02$) following reocclusion of the coronary artery, and arterial concentration of FFA rose from an average of 238 $\pm$ 26 to 324 $\pm$ 50 µEq/1 (p<0.025). Inhibition of lipolysis with Ronicol, however, abolished the rise in ΣST and plasma-FFA induced by nicotine (Ilebekk and Mjøs, in press).

It is concluded that nicotine increased severity of acute myocardial ischemic injury probably due to increased oxygen demand by FFA, since there was no increased injury by nicotine when lipolysis was inhibited. Before inhibition of lipolysis the rise in plasma-FFA effected by nicotine in the present study is about equal to smoking and inhaling 2 cigarettes for 10 minutes (Kershbaum et al., 1961). Thus the results might be relevant to studies of cigarette-smoking in man. It might be speculated that in heavy smokers, as opposed to non-smokers, higher incidence of myocardial infarction and associated ventricular arrhythmias may be linked to increased FFA levels.

ENDOTHELIAL PERMEABILITY: FOCAL AND REGIONAL PATTERNS OF ^{131}I-ALBUMIN AND ^{131}I-FIBRINOGEN UPTAKE AND TRANSMURAL DISTRIBUTION IN THE PIG AORTA*

Frank P. Bell, Ian L. Adamson, Alexander S. Gallus, and Colin J. Schwartz

The focal nature of atherosclerotic lesions has been a consistent observation in both naturally-occurring and experimental atherosclerosis although the focal determinants of focal lesion development remain uncertain. One point of view considers that areas of arterial lesion development represent areas of increased enothelial permeability (or decreased clearance) to plasma constituents. Indeed, numerous workers (Gerö et al., 1961; Watts, 1963; Haust et al., 1964; Kao and Wissler, 1965; Smith et al., 1973) have by various means identified a wide range of plasma constituents associated with atherosclerotic lesions.

In order to define more clearly the permeability of the arterial wall to plasma proteins, we have examined both focal and regional patterns of uptake of I^{131}-albumin and I^{131}-fibrinogen and their transmural distribution and influx rates in the normal pig aorta, *in vivo*. Focal areas of the pig aortas were identified by the protein-binding azo dye Evans Blue, a dye that exhibits a spontaneous focal pattern of uptake in the arteries of pigs (Packham et al., 1967; Somer and Schwartz, 1971, 1972; Bell et al., 1972) and other animals (Friedman and Byers, 1963; McGill et al., 1957). In the pigs, these areas of dye accumulation are associated with an enhanced uptake of unesterified ^{3}H-cholesterol (Somer and Schwartz, 1971; 1972a), radio-iodinated albumin (Packham et al., 1967) and exhibit an increased endothelial cell turnover (Caplan and Schwartz, 1973). In addition, several studies have concluded that areas of Evans Blue dye accumulation coincide with areas of early atheromatous lesion development (Friedman and Byers, 1963; McGill et al., 1957).

Normal young Yorkshire pigs (14-16 kg) maintained on Purina hog chow were injected intravenously with Evans Blue dye (Somer and Schwartz, 1971) and 1 hour later injected intravenously with either 20 μCi of human I^{131}-albumin (S.A. 26 μCi/mg), (Bell et al., 1974a) or 160-218 μCi of human I^{131}-fibrinogen (S.A. 100 μCi/mg), (Bell et al., 1974b) per kg of body weight. Two hours after isotope injection, the aortas were removed intact from the valve ring to the trifurcation.

Full thickness tissue discs were punched from the thoracic arch in areas of Evans Blue dye accumulation (blue areas) and areas of no dye accumulation (while areas). Tissue was also punched from white areas in the upper abdominal aorta at the level of the 5th intercostal ostium, and from the lower abdominal aorta immediately above the trifurcation. Tissue discs of surface area 0.21, 0.40 or 0.59 cm^2 were punched out using brass cork borers. After removal of the adventitia, tissue discs were either counted directly in a crystal well counter or serially sectioned from the intima to outer media. The serial sections were cut with a cryostat at intervals of 100 μ for the first and 200 μ for succeeding sections. The serial sections were counted as above to determine the transmural distribution of isotope.

The results of Table 1 show that plasma albumin and fibrinogen are capable of entering the arterial wall of the normal pig. In addition, there are distinct regional and focal differences in the rate of entry of the proteins. Influx into the thoracic arch is 2 to 4 times greater than influx into either the upper or lower abdominal segments of the artery. Of particular interest, however, is the focal difference in influx observed within the same segment; influx into blue

---

*Supported by Medical Research Council of Canada Grants MT.3067 and MA.3067 and The Canadian Heart Foundation.

Table 1 Albumin and fibrinogen influx[a] in blue and white areas of the pig aorta in vivo

Aortic tissue	Albumin $\mu g/cm^2/h$	Fibrinogen $\mu g/cm^2/h$
Thoracic blue	27.0 ± 1.7 (4)[b]	1.73 ± 0.30 (5)
Thoracic white	16.3 ± 1.3 (4)	0.82 ± 0.13 (5)
Upper abdominal white	8.6 ± 1.4 (4)	0.46 ± 0.08 (5)
Lower abdominal white	8.8 ± 2.8 (4)	0.41 ± 0.07 (5)

[a] Influx rates were calculated by dividing the radioactivity (counts/min) in tissue by the median specific activity of plasma albumin and fibrinogen between 1 minute and 2 hours after isotope injection.

[b] Values are means of the number of animals shown ± SEM.

areas of the thoracic arch was twice that observed in adjacent white areas. The possibility that observed differences in influx reflect surface contamination of isotope was excluded by counting the arterial endothelium removed as häutchen preparations (Pugatch and Saunders, 1968). We found that only between 3 and 7% of the radioactivity was associated with the endothelial monolayer.

Fig. 1 and 2 show the transmural distribution of I^{131}-albumin and I^{131}-fibrinogen across the arterial wall, respectively. With each protein, there is a gradient of I^{131} activity that is maximal on the intimal side and least on the side of the outer media. The slopes of these gradients indicate that plasma albumin and fibrinogen enter the arterial wall from the endothelial surface and subsequently move across the arterial wall to the outer media. These results are particularly pertinent in the case of fibrinogen since the presence of fibrinogen or fibrin in atherosclerotic plaques has been taken as evidence that plaques arise from the incorporation of mural thrombi into the arterial wall (Duguid, 1946, 1948). However, our results and the recent findings of Smith et al. (1973) indicate that the presence of fibrinogen or fibrin in the arterial wall may be explained, in part, by normal endothelial permeability to fibrinogen.

The focal and regional patterns of albumin and fibrinogen uptake by the normal pig aorta reflect a broad heterogeneity in permeability properties of the arterial wall. Regional differences in permeability as observed between the thoracic arch and abdominal segments may reflect the greater distensibility of the aortic arch than the abdominal aorta (McDonald, 1960; Evans et al., 1960). Duncan et al.(1962, 1965) have demonstrated that stretching, independent of perfusion pressure, may enhance the uptake of radio-iodinated albumin in the proximal part of the canine aorta *in vitro*. It is feasible that pressure-induced stretching, occurring synchronously with the cardiac cycle would be greatest in the aortic arch, and least in the less distensible segments of the abdominal aorta. This may explain the greater uptake of the protein-binding azo dye Evans Blue in the aortic arch *in vivo*, and is consistent with the observation of Somer et al. (1972b) who observed an enhanced uptake of Evans Blue in the aortic arch proximal to, and a decreased uptake distal to, experimental coarctation in the pig.

Focal areas of Evans Blue accumulation *in vivo* have been demonstrated in the aortas of dog (McGill et al.,1957), rabbit (Friedman and Byers,1963), and the pig (Packham et al., 1967; Somer and Schwartz, 1971, 1972a; Bell et al., 1972). In the pig, these areas of dye accumulation are associated with an enhanced uptake of both unesterified ^3H-cholesterol (Somer and Schwartz, 1971, 1972a), and radio-iodinated albumin (Packham et al., 1967; Bell et al., 1974a). These areas also

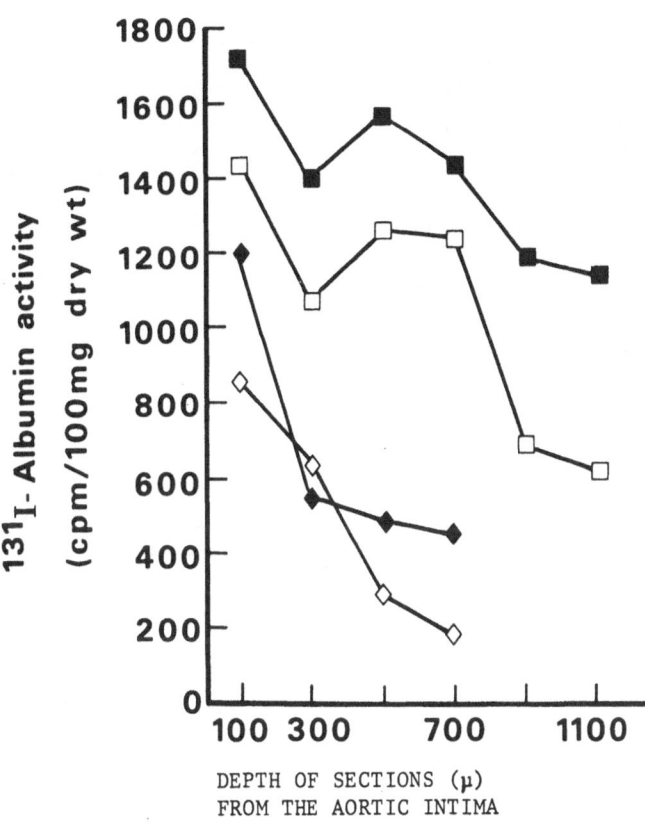

Figure 1. Transmural distribution of ^{131}I-albumin in the aorta of an individual pig 2 hours after isotope injection. Thoracic blue (—■—■—); thoracic white (—□—□—); upper abdominal white (—◆—◆—); lower abdominal white (—◇—◇—)

exhibit an increased endothelial cell turnover as determined by ^{3}H-thymidine autoradiography (Caplan and Schwartz, 1973) and are thought to represent foci of spontaneous, haemodynamically-induced endothelial injury. The present findings indicate that these foci also show an enhanced uptake of I^{131}-fibrinogen and I^{131}-albumin when compared to adjacent areas in the aortic arch showing no dye accumulation. In addition, unpublished observations from this laboratory indicate that foci of Evans Blue accumulation also accumulate cholesterol at a faster rate than adjacent areas of no dye accumulation when pigs are fed an atherogenic diet, and that I^{131}-albumin entry is enhanced in both blue and white areas after 6 weeks on an atherogenic diet.

Although one is tempted to suggest that the focal blue areas are predisposed to, or represent an early phase in atherogenesis, further studies are necessary for an understanding of the significance of such areas.

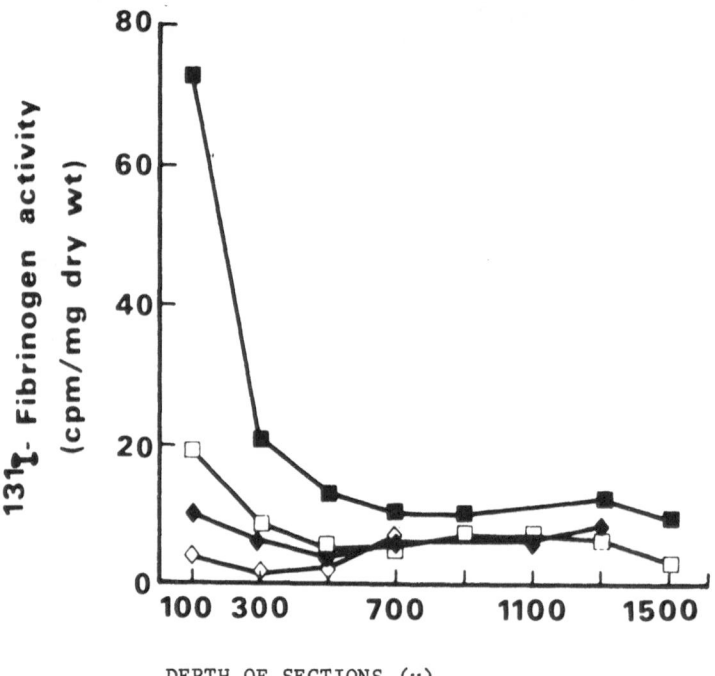

Figure 2. Transmural distribution of ^{131}I-fibrinogen in the aorta of an individual pig 2 hours after isotope injection. Thoracic blue (—■—■—); thoracic white (—□—□—); upper abdominal white (—◆—◆—); lower abdominal white (—◇—◇—)

INCREASED COLLAGEN SYNTHESIS IN EARLY RABBIT ATHEROSCLEROSIS AND ITS INHIBITION BY CIS-HYDROXYPROLINE*

Keith G. McCullagh and Irvine H. Page

The examination of histological section prepared from human coronary arteries, taken post-mortem from patients who have died from coronary heart disease often reveals that the occlusive or stenosing aspect of atherosclerotic lesions is not lipid but dense fibrous connective tissue. This facet of the disease is not always recognized in experimental animal lesions but has been well described in human atherosclerosis (Constantinides, 1965; Friedman, 1964; Smith, 1965; Levene and Poole, 1962).

We have recently been measuring rates of collagen synthesis in a variety of arterial tissues *in vitro*. Segments of canine arteries containing advanced fibrous plaques which had been induced by a semi-synthetic atherogenic diet were found to synthesize collagen at a rate 5 to 20 times that of healthy segments (McCullagh and Ehrhart, 1973). This stimulation of collagen synthesis was relatively specific with respect to other proteins and may well be the reason for the accumulation of collagen in the sclerotic intima.

Whether increased collagen synthesis is a universal feature of atherosclerotic lesions has not been established. Fuller and Langner (1970) have demonstrated increases in the levels of protocollagen proline hydroxylase in rabbit aortas made sclerotic by repeated injections of epinephrine and thyroxine, but it might be argued that this more closely resembles repair fibrosis than atherosclerosis. We would like to present here the results of two experiments in which we have measured collagen synthesis in segments of rabbit aortas made atherosclerotic by feeding a diet of 2% cholesterol for 4 months.

Experiment I

The thoracic aortas were removed from normal rabbits and from rabbits fed 2% cholesterol for 4 months and cut into segments measuring approximately 2 cm in length. Segments from cholesterol fed rabbits had 10 to 30% of the intimal surface area covered by slightly raised fatty lesions which had a typical foam cell appearance when examined histologically. Segments from atherosclerotic aortas were paired with equivalent segments from normal rabbits and suspended in 5 ml Earle's buffered salt solution containing 10 µC [^{14}C-U]L-proline + 2.5 µmoles each of unlabeled L-proline and L-glycine. Each flask was gassed with 95% O_2 and 5% CO_2, capped, and incubated for 3 hr at 39°. The segments were then transferred to ice-cold saline containing 100 µg/ml cycloheximide and 1 mM a,a^1-dipyridyl to halt further protein synthesis and hydroxylation. The adventitia was stripped off and the segments weighed before the aortic collagen was extracted by autoclaving with distilled water. Peptide bound ^{14}C-hydroxyproline was determined in the dialyzed collagen extracts as previously described (McCullagh and Ehrhart, 1973). The amounts of collagen synthesized in 3 hr were calculated on the basis that 14.0% of the weight of collagen is due to hydroxyproline and assuming that the specific activity of free ^{14}C-proline in the tissue was identical with that of the incubation medium.

The results of this experiment are shown in Table 1 in terms of nanograms collagen synthesized per gram of aortic intima-media. In every case, the collagen formed by the atherosclerotic segment exceeded that synthesized by the normal

*Supported by Program-Project grant no. HL 6835 from the USPHS.

239

segment, the mean increment being 70% of the control value. Details of the paired t-test are given in the table and show that the increased rate of synthesis in the segments containing fatty streaks was significant at the 5% level.

Table 1. Collagen synthesized by normal and atherosclerotic segments of intima-media during 3 hour incubation. ng collagen[a]+g wet wt

Pair	Normal	Athero	Difference
1	738	1398	+ 660
2	791	1440	+ 649
3	918	1416	+ 498
4	617	1551	+ 934
5	910	1266	+ 356
6	965	1329	+ 364
Mean	823	1400	+ 577

$S_{\bar{D}}$ = 219, t = 2.63, p < 0.05

[a]Calculated from peptidyl-^{14}C-hydroxyproline formation assuming complete equilibration of medium ^{14}C-proline with collagen precursor pool.

Experiment II

In view of the clinical significance of excess collagen accumulation in arteries, we have been interested in testing potential inhibitors of fibrosis for their effect on arterial collagen production. One such inhibitor is cis-4-hydroxyproline, whose chemical and three-dimensional structure are depicted in Fig. 1. Cis-hydroxyproline is a structural isomer of the natural form of hydroxyproline occurring in collagen and is treated by the cell as an analogue of proline (Rosenbloom and Prockop, 1971). Unlike natural hydroxyproline, the cis-isomer is incorporated into collagen, in positions normally occupied by proline, where it is thought to interfere sterically with the normal triple-helical arrangement of collagen peptides (Uitto et al., 1972). Collagen containing this analogue appears to be extruded from cells at a reduced rate (Rosenbloom and Prockop, 1971) and the addition of this analogue to tendon cells *in vitro* has been shown to result in a substantial decrease in collagen synthesis (Uitto et al., 1972).

In order to investigate whether cis-hydroxyproline could also be utilised as an inhibitor of arterial fibrosis we conducted an experiment similar to that just described but in which normal and atherosclerotic rabbit aortic segments were incubated in either the presence or absence of cis-4-hydroxy-L-proline (Calbiochem) at a level of 250 µg/ml. Other details of the incubation and analysis were similar to those of Experiment I.

The results of this investigation are shown in Table 2. Under control conditions, aortic segments containing fatty streaks synthesized more labeled collagen than undiseased segments, the mean increment in this experiment being 697 ng/g or 153% of the control. When incubated in the presence of 250 µg/ml cis-4-hydroxyproline, both normal and atherosclerotic segments showed substantial depression of collagen synthesis. The depression was somewhat greater in atherosclerotic segments, there being a mean inhibition of 61% in undiseased segments and 79% in those with fatty streaks.

trans-4-hydroxy-L-proline
(natural form)

cis-4-hydroxy-L-proline
(allo-4-hydroxy-L-proline)

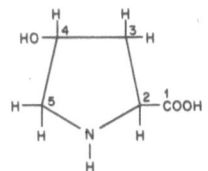
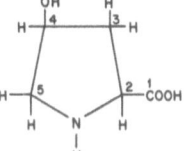

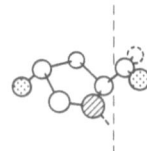
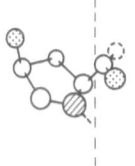

Figure 1. Comparison of the structures of the trans- and cis-forms of 4-hydroxy-L-proline. Top: diagrammatic formulae. Bottom: drawing of three-dimensional models aligned as if in peptide linkage in a collagen α-chain. Vertical dashed line represents long axis of the peptide

Table 2. Collagen synthesized by normal and atherosclerotic segments of intima-media in the presence of cis-hydroxyproline. ng collagen[a]/g wet wt

Conditions	n	Normal mean ± SD	Athero mean ± SD
No additive	4	455 ± 235	1152 ± 892
+250 µg/ml cis-4-hydro	4	176 ± 77	244 ± 64

[a]Calculated from peptidyl-^{14}C-hydroxyproline formation assuming complete equilibration of medium ^{14}C-proline with collagen precursor pool

Conclusion

These studies show that increased collagen synthesis is a part of the metabolic derangements that occur in atherosclerotic arteries, even in the early foam cell lesions of the cholesterol fed rabbit. The increments in formation of peptidyl-^{14}C-hydroxyproline in atherosclerotic rabbit aortas were not as large as those seen in canine experimental fibrous plaques. However, it must be emphasized that these rabbit lesions were relatively mild and occupied no more than 30% of the intimal surface area. Rates of synthesis higher than those measured here might well be encountered in more severe lesions.

This preliminary investigation also shows that the proline analogue cis-4-hydroxy-proline is a potent inhibitor of collagen synthesis by arteries *in vitro*. Other studies with this compound *in vivo* have shown that it is also effective in preventing granuloma formation due to carrageenan (Jimenez and Prockop, 1970) and the scarring that occurs after tendon injury (Lane et al., 1972) in rats. Such investigations have revealed no short term toxicity from the analogue and indicate that this agent could be a successful non-pharmacolgic inhibitor of arterial fibrosis *in vivo*.

BASEMENT MEMBRANES IN MUSCLE CAPILLARIES OF PATIENTS WITH HYPERLIPIDEMIAS

Nepomuk Zöllner and Herbe Herrlinger

The importance of the capillary basal lamina as a microskeleton of capillaries and an ultrafilter for metabolic exchange between blood and tissue is well established (Vollrath, 1968). An entire spectrum of abnormal thickening of the basal lamina, from minimal to extreme, can be seen in certain pathologic states such as polymyositis, scleroderma and systemic lupus erythematosus, and most notably, in patients with diabetes mellitus.

In this report we will describe findings in patients with otherwise asymptomatic hyperlipidemia. We shall also mention the findings in a case of alcoholic myopathy which will be reported elsewhere in detail.

Methods

Needle biopsy of quadriceps muscle was obtained with a Vim-Silverman biopsy needle as described by Seperstein et al. (1968). Tissue was immediately fixed in 6,5% phosphate-buffered glutaraldehyde, pH 7,4 for two hours, rinsed in phosphate buffer at least two times, postfixed in 2% osmium tetroxide pH 7,4 for two hours, block-stained for 20 min. with uranyl acetate pH 5,0, dehydrated in ethyl alcohol, and embedded in Epon 812 via propylene oxide. Thin sections were cut with a "Ultrotome" LKB and double stained with uranyl acetate and lead citrate. Electron micrographs were taken at an original magnification of ca. 7200 with a Siemens "Elmiskop I"; exact magnification was determined with a carbon grating replica. Plates were enlarged three times.

To estimate the basal lamina thickness we first employed the method of Williamson et al. (1969), measuring with a magnifying lens the minimum basal lamina thickness of each capillary at two points on its circumference. Then we remeasured the basal lamina thickness with a slide gage according to the method of Siperstein et al. (1968), at least at twelve points around the capillary circumference.

Results

Minimum basal lamina thickness of muscle capillaries in eleven normal weight controls with normal glucose tolerance curves and no known vascular disease measured 913 ± 67 Å (mean ± s.e.m.), the individual means varying from 758 ± 51 Å to 1211 ± 124 A. Table 1 summarizes the pertinent data on the basal lamina measurements of the control patients.

Minimum basal lamina thickness of the alcoholic patient measured 2460 ± 119 Å, i.e. nearly three times the normal thickness.

Single capillary basal lamina thickness of all controls ranged from 485 to 1526 Å, whereas the thinnest basal lamina in the patient measured 1364 Å, the thickest 3885 Å. Only about 15 per cent of his basal lamina values fall within the normal range.

In addition to a simple basal lamina thickening we frequently encountered duplication or splitting of basal lamina into several lamellae with an electron-lucent space between them. The width of a single lamella often measures about 800 Å.

Endothelial cells and the pericytes generally had a normal appearance; between the endothelial and the pericyte cells basal lamina thickening was generally not seen.

Table 1. Minimum thickness of basement membranes ($\bar{x} \pm s_{\bar{x}}$) of controls (weight and OGTT normal)

Age	Sex	Chol.	Tgl.	B.P.	B.M.
6	f	90	65	105/65	758 ± 51
17	f	180	70	125/80	830 ± 63
26	m	195	140	130/85	973 ± 86
30	m	87	47	120/70	960 ± 100
36	m	185	135	140/90	838 ± 23
40	f	135	85	135/85	1005 ± 83
42	m	180	55	130/70	838 ± 50
45	m	200	120	150/90	897 ± 17
46	f	170	135	140/95	1211 ± 124
53	m	160	60	120/70	911 ± 78
81	m	190	85	145/75	825 ± 61
				average	913 ± 67

Table 2 summarizes the measurements of basement membranes in patients with hyperlipidemias, Fredrickson's types II and IV. (The last case could not be typed definitely, not an uncommon occurence.) It can be seen, that all values obtained fall into the normal range.

Table 2. Minimum thickness of basement membranes ($\bar{x} \pm s_{\bar{x}}$) of patients with hyperlipidemia (controls from the same range of age)

Age	Sex	OGTT	Chol.	Tgl.	Type	B.P.	B.M.
31	m	n	360	100	II	145/100	763 ± 56
28	f	n	316	71	II	120/ 75	853 ± 58
30	m	path.	220	355	IV	140/ 90	1129 ± 148
36	m	path.	200	825	IV	145/ 90	1073 ± 74
40	m	path.	410	3600	IV	130/ 90	809 ± 77
52	m	n(i.v.)	500	405	IV	120/ 80	967 ± 94
63	m	path.	285	420	IV	170/100	1011 ± 116
65	f	path.	445	300	IV/II/V	210/ 90	778 ± 66
					age matched controls:		951 ± 68

However, in the group of patients with hyperlipidemia type IV the standard error of the mean is comparatively large. Since the number of measurements taken was the same in all cases and controls this indicates increased spread of single measurements. We do not think that this minor deviation from normal can be related to the hyperlipidemia. If at all, a relationship to the deranged oral glucose tolerance may be considered.

No differences between the ultramicroscopic appearance of muscle capillaries from controls and hyperlipidemic patients could be discerned.

The findings described suggest that neither the metabolic disorders producing the various forms of hyperlipidemia nor hyperlipidemia itself influence the capillary wall. Tissue reactions to hyperlipidemia (cf. Braun-Falco et al., 1972), so well known for the arterial wall, the skin, the heart valves and the cornea thus presumably are not mediated by deposition of increased or altered lipoproteins at the capillary level.

In contrast to the normal findings in hyperlipidemia our patient with chronic hyperethanolemia shows gross thickening and laminating of the basal lamina of nearly all capillaries evaluated. In nine patients suffereing from alcoholic pancreatitis Siperstein et al. (1968) described thickening of the basal lamina in only two; they were hyperglycemic. Danowski et al. (1971) found basal lamina thickening in six of eight alcoholic patients, ranging in severity from moderate to maximal.

There exist studies on thiamine-deficient rats which have shown a general widening and disarray of the structural organization of the vascular basal lamina in the brainstem (Collins, 1967; Manz et al., 1972).

EFFECT OF ADRENOCORTICAL HORMONES ON THE INTEGRITY OF RAT AORTIC ENDOTHELIUM

Sören Björkerud

More than a century ago Virchow postulated that increased arterial permeability could be an atherogenic factor. Zilversmit and Newman (1966) concluded from their own and other data that a "permeability barrier" might exist in the arterial wall, and that such a hypothetical barrier might protect the artery against atherogenic serum factors. We have studied the transfer of albumin and serum lipoproteins between the blood and the arterial wall and the relationship of this transfer to the structural and functional integrity of the endothelium (Björkerud and Bondjers, 1971, 1973; Bondjers and Björkerud, 1973 a; 1973 b). In regions with intact endothelium the transfer rate was much lower than in regions with spontaneously or experimentally injured endothelium. This indicates strongly the endothelium as the structural correlate to the arterial wall permeability barrier.

Traditionally, the arterial endothelium is conceived as a continuous lumenal lining. However, with the use of refined techniques as interference contrast microscopy of arterial segments made transparent (Björkerud and Bondjers, 1972) and scanning electron microscopy (Björkerud, Bondjers and Hansson, in preparation) we found a varying proportion of the arterial surface to contain large numbers of apparently injured endothelial cells even in unmanipulated rats and rabbits.

Material and Methods

The inability of injured or dead cells to prevent the uptake of, *i.e.* to exclude, certain vital dyes (Claesson, 1971) was used as a basis for estimation of the extent and degree of arterial endothelial injury. The aorta of the anesthetized animal was cannulated via the left ventricle. The blood was eliminated by an introductory perfusion with Ringer's solution at a pressure of 100 mm of mercury. The pressure was successively decreased to 9 mm of mercury. The Ringer's solution was exchanged for a solution of 0.3 per cent of Evan's blue in Ringer's solution, and the perfusion continued for 6 minutes. The perfusion was again changed to Ringer's solution to eliminate excessive dye. The aorta was finally fixed with formalin at a perfusion pressure corresponding to the systolic blood pressure, removed, cut open, and mounted flat.

The extent of endothelial staining was estimated semiquantitatively with densitometry of the mounted aorta, using a thin-layer chromatogram densitometer. Markedly stained areas regularly present in the aortic arch were used as a 100 per cent injury reference standard and a segment of an unstained aorta as nought per cent reference standard.

Results

In preliminary explorations for factors influencing endothelial integrity, the degree of injury was inversely related to thymus weight in unmanipulated rats (Fig. 1). This suggests that corticosteroids might promote arterial endothelial injury.

This hypothesis was tested in a second experiment. Specific pathogen-free male rats, weighing ca. 280 grams, were reared in a low-stress environment. Four groups were adrenalectomized and a fifth group was sham-operated. The sham-operated

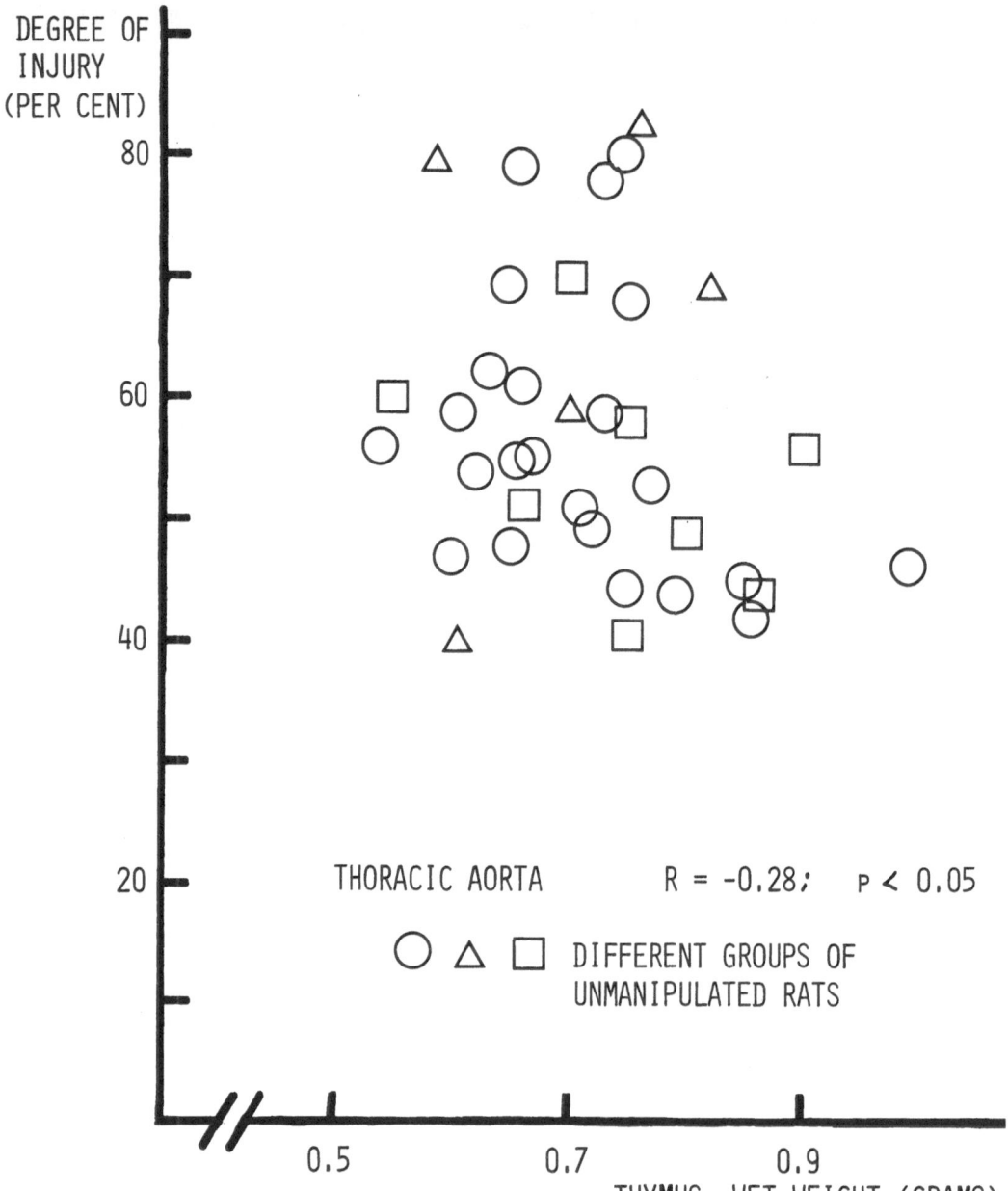

Figure 1

group and one of the adrenalectomized groups did not receive any treatment. The other adrenalectomized groups received aldosterone – 45 µg per day; dexamethasone – 15 µg per day; and corticosterone – 6 mg per day, respectively. The doses of dexamethasone and corticosterone were decreased to 2.5 µg and 1 mg, respectively, after 8 days, as there was a tendency for retardation of growth. After the adjustment the growth curves of all groups were parallel. All animals had water and saline to drink. The animals were killed and subjected to the procedure described above 15 days after the adrenalectomy or sham-operation.

Effect of Adrenalectomy (ADE) and Therapy with Different Adrenocortical Hormones on the Degree of Endothelial Injury in the Descending Thoracic Aorta in Rats

Exptl Group	Degree of Injury %			
ADE	40	56	M̄ 51.7	
	74	37	S.E.M. 4.2	
	74			
ADE PLUS				
ALDOSTERONE	39	46		M̄ 47.2
	48	54		S.E.M. 2.4
	49			
			P < 0.01	P < 0.01
CORTICOSTERONE	55	67		
	54	58		
	50			
DEXAMETHASONE	85	49		
	55	68		M̄ 62.5
	84			S.E.M. 4.2
SHAM-OP	49	67	M̄ 59.7	
	51	44	S.E.M. 3.4	

Figure 2

The degree of injury was significantly higher in the dexamethasone- and corticosterone-treated than in the aldosterone-treated animals both in the thoracic (Fig. 2, right column) and distal abdominal aorta (Fig. 3, right column). The degree of injury was higher for the groups having endogeneous, *i.e.* sham-operated, or exogeneous glucocorticoids (Fig. 2 and 3, middle columns). Similar differences were found for the proximal abdominal aorta (not shown). This study did not include dose-response experiments and, strictly, the results may only be valid at the dose levels specified.

Effect of Adrenalectomy (ADE) and Therapy with Different Adrenocortical Hormones on the Degree of Endothelial Injury in the Distal Abdominal Aorta in Rats

Exptl Group	Degree of Injury %			
ADE	43 76 65	49 56	$\bar{M}$ 49.2 S.E.M. 4.2	
ADE plus ALDOSTERONE	33 43 48	42 37		$\bar{M}$ 40.6 S.E.M. 2.6
			P < 0.01	P < 0.01
CORTICOSTERONE	55 43 30	69 52		
DEXAMETHASONE	81 47 81	47 66		$\bar{M}$ 57.1 S.E.M. 5.3
SHAM-OP	39 41	77 36	$\bar{M}$ 54.6 S.E.M. 4.6	

Figure 3

Discussion

Increased numbers of injured or dead endothelial cells were found in a large proportion of the aortic surface even in the unmanipulated rat. The location of
injured areas corresponded to sites where increased hemodynamic strain can be
expected. That these regions probably have an increased turnover of endothelial
cells is indicated by a similar distribution of increased endothelial cell replication rate as shown by Wright (1968).

The very large area of the aorta which had increased number of injured cells would
suggest that what we observe is a reflection of the normal turnover of endothelial
cells and a marginal increase of dead or injured cells by the action of glucocorticoids. It does not seem probable that this effect would be atherogenic *per se*.

However, it could be atherogenic in combination with factors restricting endothelial growth, increasing endothelial injury, or if combined with hyperlipidemia.

A study of the mechanism for the hormone effect was beyond the scope of the present work. However, it is reasonable to propose that the mechanism could either be indirect due to increased hemodynamic strain from corticoid-induced hypertension or, direct, by influence on the growth properties of the endothelium, as is the case for thymus tissue.

Whatever the mechanism may be, if applicable to man, the endothelial injury-promoting effect of glucocorticoids may be an important factor for the formation of human arterial disease, a suggestion which is justified because cases with untreated Cushing's syndrome develop severe atherosclerosis early (Katz and Stamler, 1953; P. Bastenie, personal communication, 1973). Cushing's syndrome is an extreme situation. However, it is possible that the same mechanism(s), but on a less dramatic level, underlies the relationship between ischemic heart disease and psychosocial stress. Furthermore, the results of this study suggest that this relationship, at least partically, could be mediated by hormonal influence on the arterial endothelium.

VII
Platelets-Thrombogenesis-Fibrinogen-Fibrinolysis

THROMBOSIS AND ATHEROSCLEROSIS

J.F. Mustard, M.A. Packham, S. Moore, and R.L. Kinlough-Rathbone

Thrombosis is one of the principal responses of the blood to injury. The injury
stimulus can be damaged endothelium, exposed components of the vessel wall, or
intravascular agents such as antigen-antibody complexes, bacteria or viruses.
Because vessel injury is thought to be involved in the development of atherosclerosis and its complications, there is ample reason to believe that thrombosis
also plays a part in this process. There are several aspects of this problem to
be considered:

1. The response of the blood to vessel injury.
2. The relation among early vessel wall injury, thrombosis, and the early lesions
   of atherosclerosis.
3. The relation among repeated vessel injury, mural thrombi, and the development
   of atherosclerotic lesions.
4. The relation among thrombosis, atherosclerosis, and the clinical complications
   of atherosclerosis.
5. The influence of diet, smoking, and oestrogens on platelets and thrombosis.

Before considering these problems in detail it is useful to review what is now
known about the interaction of blood constituents with the vessel wall when the
endothelium is damaged.

Response of Blood to Vessel Injury

When the endothelium is lost, subendothelial structures such as collagen, base-
ment membrane, elastin, and the microfibrils associated with elastin are exposed.
Collagen activates factor XII which initiates the blood coagulation sequence.
Activated factor XII also causes the conversion of plasminogen to plasmin and the
formation of plasma kinins (Webster and Ratnoff, 1961; Niewiarowski et al., 1966;
Ogsten et al., 1969; Harpel, 1972; Kaplan et al., 1972).

Injured endothelial cells may also affect blood coagulation. When endothelial
cells are stimulated they release an activator of plasminogen (Nilsson and Pandolfi, 1970). Recently Nemerson and Pitlick (1972) have observed that there is a
considerable amount of tissue thromboplastin associated with the surface of the
endothelial cells; this may be involved in initiating coagulation when the endothelial cells are injured. Ashford and Freiman (1968) found that mild injury of
the vessel wall did not cause loss of endothelium, but in the presence of inhibitors of fibrinolysis fibrin formed in association with the damaged endothelium.
Platelets were found adherent to the fibrin and endothelium at such sites. Since
platelets readily adhere to polymerizing fibrin (Niewiarowski et al., 1972) this
may provide a means for the initiation of thrombi at a site of endothelial injury.

As well as affecting plasma proteins, constituents of the vessel wall can also
interact with platelets. Platelets adhere to collagen, basement membrane and the
microfibrils around elastin (Hugues, 1962; Hovig, 1963; Tranzer and Baumgartner,
1967; Stemerman et al., 1971; Baumgartner, 1973). When platelets adhere to collagen they are stimulated to release their granule constituents (Hovig, 1963).
These include adenosine diphosphate (ADP) which causes platelets flowing past the
injury site to change shape and stick to each other and to the platelets which
have adhered to the vessel wall. This results in the formation of a mass of

aggregated platelets at the injury site. There is no evidence available concerning the question of whether the microfibrils and basement membrane stimulate platelets to release their constituents.

The growth of a thrombus is related to the effects of blood flow, the local concentration of ADP in the plasma, and the generation of thrombin. The generation of thrombin and the resulting fibrin formation around the platelet aggregate is thought to be important in the growth and stabilization of the thrombus. Platelet aggregates facilitate the generation of thrombin primarily by providing platelet phospholipoprotein for the acceleration of the coagulation sequence (Papahadjopoulus and Hanahan, 1964; Hemker and Kahn, 1967; Joist et al., 1972). In addition, many clotting factors are absorbed on the surface of the platelets (Nachman, 1968) and there is some evidence that the natural anticoagulants in the blood have much less effect on the clotting factors that are associated with the platelet surface (Walsh and Biggs, 1972). The thrombin that is generated on the surface of the platelets can cause the platelets to release their granule constituents including ADP; this ADP causes platelets flowing past to adhere to the platelet mass at the injury site.

An important effect of thrombin is stabilization of the platelet mass by causing fibrin polymerization (Hirsh et al., 1968). Platelet aggregates induced by ADP deaggregate within minutes in a stirred system and most of the experimental evidence indicates that in vivo ADP-induced aggregates break up rapidly unless they are stabilized by the formation of fibrin around them (Mustard et al., 1966). Because platelet aggregates promote the coagulation reaction, polymerizing fibrin forms in close proximity to the surface of the platelets, particularly those platelets at the perimeter of the initial aggregate. The polymerizing fibrin readily adheres to platelets (Niewiarowski et al., 1972) and prevents the break-up of the aggregate. The platelet mass generates factors which are chemotactic for polymorphonuclear leucocytes (Weksler and Coupal, 1973; Kay et al., 1973) and white blood cells accumulate around and in the thrombus. The amount of material deposited in a thrombus will be greatest in areas of disturbed blood flow. The forces that govern this are well described by Goldsmith (1972). In areas of stagnant or disturbed flow, extensive fibrin formation may occur and red cells will be trapped.

Materials released from the platelets affect not only the formation of the thrombus but also affect the vessel wall. Table 1 lists a number of agents which stimulate platelets to release their granule constituents and also lists the materials which are released or formed when platelets are exposed to these agents. Among the released materials are ATP, ADP, serotonin, adrenaline, lysosomal enzymes, cationic proteins, and mucopolysaccharides (Holmsen et al., 1969; Mustard and Packham, 1970). Platelets also release factors which can increase vessel permeability (Packham et al., 1967) and alter elastic tissue (Robert et al., 1971) and collagen (Chesney et al., 1974). In addition, when platelets are stimulated by release-inducing stimuli, they form the prostaglandins PGE_2 and $PGF_{2\alpha}$ (Smith and Willis, 1971; Kocsis et al., 1973). These prostaglandins are lost into the fluid surrounding the platelets and PGE_2 has been shown to increase vascular permeability (Crunkhorn and Willis, 1971). Some of these materials that are released or formed by the platelets when they are stimulated may be responsible for producing the vessel wall changes and vasculitis that can develop in association with platelet aggregates (Jørgensen et al., 1970).

In vivo observations indicate that a thrombus is not a static structure. Studies of the microcirculation have demonstrated quite conclusively that although a platelet-rich thrombus forms rapidly at a site of vessel injury, the mass is unstable, tends to break down, and then reforms (Fulton et al., 1953; Honour and Ross-Russell, 1962). Baumgartner (1973) has shown in the rabbit aorta that removal of the endothelium with a balloon catheter leads immediately to the formation of masses of platelets on the denuded surface. If the vessel is examined 40 minutes or more after the injury, the amount of thrombus material found on the surface is

Table 1a. Agents that cause release of platelet granule contents

---

Collagen

Thrombin, plasmin, trypsin, papain, pronase, subtilisin, elastase

Antiplatelet antibodies

Antigen-antibody complexes

Aggregated gamma globulin

Gamma globulin-coated surfaces and particles

Foreign particles

Some viruses

Some bacteria

Endotoxin and **staphylococcal toxins**

Some snake venoms

Adrenaline and noradrenaline

Long chain fatty acids, particularly saturated fatty acids

Arachidonic acid

Ristocetin

ADP (in citrated platelet-rich plasma of some species)

Vasopressin

---

much less. Only a thin coating of platelets remains. Presumably the effect of ADP on the platelets gradually diminishes and the flowing blood shears emboli off the mass of platelets leaving only those which are closely adherent to the vessel wall. In contrast, in a region of disturbed blood flow where ADP is diluted less rapidly and thrombin forms, the tendency for a platelet mass to grow and persist is much greater. One of the important points that was emphasized by Baumgartner (1973) was that although there may be a considerable mass of platelets at an injury site, examination of the site at a later time may reveal little evidence of the initial thrombus material. Therefore, it is not surprising that areas of vessel injury can be found that do not appear to have platelet material or fibrin associated with them (Jørgensen et al., 1972; Gutstein et al., 1973; Björkerud and Bondjers, 1973).

The importance of the dynamics of thrombus formation is illustrated by the recent work of Cade et al. (1972). Emboli labelled with ^{125}I-fibrinogen were injected into the pulmonary circulation of dogs. In untreated animals the emboli decreased in weight and lost radioactive fibrin, but they took up radioactive fibrinogen from the plasma. If heparin were given to the animals, the rate of dissolution of the emboli was increased because the fibrinogen from the plasma was not converted to fibrin that normally would have become associated with the emboli. When the fibrinolytic mechanism was activated, the loss of radioactivity from the emboli was increased but the uptake of labelled fibrin formed from fibrinogen in the plasma was not blocked. A combination of heparin and a fibrinolytic agent caused a marked reduction in the size of the emboli because the production of labelled fibrin around the emboli was inhibited and the loss of radioactive material from them was enhanced. These observations demonstrate that even in a fibrin-rich mass, fibrin is being constantly lysed and fresh fibrin is being formed. This concept is relevant to the consideration of the relation between thrombosis and the clinical complications of atherosclerosis. In studies with ^{125}I-fibrinogen, the amount of radioactivity in a thrombus may be more dependent on its rates of formation

Table 1b. Materials released, made available, or lost when platelets undergo the release reaction

---

Adenine nucleotides (ATP and ADP)

Serotonin

Calcium or magnesium (depending on species)

Histamine

Adrenaline

Mucopolysaccharides

Fibrinogen

Platelet factor 4 (antiheparin factor)

Potassium

Free amino acids, small amounts of protein and lipoprotein

Lysosomal enzymes –

>acid phosphatase
>B-galactosidase
>a-mannosidase
>ß-glucuronidase
>ß-N-acetyl glucosaminidase
>cathepsin
>aryl sulphatase
>phospholipase A_1

Elastase, collagenase

Platelet factor 3 (a phospholipoprotein that becomes available on the membrane)

Prostaglandins E_2 and F_{2a} (formed and lost into the surrounding medium)

Factor that increases vessel permeability (cationic protein?)

Factor that is chemotactic for leukocytes

Factor that stimulates proliferation of smooth muscle cells

---

and dissolution than on its age. Thus studies of arterial thrombosis with ^{125}I-fibrinogen should be interpreted carefully and should not be interpreted as in some studies (Erhardt et al., 1973) as establishing the age of thrombi.

Vessel Injury, Thrombosis, and Early Vessel Wall Changes

In 1957, McGill and Geer observed focal areas of Evans blue accumulation in the aorta of dogs injected with Evans blue. The dye accumulated at sites of lesions caused by parasites. Magnani and Coccheri (1960) reported that in the aorta of pigs there were areas of focal protein accumulation as determined by the use of Trypan blue. Evans blue labelling of plasma proteins has been extensively used for studying increased permeability of vessels in the microcirculation (Burke et al., 1964). We have used this method to study the pattern of accumulation of labelled proteins in the intima of pigs and rabbits (Packham et al., 1967; Jørgensen et al., 1972). Evans blue bound to plasma albumin accumulated at the same sites as ^{131}I-labelled albumin. Histologic examination of the blue areas demonstrated that the endothelium was lost or damaged and frequently the intima was edematous. In association with these injury sites, white blood cells, platelets, and small thrombi (some of which contained fibrin) were found. In studies of equivalent sites in the vessels of young humans who had died suddenly, similar patterns of endothelial change, white cell accumulation and small mural thrombi were also found (Jørgensen et al., 1972). This evidence is in keeping with the concept that early vessel wall changes occur at sites of vessel injury. Recently Gutstein et al., (1973) have confirmed these observations in pigs. In areas of highly disturbed flow patterns, particularly around the ilio-aortic junctions, they found marked ultra-structural degenerative changes of the endothelium and at some sites a total loss of endothelial cells. In an extension of the earlier work, Somer and Schwartz (1971, 1972) have provided further evidence of the accumulation of labelled protein and cholesterol at these sites in pigs. They have shown that there is a gradient of labelled cholesterol extending from the intima to the adventia with the greatest amount of radioactivity in the intima.

Because these are areas of injury, increased endothelial turnover might be expected at them. A number of investigators have reported increased incorporation of tritiated thymidine into the endothelial cells at sites where injury may occur (Thomas et al., 1968; Wright, 1968; Stary and McMillan, 1970; Caplan and Schwartz, 1973).

Mechanisms that might account for focal injury in the aorta may be related to the effects of blood flow. One possibility that has been considered is the effect of blood flow on the constituents of the blood (Mustard et al., 1972). Fry (1968) has presented evidence that in areas of high shear the mechanical effects of flow are sufficient to cause endothelial injury. However, some investigators consider that the early changes in the vessel wall actually occur in areas of low shear (Caro et al., 1971). Vibrational phenomena also have been suggested as a possible source of vessel and endothelial damage (Stippes et al., 1961; Fry, 1969). In addition, the pulsatile nature of blood flow must be considered. As well as affecting the vessel wall, disturbed blood flow may facilitate the interaction of the formed elements and promote the generation of active clotting factors (Goldsmith, 1972). In areas where there is either separation of flow or vortex formation, the prolonged time that the platelets and plasma components remain within the vortex facilitates the formation of platelet aggregates. Within the vortex agents which promote platelet aggregation and blood coagulation can accumulate. There is considerable evidence that the formed elements can induce and contribute to vessel injury (Hughes and Tonks, 1962; Moore and Lough, 1970; Lough and Moore, 1972; Jørgensen et al., 1972). Intravascular platelet aggregates have been observed in association with vasculitis (Jørgensen et al., 1970). In serum sickness it has been found that the immune complexes that form in the circulation cause focal injury at the same sites in the aorta of the rabbit as those where the early changes of atherosclerosis occur. Platelets are involved in this reaction (Kniker and Cochrane, 1968). Presumably the antigen-antibody complexes cause platelet aggregation and the release of platelet constituents. Margaretten and McKay (1971) found that platelets were important in inducing the vascular lesion in the direct active Arthus reaction. Graham and Griffin (1972) also concluded that platelets played a key role in the development of this reaction in the synovial membranes of rabbits. Howse et al. (1973) found that platelets contributed to the endotoxin-induced increase in vascular permeability of the ocular vessels of the rabbit. Recently, Tsal et al. (1973) reported that in the Forssman reaction the vessel wall changes are at least partly caused by material released from the platelets.

It scarcely needs to be emphasized that in areas where the endothelium is altered and the permeability of the wall is increased, plasma constituents will accumulate in the vessel wall. If there is an increased amount of low density lipoprotein in the plasma, its accumulation at such sites will be enhanced.

Endothelial Injury and Intimal Changes. The relation between vessel injury and intimal changes deserves attention. Among the more significant observations in the last few years is that when the endothelium is removed from the surface of an artery, the smooth muscle cells in the media migrate into the intima and proliferate in it (Stemerman and Ross, 1972; Björkerud and Bondjers, 1973). Ross and

Glomset (1973) have recently reviewed the factors that appear to be involved in inducing the smooth muscle cell proliferation. These include loss of the endothelium, possibly hormones such as insulin, possibly plasma proteins and peptides, and high blood pressure. Their work indicates that low density lipoproteins enhance smooth muscle cell proliferation whereas this is not the case with the high density lipoproteins. Recently Ross et al. (1974) have observed that the constituent in serum required for the growth of the smooth muscle cells appears to be derived from platelets. This may indicate that platelet constituents released at sites of vessel injury may be involved in initiating or enhancing smooth muscle cell proliferation.

Another result of endothelial injury and intimal repair is a change in the nature of the vessel wall subendothelial constituents; they appear to provide a greater stimulus for thrombus formation than the constituents of the normal wall. Stemerman (1973) has shown that when an area of a rabbit aorta that had healed after injury with a balloon catheter was re-injured, the amount of thrombus material that accumulated was far greater than that which accumulated after a single injury.

Repeated Vessel Injury and Atherosclerosis. Vessel injury, thrombosis, and atherosclerosis occur at sites of altered vessel configuration and disturbed blood flow. These are presumably sites of repeated injury. Since sites that are subjected to repeated injury may have different properties than those exposed to a single injury, it is of some importance to consider what happens to the intima of vessels when they are repeatedly injured. Experiments carried out by Moore (1973) illustrate that repeated injury can lead to the development of atherosclerotic lesions. In studies designed to investigate the effects of thrombi in the aorta on embolization of the renal circulation of rabbits, it was observed that catheters left in the aorta caused quite extensive atherosclerotic lesions. After the catheters had been in place for several weeks, lesions similar to typical fatty streaks were produced as well as small linear edematous streaks with little lipid. In areas without thrombus where endothelium had covered the lesions, fibrous plaques rich in smooth muscle cells were found. These lesions usually contained no stainable lipid. Another type of lesion was characterized by intimal thickening and intra- and extra-cellular lipid. Cholesterol clefts and foam cells were frequently found in these lesions. This type of lesion usually had thrombi on the surface in association with areas where the endothelium was damaged or lost. The observations in these studies indicate that repeated injury can produce the full spectrum of atherosclerotic lesions in rabbits receiving a normal diet.

Loss of endothelium not only leads to stimulation of the smooth muscle cells and the influx of plasma constituents into the subendothelial area, but also has a significant effect on the lipid changes in the vessel wall. Björkerud and Bondjers (1973) found that in the rabbit aorta, after the induction of a large superficial transverse injury, in the areas where re-endothelialization was slow or non-existent the intima was thickened and lipid accumulated as fine particles in the tissue. They concluded that loss of endothelium was a basic cause of the development of hyper-elastic, lipid-containing lesions. They also suggested that the delayed re-endothelialization might be caused by the recurrent formation of mural thrombi because the platelet constituents released at such sites might impair endothelial regeneration.

Vessel wall injury in the presence of hyperlipidemia leads to more extensive lesions with a greater content of stainable lipid (Prior and Hartmann, 1956; Friedman et al., 1962; Prathap, 1973b). Recently Stemerman and Ross (1972) and Nam et al. (1973) have reported that balloon injury to the endothelium in pigs, monkeys, and other animals on a high fat diet leads to extensive proliferative lesions.

The relation among all these observations and the recent report by Bendilt and Bendilt (1973) of a monoclonal origin of human atherosclerotic plaques is not clear. If the smooth muscle cells and the connective tissue in the plaques proliferated in response to injury, or the plaques were formed by the organization of mural thrombi, one would not expect them to be monoclonal. Since, however, the smooth muscle cells in each plaque were monoclonal, the results indicate that the atherosclerotic plaque in humans may arise by some other mechanism than the response to injury with which we are familiar. The monoclonal nature of the lesions reported by Benditt and Benditt (1973) could mean that a chemical or virus-induced mutation of the cells may have occurred.

Thrombus Organization and Atherosclerosis

The other mechanism through which thrombi may be involved in the development of atherosclerotic lesions is by the persistence of mural thrombi and their incorporation into the vessel wall (Duguid, 1948; Morgan, 1956; More and Haust, 1961; French, 1966; Chandler, 1970). There is ample evidence that mural thrombi become organized and give rise to intimal thickenings rich in connective tissue. Studies of the organization of mural thrombi in the systemic arteries of swine showed that over a one month period a healed lesion became an intimal thickening rich in smooth muscle cells with little lipid (Jørgensen et al., 1967; Woolf et al., 1968). Recently Prathap (1973a) has shown that two years after healing, thrombi that had been incorporated into the aortic wall of monkeys had produced an avascular smooth muscle cell-rich intimal thickening. This evidence indicates that arterial mural thrombi formed in response to vessel injury give rise to the "hard" type of atherosclerotic plaques described by Branwood and Montgomery (1956) and Bouch and Montgomery (1970).

There have been a number of experimental studies in animals which can be interpreted as indicating that organization of certain types of thrombus material gives rise to lipid-rich lesions. The injection of blood clots or platelet-rich emboli into the pulmonary circulation of rabbits produces intimal thickening. A number of investigators (Harrison, 1948; Wartman et al., 1951; Heard, 1952; Barnard, 1954; Thomas et al., 1956) found that when fibrin-rich emboli were injected into the pulmonary circulation of rabbits, the resulting lesions were fibrous thickenings of the intima, relatively free of lipid. Heptinstall (1957) injected blood clots prepared from hypercholesterolaemic rabbits and obtained similar findings. In contrast, Hand and Chandler (1962) observed that if platelet-rich emboli were injected into the pulmonary circulation of rabbits, the resulting lesions were fibrous intimal plaques rich in foam cells. They concluded that at least part of the lipid was derived from the platelets phagocytosed by the mononuclear cells. Still (1966), in an electron-microscopic study, provided further evidence that the lipid in the lesions was derived in this way. In subsequent studies, Ardlie and Schwartz (1968) confirmed the earlier observations that emboli rich in fibrin produced fibrous intimal thickenings whereas emboli rich in platelets produced fibrous lesions containing lipid and foam cells.

Craig et al. (1973) studied the fate of emboli composed of a mixture of platelets and fibrin formed in a Chandler loop (Chandler, 1958). When these emboli were injected into the pulmonary circulation of pigs, intimal thickenings formed which were essentially fibrous with only small amounts of lipid in them. The phospholipid, fatty acid and cholesterol of the organizing lesions differed from those in fatty streaks and fibrous plaques in older pigs. Craig et al. (1973) concluded that the lipids of the atherosclerotic plaques are largely derived from a source other than organizing thrombi. It should be pointed out that all these studies involved the pulmonary circulation and the situation may be quite different in the systemic circulation. There also may be species differences in the response to the material injected into the pulmonary circulation.

Friedman and Byers (1961) inserted a magnesium-alloy coil, or a piece of polyethylene tubing into the abdominal aorta of rabbits. The resulting thrombi became organized into dense fibrous intimal plaques containing little lipid. When the rabbits were fed a high fat diet, there was an increase in the amount of lipid associated with the organizing thrombi. Scott and Hurley (1969) have shown that plasma lipoproteins are incorporated into organizing thrombi in man. However, it is difficult to be certain that the lipid has not accumulated as a consequence of the mechanisms discussed in the previous section. That is, if the endothelium is subjected to repeated injury, this might be the cause of the increased amount of lipid rather than the organization of the thrombus itself.

The importance of thrombus organization in the development of atherosclerotic lesions is not known. The majority of thrombi that occur in damaged arteries are considered to be mural thrombi rather than occlusive thrombi. Since older subjects tend to have advanced atherosclerotic lesions on which mural thrombi form, it seems likely that mural thrombosis contributes to the growth of atherosclerotic lesions in human beings (Jørgensen, 1971).

Thrombosis and Clinical Complications of Atherosclerosis

The role of thrombosis in the clinical complications of atherosclerosis appears to be more complex than the simple concept of an occlusive thrombus on an advanced atherosclerotic plaque in a major artery. In the arterial circulation, blood flow has a major effect on the site and extent of the thrombi that form (Mustard et al., 1972). It is doubtful that occlusive thrombi could form in the major human arteries unless disturbed blood flow such as occurs around a stenotic atherosclerotic plaque is present. It seems likely that mural thrombi are far more common in the arterial circulation than occlusive thrombi. Mural thrombi may be more important in the clinical complications of atherosclerosis than occlusive thrombi.

As emphasized earlier, there is a balance between the factors promoting the growth of a thrombus and those causing its dissolution. ADP-induced platelet aggregates are unstable and unless an extensive amount of fibrin forms to bind the platelets together, the bulk of the thrombus will be disrupted. Even when fibrin is forming, it is also being broken down. A number of studies, particularly in the microcirculation, have indicated that as a thrombus forms at an injury site, portions of it are disrupted and broken off by the effects of blood flow (Fulton et al., 1953; Berman, 1961; Honour and Ross-Russell, 1962; Born et al., 1964). The fragments of the thrombus that are sheared off pass into the distal parts of the circulation as microemboli. An important question, therefore, is what effect do these microemboli have on the function of an organ?

Although thrombotic occlusion of the major extracranial arteries causes strokes, there is a considerable body of evidence indicating that mural thrombi at the bifurcation of the internal carotid artery do fragment and shower the cerebral circulation with microemboli (Fisher, 1959; Russell, 1961; Gunning et al., 1964; Torvik and Jørgensen, 1966; Jørgensen, 1969). These emboli can cause transient attacks of weakness and sensory changes as well as transient monocular blindness. In the latter case, the microemboli have been observed passing through the retinal circulation.

The importance of this mechanism in causing clinical complications of carotid artery disease has been illustrated by the effects of drugs that inhibit platelet function. There are several recent reviews concerning these drugs (Mustard et al., 1972; Mills, 1972; Weiss, 1972; Packham and Mustard, 1974). At the present time it appears that the most important in terms of clinical use are those which inhibit the platelet release reaction. Aspirin, phenylbutazone, sulfinpyrazone and related drugs do not inhibit primary ADP-induced aggregation at concentrations that are achieved in the circulation, but they do inhibit the release reaction induced by collagen. This is the vessel wall constituent that seems most likely to be the one that is principally involved in the initiation of thrombi when the endothelial lining is lost. These drugs inhibit platelet adherence to surfaces such as fibrinogen-coated glass, or collagen (Jenkins et al., 1973; Cazenave et al., 1974). Aspirin also inhibits platelet adherence to the damaged surface of the rabbit aorta (Cazenave et al., 1973). Dipyridamole is another drug which has been under considerable study. Its effect on the platelet release reaction appears to be less than that of the non-steroidal anti-inflammatory drugs, but it does have some effect on the primary phase of ADP-induced aggregation (Emmons et al., 1965a; Eliasson and Bygdeman, 1969; Zucker and Peterson, 1970; Cucuianu et al., 1971). It is not as strong an inhibitor of the adherence of platelets to surfaces as the other drugs. There is evidence from experiments with animals that some of the pyrimido-pyrimidine compounds inhibit thrombus formation in response to vessel injury (Emmons et al., 1965a; Arfors et al., 1968; Didisheim and Owen, 1970; Horch et al., 1970), although there have also been negative results (Philp and Lemieux, 1968).

Several studies have been reported in which the non-steroidal anti-inflammatory drugs were administered to individuals with carotid artery disease characterized by transient attacks of cerebral ischemia. The results support the hypothesis that modifying platelet function affects the clinical manifestations of this type of thromboembolic disorder in arteries. Evans (1973) found that the administration of sulfinpyrazone to patients with transient attacks of cerebral ischemia produced a significant reduction in the frequency of the attacks. In addition, there are two reports of case studies indicating that aspirin diminished the frequency of attacks (in one of these dipyridamole was found to be ineffective) (Harrison et al., 1971; Mundall et al., 1972).

In a study of the effect of sulfinpyrazone with older patients in a hospital, Blakely and Gent (1974) found that sulfinpyrazone administration to individuals admitted with a diagnosis of vascular disease complications, caused a significant reduction in the number of deaths in comparison with the control group given a placebo over a period of five years. When they examined the fate of individuals who had a history of stroke before entering the trial, they found that sulfinpyrazone caused a significant reduction in the number of deaths from vascular causes in this group when compared with the group given the placebo. In a similar study with aspirin, Heikinheimo and Järvinen (1971) could not demonstrate that the drug had any effect.

If mural thrombi in damaged vessels can fragment and embolize in the carotid circulation, it seems quite likely that this may also occur in other parts of the arterial circulation. Evidence in relation to other sites is less conclusive. However, Moore (1964) observed that there was a relation in humans among mural thrombi, atherosclerotic lesions, and the incidence of nephrosclerosis. It was suggested that one cause of chronic renal disease and possibly of high blood pressure was the development of atherosclerosis in the aorta, the formation of mural thrombi on the lesions above the renal arteries, and the fragmentation of these thrombi into microemboli which impacted in the microcirculation of the kidney. In a number of experiments in rabbits, dogs and monkeys in which thrombi were produced above the renal vessels, Moore and Mersereau (1968) and Moore (1969) showed that these thrombi fragmented and showered the kidneys with microemboli. The result was intimal hyperplasia in the renal vessels, elevated blood pressure and nephrosclerosis. It was also shown that the embolization caused changes in plasma renin activity (Moore and Gent, 1972). It is difficult to determine how important this is in adult humans. The postmortem studies indicate that it might be of some significance in patients with atherosclerotic lesions (Moore, 1964).

When one turns to the coronary artery circulation there is very little evidence about the occurrence of such a mechanism. Detailed pathologic studies indicate that individuals who die suddenly with myocardial ischemia rarely have occlusive thrombi in their coronary arteries (Spain and Bradess, 1960; Baroldi, 1965; Roberts and Buja, 1972). Individuals who die later, after the onset of symptoms, who have full thickness infarcts, almost always have thrombi in the coronary artery supplying the area (Sinapius, 1965; Mitchell and Schwartz, 1965; Harland and Holburn, 1966; Jørgensen et al., 1968). It is important to point out that the infarct is almost always distal to the site of the thrombus. This seems to indicate that the thrombus plays a part in causing the infarction rather than occurring as a result of it. This evidence could be interpreted as indicating that there are at least two mechanisms causing death in association with coronary artery disease:

1. A mechanism or mechanisms causing sudden death which is unrelated to occlusive thrombosis.
2. A mechanism dependent upon the formation of occlusive thrombi which leads to infarction and usually does not cause sudden death.

However, if mural thrombi formed on an atherosclerotic lesion in a coronary artery fragmented and showered the microcirculation, this could cause sudden death although postmortem evidence for this mechanism might be difficult to establish. This would be particularly true if a large part of the mural thrombus were disrupted and only traces of thrombus material were left on the coronary artery wall.

Results of some animal experiments support this concept. ADP-induced platelet aggregates in the myocardial circulation were found to cause arrhythmia, myocardial infarction, and sudden death (Jørgensen et al., 1967). The cause appeared to be the transient platelet aggregates in the microcirculation distal to the coronary artery that had been infused with ADP. Moschos et al. (1973) have recently demonstrated that the induction of thrombi in a coronary artery of dogs leads to embolization of the distal circulation. Haft et al. (1973) have reported that the myocardial disorder caused by the infusion of noradrenaline may be due to the formation of intravascular platelet aggregates in the microcirculation of the myocardium. Haft and Fani (1973) have shown that similar effects are produced in rats subjected to stress. This may be important because catecholamines not only cause platelet aggregation but also potentiate the effects of other agents that cause platelet aggreation and the platelet release reaction (Ardlie et al., 1966; Mills and Roberts, 1967; Thomas, 1968). Thus stress, with an outpouring of catecholamines, might facilitate the formation of intravascular platelet aggregates and lead to microcirculatory disturbances.

Haerem (1972) has tried to obtain evidence in humans that such a mechanism might operate. He carried out detailed postmortem studies of individuals who had died suddenly from acute myocardial ischemia and of individuals who had died suddenly from other causes such as accidents. The incidence of platelet aggregates in the small vessels of the myocardium was greater in those who had died from what was believed to be myocardial ischemia. The evidence was inconclusive, however, because the differences were small. Several reasons for this can be advanced, but one important fact to be considered is that platelet aggregates break up rapidly after death. In swine in which ADP-induced platelet aggregates caused myocardial changes, if the postmortem were done ten minutes or longer after the death of the animal it was very difficult to find platelet aggregates. They were only found in large numbers if the postmortem were done immediately. Since there is a long time interval between death and postmortem studies in humans, platelet aggregates would have time to break up following death and it would be difficult to establish by morphologic criteria that this mechanism was operating. However, if it does operate, careful examination of the main coronary arteries of people who die suddenly should show evidence of vessel wall changes and traces of platelet material on the area of vessel injury. Such studies might require the application of techniques involving labelled platelet antibodies.

Although there has been no detailed study or clinical trial of the effect of the drugs that inhibit platelet function on deaths or complications in individuals with coronary artery disease, there is some evidence from studies with other drugs that relates to the question of the operative mechanism. Clofibrate has recently had two extensive trials in individuals with a history of angina and/or myocardial infarction (Arthur et al., 1971; Oliver et al., 1971). The mortality and morbidity in the patients given clofibrate who had presented with angina was significantly reduced in contrast to the group given the placebo compound. The effect appeared to be independent of the initial serum cholesterol levels or of the extent to which the serum cholesterol level was lowered by the administration of clofibrate. In the discussion of these studies the possibility was raised that the beneficial effect of clofibrate might be related to its other actions. One of the other effects of clofibrate is prolongation of platelet survival in man (Gilbert and Mustard, 1963). Although it does not appear to be a strong inhibitor of the platelet functions that are usually tested in the laboratory, there is increasing evidence that effects of drugs on platelet survival may be a clearer indication of their possible value in the management of thromboembolic disorders (Harker and Slichter, 1972; Steele et al., 1973). In animal studies, Herrmann (1973) has shown that clofibrate inhibits the interaction of platelets with damaged vessel walls that must occur during the formation of a hemostatic plug. It is possible that the effect of clofibrate in the trials may be related to its influence on the platelet thromboembolic process rather than on serum lipids.

In contrast to the effects of sulfinpyrazone and clofibrate, dipyridamole has not been found effective in reducing morbidity or mortality in patients who have had myocardial infarcts or strokes (Gent et al., 1968; Acheson et al., 1969).

It should be pointed out that any trial of a drug in coronary artery disease would probably best be done in terms of primary prevention rather than secondary prevention. The mechanisms which cause death in people who have had a myocardial infarct may be considerably different from the mechanisms which lead to the initial manifestations of ischemia and/or infarction.

Influence of Diet, Smoking and Oestrogens on Platelets and Thrombosis

Dietary Fat. The evidence that dietary fat can influence thrombosis comes primarily from animal experiments. When blood from pigs that had been given a diet enriched with egg yolk was shunted through an extracorporeal circulation containing a bifurcation, the amount of deposit which formed in the extracorporeal shunt was significantly greater than that formed if the animals had been given a low fat diet (Mustard et al., 1963). There was no association between the serum cholesterol level produced by the high fat diet and the amount of thrombus formed in the extracorporeal shunt. Rabbits fed a diet enriched with coconut oil and cholesterol showed increased deposits in extracorporeal shunts (Mathues et al., 1968). Hornstra and Vendelmans-Starrenburg (1973) have recently reported that the addition of sunflower seed oil to the diet of rats diminishes the amount of thrombus which forms at the ends of a polyethylene cannula inserted into the aorta. Thomas and Hartroft (1959) found that rats given an artificial diet containing saturated fat formed thrombi in the chambers of the heart. Renaud et al. (1970) have shown that when rats are given a diet containing some of the ingredients of the diet used in the Thomas and Hartroft (1959) study and enriched with butter or stearic acid, the extent of endotoxin-induced thrombosis in the liver is greatly enhanced. In these studies, platelets taken from the rats given the butter-fat or stearic acid diet were more sensitive to thrombin-induced aggregation than those from the animals given the low fat diet or a diet enriched with corn oil or oleic acid. The increased sensitivity of the platelets to thrombin appeared to be due to changes in the platelets themselves, because suspensions of washed platelets prepared from these rats showed the same increased sensitivity to thrombin (Renaud et al., 1970). In subsequent studies, Renard and Lecompte (1970) have found an association between the changes in the platelet phospholipids and the increased sensitivity of the platelets to thrombin-induced aggregation. The increased susceptibility of the rats given the diets enriched with butter or stearic acid to endotoxin-induced thrombosis was prevented by sulfinpyrazone, aspirin, heparin, or steroids (Renard, 1973). These observations indicate that the effect of the diet on platelets is not the sole cause of the enhanced susceptibility to endotoxin because steroids and anticoagulants have little effect on platelet reactions.

Nordöy et al. (1968) found that when rabbits were given a diet rich in saturated fat, ADP-induced platelet aggregates in platelet-rich plasma in vitro were more extensive and persisted longer than if the animals had been given a low fat diet. The precise characteristics of the lipid or lipids responsible for these effects are not known.

Saturated fatty acid have been shown to activate factor XII (Connor, 1963; Margolis, 1962; Botti and Ratnoff, 1963), and to cause platelet aggregation (Shore and

Alpers, 1963; Connor et al., 1963; Haslam, 1964; Hoak et al., 1966). However, it would appear that they have little effect on thrombosis unless the level of free fatty acid exceeds the fatty acid binding capacity of the plasma albumin (Haslam, 1964; Hoak et al., 1966). The effects on platelets and blood coagulation are inhibited by the presence of albumin. Recently it has been shown that, arachidonic acid causes platelet aggregation (Ingerman et al., 1973). This has been attributed to the formation of a labile intermediate formed during the synthesis of prostaglandin E_2 (Willis, 1973).

Hampton and Mitchell (1966) found that platelets from individuals with a history of ischemic heart disease were more sensitive to ADP than platelets from normal subjects. Sensitivity to ADP was measured by determining changes in the electrophoretic mobility of the platelets. It was suggested (Bolton et al., 1967) that the increased sensitivity was caused by lysolecithin. However, Besterman and Gillett (1971) showed that lysolecithin inhibits collagen-induced platelet aggregation and the second wave of aggregation induced by ADP or adrenaline.

Observations in man indicating that diet influences platelets and thrombosis are more limited. McDonald and Edgill (1958) found that platelets from blood taken from subjects given low fat diets showed less adhesion to glass than platelets from blood taken from subjects eating their usual diet. Platelets from subjects eating high fat meals showed increased retention in glass bead columns (Horlick, 1961). Mustard and Murphy (1962) found that when patients in a metabolic unit were given a diet rich in dairy fats and egg yolk, platelet survival was shorter and platelet turnover was increased in comparision to a period when the patients were given a low fat diet or a diet enriched with corn oil.

Hornstra et al. (1973) have reported that subjects receiving a diet containing a high proportion of saturated fat show increased platelet accumulation on filters in an extracorporeal device when compared with patients given a diet rich in polyunsaturated fat. Turpeinen et al. (1968) and Miettinen et al. (1972) have reported that the incidence of ischemic heart disease in man is diminished if the amount of linoleic acid in the diet is increased and the amount of saturated fat is reduced.

Smoking

Most of the early studies of the effect of smoking on platelet function assessed by in vitro tests have not been conclusive (Murphy, 1968). Recently, Hawkins (1972) found that smoking causes an increased sensitivity of platelets to aggregating agents. Levine (1973) has also shown that smoking a single cigarette increases the response of the smoker's platelets to ADP. Nicotine has been reported to cause platelet aggregation in vitro and to potentiate the action of ADP (Werle and Schievelbein, 1965). McDonald and associates (1973) found that nicotine caused enhanced clot retraction in rat platelet-rich plasma and that this effect was due to the action of nicotine on a plasma factor that acts on the platelets. In a study of platelet survival under controlled conditions, Mustard and Murphy (1963) observed that when the individuals stopped smoking, platelet survival was prolonged and platelet turnover was reduced. It has been suggested that prolonged exposure to carbon monoxide accelerates the development of atheroma in rabbits because of intimal accretion of platelets and fibrin and intramural lipid accumulation (Birnstingl et al., 1971). Other studies indicate that changes occur in the arteries of primates after prolonged mild carbon monoxide exposure (Thomsen, 1973). Subendothelial edema and some endothelial changes were observed.

All of this evidence is compatible with an effect of smoking either on the platelets or on the vessel wall or possibly on both. The effects of smoking on platelet survival, platelet aggregation, and possibly on vessel walls may be relevant to the fact that subjects who give up smoking show a reduced incidence of clinical complications of vascular disease (Doyle et al., 1964). Prospective studies by these investigators showed that myocardial infarction occurs three times more commonly in heavy cigarette smokers compared with non-smokers, ex-cigarette smokers or cigar or pipe smokers.

Oestrogens. There is evidence from retrospective studies that the risk of thromboembolisms is increased in women taking oestrogen-containing oral contraceptives (Vessey and Doll, 1969; Inman et al., 1970). Men taking high doses of oestrogen for carcinoma of the prostate show an increased incidence of myocardial infarction (Veterans Administration Cooperative Urological Research Group, 1967). In the clinical trial of oestrogen for the management of patients with a high risk for the development of coronary artery disease, the trial was stopped because of the increased deaths in the group given oestrogens (Coronary Drug Project Research Group, 1970). There have been a large number of studies indicating that oestrogens influence clotting (Dugdale and Masi, 1971; Shanberge et al. 1972; Zuck and Bergin, 1973) or platelets (Hilden et al. 1967; Elkeles et al., 1968; Poller et al., 1969; Sanderson and Delamore, 1973; Zahavi et al., 1973), and it has been suggested that these effects are responsible for the increase in thromboembolic complications in subjects taking oestrogen. However, the data are not conclusive. Recently it has been suggested that this hormone may affect the vessel wall leading to intimal proliferation, alterations in blood flow, and thrombosis (Irey and Norris, 1973).

Gaynor (1973) has recently reported that testosterone treatment of rabbits decreased the number of subendothelial microfibrils of rabbit iliac arteries, whereas oestradiol increased the number of microfibrils. However, when the endothelium was removed with a balloon catheter, the vessels from the testosterone-treated animals were more thrombogenic.

The results from prospective studies do not indicate an adverse effect of oral contraceptives on thromboembolic disease in women (Drill, 1972). The normal incidence in these studies was derived from various segments of the population rather than by using a matched control group. Because of this the results from these analyses have been criticized (Hougie, 1973). However, the study by Fuertes-de la Haba et al., (1971) with a treated and a control group did not show an increased incidence of venous thromboembolic disorders among the women taking the contraceptive pill. The retrospective studies also suffer from potential sampling problems and the question of the significance of an association found in retrospective studies. They certainly do not prove cause and effect as claimed by Inman and Vessey (1968). The inconclusive relationship among platelets, blood coagulation tests, and thrombosis make it difficult to conclude that we have good evidence that oestrogens enhance the risk of developing thromboembolic disorders.

Platelet Survival Studies as a Method of Measuring Changes in Platelet Function

Although it is difficult to demonstrate that in vitro tests of platelet function are relevant for the detection of clinical thrombosis, there is some evidence that measurement of platelet survival and turnover may be of some value. Murphy and Mustard (1962) originally demonstrated that subjects who had a history of clinical manifestations of atherosclerosis had shorter platelet survival times (using $DF^{32}P$) than subjects with a negative family and clinical history for complications of atherosclerosis. Abrahamsen (1969) reported subsequently that some subjects with a history of arterial thrombosis showed a shorter platelet survival than normal subjects, as measured by ^{51}chromium-labelling of platelets. Recently, Harker and Slichter (1970) and Weily et al. (1972) have found that some subjects with prosthetic heart valves show a shortened platelet survival in comparison to controls. The subjects with a shortened platelet survival appear to have an increased incidence of thromboembolic manifestations. Genton et al. (1973) have found that subjects who show shortened platelet survival values before heart valve operations are those most at risk of developing thromboembolic disorders.

Smythe et al. (1965) found that sulfinpyrazone (a drug which inhibits collagen-induced platelet aggregation) prolongs platelet survival and reduces platelet turnover in man. Harker and Slichter (1972) and Steele et al. (1973) have also demonstrated that drugs which influence platelet function prolong platelet survival values before treatment. Dipyridamole in the presence of anticoagulants has been found to reduce the clinical manifestations of thromboembolic episodes in subjects with prosthetic heart valves (Sullivan et al., 1971), as well as restoring platelet survival values to normal in such patients (Harker and Slichter, 1972). Harker and Slichter (1973) found that homocystine, which is known to cause endothelial injury, causes shortened platelet survival when it is given to baboons. The endothelial injury caused by homocystine could be the cause of the increased thrombosis found in subjects with homocystinuria.

Harker and Slichter (1972) have one piece of evidence which indicates that not all drugs which inhibit platelet function (as judged by in vitro tests) prolong platelet survival. They could not show in man that aspirin at a dose of 1.2g/day affected platelet survival even though this dose of aspirin inhibited the platelet-collagen reaction. In rabbits much higher doses of aspirin were found to prolong platelet survival and reduce platelet turnover (Evans et al., 1968). As discussed earlier, sulfinpyrazone in doses which affect platelet survival in man appears to reduce the incidence of thromboembolic episodes in a number of arterial disorders whereas aspirin (which does not affect platelet survival in the doses used) does not seem to have much effect on the manifestations of arterial thrombosis.

Summary

Vessel injury may initiate some of the early vessel wall changes related to atherosclerosis. Thrombosis could contribute to these early vessel wall changes because platelets are an important early component of arterial thrombi and are known to release factors which can alter the vessel wall.

Repeated vessel wall injury leads to extensive lipid-rich atherosclerotic lesions. Over most of these lipid-rich lesions there are breaks in the endothelium and sometimes thrombotic material can be found on the surface. It is unlikely that such lesions are the result of the organization of mural thrombi. However, some of the changes in the intima may be caused by materials released from platelets which damage the vessel wall and cause the proliferation of smooth muscle cells.

Mural thrombi can be organized into the vessel wall, giving rise to fibrous intimal thickenings. This mechanism is of some importance in the progression of aherosclerosis.

In many situations the clinical manifestations of atherosclerosis may be the consequence of mural thrombi in major arteries; these thrombi fragment and shower the distal circulation with microemboli. Such a mechanism has been shown to occur in carotid artery disease and there is good evidence that embolization of the kidney from mural thrombi in the aorta above the renal arteries causes nephrosclerosis and high blood pressure. It seems very likely that such a mechanism may occur in the coronary circulation. This could account for sudden death without evidence of occlusive thrombi in a major coronary artery.

Some of the drugs which influence platelet function have proved to be useful in the managment of transient attacks of cerebral ischemia. If thromboembolism is an important cause of the clinical manifestations of coronary artery disease, these drugs may prove to be beneficial in the prevention of sudden death and myocardial infarction.

Dietary fat (particularly saturated fatty acids), as well as influencing serum lipids and development of atherosclerosis, has been found to make animals more susceptible to thrombosis. Humans given a diet rich in unsaturated fatty acids show a decreased incidence of myocardial infarction. Cigarette smoking is associated with increased incidence of **cardiovascular deaths** and has been found to enhance platelet reactions. The only test of platelet function which appears to show a relation to the clinical problems of thrombosis and the effects of drugs on platelets is the estimation of platelet survival.

THE NATURAL HISTORY OF EXPERIMENTALLY INDUCED MURAL THROMBI IN SYSTEMIC ARTERIES OF NORMOCHOLESTEROLAEMIC AND HYPERCHOLES - TEROLAEMIC MONKEYS

Kesavan Prathap

The natural history of arterial thrombi has been studied many times with the hope that the end result would be morphologically identical to atheromatous plaques. However, these studies have led to conflicting results (Harrison, 1948; Friedman and Byers, 1961; Hand and Chandler, 1962; Ardlie and Schwartz, 1968), and have been subject to the criticism that the experimental animal used has been a small animal which has little similarity to man. Also, many of the earlier workers had used emboli derived from blood clot rather than platelet-rich thrombi, and most of the observations had been made on the pulmonary arteries where the arterial pressure is much lower than in systemic arteries. There are two reports of thrombi in systemic arteries of swine (Jorgensen et al., 1967; Woolf et al., 1968) but these include only the early natural history, the oldest thrombi being four months and one month respectively.

This paper summarizes the natural history of platelet-rich thrombi in femoral and carotid arteries of the *Macaca irus (Macaca fascicularis)*, a subhuman primate species which is susceptable to spontaneous (Prathap, 1973a) and experimental (Prathap 1972) atherosclerosis.

Materials and Methods

Ninety-nine platelet-rich mural thrombi were produced in femoral and carotid arteries of 50 adult male monkeys, by the intraluminal insertion of catgut sutures. Thirty-eight of the monkeys were maintained on a low fat, cholesterol-free diet, while the remaining twelve were rendered hypercholesterolaemic by feeding a high fat, cholesterol-enriched diet. The morphology of the thrombi was studied by light and electron microscopy at intervals ranging from one hour to three years.

Results and Conclusions

In monkeys maintained on a low fat diet, blood cholesterol levels ranged from 70-220 mg per 100 ml throughout the course of the experiment. This is within the normal range for free-ranging *Macaca irus* (Prathap, 1973a). The twelve monkeys that were fed the high fat, cholesterol-enriched diet developed a sustained elevation of their average serum cholesterol levels in the range of 300-450 mg per 100 ml.

Platelet-rich thrombi were present in every specimen studied one hour after insertion of the suture. By the fourth day the thrombi consisted mainly of fibrin and were largely covered by a surface layer of cells. By ten weeks all thrombi in normocholesterolaemic monkeys were replaced by fibromuscular intimal thickenings in which lipid droplets were few and inconspicuous. When observed two years later, no further change had occured. In every instance, the lesions consisted of eccentric, relatively avascular fibromuscular intimal plaques lined by a single layer of endothelium. Macrophages were not seen and no lipid was demonstrable in frozen sections stained with oil red O. There was no calcification, haemorrhage, or necrosis.

In monkeys with raised blood cholesterol levels, the early natural history of the thrombi was similar to that in normocholesterolaemic monkeys. There were, however, collections of lipid especially at the angles of the plaques and within their depths. Two and three year old plaques contained less lipid than during the phase of organisation, despite persistent moderate hypercholesterolaemia which caused the development of advanced lipid-rich atherosclerotic lesions elsewhere in the arterial system. However, foam cell aggregates morphologically similar to fatty streaks developed *on the luminal surface* of a few healed thrombi. Calcification was sometimes present, but there was no evidence of haemorrhage, ulceration, central necrosis or fatty gruel. A detailed illustrated account of the light and electron microscopic appearances of these lesions is presented elsewhere (Prathap, 1973 b,c).

It is concluded that the healing of mural thrombi in systemic arteries of normo-cholesterolaemic monkeys results in relatively stable, hard, fibromuscular plaques lacking in the fatty gruel that is typically seen in "soft" atheromatous plaques. The lipid content of the plaque is increased slightly if the blood cholesterol level is raised during the phase of organisation. Nevertheless, the "soft" lipid-rich atheromatous plaque cannot be explained on the basis of organisation of mural systemic arterial thrombi even in the presence of persistent hypercholesterolaemia.

BEHAVIOR OF FIBRINOGEN AND FIBRINOLYSIS IN TYPE II AND TYPE IV HYPERLIPEMIC SUBJECTS AND IN PATIENTS WITH CORONARY HEART DISEASE

A. Pagnan, W. Donadon, E. Tonolli, and C. Dal Palù

Introduction

Since the hypothesis of Duguid (1946) that atheroma may be derived from "mural fibrin thrombi", the attention of many investigators has been focused on the possible significance of changes in fibrinolytic activity and plasma fibrinogen in the pathogenesis of CHD (coronary heart disease). The interest in the possible relationship between elevated serum lipid levels, increase of fibrinogen and/or defective fibrinolysis, and CHD, encouraged us to investigate the behavior of fibrinogen and fibrinolytic activity in hyperlipemic (type II A-B and type IV) subjects without CHD and in hyperlipemic and normolipemic patients with CHD, compared with subjects free from CHD and lipid abnormalities (controls).

Material and Methods

The subjects of this study (397 cases), 238 males and 159 females, were divided into 3 groups: 1. healthy normolipemic subjects (n = 152) free from clinical symptoms and ECG signs of CHD and without recent infection or other illness (controls); 2. hyperlipemic subjects without CHD (n = 89); 3. hyperlipemic and normolipemic patients with CHD (n = 79; 53 with ischemic heart disease (IHD) and 26 who had myocardial infarction at least 3 months before the examination); clinical diabetes was found in 9 CHD patients. These groups were then subdivided by age: 20-34; 35-49; 50-64; the distribution within these latter was sufficiently homogeneous for number and sex. Diagnostic criteria for CHD were based on: history of angina, typical ECG changes, serum enzymes (for myocardial infarction), and coronary arteriography (in 22 cases of IHD). The diagnosis of hyperlipoproteinemia was supported by electrophoretic pattern and chemical determination of TC (total cholesterol) and TG (triglycerides). Normal values, according to our laboratory standards, were: TC ≤ 250 mg% and TG ≤ 180 mg%. According to these diagnostic criteria we were able to separate type II A-B (77 cases) and type IV (53 cases). TC, TG, plasma fibrinogen (F), and euglobulin lysis time (ELT) were measured according to the methods of Levine and Zak (1964), Kessler and Lederer (1966), Lempert (1962), and Buckell (1958). Lipoprotein electrophoresis was performed on agarose-gel according to Noble's method (1968) modified by Pagnan et al. (1971).

Results

In hyperlipemic subjects (without CHD) and in hyperlipemic and normolipemic patients with CHD mean F levels were significantly higher (p <0.001) than in controls, only for the first two age groups (Table 1). CHD patients, both normolipemic and hyperlipemic, exhibited mean ELT values significantly higher (p <0.05) than in controls in all age groups: hyperlipemic subjects without CHD showed significantly higher values (p <0.05) only in the first two age groups (Table 2). No significant differences were found in F and ELT values between normolipemic and hyperlipemic CHD patients. Mean F and ELT values did not differ in type II compared with type IV hyperlipoproteinemia (Table 3). No statistical correlation was found by matching separately TC and TG with F and ELT.

Table 1. Mean fibrinogen levels .(mg%)

	Age groups (yr)	20-34	35-49	50-64
Non C.H.D.	Controls	336 *81*	352 *87*	388 *90*
	Hyperlipemics	376 *67*	422 *81*	390 *52*
C.H.D.	Totals C.H.D.	–	412 *100*	412 *86*
	Hyperlipemics C.H.D.	–	428 *118*	411 *81*
	Non hyperlipemics C.H.D.	–	40Q *93*	403 *86*

M = Mean (large number).   SD = Standard deviation (small number)

Table 2. Mean euglobulin lysis time (minutes)

	Age groups (yr)	20-34	35-49	50-64
Non C.H.D.	Controls	232 *47*	231 *52*	236 *47*
	Hyperlipemics	259 *34*	262 *41*	242 *47*
C.H.D.	Totals C.H.D.	–	265 *27*	263 *48*
	Hyperlipemics C.H.D.	–	266 *26*	274 *36*
	Non hyperlipemics C.H.D.	–	264 *29*	260 *42*

Table 3. Mean fibrinogen and euglobulin lysis time values in type II and IV hyperlipoproteinemia

	Type II	Type IV	p
Euglobulin lysis time (m')	253 *50*	259 *33*	N.S.
Fibrinogen (mg%)	414 *83*	401 *84*	N.S.

Discussion

Hyperlipemic and normolipemic patients with CHD, and hyperlipemic subjects without CHD, exhibit a significant increase of mean F levels, compared with controls in younger age groups (20 to 49), but not after the age of 50. This finding is consistent with those of Ogston and Ogston (1966) and emphasizes the possible atherogenic role of raised plasma fibrinogen in younger age. It is also of interest that both hyperlipemic and normolipemic patients with CHD and hyperlipemic subjects without CHD exhibit a similar increase of mean F levels and ELT values as the controls. The increase found in CHD patients is not dependent on hyperlipemia, since both normolipemic and hyperlipemic subjects of the CHD group exhibited similar values of F and ELT. Therefore, the abnormalities found in this group seem to be related to the atherosclerotic process. As far as hyperlipemic non-CHD patients are concerned, the increase of F and ELT might be due to a subclinical atherosclerosis: however, some abnormalities of blood coagulation related to hyperlipemia are well-known. Most of the previous reports in this field, especially on fibrinolysis behavior, are based on the evaluation of fibrinolytic activity after fatty meal ingestion in normal subjects (Greig, 1956; Kwaan and MacFadzean, 1957). The common opinion is that fats do inhibit fibrinolysis, but there is disagreement about the type of lipid directly responsible for this behavior. Spöttl et al. (1967) found a longer fibrinolysis time in a group of patients with "endogenous" hypertriglyceridemia, compared with control normolipemic subjects. On the contrary, Nitzberg et al. (1959), comparing 19 fasting hyperlipemic subjects (10 with hypercholesterolemia and 9 with "idiopathic" hyperlipemia) with controls, were unable to find any significant difference between these two groups or between the two different types of hyperlipemia. We too failed to find any significant difference in the abnormal levels of F and ELT between type II and type IV hyperlipoproteinemia, nor did we find any by matching separately TC and TG with fibrinogen and ELT.

CONTROL OF PLATELET FUNCTION IN POSTMYOCARDIAL INFARCTION PATIENTS DURING A TWO YEAR ASPIRIN STUDY*

Erhard Walter, Theo Pfleiderer, and Ellen Weber

The Department of Medicine of the University of Heidelberg takes part in a two-year trial for secondary prevention of myocardial infarction. This is a multicenter, prospective, randomized, double-blind study. The question to be answered is: Can aspirin reduce the number of reinfarctions? The study has been running now for nearly 2-1/2 years. The collecting period will soon be finished.

Males and females between 45 and 70 years, who have suffered at least one myocardial infarction are allocated to one of three groups. They receive either phenprocoumon or 1.5 g aspirin a day or placebo. The two last groups are running double-blind. The observation period and the special medications are started 6-8 weeks after the acute event and last for 2 years. Patients with acute myocardial infarction, diagnosed by cardiac complaints; ECG alterations; elevation of CPK, transaminases, and LDH are asked to take part in this study. Nearly 80% of them accept this. The patients are seen every 4 weeks. They are questioned about their complaints. Furthermore, aspirin or placebo tablets or the anticoagulant schedule are handed out to them. Controlled are the arterial pressure, pulse rate, Quick prothrombin time in the phenprocoumon group, and platelet function tests in all 3 groups. If there is no need for earlier examination caused by any symptoms, ECG, serum uric acid, serum triglycerides, and cholesterol, as well as blood sugar are checked every 6 months. In the case of reinfarction the study ends for this patient. Other reasons for canceling patients before term are: if the therapy was stopped for more than 21 days; if the patient needs, besides the therapy of his group, ASA-containing preparations, anticoagulants, dipyridamole, or phenylbutazone; if the key was broken; finally in the case of death.

For the control of platelet function we used four different tests: the rotating bulb technique according to Wright (Wright, 1941), the glass bead filter method of Hellem in the modification of Rosner et al. (1967), the platelet aggregation test (PAT) of Breddin (1968), and the fibre test of Jacobi et al. (1971). In these tests thrombocytes face foreign surfaces and forces which cause adhesion and/or aggregation. In the tests of Wright and Hellem the decrease in platelet count, expressed in % of the initial value, indicates platelet stickiness. In the PAT we control the behavior of thrombocytes on plastic slides after having rotated them in platelet-rich plasma. The degree of aggregation is classified in 5 grades. In the fibre test of Jacobi we determine the quantity of platelet protein deposited on nylon fibres within a perfused glass capillary. As can be seen from Fig. 1, the platelet deposits on the nylon fibres look like the deposits on injured vessel wall intima.

There are quite a variety of platelet function tests. But we think they measure different parameters, even if we compare those measuring platelet aggregation apart from the adhesion tests. If we try to depress raised platelet stickiness and if we want to control this effect, we must find a test system that detects this increased platelet stickiness. We therefore carried out the four different tests simultaneously after one venepuncture with blood of two groups (Fig. 2). The first group consisted of 25 healthy volunteers with an average age of 28 years.

*These studies were supported by the German Research Foundation within the SFB 90 'Cardiovasculäres System' and by the 'Paul-Martini-Stiftung'.

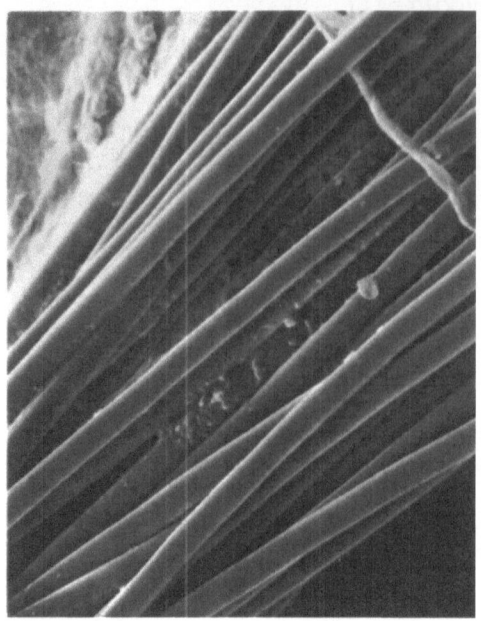

Figure 1. Scanning electron microscopic picture of the bundle of nylon fibres with clusters of thrombocytes, especially in center of bundle (X 246). We thank Prof. H. Fritsch for preparing the SEM-photograph

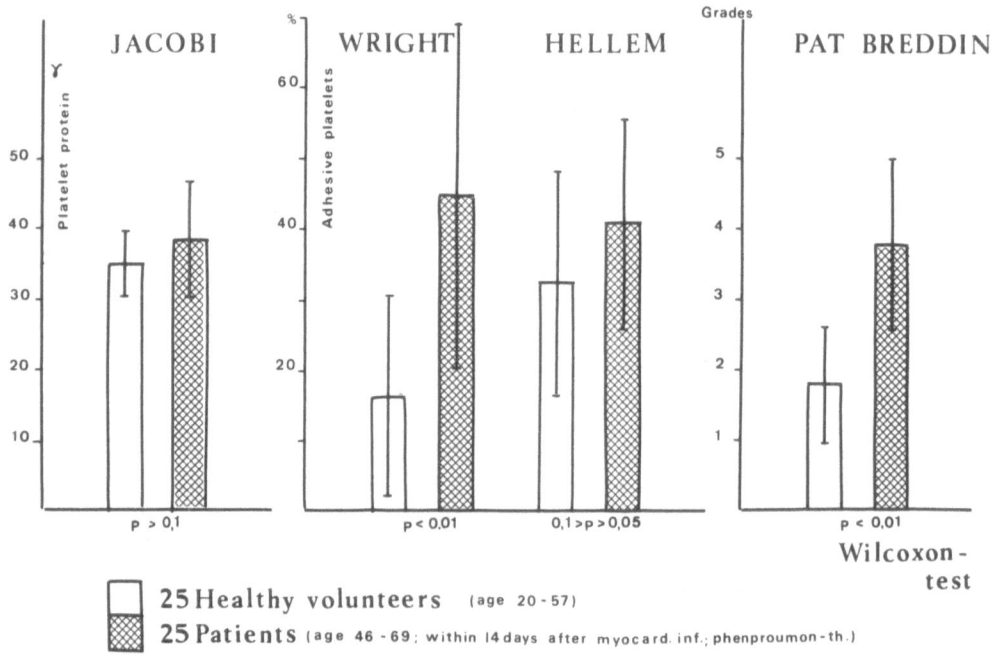

Figure 2. Platelet function measured by 4 different tests (mean ± SD). All 4 tests were performed simultaneously after one venepuncture

The sex ratio was 60% females and 40% males. The second group consisted of 25 patients with myocardial infarction which was not older than 14 days, and treated with phenprocoumon. The average age was 60 years, the sex ratio 30% women and 70% men. Using Jacobi's test, the mean value in the first group lies within the normal range of 30-50 γ as indicated by the author (Jacobi et al., 1971). The fact that there is no increase with age and in patients with myocardial infarction except during the first day corresponds very well with Jacobi's own results (Jacobi et al., 1973). The normal value for the Hellem I test was given as 42 ± 8% (Lechner et al., 1971). The value for our group of healthy volunteers is lower and has a higher standard deviation. This test shows increased platelet stickiness in patients with myocardial infarction but with no statistical significance. A statistically significant difference between both groups could be measured by the method of Wright and by the PAT of Breddin. For the Wright test this fact was already shown by Zebe (Zebe et al., 1970). Breddin found pathological PAT values in 70-80% of patients with myocardial infarction (Breddin, 1968).

In 1964 Gast measured with the rotating bulb technique of Wright a decrease of platelet stickiness in patients treated with ASA (Gast, 1964). Scharrer demonstrated the efficacy of ASA with the PAT (Scharrer et al., 1969), Jacobi with the fibre test (Jacobi et al., 1973). When we controlled 26 patients of our placebo group and 23 patients of the ASA group 3 to 4 times with all 4 tests simultaneously, we found that the efficacy of ASA was detectable in three of them. With the rotating bulb technique of Wright the mean value was 23.26% in the placebo group and 14.67% in the ASA group. Similarly significant was the result with the PAT. Grade 3.11 in the placebo and 2.06 in the ASA group. Only a minimal, non-significant decrease was shown in the fibre test. Nearly identical mean values were found with the glass bead column test of Hellem.

An important question is: Does platelet stickiness change during long-term treatment with aspirin? In spite of further ASA therapy Jacobi found in patients with polycythemia vera, after an initial decrease of platelet stickiness, a steady increase which surmounted even the value before therapy (Lechner et al., 1971). Also, patients with myocardial infarction who were treated with ASA had pathological values on the 9th day after the infarction (Jacobi et al., 1973). Fig. 3, 4, 5 show the mean values of 20-24 patients of the anticoagulant, the ASA and the placebo group, whose platelet function was controlled up to 84 weeks. For the ASA and the placebo group the standard deviations are also shown. ASA therapy began after the 4 weeks value.

Fig. 3 shows the curves of the platelet adhesion test of Hellem. The lowest are the values of the phenprocoumon group. The curves of the ASA and the placebo group cross. As already mentioned before, there is no difference between ASA or placebo treatment. All three curves show a decrease till the 50th week. This means that there is a normalization of this test within one year after myocardial infarction. Bouvier reported a tendency to normalization of the initially raised Hellem I values of myocardial infarction patients. They did not continue for more than 4 weeks after the acute event (Bouvier et al., 1967).

The initial values of the Wright test of all three groups lie close together (Fig. 4). ASA therapy brings down these increased values to normal. This effect lasts continously over 84 weeks. Similar to the results of the Hellem test, there is a tendency to normalization within one year in the placebo group and in the group treated with anticoagulant.

Also the initial values of the PAT are close together (Fig. 5). The decrease of platelet stickiness after starting ASA therapy in the ASA group is statistically significant with p<0.01, using the Wilcoxon test. As already shown with the rotating bulb test, this effect is stable during the whole medication period. But in contrast to the two other tests, the values of the anticoagulant and of the placebo group show no decreasing tendency. From the curves of the ASA-treated patients we can also deduce that tablets were taken regularly.

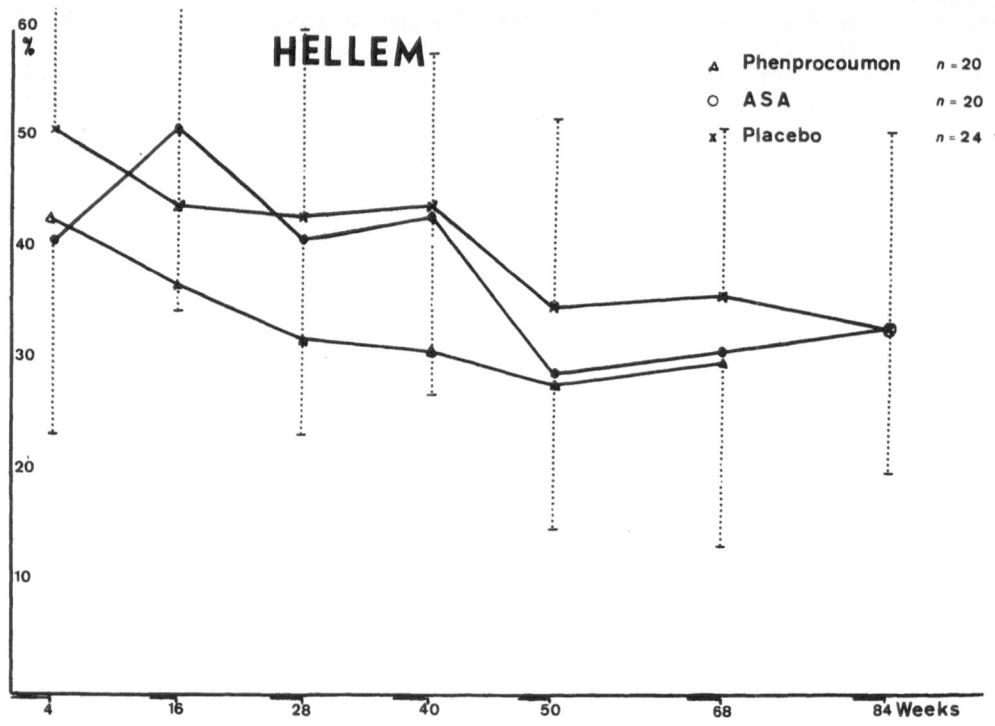

Figure 3. Effect of long-term treatment with phenprocoumon, ASA, or placebo on platelet stickiness measured by the Hellem I test (mean ± SD)

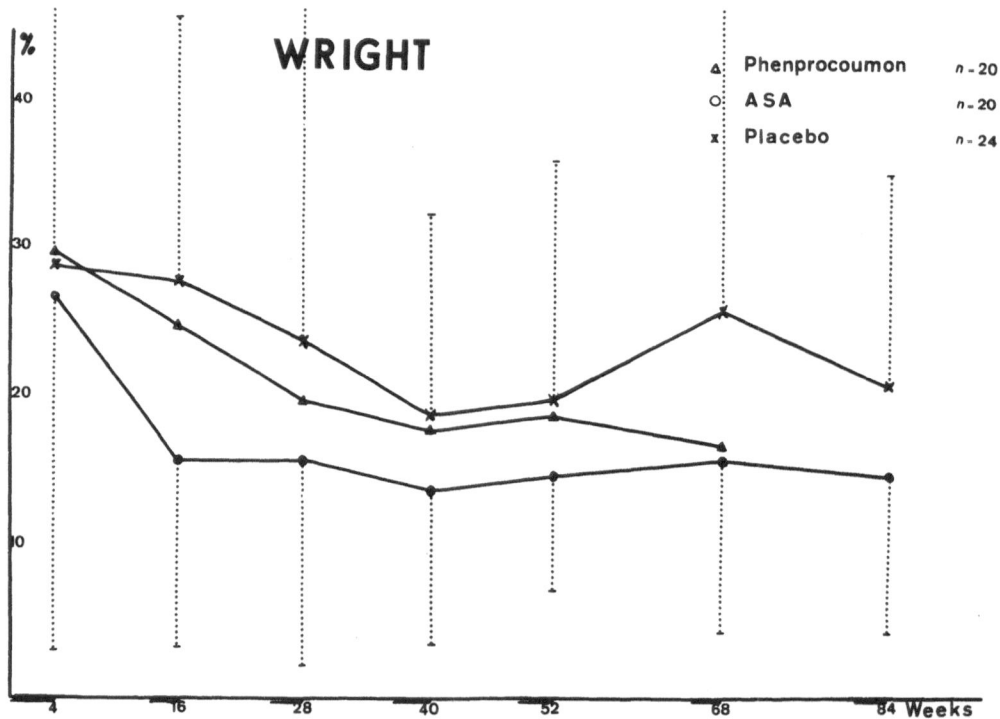

Figure 4. Influence of long-term treatment with phenprocoumon, ASA, or placebo on platelet stickiness measured by the test of Wright (mean ± SD)

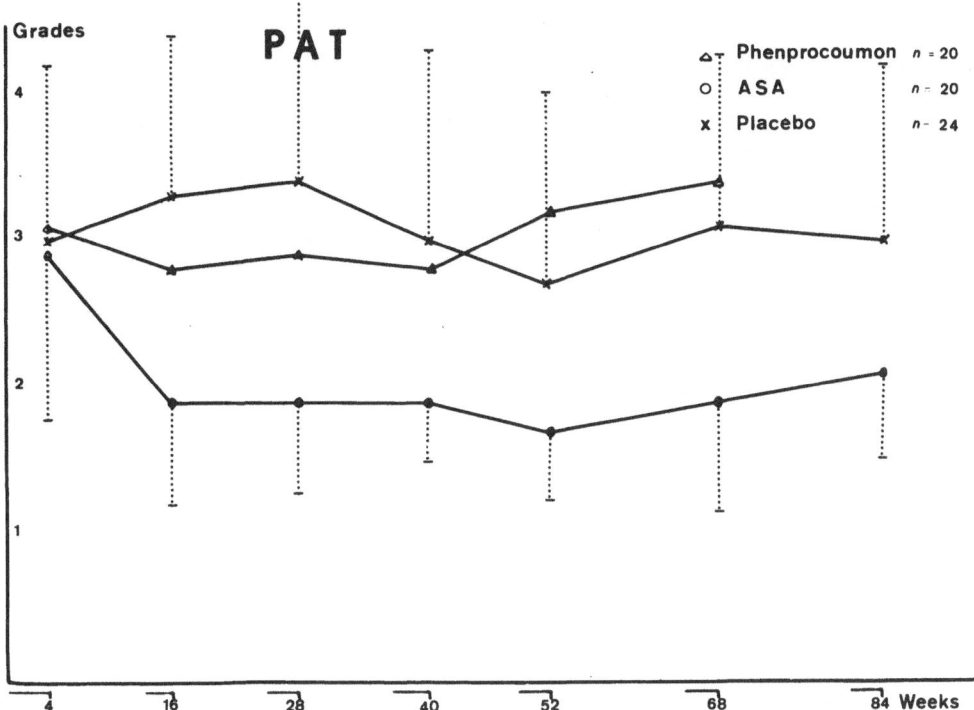

Figure 5. Effect of long-term treatment with phenprocoumon, ASA, or placebo on platelet aggregation measured by the PAT of Breddin (mean ± SD)

What happens when we stop ASA medication after 2 years? Elevated platelet sticki- ness returns when the therapy is stopped, even after 2 years of medication (Fig. 6).

Up to now we have seen only very few ASA-induced complications, which could be overcome by changing the time of intake or by discontinuing therapy for a short time.

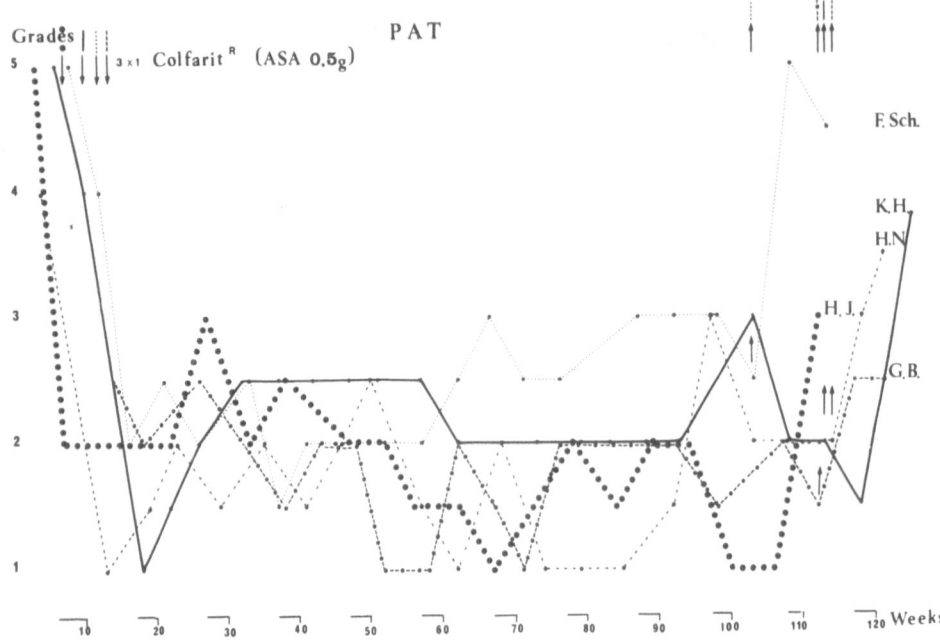

Figure 6. Long-term treatment with 1.5 g of acetylsalicylic acid per day (Col-
farit^R, Bayer) of patients with elevated placelet stickiness. Normalized platelet
aggregation increases again after stopping therapy

DIETARY FAT, PLATELET FUNCTION AND CORONARY HEART DISEASE IN MAN

G. Hornstra

Coronary heart disease (CHD) is the result of progressive atherosclerosis in the coronary arteries. In the atherosclerotic process, arterial thrombosis is of great importance, both as an initiating as well as a complicating factor. In arterial thrombosis, blood platelets play a key role since they are involved in the formation of mural and circulating thrombi.

It is now generally accepted that the type and amount of the dietary fat influences the development of atherosclerosis. Therefore, we thought it important to study the effects of these fats on platelet function and arterial thrombosis. From work we did on rats (Hornstra, 1973) we could conclude that

- saturated fats with 14 or more carbon atoms are thrombogenic;
- oleic acid, and probably other monoenoic acids, are neutral as to arterial thrombus formation;
- linoleic acid, and most probably linolenic acid, have a specific anti-thrombotic effect.

It should be noted that these conclusions are only valid in rats and that it remains questionable whether they also apply to man. To establish this, it is necessary to repeat the experiments with rats also in man, for which a suitable technique to quantify thrombosis tendency in humans is needed.

After it became evident that in rats a high tendency to thrombosis is associated with a high amount of circulating platelet aggregates (Hornstra, 1973), we assumed that determination of the degree of intravascular aggregation in man might be a suitable technique to measure their thrombosis tendency.

Through the courtesy of Prof. Turpeinen and Prof. Karvonen of Helsinki, Finland, we were given the opportunity to test this hypothesis and moreover, to investigate the effect of the dietary linoleic acid level in man. Measurements were carried out in 2 groups of male patients of two mental hospitals in Finland. In one hospital the normal Finnish diet was given which contains only 4 cal% linoleic acid, and in which the ratio of polyunsaturated to saturated fatty acids (P/S-ratio) was about 0.25. In the other hospital the diet was modified in such a way that a linoleic acid content of 12 cal% and a P/S-ratio of about 1.60 were obtained. In a 12-year study in these hospitals, it was shown that in man, the use of the high linoleic acid diet was associated with considerably and significantly reduced mortality from CHD (Miettinen et al., 1972). In fact our patients were an at random selection from their experimental groups. There were no differences between the two groups in age, body weight and smoking habits. Moreover, no appreciable differences in blood pressure and medication existed.

As might be expected, the serum cholesterol content was significantly lower in the high linoleic acid group (5.8 vs 6.5 mmol/1, $P_2 < 0.001$) whereas no significant difference existed in the serum triglyceride content (1.90 vs 1.83 mmol/1).

Platelet-to-glass adhesion was measured by the rotating-bulb technique, originally devised by Wright (Wright, 1941). In our experiment no significant effect of the diet could be found (35.5 vs 31.5% retention).

The same holds for the template bleeding time (268 vs 266 s) which was determined by a recently described automatic device (Praga et al., 1972). Significant differences were found neither in platelet nor in red cell concentration, which were within the physiological range.

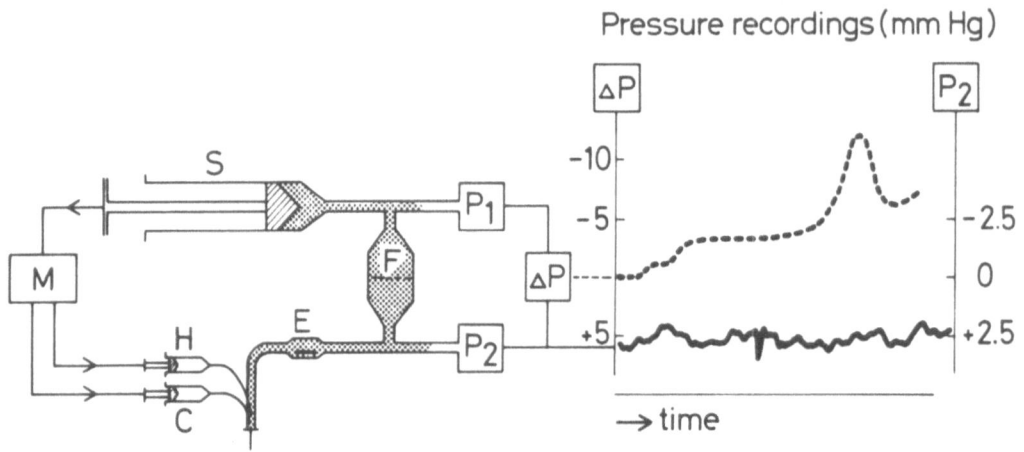

Figure 1. Diagram of Filtragometer

Fig. 1 shows a diagram of the newly developed apparatus, by which the platelet aggregation was measured (Filtragometer). With a motor (M) driven syringe (S) blood from a forearm vein is drawn through a microfilter (F) at a constant rate of 2.25 ml/min. The filter consists of a nickle plate with pores of 20 µm in diameter. This filter permits passage of red- and white cells and of single platelets but it is occluded by platelet aggregates. Pressures proximal (P_2) and distal (P_1) to the filter are measured and subtracted electronically to obtain the pressure difference across the filter (ΔP), which is monitored. The pressure between arm and filter (P_2) is also recorded to check blood supply.

Heparin (H), infused just distally to the needle at an end concentration of 5 U/ml, anticoagulates the blood. Moreover, it stabilizes occurring intravascular aggregates which therefore obstruct the filter, resulting in a change in ΔP. At a ΔP value of 5 mm Hg, heparin is replaced by sodium citrate (C) and after some time partial disaggregation takes place. Fig. 2 shows the ΔP-tracing in more detail.

The start of the experiment is indicated by an upward deflection of the tracing. A downward deflection marks the moment when ΔP equals 5 mm Hg.

From this tracing the following parameters are calculated:

- the aggregation time, AT, (s), necessary to reach a ΔP value of 5 mm Hg.
- the aggregation slope T_s, which is the slope of the tangent to the curve where ΔP equals 5 mm Hg.
- the maximum aggregation, A_{max}, that is the maximum height of the aggregation curve in mm Hg.
- the disaggregation induction time, DIT, being the time between termination of the heparin infusion (at ΔP = 5 mm Hg) and the beginning of disaggregation.

Fig. 3 shows the results of the aggregation measurements. In the high linoleic acid group the aggregation time is longer, the aggregation slope is flatter and the maximum height of the aggregation curve is lower. Finally the disaggregation

280

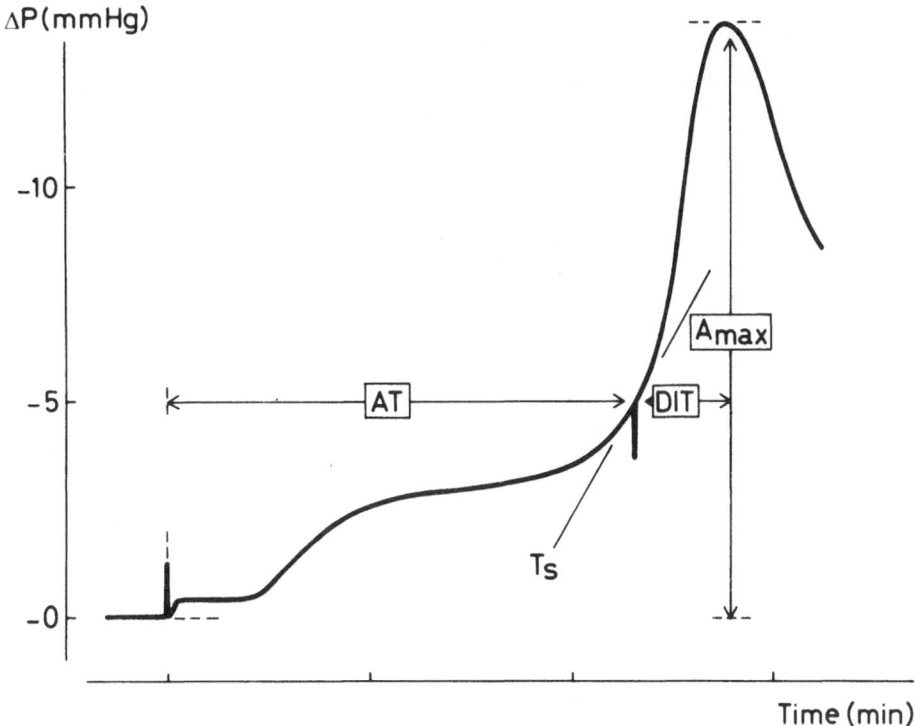

Figure 2. Schematic recording of the pressure difference (ΔP) over the filter

induction time is shorter. These results indicate a decreased platelet aggregatability and enhanced disaggregatability in the high linoleic acid group as compared to the subjects receiving the normal, low linoleic acid diet.

As mentioned before, in the high linoleic group the mortality from CHD was considerably reduced. Since CHD-mortality has repeatedly been reported to be associated with occlusive thrombi in the coronary arteries (Harland, 1966; Haerem, 1971) it is conceivable that the lower platelet aggregation we observed has contributed to this lower mortality.

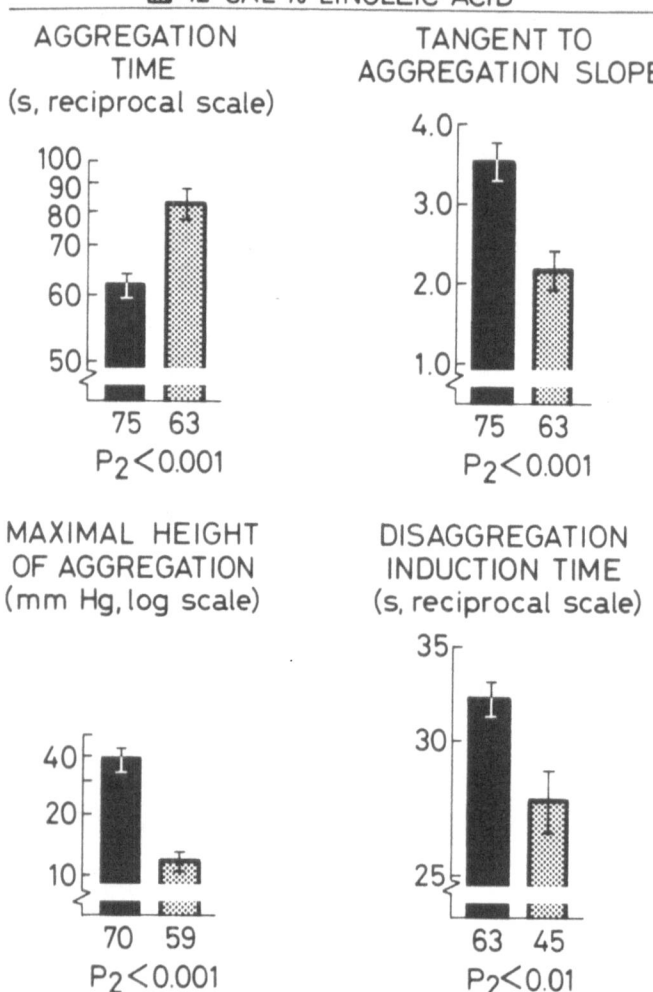

Figure 3. Effect of dietary linoleic acid content on platelet aggregation (Filtragometer). Mean values ± S.E.M. Figures under bars represent number of observations

ENHANCED PLATELET AGGREGATION AS A RISK FACTOR FOR THROMBOEMBOLIC COMPLICATIONS IN ATHEROSCLEROSIS

H.J. Krzywanek, K. Breddin, I. Scharrer, and J. Kutschera

In recent years great emphasis has been laid upon the importance of so-called risk factors in the progression of atherosclerotic disease and its thromboembolic complications. In the past decade we have been collecting data on the spontaneous platelet aggregating activity in normal subjects and in patients with a wide variety of internal diseases, a total of about 5000 persons have been studied.

Methods

Platelet aggregating activity was assessed using the Platelet Aggregation Test (PAT) (Krzywanek and Breddin, 1972), which was first described by Breddin et al. (1963). In some aggregation tests (Born, 1962; O'Brien, 1961) platelet clumping has to be induced by addition of ADP, collagen, or epinephrine to PRP. With the PAT we are able to study the *spontaneous* aggregation of thrombocytes in their normal plasma environment, and the addition of inducing substances is not necessary.

Selection of Patients

A group of 545 "healthy" subjects included nurses, students, members of the medical staff and other personnel of the Frankfurt University Medical Center and almost 300 policemen of the City of Frankfurt with no apparent disease. These persons stated that they felt to be in good health and had no medical treatment at the time of the study. They were not examined whether they had symptoms of manifest atherosclerosis or its complications. The other group were in- and out-clinic patients of the University Medical Center, Frankfurt/Main, with a variety of acute and chronic internal diseases.

A number of patients, who were seen for other reasons, had a thromboembolic accident in the weeks or months following the performance of an aggregation test. In this way data were obtained of 148 patients "prior to a thromboembolic event".

Results

1. In an apparently "healthy" population an increasing number of individuals with enhanced platelet aggregation (PAT grades 4 and 5) was found with rising age (Fig. 1). In the age group 50-59 years one third of the normals showed a markedly enhanced spontaneous aggregation.
2. In 2826 medical patients with various diseases - peripheral atherosclerosis, diabetes mellitus, myocardial infarction and thrombosis were excluded - the incidence of PAT grades 4 and 5 was roughly doubled in comparison with normal controls of the matching age groups.
3. Two groups of diabetics were studied (Fig. 2): 388 patients in whom the duration of the disease was unknown, and 472 patients with diabetes of more than 5 years' duration. Throughout the various age groups the incidence of enhanced platelet aggregation was markedly higher in diabetics than in the control group, which was most evident below 40 years of age. If the disease was known for more than five years, there was another 10-15% increase of PATs grade 4/5 as compared with the unselected group of diabetics.

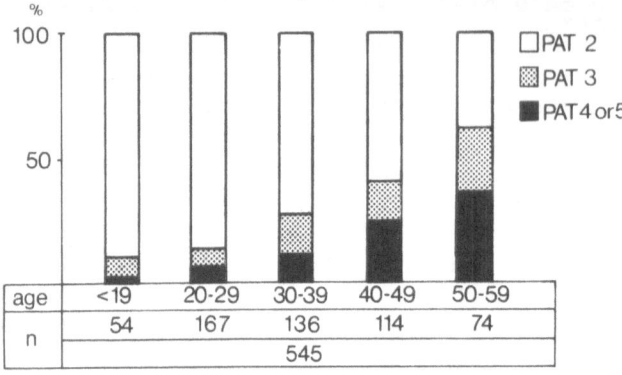

Figure 1. Incidence of enhanced platelet aggregation in "Healthy Subjects"

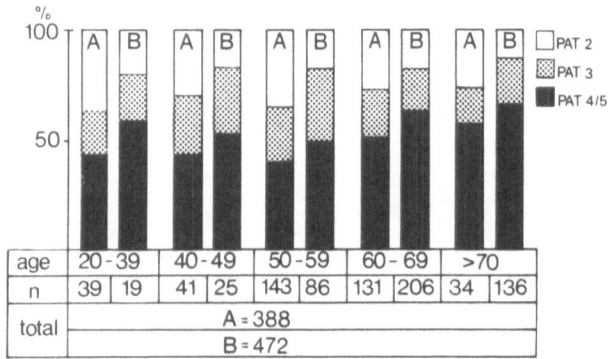

Figure 2. Incidence of enhanced platelet aggregation in "Diabetes Mellitus" of unknown duration (A) and of > 5 years' duration (B)

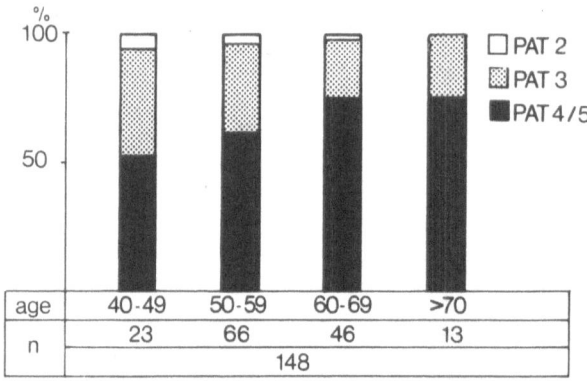

Figure 3. Incidence of enhanced platelet aggregation in persons prior to "Thromboembolic Disease"

4. In a follow-up study of 401 patients in whom a PAT was performed between 5 days and 3 years after they had suffered a myocardial infarct, more than half of them had enhanced platelet aggregation in all groups over 40 years of age.
5. The incidence of PAT grades 4 and 5 in 273 patients with peripheral arterial occlusive disease was between 45 and 60%.
6. In 148 patients a PAT had been done within 6 months prior to a thromboembolic episode (Fig. 3), like myocardial infarction, arterial thrombosis or embolism, venous thrombosis, thrombophlebitis, pulmonary embolism and cerebral vascular occlusions. The incidence of normal platelet aggregation was strikingly low in all age groups (40 to >70 years), PAT grades 4 and 5 were found in 54-78% of these patients.

Discussion

The number of "healthy" persons with enhanced platelet aggregation is growing with age. In our opinion this is correlated with the progression of atherosclerosis with advancing years.

In patients with complications of atherosclerosis like recent myocardial infarction, peripheral occlusive disease, but also in diabetics the incidence of abnormal platelet aggregation was significantly higher than in "healthy" subjects and in patients with various other internal diseases. The highest incidence of PAT grades 4/5 was observed *prior* to thromboembolic attacks in atherosclerotic patients, the frequency comparable only with diabetes of more than 5 years' duration and recent myocardial infarction. These groups were not different in statistical analysis, but altogether varied from "healthy" persons and from patients with various internal diseases.

Following these findings it might be permissive to postulate that enhanced platelet aggregation, repeatedly evident as indicated by PAT grades 4 and 5, by itself represents an important risk factor for thromboembolic disease, especially in patients with advanced atherosclerosis. This postulate will have to be proven by a large scale prospective study, which should lead to a more precise predictability of the presence and progression of atherosclerosis and its threatening complications in an individual patient. Such a study will also yield more basic information to substantiate the rationale of an antiaggregating therapy as prophylaxis of atherosclerotic and thrombotic disease.

VIII
Animal Models of Atherosclerosis

WORKSHOP: Animal Models of Atherosclerosis

Chairmen: Th.B. Clarkson, USA
          J.P. Strong, USA

Participants: C.R. Minick, USA
             G.A. Gresham, Great Britain
             R.F. Scott, USA
             M.L. Armstrong, USA
             M.R. Malinow, USA

THE HUMAN LESION

Jack P. Strong

The importance of comparing the morphology and natural history of human atherosclerosis with that seen in animal models was stressed. It was also pointed out
that communication of observations could be improved if efforts were made to use
common terminology in describing the lesions of animals and human beings. The
following operational definitions of types of atherosclerotic lesions were proposed: *Fatty Streak:* Any intimal lesion that is stained distinctly by Sudan IV
and does not show any other underlying change. *Fibrous Plaque:* A firm, elevated
intimal lesion which in the fresh state is pale gray, glistening, and translucent.
After staining, it may be partially or completely covered by sudanophilic deposits.
If a lesion shows hemorrhage, thrombosis, ulceration, or calcification, that portion is classified under that category. *Complicated Lesion:* A lesion in which
there is hemorrhage, ulceration, or thrombosis with or without calcium. *Calcified
Lesion:* A lesion in which calcium is visible or palpable without overlying hemorrhage, ulceration, or thrombosis.

Fatty streaks begin in the arteries of children as accumulations of fat in s
slightly thickened intima (Strong and McGill, 1969). On the basis of a large number of autopsied persons in New Orleans, it was established that aortic fatty
streaks are present in many children under age three and in all children over age
three (Holman et al., 1958; Strong and McGill, 1963). Fatty streaks of the coronary arteries are rare before age ten and are nearly always present after age
twenty (Strong and McGill, 1962). The anatomic distribution of the fatty streaks
was stressed. In the aorta, lesions are more pronounced in the abdominal as compared with the thoracic aorta, and the aortic arch is relatively spared (Fig. 1
and 2). In the coronary arteries, lesions affect the proximal main branches with

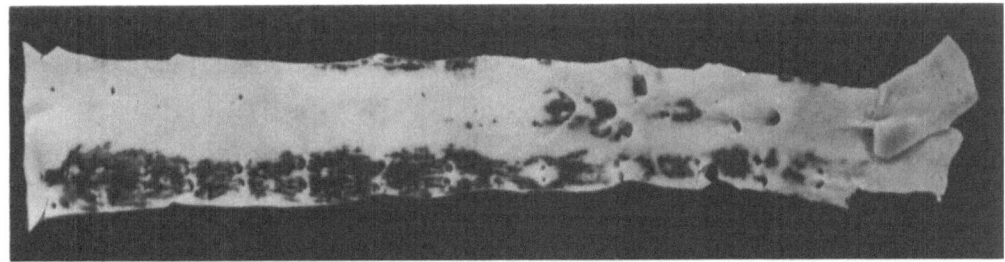

Figure 1. Aorta from a 22-year-old black man who died as a result of an accident.
This Sudan IV-stained specimen contains typical fatty streaks which are black in
this photograph

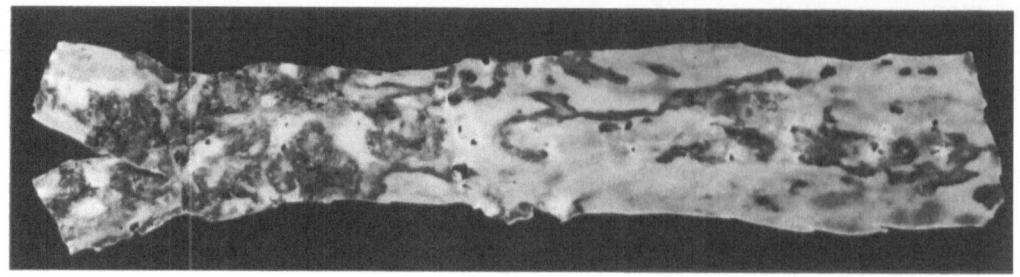

Figure 2. Aorta from 52-year-old white man who died as a result of coronary heart disease. This Sudan IV-stained specimen contains fatty streaks and fibrous plaques in the descending thoracic aorta and fatty streaks, fibrous plaques, and complicated plaques in the abdominal aorta

the small intramyocardial arteries being rarely effected (Fig. 3 and 4). The ultrastructural feastures of aortic and coronary atherosclerosis are not different both containing monocytes, smooth muscle cells with lipid, foam cells and connective tissue elements (Fig. 5).

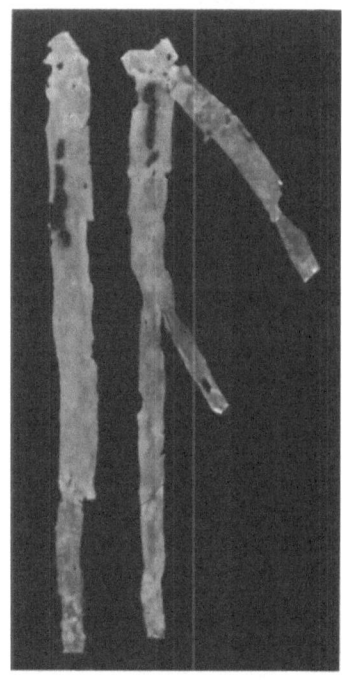

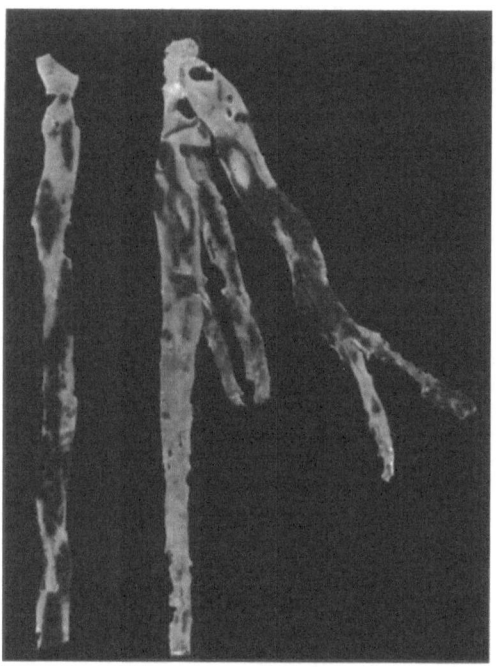

Figure 3. Coronary arteries from a 25-year-old white man who died as a result of an accident. The arteries have been dissected from the heart, opened longitudinally, flattened, and stained with Sudan IV. They contain typical fatty streaks which are black in this photograph

Figure 4. Coronary arteries from a 31-year-old black man who died of cirrhosis of the liver. The Sudan IV-stained arteries contain fatty streaks and fibrous plaques

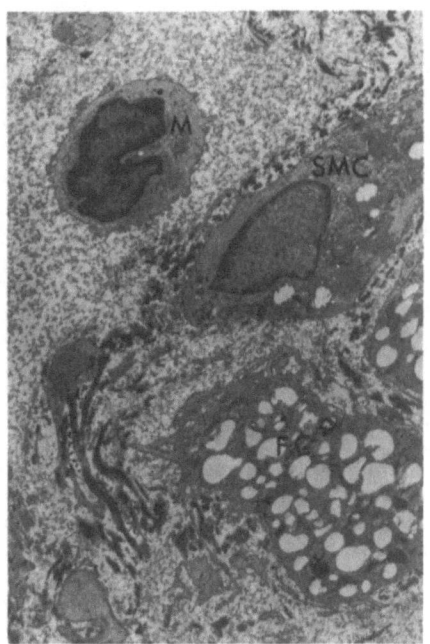

Figure 5. Electron micrograph taken from a section of aorta of a 19-year-old black man who died as a result of an accident. This micrograph shows a portion of the intima containing a monocyte (M), smooth muscle cell with many lipid droplets (SMC) and a lipid filled foam cell (FC). These cells are surrounded by connective tissue

There has been considerable emphasis placed on the geographic pathology of atherosclerosis (Strong et al., 1971). These studies have provided evidence to indicate that there is little difference in the extent of aortic fatty streaks among groups from different geographic locations. Racial differences, however, were observed with Negroes having more extensive fatty streaking in early life than other groups. In contrast, aortic fibrous plaques and complicated lesions tend to parallel differences in the incidence of ischemic heart disease among the populations studied. These observations suggest that species and racial differences among animal models should be expected and will be useful in providing a better understanding of these differences among human beings.

In considering the comparative aspects of natural history of atherosclerosis it should be recalled that the extensiveness of human coronary atherosclerosis varies with age, sex, geographic location, race, plasma cholesterol concentration, and is markedly influenced by such disease as hypertension and diabetes mellitus.

ARTERIOSCLEROSIS OF AFRICAN GREEN AND STUMP-TAILED MACAQUE MONKEYS

Thomas B. Clarkson

Because of their close phylogenetic relationship to man, nonhuman primates have become of considerable interest in a search for animal models in which metabolic and pathologic processes thought to be related to atherosclerosis simulate the situation in man. During the past decade, primary emphasis has been on rhesus monkeys *(Macaca mulatta)*, squirrel monkeys *(Saimiri sciureus)*, and baboons *(Papio cynocephalus)* (Clarkson, 1972). While all of these species have some characteristics that closely resemble man, most of the arterial lesions that have been induced by diet have more nearly resembled fatty streaks of man than human fibrous plaques. A possible exception to this general statement may be the finding of Wissler and his coworkers (1967) indicating that the kind of dietary fat fed affects the histologic characteristics of the arteriosclerotic lesions induced. In their studies, peanut oil was found to induce lesions with fibromuscular caps that did bear a striking resemblance to the fibrous plaques of man.

We have recently studied the pathologic characteristics of diet induced atherosclerosis of two nonhuman primates that have so far received little attention; the African green monkey *(Cercopithecus aethiops)* and the stump-tailed macaque *(Macaca arctoides)* (Bullock *et al.*, 1972; Bullock 1973). In these studies, adult male monkeys were fed a semipurified diet with 45% calories being provided by lard and containing 1 mg of cholesterol/Cal. The total serum cholesterol concentrations of the African green monkeys fed this diet averaged about 400 mg/dl while those of the stump-tailed macaques averaged 700 mg/dl. We examined the arterial lesions of these two species after they had consumed the atherogenic diet for 42 months.

The distribution of aortic lesions among the African green monkeys fed the atherogenic diet was of interest. The extensiveness of fatty streaking was about the same in the thoracic and abdominal aorta, however, there was about twice as much of the abdominal aorta covered by plaques. The gross appearance of the aortic lesions in the African green monkeys was consistent with what has been described as the pearly or fibrous plaques of man (Fig. 1). Microscopically, the plaques of African green monkeys had a pool of lipid, usually near the intima media junction that was covered by a fibromuscular cap (Fig. 2). Extensive mineralization with some hemosiderin deposits were found in the larger plaques.

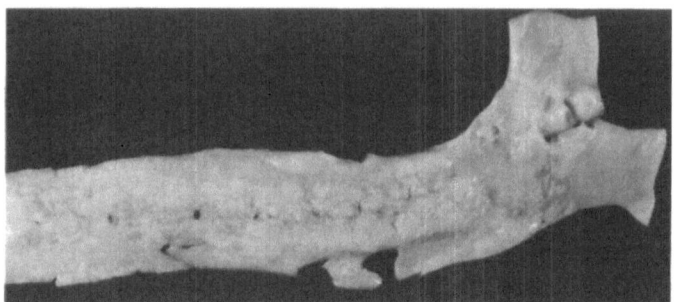

Figure 1. The thoracic aorta from an African green monkey fed an atherogenic diet for about 40 months. Many of the plaques have a glistening white surface

The coronary artery atherosclerosis of the African green monkeys affected the proximal main branches with the main truck of the coronary artery being more commonly affected. The plaques occupied about 10 to 15% of the lumen, were focally distributed and did not extend into the small intramyocardial branches. The atherosclerotic plaques of the coronary arteries in this species had a well defined fibromuscular cap, gruel, lipid clefts, vascularization, and medial thinning.

The stump-tailed macaques had more extensive aortic atherosclerosis. Grossly, they too had plaques that resembled fibrous or pearly plaques of human beings (Fig. 3). Histologically, mineralization, vascularization, medial thinning, lipid clefts, and fibromuscular caps were found in all sections examined from the lesions. The lesions in this species had a multilayered, interlacing and overlapping appearance that gave the impression of the lesions being formed in successive layers.

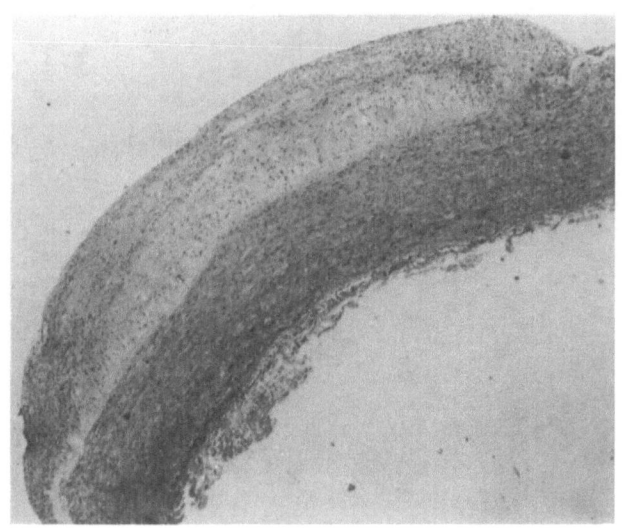

Figure 2. An aortic plaque from an African green monkey. There are many lipid clefts near the intima-media junction covered by a fibromuscular cap. H & E original magnification X 8

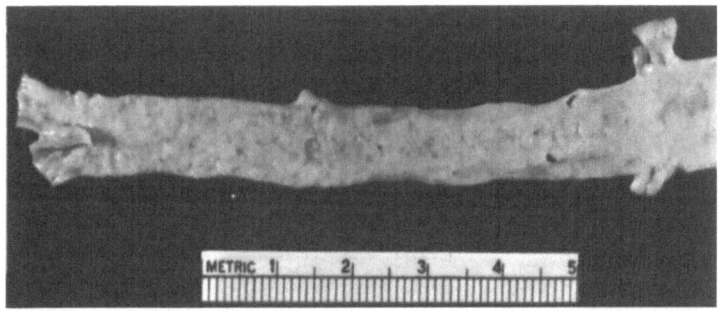

Figure 3. The abdominal aorta from a stump-tailed macaque fed an atherogenic diet for about 40 months. There are confluent plaues covering most of the intimal surface. Some plaques have a glistening white surface

Similarly, the stump-tailed macaques had the more extensive coronary artery atherosclerosis of the two species. The major coronary arteries and their extramural branches were sclerotic from the ostia to the point where smaller branches originated. The affected arteries were yellow, nodular, and had rigid walls. The lesions tended to occupy about 75% of the lumen of the coronary arteries (Fig. 4). In this species the media of the coronary artery was rather markedly affected. The smooth muscle cells of the media were decreased in number and usually separated by or replaced by collagenous tissue.

In summary, these two species of nonhuman primates would appear to be useful models for studying the transformation of fatty streaks to fibrous plaques.

293

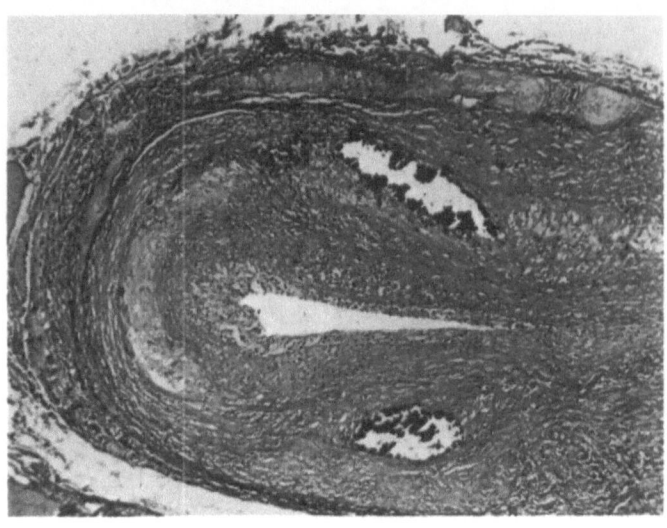

Figure 4. The left anterior descending coronary artery from a stump-tailed macaque. The lumen is markedly narrowed and the media is thin and fibrotic at bottom
of the photomicrograph. There is a relatively amorphous pool of lipid to the left
and two dark areas of mineralization. Verhoeff van Gieson original magnification
X 21)

RABBIT ARTERIOSCLEROSIS - THE DIET IMMUNOLOGIC INJURY MODEL

C. Richard Minick

Rabbits have been used for many years as animal models for the study of atherosclerosis. However, many have felt that both the morphology and anatomic distribution of the lesions were somewhat unlike the human disease. It has been shown
recently that the synergy of immunologic injury and hypercholesterolemia can lead
to atherosclerosis in rabbits which shares many characteristics with human atherosclerosis (Minick et al., 1966; Hardin et al., 1973; Minick and Murphy, 1973).

In these experiments, immunologic injury to arteries is induced by intravenous
injections of horse serum for intervals of 16-18 days. The diets used to study
the synergy with hypercholesterolemia have been modest, inducing serum cholesterol
concentrations between 200 and 250 mg/dl.

Rabbits fed a lipid-rich cholesterol-poor diet, and given concomitant injections
of foreign protein over a period as long as 17 months developed coronary artery
lesions that consisted both of a proliferative fibromuscular intimal thickening
(much like the thickened intimas commonly seen in man) and fatty-proliferative
fibromuscular intimal thickenings that bore a striking resemblance to coronary
atherosclerosis of human beings. Subsequent experiments provided evidence that
immunologically induced fibromuscular intimal lesions induced in rabbits would in
later life preferentially accumulate lipids in the presence of hypercholesterolemia.

Examples of the striking similarity of the lesions produced by the combined action
of diet and immunologic injury with those of man are presented in Fig. 6.

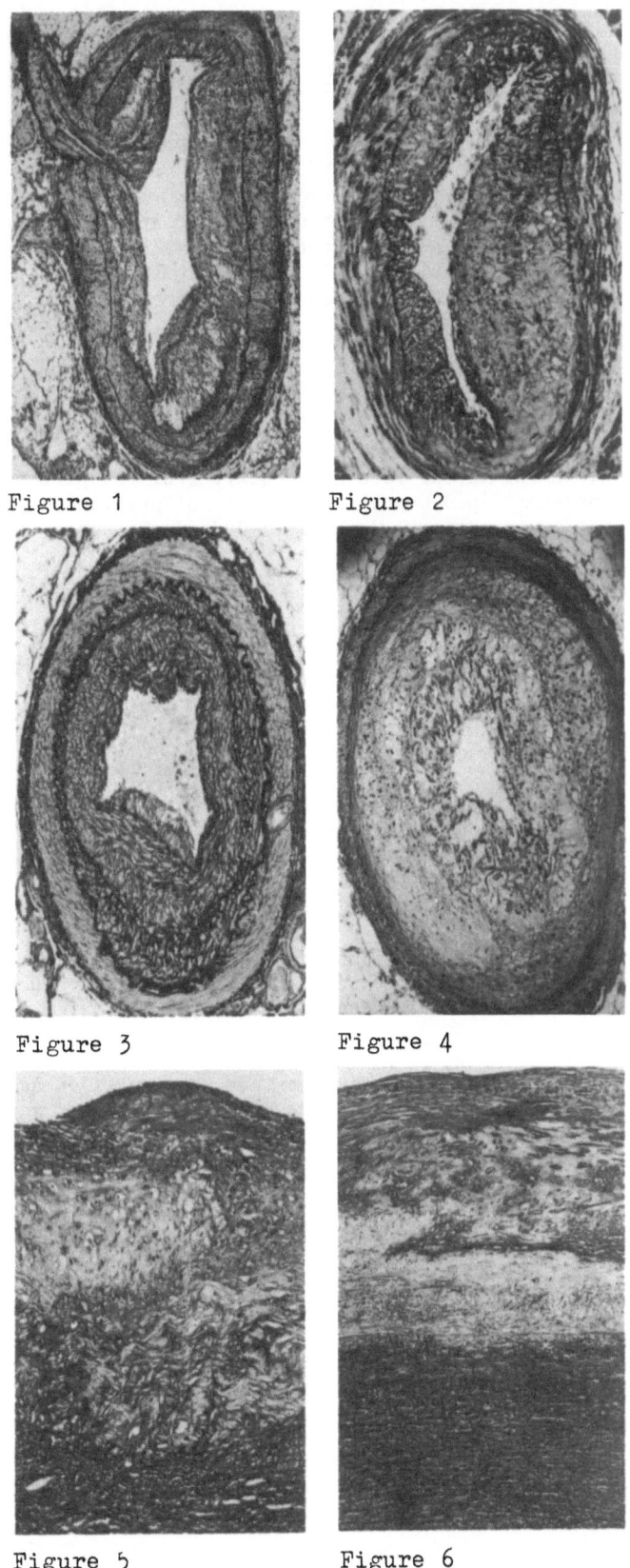

Figure 1

Figure 2

Figure 3

Figure 4

Legends see page 296

Figure 5

Figure 6

Figures see page 295

Figure 1. Atherosclerosis of left coronary artery of a rabbit that received a
semi-synthetic lipid-rich diet and 13 injections of foreign serum protein over
a period of 13 months. Fatty-proliferative changes with pooling of lipid overlie
a layer of musculo-elastic intimal thickening. Weigert-hematoxylin and eosin x 28,8
(Reproduced with permission from Minick, C.R. and Murphy, G.E. Am.J.Path. *73*: 265,
1973)

Figure 2. Atherosclerosis of left coronary artery of a rabbit that received a
semi-synthetic, lipid-rich diet and 13 injections of horse serum over a period of
16 months. Proliferative, fatty-proliferative and hyaline thickening of the
intima with cholesterol clefts deep in the intima. Fatty-proliferative intimal
thickening in the left upper quarter of the picture and right lower portion may
represent lipid deposit in regions of preexisting intimal change like that in the
left lower quarter. Verhoeff X 115 (Reproduced with permission from Minick, E.R.
and Murphy, G.E., Am.J.Path. *73*: 265, 1973)

Figure 3. Arteriosclerosis, without manifest lipid, of superior mesenteric artery
of a rabbit that received lipid-poor diet and 5 injections of horse serum over a
two month period. Cholesterol-supplemented diet was instituted 40 days after last
serum injection and continued for 80 days. Weigert-hematoxylin and eosin X 72
(Reproduced with permission from Hardin, N.J., Minick, C.R. and Murphy, G.E., Am.
J.Path. *73*: 301, 1973)

Figure 4. Atherosclerosis of a nearby segment of the artery referred to in
Fig. 3. Data from this experiment indicate that rabbit atherosclerosis like that
shown in Fig.4 evolved as follows: 1. that in the presence of normal serum
cholesterol sites of immunological arterial injury healed to evolve as fibromuscular intimal thickening like that shown in Fig.3, and 2. that later, in the
presence of hypercholesterolemia, some of these immunologically induced fibromuscular intimal lesions preferentially accumulated lipid. Weigert-hematoxylin
and eosin X 72 (Reproduced with permission from Hardin, N.J., Minick, C.R. and
Murphy, G.E., Am.J.Path. *73*: 73-301, 1973)

Figure 5. Arch of aorta of rabbit that received semi-synthetic, lipid-rich diet
and 12 injections of foreign serum protein over a period of 15 months. Note close
resemblance of rabbit arteriosclerosis to human arteriosclerosis shown in Fig.6.
Hematoxylin and eosin X 45 (Reproduced with permission from Minick, C.R. and
Murphy, G.E., Am.J.Path. *73*: 265, 1973)

Figure 6. Aortic arteriosclerosis in 62 year old man. Fatty-proliferative and
fatty-hyaline intima and medial change. Note close resemblance of human aortic
arteriosclerosis to rabbit atherosclerosis in Fig. 5. Hematoxylin and eosin X 36
(Reproduced with permission from Minick, C.R. and Murphy, G.E., Am.J.Path. *73*:
265, 1973)

NATURALLY OCCURRING AND INDUCED ARTERIAL LESIONS IN ANIMALS

G. A. Gresham

Professor Gresham pointed out one of the difficulties in the study of the morphology of atherosclerosis in both man and animals as being the great diversity in lesions. By the proper selection of examples from either man or an animal model almost any point could be made. Since the first International Symposium on Atherosclerosis, much work has been done both on the light and electron microscopic structure of the lesions of animals but it is as yet unclear whether major emphasis should be on the fatty streak, fibrous plaque, the complicated plaque, or perhaps changes that go on in the arterial wall even before the appearance of fatty streaks.

In order to illustrate the diversity of lesions that occur among the animal species, observations made by Professor Gresham and Dr. Alan Howard that dealt both with naturally occurring and induced atherosclerosis were discussed. In selecting examples from animals, Professor Gresham attempted to provide support for the notion that the pathogenesis of atherosclerosis involves first some transudation of plasma constituents into the arterial wall, and then a reactive proliferation by the arterial wall itself.

The first example to be cited was the arteriosclerosis that occurs in the abdominal aorta of rapidly growing Broad-Breasted Bronze and Beltsville White turkeys (Gresham and Howard, 1961). Both of these breeds of turkeys are hypertensive as compared with wild turkeys and other breeds of turkeys in which arteriosclerosis does not occur, and among the Broad-Breasted Bronze and Beltsville White dissecting aneurysms of the aorta occur frequently at the site of the arterial lesion and deaths due to this disorder are common (Clarkson et al., 1965). The intimal lesion seen in turkeys is one with marked proliferation of smooth muscle cells and ground substance material with rather minimal amounts of lipid. In order to better understand the pathogenesis of the turkey lesion, Professor Gresham and his coworkers examined the aortas of newly hatched and embryonic turkeys using electron microscopy. These studies suggested that intracytoplasmic inclusions of lipid within the smooth muscle cells of the intima shortly after hatching was the earliest change seen.

Thinking that this observation suggested that the earliest change might be an insudation or a transudation of plasma lipid, Professor Gresham and his group extended their observations to certain of the nonhuman primates (Gresham and Howard, 1965). The first baboon *(Papio cynocephalus)* studied by their group, was one that had been used earlier at Cambridge in immunologic studies. The animal that was being studied had been given several intravenous injections of Evans Blue as a part of the immunologic study, and it was of interest to them to note that the accumulation of the Evans Blue in the intima was generally in the area where fatty streaks were occurring, suggesting an altered permeability. Additional lesions from baboons were illustrated to point out the variety and morphology. Lesions in both the aorta and the coronary arteries varied from focal accumulations of foam cells to other lesions that were predominatly proliferated smooth muscle cells with little or no demonstrable lipid.

For comparison the gross distribution of aortic atherosclerosis in swine was illustrated, and it was pointed out that the areas affected by lesions are the same areas in which platelet thrombi occur when these aortas are profused *in vitro*, suggesting, at least in this model, the possibility of mural thrombi being involved in the early pathogenesis. Once again, it was pointed out that pigs like the nonhuman primates are quite variable, with the amount of cellular material in plaque varying from a little to a large amount. In the experience of the Cambridge group the accumulation of foci of medial calcification among the swine was not uncommon but was believed to have little to do with their atherosclerosis.

In summarizing, Professor Gresham put forth a hypothesis that the early lesion was a transudation of plasma constitutents into the subendothelial spaces giving rise to a proliferative process, and that perhaps more emphasis should be given to the metabolism of the cells rather than their precise identity or morphology.

SWINE AS A MODEL FOR ATHEROSCLEROSIS

R. Foster Scott

It is well established that swine, either the miniature strain or the more common Yorkshire strain, are satisfactory models for use in atherosclerosis research. Purely dietary methods of producing atherosclerotic lesions and the characteristics of the lesions themselves have been well covered in previous reports. In this workshop two new swine models will be described, and emphasis will be placed on what has been learned from these models.

Recently severe coronary atherosclerosis with occlusive lesions has been induced in swine within 5 to 6 months by two different procedures. Both procedures use an atherogenic diet high in cholesterol fed for 5 to 6 months. In one of the models on day 90 and 120 of the diet the swine receive 1500 rads of radiation to the precordium (Lee et al., 1971). In the other method, just before being placed on the atherogenic diet, the coronary arteries are ballooned for a distance of 1-2 cms from the ostia (Nam et al., 1973). A Fogarty catheter is inserted into the coronary arteries, the balloon inflated and then the catheter is withdrawn, denuding the coronary artery endothelium. The results of the two procedures are similar. The resultant arterial lesions resemble the occlusive atheroma lesions seen in human coronary arteries and often cause large through and through myocardial infarcts. Most of the swine die suddenly. In some cases it has been possible to assess the electrical activity of the heart in the agonal phase. In such cases, more than two thirds of the swine have died in ventricular fibrillation, sometimes preceded by bradycardia and premature ventricular contractions.

Now to turn to some of the things learned from using swine as models for atherosclerosis research. The work to be described deals with the bioenergetic state of the ischemic myocardia of swine with advanced coronary atherosclerosis, and myocardial infarcts prone to sudden death. In one study we used the above described diet - x-irradiated model and measured levels of high energy phosphate compounds and lactate in the ischemic myocardium. In addition, acceptor control ratios (ACR), O_2 uptake, and cytochrome oxidase activity were measured in mitochondria from myocardia of swine with advanced atherosclerosis. To determine if the hypercholesterolemia or x-irradiation alone affected myocardial mitochondrial function, swine receiving these regimens alone were investigated. In the myocardia served by atherosclerotic coronary arteries, the high energy compounds adenosine triphosphate (ATP) and creatine phosphate (CP) were significantly lower than in stock swine while lactate levels were higher (Table 1). Studies of myocardial mitochondrial function in these same animals showed decreased acceptor control ratios (ACR) or O_2 uptake or both using glutamate, ß-OH butyrate or succinate as substrate; when pyruvate malate was used as substrate, no abnormalities were found (Table 2). Measurements of cytochrome oxidase, an enzyme specific to mitochondria, showed a significantly lower amount of this enzyme in whole heart tissue, as well as a decreased yield of mitochondria recovered from the ischemic myocardia. Studies of swine made hypercholesterolemic or swine receiving x-irradiation alone revealed no abnormalities of ACR or O_2.

Table 1. High energy phosphate compounds[a], and lactate in normal and ischemic myocardia

	Normal 4		Ischemic 4
ATP	4.54 (± 0.10)[b]	←——→ [c]	3.42 (± 0.41)
ADP	0.66 (± 0.04)		0.49 (± 0.07)
AMP	0.04 (± 0.005)		0.07 (± 0.019)
C.P.	8.41 (± 0.52)	←——→	3.71 (± 0.76)
Lactate	2.16 (± 0.40)	←——→	5.95 (± 1.33)

[a] $\mu mol/g$ wet wt of myocardium.   [b] ± = S.E.M.   [c] ←——→ = significantly different at $p < 0.05$ or less.

Table 2. Mitochondrial ACR and O_2 uptake in normal and ischemic myocardia of diet-fed x-irradiated swine

Substrate	Normal 6		Ischemic 6
Glutamate			
ACR	21 (± 2.0)[a]	←——→ [b]	12.2 (± 1.9)
QO_2	232 (± 17)	←——→	151 (± 22)
ß-OH Butyrate			
ACR	12.8 (± 0.7)	←——→	7.7 (± 1.3)
QO_2	162 (± 15)	←——→	99 (± 25)
Succinate			
ACR	2.85 (± 0.2)		2.77 (± 0.16)
QO_2	258 (± 22)	←——→	186 (± 14)
Pyruvate-Malate			
ACR	8.8 (± 0.8)		7.0 (± 0.7)
QO_2	151 (± 10)		133 (± 24)

[a] ± = S.E.M.   [b] ←——→ = significant at $p < 0.05$ or less.

The conclusions from this study were that in the ischemic myocardium of this particular swine model with advanced coronary atherosclerosis, there was mitochondial damage with both uncoupling of mitochondria and decreased O_2 uptake. The damage was so severe that there was a significant fall in high engergy phosphate compounds, with the myocardium switching to anaerobic glycolysis.

It was thought important to investigate mitochondrial function in another atherosclerotic swine model, and attempt to confirm the findings in the diet x-irradiated swine. We, therefore, conducted studies of myocardial mitochondrial function in swine fed an atherogenic diet after their coronary arteries had been ballooned. No x-irradiation was used. Either ACR or O_2 uptake or both were abnormal in myocardial mitochondria from the ballooned atherosclerotic swine using glutamate, succinate or ß-OH butyrate as substrates. As in the atherogenic x-irradiated swine, no mitochondrial abnormalities were found with pyruvate-malate as substrate (Table 3). In addition, cytochrome oxidase activity in the ballooned atherosclerotic swine were significantly lower in whole tissue and in isolated mitochondria. Despite the damage to mitochondria, however, the high energy phosphate compounds and lactate levels were not altered.

Table 3. Mitochondrial ACR and O_2 uptake in normal and ischemic myocardia of diet-fed ballooned swine

Substrate	Normal 7		Ischemic 7
Glutamate			
ACR	16.1 (± 1.3)[a]	←——→[b]	12.6 (± 1.5)
QO_2	183 (± 12)	←——→	153 (± 13)
ß-OH Butyrate			
ACR	12.4 (± 0.7)		10.4 (± 1.4)
QO_2	144 (± 16)	←——→	112 (± 15)
Succinate			
ACR	3.6 (± 0.4)		3.4 (± 0.4)
QO_2	255 (± 21)	←——→	208 (± 18)
Pyruvate-Malate			
ACR	10.9 (± 0.6)		7.8 (± 0.7)
QO_2	151 (± 8)	←——→	108 (± 8)

[a] ± = S.E.M.   [b] ←——→ = significant at $p < 0.05$ or less.

In summary, in both of these swine models then with advanced coronary artery atherosclerosis, there appear to be damage to myocardial mitochondria, presumably due to anoxia. Whether or not this is related to the findings of sudden death in these swine (and in humans with coronary atherosclerosis) is difficult to judge One possibility, however, is that the abnormalities of mitochondrial function impairs the function of the cardiac ion transport system, thus enhancing ventricular fibrillation.

ATHEROSCLEROSIS REGRESSION IN ANIMAL MODELS - MESENCHYMAL COMPLICATIONS

Mark L. Armstrong

Professor Mark Armstrong pointed out that diet induced atherosclerosis of rhesus monkeys and perhaps other species can be favorably influenced by dietary changes. However, there are other pathologic processes involving the mesenchymal elements of arteries that may not be so favorably influenced. An experiment conducted at the University of Iowa was described (Armstrong et al., 1970; Armstrong and Megan, 1972). In that experiment, rhesus monkeys were fed a cholesterol containing diet for 17 months (with serum cholesterol concentrations of about 700 mg/dl), the baseline extent of atherosclerosis determined in a representative group of monkeys, and the remaining animals fed a control ration for 40 months that maintained their serum cholesterol concentrations at about 135 mg/dl. After 40 months, stenosis of the lumens of coronary arteries was markedly decreased, stainable lipid as observed microscopically was decreased, as well as free and ester cholesterol concentrations as determined analytically. Similarly, changes were noted in other muscular arteries such as the tibial artery.

It was pointed out that although the size of the plaques was smaller and they contained less lipid, the calcium and collagen concentrations of the remaining plaques appeared increased. The problems that remain after achieving the early stages of regression were enumerated, the residual intimal thickening may continue to obliterate 50 to 75% of the affected artery, physiologically there is reduced compliance of the artery, and stimuli may remain for continued fibrogenesis or perhaps for the continued stimulation of smooth muscle proliferation.

In summary, there was a brief discussion of the use of such agents as penicillamine and colchicine in preventing fibroblastic activity during regression. While it was viewed as a highly promising research direction, their value in the treatment of atherosclerosis remains to be demonstrated.

CHOLESTEROL METABOLISM. ACUTE CHANGES IN THE HEPATIC DEGRADATION OF CHOLESTEROL

M.R. Malinow

In research on atherosclerosis, animal models are useful for studying not only arterial lesions, but also cholesterol metabolism. Unlike most studies of cholesterol metabolism, which deal with long-term changes, our investigations have focused on some mechanisms which induce acute changes in the degradation of cholesterol by the liver.

In the experiments to be reported here adult male Sprague-Dawley rats were fed Purina rat chow pellets and water *ad libitum* up to the time of the experiment. Eight animals were randomly assigned to each of the groups shown in Tables 1 through 3, which also describe the experimental design. On any given day, one or more rats from each group in a series were studied. Since methods have been reported elsewhere (Malinow and McLaughlin, 1972), only the main features will be discussed here.

Rats were anesthetized with sodium pentobarbital i.p. (4 mg/100 g); additional anesthesia was injected intravenously as needed. Saline was infused with a Harvard Infusion Pump into a cannulated lateral tail vein at the rate of 0.034 ml/min. The abdomen was then opened, and in the appropriate groups of animals, the adrenal glands were resected; in sham-operated controls, they were exposed and handled. Both the adrenalectomized and the sham-operated rats were injected subcutaneously with 5 mg of cortisone (Cortisone acetate, Upjohn) or 0.2 ml of saline. The bile duct was ligated and cannulated with polyethylene tubing (PE 10). The distal end of the bile duct was also cannulated and the tubing advanced about 1 cm into the intestine; bile obtained from donor rats was infused by means of a Harvard Pump at the rate of 0.009 ml/min. At 20-minute intervals, the volume of bile that had collected in a graduate tube was recorded and the difference between the amount infused and the amount secreted was injected through the distal cannula. Animals with bile flows lower than 1 ml/90 min were eliminated and replaced.

Infusion of ascorbic acid in saline, with or without added drugs, as well as hindleg stimulation by repeated electrical pulses (Malinow and McLaughlin, 1972), was begun 15 minutes before the cholesterol injection and continued throughout the observation. At 0 time, about 2µCi of $1a$, $2a$, ^{3}H-cholesterol incorporated into

Table 1. Effect of adrenalectomy on the incorporation of radioactive cholesterol into bile acids. Each group consists of 8 rats; all animals infused with saline (0.034 ml/min) (Mean ± S.E.)

Series, group		Experimental	Subcutaneous injection		Body Weight	Bile flow	Bile acid radioactivity	
			Cortisone (5 mg)	Saline (0.2 ml)		(ml/90 min)	(% injected dose/ 90 min)	(relative secretion)
I	a	sham operation		X	286 ± 6	1.38 ± 0.10	1.60 ± 0.09	100
	b	adrenalectomy	X		288 ± 4	1.46 ± 0.07	1.08 ± 0.10[a]	67
	c	stimulated, sham operation		X	281 ± 4	2.04 ± 0.12[b]	2.67 ± 0.14[b]	167
	d	stimulated, adrenalectomy	X		292 ± 4	1.91 ± 0.16[c]	1.62 ± 0.24 N.S.	100
II	a	sham operation	X		292 ± 6	1.42 ± 0.09	2.15 ± 0.17	100
	b	sham operation	X		304 ± 8	1.60 ± 0.11	1.98 ± 0.25 N.S.	92
	c	adrenalectomy		X	305 ± 7	1.71 ± 0.12	1.61 ± 0.14[d]	74
	d	adrenalectomy	X		304 ± 9	1.52 ± 0.14	1.46 ± 0.16[c]	68

Student's "t" test (vs. corresponding controls (a)) N.S. non significant

[a] p <0.01. [b] p <0.001. [c] p <0.02. [d] p <0.05.

1 ml of rat plasma lipoproteins (Malinow and McLaughlin, 1972) were injected into the tail vein. The amount of labeled plasma injected was determined by weighing the syringe before and after use; the average density of rat plasma had been previously determined.

An alcohol:acetone (1:1, v/v) extract of the plasma was used to measure the radioactivity of the cholesterol. The free cholesterol was precipitated with digitonin and after drying, the washed precipitate was dissolved in dioxane and transferred to counting vials by use of the scintillator fluid (Malinow and McLaughlin, 1972). Free cholesterol radioactivity constituted 80-90% of total plasma radioactivity (Malinow and McLaughlin, 1972).

After the injection of radioactive cholesterol, bile was collected for 90 minutes in a graduated glass-stoppered centrifuge tube, and the volume was recorded and adjusted to 5.0 ml with distilled water. After the addition of Bio-Solv:toluene scintillator fluid (1:10), the radioactivity in duplicate 0.2 ml aliquots was assayed. The radioactivity of the digitonin precipitable fraction of the bile was determined on a suitable aliquot of a methanol:acetone (1:1, v/v) extract by basically the same procedure that was used for plasma.

The radioactivity incorporated into bile acids was calculated as the difference between the total radioactivity of bile and the digitonin-precipitated radioactivity (Malinow and McLaughlin, 1972). This method gives values which correspond closely to the values determined in bile acids separated by thin-layer chromatography (Malinow and McLaughlin, 1972). The results were expressed as the percent of injected labeled, nonesterified cholesterol since the free fraction apparently is the precursor of bile acids (Ogura et al., 1971).

Assays of radioactivity were carried out with a Packard Tri-Carb Liquid Scintillator Spectrometer, Model 3003. The figures were computed according to concurrent standards as disintegrations/ min by an automatic external standardization method. The data were punched directly from the scintillation spectrometer onto IBM cards and fitted to appropriate regression curves by a special program on XDS 902 computer.

For greater clarity, the observations in all animals have been rearranged without regard to chronological order (Tables 1 through 3).

Variations Between Control Groups

The results of five control groups from series III through VII were tested with one-way analysis of variance. These groups differed significantly (p "F" test <0.005) in the incorporation of cholesterol into bile acids. The variations probably represent intraspecies heterogeneity as well as nonuniformity in body weight (p "F" test < 0.005) and bile flow (p "F" test < 0.005). However, when two groups of control rats were studied in the same series (series VII, groups a and j), no differences in the secretion of labeled bile acids were observed. Similar results were obtained when these animals were rearranged in two groups, one corresponding to rats studied early in the morning and the other rats studied later in the day. Moreover, no differences in the secretion of radioactive bile acids were observed between rats infused with saline or with 0.1% ascorbic acid in saline (series III, groups a and f).

Effect of Adrenalectomy

In the animals of series I, adrenalectomy depressed by one-third the incorporation of cholesterol into bile acids but without changing the bile flow (Table 3). Repeated stimulation of the hind legs increased the secretion of radioactive bile acids by 67% and of bile flow by 39%, but adrenalectomy prevented the increase in bile acids even with an elevated bile flow. In similar experiments in series II,

Table 2. Effect of catecholamines and an adrenergic drug on the incorporation of radioactive cholesterol into bile acids in rats receiving 0.1% ascorbic acid in saline (0.034 ml/min). Each group consists of 8 animals (Mean ± S.E.)

Series, group		Drug infused	Dose (ug/min)	Body Weight (g)	Bile flow (ml/90 min)	Bile acid radioactivity (% of injected dose/90 min)	(relative secretion)
III	a	control		243 ± 7	1.29 ± 0.08	2.75 ± 0.13	100
	b	Epinephrine	0.25	238 ± 6	1.32 ± 0.08	3.81 ± 0.16^a	138
	c	Norepinephrine	0.07	239 ± 7	1.29 ± 0.08	2.89 ± 0.18 N.S.	105
	d	Dopamine	2.8	238 ± 5	1.61 ± 0.14	4.04 ± 0.31^b	147
	e	Mephentermine	0.68	242 ± 6	1.23 ± 0.09	2.81 ± 0.11 N.S.	102
	f	saline infused		238 ± 8	1.27 ± 0.07	2.71 ± 0.09 N.S.	
IV	a	control		279 ± 3	1.55 ± 0.09	3.75 ± 0.18	100
	b	Epinephrine	0.25	273 ± 4	1.46 ± 0.06	4.44 ± 0.19^c	118
V	a	control (7)^e		276 ± 4	1.32 ± 0.05	2.38 ± 0.09	100
	b	Norepinephrine	0.25	276 ± 4	1.56 ± 0.05^b	3.33 ± 0.23^b	139
	c	Dopamine (7)^e	2.8	276 ± 5	1.74 ± 0.15^c	3.13 ± 0.27^d	131
VI	a	control		254 ± 3	1.22 ± 0.05	2.39 ± 0.14	100
	b	Dopamine	2.8	252 ± 4	1.32 ± 0.05	2.99 ± 0.18^c	124
	c	Epinephrine plus Mephentermine	0.25, 0.68	257 ± 3	1.37 ± 0.10	3.02 ± 0.17^c	126

Student's "t" test (vs. corresponding controls (a)) N.S. non significant

^{a} $p < 0.001$. ^{b} $p < 0.01$. ^{c} $p < 0.02$. ^{d} $p < 0.05$.

304

Table 3. Effect of different amounts of catecholamines on the incorporation of radioactive cholesterol into bile acids in rats receiving 0.1% ascorbic acid in saline (0.034 ml/min). Each group consists of 8 animals (Mean ± S.E.)

Series, group	Drug infused	Dose (µg/min)	Body weight (g)	Bile flow (ml/90 min)	Bile acid radioactivity (% injected dose/90 min)	(relative secretion)
VII a	control		309 ± 9	1.58 ± 0.08	1.75 ± 0.09	100
b	Epinephrine	0.25	312 ± 8	1.46 ± 0.06	2.32 ± 0.06[a]	133
c	Epinephrine	0.125	312 ± 7	1.32 ± 0.09	2.15 ± 0.14[b]	123
d	Epinephrine	0.062	319 ± 7	1.52 ± 0.09	2.07 ± 0.17 N.S.	118
e	Norepinephrine	0.15	310 ± 8	1.65 ± 0.10	2.12 ± 0.15[b]	122
f	Norepinephrine	0.075	317 ± 8	1.61 ± 0.11	2.03 ± 0.10[b]	116
g	Dopamine	2.8	313 ± 11	1.81 ± 0.17	2.03 ± 0.12 N.S.	116
h	Dopamine	1.4	316 ± 9	1.67 ± 0.10	2.26 ± 0.14[b]	130
i	Dopamine	0.7	310 ± 12	1.57 ± 0.11	1.96 ± 0.14 N.S.	112
j	repeat control		319 ± 6	1.68 ± 0.09	1.78 ± 0.11 N.S.	100

Student's "t" test (vs. control a) N.S., non significant

[a] $p < 0.001$.   [b] $p < 0.05$.

the effect of cortisone injection was studied and the animals of groups (a) and (b) were compared. Cortisone did not change the parameters measured here in either group. On the other hand, adrenalectomy with or without added cortisone depressed by 25% to 32% the incorporation of cholesterol into bile acids. Bile flow in the experimental groups did not differ from that in the controls II (a).

Effect of Catecholamines and of Mephentermine

Epinephrine (0.25 µg/min), norepinephrine (0.25 µg/min), and dopamine (2.8 µg/min) increased the secretion of radioactive bile acids (Table 2). These effects were not observed with norepinephrine at a lower dosage (0.07 µg/min) or with mephentermine (0.68 µg/min). The effect of this last drug used with epinephrine was not different from that of epinephrine alone. Dopamine (0.68 µg/min) and norepinephrine (0.25 µg/min), but not the other substances tested in this series, increased bile flow.

Table 3 shows the results of infusing different amounts of catecholamines. Epinephrine (0.25 and 0.125 µg/min) increased the incorporation of cholesterol into the bile acids, but not when given at the rate of 0.062 µg/min. Norepinephrine increased the biliary secretion of radioactive bile acids at the two levels tested, and dopamine did so at the 1.4 µg/min level; the results observed with 2.8 µg/min were at the margin of statistical significance. The increases varied between 16 and 33% of the control levels. No consistent changes in bile flow were detected in the experimental groups.

In summary, our results indicate that removal of the adrenal glands decreased the incorporation of radioactive cholesterol into bile acids in resting animals and prevented the rise observed with repeated contractions of the skeletal musculature (Malinow and McLaughlin, 1972; Malinow et al., 1968). These results agree with previous findings in rats injected with ^{14}C-26-cholesterol in which adrenalectomy decreased the amount of expired $^{14}CO_2$ (Malinow et al., 1969). Both experiments were performed immediately after adrenalectomy; since the animals also received cortisone, there was no lack of adrenal corticoids. Consequently, the observed effects of adrenalectomy are apparently due to the lack of medullary hormones. That these effects resulted from adrenalectomy and not from the administration of cortisone was demonstrated in the animals of series II, where cortisone in sham-operated and in adrenalectomized rats had no effect on the incorporation of radioactive cholesterol into bile acids. Moreover, adrenalectomy depressed the incorporation in rats with and without cortisone injection. The increased secretion of radioactive bile acids after the infusion of catecholamines—epinephrine, norepinephrine, and dopamine—offers additional evidence that the medullary hormones are involved in the incorporation of cholesterol into bile acids. Our observations also indicate that catecholamines modify the incorporation of cholesterol into bile acids independently of any choleretic effect. Since mephentermine at the dosage used did not modify the secretion of labeled bile acids, the results seem restricted to catecholamines; other substances with adrenergic activity should be studied to establish a correlation between the structure of these compounds and their effect on bile acids.

Whether the effects of the catecholamines used here were physiologic or pharmacologic is difficult to decide. However, the fact that adrenalectomy depressed the incorporation of cholesterol into radioactive bile acids suggests that the catecholamines play a role in controlling the degradation of cholesterol in the liver of the intact animal. How they do so is not yet known.

When adrenalin is injected with oil, cholesterolemia is elevated in several species (Kaplan et al., 1957; Shafrir et al., 1959, 1960). Moreover, epinephrine stimulates heptatic HMG-coA reductase (Edwards, 1973), and thus, probably accelerates the synthesis of cholesterol. Long-term experiments are needed to establish the effects of administering various levels of specific catecholamines on bile acid secretion; moreover, even these short-term observations suggest that catecholamines could lower levels of plasma cholesterol by increasing its conversion into bile acids. However, the effect of catecholamines on the mass of cholesterol pools may depend on their ability to modify processes that tend to stimulate the synthesis and degradation of cholesterol.

ANIMAL MODELS OF ATHEROSCLEROSIS AND/OR MYOCARDIAL INFARCTION

A.N. Howard

Spontaneous Disease

Many species exhibit spontaneous arterial disease of the aorta and coronary arteries (Clarkson, 1972) and these provide useful models for study. Among the species which are of special interest are the carneau pigeon, chicken and turkey; many types of primates (Stout and Lemmon, 1969; Lehner et al., 1971) and pigs (Ratcliffe and Luginbuhl, 1971). Whilst animals with spontaneous disease provide valuable material for biochemical and pathological study, they are often of limited use for an investigation of numerous factors which may aggravate or ameliorate the disease such as diet, hormones, exercise. The reason for this is that the extent and incidence of lesions between individual animals is often extremely varialbe, requiring large numbers for statistical analysis.

Often spontaneous disease is only manifest in mature animals whose availability may be limited and often whose size pose additional problems of housing and expense. Among primates, those caught in the wild are often of unknown history and age, the extent of arterial disease being indeterminant. Whilst not ignoring the contribution which a study of spontaneous disease can make, this review will be concerned chiefly with experimental methods for the induction of atherosclerosis, and techniques which are strongly favoured by current investigators in the field.

The Rationale Behind Experimental Techniques

In his monograph, Constantinides (1965) postulated that the extent of atherosclerosis could be explained on the basis of the following equation:

$$A = \sum (LI)\ pd + \sum t$$

where A = atherogenesis, L = lipaemia (excess over a minimal value), I = injury, p = arterial pressure, d = duration, t = thrombosis.

The object of various experimental techniques is to employ one or more of the above mentioned factors to provoke or intensify the disease. Namely, by creating hyperlipaemia, causing vessel injury, hypertension or thrombosis, the extent of the disease depending on the magnitude of the factors employed. A typical illustration of this concept can be seen in the baboon (Howard et al., 1971). Giving these animals a diet of egg yolk and butter caused only a moderate rise in serum cholesterol to 280 mg/100 ml (Table 1) and in the space of six months no aortic disease was evident. Likewise the injection of bovine serum albumin (BSA), a substance which causes immunological injury, into control animals, had no demonstrable effect on vascular pathology. However, the combination of hypercholesterolaemic diet and BSA produced extensive aortic sudanophilia and atherosclerosis. Neither the mild lipaemia nor injury alone were sufficient but both factors acted synergistically.

According to the Constantinides equation, injury must always be present for the first term to exist. Yet arterial disease is produced in many species purely by the induction of hypercholesterolaemia alone. The explanation is that hyperlipaemia is itself an injurious factor. Supporting evidence for this concept has been obtained recently using a variety of anti-inflammatory drugs. Cortisone, prednisone, phenylbutazone, fenflunamic acid all greatly reduced the extent of atherosclerosis in the cholesterol fed rabbit (Bailey and Butler, 1973). The activity of each of these compounds was in direct relation to their anti-inflammatory ability.

Also, it is not necessary for hyperlipaemia to be present for atherosclerotic lesions to be manifest. Where the type of injury is large extensive pathological changes occur even in normolipaemic animals (Bjorkerud and Bondjers, 1973). Nevertheless, other factors being equal, there is a correlation between plasma cholesterol and the extent of atherosclerosis. In the chicken the threshold for coronary atherosclerosis to appear is estimated to be 80 mg/100 ml plasma cholesterol (Kakita et al., 1972).

Table 1. Effect of hypercholesterolaemia and immunological injury in baboons (Howard et al., 1971)

Group	Diet[a]	Bovine[b] serum albumin	No.	Aortic Atherosclerosis		Mean plasma cholesterol
				No. affected	% area	
1	Hypercholesterolaemic	+	8	8	44	262
2	Hypercholesterolaemic	−	5	0	0	299
3	Control	+	5	0	0	122
4	Control	−	5	0	0	116

[a]250 mg/kg wt. i.v.
[b]Atherogenic diet: 15% egg yolk and 15% butter for 6 months.

Induction of Atherosclerosis by Dietary Cholesterol

1. New Species. Few species when challenged by dietary cholesterol will not respond and develop arterial lipid deposition. Thus the cat which was previously thought to be resistant (Manning and Clarkson, 1973) can be rendered hypercholesterolaemic by adding 2% dietary cholesterol; a level of 0.5% has little effect. After four months at the higher level, extensive aortic and coronary disease was found. Since the cat is of a convenient size and can be accommodated easily in large numbers, its experimental use warrants further investigation.

Calves fed 250 mg cholesterol/kg body weight for 24 weeks, particularly when included in milk, also showed similar disease (Wiggers et al., 1973). Whilst the expense of maintaining large animals might preclude their widespread use, the provision of large quantities of fresh diseased tissue, as in the case of the calf, is often needed in metabolic and analytical studies.

The versatility of the Japanese quail in consuming manifold hypercholesterolaemic diets has been demonstrated (Smith and Hilker, 1973). This species has a short life span, breeds rapidly and can be housed in large numbers. For experimental research in genetics and ageing there are advantages.

Although the rat is resistant to cholesterol feeding and requires dietary adjuvants (Howard and Gresham, 1968) for the induction of hypercholesterolaemia, some other rodents are more susceptible (Dieterich et al., 1973), as is also the guinea pig (Fujinami et al., 1971). Among primates, the spider monkey has been added to the list of those responsive to cholesterol feeding (Srinivasan et al., 1972; Pucak et al., 1973).

2. *Response to Cholesterol Genetics*. Even among different animals of the same species, a difference in response to dietary cholesterol is common. Thus, for a given dietary intake of cholesterol, New Zealand white rabbits develop a greater serum cholesterol than the Dutch strain (Adams et al., 1972). The Winston Salem group were able to divide squirrel monkeys into two groups:- hyper- or hypo-responders according to their ability to attain a serum cholesterol of 400 mg/100 ml, whilst consuming a standard cholesterol diet (Clarkson et al., 1971).

By cross breeding of hypo- and hyper-responders, about 92% of the individual variability could be attributed to genetic factors as illustrated by the figures in Table 2. Hyper-responsive monkeys had more advanced atherosclerosis. The ability to breed primates responding to lower levels of dietary cholesterol, presents distinct advantages - the levels may approximate those consumed by man. Moreover, a study of cholesterol metabolism in hyper- and hypo-responders can provide much information about the control of cholesterol turnover in a uniformly bred strain.

A small number of rats are moderately susceptible to cholesterol feeding. This trait is also genetic and a strain of highly susceptible rats is now a distinct possibility (Imai and Matsumura, 1973). Their general availability could have a significant effect on the future use of the rat in experimental atherosclerosis.

Table 2. Genetics and hypercholesterolaemia squirrel monkeys (Clarkson et al., 1971)

Parents	No. of offspring	
	Hyper	Hypo
HYPER x HYPER	5	0
HYPER x HYPO	4	7
HYPO x HYPO	1	9
Dietary cholesterol 0.5%		

Serum cholesterol
Hyper-responder > 400 mg/100 ml
Hypo-responder   <   "

3. *Nutritional Factors*. Enhancement of hypercholesterolaemic activity is commonly achieved by a concomitant deficiency of essential fatty acids EFA). In confirmation of earlier work (Malmros and Sternby, 1968), Robertson et al. (1972) found that 16% hydrogenated coconut oil and 5% cholesterol gives advanced atherosclerosis in the dog after 12 - 16 months. EFA deficiency was evidenced by the presence of increased amounts of eicosatrienoic acid.

The abnormal properties of peanut oil were referred to in the last symposium (Howard, 1969). Kritchevsky et al. (1973) have attempted to characterise the atherogenic factor in peanut oil with only partial success. In rabbits given 1% cholesterol and 6% oils, the amount of aortic atherosclerosis was markedly higher in those fed peanut oil compared with corn oil (Table 3). Randomisation of the fatty acids abolished the effect. A synthetic fat resembling peanut oil was prepared by randomising a blend of olive oil, cotton seed oil, safflower oil, arachidic and behenic acids. This also showed an enhancing effect but not so marked as with native peanut oil. It is suggested that the position of the fatty acids in the glycerol molecule may be of importance. Native peanut oil has 54% linoleic acid in the 2-position compared with 33% for randomised oil.

Table 3. Peanut oil and rabbit atherosclerosis (Kritchevsky et al., 1973)

Dietary oil	Contained arachidic + behenic acid	Randomised	Atherosclerosis aortic grade
Peanut	+	-	1.59
Peanut	+	+	1.18
Corn	-	-	1.28
Corn	+	+	1.34
Olive) Cotton seed)PGF Safflower)	+	+	1.41
PGF	-	-	1.17

Diet: cholesterol 2%)
      oil   6%) for 8 weeks

The possible importance of dietary fibre has been emphasised by Trowell (1972), who drew attention to the low incidence of coronary heart disease among people consuming a high fibre diet. In a consideration of Indian pulses and cereals, Vijayagopal et al. (1973) came to the conclusion that those which showed high hypocholesterolaemic activity in the cholesterol - cholic acid fed rat were also high in fibre content. Although the experimental system is highly artificial, the correlation is high and the examination of more susceptible species is indicated.

The relationship between vitamin C remains a controversial topic. Scorbutic guinea pigs fed cholesterol show more lesions (Fujinami et al., 1971) but vitamin C when added to rabbits given atherogenic diets have no preventative effect, nor could earlier reports be confirmed that biotin was effective (Pool et al., 1971).

4. *Exercise*. Very few problems have provided such conflicting experimental results as the relationship between exercise and atherogenesis. However, the recent experiments of Link et al. (1972) in miniature pigs are particularly convincing. Two groups of animals were given an atherogenic diet containing 1% cholesterol and 10% cotton seed oil for 22-1/2 months. One group was exercised daily for approximately 10 minutes on a treadmill at about 10 miles/hour (16 km/hr), the other was not exercised. At the end of the experiment the numbers of pigs showing lesions was far greater in the non-exercised group (Table 4) and the disease was more severe. During the experiment, serum lipid levels were not excessively high being 120 mg/100 ml and 250 mg/100 ml serum cholesterol for males and females respectively. For males, this level was not much higher than pre-experimental controls on a normal diet. There was no difference in the serum lipids between the exercised and non-exercised groups. Such an important result needs confirmation and a renewed examination in other species.

5. *Species Differences*. The composition of serum lipoproteins in normal and hypercholesterolaemic baboons and chimpanzees has been studied in detail (Howard et al., 1972; Blaton et al., 1972; Peeters and Blaton, 1972) and compared with man. There

Table 4. Atherosclerosis and exercise in pigs (Link et al., 1972)

Sex	Exercise	Serum cholesterol	No.	Incidence of lesions				
				Aorta			Coronary	
				Thoracic	Abdominal		Left	Right
Male	+	120	8	2	3		1	0
	−	120	9	8	9		9	3
Female	+	250	9	3	7		2	0
	−	250	9	7	7		9	4

Exercise = 1.75 miles/day;
Diet: 1% cholesterol, 10% cotton seed oil;
Time: 22-1/2 months.

is a great similarity between the hyperlipoproteinaemia induced in these animals and type IIa disease in man, low density lipoproteins being chiefly elevated (Table 5). Among important similarities was that cholesterol oleate was increased more than linoleate and sphingomyelin was also increased. There was a greater similarity between chimpanzee and man, the baboon showing several important differences.

Table 5. Percentage lipid distribution in plasma α- and β-lipoproteins in man, baboon and chimpanzee (Howard et al., 1972)

Lipid	Sample	% Total lipid in sample					
		Man		Baboon		Chimpanzee	
		N	II	C	A	C	A
CE	plasma	41	46	47	50	44	52
	α-Lp	34	37	43	51	32	34
	β-Lp	46	50	52	50	52	57
F.chol.	plasma	12	12	6	7	9	11
	α-Lp	8	8	6	7	9	9
	β-Lp	14	13	6	7	9	12
TG	plasma	8	10	11	6	8	4
	α-Lp	9	12	7	4	6	6
	β-Lp	7	9	16	7	9	4
PL	plasma	39	33	36	37	40	33
	α-Lp	50	44	44	38	53	51
	β-Lp	33	28	26	36	30	27

N = normal; II = Type II hyperlipoproteinaemia; C = control; A = atherogenic diet;
CE = cholesterol ester; F.chol. = free cholesterol; TG = triglycerides;
PL = phosphatlipids.

The resistance of the rat to the development of atherosclerotic lesions, even in the presence of high serum cholesterol, remains an anomaly (Howard and Gresham, 1968). Presumably the rat arterial wall has protective properties. In an analysis of the aortic lysomal enzymes in several species (Fig. 1), Bonner et al. (1972) found that the activity was much higher in the rat than other more susceptible species. This resistance could be related to the ability of the aorta to metabolise and remove lipids and prevent deposition.

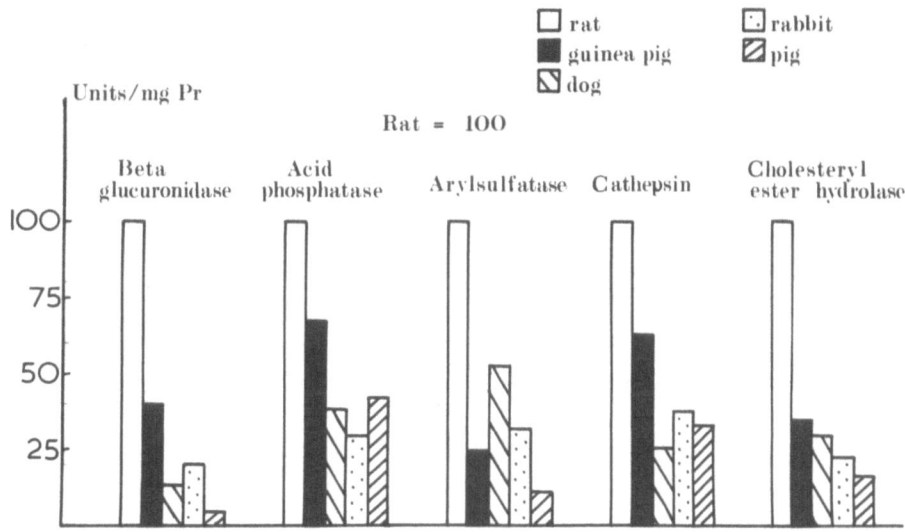

Figure 1. Lysosomal enzyme activity in aortas (Bonner et al., 1972)

Hypercholesterolaemia and Atherosclerosis Without Dietary Cholesterol

Rabbits, when given a semi-synthetic diet, develop hypercholesterolaemia and atherosclerosis. Although Malmros and Wigand (1959) claimed that the syndrome could be explained on the basis of an essential fatty acid deficiency, this appeared not to be the whole explanation (Howard, 1969). The situation has been clarified by Carroll (1971), who compared commercial and semi-synthetic diets to which were added fat of different unsaturation (Fig. 2). Saturated fat only increased hypercholesterolaemia in a semi-synthetic diet. Such an effect was also seen when casein was added to the commercial diet. Thus, the hypercholesterolaemia is due to a combination of factors: low polyunsaturated fatty acids and a high animal protein content. It should also be noted that vegetable protein will also show the same potentiating effect when in high concentration (25%, see Howard et al., 1965).

The mechanism of the hypercholesterolaemia is not clear. There is little cholesterol in the diet so the accumulation must result from body synthesis. Liver cholesterol synthesis is decreased (Fig. 2) but intestinal synthesis is unaffected (Kyd and Bouchier, 1972). The most likely defect is the ability of the animal to excrete cholesterol or its metabolites (Howard, 1969).

Saturated fat when added to commercial rations has also been reported to increase aortic and coronary atherosclerosis in miniature pigs (Dahme et al., 1971) but here the serum cholesterol levels are not markedly elevated

Injections of diethyl stilbestrol cause hyperlipaemia and atherosclerosis in the turkey (Simpson and Neilson, 1973; Krista et al., 1969) and chicken (Nichols et al., 1971). The elevation of serum lipids is due to increased very low density and chylomicrons, thus the syndrome resembles type V hyperlipoproteinaemia in man.

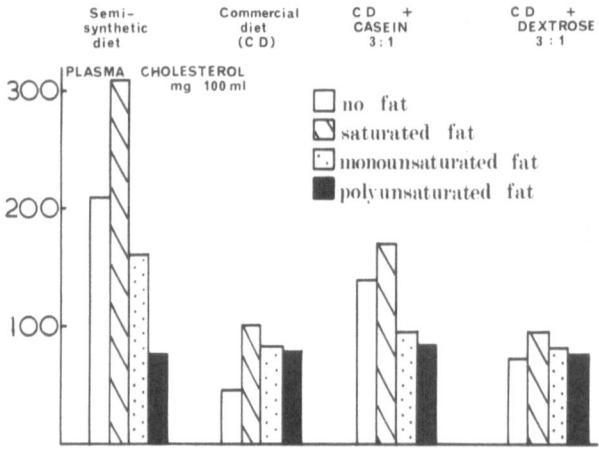

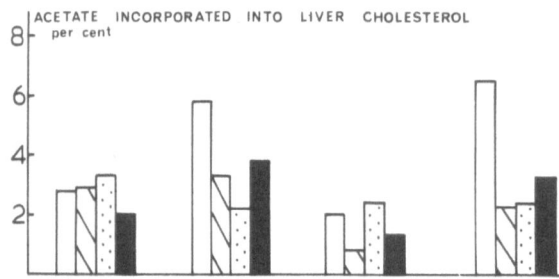

Figure 2. Plasma cholesterol and liver cholesterol biosynthesis in rabbits (Carroll, 1971)

Vessel Wall Injury

Numerous methods for inducing injury have been studied in recent work (Table 6). Certain types of mechanical injury are of special interest since lesions resembling early and late atherosclerosis and deposits of lipid can be seen even in normo-cholesterolaemic animals. The most extensive investigations are those of Bjorkerud and Bondjers (1971-73) using a diamond cutting instrument inserted into the aorta via the femoral artery. According to the type of cut, differences in pathology are seen (Fig. 3) and many of the features of human atherosclerosis reproduced. The system is a particularly valuable one since a study can be made of lesions at different stages. Their technique is easier to standardise than the similar injury due to inflated balloons (Stemmermann et al., 1972; Helin et al., 1971; Nam et al., 1973) based on the original technique devised by Baumgartner and Studer (1963).

Hypervitaminosis causes deposition of calcium in the media, and this combined with hypercholesterolaemia leads to severe atherosclerotic lesions in the rat. This system has been used to study the anti-arteriosclerotic properties of chondroitin sulphate (Morrison et al., 1972).

The damage caused by carbon monoxide is of great importance, since this has been implicated as the atherogenic factor in cigarette smoke. Kjeldsen et al. (1972) find that even short exposure of normolipaemic rabbits to carbon monoxide can

Table 6. Injury and atherosclerosis

Type	Species	Hyperlipaemia	Authors[a]	
Mechanical				
aortic dilation	rabbit, rat	−	Helin	(1971)
	pig	+	Jamolych	(1973)
cutting	rabbit	−	Bjorkerud	(1971-3)
polyethylene tubing	rabbit	−	Sumiyoshi	(1973)
Biochemical				
carbon monoxide	rabbit	−	Kjeldsen	(1972)
vitamin D	rat	+	Morrison	(1972)
Immunological				
protein antigens	baboon	+	Howard	(1972)
cardiac allographs	rat, rabbit	+	Laden	(1972)
Radiation				
X-rays	pig	+	Lee	(1971)
Infection				
Coxsackie virus	mice	−	Burch	(1971)
Thromboembolic				
autologous thrombi	pig	−	Craig	(1973)
Hypertension				
cellophane	rabbit	+	Campbell	(1973)
DOCA	rat	+	Still	(1970)
renal clip	rat	+	Daly	(1972)

[a]First named only; for complete list see references.

cause considerable damage to the endothelium leading to increased permeability, as judged by their electron microscope observation.

There is a renewed interest in injury caused by immunological damage. Injections of bovine serum albumin precipitates atherosclerosis in moderately hypercholesterolaemic baboons (Howard et al., 1971). The subject is of importance because of severe atheroma seen in human transplants (Kosek et al., 1971) which can be reproduced experimentally in hypercholesterolaemic rats and rabbits by cardiac allographs (Laden, 1972). It is not clear whether immune phenomena may play a part generally. Infection of mice with the coxsackie virus, for instance, will cause endothelial cell degeneration in the aorta and coronary arteries (Birch et al., 1971); as will also LCM virus (Kajima and Pollard, 1969). Complement is also implicated (Geertinger and Sorensen, 1972).

Other diverse types of injury employed were radiation with X-rays in pigs (Lee et al., 1971), injections of noradrenaline (Helin et al., 1970) autologous thrombi for causing pulmonary atherosclerosis in pigs (Craig et al., 1973) cerebral ischaemia in the rabbit (Tomus et al., 1971) injections of allylamine and egg yolk emulsions in the rabbit (Giordano et al., 1970), and insertion of polythene tubing (Sumiyoshi et al., 1973).

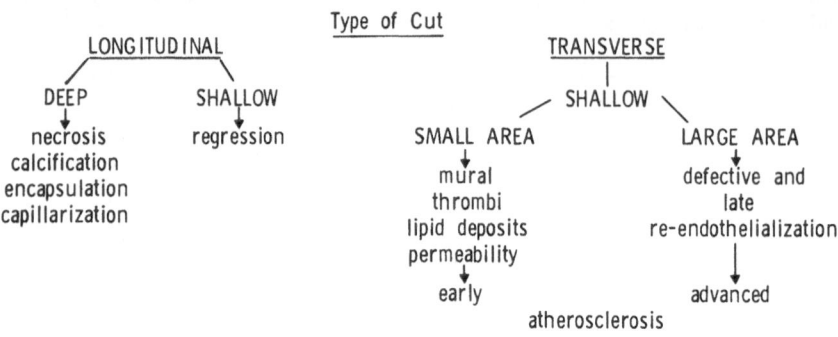

Figure 3. Mechanical injury in normal rabbit aorta (Björkerud and Bondjers, 1971-1973)

Hypertension is a valuable adjunct for intensifying atherosclerosis caused by hypercholesterolaemia. As might be predicted, the greater lipid accumulation is caused by a greater rate of entry. Techniques include nephrectomy and DOCA implantation (Still, 1970) wrapping the kidneys with cellophane in the rabbit (Campbell et al., 1973) and constricting the renal artery with silver clips (Daly, 1972).

Diabetes, Insulin and Atherosclerosis

The increased incidence of coronary heart disease in diabetics has stimulated a number of workers to examine the inter-relationship between diabetes, insulin and atherosclerosis in experimental animals. Rather surprisingly alloxan diabetic rabbits fed cholesterol show less atherosclerosis (Duff and McMillan, 1949; McGill and Holman, 1949). In contrast, disease is greater in the alloxan diabetic rat (Kalant et al., 1964; Still et al., 1964; Wexler, 1971) and squirrel monkey (Lehner et al., 1972).

Table 7. Effect of insulin in chickens (Stout et al., 1973)

| Injection | Serum | | Plasma | Intimal |
| | cholesterol   triglyceride | | glucagon | aortic grade |
	mg/100ml		ng/ml	
Control	161	119	0.9	0.4
Insulin (10 i.v./day)	210	186[a]	1.4[a]	2.1[a]

[a]Significant.

Recent interest has arisen because of the hypothesis of Stout et al. (1973) that insulin can stimulate lipid synthesis in the arterial wall. Studies with tissue culture of intimal cells have shown that insulin can enhance the incorporation of glucose into arterial lipids (Mahler and Parkes, 1970). In a continuation of these studies, chickens on a normal diet were injected with long acting insulin for 19 weeks, the occurrence and severity of spontaneous lesions was greatly increased (Table 7). However, the increased lipid deposition could be due to the elevated serum lipids rather than the direct action of insulin on arterial wall metabolism.

Other studies in hypercholesterolaemic chickens (Stamler et al., 1960) showed no differences with insulin injections, and in these experiments serum lipids were unaffected. Further work in this field is indicated since many diabetic subjects have elevated plasma insulin (Peters and Hales, 1965) in addition to that given in the course of treatment.

Regression of Atherosclerotic Lesions

The regression of lesions has tended to be neglected because of the long periods required to achieve results and there has been considerable doubt as to whether established aortic and coronary lesions could regress. In rabbit atheroma no regression can be seen after one year of transferring the animals to a normal diet (Adams et al., 1973) but some histological changes were noted (Gupta, 1970). However, this situation does not apply to other species. Armstrong (1972) gave rhesus monkeys a cholesterol containing diet for 17 months and then changed some of the animals to a control diet for 40 months. As shown in Table 8, there was considerable regression of the induced lesions and a decrease in both free and ester cholesterol. Such was the impression gained by Tucker et al. (1971) in a similar but shorter experiment. Lesions in carneau pigeons have also been demonstrated to regress (St. Clair, 1972). It is hoped that the situation in man is similar to the rhesus monkey and carneau pigeon rather than the rabbit.

Table 8. Regression of lesions in atherosclerotic rhesus monkeys (Armstrong and Megan, 1972)

	Lipid content of coronary arteries, mean mg/g dry wt.		
	Control	Atherosclerotic[a]	Regression[b]
Cholesterol			
Total	6.8	51.2	18.1
Ester	1.8	37.6	11.8
Free	5.1	13.6	6.3
Triglycerides	15.8	30.6	24.1
Phospholipids	27.1	36.6	34.2

[a]Atherogenic diet – 40% egg yolk lipids for 17 months.
[b]Regression diet – 40% calories corn oil for 40 months.

Experimental Myocardial Infarction

An early report of myocardial infarction in one rhesus monkey fed cholesterol aroused considerable interest (Taylor, 1959). However, extensive use of this species has not been characterised by a high incidence. Infarction in one chimpanzee has also been reported (Vastesaeger et al., 1972). The species Macacca Iris (cynamolgus monkey) is much more susceptible. Of some 40 monkeys fed a diet containing 2% cholesterol for 12-18 months, 27 developed myocardial fibrosis and necrosis, and all had severe coronary atherosclerosis (Kramsch et al., 1970). Serum cholesterol was not excessively high being about 350 mg/100 ml.

Other techniques, although inducing myocardial infarction employ more bizarre methods. The Hartroft-Thomas thrombogenic diet of butter, cholesterol, cholic and thiouracil still receives some attention in the rat (Ruckdeshel et al., 1972; Wilson and Hartroft, 1970) and pig (Lee et al., 1971). In the latter, X-rays in addition to the diet leads to sudden death and myocardial infarction in 6 months. A relatively new development with this diet is that in dogs, cerebral atherosclerosis can be achieved by 36 months feeding (Suzuki et al., 1973); an interesting and unexpected result. Injections of isoproterenol, which increases the heart rate dramatically and leads to myocardial anexia, has been found useful in rabbits for metabolic studies (Wexler and Lutmer, 1972; Wexler, 1973).

Conclusions

There is no dearth of experimental techniques for producing atherosclerosis and/or myocardial infarction in a number of species. Most depend on the induction of lipaemic and/or injury to the vessel wall. The choice of method and species is governed largely by time and finance. Most of the recent experiments which have given information of great value have been with relatively expensive animals, viz. primates or pigs studied for long periods of time, up to 4-5 years in some instances. Often relatively simple changes of diet and mild hypercholesterolaemia have been employed, and the similarity to human disease has been striking. So far no one has reproduced in animals the exact model of coronary heart disease in man. Since this is a multifactorial disease, it may be necessary to combine more than one technique before such an aim is achieved.

DIFFERENCES BETWEEN HUMAN AND ANIMAL ATHEROSCLEROSIS

Robert W. Wissler and Dragoslava Vesselinovitch[*]

Introduction

Atherosclerosis, perhaps more than any other widespread and life-threatening pathological process of modern times, needs to be studied using experimental models. It is very difficult to study the pathogenesis of this disease process adequately in man because it has a complex, multi-faceted set of initiating and augmenting factors; it comes on slowly over a long life span; and it produces essentially no clinical effects until it is far advanced. Furthermore, it is very difficult, short of relatively risky invasive techniques, to document the severity of atherosclerosis in any part of the arterial tree until it produces clinical effects (McGill et al., 1963).

For those of us who are interested in prevention, therapy and reversal of the lesions of atherosclerosis, reliable experimental models are essential. Modern man, with his highly variable diet and life habits and his high degree of mobility, is very difficult to study over a period of years in a controlled and useful way. It is especially difficult to study human beings when the pathological process one is studying probably involves diet and other living habits, and when prevention, treatment or reversal can only be adequately evaluated by quantitative methods applied to the diseased arteries at autopsy.

In response to this need a remarkable number of animal models of atherosclerosis has been developed during the past 65 years (Ignatowski, 1909; Anitschow, 1933; Katz and Stamler, 1953; Constantinides, 1965; Roberts and Straus, 1965). It is the purpose of this paper to evaluate the pathological characteristics of the most commonly used experimental models and to point out the troublesome differences (as well as the helpful similarities) which some of them present.

The Characteristic Features of Atherosclerosis in Man (Fig. 1)

As a background for the study of atherosclerosis in man or in experimental animals one must recognize that the fully developed pathological process and its clinical effects are absent in most of the members of many populations, even though the fatty streak or the mild fatty plaque seems to be present in almost all members of all human populations (and in almost all animal species).

Furthermore, one must be cognizant of the relative sensitivity of human beings (especially males) to the development of this disease. This sensitivity seems to be correlated with certain genetic and environmental conditions.

In general this disease process in man is largely confined to the large and medium elastic and muscular arteries. It usually exhibits greater severity in the abdominal aorta than in the thoracic aorta; it is more severe in the aorta than in the

[*]The authors wish to acknowledge the valuable help of Miss Lee Gatewood, Miss Georgia Mohr, and Miss Nada Devetak in preparing this paper. Some of the work originating in this laboratory and included in the paper was for the most part supported by grants from the National Heart and Lung Institute, HE 2174, HL 6894 HL 12487 and HL 15062.

coronary arteries, which are in term more seriously affected than the renal or mesenteric arteries (Glagov et al., 1961). It is also likely to affect the proximal portions of the coronary arteries much more than the distal parts (Montenegro and Eggan, 1968). In fact, the classical features of atherosclerosis are usually absent in the intramural coronary artery branches and in other small arteries elsewhere in the body. The smooth muscle medial cell proliferation that is sometimes seen in these small arteries is probably a different process with a different etiology and pathogenesis.

1. LITTLE SPONTANEOUS DISEASE OF ANY SIGNIFICANCE WITHOUT ELEVATED BLOOD CHOLESTEROL I.E. ABOVE 150 M.G. %.

2. DEFINITE CORRELATION OF DISEASE WITH DIET INDUCED HYPERCHOLESTEROLEMIA.

3. GROSS DISTRIBUTION OF LESIONS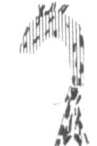

4. CHARACTERISTIC MICROSCOPIC APPEARANCE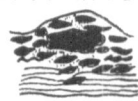

5. LITTLE OR NO SMALL ARTERY INVOLVEMENT.

6. LITTLE OR NO LOADING OF RES WITH LIPID.

Figure 1. Characteristics of atherosclerosis in man

The principal histopathological features of atherosclerosis in man (Fig. 1) can be listed as follows:

1. Lipid deposition in, on or between cells of the artery wall, including localization in or on their products - the fiber proteins (collagen and elastin) and acid mucopolysaccharides.
2. A necrotic center made up of lipid and other cell breakdown products.
3. A variable but often very important element of cell proliferation, mostly of medial multifunctional cells that may in turn produce a rather remarkable amount of new collagen, elastin and mucopolysaccharide.

Except for notable exceptions of extreme hypercholesterolemia of genetic origin, human atherosclerosis generally shows little or no involvement of the reticuloendothelial system by lipid accumulation.

The Characteristics of Atherosclerosis in the Most Commonly Used Experimental Animal Models

Fig. 2 represents a summary of the major features of atherosclerosis in species that have been commonly employed to study this experimental disease process. In general, it is apparent that it is relatively easy to produce lesions in the rabbit by means of commonly employed dietary approaches. There is relatively little spontaneous disease. It is also evident that the lesions are distributed differently from human lesions, i.e. they are more frequently encountered in the thoracic aorta than in the abdominal aorta. Furthermore, the lesions are much more likely to be composed of foam cells, which are in turn likely to be of monocyte or macrophage origin (Imai et al., 1966). Perhaps the most important changes noted in the rabbit that are not usually seen in man are the widespread involvement of small arteries by lipid rich lesions and the remarkable loading of the reticuloendothelial system that accompanies the arterial lesions.

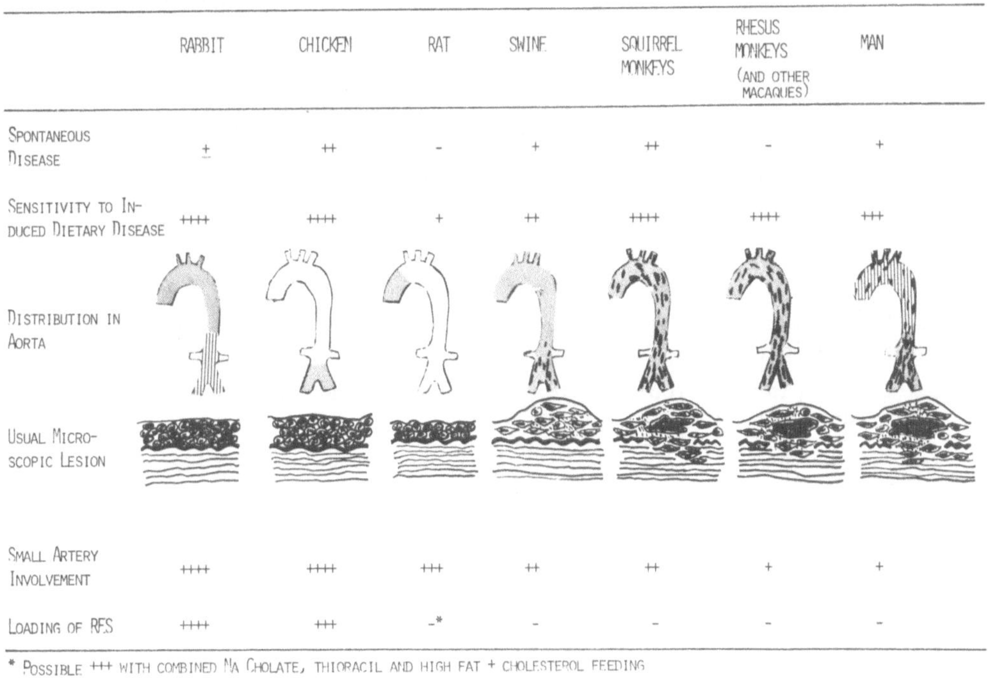

	RABBIT	CHICKEN	RAT	SWINE	SQUIRREL MONKEYS	RHESUS MONKEYS (AND OTHER MACAQUES)	MAN
SPONTANEOUS DISEASE	±	++	-	+	++	-	+
SENSITIVITY TO IN-DUCED DIETARY DISEASE	++++	++++	+	++	++++	++++	+++
DISTRIBUTION IN AORTA							
USUAL MICRO-SCOPIC LESION							
SMALL ARTERY INVOLVEMENT	++++	++++	+++	++	++	+	+
LOADING OF RES	++++	+++	-*	-	-	-	-

* POSSIBLE +++ WITH COMBINED Na CHOLATE, THIORACIL AND HIGH FAT + CHOLESTEROL FEEDING

Figure 2. Characteristics of atherosclerosis in commonly used species

Fortunately it is now possible to utilize the rabbit model in such a way that the lesions in the medium and large arteries show a much closer resemblance to those in man. This can be done by intermittent feeding of an atherogenic diet; can also be achieved by combining a cholesterol-containing diet with epinephrine adminis-tration or with other substances that damage arteries (Constantinides, 1965). Serum sickness and other immunological processes can also convert the usual foam cell lesions to complicated lesions that have a striking resemblance to the advanced atherosclerosis seen in man (Minick et al., 1966).

Fig. 3 summarizes some of the advantages and disadvantages of the rabbit athero-sclerosis model as it has usually been utilized during the past 65 years. It is apparent that it has many advantages in terms of availability, ease of utiliza-tion and size. These make it worthwhile to continue to modify the model so that its lesions are more comparable to those in man in terms of pathogenesis, topo-graphy and morphology. In the meantime, care must be exercised in applying know-ledge learned in the rabbit directly to man.

The chicken model has many of the same advantages and disadvantages as the rabbit. In addition, the chicken (and probably other fowl as well) seems to have a strong tendency to develop unusually severe disease in the lower aorta (Katz and Stamler, 1953).

This focal area of predilection appears to be even more prominent in the pigeon (Clarkson et al., 1959). Further study of it may yield insights into the way in which the arterial wall can be exquisitely sensitive to atherosclerosis.

The rat, which is normally very resistant to the development of atherosclerosis (Wissler et al., 1954) can be made into a very susceptible animal by feeding Na cholate with or without thiouracil, along with usual forms of the atherogenic diet (Thomas and Hartroft, 1959). However, induction of rat lesions involves an increase in blood cholesterol levels, which produces lesions usually consisting

Advantages

1. Easily available.

2. Easy to cage, handle and feed.

3. Size permits most manipulation, tissue and blood studies.

4. Easy to produce advanced lipid-rich arterial lesions quickly.

Disadvantages

1. Vegetarian, lesions develop with little lipid in diet. Cholesterol mainly responsible.

2. Lesion distribution not like man (small arteries involved, thoracic aorta predominant, etc.).

3. Mostly foam-cell lesions with little progression to complicated plaque[a] with necrosis etc.

4. Usual clinical effects seen in human are rare, i.e. myocardial ischemia, thrombosis, aneurysms, etc.

5. Lipid metabolism not like human, RES overloading with lipid and cholesterol usual.

6. Polyunsaturated food fat protection not usually observed.

[a]Plaque can be produced by combining cholesterol feeding with serum sickness or epinephrine. Also intermittent feeding, vitamin D, etc.

Figure 3. Evaluation of *rabbit* for study of experimental atherosclerosis

of intimal foam cells. These lesions may also have a large component of lipid-laden monocytes or macrophages (Suzuki and O'Neil, 1964). The rat, like the rabbit and the fowl, shows a rather remarkable involvement of small arteries (especially in the heart and kidney). It is also noteworthy that when the aorta is involved, it is usually affected at the root (O'Neal et al., 1959). The rat offers many tempting advantages as an experimental subject for atherosclerosis. It is small, easily acquired, and the disease is relatively easy to study in large numbers of fairly standardized and uniform animals. Furthermore, its nutritional requirements and metabolic processes have been rather thoroughly studied.

Like many others, we have tried to exploit the rat for the study of experimental atherosclerosis. It is probably fair to say that although much of value concerning lipid metabolism has been learned in this species, the rat does not at present offer a very satisfactory model of atherosclerosis in man.

Swine are being widely utilized for the study of atherosclerosis and its effects. They are also gaining popularity for the study of prevention, therapy and reversal of this disease. In general the advanced disease in the larger arteries resembles that in man, and so does much of the swine anatomy and cardio-respiratory physiology (Fig. 4). Unfortunately, there is evidence that in some strains or populations of swine a rather remarkable degree of proliferative small artery disease may develop spontaneously under conditions which are still poorly understood (Luginbühl et al., 1969). Other strains or populations of swine appear to be extremely resistant to the development of any type of arterial disease. Another real disadvantage to this model at the present time is that advanced clinically important atherosclerosis seems to be difficult to produce without inducing rather remarkable lipid metabolic alterations (Florentin and Nam, 1968) or arterial injury (Lee et al., 1971). Nevertheless, the swine is a relatively inexpensive and available animal; and its size, its acceptance of experimental rations and the relatively atherosclerosis-free baseline make it very attractive as an experimental model. As more is learned about the genetic pattersn of susceptibility in this species, it will probably be possible to select a strain of swine offering many of the advantages and fewer of the disadvantages. It is noteworthy that swine have furnished a rather remarkable example of advanced cerebral atherosclerosis occuring "spontaneously" in a group of aging animals fed human garbage for many years (Luginbühl and Jones, 1965).

Advantages

1. Omnivore. Readily eats experimental rations.

2. Many features of the lesions similar to human.

3. Known nutritional and metabolic patterns. Purebred lines available.

4. Thoracic, cardiac and coronary artery anatomy and cardio-respiratory physiology similar to human.

5. Size of animal often helpful.

6. Spontaneously occurring cerebral atherosclerosis in old animals (with cerebral infarction).

7. Little spontaneous atherosclerosis in younger animals.

Disadvantages

1. Expensive. Hard to manipulate. Special facilities required.

2. Advanced progressive atherosclerosis difficult to induce unless special rather artificial measures used.

3. Consumes large amounts of diet and other material used in experiments.

4. Sex differences in severity of disease not evident.

Figure 4. Evaluation of *swine* for study of experimental atherosclerosis

In recent years the non-human primate has been studied with increasing frequency. It has become evident, largely through the pioneering efforts of Taylor et al., that the Rhesus monkey is quite susceptible to the development of advanced atherosclerosis and to some of its clinical complications (Taylor et al., 1962; 1963a; 1963b). Squirrel monkeys have also developed rather remarkable atherosclerotic lesions, exhibiting most of the features of human lesions (Middleton et al., 1964; Clarkson et al., 1969). The only disadvantages offered by the squirrel monkey are that it seems to be prone to develop rather substantial atheromatous disease without any experimental intervention, and it is rather small for some types of studies.

Even though the Rhesus monkey atheromatous lesions are substantial and show most, if not all, of the features of advanced atherosclerosis observed in man, other macaques are presently being studied which also seem to have characteristic features that may be advantageous. For example, the stump-tailed macaque (Macaca Speciosa) appears to be equally susceptible to dietarily induced atherosclerosis, and its more docile behavior and larger size may be very positive features in some types of studies (Wissler et al., 1972). The Macaca Irus also seems to be particularly valuable; recent studies (Kramsch et al., 1970) indicate that it is very susceptible to coronary occlusion and myocardial infarction occurring in relation to advanced coronary atherosclerosis.

Advantages

1. Omnivore. Readily eats experimental rations.

2. Most features of lesions similar to man from "early" to "advanced" stages. Histogenesis seems similar.

3. Nutritional and metabolic patterns similar to human. Disease develops on same diet as human.

4. Thoracic, cardiac, coronary artery, anatomy and cardiac pulmonary physiology similar to human.

5. Animal size often preferable to rat, chicken, and rabbit.

6. Atherosclerosis-free baseline.

7. Complicated advanced lesions lead to same clinical effects as in atherosclerosis in human.

8. Distribution of lesions similar to human.

Disadvantages

1. Expensive. Hard to handle. Special cages and facilities needed.

2. Uniform, disease-free adult animals hard to obtain.

3. Sex differences in severity of disease not evident.

Figure 5. Evaluation of *rhesus monkey* (and other macaques) for study of atherosclerosis

The "advantages" and "disadvantages" of these macaque models are summarized in Fig. 5. Of the "advantages", there may be some debate about 2, 6 and 8. The similarity of the early histogenesis to that of man has been questioned because of the rather substantial amount of lipid that appears in the inner medial smooth muscle cells of the arteries. It is our opinion that this feature is characteristic of the lesions in younger men as well as monkeys, and we are conducting a study to throw light specifically on this point. The question of the atherosclerosis-free baseline in the Rhesus monkey has also been raised. It appears that even though occasional fatty streaks may be encountered, they are not any more frequent than in many other species that do not develop spontaneously progressive disease. It has been said that the distribution of the lesions in the aorta of the Rhesus monkey is more severe in the thoracic aorta. This may be true in most cases of relatively mild disease; but our observations in 42 adult male animals subjected to a coconut-oil, butterfat, cholesterol-rich ration for 9 months indicate that when the lesions are advanced, they are usually more numerous and more severe in the abdominal aorta, and they are frequently almost completely absent in the proximal aorta adjacent to the aortic valve.

Using this model a number of rather useful studies have been or are being conducted. Some of the characteristics of atheromatous lesions that seem to be related to specific food fats have been delineated (Vesselinovitch et al., in press in Atherosclerosis). Furthermore, rather close confinement in cages that are ample for free movement and well within the guidelines set up in the "Guide for the Care and Use of Laboratory Animals" seems to augment the severity of coronary artery atherosclerosis without much influence on the severity of aortic lesions in otherwise comparably treated animals (Wissler et al., 1969). It has also been demonstrated that a prudent human table-prepared diet modeled after the kind of ration recommended by many heart disease prevention groups - a diet relatively low in calories, cholesterol and saturated fat - will produce substantially less atheromatous disease in a 2 year period than a ration composed of the ingredients present in similar quantities in the average American table prepared diet (Wissler et al., 1971).

The Rhesus model is also proving to be useful in studying regression of atherosclerotic lesions (Armstrong et al., 1970). Armstrong et al., have produced impressive evidence that a sustained lowering of the blood cholesterol to initial levels (about 135 mg%) will lead to a substantial enlargement of the lumenal diameter of coronary arteries which were presumably markedly narrowed from diet-induced atherosclerosis (Armstrong et al., 1970). Vesselinovitch et al., have recently confirmed many of the results of this study (Vesselinovitch et al., 1973), and additional studies investigating other aspects of lesion regression are being carried out in this species in our laboratory and at other centers.

This species is also proving to be very useful in a study being carried out by Harold Brooks and ourselves; standardized myocardial infarcts in severely atherosclerotic Rhesus monkeys are being compared with similar infarcts in monkeys with normal coronary arteries.

Many aspects of atherosclerosis are still unexplained, and it is likely that this model and others not yet developed will be utilized to evaluate numerous dietary variables; to study interrelationships with hypertension, diabetes and other endocrine imbalances; and to evaluate new methods of prevention and treatment.

In conclusion, it is evident that no animal model perfectly duplicates the human disease or satisfies all desirable requirements. In fact, most experimental models of most diseases are not absolutely identical with the human disease. However, they still serve a very important purpose, and this is particularly true for atherosclerosis. At present it appears that the most useful models of human atherosclerosis are those induced in the non-human primate and in the swine.

EXPERIMENTAL ATHEROSCLEROSIS DUE TO ASCORBIC ACID DEFICIENCY

Takao Fujinami and Kota Okado

To account for capillary hemorrhage by scurvy, various investigators have inferred alterations in the vascular endothelium, the intercellular cement, or the supporting tissues of the vessel wall. Gore and Fujinami (1965 a,b) have reported upon altered endothelium of the aorta of scorbutic guinea pigs, and also a decrease of aortic collagen and an increase of acid mucopolysaccharides. Willis (1957) has reported on the stainable lipid deposition along the internal elastic membrane of the aorta as well as capillaries. Present studies are intended to elucidate the role of ascorbic acid on atherosclerosis.

Short Period Experiments

Male guinea pigs weighing about 300 grams each were employed for the studies. Animals of group 1 were made ascorbic-acid deficient by scorbutic-diet feeding for two weeks. Animals of group 2 were fed with the same scorbutic diet with a supplement of 25 mg ascorbic acid daily. Guinea pigs of group 3 were maintained on the scorbutic diet with added 5% coconut oil by weight, and group 4 received the same high-fat scorbutic diet with a supplement of 25 mg ascorbic acid daily for two weeks. The scorbutic diet was supplied by Clea Company in Tokyo. The ascorbic acid content in the blood was estimated with 2,4 -dinitrophenylhydralazine (Roe and Kuether, 1943), and serum cholesterol and triglycerides were determined by the usual methods (Fujinami et al., 1971; Yoshiuawa, 1960; Van Handel and Zilversmit, 1959). Lipoprotein lipase (LPL) activity in the plasma after heparin injection was determined by the turbidity method of Hara and Kuzuya (1967).

Blood ascorbic acid content at the end of 2 weeks feeding is shown in Table 1. The level of group 1 was practically scorbutic, although remaining apparently normal in group 2. The content in group 4 was as low as in group 3, even though ascorbic acid was supplemented. This phenomenon suggests that ascorbic acid was consumed by much lipid loading. Serum triglyceride and cholesterol were moderately elevated by ascorbic acid deficiency. Administration of coconut oil caused a greater increase of serum lipid, but this increase was reversible by ascorbic acid supplement, as observed in group 4. LPL activity was markedly suppressed in group 1 and 3.

Histological examination of the aorta revealed edematous swelling of the intima and media with tortuous lamination of the elastic membrane and subendothelial accumulation of lipid in the aorta of group 1. The aorta of group 2 was apparently normal. Swelling of ground substance in the media, indicating accumulation of mucopolysaccharides, appearance of foam cells in the intima, and increased infiltration of lipid into deep layers of the media were observed in the group 3, but were minimal in the aortas of group 4.

Prolonged Experiments

Following observations in short-period experiments, ascorbic acid deficiency was supposed to be one of promotive factors of atherosclerosis. The effect of covert ascorbic acid deficiency without high-fat diet was studied in prolonged experiments.

Table 1. Content of blood ascorbic acid and serum lipids

	Number of animals	Ascorbic acid mg%	Cholesterol mg%	Triglyceride mg%
Short period experiment				
Group 1	7	0.28 ± 0.09	122 ± 17	47 ± 14
Group 2	11	0.67 ± 0.20[a]	79 ± 10[a]	33 ± 8[b]
Group 3	6	0.37 ± 0.06	155 ± 34	86 ± 18
Group 4	8	0.38 ± 0.05	108 ± 17[a]	72 ± 20
Prolonged experiment				
Deficient	8	0.39 ± 0.08	110 ± 18	104 ± 19
Control	8	0.78 ± 0.13[a]	101 ± 17	88 ± 12

Mean + standard deviasion statistical difference. [a]$p < 0.01$, [b]$p < 0.05$.

Guinea pigs were kept on the scorbutic diet with a twice-a-week supplemtn of 5 mg ascorbic acid for eight weeks. The controls were fed the same diet supplemented with 50 mg of ascorbic acid every other day. Increase of their weight was practically the same. The animals were sacrificed at the end of the eighth week by decapitation after 24 hours fasting. Methods employed for determination of ascorbic acid, triglyceride, and cholesterol were the same as for the short period experiment. The aorta was divided into three segments: arch, thoracic, and abdominal, and homogenized with distilled water or buffer for enzyme studies. Lipid content was estimated on the extract by Folch's (1957) method from aqueous homogenate. Several kinds of hydrolase activities in the aorta were estimated to elucidate metabolic alteration of the arterial wall (Table 2). Esterase and lipase activities were determined by the method of Seligman, alkaline and acid phosphatase by Sigma procedure (1961), 5'-nucleotidase activity by the method of Kirk (1959) and ß-glucuronidase by that of Masuya et al. (1961). Segments of the aorta were examined histologically and ß-glucuronidase activity determined by the method of Hayashi et al. (1964).

The ascorbic acid contents in the blood, spleen and adrenal were suppressed in ascorbic acid deficient animals. Serum cholesterol and triglyceride were slightly elevated in the scorbutic animals but the difference from the controls was not significant. In about one third of the scorbutic animals, small white patchy plaques, solitary or grouped, were observed in the proximal portion of the aorta. Histological examination revealed that the lesions were primarily localized in the center of media and intima. The elastic membranes lost their induration and showed splitting and fragmentation at the lesion. Degenerative changes in the smooth muscle cells and accumulation of the amorphous ground substance with deposition of calcium, and intimal fibrous thickening were observed in the aorta of chronic scurvy. Stainable lipids were demonstrated in the intima and in the medial lesion. Contents of cholesterol and triglyceride in the aorta were significantly elevated in the arch of the deficient, but not significant in the thoracic and abdominal aorta. There were increased activities in esterase, lipase, acid phosphatase and 5'-nucleotidase in the proximal portion of the aorta of the ascorbic-acid deficient. Significant elevation of ß-glucuronidase activity was observed in the whole aorta of the deficient and was localized mainly in the medial lesion as demonstrated by histochemistry.

Since the aortic lesion induced by chronic ascorbic acid deficiency was similar to the lesion induced by epinephrine, and a large amount of ascorbic acid was contained in the adrenal gland, influence of ascorbic acid deficiency on catecholamine in the adrenal gland and urinary output were studied. Total catecholamine content in the adrenal gland estimated by the method of Lund (1950) was moderately decreased. Urinary output of catecholamine estimated by ion-exchange separation and fluorometry (Bio-Rad Laboratories), and of vanilmandelic acid determined by the method of Pisano et al. (1962) showed no difference between chronic scurvy and the controls.

Table 2. Content of lipids and hydrolase activities in the aortic wall

	Number of animals	Arch	Thoracic	Abdominal
Cholesterol (mg/mgN)				
Deficient	8	0.73 ± 0.23	0.39 ± 0.13	0.69 ± 0.24
Control	8	0.38 ± 0.15[a]	0.45 ± 0.16	0.53 ± 0.25
Triglyceride (mg/mgN)				
Deficient	8	0.72 ± 0.41	0.27 ± 0.11	0.52 ± 0.30
Control	8	0.24 ± 0.10[a]	0.31 ± 0.15	0.32 ± 0.11
Esterase (ß-naphthol μg/mgN/h)				
Deficient	9	102 ± 36	66 ± 24	62 ± 24
Control	9	39 + 17[a]		
Lipase (ß-naphthol μg/mgN/h)				
Deficient	9	43 ± 23	25 ± 9	28 ± 18
Control	9	16 ± 9[a]	20 ± 7	20 ± 16
Alkaline Phosphatase (mMol p-nitrophenol/mgN)				
Deficient	8	0.62 ± 0.41	0.61 ± 0.24	1.11 ± 0.75
Control	7	0.56 ± 0.23	0.98 ± 0.41	0.84 ± 0.43
Acid Phosphatase (mMol p-nitrophenol/mgN)				
Deficient	7	5.46 ± 1.28	3.29 ± 1.26	3.59 ± 2.12
Control	6	2.37 ± 1.21	3.44 ± 1.22	2.97 ± 2.23
5'-Nucleotidase (μg P/mg N)				
Deficient	7	41.51 ± 22.22	43.64 ± 29.07	50.62 ± 31.76
Control	7	31.10 ± 14.74	29.94 ± 16.38	41.48 ± 30.97
ß-Glucuronidase (μg p-nitrophenol/g of tissue/hr)				
Deficient	7		407 ± 98	
Control	7		220 ± 45[a]	

[a]Statistical difference $P < 0.01$.

The results of these experiments indicate that ascorbic acid deficiencies cause endothelial changes probably with altered permeability of the vascular wall, metabolic alteration of the arterial wall, and also lead to changes in lipid metabolism, and subsequently induce atherosclerosis. Catecholamines possibly do not contribute to atherosclerosis in this study. Since primates are dependent on external sources of ascorbic acid as is the guinea pig, ouvert ascorbic acid deficiency in humans is supposed to be one of contributing factors of atherosclerosis.

ON PATHOGENETIC FACTORS CONCERNED WITH VASCULAR LESIONS INDUCED BY HIGH SUCROSE DIET IN MONKEYS

M. Murakami, H. Sekimoto, I. Nakada, K. Nakamura, and M. Takaori

In 1963 we found that vascular lesions resembling human diabetic vascular changes had been induced in rabbits by feeding high sucrose diets, and we subsequently succeeded inducing the same arterial lesions in rats and beagles. The purpose of the present investigation was to study the effect of high sucrose diets on the development of vascular lesions in non-human primates. This was of importance, not least because they were phylogenetically closer to man.

Seven male crab-eating monkeys were fed a full semi-synthetic diet (Oriental A) and sucrose (40-80 g/day). The monkeys were sacrificed at the end of the experimental period. Blood and organs were examined for biochemically histologically respectively. Remarkable changes were found in the kidneys of all experimental monkeys.

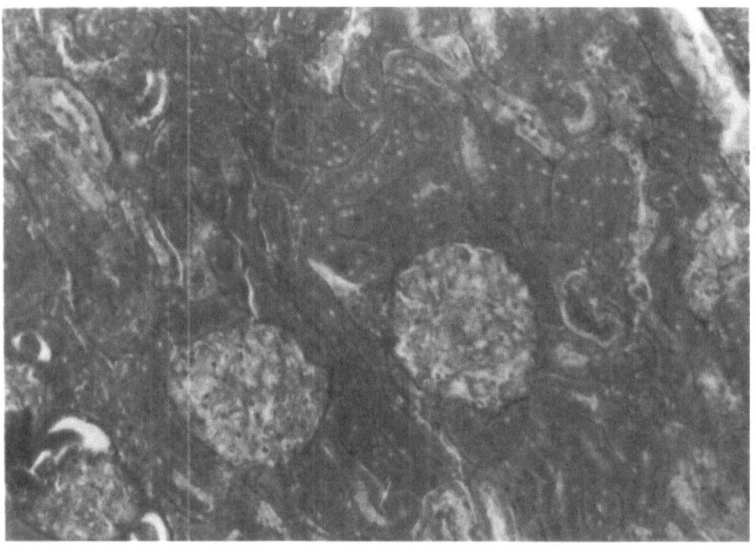

Figure 1. Glomerulus containing swollen and vesicular mesangial cells (Azan stain)

Sections stained by Azan showed a glomerulus containing markedly swollen and vesicular mesangial cells with small pycnotic nuclei. The basement membrane of the tufts was not thickened. The convoluted epithelium was normal (Fig. 1).

Some of the glomeruli showed slight swelling due to a thin amorphous exudate in Bowman's space. The glomerular tufts were somewhat irregularly thickened with slight mesangial proliferation. Bowman's epithelium was focally swollen. The medium-sized interlobular artery presented a slight thickening of the wall with focal fibrosis.

Arteriosclerotic changes were found in the coronary artery. A moderately large-sized coronary artery showed focally a markedly thickened wall replaced by edematous and myxomatous fibrous tissue.

The degenerated portion was mainly in the intima. The endothelium overlying the thickened area was slightly proliferated (Fig. 2).

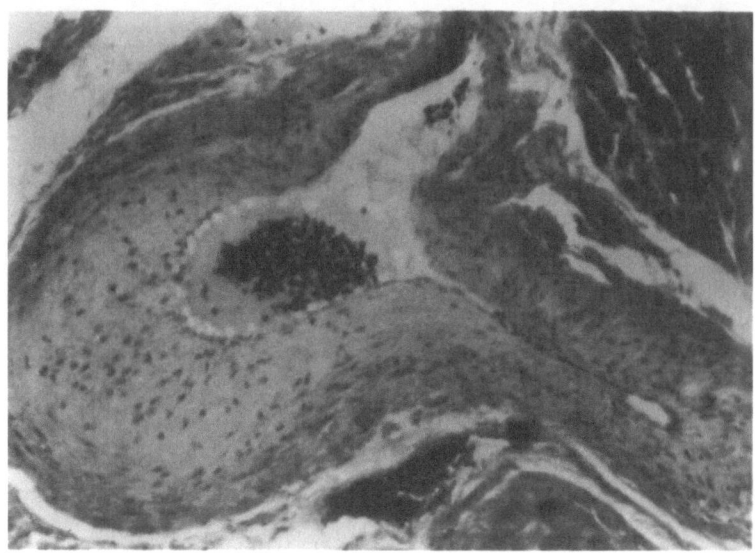

Figure 2. Arteriosclerotic changes in coronary artery

There were small degenerated foci of the myocardial fibers. The sarcoplasmar was basophilic and nuclei staining was faint. It might suggest minute early myocardial ischemic changes.

Atheromatous plaques of the aorta were found in two of seven experimental monkeys. Foam-cell plaques and remarkable intimal thickening were found.

In some cases, spotty small sclerotic lesions were found. On close examination of the lesion, a few monolayered foam cells were lined outside the endothelial surface, which might suggest breaking of endothelial lining (Fig. 3). These changes did not display arterosclerotic lesions seen in rabbits, rats, and beagles previously reported by us.

To sum up, the following results were obtained in monkeys:
1. Arteriosclerotic lesions by feeding of high sucrose diets developed in aorta, kidney, and coronary artery.
2. Platelet aggregation was enhanced.
3. Serum enzyme activities, such as creatine phosphokinase, aldolase, alkaline phosphatase were increased.
4. High sucrose diets play an important role in the development of vascular lesions resembling human diabetic vascular changes.
5. These results suggested that very high sucrose intake might induce vascular lesions in humans.

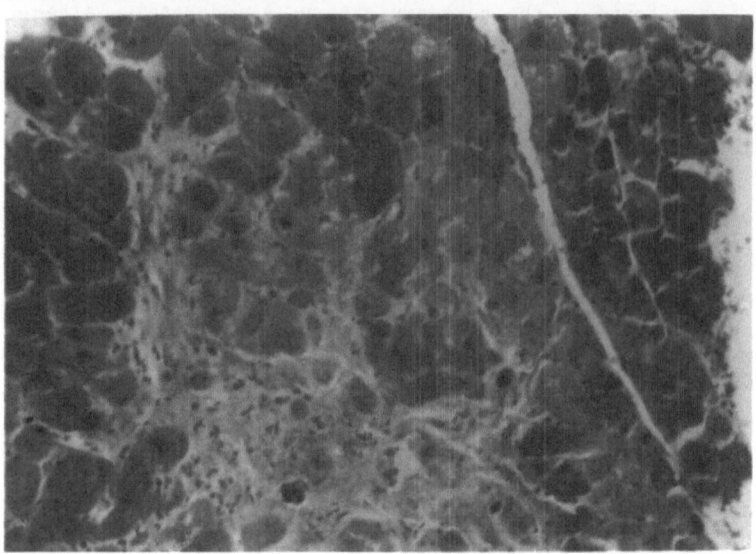

Figure 3. Sclerotic lesion of the aorta

ULTRASTRUCTURAL CHANGES IN THE CORONARY ARTERIES OF PRIMATES (MACACA IRIS) AFTER A PROLONGED, MILD CARBON MONOXIDE EXPOSURE

Henrik Klem Thomsen

Introduction

In 1967 Astrup et al. found that carbon monoxide (CO) enhanced the atherogenic effect of cholesterol feeding on the rabbit aorta. These results were later reproduced in primate coronary arteries (Webster et al., 1970).

In 1972 Kjeldsen et al. demonstrated that exposure of rabbits to a moderate dose of CO for two weeks, produced aortic intimal edema.

The present study was carried out to elucidate, if such changes could be induced in coronary arteries of primates after a similar CO-exposure.

Material and Methods

20 juvenile macaca irus monkeys were used in the experiment. All animals were placed in exposure chambers. They were fed standard pellets, fruit, and tap water. 6 animals were exposed to 250 ppm CO in atm. air continuously for two weeks, while 6 other animals were exposed intermittently for 12 hours a day to the same gas-mixture and 8 animals served as controls. After sacrificing the animals the coronary arteries were excised and cut into pieces and fixed either in 10 per cent acrolein or 2 per cent glutaraldehyde in 0,1 M Na-cacodylate buffer with 0,05 M $CaCl_2$ (pH u,4). Postfixation was carried out in 2 per cent osmium tetraoxide in the same buffer. The tissue was embedded in araldite (Durcupan ACM). Ultrathin sections were contrasted with uranyl acetate and lead citrate.

Results

One control animal and two animals from the exposed groups suffered from fibro-muscular intimal thickening and were excluded from the study.

In the control animals the endothelium appeared flat, the subendothelial space was narrow and the internal elastic membrane was unbroken. Occasionally a few myocyte-like cells were found in the subendothelial space.

All animals in the continously exposed group showed more or less pronounced sub-endothelial edema in the main coronary arteries. In some areas the edema was present as blisters beneath the endothelial cells, but more common was a regular sub-endothelial edema in which cells with or without lipid-droplets were accumulating (Fig. 1). None of these cells had the characteristic of myocytes - myofibrils, dense bodies or pinocytotic vesicles - but were rather monocyte-like with short pseudo-podies (Fig. 2). These lipid-laden subendothelial cells contained occasionally myelin-bodies. The internal elastic membrane could be broken, but an intact membrane was the typical finding. In a few slices a gap between the endo-thelial cells was seen (Fig. 3). A lipid-containing cell was always present beneath such a gap.

No intimal changes were seen in the intermittently exposed group, but two animals suffered from media-edema.

The smaller intramural coronary arteries were quite normal in the exposed groups.

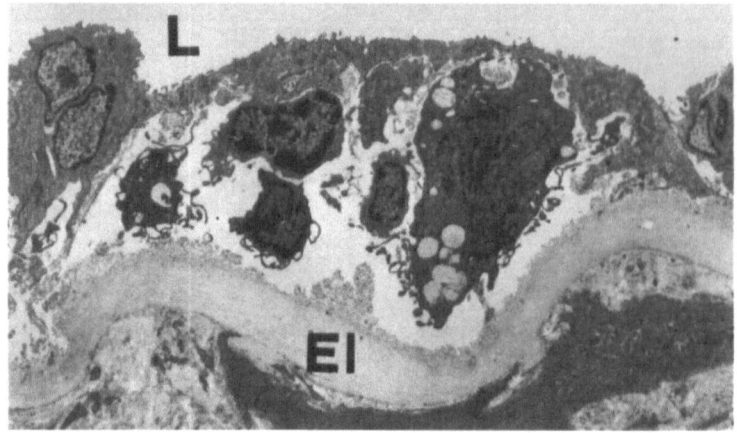

Figure 1. Coronary artery from a CO-exposed animal. The subendothelial space is widened. Monocyte-like cells are seen between the endothelium and the internal elastic membrane. L = lumen, El = internal elastic membrane

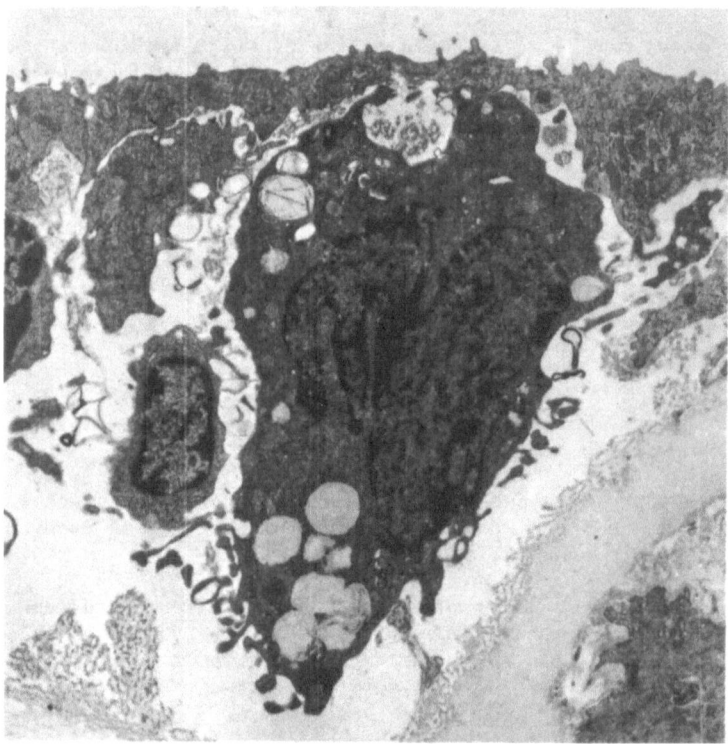

Figure 2. Coronary artery from a CO-exposed animal. The lipid-containing cell has neither myofilaments, dense bodies nor pinocytotic vesicles, but numerous short pseudo-podies

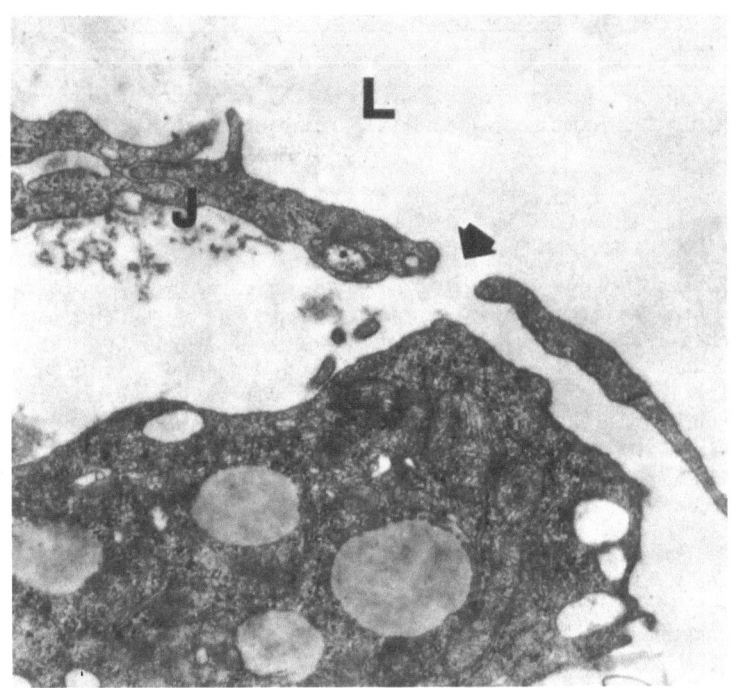

Figure 3. Coronary artery from a CO-exposed animal. A gap (arrow) is seen between the endothelial cells. A lipid-containing cell is present just beneath the gap. Note the intact junction (J) to the left. L = lumen

Discussion

In two respects the results are differing from what could be expected from earlier studies in CO-exposed rabbits:

First, lipid-laden cells have never been seen in the subendothelial space of rabbit aorta after CO-exposure. The findings indicate either, that monkeys are more sensible to CO-exposure than rabbits, or that the coronary arteries are more vulnerable than the elastic arteries.

Secondly, we expected the intermittently exposed group to react more vigorously than the continously exposed group, because it has been demonstrated in our laboratory, that the rabbit aorta acts in this way in cholesterol fed animals. In fact, this was not at all the case with the monkeys, where no intimal changes were seen in the intermittently exposed group.

It can be safely stated then that species differences exist in the reaction of the arterial wall to CO-exposure.

The findings in the continously exposed group was quite clear and since this early lesion, which could proceed to a fatty streak, was characterized by edema, monocyte-like lipid-laden cells, and an intact internal elastic membrane, beneath which normally structured myocytes were seen, we conclude that this study supports the theory, that infiltration of blood-elements - plasma constituents and monocates - into the subendothelial space is one of the very early steps in atherogenesis.

Furthermore, this study supports the idea, that CO in tobacco smoke is a main factor responsible for the increased incidence of atherosclerotic diseases seen in heavy smokers.

RESPONSES OF TWO MACAQUE SPECIES TO ATHEROGENIC DIET AND ITS WITH-DRAWAL

Mark L. Armstrong and Majorie B. Megan

Rhesus monkeys (*M. mulatta*) given diets high in cholesterol and fat for many months develop prominent atheromas in the aorta and its elastic and muscular branches (Mann et al., 1956; Taylor et al., 1962; Scott et al., 1967; Wissler, 1968; Younger et al., 1969; Armstrong and Warner, 1971; Manning and Clarkson, 1972). In cynomolgus monkeys (*M. fasicularis*) similar diets induce lesions of the same general morphology (Kramsch and Hollander, 1968), characterized by accumulations of intimal lipid and reactive mesenchymal tissue, but apparently with more variation in the distribution of atheroma formation within the arterial tree, depending on the subspecies studied and the observation period.

We compared the responses of the two species as to the hyperlipidemic and atherogenic effects of a standard high-fat, high-cholesterol diet (Armstrong et al., 1967) and as to the subsequent arterial changes after a cholesterol-free diet was substituted. Adult male animals were studied; the rhesus monkeys were imported from India and the cynomolgus from Thailand.

The atherogenic diet, containing 1.2% cholesterol with 40% calories as egg yolk fat, was fed for 17 months. In both species there was prompt, marked elevation of plasma cholesterol to a plateau reached in a few months and maintained to the end of the feeding of the atherogenic diet (Table 1). Average cholesterol levels were higher in rhesus than in cynomolgus (P <0.01). Plasma triglycerides showed little change in either species. Electrophoretic determination of plasma lipoproteins showed a striking increase in both species in the low-density lipoprotein band. Correspondingly, there was a great increase of the cholesterol content in the density-defined fraction 1.019 - 1.063 of ultracentrifuged plasma.

Table 1. Plasma lipids (mg/dl) in rhesus and cynomolgus monkeys

	Baseline	Atherogenic diet	Cholesterol-free diet
Rhesus			
cholesterol	140 ± 7	782 ± 24	137 ± 9
triglycerides	69 ± 3	71 ± 6	74 ± 8
Cynomolgus			
cholesterol	148 ± 11	526 ± 21	187 ± 17
triglycerides	63 ± 7	70 ± 7	67 ± 5

At the end of the atherogenic diet atherosclerosis in cynomolgus equaled and usually exceeded that in rhesus in the aorta and the subclavian, carotid, femoral and coronary arteries. Furthermore, several features of atherosclerosis in cynomolgus, aside from a tendency toward more intimal thickening, distinguished the experimental lesions from those in rhesus. *First*, medial damage in elastic arteries was clearly greater. *Second*, the fibrotic response in the intimal lesions was more extensive. *Third*, although foam cell concentrations in the intima were not definitely greater, more sterol clefts and other evidences of extracellular lipid were present in cynomolgus. These differentiations in induced atherosclerosis are considered valid for the cynomolgus subspecies studied as compared with rhesus (in which subspecies differences have not been found).

Substitution of the cholesterol-free diet after the atherogenic diet disclosed both similarities and differences in the regression phenomenon seen in rhesus and cynomolgus. Up to twenty months of cholesterol-free diet, visible lipid decreased in both. More residual extracellular lipid was noted in the intima of cynomolgus. Several other characteristics of the regression picture in cynomolgus made it quantitatively different from that seen in rhesus. Areas of transmural replacement fibrosis of the media of elastic arteries were seen occasionally (Fig. 1) rather than rarely, and 25-50% fibrous replacement, measured from internal to external elastica, was common. Intimal collagen fibers were more densely packed.

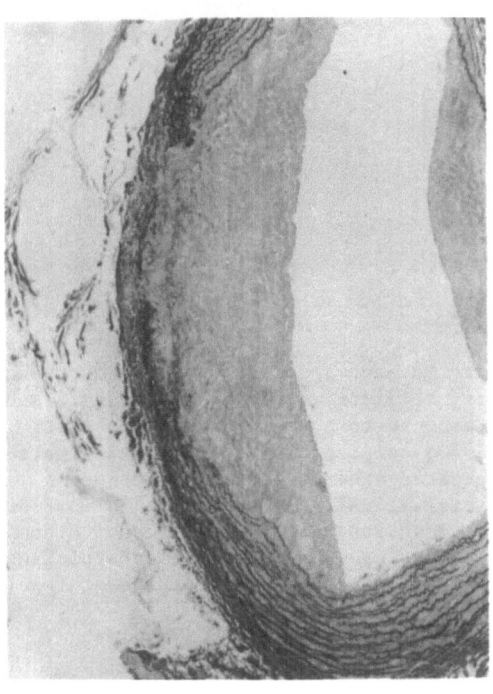

Figure 1. Transmural replacement fibrosis in carotid artery of cynomolgus. Media penetrated by collagenous mass to varying depths, with disruption and loss of stainable elastic. At region of complete replacement (10 o'clock), outermost slightly darker zone is adventitia. Verhoeff Van Gieson, X 30

Mineralization was more frequent. Areas of metaplasia of compacted fibrous tissue to discrete plates of fibrohyaline character were occasionally seen, with cells that gave these lesions a chondroid appearance (Fig. 2). They tended to lack alcianophilia (at pH 2.5), in contrast to dense Van Gieson-positive budles which typically surrounded them. Uncommonly, calcium and iron salts impregnated these metaplastic areas, with an accented line of iron demarcating the periphery of the plates. Rarely, bone formation occurred.

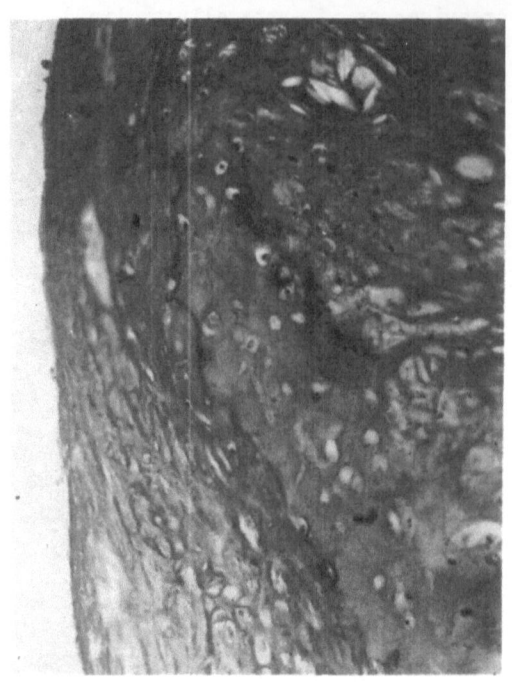

Figure 2. A discrete plate of
fibrohyaline material in aorta
of cynomolgus with altered
mesenchymal cells in apparent
lacunae. Surrounding the plate
are dense collagen bundles.
Verhoeff Van Gieson , X 82,50

Summary

Two macaque species, rhesus and cynomolgus, were compared as to their vulnerability to diet-induced hyperlipidemia and atherosclerosis and to their subsequent
response to a cholesterol-free diet. Type II-A hyperlipidemia (Beaumont et al.,
1970) occurred in both but was greater in rhesus. Conversely, equal and usually
greater atherosclerosis occurred in cynomolgus. We therefore propose that the
arterial wall of cynomolgus is more susceptible to experimental atherosclerosis.
The atherosclerotic arteries of cynomolgus showed more striking mesenchymal changes during subsequent cholesterol-free diet. In this respect cynomolgus may be
valuable in the investigation of repair processes in atherosclerosis.

PRELIMINARY RESULTS OF REVERSIBILITY OF SPONTANEOUS AND DIET-INDUCED ATHEROSCLEROSIS IN SQUIRREL MONKEYS BY CHONDROITIN-4-SULFATE

Lester M. Morrison, Benjamin H. Ershoff, Gurwant S. Bajwa, O. Arne
Schjeide, Roslyn B. Alfin-Slater, and Norbert L. Enrick

A study of the rapid turnover and "clearing" of radioactive isotope-labelled
cholesterol from the aortas of infant and adult aortic preparations, by chondroitin sulfate A (CSA) (Morrison, 1965; 1969) led to the following investigations
with CSA, a naturally occurring acid mucopolysaccharide present in human, mammalian, fish and fowl connective tissues (Meyer, 1969) (Fig. 1).

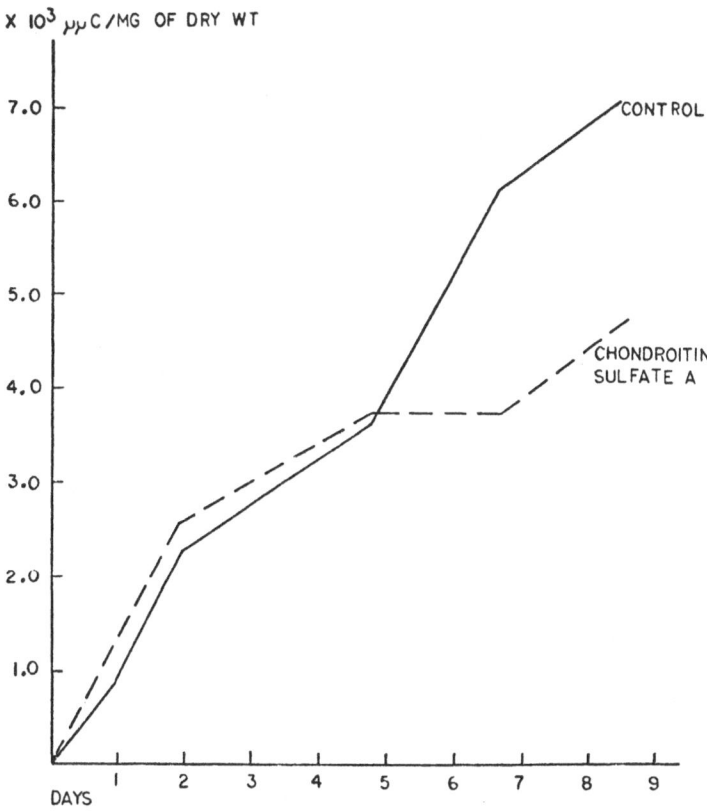

Figure 1. C^{14}-Cholesterol uptake in human aortic segments following treatment
with chondroitin sulfate A (71 year old male)

Regression studies of coronary and aortic athero-arteriosclerosis were first carried out in Wistar, Long-Evans and Sprague-Dawley rat strains by the feeding of
cholesterol and hypervitaminosis D diets. Coronary and aortic athero-arteriosclerosis was produced in 100% of a group of rats so treated within a twelve week
period.

Following the production of these vascular lesions, at twelve weeks the athero-genic diet was withdrawn, a standard laboratory diet was substituted, together with 1% feedings of CSA in the diet.

After twelve weeks of CSA feedings, both coronary arteries and aortas in this group of 18 animals was found to be free and cleared of lipids; calcium and connective tissue scars, however, remained unchanged as compared to a control group of rats (Morrison et al., 1972). In rats not treated by CSA, coronary and aortic atherosclerotic lesions were found to disappear ultimately after approximately one year on a routine rat laboratory diet.

A preventive study of the effects of CSA was carried out on dietetically accelerated athero-arteriosclerosis in squirrel monkeys (Morrison et al., 1966). Natural athero-arteriosclerotic lesions occur spontaneously in sub-human primates, squirrel monkeys (Saimiri sciurea) from South American jungles, who develop naturally occurring or spontaneous athero-arteriosclerosis following maturity. The ages of these animals were from 2-1/2 to 3 years; both sexes were equally represented.

One group of 65 monkeys was divided into sub-groups wherein one group of animals was fed a cholesterol monkey Purina Chow diet as controls, and one group was maintained on a regular monkey Purina Chow diet alone. Another group of monkeys was fed the same atherogenic diet as the first group, but given daily injections of 10 mg per kg body weight of pure, sterile, pyrogen-free CSA in saline solution for nine months.

Following the nine month study period, the aortas of all animals were examined macroscopically, microscopically and chemically analyzed for lipid content.

One control group of monkeys given the atherogenic diet and daily saline injections revealed grade II athero-arteriosclerotic lesions of the aorta on a grading basis of 0 to IV maximum macroscopic evaluation of atherosclerotic lesions. The control group of animals on non-atherogenic monkey Purina Chow diet revealed a slight degree of atherosclerotic aortic lesions, at the pre-maturity ages of 2-1/2 to 3 years, a macroscopic grade of 0.6.

In the CSA treated group, atherosclerotic lesions were absent macro- and micro-scopically. The aortas of these animals appeared grossly to be remarkably healthy by visual and palpable inspections, presenting a glistening, moist color and healthy physical appearance. Artefacts were listed in this grading, reducing the macroscopic grading to 0.4 for aortic athero-arteriosclerosis. Lipid analysis of the CSA-treated group revealed the same lipid content of aortas as the control, non-atherogenic dietary group, 9.2 vs. 95 respectively.

The above findings suggested the possiblity of regression of atherosclerosis in these pre-maturity monkeys, leading to the following study.

A group of 8 squirrel monkeys was taken from the control, non-atherogenic dietary group, at the ages of 3-1/2 to 4 years, and kept on a Purina Chow monkey diet supplemented by fruit feedings, for a five year period. The animals were maintained in good health, growth and mature development.

Following the five year observation period, the animals were divided into two sub-groups, one group of four controls of both sexes continued to receive their normal monkey chow diet plus daily subcutaneous injections of saline for 90 days (Morrison et al., 1972). The second sub-group of four animals received 20 mg daily of pure, sterile, pyrogen-free CSA for 90 days together with their normal monkey chow diet.

In both sub-groups, all hearts were sectioned through three areas, i.e. base, mid-section and apex. Random-selection sections with 10 slides each were made of each section of every heart for both sub-groups. All aortas were examined macro- and microscopically.

Table 1. Regression of naturally occurring coronary atherosclerosis in squirrel monkeys following intramuscular administration of CSA[a]

Monkey identity	Sex	Histology: Incidence of coronary atherosclerosis throughout heart						Aortic atherosclerosis
		Base		Center		Apex		Intracardiac section
		Site[b]	Severity	Site[b]	Severity	Site[b]	Severity	
Control group								
SM2 F	F	1 main 1 branch	2 1	2 main	2	1 main	1	2
SM2 G	F	0		0		0		2
SM2 H	F	2 main	2	0		0		2
SM2 I	M	2 main	1	0		0		2
CSA treated group								
SM2 A	M	0		0		0		0
SM2 B	M	0		0		0		2
SM2 C	F	0		1 branch	1[c]	0		1
SM2 D	F	0		0		0		2

[a]Chondroitin sulfate A was administered daily (6 days per week), dosage 20 mg per monkey.

[b]The site of arteriosclerotic lesions are indicated as occurring either on the main or branch coronary arteries.

[c]Probable artefact.

Grade: 0 - none, 1 - slight, 2 - moderate, 3 - marked, 4 - maximal involvement.

Every coronary artery section through the base, mid-section and apex of each animal treated with CSA, showed an absence of any macroscopic or microscopic athero or arteriosclerotic lesions. In the controls only two instances of lesions occurred in the mid-section and apex of the heart, as compared to one instance (probable artefact) in the mid-section of a CSA-treated animal; no particular significance is attached to the latter finding. In the aortas of each sub-group these differences, however, did not appear to be significant and are thus considered to be only somewhat less in severity of lesions by CSA treatment (Table 1).

Since most human coronary atherosclerotic disease is found in the base part of the heart, this 90 day short-term treatment with injectable CSA is of especial interest. The findings suggest that a longer period of treatment such as the 9 month daily CSA injections previously reported by the authors may possibly have produced a similar clearance of athero-arteriosclerotic lesions in the aortas of these sub-human primates.

In four experiments with rats, the authors noted an increase in coronary collateral circulation of animals treated by CSA, in whom regression of coronary athero-arteriosclerosis was observed and in rats with hyocardial infarction induced by isoproterenol; in the latter regression of ischemic and degenerative myocardial tissue was induced by CSA and accompanied by a striking increase in coronary collateral circulation (Morrison et al., 1973).

Table 2. Increase in coronary artery collateral circulation in hearts of 7-1/2 to 8 year old monkeys following intramuscular administration of CSA[a]

Monkey identity	Sex	Histology: coronary count	
		Main coronaries and principal branches	Small branches and arterioles
Control group			
SM2 F	female	12	126
SM2 G	female	14	110
SM2 H	female	11	104
SM2 I	male	11	106
	Average	12	111.5
CSA treated group			
SM2 A	male	17	136
SM2 B	male	13	165
SM2 C	female	14	137
SM2 D	female	12	134
	Average	14	143

Tests of significance indicate highly significant differences between the controls and the CSA treated monkeys $p < 0.01$ (Lord, E. Biometrika 34:41, 1947)

[a]Chondroitin sulfate A was administered daily (6 days per week), dosage 20 mg per monkey.

Similar increases in coronary artery collateral circulation was found in the sub-group of squirrel monkeys treated by CSA in whom absence or regression of coronary basilar lesions was found.

Table 2 shows the statistically significant increases in the small brances and arterioles of the coronary collateral circulation of CSA treated animals as compared to control animals.

In summary, preliminary findings are noted of 1. clearance of cholesterol from human aortas and tissues by CSA in tissue, organ and whole aorta section preparations, 2. regression effects on athero-arteriosclerosis in rats by CSA feedings, 3. regression of atheromatous aorta lesions in squirrel monkeys during preventive studies over a 9 month treatment period with daily injectable CSA, 4. absence or regression of atherosclerotic lesions in the coronary arteries of squirrel monkey hearts treated for 90 days by daily CSA injections and 5. significant increases in the coronary collateral circulation by CSA feedings and injections in rats as well as by injections of CSA in squirrel monkeys.

These five parameters suggest further, long-term regression studies in sub-human primates with naturally or spontaneously occurring athero-arteriosclerosis lesions analagous to those found in man.

NECROGENIC AGENT OBTAINED FROM CHOLESTEROL USED IN DIETARY EXPERIMENTS[*]

K.T. Lee, H. Imai, N.T. Werthessen, and C.B. Taylor

Necrosis of arterial smooth muscle cells is one of the important anatomic manifestations of atherosclerosis. We have in the past conducted a short-term experiment of five days in the swine and rhesus monkey and ascertained the necrogenic effect of crystalline cholesterol on the arterial smooth muscle cell. The objective of the current study was to determine if these short-term necrogenic effects could be due to cholesterol *per se* or to contaminants of the cholesterol, such as spontaneous oxidation products.

Four separate cholesterol samples have been used in these studies. Two were old and two were fresh. All provided potent "extracts" by the following procedure:

A kilo or less of the cholesterol was placed in an appropriate large Erlenmeyer, and methanol was added in sufficient quantity to cover the cholesterol. The mixture was heated for an hour or more on the steam bath, cooled and the liquid filtered off. The procedure can be repeated to improve the yield, particularly if the cholesterol is old.

The methanol solution was then cooled to produce a crop of crystals. The crystals were removed, and the methanol was reduced under N_2 and heat. Upon cooling further crystals were formed and removed. The process was repeated until the cholesterol crystals were obviously of poor quality and contaminated by substances concentrated in the mother liquor.

At this point the methanol was removed as above until a liquid tar formed. High vacuum desiccation removed all the methanol and produced a dry porous mass which crumbled into a powder. It obviously contained cholesterol plus what were presumed to be, from analyses in progress, a multitude of oxidation products.

The experimental animals used were male New Zealand white rabbits, 2-3 kg, with free access to commerical pellets and water except for the 24-hour period prior to the gavage of the test substance. Light and electron microscopy studies were carried out on rabbits given the methanol concentrate tar. Methanol-free tar was pulverized and suspended in 2% aqueous gelatin, then administered by gastric tubing to rabbits. At the end of the experimental period, the rabbits were deeply anesthetized with pentobarbital sodium and exsanguinated. Immediately after exsanguination from the iliac artery, the left ventricle was cannulated and 3% glutaraldehyde (in 0.05 M Sorensen's phosphate buffer with 7.5% sucrose, pH 7.4) was perfused for one half to one hour at the pressure gradient of 20-25 mm/Hg. Tissue blocks were taken from the proximal descending aorta at the level of atrioventricular groove and processed for electron microscopy (1% Dalton's three hours, dehydration with hexylene glycol, Spurr's low viscosity embedding medium, double straining with acetate and lead citrate).

For the study of an acute effect of the methanol extract, 250 mg/kg body weight of the methanol extract was given to rabbits by gastric tubing and they were sacrificed 18 hours later. The characteristic changes as observed by light microscopy were scattered focal areas of hydropic, but not fatty, changes adjacent to viable smooth muscle cells. By electron microscopy, these areas were scattered foci of

[*]Supported by PHS Grant HL-14177 and BSSG-PHS Grant RR 07085.

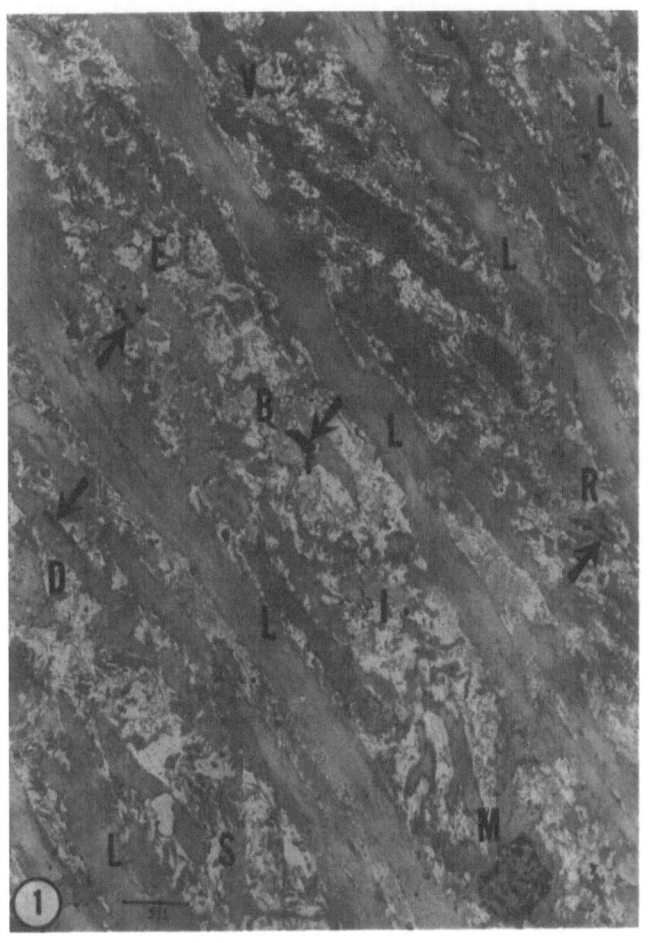

Figure 1. Methanol extract, 250 mg/kg, by gavage, 18 hours, media of thoracic aorta. Lamellae of elastica (L) appear intact and regularly spaced. Viable smooth muscle cells are at V and M. Groups of degenerated smooth muscle cells are indicated by D, E, B, R, I and S illustrating severe and extensive medial necrosis. Arrows indicate dense bodies representing nuclear debris

separation of structure which we interpreted as focal edema in the media. Groups of smooth muscle cells appeared degenerated in successive layers (Fig. 1). These changes were scattered throughout the media, apparently at random.

The typical ultrastructural changes of affected smooth muscle cells varies greatly from minimal degenerative changes to frank necrosis (Fig. 2) of the cell. In many places, exposing cytoplasmic components to the stroma. At places the membrane appeared segmented and dense. The nuclei showed various stages of pyknosis and karyorrhexis. In some cells, the perinuclear cistern was focally distended and aggregates of vesicles, possibly the remnant of the Golgi or endoplasmic reticulum, were present. In these degenerated cells, recognizable mitochondria were quite rare. Instead, dense bodies with markedly electron dense particles, probably metallic, and some suggestions of double membrane structure, were present.

When three administrations 100 mg/kg of the methanol extract were given to rabbits once every other day, and killed on the sixth day, the changes observed were similar in character and more severe than those seen after single administration.

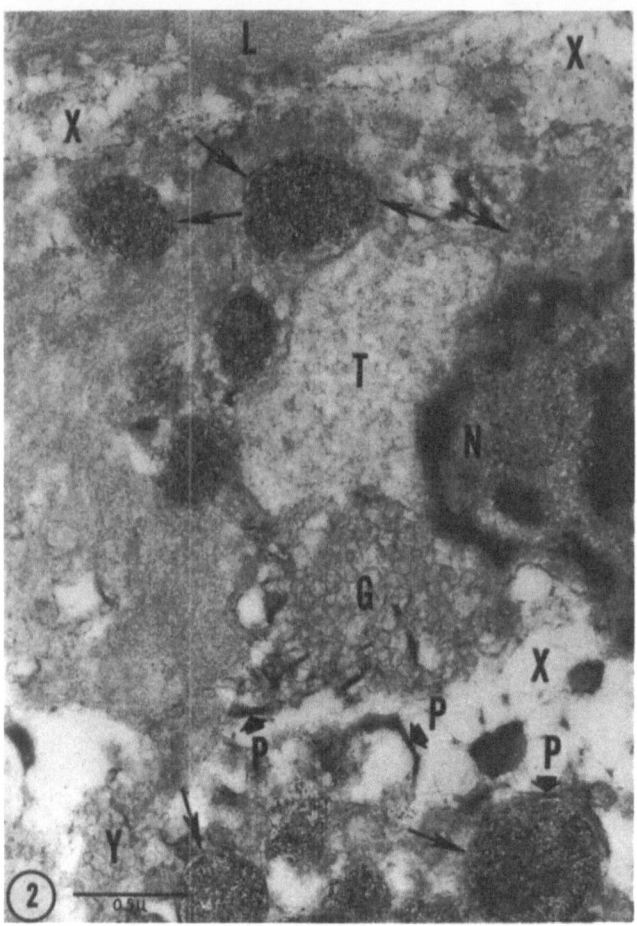

Figure 2. Methanol extract, 250 mg/kg, by gavage, 18 hours, media of thoracic aorta. N: pyknotic nucleus. T: distended perinuclear cisterna. G and Y: collection of vesicles, Golgi or E.R. Myofilaments are obscure and distorted. P: abnormally dense segments of plasmalemma. The rest of plasmalemma and basement membrane are indistinct. Mitochondria near the nuclear pole are conspicuously absent. Instead, dense bodies with granular to needle-like deposits and sporadic double membranes (arrows) are noted

The aortae of rabbits given the same dosage of cholesterol purified via dibromination in the same fashion did not show any of the above-mentioned necrotic changes of the aortic cells. The cholesterol recipients' aortae were indistinguishable from those of untreated controls.

In a study of the long-term effect of methanol extract administration, a total of 1.0 g of the methanol extract or purified cholesterol was given to two groups of 12 rabbits. The substances were administered three times a week; 250 mg were given by gavage initially and 100 and 50 mg/kg later. The experimental period was five weeks.

The aortae of pure cholesterol-fed rabbits were indistinguishable from untreated controls. Only so-called spontaneous lesions characterized mainly by the medial calcification and distortion were occasionally present. Methanol extract-fed rabbits exhibited accentuated cushions at the branching sites and, in addition, slightly elevated focal intimal lesions (Fig. 3). These methanol extract-induced lesions were characterized by frequent presence of poorly differentiated intimal

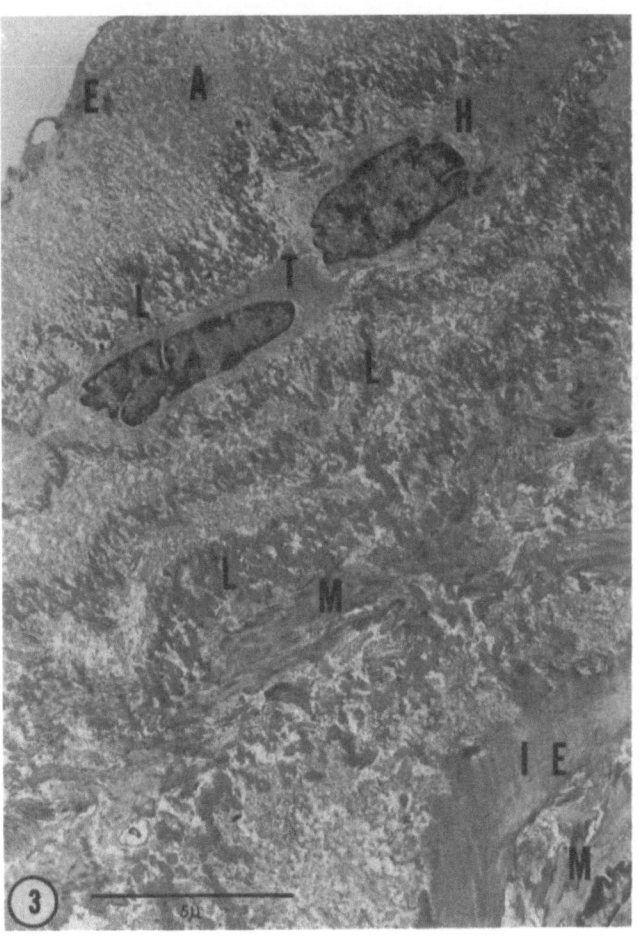

Figure 3. Intimal proliferative (not foam cell) lesion induced by a total of 1.05 g/kg methanol extract, 36 days, thoracic aorta. E: endothelium. A: redundant basement membrane densities. L: layers of fragments of elastica. H: poorly differentiated, intimal Langhaas' cell. T: transitional cell with minimal resemblance to mature smooth muscle cell (M). IE: internal elastica

cells as described by Langhaas in 1868. These Langhaas cells do not have specialized structure such as basement membrane, fusiform densities and myofilaments. The most interesting observation was that, unlike the usual cholesterol-induced lesions in the rabbit, methanol extract-induced lesions were characterized by the conspicuous absence of foam cells. The major components were modified smooth muscle cells and connective tissue.

Our preliminary studies also show that a chloroform methanol extract of commercial dry whole milk powder such as that used for dietary experiments can induce similar changes in aortic cells of rabbits.

As a result of the above observations, the following salient points can be noted: 1. necrosis and degeneration of arterial smooth muscle cells is evident at 18 hours after administration of the extract *per os*; 2. an increase in severity after further treatment is observable at 144 hours; 3. total dosage of one gram over five weeks produces a nonfatty proliferative lesion; and 4. controls given equal quantities of pure cholesterol show no such response. Therefore one can conclude that the necrosis observed when cholesterol is used in dietary experiments cannot be attributed to it, but rather to contaminants, presumably oxidation products.

PRODUCTION OF ADVANCED ATHEROMATOUS LESIONS IN AN ALLOGRAFTED SEGMENT OF AORTA IN A NORMOCHOLESTEROLAEMIC RABBIT

David E. Bowyer, David Dunn, and G. Austin Gresham

Many forms of arterial injury exacerbate the formation of atherosclerotic lesions (Constantinides, 1965) especially in the presence of hypercholesterolaemia. Well known example of methods, which have been used for injuring the arterial wall, include freezing (Taylor et al., 1950), mechanical abrasion of the intimal surface (Björkerud, 1969), application of chemicals such as allylamine (Giordano et al., 1970), and deposition of immune complexes in serum sickness (Roberts, 1960; Minick, 1966). It is also apparent that the damage caused by immune rejection of transplanted vessels leads to atherosclerotic lesion formation. Indeed, soon after the techniques of vascular surgery had been perfected by Carrell and others (Carrel, 1902; Von Decastello, 1902; Hoepfner, 1903; Carrel, 1910), Yamanouchi (1911) demonstrated that in arterial homografts, but not autografts, there was proliferative intimal thickening accompanied by medial thinning and fragmentation of the elastic lamellae. When the practical needs of reparative vascular surgery, occasioned by the Second World War, stimulated more research into arterial transplantation, the findings of Yamanouchi were confirmed (Miller et al., 1951; Sauvage and Harkins, 1953) and Fisher and Fisher (1956) showed that in hypercholesterolaemic rabbits, atherosclerosis is more severe in fresh aortic homografts than in the recipient aorta.

During the last decade, many studies of the vasculature of transplanted organs in man, have also shown increased susceptibility of the rejecting artery to the formation of lesion resembling atherosclerosis (for example in heart, see Thomson, (1969) Kosek and Bieber (1970) and, although lipid filled lesions are not always found (Kennedy et al., 1971), they often occur even in the absence of hypercholesterolaemia (Thomsen, 1969). In order to try to find a model of advanced atherosclerotic lesions, we therefore, investigated the formation of lesions produced in a normo-cholesterolaemic rabbit by immune rejection of a transplanted artery. The aorta was chosen because it would provide sufficient tissue for lipid analysis and might allow investigation of the role of haemodynamic factors in lesion formation.

The donor rabbit, a male New Zealand White, was killed by cervical fracture, the side branches of the aorta, from the diaphragm to the bifurcation, ligated and the segment removed with as little adventitial fat as possible. This took about 10 minutes. The artery was then kept at 4°C in Hank's buffered salt solution, whilst the recipient was prepared. The recipient rabbit, a male New Zealand Black, was sedated with Hypnorm (Jansen, 0.2 ml/kg im) and then anaesthetised with halothane. In order to try to inhibit aortic thrombosis, 0.9% sodium chloride containing Heparin (10 iu/ml) was infused intravenously (1 ml/min) during the operation. A mid-line incision was made and the viscera reflected to the right. The aorta was mobilised 2 cm below the renal arteries, care being taken to preserve a lumbar branch at this level. Narrow umbilical tape was threaded around the aorta proximal and distal to the mobilised segment, the aorta cross-clamped by tension on the tapes and transected. The donor segment was then inserted as a loop in series with the recipient aorta by end-to-end anastamosis using Virgin 7/0 ophthalmic silk as a continuous suture. The rabbit was killed after one year and had a serum cholesterol concentration of 70 mg/100 ml.

At autopsy, the transplanted loop was covered with a layer of fibrous tissue. When the aortas were opened, the loop was found to be distended compared with the recipient aorta and contained atheromatous lesions which were severe on the curve

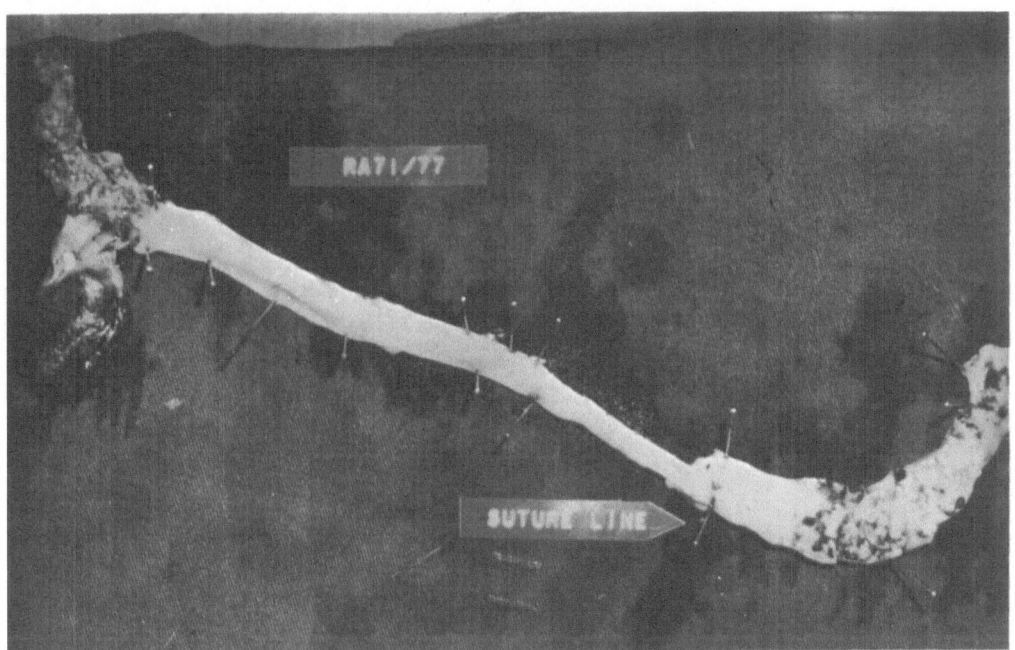

Figure 1. Macroscopic appearance of the recipient heart and aorta and the donor loop. Notice the distention of the loop and the atheromatous lesions on the curve, with relative sparing of the straight part of the segment

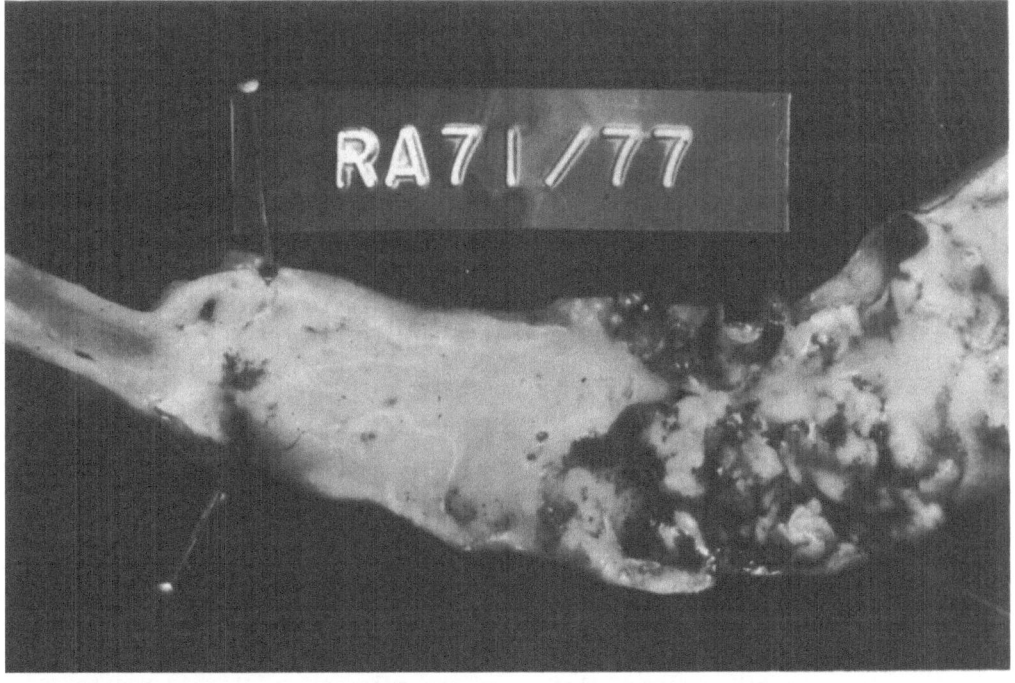

Figure 2. Detail of the transplanted loop, showing relative sparing of straight part of the segment

of the loop with relative sparing of the straight sections joining the segment to the recipient aorta. There was fibrin in some parts of the intima. The recipient aorta was undiseased (Fig. 1 and 2).

The areas of aortas adjacent to the proximal suture line were stained with silver and viewed by the scanning electron microscope (Garbarsch and Christensen, 1970). The endothelium was a continuous sheet covering the anastamosis, and had probably grown out from the recipient aorta (Lautsch et al., 1959).

Histological studies revealed that the general architecture of the loop was distorted, with thickening of the intima by fibrous connective tissue, medial thinning and fragmentation of the elastic lamellae (Fig. 3). Throughout the loop there were many 'foam cells' (Fig. 4) and the atheromatous lesions contained extracellular lipids with many cholesterol clefts. Sections stained by the Picro-Mallory method showed fibrin accumulation both on the intimal surface and within lesions None of the lesions contained haemosiderin as judged by Perl's method for ferric iron.

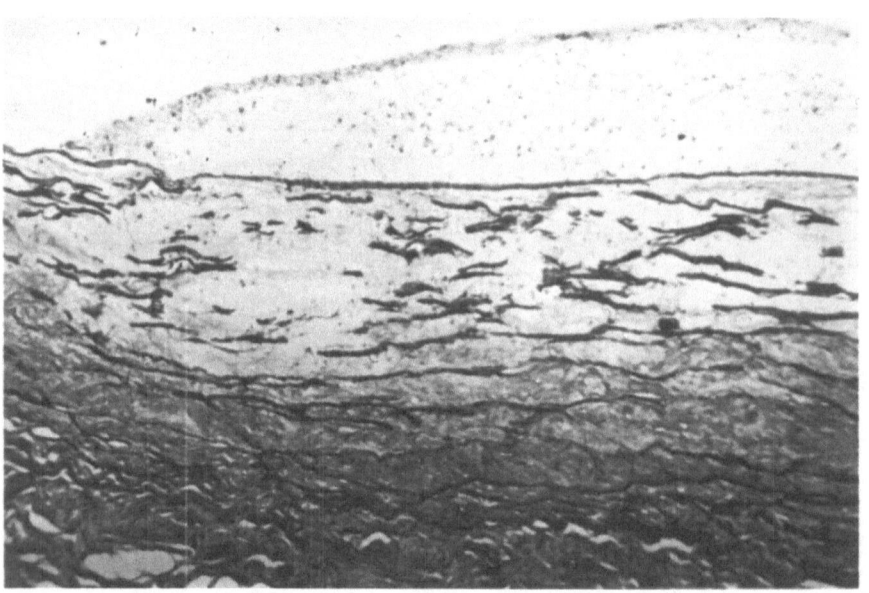

Figure 3. General architecture of an atheromatous lesion showing fragmentation of the underlying elastic lamellae. Stained with Weigert's resorcin fuchsin stain (X 10,50)

In some areas, the loop was heavily infiltrated by polymorphonuclear leukocytes (heterophils) and it was suspected that this may have been due to an infection of the graft. This was not thought to have been of long standing, because the animal had been in good health. In some areas the infiltrating polymorphs were clustered around cholesterol clefts.

The lipid composition of the arteries was also studied by micro-thin layer chromatography and chemical assay (Bowyer and King, unpublished).

A small pultaceous atheromatous plaque and the adjacent relatively undiseased tissue of the loop were analysed and the composition compared with an intima-media sample of recipient aorta. The results are shown in Table 1 and compared with an analysis of an aortic atheroma and adjacent undiseased intima from a man aged 56 years.

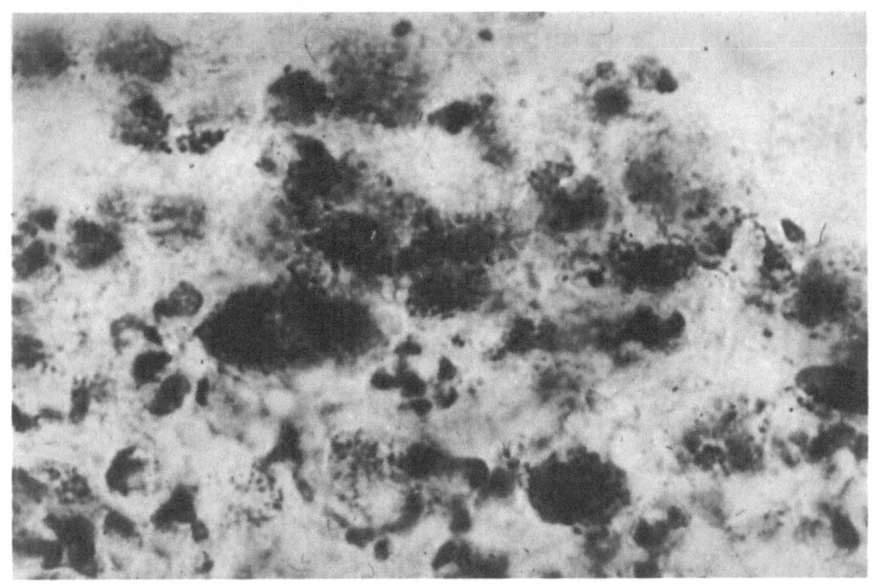

Figure 4. Foam cells in the atherosclerotic lesion, stained with Sudan III/IV mixture (X 210)

Table 1. Lipids mg/g dry defatted tissue

	LPC	SPH	PC	PS	PI	PE	FFA	TG	C	CE
Recipient	0.7	4.7	6.7	3.9	1.5	3.3	0.5	21.9	5.7	0.7
'Undiseased' donor	1.1	4.0	4.8	2.6	0.7	2.0	0.7	18.1	7.7	10.6
Atheroma	4.6	9.9	8.2	5.4	2.6	4.8	6.3	22.1	13.6	14.1
Man aged 56										
'Undiseased'	1.7	6.0	10.0	3.4	–	1.7	1.5	7.9	9.7	51.3
Atheroma	5.8	21.9	19.7	5.0	–	2.6	3.1	30.4	89.5	338.7

In the rabbit, the most marked difference in lipid composition, between the normal recipient aorta and the transplanted loop is in the concentration of free and esterified cholesterol. This parallels the situation in the human atheroma, although in that case there is a vastly greater amount of cholesteryl ester, probably because of the greater age of the lesion. In both species, in the atheroma there was more phospholipid, especially lyso-lecithin and sphingomyelin, and slightly more free fatty acid. Triglyceride accumulation in the rabbit lesion was, however, negligible.

We have concluded from this single long-term experiment, that advanced atheromatous lesions can be produced in the normo-cholesterolaemic rabbit, following immune rejection. It is known that lesions resembling atherosclerosis can even occur in synthetic vascular grafts and possibly they are formed by hyperplasia and lipid accumulation in cells of host origin which grow to line the grafts

(Tarizzo et al., 1961). It cannot be stated from this one experiment whether the immune rejection is necessary for the production of advanced lesions. Haemodynamic forces certainly play a role, in that the lesions were more severe on the curve of the loop than on the straight sections adjacent to the anastamoses.

The model provided sufficient material for chemical analysis of all of the major lipids and shows the expected accumulation of cholesterol esters in the atheroma.

It is considered that this technique would be useful in studies of the factors which contribute to atheroma formation in normo-cholesterolaemic animals and also for investigation of alterations of lipid composition, lipid metabolism and vascular permeability during acute rejection.

RAT HOMOGRAFTS OF ARTERIAL WALL FRAGMENTS
A CONTRIBUTION TO THE UNDERSTANDING OF EXPERIMENTAL ATHEROSCLEROSIS

Jacky Larrue, Jean J. Berjon, Claude Desgranges, Jean M. Meunier, and Henri Bricaud

Several mechanisms may be involved in the genesis of atherosclerotic disease: extrinsic factors, related to the contents of the arterial surroundings, intrinsic factors related to the arterial wall itself. The assessment of the role of any single factor in the pathogenesis of atherosclerosis by means of in vivo studies is extremely difficult because of the complexity of the disease. In order to suppress factors related to the circulation and for better definition of the parietal factors, we designed two systems, namely: the graft of aortic fragments into different organs and a true organotypic culture in a semisynthetic gelosed medium. The essential feature of these two techniques was the appearance of the maintenance of the morphologic integrity of the explants under standard conditions (Larrue et al., 1973 a and b). The present report deals with the data obtained by the differential or simultaneous use of these two systems.

Material and Methods

Adult male Wistar rats weighing about 150 g, born in the laboratory, and belonging to the same litter, were used. They were kept under standard conditions. The animals were killed with ether, the aorta was quickly removed and washed in an isotonic medium. The conditions of explant preparation for grafts or cultures were the same as described earlier (Larrue et al., 1973 a). The cultures were performed according to the following technique: "total explants" (5 mm x 1 mm) including the three layers (intima, media, externa) were put on 1 ml of semisynthetic gelosed medium (modified T 8 of Trowell, explant donor rat plasma, 1% agar and phenol red, without antibiotics) in a micrographic glass flask during two to five days at 37°C. In some experiments, tissue extracts were added. Other explants were grafted under the kidney capsule, or in the testis or pancreas for 1 to 15 weeks from the day of removal or after a few days of culture. At the end of the experimentation, one explant in each group was reserved for microscopy. Light microscopic preparations included sections stained with hematoxylin and eosin, Weigert's resorcin fuchsin, Masson's trichrome, and Alcian-blue PAS. Histoenzymologic study included the following enzymes: LDH, MDH, G-6-PDH according to the method of Hess et al. (1958), ATPase (Padykula and Herman, 1955), alkaline phosphatase (Gomori, 1941), ß-glucuronidase according to Seligman et al. (1954).

Results

1. Development of the Explant System in Culture (Fig. 1)

Under standard conditions, the morphologic integrity of the explant was correctly preserved. The cultures gave consistent results for 4 days, at least. There was no real increase in the number of cells in the explant nor cellular growth at the periphery. The dehydrogenase activities disappeared about 5 days later, followed by weak cell necrosis which increased later; but ATPase was partially maintained in the same way as alkaline phosphatase.

The organotypic cultures with pancreatic or testicular extracts of the same animal supplying the explant added to the medium, yielded different results according to the origin of extract used. With pancreatic extract, the culture showed generally a weak cellular growth outside and into the explant, the elastic framework

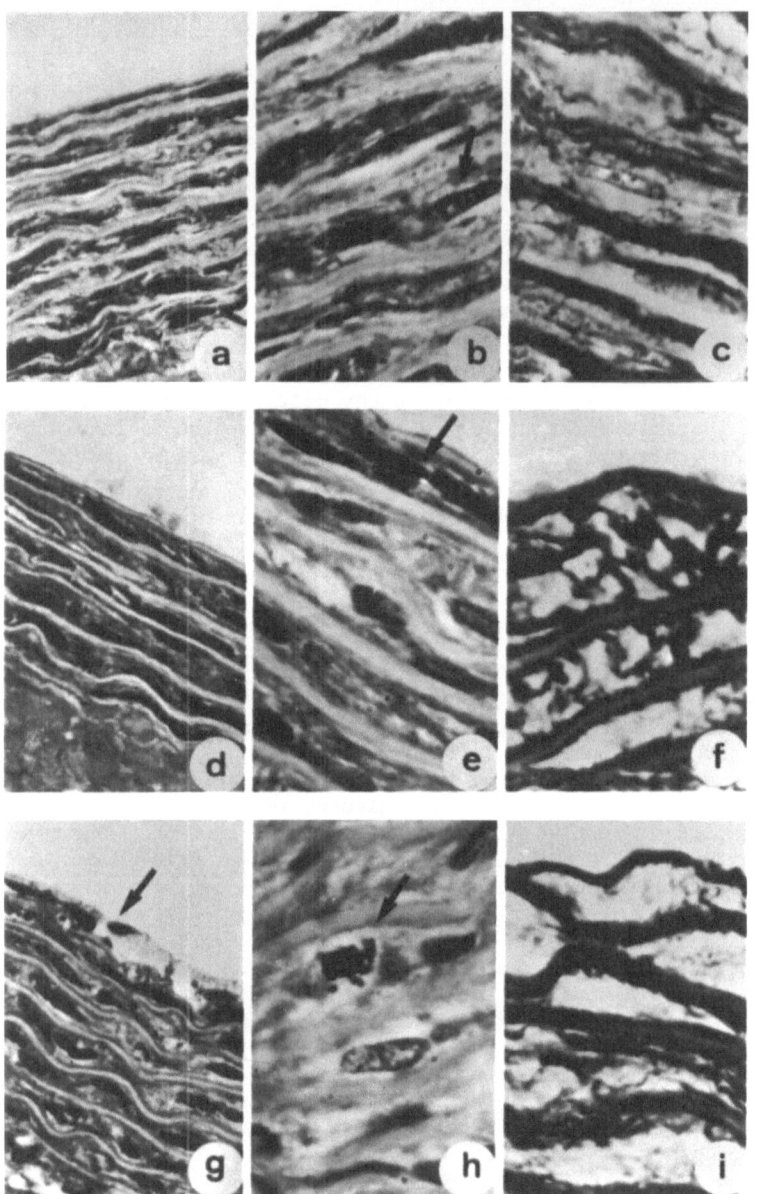

Figure 1. Modifications of the explants in culture after 4 days. Upper row: maintenance of the morphologic integrity under standard conditions. Masson's trichrome
X 328 (a), X 820 (b), Weigert's resorcin fuchsin X 820 (c). Middle row: culture
in the presence of testicular extract. Pyknotic nuclei (arrow). Masson's trichrome
X 328 (d) and X 820 (e). The elastic membranes in the inner half of the tunica
media are seen to be fragmented. Weigert's resorcin fuchsin X 820 (f). Bottom
row: culture in the presence of pancreatic extract. Cellular growth out of the
explant (arrow) (g) and mitosis in the explant (arrow) (h). Masson's trichrome
X 328 (g) and X 820 (h). Normal elastic membranes. Weigert's resorcin fuchsin x
820 (i)

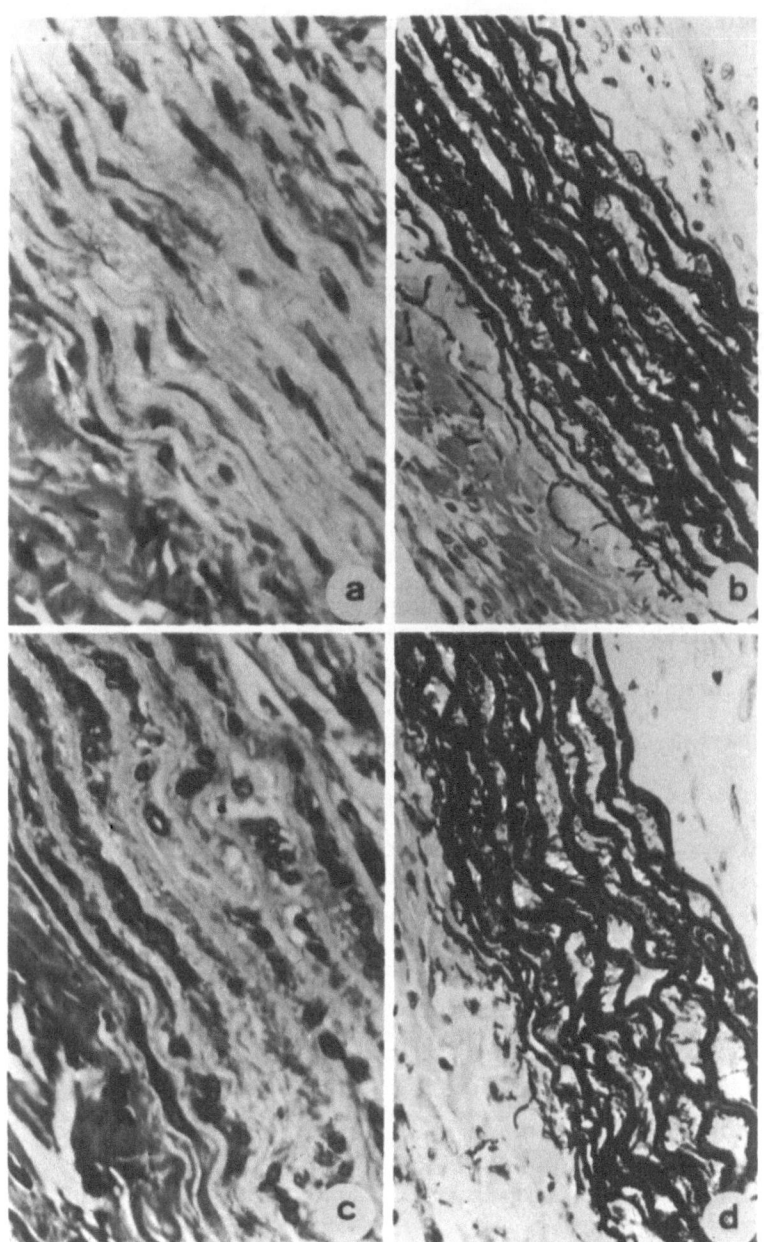

Figure 2. Evolution of the explant in graft. Upper row: graft under the kidney capsule on the 8th day. Maintenance of normal organization of the explant. Masson's trichrome (a) and Weigert's resorcin fuchsin (b) X 328. Lower row: graft in pancreas on the 8th day. Cellular proliferation and disarrangement in the tunica media (c), maintenance of the elastic framework (d). Masson's trichrome (c), Weigert's resorcin fuchsin (d) X 328

being quite normal. On the contrary, cultures on a medium with testicular extract had no peripheral growth, but inside the explant there was cellular necrosis with numberous pyknotic nuclei; the elastic lamellae were thick, rigid, and often torn.

2. *Development of the Explant System in Graft (Fig. 2)*

a) The graft under the kidney capsule preserved in our experimental conditions, without any rejection, normal organization of the aortic wall at least 60 days after grafting. The externa kept all these characteristics and normal vascularizatiqn. The media showed no modification. We could observe the same organized features and the same relations between fibrous and cellular constituents as in the "in place" organ. Nevertheless, the intima seemed to be disorganized in front of kidney parenchyma. Histoenzymatic activities were normal for all the enzymes studied, except alkaline phosphatase activity which disappeared quickly from the media externa junction (Fig. 3a).

b) The graft in both testis and pancreas produced several modifications of the explant structure. The externa remained intact but the media, on the contrary, showed cellular proliferation and disarrangement in relation to the fibrous framework, with cell dedifferentiation. In some grafts, these phenomena were located exclusively from the internal half of the media, the external half being free of cells. Elastic structures did not seem altered in the pancreatic graft, but had microfibrillar expansions in the testicular graft. The intima presented the same modification as in the kidney graft. These morphological alterations were constantly and significantly accompanied by histometabolic variations.

The dehydrogenase activities (LDH, MDH, G-6-PDH) and ATPase are irregularly distributed but of normal intensity. The ß-glucuronidase was always extremely increased. In these two cases (graft and culture alone), we saw parietal alterations due to the effect of the medium; (nature of the receiver organ used in graft, nature of the medium for cultures). These alterations could be used as reference of a modification of intrinsic metabolism of the arterial wall (Fig. 3b).

3. *Development of the explant system previously cultivated, then grafted*

If the graft was performed after 4 days of culture (the explants had kept their enzymatic activities), we observed good maintenance of both histometabolic and structural features 15 days later. On the other hand, if five-day-culture explants (which had lost the major part of their enzymatic activities) were grafted under the kidney capsule, we noticed without any sign of rejection complete disorganization of the graft 75 days later. Elastic lamellae were calcified with mesenchymal cells arranged around them, and numerous macrophages were found. All these characteriestics suggested ossification processes.

Conclusion

The utilization of both organotypic culture and graft techniques alone or associated, in different surroundings, is able to produce numerous and specific alterations in both metabolism and structure of the arterial wall. It seems very important to notice that these alterations, which have many of the features of early atherosclerosis, are obtained in a short time (a week) in species with a high resistance to the disease.

Furthermore, the true organotypic culture of the aorta may be considered a suitable standard system for studies of factors in tissue extract, drugs, or serums, which may be related to the atherogenesis.

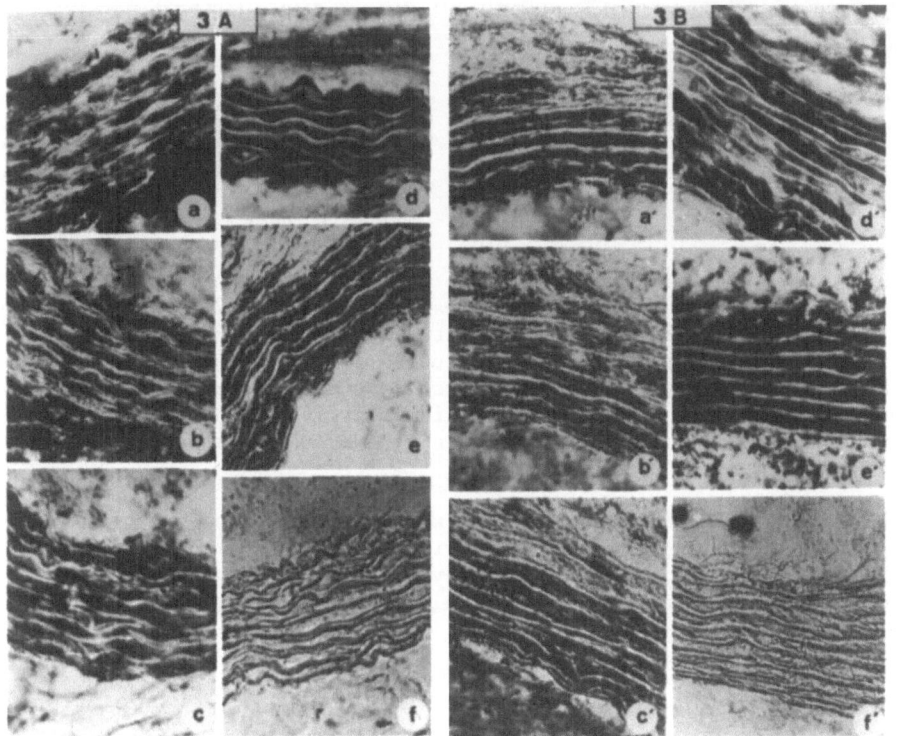

Figure 3. Histoenzymologic study of the graft under the kidney capsule on the 15th day (3a). Normal distribution of dehydrogenase activities, cells reacting positively to LDH (a), MDH (b), and G-6-PDH (c). ATPase (d) and ß-glucuronidase (e) are normal. Alkaline phosphatase is inactive (f). Histoenzymology of the graft in the testis on the 15th day (3b). Irregular distribution of enzyme activities in the tunica media. LDH (a'), MDH (b'), G-6-PDH (c'), ATPase (d'). Increase of ß-glucuronidase activity (e'). No reaction of alkaline phosphatase (f'). Frozen sections x 400

Also, the graft constitues a fertile step before experimenting on the whole animal. With its characteristics, the graft may be regarded as a true "in vivo culture", and it is able to contribute to the understanding of arterial wall behavior in pathological conditions.

The cultures were performed in the Laboratory of Biology, Hopital Xavier Arnozan Bordeaux. We again wish to thank Mrs. F. Drouillet, Misses D. Dabernat and J. Demond, and Mr. H. Gomez for their technical assistance.

H. Hess, M. Marshall, and M. Mallasch

The scanning electron microscope in combination with a multichannel analyser proved to be a many-sided instrument for studies on the reactions in and on artery walls. This combination enables us to demonstrate at the same time the morphology of the surfaces and to perform histochemical studies in the same areas. The principle of this technique is, in short, as follows: a primal electron beam is scanning in a high-vacuum line by line as a television monitor over a chosen area of a slide. Thus the relief of the surface is drawn by the emitted secondary electrons and the backscattered electrons.

The primal radiation simultaneously induces an x-ray emission. The spectrum of this radiation consists of the nonspecific slowing continuum and characteristic lines specific for the elements within the analyzed area. By means of special histochemical reactions, elements from outside can be made to precipitate on

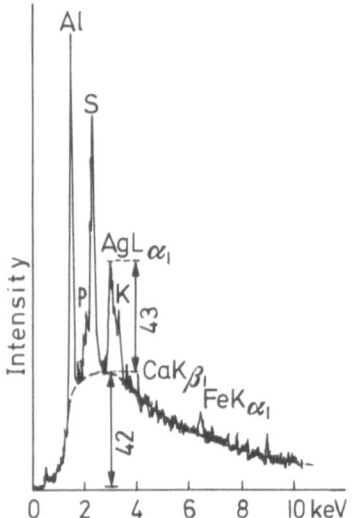

Figure 1. Integral x-ray spectrum of a segment of the femoral artery of a minipig after argentaffin reaction with epinephrine and norepinephrine. Above the background (drawn into the original graph subsequently with interrupted line) maxima of intensity are to be seen, the energies of which are characteristic for aluminum K | (1.49 keV), phosphorus K | (2.01 keV), sulphur K | (2.31 keV), silver L | (2.98 keV), potassium K | (3.31 keV), calcium K | (3.69 keV) and iron K | (6.40 keV).

The quotient – $\dfrac{\text{intensity Ag}_L \mid \text{above background}}{\text{intensity background}}$ = 43:42 = 1.02.

(From: M. Marshall, H. Hess, and M. Mallasch: On the Content of Biogenous Amines in Several Arteries of the Miniature Pig. Res.exp.Med., 161, 210–223 (1973))

---

[*]Mit Unterstützung der Deutschen Forschungsgemeinschaft.

biologicals. The different biogenous amines for instance react more or less argentaffin or chromaffin dependent on the fixation method and incubation time in
solutions of silver or chromium (Geyer, 1969). The thus precipitated amount of
silver or chromium depends on the amount of reacting biogenous amine and can be
demonstrated semi-quantitatively by x-ray microanalysis (Fig. 1) (Hess et al.,
(1972).

Results

1. The inner layer of the in vivo extirpated femoral artery of man and miniature
pig are identical in morphology. We did not by any means find adhesions of particles of the streaming blood, especially platelets or fibrin, on the arterial
endothelium of healthy people and so far nonirradiated miniature pigs (Hess and
Frost, 1969).

2. The innermost layers of the femoral artery of man and minipig contain equal
amounts of norepinephrine, dopamine and serotonin. In both vessels no epinephrine
at all or only very little could be demonstrated.

The thoracic aorta of the miniature pig contains much less norepinephrine than
the abdominal aorta or the femoral, carotid, or coronary artery (Fig. 2) (Marshall
et al., 1973).

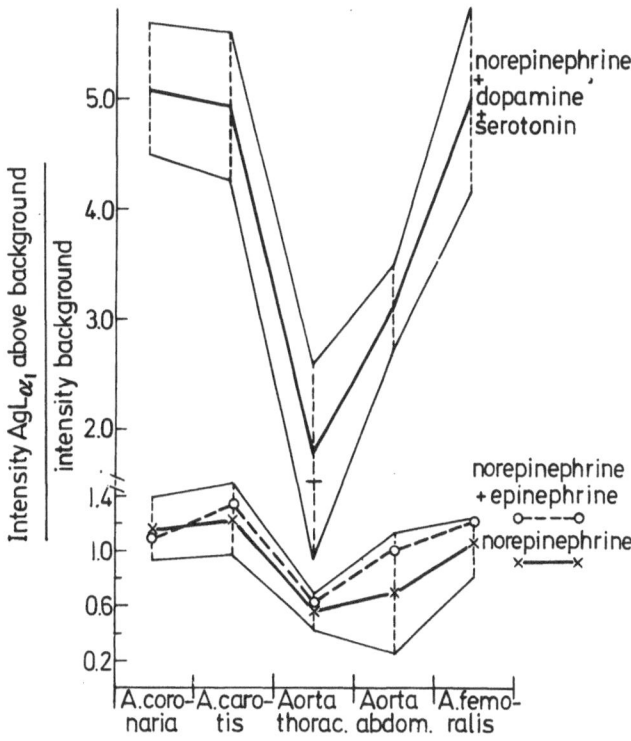

Figure 2. Comparison of catecholamine content of inner wall layers of different
artery segments of three minipigs. For epinephrine and norepinephrine the average
value only of the quotient is drawn out, for the argentaffin reactions with norepinephrine alone, for norepinephrine plus dopamine plus serotonin the deviations
are also shown. (From: M. Marshall, H. Hess, and M. Mallasch: On the Content of
Biogenous Amines in Several Arteries of the Miniature Pig. Res.exp.Med., 161,
210–223 (1973))

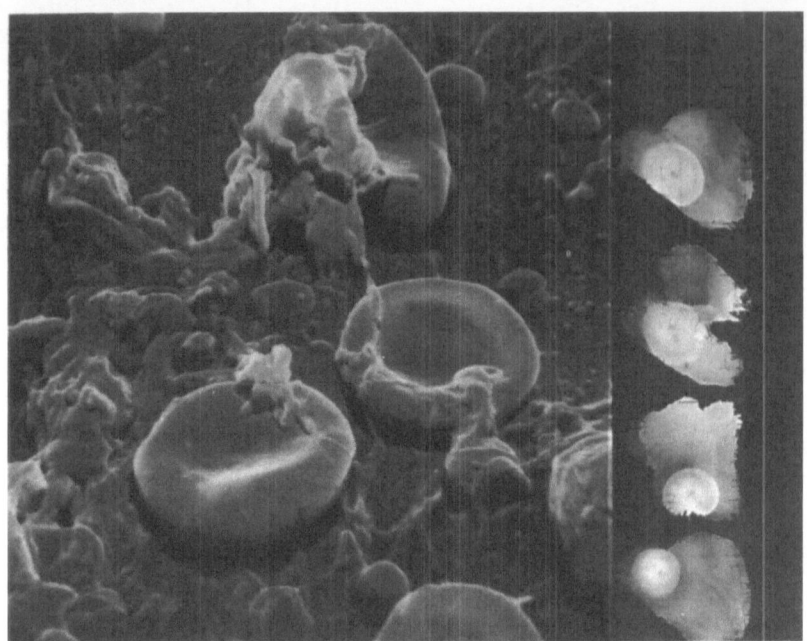

Figure 3. Inner surface of the femoral artery extirpated during amputation of the right leg of an 83-year-old man with arteriosclerosis obliterans. Adhesions of platelets and fibrin-surrounded erythrocytes are seen. Scanning electron microscopic enlargement 5000:1, Registration No. 9470

3. On the endothelium of patent femoral arteries extirpated in vivo from patients with obliterative arteriosclerosis, adhesions of platelets or fibrin or included erythrocytes can be found regularly (Fig. 3).

4. There were further minipig experiments in order to answer the question whether these adhesions of particles of the streaming blood on the arterial wall are early changes in the developing obliterative angiopathy or late complications of this disease, which imitated conditions leading to obliterative arteriosclerosis in man.

a) *Cold Angiitis.* A ten-minute contact with ice of a minipig carotid or femoral artery always leads to adherence of platelets on the intact looking endothelium within the exposed segment, as it does in man.

Within a few hours, the first spherical platelets with pseudopods change by continuous metamorphosis into coherent covers which stick together like wallpaper.

The cold angiitis of man does not histologically differ at all from the endangiitis obliterans which is induced mainly by smoking.

b) *Thrombangiitis Obliterans.* In two experiments in which minipigs inhaled cigarette smoke in the respired air at intervals, adherent platelets were found on the endothelium of the femoral and carotid as well as on the coronary artery in all biologicals.

After the smoking experiments the content of the innermost vascular layers of the carotid and femoral arteries was ten per cent higher than before.

c) Arteriosclerosis in Hyperlipidemia. Similar adhesions of platelets can be demonstrated in the pig already a few days after ingesting dried food containing five per cent cholesterol. In the rabbit the same could be demonstrated already after one such feeding.

With the models demonstrated so far, in which the vessels were studied from a few minutes to six days after irritation, only platelet adhesions were found. But on the endothelium of rabbit arteries, platelets as well as clots could be seen after a four-month high cholesterol diet. In these cases the wall-adherent thrombi are already partly covered by endothelium and thus incorporated in the vessel wall.

Similar pictures of human obliterative arteriosclerosis plead for the idea that here also platelet adhesions and secondary clots are early changes in the course of the vascular disease and not late complications (Hess, 1970).

EFFECT OF EXERCISE ON COLLAGEN AND ELASTIN IN AORTAS OF COCKERELS WITH INDUCED ATHEROSCLEROSIS

Harry Y.C. Wong, Stanley N. David, and Simeon O. Orimilikwe

To our knowledge no report exists on the influence of exercise on arterial wall connective tissue as related to atherosclerosis. It has been reported by Fischer and Llaurado (1966) that the combination of collagen and elastin comprise over one-half the dry weight of the arterial wall. Fischer (1972) reported that in rats without estrogen treatment, the level of arterial collagen was likely to be elevated. This resulted in a marked rise in collagen to elastin ratio which is an index of the rigidity of an artery. Burton (1954) indicated that the passive tension of the wall is largely due to collagen and elastin. A low collagen to elastin ratio (C/E) increases distensibility in blood vessels like the aorta with high concentration of elastin fibers. Conversely, the relatively stiff coronary artery has a high proportion of collagen fibers and is inclined toward atherosclerosis. Therefore, any substance or factor which will change the collagen and elastin ratio in arteries would affect the rigidity of the wall and thus be implicated in the pathogenesis of atherosclerosis. The present study was undertaken to determine the effects of exercise upon the hydroxyproline concentration of collagen and elastin in aortas of cockerels with atherosclerosis induced by and maintained on a high cholesterol regimen.

Materials and Methods

This experiment was performed in two parts. *Part one:* One hundred and twenty-four 50-week-old Hy-line cockerels were divided into two groups of 62 birds each. One group was maintained on a commercial plain mash (P.M.) diet while the other group was fed an atherogenic diet (A.D.) consisting of a mixture of P.M. plus 2% cholesterol and 5% cottonseed oil by weight. After fasting overnight the body weight and plasma samples were taken at the beginning of the experiment and every two weeks thereafter. Total plasma cholesterol was determined by the method of Wong et al. (1965). After eight weeks on these diets, seven birds from each group were sacrificed at random to determine the degree of aortic atherosclerosis according to the method of Katz and Stamler (1953). All birds on a cholesterol regimen had aortic lesions averaging 2.1 while birds on plain mash had none. *Part two:* Nine birds from each diet were exercised while nine others served as controls. Groups thus formed were: I. Controls, P.M.; II. P.M. + exercise; III. A.D.; and IV. A.D. + exercise. Exercise consisted of running in a circular treadmill 20 minutes twice daily, 5 consecutive days a week at a rate of approximately 750 yards daily. At the end of an additional eight weeks, these cockerels were sacrificed. The hearts, adrenals and thyroids were excised and weighed. The aortae were rapidly removed, trimmed of extraneous tissue and opened longitudinally to be grossly graded by the method vide supra. The aortae were blotted with filter paper and weighed. A section of the thoracic aorta was removed, weighed and minced. The hydroxyproline concentration for collagen and elastin was determined according to the method of Newman and Logan (1950). The level of nitrogen in the collagen extract was analyzed by the procedure of Houck and Jacob (1958).

Results

Table 1 summarizes the plasma cholesterol levels and severity of aortic atherosclerosis of cockerels selected from plain mash or the atherogenic diet prior to the beginning of the second part of the experiment. There were no significant differences between the initial and final plasma cholesterol values of the controls

Table 1. Effect of exercise on plasma cholesterol and severity of aortic athero-sclerosis of cockerels with induced atherogenesis

| Groups | No. of birds | Plasma cholesterol | | Aortic grading | | |
		Initial mg/100 ml	Final mg/100 ml	No. with lesions	%	Avg.
Before experiment						
Controls, plain mash (P.M.)	7	92 ± 2[a]	95 ± 3	0	0	0[d]
Atherogenic diet (A.D.)[b]	7	90 ± 3	874 ± 206	7	100	2.1
After experiment						
Controls, P.M.	9	91 ± 3	93 ± 3	0	0	0
P.M. + exercise[c]	9	84 ± 3	87 ± 4	0	0	0
A.D.	9	1276 ± 173	1195 ± 154	9	100	2.9
A.D. + exercise	9	953 ± 34	906 ± 32	5	55	0.3

[a] Standard error of mean.
[b] 2% cholesterol + 5% cottonseed oil added to mash.
[c] 750 yds. daily, 5 days per week.
[d] Based on zero to four.

on plain mash. Birds fed a cholesterol regimen showed a ten fold increase in plasma cholesterol by the end of the first eight weeks. The data show that exercise had no effect on plasma cholesterol of cockerels on either plain mash or on an atherogenic diet. Prior to the second part of the experiment, no gross aortic lesion was observed in any of the controls on plain mash while all birds in the atherogenic fed groups had lesions with an average gross grading of 2.1 based on a scale of zero to four. After eight weeks of exercise, no lesions were noted in any of the controls on plain mash. In the group fed an atherogenic regimen only, all cockerels had aortic lesions with a grading of 2.9 which was more severe than the 2.1 grading of a similarly fed group before the second part of the experiment began. Five of nine of the cholesterol fed birds which were exercised had lesions with an average grading of 0.3. This severity was lower than the 2.9 of the similarly fed non-exercised group. It was also lower than the initial grading of 2.1 for the cholesterol fed group even though these birds were continued to be fed an atherogenic regimen for another eight weeks. Before the experiment began, the adrenal and thyroid weights of the birds fed either plain mash or a cholesterol regimen were not statistically different. After exercising for eight weeks, our data indicate that physical activity did not have a marked effect on either adrenal or thyroid weights of any of the exercised groups (Table 2). The adrenal glands of the atherogenic group with exercise were much heavier than the controls on plain mash ($p < .01$). Exercise had no effect on thyroid weights, but the thyroids of the group fed a cholesterol diet only were significantly heavier than the exercised controls on plain mash ($p < .001$).

Table 3 depicts the changes in the hydroxyproline concentration of collagen and elastin as well as the C/E ratio in the thoracic aortas of these birds with induced atherosclerosis. There were no significant changes in the hydroxyproline content of collagen in any of the birds except the atherogenic fed group with exercise. This group was markedly lower in collagen than the plain mash group with

Table 2. Influence of exercise on adrenal and thyroid weights of cockerels with induced atherosclerosis

Groups	No. of birds	Adrenal wt. (mg)	Thyroid wt. (mg)
Before experiment			
Controls, plain mash (P.M.)	7	205 ± 10[a]	215 ± 21
Atherogenic diet (A.D.)[b]	7	222 ± 22	198 ± 29
After experiment			
Controls, P.M.	9	194 ± 11	200 ± 17
P.M. + exercise[c]	9	227 ± 16	187 ± 8
A.D.	9	233 ± 12	247 ± 12[e]
A.D. + exercise	9	243 ± 7[d]	210 ± 14

[a] Standard error of mean.
[b] 2% cholesterol + 5% cottonseed oil added to mash.
[c] 750 yds. daily, 5 days per week.
[d] $p < .01$ - controls, P.M. vs A.D. + exercise.
[e] $p < .001$ - controls, P.M. vs A.D.

exercise or the group fed an atherogenic diet only. Exercise did not have any effect on the concentration of hydroxyproline of elastin in the thoracic aorta. Of these changes, the most important factor was the C/E ratio. Exercise had no influence on the collagen to elastin ratio of the controls on plain mash. However, the ratio of the atherogenic fed group with exercise was significantly lower than that of the non-exercised birds fed a similar diet ($p < .05$). It was also observed that the ratio of the exercised group fed an atherogenic regimen was markedly lower than similarly fed exercised birds on plain mash ($p < .005$) (Table 3). Further analyses were undertaken to determine the amount of hydroxyproline and nitrogen in the collagen extract of 100 mg. of dry, lipid-free aortic tissue. There were no marked differences in any of the groups with the exception of the birds on an atherogenic regimen with exercise. The amount of hydroxyproline in the group on an atherogenic diet was significantly reduced by exercise when compared to similarly exercised birds on plain mash ($p < .01$). The concentration of nitrogen in collagen extract was statistically different for only the exercised group on a cholesterol regimen. The content of nitrogen in this group was markedly lower ($p < .001$) than the exercised group on plain mash. Changes in both levels of hydroxyproline and nitrogen further confirm the significant difference observed in the C/E ratio of the exercised birds on an atherogenic diet as compared to the other groups.

Discussion

In this study the exercise employed was not sufficiently severe to lower the plasma cholesterol levels of cockerels on an atherogenic diet with induced aortic atherosclerosis. That the physical activity was not stressful was further indicated by the slight increase in the adrenal weights of the birds on plain mash or on an atherogenic diet. Results from this study indicate that the hydroxyproline concentration of collagen was not influenced by exercise and the only decrease was observed in the atherogenic fed group with exercise. Our values are lower than

Table 3. Hydroxyproline concentration of collagen and elastin in thoracic aortas of cockerels with induced atherosclerosis

Groups	No. of birds	Percentage hydroxyproline due to collagen	Percentage hydroxyproline due to elastin	C/E ratio
Controls, P.M.	9	1.64 ± 0.12[a]	1.32 ± 0.07	1.31 ± 0.16
P.M. + exercise[b]	9	1.71 ± 0.55	1.20 ± 0.01	1.39 ± 0.05
A.D.[c]	9	1.70 ± 0.02	1.19 ± 0.04	1.46 ± 0.14[d]
A.D. + exercise	9	1.42 ± 0.08	1.24 ± 0.07	1.15 ± 0.06[e]

[a] Standard error of mean.
[b] 750 yards daily, 5 days a week.
[c] 2% cholesterol + 5% cottonseed oil added to mash.

$$C/E = \frac{\text{Percent of hydroxyproline due to collagen}}{\text{Percent of hydroxyproline due to elastin}}.$$

[d] $p < .05$ A.D. vs A.D. + exercise.
[e] $p < .05$ A.D. + exercise vs P.M. + exercise.

those reported by Cembrano et al. (1960) and Nichols et al. (1971). The former also reported that the collagen and elastin of aortas of five to six month old chickens was significantly higher in cockerels than pullets. The latter investigators reported that the hydroxyproline concentration of collagen in the thoracic aorta of cockerels fed a diet containing 0.5% cholesterol at the end of five months was elevated as compared to the controls on plain mash. They observed that the total hydroxyproline concentration in the abdominal aorta of controls and treated birds was higher than the values determined in the thoracic segments. Exercise had no effect on the elastin concentration of the thoracic aorta for our plain mash controls which is similar to the data reported by Cembrano et al. (1960) and Nichols et al. (1971). Exercise had no effect on the collagen to elastin ratio of cockerels on plain mash, while the cholesterol fed group which was exercised had a significantly lower C/E ratio as compared to a similarly fed non-exercised group. It has been suggested by Kramsch and Hollander (1973) that the mechanism involved in the deposition of lipids in arterial elastin may be due to an interaction of the elastin protein to LDL or VLDL lipoproteins. Since a decrease in the C/E ratio also indicates a lower concentration of collagen and elastin, we can only speculate that this may explain the phenomena observed in our study whereby there was a reversal in the severity of aortic atherosclerosis of exercised cockerels with induced atherosclerosis when compared to a similarly fed sedentary group even though the plasma cholesterol of these two groups was not significantly different.

THE ROLE OF HYPERTENSION AND HYPERLIPEMIA IN THE MORPHOGENESIS OF EXPERIMENTAL ATHEROSCLEROSIS[*]

Alberto Trillo, Serge Renaud, and M. Daria Haust

Introduction

Data accumulating from extensive investigations into the nature of both human and animal experimental atherosclerosis during the past decades suggest that this disease may represent the end result of many factors acting upon, or operating within, the structurally and metabolically complex arterial wall. These various factors may be acting either singly or synergistically and may be playing either an initial, aggravating, or complicating role with respect to the underlaying intimal lesion, or may precipitate the clinical manifestations and their sequelae (Haust and More, 1972).

Among the factors often related to either one or several levels of atherosclerosis are hyperlipemia and hypertension. Whereas intimal lipid accumulations in general are related to, or regarded as a consequence of hyperlipemia, hypertension has been thought to enhance the lesions possibly by several means (Hass, 1955; Hess and Stäubli, 1963; Koletsky and Rivera-Velez, 1968; Still, 1970; McGill et al., 1961; Esterly, 1965; Still, 1967; 1968; Hüttner et al., 1970). However, it has not been established with certainty how either of the above implicated factors operates, and whether the mode of operation is always identical.

To study some of these unresolved problems the present experiments were carried out.

Material and Methods

Four groups each consisting of 12 Holzman male rats were utilized in the present experiments. The total length of the experiments was 26 weeks and the experimental procedures were as follows: Group I. Metacorticoid hypertension was induced by subcutaneous administration of desoxycorticosterone acetate at the dosage of two milligrams per day during four weeks. In addition, the animals had one per cent sodium chloride added to their drinking water for an additional week. The animals of group II, on an identical hypertensive regime, were fed a hyperlipemic diet (Renaud et al., 1966) for the remaining 21 weeks. The rats in group III were kept exclusively on the same hyperlipemic diet for 21 weeks. Group IV consisted of animals fed Purina Chow pellets and water ad libitum, and served as the normal control group.

All animals were killed and their aortae, hearts and brains removed and processed for the study of arterial lesions. This report is concerned with the results of morphological examinations of the aortae only. The extent of involvement of the aortic surface with atherosclerotic lesions was graded from 0 to ++++. Sections removed from standard sites of the aortae from all 48 animals were processed for light and electron microscopy by well established conventional techniques.

---

[*]Presented in part at the 54th Annual Meeting of the Federation of American Societies for Experimental Biology, Atlantic City, N.J., April, 1970 (Trillo et al., 1970).

Results

In normal control animals the intima consisted of a continous layer of endothelial cells separated from the internal elastic lamina by a narrow subendothelial space containing scanty connective tissue elements.

In hypertensive normolipemic animals the intimal alterations considered to represent the earliest lesions consisted of the formation of gaps at the endothelial cell junctions. Often, membrane-bound vesicles containing a particulate matter occupied these gaps. In somewhat more progressed lesions, the intima was considerably thickened and contained smooth muscle cells, pools of a fibrogranular proteinaceous material, fibrin and strands of basement lamina-like material. In the media, the intercellular spaces were widened and occupied by aggregated strands of basement lamina-like material and newly formed elastic elements (Fig. 1).

In hyperlipemic rats, the early lesions were characterized by a widened intima containing smooth muscle cells with intracytoplasmic lipid droplets and by the presence of osmiophilic bodies in the subendothelial space. At a later stage, the thickened intima and inner media were largely occupied by lipid laden cells, many osmiophilic bodies and lipid droplets laying freely in the interstitial spaces (Fig. 2).

In hypertensive hyperlipemic animals, the endothelial cells appeared thinned out and in many instances showed degenerative and necrotic features. Lipid droplets and osmiophilic bodies were largely increased in the subendothelial space. Pools of proteinaceous material and fibrin were also a prominent feature in the interstitial spaces. Advanced lesions showed large areas of the intima devoid of endothelial lining and containing large amounts of proteinaceous material, lipids, red blood cells, cellular debris and a few cholesterol clefts. There were numerous areas of rupture and splitting in the internal elastic lamina. In the media, the widened interstitial spaces contained large amounts of lipid in various forms, and proteinaceous material (Fig. 3). Intracytoplasmic lipid droplets and occasional small cholesterol clefts were also present in some smooth muscle cells. Other medial smooth muscle cells were in various stages of necrosis.

Comments

Aortic lesions were found in all animals of the three experimental groups. The type and severity of the lesions depended upon the experimental regime.

In normolipemic hypertensive rats, the lesions were predominantly of insudative nature and contained varying amounts of nondescript proteinaceous material and identifiable fibrin. The formation of gaps and thinning of the endothelial cytoplasm indicated overstretching of the intimal surface. This type of arterial lesion is comparable to the grey gelatinous elevations considered to represent early or potential atherosclerotic lesions (Haust, 1971).

In hyperlipemic normotensive animals, the aortic alterations were characterized by intra- and extracellular deposition of lipid material and cellular degeneration. The latter may well have resulted from overdistention with intracellular lipid accumulation or impaired metabolism. The microscopic appearance of these especially early lesions is comparable to that of the fatty dots and streaks.

The more severe and complex lesions were observed in hypertensive hyperlipemic animals and represented a combination of processes of insudation of blood components, lipid accumulation and cellular degeneration. In addition, cholesterol clefts, not observed in either of the two other groups of animals, were present. Strands of basement lamina-like material, collagen and elastic tissue elements were also present in the lesions and were particularly prominent in the media.

It may be stated in conclusion that under our experimental conditions, hypertension not only aggravates atherosclerotic lesions but per se seems to have resulted in focal alterations resembling in several aspects the gelatinous elevations, i.e., that is one of the three forms considered to represent early atherosclerotic lesions.

▶

Figure 1. Electron micrograph of the aortic intima from a hypertensive normolipemic rat. The endothelium (en) is thinned out. The widened subendothelial space contains pools of fibrogranular material (gm), elastic tissue (el), and strands of basement lamina-like material (arrows). The internal elastic lamina (iel) is ruptured and the gaps occupied by smooth muscle cells (sm) (x 4.800)

Figure 2. Electron micrograph of the aorta from a hyperlipemic normotensive rat. The subendothelial space is considerably widened and contains many lipid droplets (li) and osmiophilic bodies (ob). The internal elastic lamina (iel) shows numerous gaps (arrows). In the media, the intercellular spaces contain osmiophilic bodies (ob) (x 5.000)

Figure 3. Electron micrograph of the aorta from a hypertensive hyperlipemic rat. Large areas of the intima are devoid of endothelial lining and contain large amounts of fibrogranular proteinaceous material (gm), lipid droplets (li), osmiophilic bodies (ob), fibrin (f), red blood cells (rbc), and cell debris (d). In the media, there are accumulations of osmiophilic bodies (ob) and cholesterol clefts (cc) (x 4.900)

Figure 1

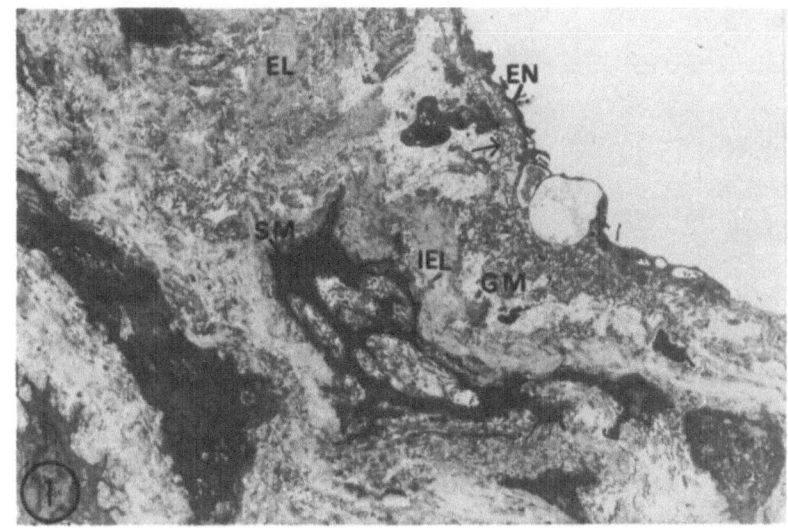

Figure 2

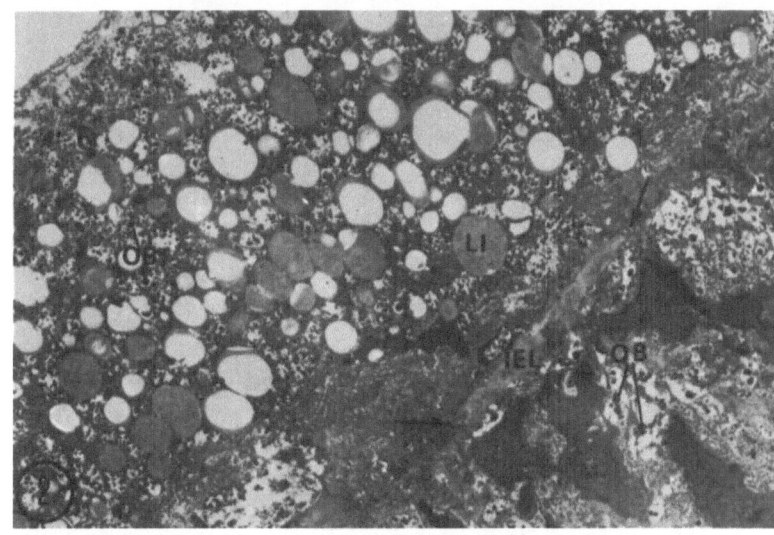

Figure 3

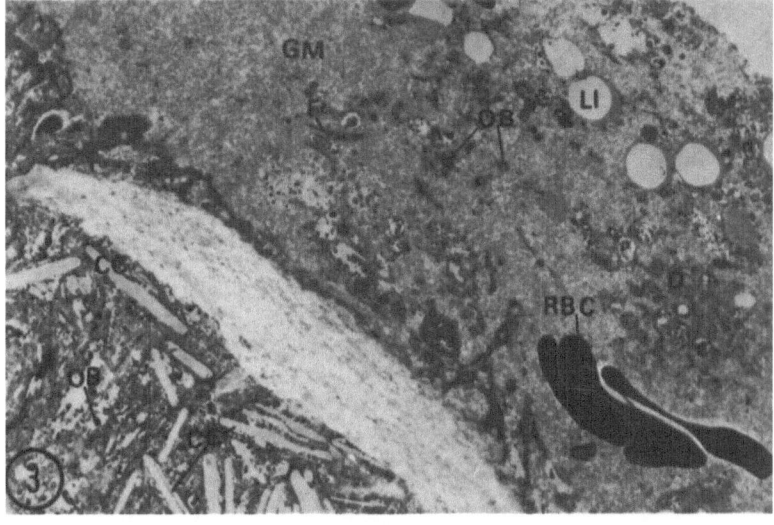

IX

Lipoprotein and Lipid Metabolism
in Experimental Animals

WORKSHOP: Lipid Metabolism in Primates

Chairmen: H.B. Lofland, USA
          O.W. Portman, USA

Participants: M.D. Morris, USA
             G.S. Getz, USA
             R.W. Wissler, USA
             D. Kritchevsky, USA

The program for the workshop was planned to encompass some areas in which substantial progress was possible because of the use of nonhuman primates. The premise for using nonhuman primates is that, despite important differences among different species of primates, the results can be more easily extrapolated than those with nonprimates to the condition in man. Some vital experiments cannot easily be performed on human beings, a limitation that provides another incentive for the use of nonhuman primates.

The difficulty in determining the role of genetic factors in the development of atherosclerosis in a human population affected by a wide range of environmental factors has been partly circumvented by experiments on genetically determined hyperlipoproteinemia in monkeys. In their studies of genetic influences on plasma lipid and lipoprotein concentrations and on the development of atherosclerosis, Drs. Morris and Lofland used colonies of rhesus and squirrel monkeys in a defined environment. Drs. Getz and Wissler discussed the structure of lipoproteins in the plasma and the role of lipids and lipoproteins in the arterial walls of rhesus monkeys, the most widely used nonhuman primate species. Although nonhuman primates do not usually develop atherosclerosis spontaneously, they can be subjected to nutritional regimens which result in the formation of lesions. Once such lesions are established, treatments to induce regression can be tested. Obviously, the progression and regression of hyperlipemia and atheroma are difficult to study in human beings. Therefore, Dr. Kritchevsky approached the question by studying nutritional influences on atherogenesis in the baboon.

Lastly, Drs. Portman and Lofland reported on the relationship between cholesterol gallstones and atherosclerosis in squirrel monkeys. Like atherosclerosis, cholesterol gallstones involve the ectopic deposition of crystalline cholesterol, and yet the human populations and individuals most severely afflicted with atherosclerosis do not have the highest predisposition to gallstones. It is possible that treating one of these diseases increases the likelihood of aggravating the other. This same dichotomy may be seen in squirrel monkeys, and recent studies with this species have introduced a new view of the factors that determine cholesterol deposition.

SERUM LIPIDS AND LOW DENSITY LIPOPROTEINS: SPONTANEOUS HYPERCHOLES-TEROLEMIA VS. CHOLESTEROL FEEDING IN RHESUS MONKEYS[*]

M.D. Morris and J.A. Lee

Introduction

It is generally recognized that an important feature of the development and sever-ity of atherosclerosis is the concentration and types of circulating lipoproteins. The increased use of subhuman primates in atherosclerosis research and the ob-served differences in species susceptibility to atherosclerosis suggest that spe-cial attention be given to the metabolism of serum lipoproteins. Rhesus monkeys have been used as an experimental model in the development and regression of ath-erosclerosis (Cox et al., 1958; Armstrong et al., 1967; 1970; Stary, 1972). Our knowledge of the lipids and lipoproteins which are present in the blood of such animals is only fragmentary.

We have had a unique opportunity to study the serum lipids and lipoproteins in two male rhesus monkeys in which very low density lipoproteins (VLDL) and low den-sity lipoproteins (LDL) are markedly increased when these two monkeys ingest a very low cholesterol diet (Morris and Fitch, 1968). For comparison, we have also fed normal rhesus monkeys a high cholesterol diet. Because of the important rela-tion between atherosclerosis and low density lipoproteins, we have studied the serum lipids and the lipids in the purified LDL from these two groups of hyper-cholesterolemic rhesus monkeys and of control monkeys fed a low cholesterol diet.

Care of Monkeys and Analytical Methods

The monkeys were caged individually and water was available at all times. The con-trol monkeys and the two male animals with spontaneous hypercholesterolemia were fed twice a day, a commercial chow (Purina 25). Those monkeys in which hypercho-lesterolemia was induced by cholesterol feeding were fed 120 grams of diet daily. After feeding the high cholesterol diet 28-42 days, the blood lipid studies were initiated. Blood was obtained after a 14-16 hour fast and serum lipids were mea-sured as previously described (Morris and Fitch, 1967). Low density lipoproteins were isolated between densities 1.019 and 1.063 and were pure by the criteria of agarose electrophoresis and immunoelectrophoresis.

Results

When compared with the controls, the hypercholesterolemic animals have signifi-cantly lower alpha-lipoprotein cholesterol (Table 1). The monkeys with spontaneous hyperbetalipoproteinemia have increased triglycerides when compared with the other two groups. Even though the serum total cholesterol concentration is simi-lar in the two groups with hypercholesterolemia, there is a mean difference of about 100 mg/dl in the phospholipids. As shown in the last column of Table 1, the cholesterol/phospholipid ratio is increased in both hypercholesterolemic groups when compared with the controls. However, this ratio is higher in the cholesterol-fed group than in the monkeys with spontaneous hypercholesterolemia.

The lipid composition of the LDL is shown in Table 2. The percent distribution of lipids in the control and spontaneous hypercholesterolemic groups was similar.

---

[*]Supported by the U.S. Public Health Service, National Institutes of Health, HE-11811.

Table 1. Serum lipids of control and hypercholesterolemic rhesus monkeys

Animals	Total Cholesterol	Alpha[a] Cholesterol	Phospho-lipids	Trigly-cerides	Cho/PL[b]
Controls [10]	143	72	240	35	0.6
	(105–186)	(57–84)	(225–310)	(20–52)	
Hypercholesterolemic					
Spontaneous [10]	525	38	470	162	1.1
	(470–675)	(25–55)	(405–540)	(105–212)	
Cholesterol-fed [10]	525	45	370	30	1.4
	(475–650)	(18–62)	(330–450)	(15–45)	

Values are averages with ranges given in parentheses. Number of samples is given in brackets. [a]Alpha cholesterol = alpha lipoprotein cholesterol. [b]Cho/PL = cholesterol/phospholipid ratio.

Major differences were observed in the composition of the cholesterol fed monkeys when compared with the other groups. The data in Table 2 clearly demonstrate a significant increase in the cholesteryl esters in the cholesterol-fed animals. This increased content of cholesteryl esters, with no apparent change in free cholesterol or phospholipids, resulted in a much higher cholesterol/phospholipids ratio. There was also a decrease in the percent of triglycerides in the LDL of the cholesterol-fed monkeys.

Table 2. Lipid composition (%) of low density lipoprotein of control and hyper-cholesterolemic rhesus monkeys

Animals	Free Cholesterol	Cholesterol Esters[a]	Phospho-lipids	Trigly-cerides	Cho/PL[b]
Controls [10]	9.6	40.3	28.4	11.3	1.34
Hypercholesterolemic					
Spontaneous [7]	8.2	44.6	29.8	13.1	1.24
Cholesterol-fed [21]	10.4	56.0	26.9	3.3	1.69

Number of samples is given in brackets. [a]Ester cholesterol x 1.67 = cholesterol esters. [b]Cho/PL = cholesterol/phospholipid ratio.

Discussion

In this study we compared the serum lipids of two groups of rhesus monkeys with the same degree of hypercholesterolemia. Increased serum triglycerides were found only in the monkeys with spontaneous hypercholesterolemia. This finding is indicative of increased VLDL. We have separated the VLDL by ultracentrifugation at D = 1.006 and have found a 4- to 6-fold increase in the concentration of VLDL cholesterol in each monkey with spontaneous hypercholesterolemia. We previously reported an increase in the S_f 0-12 lipoproteins in these monkeys (Morris and Greer, 1970). Thus, these two animals have combined hyperlipoproteinemia (Type IIb). The serum triglycerides of the cholesterol-fed monkeys were not elevated.

An additional difference between the two groups of hypercholesterolemic monkeys was the ratio of cholesterol to phospholipids. In most samples, the ratio was higher in the cholesterol-fed monkeys than in these with Type IIb hyperlipoproteinemia. This finding suggested an altered lipoprotein composition or abnormal lipoproteins in the serum. Since the LDL comprised the major lipoprotein species in the serum of the hypercholesterolemic monkeys, we carried out lipid composition studies on purified LDL.

It is significant that the lipid composition of the LDL isolated from the two male monkeys with spontaneous hypercholesterolemia is not different from that isolated from normocholesterolemic monkeys. The LDL isolated from patients with primary hyperbetalipoproteinemia (Type II) may or may not have an altered lipid composition (Levy and Fredrickson, 1971; Slack and Mills, 1970). To our knowledge there have been no reports of the lipid composition of LDL from Type IIb human beings.

Our present data suggest that an LDL of altered lipid composition may be an important component in the plasma of cholesterol-fed rhesus monkeys and raises the question of its relative atherogenesis.

An additional difference between the monkeys with spontaneous hypercholesterolemia and cholesterol-fed animals is in the appearance of xanthomas. Armstrong et al. (1967) reported the appearance of xanthomas in a high percent of monkeys fed a 1.2% cholesterol diet for 10-12 months, whereas the monkeys with spontaneous hypercholesterolemia have had a plasma cholesterol level of about 525 mg/dl for more than seven years, with no obvious xanthomas.

The present observations suggest that additional studies be conducted relating distribution and types of serum lipoproteins in cholesterol-fed animals. It is noteworthy that cholesterol feeding in rabbits is also associated with the appearance of cholesteryl ester rich lipoproteins (Dury, 1957).

CERTAIN ASPECTS OF LIPID METABOLISM IN THE YOUNG SQUIRREL MONKEY (SAIMIRI SCIUREUS)[*]

Hugh B. Lofland, Richard W. St. Clair[**], and Dianne G. Greene[***]

Shortly after weaning, two groups of squirrel monkeys (20 per group) were fed diets in which the fat was either butter or safflower oil. Fat comprised 40% of calories, and the diet contained cholesterol at a level of 0.75 mg/cal. Each dietary group included equal numbers of animals whose parents were known to be either hyper- or hyporesponders to exogenous cholesterol (Clarkson et al., 1971).

[*]This work was supported by grants from the U.S.P.H.S. (HL14164 and RR00180).
[**]Established Investigator, American Heart Association.
[***]Predoctoral trainee, U.S.P.H.S. Training Program HL5883.

Table 1. Composition of the diets

	Components of the diet		Fatty acid composition (% total fatty acid)		
	Safflower oil (g)	Butter (g)	Fatty acids[a]	Safflower oil	Butter
Dry milk solids	6720	6720	14:0	0.17	12.90
Complete vitamin mixture	480	480	16:0	8.88	34.83
Salt XIV	480	480	16:1	0.00	2.84
Sucrose	4800	4800	17:0	0.19	0.51
Gelatin	320	320	18:0	2.89	14.64
Fat (S or B)	3200	3952	18:1	16.34	30.76
Cholesterol[b]	55.6[b]	46.0[b]	18:2	70.60	0.46
Vitamin D$_3$	9.9	9.9	20:0+18:3	0.30	2.06
ß-sitosterol	–	9.6	20:1	0.32	0.08
			20:4+22:1	0.02	0.00
			Unidentified	0.29	0.92

[a]Expressed as chain length:number of double bonds. [b]0.75 mg cholesterol/cal.

After the animals had consumed the diets for approximately one year, cholesterol turnover was studied by injecting an emulsion of cholesterol-4-[14]C (50 µCi/animal) and plasma cholesterol specific activity was followed for a period of 84 days. During this period, the lipoprotein composition of the plasma was determined by heparin-manganese precipitation (Burstein et al., 1970) and by ultracentrifugal analysis. At the end of this time, the animals were killed and the cholesterol content of the entire body (minus brain and spinal cord) was determined by digesting the whole animal in alcoholic KOH (Lofland et al., 1970).

The composition of the diets is shown in Table 1. As would be expected, they differ markedly in fatty acid composition, and especially in linoleic acid content. Table 2 shows the plasma cholesterol concentrations resulting from the two diets. It is apparent that there are both dietary and phenotypic differences. On the other hand, there were only negligible differences among the groups in the relative amounts of cholesterol transported as either high or low density lipoprotein.

The composition of the fatty acids of the various lipoprotein classes of plasma phospholipids is shown in Table 3, and of cholesteryl esters in Table 4. It is apparent that the fatty acid composition of both lipid classes resembles that of the diet which the animals were consuming, and also that there are marked differences between the dietary groups, especially marked in the cholesteryl ester fraction. The turnover rates of the labeled cholesterol being transported by these strikingly different lipoproteins, however, are virtually identical, as shown by Fig. 1.

From the cholesterol turnover data obtained, we have calculated the following kinetic parameters (Table 5): the mass of the rapidly miscible pool (Goodman and Noble, 1968), the traced mass (Perl and Samuel, 1969), and the turnover rate (Goodman and Noble, 1968). As suggested by the dieaway curves, turnover rates for

Table 2. Distribution of lipoproteins in plasma by heparin-manganese precipitation

Phenotype and diet	Total cholesterol (mg/dl)	Low density lipoproteins (mg/dl)	High density lipoproteins (mg/dl)
Hyper-[a]			
butter	412 ± 49[d]	280 ± 38	133 ± 12 (33%)[b]
Hypo-[c]			
butter	272 ± 21	174 ± 18	99 ± 6 (37%)
Hyper-			
safflower	327 ± 18	213 ± 13	114 ± 8 (35%)
Hypo-			
safflower	245 ± 9	144 ± 9	101 ± 7 (41%)

[a]Progeny of hyperresponder parents. [b]Per cent of total cholesterol in HDL in parentheses. [c]Progeny of hyporesponder parents. [d]Mean ± standard error of the mean.

Table 3. Average fatty acid compositions of lipoprotein phospholipids

Lipoprotein fraction (g/ml)	Diet group	Fatty acids[a]				
		16:0	18:0	18:1	18:2	20:4
d 1.006	Safflower	30	24	7	39	0[d]
	Butter	47	27	16	6	4
d 1.019–1.063	Safflower	33	25	7	29	6
	Butter	38	25	23	8	6
d 1.063–1.21	Safflower	27	19	12	32	10
	Butter	35	24	26	10	6

[a]Fatty acids designated by carbon chain length:number of unsaturated bonds. [b]Includes both hypo- and hyperresponders. [c]Per cent of these five fatty acids. [d]Because the small sample size of arachidonic acid did not allow quantitation by GLC.

the dietary and phenotypic groups showed only slight and non-significant differences. In both the mass of pool A, and the total traced mass, there are differences between hyper- and hyporesponders when the animals consumed butter, but not when the dietary fat was safflower oil. It is also of interest that the traced mass measurement underestimates the size of the whole body cholesterol pool determined by carcass analysis, in some cases rather grossly. We are unable at present to explain this discrepancey.

Table 4. Average fatty acid composition of lipoprotein cholesteryl esters

Lipoprotein fraction (g/ml)	Diet[b] group	Fatty acids[a]			
		16:0	18:0	18:1	18:2
d 1.006	Safflower	10	2	15	72
	Butter	29	10	56	5
d 1.019–1.063	Safflower	14	4	20	62
	Butter	23	6	52	18
d 1.063–1.21	Safflower	10	2	23	65
	Butter	24	5	54	17

[a]Expressed as chain length:number of double bonds. [b]Includes both hypo- and hyper-responders. [c]Per cent of these four fatty acids.

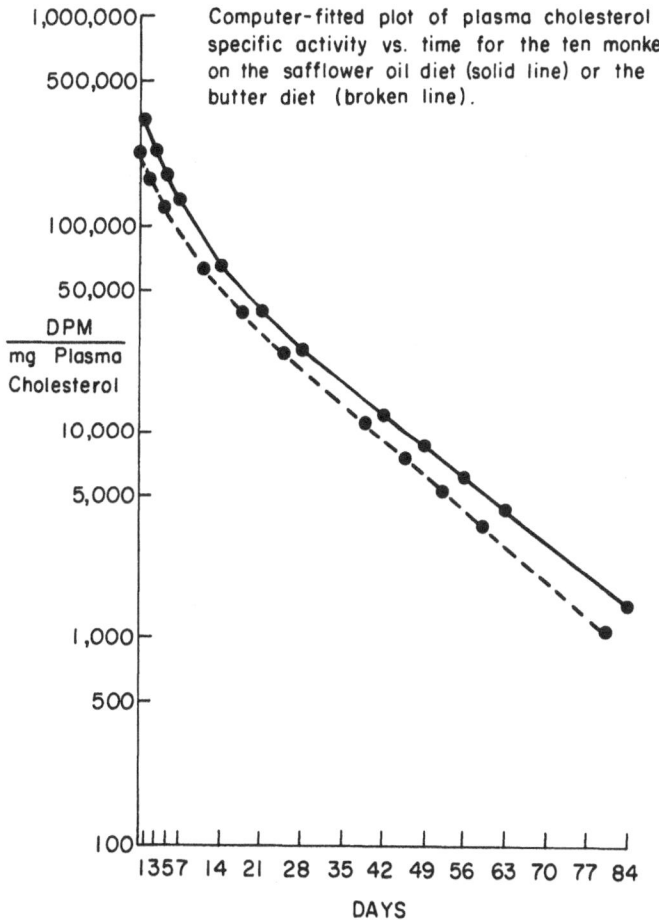

Computer-fitted plot of plasma cholesterol specific activity vs. time for the ten monkeys on the safflower oil diet (solid line) or the butter diet (broken line).

Figure 1. Plot of mean plasma specific activity versus time in monkeys fed either butter or safflower oil

Table 5. Kinetic parameters from dieaway studies

Phenotype and diet	Mass pool A[a] (mg)	Total traced mass (mg)	Turnover rate (mg/day)	Whole body pool[b] (mg)
Hyper-[c] butter	713 ± 11[d]	950 ± 63	67 ± 5	1806 ± 454
Hypo-[e] butter	435 ± 26	737 ± 38	61 ± 2	1178 ± 29
Hyper- safflower	562 ± 67	883 ± 49	60 ± 3	1484 ± 135
Hypo- safflower	498 ± 41	790 ± 35	59 ± 5	1261 ± 40
	[d]$P < 0.05$	$P < 0.01$	N.S.[f]	N.S.

[a]Rapidly miscible pool (Goodman and Noble, 1968). [b]Analytical determination by carcass analysis. [c]Progeny of hyperresponder parents. [d]Mean $\pm$ standard error of the mean. [e]Progeny of hyporesponder parents.

STUDIES ON PLASMA HIGH DENSITY LIPOPROTEIN OF NORMAL RHESUS MONKEYS

Godfrey S. Getz and Angelo M. Scanu

One of our major objectives is the elucidation of the pathogenesis of atherosclerosis and for this we need an animal model in which the human disease is most closely simulated. Much attention has hitherto been given to a comparison of the human lesion and its experimental counterparts. Although an important role is attributed to plasma lipoproteins in the pathogenesis of atherosclerosis, the kind of comparative information available on the lesion is certainly not matched by what we know of plasma lipoproteins. Until recently, knowledge of these molecules in various experimentally susceptible species barely extended beyond the lipid composition and proportion of various lipoprotein classes found in their plasmas. However with the rapid application and development of new techniques, this deficiency is fast being remedied. And this is important not only for our understanding of the relationship of the lipoproteins to the development and sustenance of the lesion but also as a basis upon which to study their biosynthesis and metabolism - which cannot be adequately done in man. An understanding of these aspects of lipoprotein behavior is essential if we are to control the hyperlipidemias, recognized to be so significant a risk factor.

We believe that the rhesus monkey comes closest to ideal of those species currently in use for studies of atherosclerosis. So in order to remedy the deficiency I spoke of, a study of rhesus lipoproteins has been initiated (see Edelstein et al., 1973).

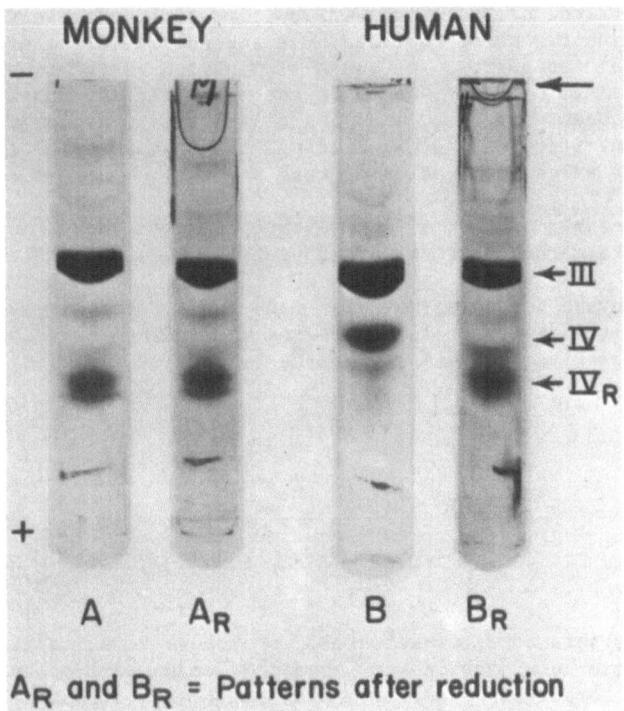

Figure 1. SDS-polyacrylamide gel electrophoresis of monkey and human high density lipoprotein performed according to Weber and Osborn (1969). Gels were stained with Coomassie Blue according to Fairbanks et al. (1971). ß-mercaptoethanol was the reducing agent. 20-40 µg of protein was applied to each gel (from Edelstein et al., 1973)

The distribution of lipid classes in the HDL of rhesus and man is similar. Whereas in man the ratio of HDL_2/HDL_3 is 1:3, in rhesus monkeys it is 2:1. The overall molecular parameters, namely size and particle weight, of HDL_2 and HDL_3 resemble one another in man and monkey. In rhesus, both classes of HDL have a lower sphingomyelin (4% vs 9-14%) than in human HDL but a higher lecithin content. A similar but not quite so marked difference in α-lipoprotein sphingomyelin was observed in a comparison of baboon and human lipoproteins by Blaton and Peeters (1971).

For the rest of this discussion, I will concentrate on the major apoproteins of HDL (Fig. 1), A-I and A-II - frequently referred to previously as fractions III and IV. Fraction III (A-I) is very closely similar in the two species. It has a similar amino acid composition, approximately the same molecular weight (27,000), the same NH_2 terminal, aspartic acid, and COOH terminal glutamine. While there are small but significant differences in amino acid composition between the peptide A-I of monkey and man, the two proteins cross-react immunologically.

A-I or Fraction III of both species has no cysteine and hence no reducible S-S bond as shown in Fig. 1 in which it is seen that reduction and alkylation had no effect upon its electrophoretic mobility. The figure also shows a well known phenomenon of human A-II - it exists as a dimer of identical monomers linked by an S-S bond so that its electrophoretic mobility is increased by reduction and alkylation. On the other hand the monkey band is not so affected, having a mobility with or without reduction equal to that of the reduced and alkylated human peptide. Its molecular weight determined from SDS polyacrylamide electrophoresis or amino acid composition is ± 8,500, almost exactly half that of the native human peptide. In both species the NH_2 terminus is blocked with pyrrolidone carboxylic acid and the COOH terminus is glutamine. Amino acid analysis reveals the absence of the single 1/2 cystine residue present in the human monomer at position 6 - being replaced by a serine. There are other small differences in amino acid composition of the A-II peptides of the two species which also cross-react immunologically. Hence in the rhesus monkey and also in preliminary studies of baboon, dog, cow, and rabbit A-II exists as the monomer. This does not apparently interfere with lipid binding, although more subtle differences may emerge on more detailed examination of this property.

Neither A-I nor A-II in either human or rhesus monkey contains any carbohydrate. The carbohydrate of HDL appears to be mainly on the C peptides.

Thus a beginning has been made and further extension of this work particularly with respect to lipid binding promises to be rewarding, especially when the comparative analysis is applied to the lower density classes of lipoproteins.

LIPIDS IN THE ARTERIAL WALL[*]

Robert W. Wissler, Katti Fischer-Dzoga, and Robert Chen

In this brief presentation we propose to summarize a series of observations that have been made in our laboratory using cell culture systems to investigate the interaction of aortic medial cells with lipoproteins and with hyperlipemic serum.

During atherogenesis in primates, including man, lipid accumulates in the arterial intima and media. Fig. 1 illustrates diagrammatically that these lipid deposits may be found in a number of areas and in various physical states. As noted in the diagram, much of this lipid accumulates inside cells, usually as visible and stainable droplets. A substantial amount of lipid may also be found interstitially either "free" in the spaces between cells or fibers or bound to acid mucopolysaccharides and/or elastin or collagen. In the advanced plaques one usually finds areas of necrosis containing lipid-rich "atheromatous gruel" often associated with abundant cholesterol crystals. All of these lipid deposits are added to the normal cell lipids that are always present, mostly in cell membranes and organelles.

It is evident from microscopic examination of accumulated lipid in the artery wall of primates that biochemical analysis of each rather small sample of diseased arterial tissue will yield complex and misleading results. The atheromatous lesion contains a variable mixture of lipid; some may be derived from partially metabolized intracellular lipid, some will come from extracellular lipid released by dying lipid-filled cells, and some of it may come from lipoproteins that have been "trapped" interstitially in the extracellular parts of the lesion.

The complexity of lipid metabolism in the artery walls during primate atherogenesis is further indicated in Table 1 which lists the ways in which the artery wall and lipids from the lumen (mostly in the form of lipoproteins) interact. There are still many areas of incomplete knowledge. Where evidence indicates that several processes are going on simultaneously, further work must be done to clarify the relative importance of each mechanism.

---

[*]Most of the studies that are summarized in this paper were carried out with the support of grants from the U.S. Public Health Service, HE 2174, HE 6894, HL 15062.

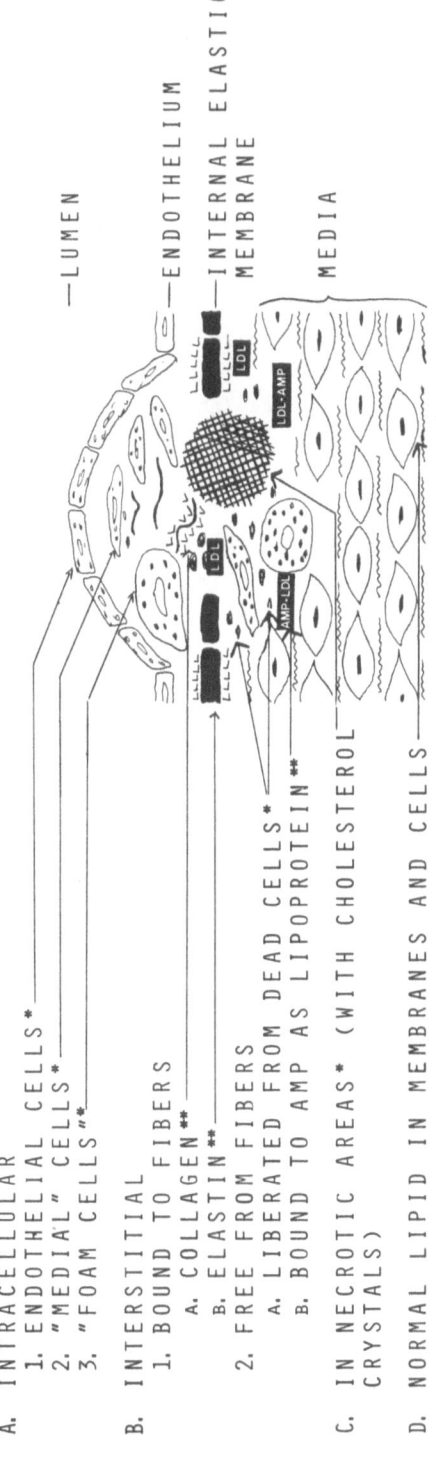

—LUMEN

—ENDOTHELIUM

—INTERNAL ELASTIC
MEMBRANE

MEDIA

A. INTRACELLULAR
  1. ENDOTHELIAL CELLS*
  2. "MEDIAL" CELLS*
  3. "FOAM CELLS"*

B. INTERSTITIAL
  1. BOUND TO FIBERS
    A. COLLAGEN**
    B. ELASTIN**
  2. FREE FROM FIBERS
    A. LIBERATED FROM DEAD CELLS*
    B. BOUND TO AMP AS LIPOPROTEIN**

C. IN NECROTIC AREAS* (WITH CHOLESTEROL
  CRYSTALS)

D. NORMAL LIPID IN MEMBRANES AND CELLS

  * LIKELY TO BE SUBSTANTIALLY ALTERED FROM THAT FOUND
  IN BLOOD BY CHOLESTEROL ESTER REMOVAL, ESTERIFICA-
  TION WITH NEW FATTY ACIDS, PHOSPHOLIPID SYNTHESIS

  ** MAY RETAIN MOST OF THE CHARACTERISTICS OF THE CIRCU-
  LATING LIPOPROTEINS (ESPECIALLY LDL)

Figure 1. The nature of lipids in the lesions

Table 1. The function of the artery wall in atherogenesis

A. *Transports lipid*

    1. From artery lumen across endothelium

        a. Through normal "pores"
        b. Through areas of injury
        c. Between cells
        d. Through cells
        e. In cells[a]

    2. From interstitium into "MM"[b] cells or foam cells

        a. Across cell membrane
        b. Through pinocytotic vacuoles (as intact LDL)
        c. By phagocytosis

B. *Traps (accumulates) lipid from blood*

    1. As intact lipoprotein interstitially

        a. Bound to AMP or elastin or collagen

    2. As cholesterol ester inside cells

C. *Shows cell proliferation in response to hyperlipemic LDL*

D. *Shows cell necrosis in response to hyperlipemic LDL*

E. *Metabolizes and synthesizes lipid*

    1. Breaks down lipoprotein components

    2. Hydrolyzes cholesterol esters

    3. Synthesizes cholesterol esters

    4. Uses fatty acids for energy

    5. Makes phospholipid

    6. Makes fatty acids

    7. Makes cholesterol (?)[c]

    8. Makes a low density lipoprotein (??)[d]

---

[a]The carrying of lipid into the artery wall from the lumen by lipid-filled cells and the entrance of lipid into "Foam" cells by phagocytosis probably occurs to a much greater extent in rabbit or fowl atherogenesis than in primate atherogenesis (Wissler and Vesselinovitch, 1968).
[b]Refers to multifunctional medial mesenchymal (MMM) cells, the major cell involved in primate atherogenesis (Wissler, 1968).
[c]Although there is no doubt that normal arterial wall cells can synthesize small amounts of cholesterol for structural membranes, it is unlikely that this contributes very much of the cholesterol to the atherosclerotic plaque.
[d]Thus far demonstrated only with cell components and not with intact arterial wall cells (Hollander and Paddock, 1973).

Table 2. Current status of tissue culture studies involving arterial medial cells and lipoproteins

---

A. *Effects of hyperlipemic serum and its fractions on primary explants of monkey aortic media*

1. Cells grown out from these primary explants can be stained by antibodies to smooth muscle myosin or actomyosin (Kao et al., 1968; Dzoga et al., 1970; Fisher-Dyoga et al., 1973a).

2. When these cells are exposed to monkey hyperlipemic serum, they accumulate lipids promptly. These intracellular lipid droplets can be stained by oil red 0 and antibodies to serum LDL (Kao et al., 1968; Dzoga et al., 1970; Fisher-Dzoga et al., 1973a).

3. Hyperlipemic LDL stimulates these cells to proliferate as demonstrated by both outgrowth measurement and ^{3}H-thymidine pulse labeling. HDL, lipid-free serum, and LDL from normal serum do not show such an effect. The evidence thus far indicates that this stimulatory effect is not due to the cholesterol content of the LDL from hyperlipemic serum (Kao et al., 1968; Dzoga et al., 1971; Fisher-Dzoga et al., 1973; 1973b).

B. *Chemical effects of hyperlipemic serum on subcultures of aortic media*

1. Cells exposed to hyperlipemic serum not only show a higher proliferative activity but also a higher death rate, an increase both in cell size and protein content as compared with cells remaining in normal serum (Chen, 1973; Chen et al., 1974).

2. When these cells are exposed to hyperlipemic serum, they show prompt accumulation of lipids. The accumulation of cholesterol esters is most prominent and appears to come largely from the LDL (Chen, 1973; Chen and Dzoga, 1973; Chen et al., 1972).

3. These accumulations of lipids are time dependent and reversible. Some of the cholesterol esters from the culture medium are apparently hydrolyzed in the cells and the free cholesterol excreted into the medium (Chen, 1973; Chen and Dzoga, 1973).

4. Cells grown in hyperlipemic serum show suppressed biosynthesis of cholesterol and increased efflux of most of the lipid subclasses as indicated by ^{14}C-acetate tracing. Based on suppressed biosynthesis and increased excretion, it is assumed that the accumulation of cholesterol in these cells is largely the consequence of increased uptake from the serum (Chen, 1973; Chen et al., 1973).

For the past five years we have been studying some of these lipoprotein arterial wall interactions in vitro utilizing cell cultures of medial cells grown either as primary cultures from medial explants of monkey aortas or as subcultures from trypsinized monkey or rabbit primary cultures. Some of our results, the first of which were reported in 1968 (Kao et al., 1968), are summarized in Table 2. These studies indicate that the in vitro approach is valuable in the study of atherogenesis, particularly for investigating the lipid metabolism of artery wall cells and the effects of lipid on these cells. Although conditions are not the same as in the intact artery in vivo, results from controlled in vitro studies may give insight into how serum lipids and lipoproteins interact with the arterial medial multifunctional mesenchymal (MMM) cell. The system may now be extended to study blood lipid-endothelial cell interactions.

Even though this approach has only begun to be applied to problems of lipids in the artery wall, results obtained thus far indicate that hyperlipemic monkey or rabbit serum added to this cell system produces effects on cell proliferation and/or lipid metabolism that are not seen when normal serum is added to the cultures. Furthermore the studies conducted by Dr. Fisher-Dzoga and Dr. Chen in this laboratory indicate that the increased cell proliferation that is observed in stationary arterial cell cultures when hyperlipemic serum is added can be largely reproduced by the LDL fraction of hyperlipemic serum. This effect cannot be reproduced by increasing the concentration of lipid, specifically of cholesterol, in cultures to which normal serum is added.

Insofar as the studies have progressed it also appears that the prompt and rather remarkable increase in cholesterol esters in the arterial medial cells that occurs when 2% of hyperlipemic serum is added to the tissue culture medium is not produced by 5%, 10%, 20%, or 40% of normal serum. It is noteworthy that the two latter amounts of normal serum in the media yield a concentration of serum lipids that is as high or higher than that obtained when 2% hyperlipemic serum is added to the media.

Hopefully with further work this type of in vitro system will yield knowledge regarding a number of aspects of atherogenesis that have been difficult to study in vivo. For example, it should be possible to find out more about how lipoproteins or their chemical components enter or interact with both endothelial and arterial medial cells. It should be feasible to learn more definitively how lipoproteins of various types are bound to and accumulate on or near to elastin or collagen, as well as how and why they are complexed with arterial wall mucopolysaccharides and proteoglycans. The mechanisms of cell proliferation and cell death in the atherosclerotic lesion may be clarifed by in vitro studies of this type. Perhaps most important of all, the details of lipid metabolism and lipid synthesis by artery cells should be considerably clarified by sustained study of these cells in well-defined media which contain blood serum and cellular components.

EFFECT OF DIETARY CARBOHYDRATE ON AORTIC SUDANOPHILIA IN BABOONS[*]

David Kritchevsky

Lambert et al. (1958) and Malmros and Wigand (1959) reported that a high carbohydrate, high saturated fat, cholesterol-free diet was atherogenic for rabbits. We have found (Kritchevsky et al., 1968; 1973) that the type of carbohydrate used in the diet could affect the severity of atherosclerosis. We have now investigated the influence of this diet on lipid metabolism and atherosclerosis in baboons. The diet consisted of 40 parts carbohydrate, 25 parts casein, 14 parts hydrogenated coconut oil, 15 parts cellulose, 1 part vitamin mix, and 5 parts salt mix IV. Five groups of baboons (3 male, 3 female) were used. One group was fed a control diet consisting primarily of bread, yams, and oranges. The other four groups were fed the semisynthetic diet containing fructose, sucrose, starch, or glucose. After one year, the baboons were killed, the liver and bile analyzed for lipids and bile acids respectively, and the aortas removed, coded and sent to Dr. T.B. Clarkson (Bowman Gray Medical School, Winston-Salem, N.C.) for histopathological analysis.

[*]This work was supported in part by U.S.P.H.S. Grant HL05209 and Research Career Award, N.I.H. HL-734.

Table 1. Average serum lipid values of baboons fed special diets for 12 months

Diet	Cholesterol (mg/dl) (121)[a]	Triglycerides (mg/dl) (75)	ß-Lipoprotein cholesterol (%) (55)
Fructose	162 ± 10[b]*	129 ± 11*	66 ± 1.1*
Sucrose	152 ± 9*	116 ± 8*	65 ± 1.3*
Starch	156 ± 8*	108 ± 5*	64 ± 1.0*
Glucose	151 ± 11**	105 ± 7*	63 ± 1.0*
Control	113 ± 3	78 ± 4	57 ± 1.0

[a]Average starting levels, all animals. [b]Standard error.
Significance, diet vs. control: *P <0.001; **P <0.01.

Table 2. Percent of aorta area stained with Sudan IV

Sex	Fructose	Sucrose	Starch	Glucose	Control
F	35.0	30.0	15.0	1.0	0.0
F	10.0	3.0	0.1	0.5	0.0
F	0.5	1.0	0.0	0.2	0.0
M	20.0	3.0	25.0	30.0	0.1
M	1.0	3.0	15.0	5.0	0.0
M	0.5	1.0	0.5	0.5	0.0
Avg ± S.E.M.	11.2 ± 5.7	6.7 ± 4.7	9.3 ± 4.3	6.2 ± 4.8	0.02 ± 0.02

The average lipid levels observed over the feeding period are presented in Table 1. It is evident that the diet caused hypercholesteremia and hypertriglyceridemia. The level of increase of serum cholesterol was similar for all four dietary groups. The increase in serum triglycerides was slightly greater for the fructose and sucrose groups than for the glucose and starch groups. The extent of sudanophilia in the aortas of the animals used in this experiment is shown in Table 2. The most sudanophilic diet was the fructose diet and the least was the glucose diet. When ranked by the method of Wilcoxon (1945) the order of decreasing involvement (rank in parentheses) was: fructose (66.5); sucrose (64.5); starch (87.0); glucose (86.0); and control (161.0). The fructose and sucrose diets were more sudanophilic for female baboons and the starch and glucose diets for males.

One question that has been posed by the use of these semisynthetic diets is the source of the hypercholesteremia. At the beginning and end of this experiment two animals in each group were injected intravenously with mevalonic acid labeled with either tritium or carbon-14. The extent of incorporation of this precursor into cholesterol was unchanged or slightly increased in the intervening year. Examination of the radioactivity present in biliary cholesterol and tauro- and glycocholanoic acids (Table 3) reveals that whereas the biliary cholesterol specific

Table 3. Specific activity (dpm/mg x 10^3) of bile lipids of baboons given [5-^{3}H] mevalonate

Product	Dietary group				
	Fructose	Sucrose	Starch	Glucose	Control
Cholesterol	88	30	47	47	59
Taurocholanoic acids	3	3	2	2	15
Glycocholanoic acids	5	3	3	5	15

Table 4. Ratio of primary/secondary bile acis (P/S)[a]

Dietary groups	P/S ratios		
	Taurine conjugates	Glycine conjugates	Total bile acids
Fructose	0.57	0.43	0.56
Sucrose	0.68	0.20	0.61
Starch	1.36	0.63	1.33
Glucose	0.83	0.46	0.81
Control	1.71	0.88	1.67

[a]Primary bile acids = cholic and chenodeocycholic; secondary bile acids = lithocholic and deocycholic.

activity in the test groups was similar to or higher than that of the controls, the bile acid specific activities of the test animals was one third to one seventh that of the controls. These data suggest reduced conversion of cholesterol into bile acids. A similar conclusion is suggested by the ratio of primary to secondary bile acids in the pooled biles of the various groups (Table 4).

An explanation of these data is that reduced conversion of cholesterol to bile acids, in the face of continued cholesterogenesis, makes more of this sterol available to the circulation. Kyd and Bouchier (1972) made a similar suggestion based on data derived from their experiments in rabbits. More work must be done to determine the source of the hypercholesteremia in animals fed these semisynthetic diets. Further information will be gained through experiments in which the sources of protein and fiber in these diets will be varied.

NUTRITIONAL INFLUENCES ON GALLSTONES, BILE LIPIDS, AND ARTERIAL LIPIDS[*]

Oscar W. Portman, Toshiaki Osuga, and Manfred Alexander

Different species of primates vary widely in their susceptibility to nutritionally induced hyperlipemia and atherosclerosis. Because of their exceptional vulnerability to atherosclerosis, squirrel monkeys have been used more than any other species for our studies of the relationship between nutrition, plasma and arterial composition and arterial metabolism (Portman and Andrus, 1965; Portman, 1970). Within the last few years, we have documented the presence of gallstones in squirrel monkeys and have studied the nutritional, endocrine, and individual factors that influence gallstone incidence, bile composition, and the metabolic kinetics of the principal constituents of bile (Osuga and Portman, 1971, 1972) as well as the mechanism of crystal assembly and stone growth (Osuga et al., 1974). We have also investigated the relationship between the development of atherosclerosis and gallstones, which seemed particularly important in light of two recent papers. Sturdevant et al. (1973) reported an increased incidence of gallstones in human beings fed a highly unsaturated fat diet, and Melchior and associates (1972) made a similar observation in squirrel monkeys.

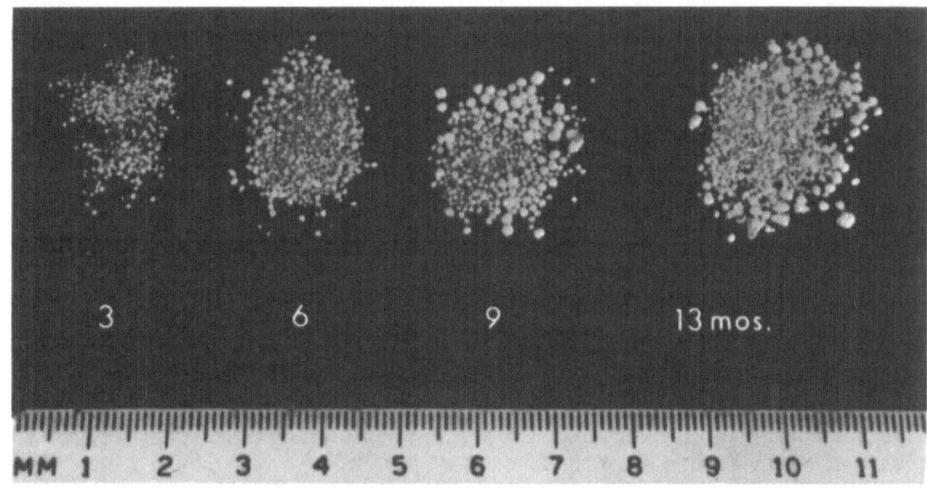

Figure 1. The relative size and number of gallstones from single gallbladders of susceptible squirrel monkeys which had been maintained on diets containing 45% of calories as butter and with 0.1 g cholesterol/100 Kcal for 3, 6, 9, and 13 months (from Osuga and Portman, 1971)

[*]The work described in this report was supported by grants in aid from the National Institutes of Health (HL 09744), Bethesda, Md. This is publication No. 698 from the Oregon Regional Primate Research Center which is supported in part by grant RR 00163 from the National Institutes of Health, United States Public Health Service.

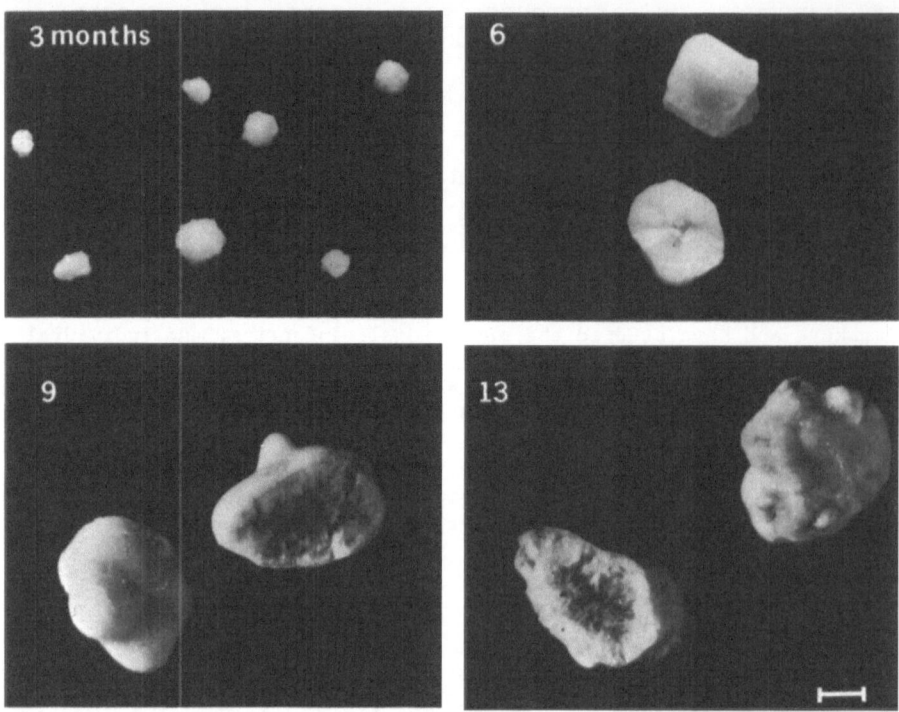

Figure 2. The relative size and shape of the gallstones of Fig. 1. Seven unbroken
stones are shown at 3 months. Single stones broken through the approximate center
are shown for 6, 9, and 13 months. Line = 1 mm (from Osuga and Portman, 1974)

When squirrel monkeys were fed a semipurified diet which supplied 45% of calories
as butter and 0.1 g cholesterol/100 Kcal, about half of them developed cholesterol gallstones. Fig. 1 shows the stones from representative susceptible monkeys
which were on this diet for 3, 6, 9, and 13 months. With time, the total weight
of the stones and the size of the largest ones increased. This figure suggests
that new small stones were continuously attaining macroscopic size over a period
of almost 3 months and that older ones were growing and aggregating. Fig. 2 shows
in more detail the development of the largest stones from fine, irregular stones
at 3 months to the mulberry form at 13 months. When the gallbladders of some monkeys that had been on the butter diet for 13 months were completely emptied, only
some of them had stones. After 4 more months on the diets, those with stones at
the first cholecystotomy had small irregular stones similar to those shown in the
3-month frame of the figure. The monkeys without stones at the first cholecystotomy were still free of them.

The incidence and mean weights of stones for males and females from 3 diet groups
are shown in Table 1. Only the monkeys fed the Purina chow (Commercial mix of
grains) were free of gallstones. Those fed the butter + cholesterol diet had a
higher incidence of gallstones and a greater mass of stones per animal than those
on a diet containing low levels of corn oil. All of the numerous variations of
semipurified diets we tried were associated with some gallstone formation. Sub-
stituting a complex carbohydrate or adding cellulose to the diet did not prevent
the condition. Adding butter and cholesterol to the commercial chow also resulted
in gallstone formation. There were no obvious sex differences in susceptibility
to gallstones.

Table 1. Incidence and weight of cholesterol gallstones of monkeys on the indicated diets for 6 months or more

Diet	Females	Males
Commercial chow	0/16[a]	0/21
Semipurified: corn oil = 15% of cal.	6/27 (21.0)[b]	3/9 (21.1)
Semipurified: butter = 45% of cal. + cholesterol (0.1 g/100 Kcal.)	20/41 (82.0)	5/9 (147.1)

[a]Number of animals with stones/total number of animals. [b]Number in parentheses = mean weight of stones (mg) in those animals with stones.

Table 2. Effect of mean plasma cholesterol on gallstone incidence, mean weight of gallstones in animals with gallstones, and cholesterol in the aortic intima + inner media.

Squirrel monkeys were on a single hyperlipemia-inducing diet containing butter and cholesterol for 6+ months. 20 monkeys had a mean plasma cholesterol less than 300 mg% and 20 had values greater than 300 mg%

Mean plasma cholesterol	Gallstone incidence	Mean weight gallstones (mg)	Intima + inner media cholesterol (mg/g)
< 300 mg%	9/20[a]	104.8	13.0
> 300 mg%	12/20	72.6	21.8

[a]Number of animals with stones/total number of animals. r, plasma cholesterol vs. arterial cholesterol = 0.349; P = 0.03. r, plasma cholesterol vs. weight of gallstones = -0.020.

Since only half the monkeys on the butter and cholesterol diet for 6 months or longer had gallstones, we compared the concentrations of cholesterol in plasma and aortic intima plus inner media with the presence and quantity of gallstones in that group (Table 2). A mean plasma cholesterol of 300 mg% divided the group exactly in half. In the animals with a mean plasma cholesterol of more than 300 mg%, the incidence of gallstones was slightly increased, but the mean weight of stones was slightly less than for the monkeys with a mean cholesterol of less than 300 mg%. The correlation coefficient for plasma cholesterol vs. weight of gallstones was a small and insignificant negative number. On the other hand, a high plasma cholesterol level was associated with a high cholesterol content in the aortic intima plus inner media. This relationship, significant even for animals fed a single diet, was much more striking when monkeys fed a variety of diets were evaluated together.

Since the plasma cholesterol concentration was a good indicator of the quantity of cholesterol in the arterial wall but not in gallstones, we looked for other predictive indices of cholesterol gallstones. We have observed 4 kinds of measurements which tend to differ for animals with and without a tendency to form gall-

stones. In squirrel monkeys with gallstones, 1. after an 18-hour fast, hepatic
and gallbladder biles had higher concentrations of cholesterol relative to phospholipids and bile salts than biles of nonsusceptible animals; 2. bile salt pools
and production rates were low; 3. a low proportion of the bile salt pool was outside the gallbladder; and 4. after surgical interruption of the enterohepatic
circulation, the bile became supersaturated with cholesterol unusually rapidly.

Clearly the pathogenesis of cholesterol gallstones in squirrel monkeys is at
least as imperfectly understood as the development of atherosclerosis. We believe,
however, that it is desirable to study both of these processes in the same experimental animal.

CHOLESTEROL GALLSTONES IN NONHUMAN PRIMATES[*]

Hugh B. Lofland, Thomas B. Clarkson, and George W. Melchior

It has been known for some time, from the work done in Dr. Portman   laboratory,
that squirrel monkeys respond to cholesterol ingestion with the formation of gallstones. Similar observations have been made in our laboratories, and will be described herein.

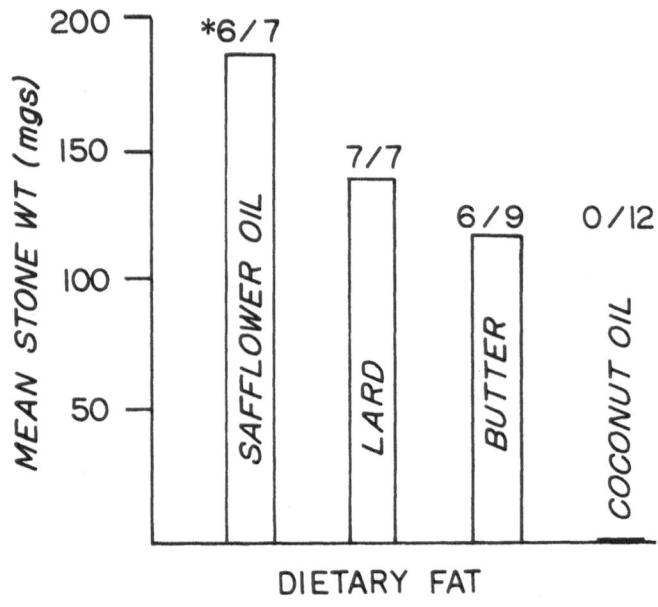

Figure 1. Stone frequency and stone weight in squirrel monkeys fed four different
fats, with cholesterol

[*]Supported by grants from the U.S.P.H.S. (HL-14164 and RR00180). Predoctoral
trainee, U.S.P.H.S. Training Grant HL-5883. Presented in part at the meeting of
the Council on Arteriosclerosis, American Heart Association, in Dallas, Texas,
November, 1972 (Melchior et al., 1972).

We fed a diet containing cholesterol at a level of 1 mg/cal, and 45% of calories came from fat (safflower oil, lard, butter, or coconut oil). Mean plasma cholesterol concentrations for the four groups were, respectively, in mg/dl, 420, 525, 671, and 478. The animals were fed the diets for approximately one year. Fig. 1 shows the results in terms of stone frequency and mean stone weight. As can be seen, with the exception of coconut oil, the frequency of cholelithiasis ranged from 67 to 100 per cent. When the extent of cholelithiasis was expressed as the mean weight of the gallstones, it was greatest among animals fed safflower oil, followed by butter and lard. No explanation has been found for the lack of gallstones in the coconut oil group.

Frequency of cholelithiasis in non-human primates fed an atherogenic diet

Species	No. examined	No. with stones
Sq. Monkeys	17	15
Rhesus	20	0
Cebus	35	1
Spider	8	0
St. Macaque	7	0
African Green	7	1

Figure 2. Frequency of cholesterol gallstones in six species of nonhuman primates

Also of interest were the marked differences found in the frequency of cholelithiasis when squirrel monkeys were compared to other nonhuman primate species (Fig. 2). All of these animals had been fed the same lard-containing diet. It is apparent that cholelithiasis is much more frequent in squirrel monkeys than in the other species examined.

In an attempt to gain some insight into these species differences, bile was collected from squirrel monkeys, African green monkeys, and stumptail macaques, and was analyzed for cholesterol, phospholipid, and bile salts, essentially as described by Admirand and Small (1968). The sample of bile was divided into two portions, on one of which cholesterol and phospholipid were isolated and quantified using standard procedures. The other portion was diluted, deconjugated enzymatically, and the bile acids were methylated, converted to their trifluoroacetate derivatives and quantified by gas-liquid chromatography. The molar ratios of cholesterol, phospholipid, and bile salts were then calculated. The data were plotted on triangular coordinates as suggested by Admirand and Small (1968); any points that fell within the curve indicating maximum cholesterol solubility were considered "nonlithogenic". Those falling outside the curve were considered as having a high potential for stone formation. The results were as follows: bile of six of seven squirrel monkeys (Fig. 3) fed the cholesterol-containing diet fell on or above the line of maximum solubility; nine of nine animals fed the diet devoid of cholesterol fell in the nonlithogenic zone. Among the animals fed cholesterol, five of seven had stones.

Among African green monkeys (Fig. 4), bile from six of seven animals fell on or within the nonlithogenic zones, as did all of the control animals. Only one animal of this species had cholelithiasis, and the composition of its bile was such that it fell well into the zone of lithogenicity.

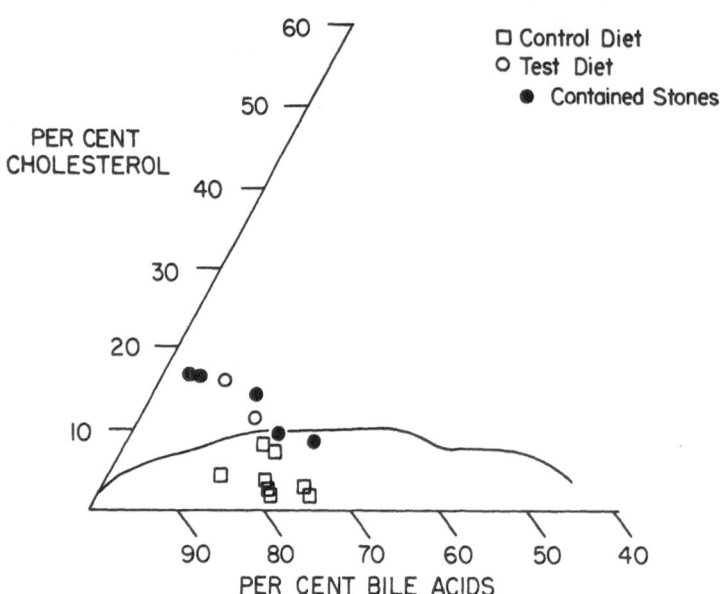

Figure 3. Bile composition in squirrel monkeys plotted on triangular coordinates

All of the stumptail macaques (Fig. 5), regardless of the presence o absence of cholesterol in the diet, had bile that was nonlithogenic. None had gallstones.

Metzger et al. (1972) have demonstrated that the points representing bile composition can be represented numerically. They have designated this as the "lithogenic index", in which a value greater than one indicates a bile the composition of which is such that it has a high potential for gallstone formation. Fig. 6 shows our data calculated in the same way. As expected, squirrel monkeys had the highest

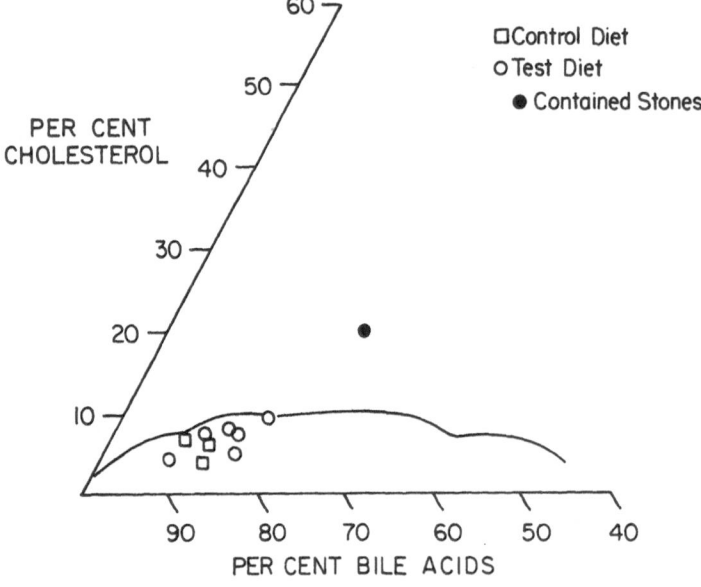

Figure 4. Bile composition in African green monkeys plotted on triangular coordinates

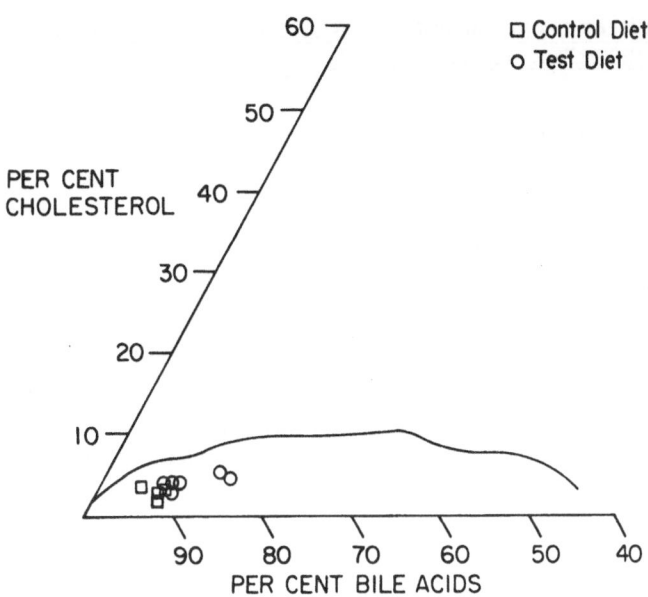

Figure 5. Bile composition in stumptail macaques plotted on triangular coordinates

SPECIES		CHOLIC	DEOXY	CHENO	ALL OTHERS	LITHOGENIC INDEX
SQ. MONKEYS	TEST	36	14	29	21	1.87
	CONTROL	41	13	21	25	.45
AFRICAN GREEN	TEST	7	58	23	11	.96
	CONTROL	43	24	16	17	.69
ST. MACAQUE	TEST	9	58	21	12	.57
	CONTROL	47	18	19	16	.44

Figure 6. Lithogenic index and individual bile acid (molar ratio) content in three species of monkeys

mean index, and stumptail macaques the least; African green monkeys were inter-mediate. Fig. 6 also shows the composition of the bile samples in terms of indivi-dual bile acids. It is of interest that those animals which do not form gallstones appear to have significantly more deoxycholic acid than do stone-formers - i.e., squirrel monkeys.

In summary, we feel that these studies show that major differences in bile acid metabolism exist among the primate species, and that the squirrel monkey is a promising model for further studies on cholelithiasis.

UPTAKE AND AUTORADIOGRAPHIC LOCALIZATION OF VERY LOW DENSITY LIPO-PROTEINS IN RAT LIVER

O. Stein, D. Rachmilewitz, S. Eisenberg, L. Sanger-Gabay, and Y. Stein

The liver is the main source of plasma very low density lipoproteins (VLDL) which are discharged by the process of exocytosis in the form of particles 300-800 A in diameter (Stein and Stein, 1967a). A similar mechanism is used by the small intestine to release chylomicrons and under fasting conditions some VLDL. Secretion of high density lipoproteins (HDL) from both the liver and small intestine has been demonstrated in a perfusion system (Windmueller et al., 1973), but the mode of secretion of these lipoproteins has not been elucidated so far. The main role

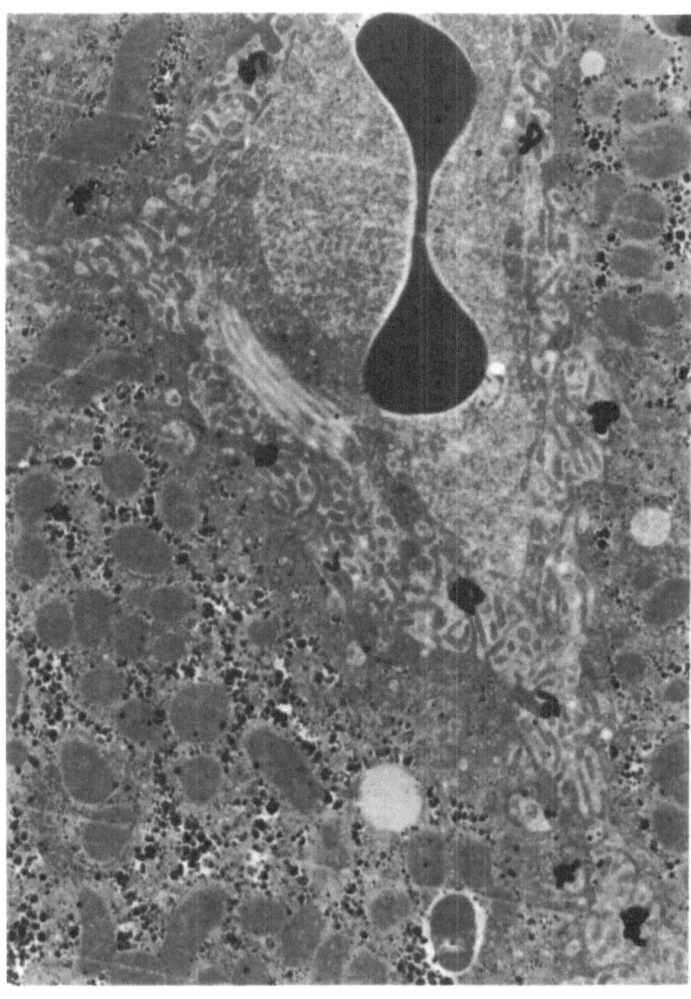

Figure 1. Section of liver 30 min after injection of ^{125}I-VLDL. The radioautographic reaction is concentrated over the sinusoidal cell boundary (X 10,500)

of the VLDL and chylomicrons is triglyceride transport and following release into the circulation most of the triglyceride is removed by adipose tissue and muscle, after hydrolysis catalyzed by lipoprotein lipase (Robinson, 1970). Following injection of chylomicrons labeled in their triglyceride moiety, only 20% of the injected label was recovered in the liver 5 min after injection. The labeled triglyceride could be demonstrated, with the help of radioautography, over both hepatocytes and Kupffer cells (Stein and Stein, 1967b). When the label was introduced into the cholesterol ester moiety of the chylomicrons, up to 80% of the injected label was recovered in the liver. During the first 30 min, while most of the radioactivity was in the form of cholesterol ester, the label as visualized with the help of radioautography, was concentrated mostly at the sinusoidal cell boundary. At later time intervals the label, then due to free cholesterol, was truly intercellular (Stein et al., 1969). Presently, VLDL, isolated from rat plasma were iodinated with ^{125}I and 70-80% of the label was in the protein portion. Rats were injected with 0.8 - 3.0 mg of VLDL protein and the livers were removed 5 - 120 min thereafter. Eight to 30% of the injected dose were recovered in whole liver, 90% of the label was TCA-precipitable and 25% extractable by chloroform methanol (2:1). Seventy-five to 92% of the radioactivity was extractable by 1% sodium cholate. At 5 and 30 min, 60-90% of the solubilized lipoprotein was recognized by a specific antibody. Liver tissue was prepared for radioautography using conventional procedures which removed about 26% of the label, which was mostly lipid. On light microscopic radioautography most of the autoradiographic reaction was associated with parenchymal liver cells and some Kupffer cells. On electron microscopic radioautography 5 and 30 min after injection many of the autoradiographic silver grains were associated with sinusoidal cell surface (Fig. 1), while at 120 min the radioautographic reaction was predominantly intracellular, and some grains were concentrated over secondary lysosomes. The mode of uptake of the injected VLDL resembled to some extent the uptake of the cholesterol labeled chylomicrons, as in both instances the radioautographic reaction was localized initially to the sinusoidal cell boundary, suggesting that a lag period exists between possible attachment and interiorization. It has been proposed that the chylomicron derived cholesterol ester is delivered to the liver in the form of a remnant particle (Redgrave, 1970). It seems plausible that in the present experiments the uptake of label by the liver represents also uptake of VLDL remnants. In analogy to the findings with chylomicrons (Stein and Stein, 1967b; Stein et al., 1969) the uptake of VLDL by Kupffer cells was by means of phagocytosis, but no labeled intact VLDL were seen in the parenchymal cells. In the experiments with chylomicrons the delay in the interiorization encountered with respect to cholesterol ester was interpreted to mean that hydrolysis of the ester bond preceded uptake into the cell. One might speculate that a similar process occurs also during the uptake of the VLDL or its remnant, however the exact mode of entry has not been elucidated so far. Two hours after injection, the presence of the label over secondary lysosomes resembled that encountered 6 h after injection of labeled HDL (Rachmilewitz et al., 1972) and thus it seems that the liver participates in the catabolism of the protein moiety of serum VLDL.

CHARACTERIZATION OF EXPERIMENTAL TYPE II HYPERLIPOPROTEINAEMIA IN GUINEA PIGS

Gervase L. Mills and Fergus McTaggart

When guinea pigs are fed for six days on a diet containing 15% corn oil and 1.6% cholesterol by weight, they generate a high level of a low density lipoprotein (LR-LDL) which is unusually rich in cholesterol and its ester, but is deficient in triglyceride and protein (Mills et al., 1972). This report is concerned with the changes in lipoprotein metabolism which lead to the production of these abnormal compounds, which are particularly interesting in view of their analogy with the anomalous LDL of human familial hyperbetalipoproteinaemia (Slack and Mills, 1970).

Low density lipoproteins from the serum of both fat-fed and normal guinea pigs have been isolated centrifugally, as the fraction of density between 1.007 and 1.100 g/ml. These preparations, which will be called LR-LDL and N-LDL respectively, were labelled with radioactive iodine to the extent of 1-2g.atom/3x10^{6}g of lipoprotein, using the method of Hunter (1970). In some experiments N-LDL was labelled with I^{131}, while LR-LDL was labelled with I^{125}. The purified products were mixed, and equal amounts were injected *via* the heart into normal and fat-fed animals. The disappearance of this labelled LDL from the serum was followed over a period of 100 hours. In an alternative design, the N-LDL and LR-LDL were each labelled with I^{125}, and were injected separately into different recipients.

Table 1. The fractional catabolic rates (mean ± std. devn.) of normal guinea pig LDL (N-LDL), and LDL from animals fed on a lipid enriched diet (LR-LDL), when determined in both normal and fat-fed guinea pigs

	Mean fractional catabolic rate (hr^{-1})	
	N-LDL	LR-LDL
Determined in guinea pigs fed on normal diet	0.0925 ± 0.0124[a] (6 expts)	0.0757 ± 0.0079[b] (8 expts)
Determined in guinea pigs fed on lipid-rich diet	0.0586 + 0.0058[c] (4 expts)	0.0457 + 0.0061[d] (6 expts)

The comparison of these mean fractional catabolic rates by Student's test yields the following results:
[a]cf. [c] and [b]cf, [d], $p < 0.001$; [a]cf.[b], $0.01 < p < 0.02$; [c]cf.[d], $p < 0.01$.

These experiments showed that the half-life of LDL in normal guinea pigs is of the same order as that in other laboratory animals (18-19 hrs), but is significantly increased in fat-fed animals (26 hrs). Moreover, the results summarised in Table 1 show that the fractional catabolic rates (FCR) of both N-LDL and LR-LDL are considerably lower in the fat-fed animal than in the normal. In addition, the LR-LDL has a somewhat lower FCR than N-LDL, no matter what the dietary status of the recipient animal.

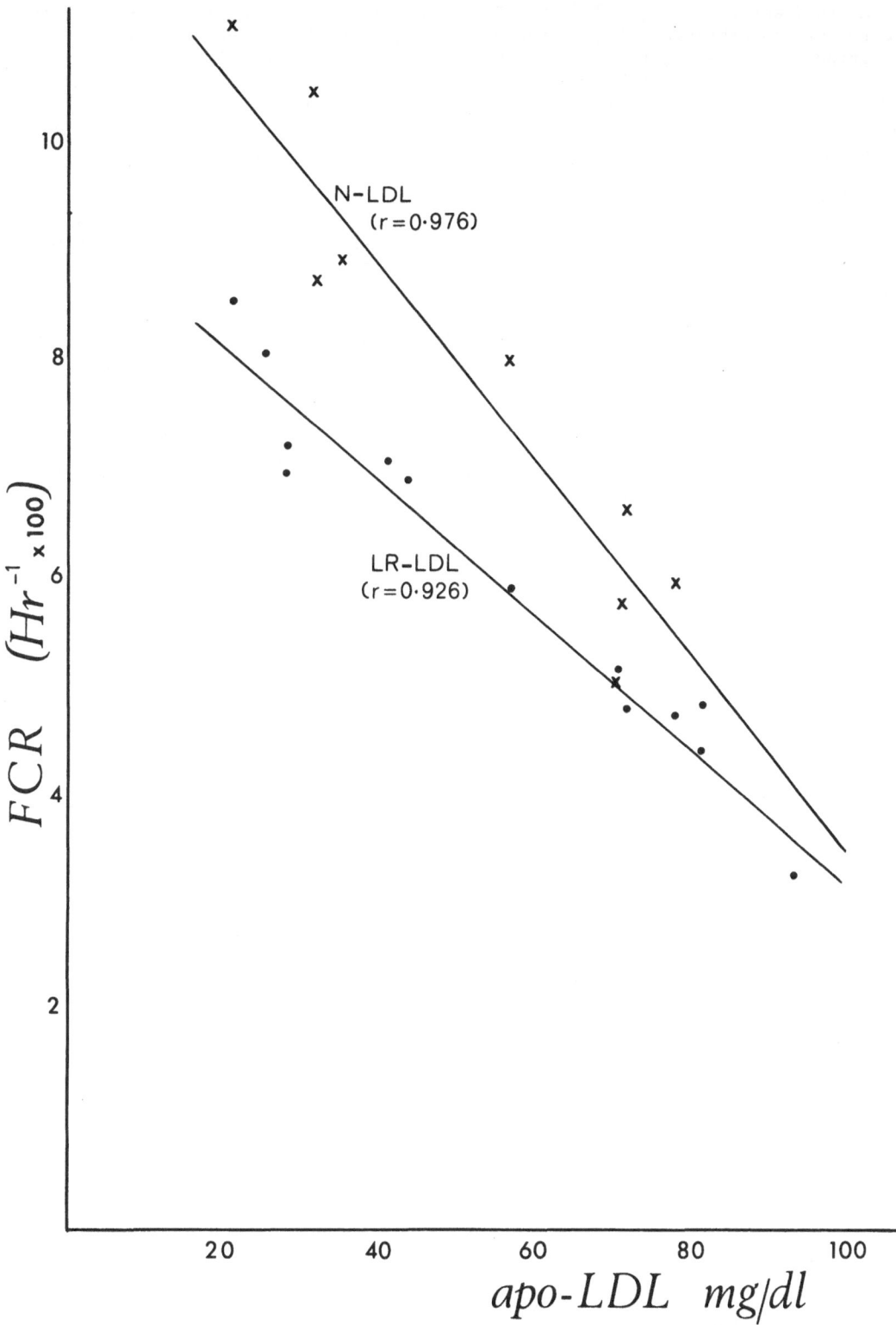

Figure 1. The relationships between the apo-LDL concentration (mg/dl serum) and fractional catabolic rate (% apo-protein pool/hr) in guinea pigs. The labelled LDL administered in these experiments was derived from control animals (N-LDL; x) and from animals which had been fed for six days on a lipid-enriched diet (LR-LDL; ●)

As in man (Langer et al., 1972), the FCR of the guinea pig LDL is inversely related to the concentration of apo-lipoprotein (apo-LDL) in the serum (Fig. 1). In
the guinea pig however, the relationship is linear over the range of concentration studied, for both N-LDL and LR-LDL, and is represented by the equations:
FCR = 0.125 - 0.000898 [apo-LDL]   (r = -0.9757; p <0.001),
FCR = 0.094 - 0.000618 [apo-LDL]   (r = -0.9256; p <0.001)
respectively, where FCR is expressed as % of intravascular pool/hr.

These two lines show that, at least up to a level of 100 mg apo-LDL/dl serum,
beyond which they may not continue to be linear, the FCR of the N-LDL is always
greater than that of the LR-LDL. Moreover, the difference in the constant terms
of the equations suggests that the catabolic mechanism in the normal guinea pig
can distinguish between these two species of LDL. However, the regression lines
differ significantly in slope (p <0.05), and their convergence suggests that any
discriminatory ability may be lost when the apo-LDL reaches very high levels in
the fat-fed animal.

An analysis of the data has shown that a fourfold increase in apo-lipoprotein concentration is accompanied by a rise in the absolute catabolic rate (ACR) by a
factor of about two. What is more, the equations quoted above imply that, over
the limited range of our experiments, the ACR is related to the apo-LDL concentration by quadratic functions of the form:
$ACR = 0.125 [apo-LDL] - 0.000898 [apo-LDL]^2........etc.$

The fat-fed guinea pig is therefore unable to increase its ability to catabolise
lipoproteins sufficiently to deal with the increased load, and this may be an important cause of the increased level of LDL in these animals.

Unfortunately, these experiments do not allow us to decide whether this catabolic
incompetence is purely an outcome of the raised lipoprotein level (e.g. through
increased competition for catabolic sites), or whether there is an essential
change in the catabolic mechanism.

A separate series of experiments on the incorporation *in vivo* of C^{14}-leucine into
guinea pig VLDL and LDL has shown that the peak of activity appears in the VLDL
after about 1 hr, whereas the LDL reaches maximum activity after 2.5 hr, when
that of the VLDL has fallen to about 30% of its peak value. This is consistent
with the hypothesis that the VLDL are the precursors from which LDL are formed by
intravascular degradation. The influence of the LR-diet on this reaction has been
studied by labelling VLDL (d <1.007g/ml) from either control or fat-fed guinea
pigs with I^{125}, and incubating the product for 2 hr at 37⁰ with post-heparin plasma which was also obtained either from normal or hyperlipidaemic animals. The products of reaction were then separated on a density gradient by centrifugation for
24 hr at 39,000 rev/min in a Spinco 41 rotor, and the distribution of the label
determined. The results of typical experiments are summarised in Table 2, in
which the separation of N-LDL and LR-LDL on the gradient is also shown. It will
be seen that the digestion degrades VLDL from the control animal into a lipoprotein with the density of N-LDL, whereas VLDL from fat-fed guinea pigs is mainly
converted into a lipoprotein with the density of LR-LDL. Moreover, the results
are the same whether the post-heparin plasma is obtained from a control or a fat-
fed guinea pig.

These results not only support the view that VLDL can be degraded within the vascular system, but also confirm that substances are formed which are ultracentrifugally indistinguishable from LDL. However, the influence of the diet upon the
nature of these products is determined, not by variation in the degradative mechanism, but by the nature of the VLDL which is the substrate. Thus, the hyperlipoproteinaemia of the fat-fed guinea pig may, like that of the human Type II lipoproteinaemia, be explained by a reduced ability to catabolise LDL, coupled with
an increased synthesis of VLDL (although the latter is not admitted by Langer et

al., 1972). The abnormal composition of the LR-LDL is the result of a change in the composition of the VLDL secreted by the guinea pig under the stress of the exogenous lipid load (cf. Chapman et al., 1973).

Table 2

Fraction	Density	N-LDL	LR-LDL	Control	N-VLDL + N-PHP	LR-VLDL + N-PHP	LR-VLDL + LR-PHP
1	1.0090	3.7	8.3	70.9	1.6	14.2	24.0
2	1.0100	0.5	1.2	3.5	1.0	2.5	3.0
3	1.0125	0.3	1.4	0.7	1.7	2.8	2.7
4	1.0150	0.2	1.5	0.4	2.4	2.8	3.0
5	1.0180	0.2	2.4	0.3	3.8	3.5	4.0
6	1.0205	0.5	3.8	0.4	5.1	5.3	4.2
7	1.0240	1.1	10.5	0.7	5.0	5.0	5.2
8	1.0275	2.0	14.8	1.1	4.6	5.7	5.7
9	1.0315	8.8	6.9	0.7	6.5	5.2	4.4
10	1.0355	12.8	2.3	1.2	8.0	4.8	2.5
11	1.0400	11.1	0.8	1.7	5.2	3.7	0.9
12	1.0445	6.1	0.3	0.5	2.3	0.9	0.4
13	1.0505	3.1	0.2	0.1	0.5	0.2	0.1
14	1.0565	0.5	0.0	0.0	0.1	0.1	0.1
15	1.0640	0.2	0.3	0.0	0.0	0.0	0.0
16	1.0730	0.0	0.2	0.0	0.1	0.0	0.0

Separation of guinea pig lipoprotein preparations on density gradients of sucrose/0.1M NaCl, buffered with 0.025M phosphate at pH 7.6, ranging from density 1.100 to 1.001g/ml. The first value in the table represents the material present in the top 0.8ml of the gradient, expressed as a percentage of the total recovered from the tube. Only the data for every alternate fraction are shown in the rest of the table, these fractions being of 0.4ml each. LDL from control guinea pigs (N-LDL) and from fat-fed animals (LR-LDL) were estimated by absorption at 280nm. N-VLDL and LR-VLDL were iodinated with I^{125}, purified, and digested for 2 hr at 37° with post-heparin plasma from either normal guinea pigs (N-PHP), or from fat-fed animals (LR-PHP). The distribution of radioactivity in the fractions was determined by scintillation counting

CHOLESTERYL ESTER ACCUMULATION IN RAT HEPATOMA TISSUE CULTURE CELLS

George Rothblat

Because of the interest in the relationship between cholesteryl ester (CE) accumulation and atherosclerosis, we have attempted to select an easily grown tissue culture cell which accumulates CE when exposed to hyperlipemic rabbit serum (HRS) and then study the mechanism responsible for such accumulation. When the sterol content of hyperlipemic serum grown cells are compared to normal rabbit serum grown cells, all cells exhibited approximately a 60% increase in free cholesterol, and from a 4 to 20 fold increase in esterified sterol. However, L, W-18, HF and numberous other cells which we have examined have an esterified cholesterol to free cholesterol ratio of 1 or less, even when grown in hyperlipemic serum. By comparison, the Fu5AH rat hepatoma cells have an ester to free cholesterol ratio of approximately 3, thus this cell was selected for more detailed studies.

Table 1. Lipid content of Fu5AH rat hepatoma cells growth on normal and hyperlipemic rabbit serum

| Lipid | µg/mg cell protein | | Hyperlipemic |
	Normal rabbit[a]	Hyperlipemic rabbit[a]	Normal
Cholesterol			
Free	12.9	22.0	1.7
Ester[b]	6.3	72.5	11.5
Total	19.2	94.5	4.9
Phospholipid[c]	4.8	4.9	1.0
Triglyceride	66.9	109.8	1.6

[a]Cells incubated 24 hr in 5% serum. [b]As cholesterol of cholesteryl ester. [c]As phospholipid P.

This increase in cholesteryl esters is rather specific, being 11 times greater in hyperlipemic grown cells (Table 1). Free cholesterol and triglycerides show about a 2-fold increase, while phospholipid remains unchanged. We have recently observed similar increase in CE in cells grown in hyperlipemic monkey and pigeon sera.

This increase in CE is often accompanied by the appearance of cytoplasmic vacuoles. The facuoles are composed primarily of CE and triglycerides and only low levels of free cholesterol and phospholipids are present. An average of 35% of CE is recovered in the cellular high speed supernate, indicating that considerable CE may be associated with cellular particulate material, as is approximately 90% of the free cholesterol.

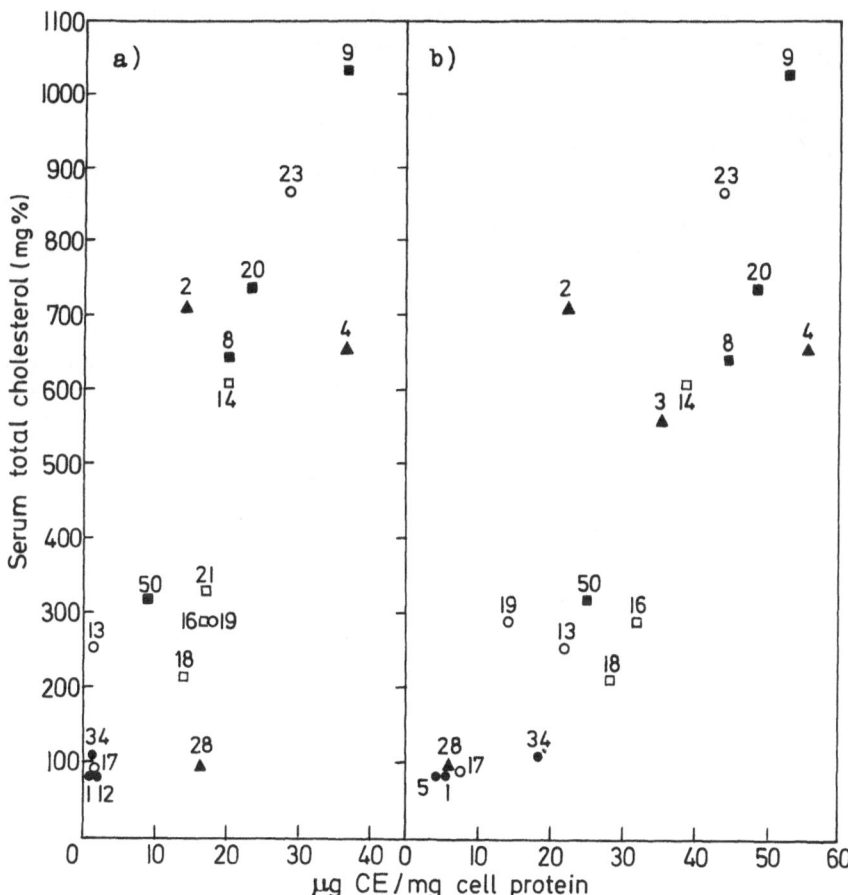

Figure 1. Cholesteryl ester content of Fu5AH cells incubated in presence of rabbit sera having varying cholesterol levels (mg %). Experiment A: sera added to
medium at constant level of 2.5%. Experiment B: sera added to equivalent total
cholesterol concentration of 300 μg/ml. Incubation time, 10 hours. Numbers on figure denote individual sera. Symbols denote number of day rabbits maintained on
cholesterol diet. o = 0 days; O = 3; ■ = 7; ▲ = 11; □ = 21

The accumulation of CE is rapid and near linear for the first 8 hrs of exposure
to hyperlipemic serum. Maximum accumulation is achieved by 24 hrs, and increasing
the incubation time beyond 24 hrs generally does not result in greater accumulation. There is a direct correlation between cellular ester content and serum concentration only at low concentrations of serum. Increasing hyperlipemic serum
concentrations above 5% does not result in greater accumulation. No accumulation
results when cells are grown in up to 40% normal rabbit serum.

Heating hyperlipemic serum or subjecting it to cycles of freezing and thawing did
not eliminate its ability to promote accumulation. If, however, it was delipidized and the proteins and lipids added to the culture medium together following
sonication at 40°, no significant accumulation was observed. Heating Fu5AH cells
eliminated the accumulation of CE while inhibiting protein synthesis with cyclohexamide resulted in an increase in CE content.

Fig. 1 shows the CE content of cells exposed to individual samples of rabbit serum obtained from rabbits maintained on hyperlipemic diets for various time period up to 21 days.

The ordinant shows the total sterol content of the individual samples of serum expressed as mg%. It does not represent sterol in the growth medium, but rather is an indication of extent of hypercholesteremia for each sample. Each serum sample is indicated by a numbered point. The abscissa is CE content of cells after 10 hrs incubation in the individual sera. In the experiment shown on the left (segment a), the serum was added to the growth medium at a constant level of 2.5%. Thus the total cholesterol concentration in the growth medium ranged from 18 to 260 µg/ml. The right segment (b), illustrates the cellular CE content when the same sera were added to the culture medium to obtain a constant concentration of total·cholesterol of 300 µg/ml. The results shown in both experiments demonstrate that the cellular level of CE can be correlated with the cholesterol level of the individual serum. This result, in the case of a constant serum dilution could be explained simply by a correlation between cellular CE and concentration of cholesterol in the medium. However, this cannot be the explanation for the results seen in Fig. 1b where cholesterol levels in the medium are similar in all samples. These data suggest the cellular CE accumulation is induced by specific serum lipoproteins, the level of which is a function of the degree of hypercholesteremia.

When lipoproteins from HRS were added to the culture medium to a level of 300 µg/ml total cholesterol, it was observed that the ability to promote cellular ester accumulation is not confined to a single lipoprotein density class, although density less than 1.006 lipoproteins appear to be most active. Lower cellular concentrations of ester were observed following exposure to LDL, while HDL provoked the least accumulation.

To gain information on the origin of cellular cholesteryl esters, balance studies were conducted quantitating both the increase in cellular esters and the level of exogenous cholesterol prior to and following a 24 hr incubation period. By the end of the incubation period, cellular ester had increased by 61 µg/mg protein in Experiment I and 44 µg/mg protein in Experiment II. In these cultures, exogenous ester decreased by 39 and 36 µg in the two experiments. Thus approximately 63% of the ester recovered from the cells could have been derived from the medium in the 1st experiment while this figure is 81% in the 2nd experiment. The most likely origin of the remaining cellular ester would be through the esterification of free cholesterol. The loss of exogenous free cholesterol from the medium in amounts greater than that recovered in the cells as free cholesterol, as was observed in these experiments, is consistent with such a mechanism. In addition, preliminary experiments using hyperlipemic rabbit serum to which had been added ^{14}C-free cholesterol have indicated that from 55 to 65% of the labeled free cholesterol incorporated by the cells in a 24 hr exposure period is recovered as esterified cholesterol. If it is assumed that the added ^{14}C-cholesterol had equilibrated with the free cholesterol in the serum, it can be calculated that from 10 to 30% of the cellular cholesteryl ester is derived through the esterification of free cholesterol after a 24 hr incubation period.

In a cellular sterol regression experiment, cells previously grown on hyperlipemic serum and containing cholesteryl esters were incubated in a medium supplemented with delipidized serum protein plus lecithin. Sterol content of both cells and medium was assayed after 24 and 48 hrs incubation. The data expressed as cholesterol/culture dish showed that the cellular pool of cholesteryl ester decreased by approximately 12%/24 hr of incubation. Thus, at the end of the two days, approximately 75% of the esters remained in the cellular compartment. The results indicate that once the cholesteryl esters have accumulated in these cells, they are relatively stable and extensive efflux or hydrolysis does not take place.

In summary, we have shown that exposure of Fu5AH rat hepatoma cells to hyperlipemic sera promotes the accumulation of cellular CE, resulting in cellular CE/FC ratio of approximately 3. The actual amount of ester present in these cells is substantially greater than has been observed in a variety of other cells we have examined, although all have exhibited an increase in cellular cholesteryl esters when grown in hyperlipemic sera.

Accumulation is rapid and serum dose dependent only at low concentrations of serum. The ability of serum to promote accumulation is correlated with the degree of hypercholesteremia. Cellular viability is required for ester accumulation but protein synthesis does not seem to be necessary. Balance studies indicate that from 60 to 90% of the cellular esters are derived from incorporation of exogenous ester while the remainder may be a product of free cholesterol esterification.

EFFECTS OF DIETARY PROTEIN ON PLASMA CHOLESTEROL LEVELS IN RABBITS FED CHOLESTEROL-FREE SEMISYNTHETIC DIETS

R.M.G. Hamilton and K.K. Carroll[*]

Plasma cholesterol levels increase several fold when rabbits are transferred from commercial diet to cholesterol-free low fat semisynthetic diets (Malmros and Wigand, 1959; Moore and Williams, 1964; Howard et al., 1965; Carroll, 1971). This increase may be due in part to the casein in the semisynthetic diet, since earlier studies (Meeker and Kesten, 1941) indicated that casein tends to cause a hypercholesterolemia in rabbits and Carroll (1971) observed elevated plasma cholesterol levels in rabbits fed a diet of one part casein and three parts commercial diet. No such increase was observed when dextrose rather than casein was added to the commercial diet. The present experiments were carried out to investigate the effects of feeding proteins from various sources in a low fat cholesterol-free semisynthetic diet and to determine how these effects may be modified by varying the fat and carbohydrate components of the diet.

The low fat control diet used for these studies had the following composition, expressed as percent by weight: Casein 27, dextrose 60, cellulose 5, salt mix 4, molasses 2 and corn oil 1, while the corresponding high fat diet contained casein 30, dextrose 42, cellulose 5, salt mix 5, molasses 2 and fat 15. Each diet contained a supplement of water soluble and fat soluble vitamins (Carroll, 1967). Groups of 5-6 male New Zealand white rabbits (initial weight 1.0-1.3 kg) were used and diets were fed for 28 days.

In the first series of experiments, the casein in the low fat semisynthetic diet was replaced by isonitrogenous amounts of protein from various animal or plant sources. The effects of these diets on weight gain and plasma cholesterol levels are shown in Fig. 1. Diets containing proteins from animal sources gave average plasma levels ranging from 105 to 230 mg/100 ml, while those containing proteins from plant sources gave lower values, ranging from 15 to 100 mg/100 ml. There seemed to be no correlation between weight gain and level of plasma cholesterol.

After most of these feeding trials had been completed, it was discovered that due to a typing error, choline was added at the level of 150 µg/kg rather than 150 mg/kg. The rabbits on diets containing soybean protein or isolated soybean protein (Promine-R), which showed the lowest plasma cholesterol levels, also had fatty livers (10-14% by weight of total fat), while animals on the control casein diet had normal liver lipid levels (3.5-4.5% by weight) in spite of the low choline intake. Increasing the level of choline to 150 mg/kg in the diets containing soybean protein or Promine-R prevented the occurrence of fatty livers and led to somewhat higher plasma cholesterol levels (averages of 35 and 66 mg/100 ml respectively).

Since methionine is the first limiting amino acid in soybean protein, the diets containing soybean protein or Promine-R were further supplemented with DL-methionine at the rate of 2% of the dietary protein level and this supplementation produced some further increase in plasma cholesterol levels (averages of 80 and 75 mg/100 ml respectively). The very low levels obtained in the initial experiments with soybean protein thus appeared to be due in part to a deficiency of choline and methionine, but supplementation did not raise the plasma cholesterol to the higher levels obtained with diets containing casein or other proteins derived from animal sources.

---

[*]Medical Research Associate of the Medical Research Council of Canada.

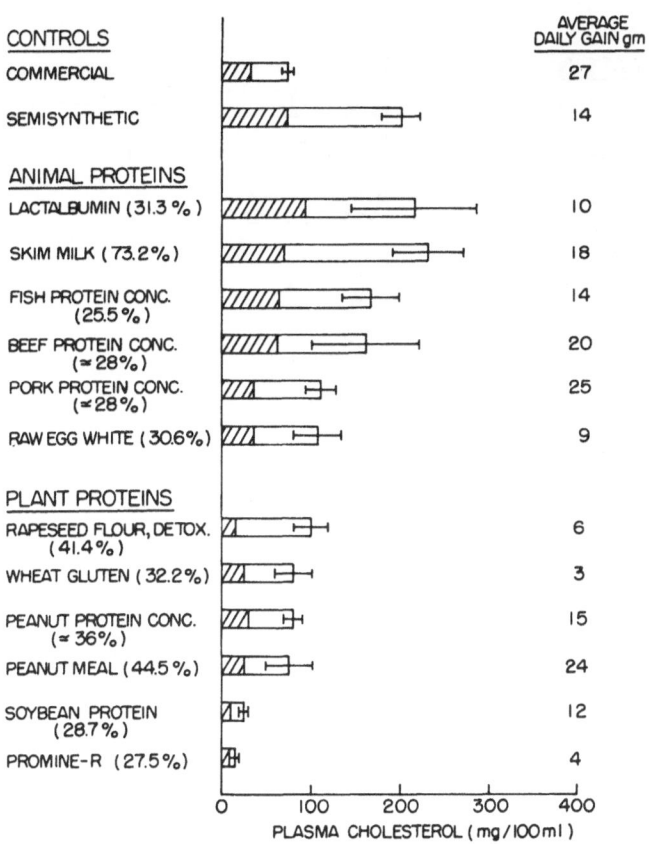

Figure 1. Plasma cholesterol levels in rabbits fed low fat, cholesterol-free semi-synthetic diets containing animal or plant proteins from different sources. The amount of material from each protein source (figures in brackets) was designed to make all diets isonitrogenous. Beef, pork and peanut protein concentrates were prepared in our laboratory, fish protein concentrate was kindly provided by Dr. Lloyd Regier, Halifax Laboratory, Fisheries Research Board of Canada, Halifax, N.S., detoxified rapeseed protein by Dr. J.D. Jones, Food Research Institute, Ottawa, Ontario, and Promine-R by Dr. E.W. Meyer, Central Soya, Chicago, Ill. Other proteins were obtained from commercial sources. Diets contained 150 µg/kg of choline, except the fish protein and rapeseed concentrate diets which contained 150 mg/kg. Plasma cholesterol values are for groups of 5-6 rabbits after 28 days on diet. Total length of bar indicates Average Total Cholesterol ± Standard Error of the Mean. Hatched portion indicates Average Free Cholesterol

Interactions of dietary protein and dietary fat were studied in a second series of experiments (Fig. 2). Corn oil reduced the level of plasma cholesterol when added as 15% by weight to semisynthetic diets containing either casein or Promine-R, but seemed to have no effect when added to commercial diet. Addition of butter to these diets at the same level had no consistent effect on plasma cholesterol.

Fig. 3 shows the effect of different combinations of dietary proteins and carbohydrates on plasma cholesterol in rabbits on low fat semisynthetic diets. Substitution of wheat starch for dextrose in the casein diet had little effect, but potato starch gave a much lower level. Diets containing Promine-R as source of protein gave consistently low plasma cholesterol levels, irrespective of the carbohydrate component.

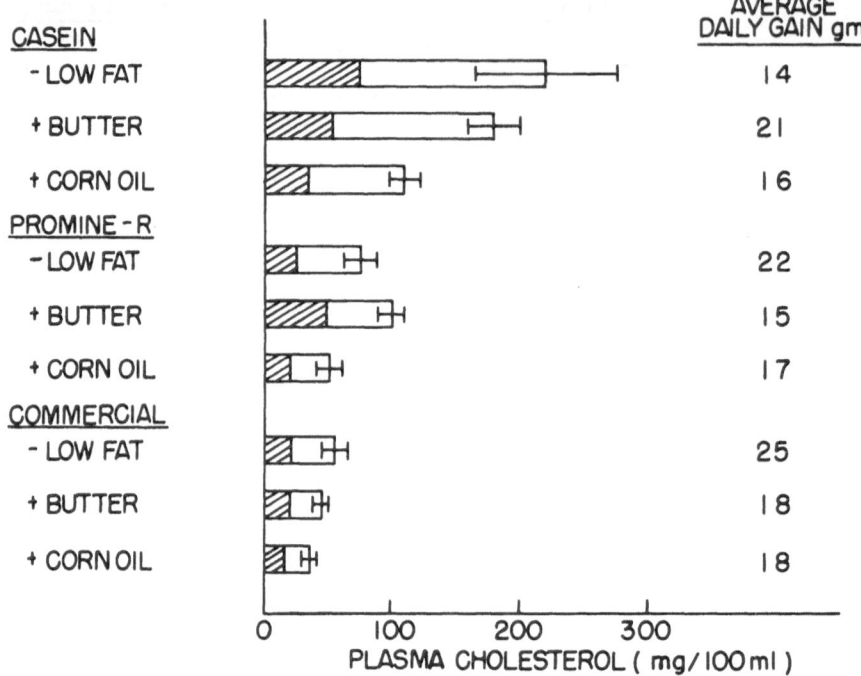

Figure 2. Effects of dietary proteins and fats from different sources on plasma cholesterol levels in rabbits. Semisynthetic diets (casein and Promine-R) contained 150 mg/kg of choline and Promine-R diets were supplemented with DL-methionine at 2% of the level of dietary protein. Design of experiments and presentation of data as in Fig. 1

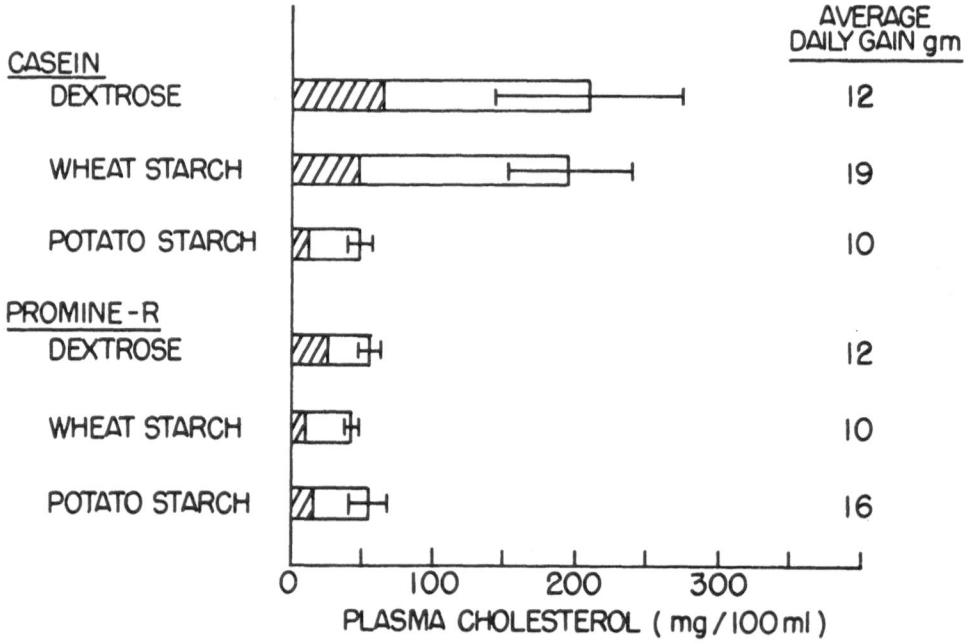

Figure 3. Effects of dietary proteins and carbohydrates from different sources on plasma cholesterol levels in rabbits. All diets contained 150 mg/kg of choline. Design of experiments and presentation of data as in Fig. 1

The results of these experiments indicate that the non-lipid components of cholesterol-free semisynthetic diets significantly effect plasma cholesterol levels in rabbits. Dietary proteins from animal sources tend to be more hypercholesterolemic than those from plant sources. The source of dietary protein should therefore be considered when effect of dietary fats and carbohydrates on cholesterol levels are being studied, because interactions may occur between these nutrients.

Acknowledgements. This work was supported by the Ontario Heart Foundation and the Medical Research Council of Canada. Technical assistance was provided by Ruth Hill, Lillian McPhee, H.E. Pedersen and R. Rasmussen.

X

Hyperlipoproteinemia and Lipoprotein
Disorders – Genetics and Epidemiology

WORKSHOP: Types and Genetics of Hyperlipoproteinemias

Chairmen: W. Fuhrmann, West Germany
W. Holmes, USA

Participants: B.M. Rifkind, USA
J. Slack, England
J.L. Goldstein, USA
M.S. Brown, USA
J. Edwards, England
J. Sobra, Czechoslovakia

NATIONAL HEART AND LUNG INSTITUTE TYPING SYSTEM

Basil M. Rifkind

The underlying concept of the National Heart and Lung Institute typing system as developed by Fredrickson, Levy and Lees (1967), and as previously emphasized by Gofman et al. (1954), is by now well known; namely, the need to translate hyperlipidemia into hyperlipoproteinemia, since it is as lipoproteins rather than as individual lipids that the major plasma lipids circulate and since different patterns of hyperlipoproteinemia are associated with characteristic features. Of the utility of the phenotyping system, there can be no doubt. Most important, it introduced a standard nomenclature where one hardly existed previously. Subsequent to the system's introduction there has been a considerable expansion of work and interest in the field of hyperlipidemia and hyperlipoproteinemia. Further, it has led to a more precise definition of several disorders in terms of their clinical, biochemical, pathological and genetic features, and therapeutic requirements.

Aspects of the typing system are periodically criticized. I believe that some, though not all, of these criticisms are related to certain misconceptions and misapplications of the system and propose to describe these. It should be emphasized from the outset that when the system was introduced it was envisaged that it almost certainly concealed heterogeneity; in this respect one thinks especially of the Type IV pattern. It was also anticipated that it would be duly replaced by a classification based on the specific metabolic defects underlying the various lipoprotein abnormalities.

Initially, the system was based on estimation of plasma cholesterol and triglyceride, and on electrophoresis of whole plasma. Electrophoresis was selected because, in contrast to other means of separating lipoproteins, it provided a rapid, simple and inexpensive means of visualizing the four major lipoprotein fractions in large numbers of subjects. The system was only semi-quantitative and shortly after its introduction the authors realized the need, in some subjects, to quantify the lipoprotein fractions. The so-called beta quantification system which measures LDL concentrations in terms of the LDL plasma cholesterol content was then introduced. Ideally this involves a combination of preparative ultracentrifugation and a simple precipitation procedure. Should the preparative ultracentrifuge not be available then the LDL cholesterol can be accurately derived, in most situations, by the formula:

$$\text{LDL cholesterol} = \text{plasma cholesterol} - \frac{\text{triglyceride}}{5} - \text{HDL cholesterol}$$

(Friedewald et al., 1972).

If necessary, a figure of 45 mg for HDL cholesterol can be used with some loss of accuracy.

There are three groups of subjects in whom it is necessary to carry out LDL quantification. Firstly, some individuals, especially females on oral contraceptives, have modest hypercholesterolemia due to a raised HDL cholesterol. They have to be distinguished from subjects with mild hypercholesterolemia and normal triglycerides due to an LDL increase. Secondly, some Type II subjects have a raised LDL cholesterol but a total cholesterol lying between the 90th and 95th percentile, i.e., below the conventional upper limit. At the NHLI about 10% of Type II subjects have proven to have fallen into this category. Thirdly, subjects with Types IIB, III or IV hyperlipoproteinemia can have identical cholesterol and triglyceride levels and some of the distinction between these various subjects is afforded by estimating the LDL cholesterol.

Another methodological modification involving preparative ultracentrifugation was necessary to acquire the VLDL (d<1.006) fraction for electrophoresis to demonstrate so-called floating beta lipoprotein required for the definite diagnosis of Type III. The original requirement of a broad beta band on electrophoresis of whole plasma is now regarded as unsatisfactory since it is not present in all Type III plasmas.

What, in fact, is the information required to allocate a subject with hyperlipidemia into the appropriate lipoprotein category? Four questions have to be answered: 1. Are chylomicrons present or absent? 2. Is LDL present in normal or increased concentration? 3. Is VLDL normal or increased in concentration? 4. Is the abnormal lipoprotein form of Type III hyperlipoproteinemia present? *Chylomicrons* can be easily detected by inspection of cold stored plasma. A raised *LDL* concentration can be inferred to be present when hypercholesterolemia of moderate to severe degree exists without hypertriglyceridemia. When the hypercholesterolemia is less pronounced, then the LDL fraction has to be quantified as just indicated. Electrophoresis seldom assists in this situation because it is too insensitive to determine whether a modest elevation of LDL exists; densitometric analysis of electrophoretic strips have not yet proven to be satisfactory in this situation. Whether plasma *VLDL* is normal or increased in concentration is determined by the plasma triglyceride levels. In the absence of other triglyceride-bearing fractions, namely chylomicrons or the abnormal lipoprotein of Type III, a raised triglyceride concentration indicates that the VLDL fraction is increased. Finally, as mentioned, *floating beta lipoprotein* is detected by electrophoresis of the appropriate plasma fraction. In summary, electrophoresis is only required for the diagnosis of Type III. Many clinical laboratories still merely provide electrophoresis for the evaluation of hyperlipidemia and misdiagnose many subjects. It is important that lipoprotein quantification procedures be built into routine clinical chemical practice for the management of appropriate hyperlipidemic subjects, and that less reliance be put on electrophoresis.

Another misconception which sometimes underlies criticism of the typing system is that it describes diseases. On the contrary, the various types consist of abnormal lipoprotein patterns. These may be *secondary* to a variety of disorders such as hypothyroidism, obstructive jaundice or some types of renal disease, or they may be apparently *primary* in etiology, a considerable proportion appearing to be genetically determined. One of the major causes of error in applying the typing system is the failure to evaluate lipoprotein status under standardized conditions. The subject should be fasting, of stable weight, on a normal Western-type diet, not be taking drugs known to alter plasma lipids, not be pregnant, and not be acutely ill. Failure to adhere to these rules often accounts for reports of the changing lipoprotein status of individuals. For example, it is well known that when subjects with Type IV hyperlipoproteinemia are being treated by appropriate diet or drugs a temporary excess of LDL may develop (Type II pattern). Similarly, under appropriate provocation, subjects with Type IV may develop a temporary Type V pattern.

A COMPARISON OF THREE RECENT REPORTS ON THE INHERITANCE OF LIPID ABNORMALITIES IN SURVIVORS OF MYOCARDIAL INFARCTION

Joan Slack

Three studies of lipid levels and lipoprotein abnormalities in survivors of myocardial infarction and their relatives have been published recently by Patterson and Slack (1972) from London, Nikkila and Aro (1973) from Helsinki and Goldstein et al. (1973) from Seattle. The findings in each study have been compared with the populations from which they were drawn, and the mode of inheritance of lipoprotein abnormalities in survivors has been examined. There are striking similarities in the findings in the three studies and some marked differences in the conclusions, and since the differences are always more entertaining, those are what I propose to examine.

Index Patients and Controls. First it may be useful to consider the populations from which the samples were drawn, and then the methods used for analysis in the three studies. Table 1 shows the size, age and sex distribution in the three samples. The sample from the United States provides the largest numbers, but unfortuneately none of the studies was able to provide information on large numbers of young female index patients. Table 2 shows the mean lipid levels among the controls in each city. While the mean serum lipid levels in the populations from London and Seattle are similar, the mean of both serum lipid levels in Helsinki are higher. Each study used adjusted scores to enable a comparison of lipid levels between different ages and sex, fortunately this also facilitates comparisons between the studies.

Table 1. Comparison of samples in three studies

	London	Helsinki	Seattle
Males under 50	37	94	111
Males 50 and over	70	0	290
Females under 50	15	7	21
Females 50 and over	70	0	78

Table 2. Lipid levels found in controls and used to identify index patients in 3 studies

	London Chol.	Tg.	Helsinki Chol.	Tg.	Seattle Chol.	Tg.
Mean level in controls	224	105	262	112	220	97
Upper 90th centile	278	145	320	210	270	147
% survivors above 90th centile	18.5	22	32	32	22	32
Cut off used to identify I.P.s	320	212	320	210	285	165

All lipid levels adjusted to male 40-50 years.

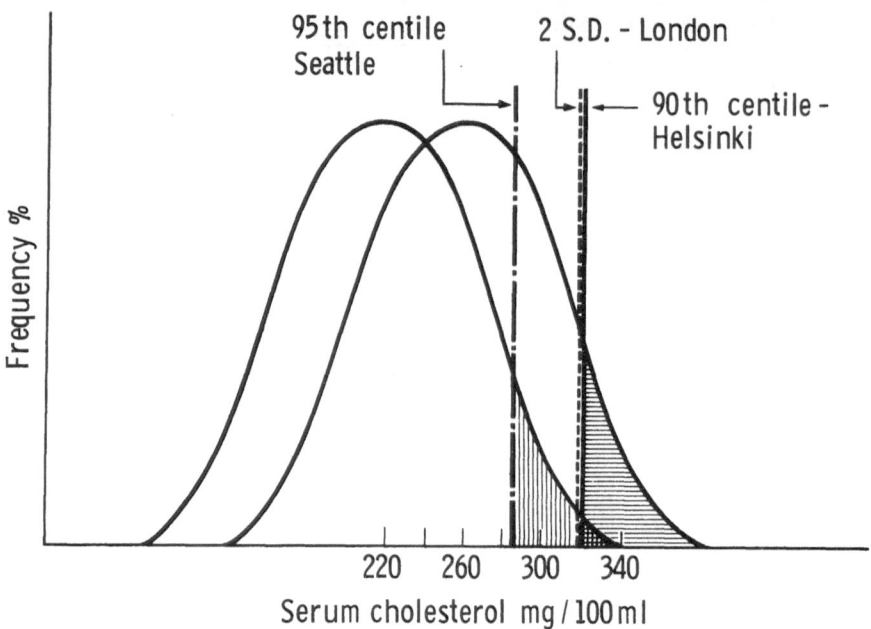

Figure 1. Serum cholesterol distributions and "cut off points" in Helsinki, Seattle and London

Fig. 1 shows a diagram of the distribution of adjusted cholesterol scores for each city. The curves are simplified and do not show the skewness found for both cholesterol and triglycerides by each study, but perhaps this is justified for comparisons. The distributions of serum cholesterol levels are shown for London and Seattle on the left and for Helsinki on the right. The different "cut off points" used for each study are indicated, and the area under the curve represents the population selected as hyperlipidaemic for each study. The London and Helsinki groups are thus working with similar levels but using different proportions of their population, the Helsinki and Seattle groups are working with different levels, but using somewhat larger proportions of their population. These differences in cut off points are likely to have an important bearing upon the findings in a genetic analysis since the most extreme outliers, and therefore probably the more genetically homogeneous, will be selected by cut off points which select the smallest proportion of the population.

Selection of Hyperlipidaemic Survivors for Study. Perhaps the most remarkable result of the three studies is that when allowance is made for the difference in population means and the cut off points selected, the results of examination of the raw material in the three studies are very similar. All three studies attempted to examine the mode of inheritance of the lipid disturbances in survivors. The differences reported can best be explained by the differences in the material selected for analysis and the methods used for analysis.

In Helsinki the families of all survivors were investigated, in London the families of all the so called "hyperlipidaemic" survivors but in Seattle the selection of hyperlipidaemic survivors above the cut off point was qualified. First there must be three or more available first degree relatives. I cannot therefore quite understand why no less than twelve published pedigrees of index patients included in the Seattle study show less than three available first degree relatives. Family 497 indeed shows none. In addition thirteen families out of presumably about thirty index patients with lipid levels between the 95th and the

92.5th centiles were specially selected for inclusion in the family studies. It is not clear to me how this selection was made.

Selection of Relatives for Study. In both Helsinki and London only first degree relatives were used for family studies, but the Seattle group studied not only 913 first degree relatives but also 643 second, 135 third and 4 fourth degree relatives. The decision to contact distant relatives was made in favour of families with one or more hyperlipidaemic first degree relatives. This selection must introduce a bias in favour of investigating a disproportionate number of hyperlipidaemic distant relatives. The authors themselves note this bias, finding more than the expected number of affected second degree relatives in the families studied. Nevertheless they include the distant relatives in their search for bimodality in the frequency distributions in relatives from the "hypercholesterolaemic" and "hypertriglyceridaemic" families.

Lipid Levels in Survivors and Relatives. It was a common finding to all three studies that there was an elevation of both cholesterol and triglycerides in relatives which was intermediate between the hyperlipidaemic index patients and the controls. All three studies agree that this finding is compatible with the hypothesis that familial factors, which may be environmental as well as genetic are contributing to the elevation of lipid levels in the survivors.

Incidence of Abnormal Electrophoretic Patterns. There was agreement by all three groups that different kinds of hyperlipoproteinaemia appear more frequently than expected within the same families of the hyperlipidaemic survivors. This finding suggests either that the use of arbitrary cut off points has favoured the selection of a heterogeneous group for family studies, or that the methods for dividing hyperlipidaemic index patients into types, nearly all IIA, IIB or IV, is inadequate to identify different phenotypes. It is most likely that both problems are involved. As a result of this observation, each group has attempted to analyse the mode of inheritance of the lipoprotein disturbances using different approaches.

Analysis of Findings. In London, we divided the hyperlipidaemic index patients into two broad groups according to the lipoprotein disturbances seen on electrophoresis. The first group contained all the index patients with predominantly hyperbetalipoproteinaemia, and the second group contained the index patients with predominantly hyperprebetalipoproteinaemia. The relatives of the hyperbetalipoproteinaemic index patients showed a shift of the distribution of cholesterol levels to the right, with 9 out of 79 appearing as outliers with serum cholesterol elevated more than 2 standard deviations above the expected mean. The nine so-called affected relatives came from five families. If the hypercholesterolaemia observed in the relatives had been caused by a dominantly inherited characteristic, 18 families would be expected to exhibit at least one "affected" first degree relative. We conclude that the hypercholesterolaemia observed in survivors of myocardial infarction is polygenically determined in the majority, but by major single gene effects in a minority (about 1 in 4 if the 2 standard deviation cut off point is used to identify hypercholesterolaemic survivors).

In Seattle a more determined attempt was made to examine the relatives without making a prior assumption that the electrophoretic pattern was useful in identifying phenotypes. An array of the findings of all lipid levels found in the relatives was used to select the lipid level most frequently elevated in each family. A family diagnosis was then made for each index patient by a majority finding in each family. If two anencephalic stillbirths in a family were followed by a live born child with spina bifida, should we diagnose anencephally in the survivor? Both conditions are apparently genetically related, but the result of this kind of analysis in a large number of families with central nervous system malformations would be to create three types, spina bifida, anencephaly and "combined". Families 332 and 458 in the Seattle study contain no individual with combined hyperlipidaemia, but the diagnosis is familial combined hyperlipidaemia. Three relatively homogeneous-looking groups *must* be identified by this diagnostic technique; the truth may be obscured. I cannot reconcile myself to the method of majority diagnosis used in Seattle.

Finally the groups in both Helsinki and Seattle divided their families into "sporadic" cases with no affected first degree relative or into "familial" cases with one or more affected. I would take issue with both groups for this manoeuvre. In Helsinki no allowance was made for the possibility that affected relatives may be dead or the probability that in small families affected relatives have never been born. But no genetic conclusions were drawn from this analysis in Helsinki.

In Seattle it was the intention to look only at families with 3 or more available first degree relatives, thus ensuring a probability of at least 7 in 8 that an affected first degree relative would be found if the condition was dominantly inherited. But it is my opinion that even in larger families, the inclusion of an affected relative as a criterion for the selection of families for analysis *must* bias the sample towards bimodality unless the affected relative is excluded from the analysis. The authors in Seattle have taken trouble to examine this possibility and have collaborated with Dr. Felsenstein to test for this bias by using a computer generated model. The model shows no bias, though the variance in the distribution of relatives of index patients appears to be greater than the variance in the distribution in relatives of controls. But the computer used families with 5 first degree relatives, while the Seattle group used families with 3 or more available first degree relatives including as we have seen 12 families with less than 3. The computer model is not really simulating the method of selection. Finally, I can see no way in which the selection of distant relatives in families where a first degree relative was affected has been tested by Dr. Felsenstein's carefully prepared model, and it is my contention that if all the biases in favour of bimodality were removed from the genetic analysis performed in Seattle, these authors too would find evidence for polygenic inheritance in the majority of hyperlipidaemic survivors of myocardial infarction, with some single genes of large effect playing an important part in the determination of hyperlipidaemia in a minority.

At present there is no way of testing or measuring the genetic defect in any of the hyperlipidaemic conditions we have seen in the survivors of myocardial infarction and we are, I think, all agreed that until these tests are found there may be no way of resolving our differences.

Discussion

Dr. Little: I have a suggestion that one might reconcile some of the differences by eliminating the biases in some of the different studies mentioned here by eliminating subjects who are used for ascertainment, e.g., in a family where one of the criteria for studying that family is that they have a first degree relative who has an abnormality, then that relative should be removed.

Dr. Goldstein: The biases that Dr. Slack mentioned are uncontrollable at the present time in the absence of knowing the basic underlying defects in these disorders, as we were careful to point out in all of our papers. It was our feeling in analyzing the data that it is a cop-out to say it is polygenic and one should try to devise some sort of approach with the least biases possible to test the model; this is what we attempted by using the method of letting the family classify the type of disorder present. Despite the biases that Dr. Slack has pointed out and which we will certainly agree to, there is no question when one looks at a large number of pedigrees, and with large numbers of relatives, on an average of 9 relatives per family, one is struck with the fact that at least 50% of these families have many relatives who are affected with hyperlipidemia. There is a pattern that tends to emerge as the syndrome of familial hypercholesterolemia with xanthomatosis. This occurred interestingly enough in 4% of Dr. Slack's material,

5% of our material, and 6% of the material from Helsinki, a remarkable similarity despite the differences in our studies. One is also struck with the fact that there are families that have pure familial hypertriglyceridemia, one does not find anything other than Type IV pattern in those relatives who are affected. The most interesting result of our study, that Dr. Slack did not find in London but which was confirmed independently by Dr. Nikkila in Helsinki, was that the majority of familial involvement in patients with coronary heart disease concerned multiple lipoprotein types within a family. We termed this "combined hyperlipidemia", the Helsinki group termed it "multiple lipoprotein type hyperlipidemia", you find Type II-A, Type II-B, Type IV and sometimes Type V. This is a remarkable finding, i.e. there are qualitatively three different types of families present in these patients with coronary heart disease. Until one determines the basic defect, one cannot be sure whether it is due to a single major gene, but our hypothesis would be that it is, and I as a medical geneticist think the data exciting enough to advise my metabolism friends to search for an underlying biochemical defect. Polygenic means many different things to different people; one interpretation of polygenic is that it means one locus with different alleles, which is really the same thing as saying it is due to a single gene, so one would have to define a polygenic interpretation very carefully. I would also mention that our data was tested for by one polygenic model which did not fit; Dr. Slack's data was not tested formally for a polygenic model – it was concluded it was polygenic because it wasn't monogenic.

Dr. Motulsky: I certainly agree that puristically in a statistical sense certain objections can be made to the analysis we did, some of which were outlined by Dr. Slack. Our concept when we started the study was strongly toward polygenic inheritance, and we tried in various ways to fit our data to polygenic inheritance, yet it did not seem to fit. We then did the analysis that was published and mentioned earlier. Using an analysis based on triglycerides and cholesterol to find these disorders is like trying to find different causes of anemia, hereditary anemias, acquired anemias, etc. by doing hematocrit or hemoglobin determination. The cholesterol and triglyceride are far removed from what these genes are doing. If we do a pure statistical analysis on all kinds of anemias, just using hemoglobins, one would get a mish-mash of data presumably suggesting some hereditary components because there would be some genetic cases present. So, in doing the analysis, one had to try some a priori knowledge about, let us say hypercholesterolemia, and there I think that everyone agrees on the evidence that such a monogenic disorder exists. The rest of the data we thought as monogenic, and you heard the argument. There are a number of other studies available now, including ours, dealing mainly with very large pedigrees, and with very large pedigrees it becomes much more difficult to mimic polygenic inheritance. Now, if one finds very large pedigrees where there is, in fact, transmission of triglyceride levels in what appears to be a Mendelian dominant manner, and if one finds this for cholesterol, which has been known for a long time, but particularly if one finds large pedigrees where the new phenotype that we call combined hyperlipidemia seems to segregate in the expected manner our conclusions appear somewhat close to what might be ultimately correct; certainly, one needs a much better marker, and I would agree and I think Dr. Goldstein would agree that there may be some misclassifications in our families, but that the distinction made has some merit.

Dr. Steinberg: It is a very difficult thing to convey to medical students or to practitioners that the term "combined hyperlipidemia" does not necessarily mean that the patient will have both an elevation of cholesterol and triglycerides because the name implies that, and I think it would be much easier if this were called something else, like "undifferentiated hyperlipidemia".

Dr. Goldstein: I think the Helsinki description is actually the best: multiple lipoprotein type.

Dr. Sobra:[*] I should like to add a short genetic case history of a family with Type II-A and IV.

In 1969 and 1970 we defined and published independently the clinical and laboratory picture of a mixed form of hyperbetalipoproteinaemia and hyperprebetalipoproteinaemia, which we termed at that time, familial hyperlipoproteinaemia type IIc (Sobra et al., 1970; Sobra, 1970). The description of this type corresponds fully of the later description of the type IIB hyperlipoproteinaemia (Beaumont, 1970).

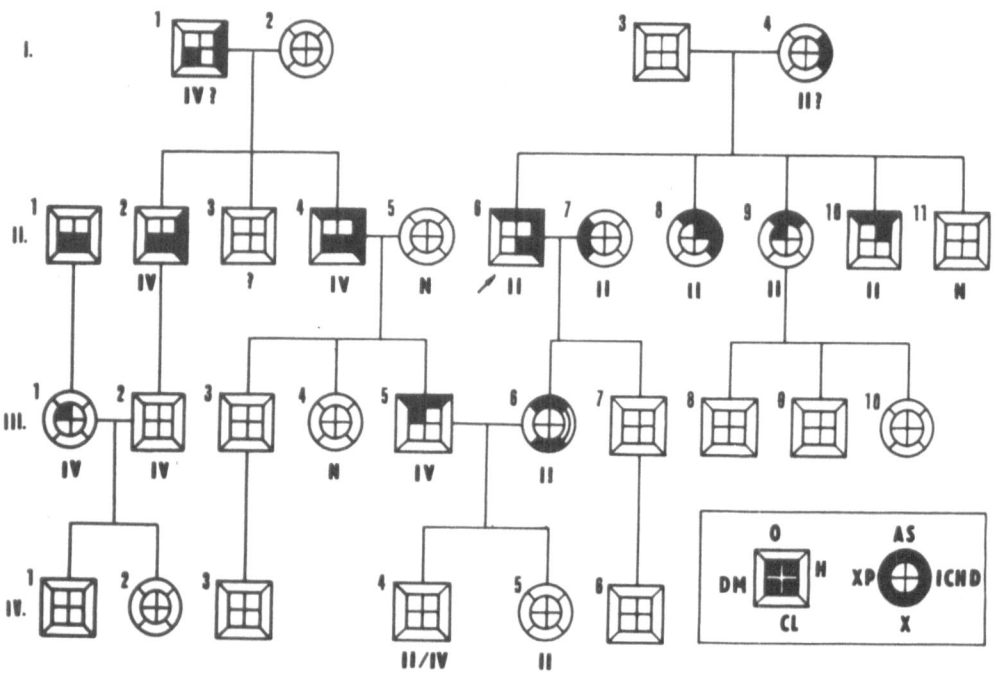

Figure 1. Family tree showing a possible explanation of the origin of familial hyperlipoproteinaemia type IIA/IV

In the family tree presented in Fig. 1 a woman of 31 (III-6) is a homozygote of familial hyperlipoproteinaemia type IIA. She has arcus lipoides corneae, and since the age of 17 has suffered from tendinous and tuberous xanthomatosis and since the age of 25 from angina pectoris. Her serum cholesterol level before treatment was 600 to 700 mg%, triglyceride levels were normal. Her father (II-6) and mother (II-7) are type IIA heterozygotes (Sobra, 1967). Three brothers (II-10) and sisters (II-8, II-9) of her father are similarly affected.

The husband of this woman (III-5) is a heterozygote type IV. Both, the father (II-4) and the father's brother (II-2) of the husband suffer from diabetes, both have recovered from myocardial infarction and suffer from intermittent claudications. Their blood cholesterol is about 300 mg% and the triglyceride level about 500 to 900 mg% with markedly increased pre-beta-lipoproteins. The laboratory findings thus correspond to type IV. No floating beta-lipoprotein was found in the supernatant.

---

[*]The family was studied together with M. Kvasilová and R. Procházková.

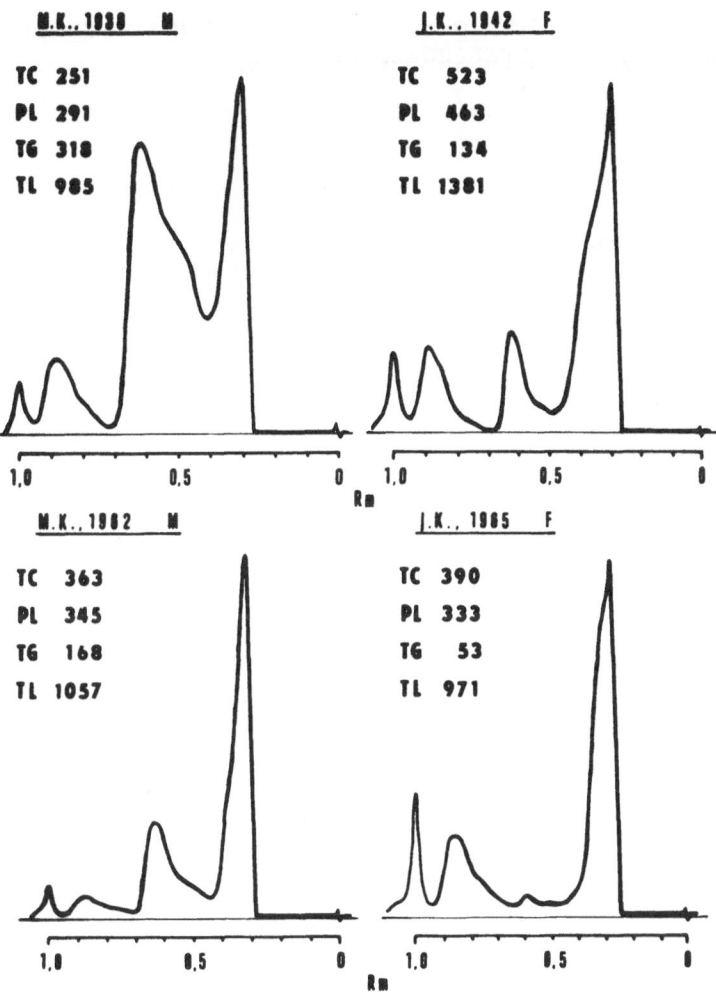

Figure 2. Densitometric curves and blood lipid levels in father (M.K., 1938 –
Type IV), mother (J.K., 1942 – Type IIA), daughter (J.K., 1965 – Type IIA) and
son (M.K., 1962 – Type IIA/IV)

Both children (IV-4, IV-5) of these parents are hyperlipoproteinaemic, but show
no clinical manifestations of disease. Laboratory findings in the daughter (IV-5)
corresponds to type IIA and in the son (IV-4) to a mixed heterozygote type IIA +
IV (Fig. 2).

We suggest that the hyperbetalipoproteinaemia descends from the mother, whereas
the hyperprebetalipoproteinaemia originates from the father. The son is assumed
to be a mixed heterozygote of types IIA and IV. It has been shown repeatedly by
many authors (Fredrickson and Levy, 1972), the genotypes IIA and IV are the most
frequent in the population. We suggest therefore, that a mixed heterozygote of
types IIA and IV may be one plausible genetical explanation of the origin of familial hyperlipoproteinaemia type IIB.

DEVELOPMENT OF A CELL CULTURE SYSTEM FOR STUDY OF THE BASIC DEFECT IN FAMILIAL HYPERCHOLESTEROLEMIA[*]

Joseph L. Goldstein[**] and Michael S. Brown

Familial hypercholesterolemia (FH) is an autosomal dominant disorder characterized by an elevated plasma level of low density lipoprotein (LDL) - cholesterol,
xanthomatosis, and premature atherosclerosis (Brown and Goldstein, 1974, in press).
The single-gene inheritance of this disorder implies that a single biochemical
abnormality underlies its pathogenesis. To date, however, very little is known
about the cellular biochemical defect.

To approach this problem, we have developed a cell culture system that allows a
comparison of the mechanism of regulation of cholesterol synthesis in cultured
fibroblasts obtained from normal subjects (Brown, et al., 1973) and patients with
the most severe form of inherited hypercholesterolemia, namely homozygotes with
FH (Goldstein and Brown, 1973). In developing our system, we relied on an earlier
observation of several groups, including those of Bailey (1973); Rothblat and
Kritchevsky (1967), and Avigan (Williams and Avigan, 1972), who demonstrated that
cultured mammalian cells synthesize cholesterol and that the rate of cholesterol
synthesis decreases when exogenous cholesterol is supplied to the culture medium.
This regulatory system in cultured cells bears some resemblance to the feedback
system that regulates cholesterol synthesis in mammalian liver. As shown by Siperstein (1970) and others, the activity of the rate-controlling enzyme in the hepatic cholesterol biosynthetic pathway, 3-hydroxy-3-methylglutaryl coenzyme A reductase (HMG CoA reductase), is regulated by the cholesterol content in the diet.
When an animal is fed cholesterol, hepatic HMG CoA reductase activity rapidly
declines and cholesterol synthesis is therefore suppressed.

We recently demonstrated that the activity of HMG CoA reductase can be measured
in extracts of cultured human fibroblasts (Brown, et al., 1973). Enzyme activity
was low in normal cells grown in standard medium containing fetal calf serum and
rose by 40-fold when the fetal calf serum was replaced by human serum from which
the lipoproteins had been removed by ultracentrifugation (Fig. 1A). The factors
in whole human serum responsible for enzyme suppression were localized to the LDL
(Fig. 1B) and very low density lipoprotein (VLDL) fractions of serum lipoproteins.
High density lipoproteins (HDL) had no effect in suppressing enzyme activity.

Since LDL and VLDL share a common protein component, apolipoprotein B, it seemed
likely that this apolipoprotein was required for the suppression of HMG CoA reductase activity of normal cells. In keeping with this hypothesis was the observation
that whole serum from a patient with abetalipoproteinemia, which is deficient in
apolipoprotein B, had no effect on HMG CoA reductase activity of normal cells
(Brown et al., 1974, in press).

When grown in the presence of fetal calf serum, cells from a homozygote with FH
had a 60-fold higher specific activity of HMG CoA reductase activity than the normal cells (Fig. 1A). This elevated activity did not increase when lipoproteins
were removed (Fig. 1A) nor did it decline when LDL was added (Fig. 1B), thus suggesting that the homozygote's cells possessed a genetically-determined resistance
to feedback suppression by LDL. Additional experiments indicated that the 60-fold
elevated level of HMG CoA reductase activity led to a similarly marked increase
in the rate of cholesterol synthesis from acetate by the homozygote's cells. We
have also shown that LDL isolated from the blood of a homozygote suppressed HMG
CoA reductase activity of normal cells in a manner identical to the LDL obtained

[*]Supported by grants from the American Heart Association (72629) and the National
Institutes of Health (GM 19258 and HL 16024).

[**]Recipient of a USPHS Research Career Development Award (GM 70, 277).

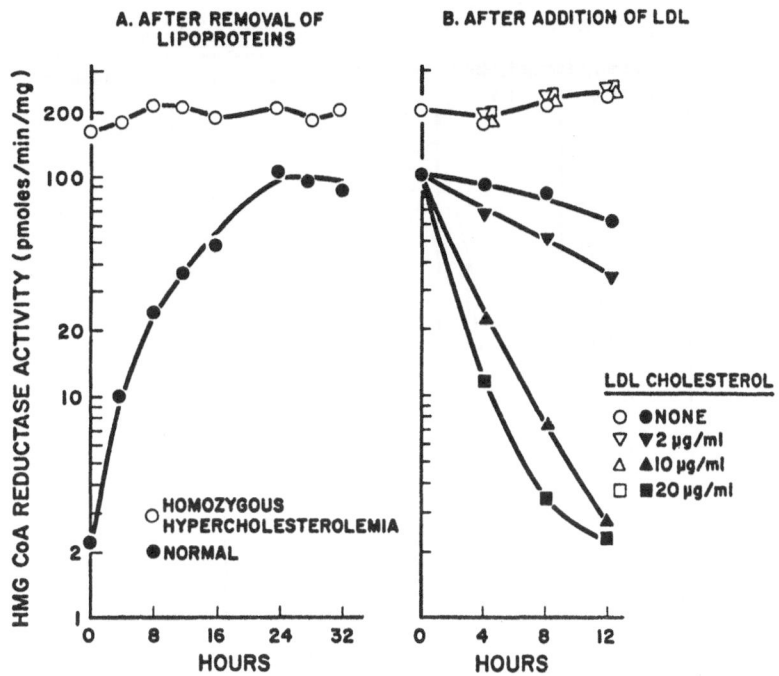

Figure 1. HMG CoA reductase activity in fibroblasts of a control subject (*closed symbols*) and a patient with homozygous familial hypercholesterolemia (*open symbols*). (A) Cells were grown in petri dishes containing standard medium and 10% fetal calf serum as previously described (Goldstein and Brown, 1973). On day 6 (O time), the medium was replaced with fresh medium containing 5% human lipoprotein-deficient serum. At the indicated time, extracts were prepared and HMG CoA reductase activity was measured. (B) 24 hrs after addition of 5% human lipoprotein-deficient plasma, 0.1 ml of buffer containing human LDL was added to give the indicated concentration: (o,•) none; (∇,▼) 2 µg/ml; (Δ,Δ) 10 µg/ml; (□,■) 20 µg/ml. HMG CoA reductase activity was measured at the indicated time (from Goldstein and Brown, 1973 with permission of *Proc Natl Acad Sci USA*)

from a normal subject, thus further indicating that the biochemical defect in FH resides in abnormal cellular metabolism rather than in abnormal serum lipoproteins (Goldstein and Brown, 1973).

The specificity of the defect in regulation of HMG CoA reductase activity in homozygotes with FH was confirmed by study of cell lines from 27 subjects. The cell lines from 8 normal controls, 4 hyperlipidemic controls (i.e., subjects with hypercholesterolemia from other causes), and 2 fetal controls showed a pattern of enzyme regulation that was both qualitatively and quantitatively different from that of the 5 homozygotes with FH (Fig. 2). The 8 heterozygotes with FH showed a partial defect in enzyme regulation with a mean ± SEM HMG CoA reductase activity in fetal calf serum (12.5 ± 3.8 pmoles/min/mg protein) that was significantly higher (p <0.001) than that of the controls (4.9 ± 0.9 pmoles/min/mg protein) and significantly lower (p <0.001) than that of the homozygotes (95.4 ± 23.9 pmoles/min/mg protein) (Goldstein et al., 1974, in press). This partial and intermediate defect in heterozygotes was more clearly demonstrated by quantitating the effect of increasing levels of LDL on enzyme activity (Goldstein and Brown, 1973).

The elucidate the mechanism by which the homozygotes' cells are resistant to the action of LDL, experiments were carried out in which the effect of cholesterol bound to LDL and cholesterol in a nonlipoprotein form were compared with regard

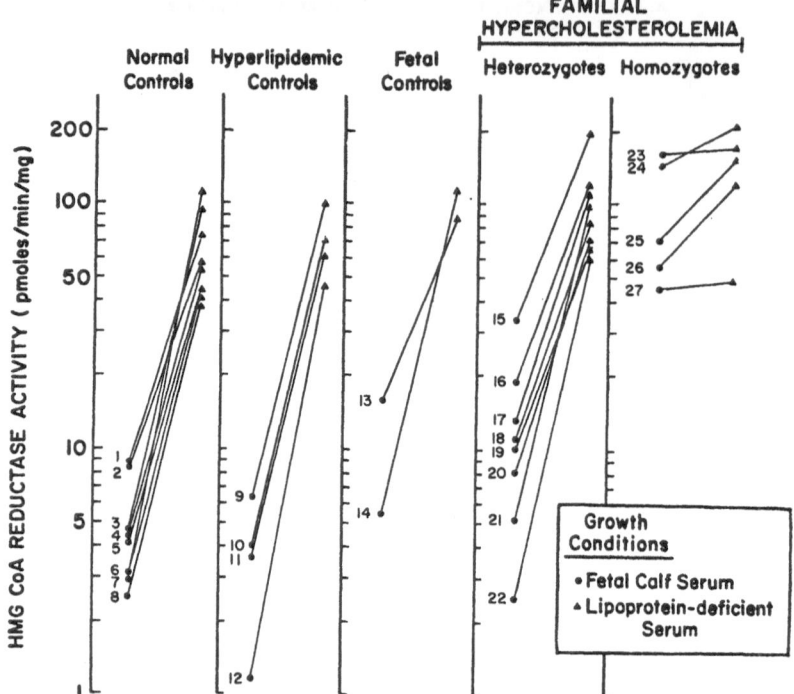

Figure 2. Regulation of HMG CoA reductase activity in fibroblasts from 27 subjects (including normal controls, hyperlipidemic controls, normal fetuses, and patients with the heterozygous and homozygous forms of familial hypercholesterolemia). Cells were grown in petri dishes containing standard medium and 10% fetal calf serum as previously described (Goldstein, et al., 1974) and on day 6 the medium was replaced with fresh medium containing either 10% fetal calf serum (•) or 5% human lipoprotein-deficient serum (▲). 24 hrs later, extracts were prepared and assayed for HMG CoA reductase activity (from Goldstein et al., 1974, with permission of *Amer J Hum Genet*)

to the ability of each sterol preparation to suppress HMG CoA reductase activity. Whereas both forms of cholesterol suppressed enzyme activity in normal cells, in the homozygotes' cells only the cholesterol in the nonlipoprotein form was effective (Brown et al., 1974). There are several important implications of these experiments. First, it would appear that cholesterol itself is the feedback regulator of HMG CoA reductase activity in normal cells and that the function of the apolipoprotein B component of LDL is to deliver cholesterol to the cell in a physiologic form. Second, since the homozygotes' cells are resistant to cholesterol bound to LDL but respond to cholesterol delivered in a nonlipoprotein form, it is likely that the mutant cells contain all the factors necessary to suppress HMG CoA reductase activity provided that cholesterol can be delivered to the proper cellular site. In this regard, we hypothesize that the primary underlying abnormality in FH involves the process by which circulating LDL interacts with the cell, presumably at the cell surface. As a result of this abnormality, cholesterol delivered to the cell as LDL does not reach its proper cellular site, HMG CoA reductase activity is not suppressed, and cholesterol is overproduced.

Although our studies of cultured fibroblasts indicate that subjects with FH carry in all cells of the body an abnormal gene that has the potential to induce excessive cholesterol production, the tissues in which this abnormal gene is expressed *in vivo* and the conditions governing its expression cannot be determined from these cell culture studies. Further studies will be necessary to relate these *in vitro* observations to the mechanism by which cholesterol accumulates in the living patient with FH.

Discussion

Dr. Steinberg: I would like to ask if you have shown that the rate of cholesterol synthesis is as high as the HMG CoA reductase activity, and also if you have looked at any other cells such as lymphocytes.

Dr. Goldstein: These studies in the homozygote are paralleled by identical studies of the incorporation of acetate to cholesterol. In a homozygote who has elevated his level to 60-fold greater than normal, the rate of cholesterol synthesis from acetate is 60-fold greater than that of normal but the rate of synthesis from mevalonate, the product of the enzymes, to cholesterol is the same in the normal and in the abnormal cells.

Question: Dr. Goldstein, the enzyme was 60 times higher in activity in the homozygous cells, yet you used the same concentrations of LDL to try to inhibit it. Do you think you might have got better inhibition if you had used an equivalent concentration of LDL, and how did your cholesterol levels, when they inhibited the enzyme, compare with the cholesterol in the LDL that you added?

Dr. Goldstein: We get inhibition at levels as low as 5 µgms/ml which is fantastically lower than the physiologic level of circulating LDL cholesterol, and we have increased this in the homozygote to as much as 2000 µgms/ml and see no inhibition. The level of cholesterol in the LDL was the same as the level of cholesterol added in ethanol to the normal cells. It turns out that in the homozygous cells there's a time lag; in other words, the response to the administration of cholesterol in ethanol in the homozygous cells takes longer than in the normal at lower doses, but at saturating doses one can get the same time effect.

Dr. Grundy: In the last few years we have been studying with Dr. Gerald Salen a sort of analogous inherited disease, cerebral tendinous xanthomatosis, and in this condition there is a definite overproduction of cholesterol as well as of cholestanol, and these patients have large accumulations of cholesterol and cholestanol in their tissues. So in some ways this may be a related disorder, although a rare one. The interesting thing about this condition is that the cholesterol level and lipoproteins in blood is actually low rather than being high despite this tremendous accumulation of cholesterol tissues. I wonder if you might speculate on just what might cause the high level of lipoproteins in the blood in patients with hypercholesterolemia?

Dr. Goldstein: It would be speculation at this point, but based on what I presented today, one possibility is that the cells are resistant to LDL, and we think the defect is at the membrane level. The fact that cholesterol itself is able to inhibit the enzyme, suggests one exciting possibility that the LDL may not be processed normally by cells yet to be identified in the body, and there may be a secondary accumulation of the LDL. This is, the cell membrane may not respond to LDL and secondarily may not metabolize it properly. That would be one hypothesis that would explain elevation of LDL in the blood and also the fact that cells would then secondarily over-produce cholesterol.

BASIC GENETIC CONCEPTS

J. Edwards

When Edward Gibbon was discussing the troubled areas around Jerusalem in the second century, he pointed out this was largely the consequence of the Monophysite and the Polyphysite heresies - the heretics, of course, being mutual with Polyphysites regarding them as Monophysites and visa versa. He pointed out how much trouble and bloodshed would have been saved if the terminology had been a little clearer, because, in fact, both sides were not clearly disagreeing, but merely thought they were disagreeing, with unfortunate consequences; to some extent this is so in this field. It may be a little obsolete to discuss statistical methods because statistical methods are only relevant if you have uncertainties and, of course, it is our primary purpose to reduce rather than to measure uncertainty: I agree with Dr. Goldstein that the computer must give way to the fibroblast. Unfortunately we have a lot of data and there are practical problems as to what to do with it.

In fact, if we cannot do anything better than has been done so far, one may as well stop collecting it because there is no point in having numerical data unless one exposes it to numerical procedures in this intervening period before the relevant enzymes, etc., can be attacked directly. It may be helpful to try and devise some sort of map showing where we are, because a lot of confusion arises from failing to appreciate that, since concepts like heritability were advanced in 1918 and variances started being split in the twenties, knowledge has advanced considerably and we no longer have a degree of ignorance about the genetic apparatus which makes it necessary to get involved in complicated probability statements; we now know the basic bits and pieces (Fig. 1).

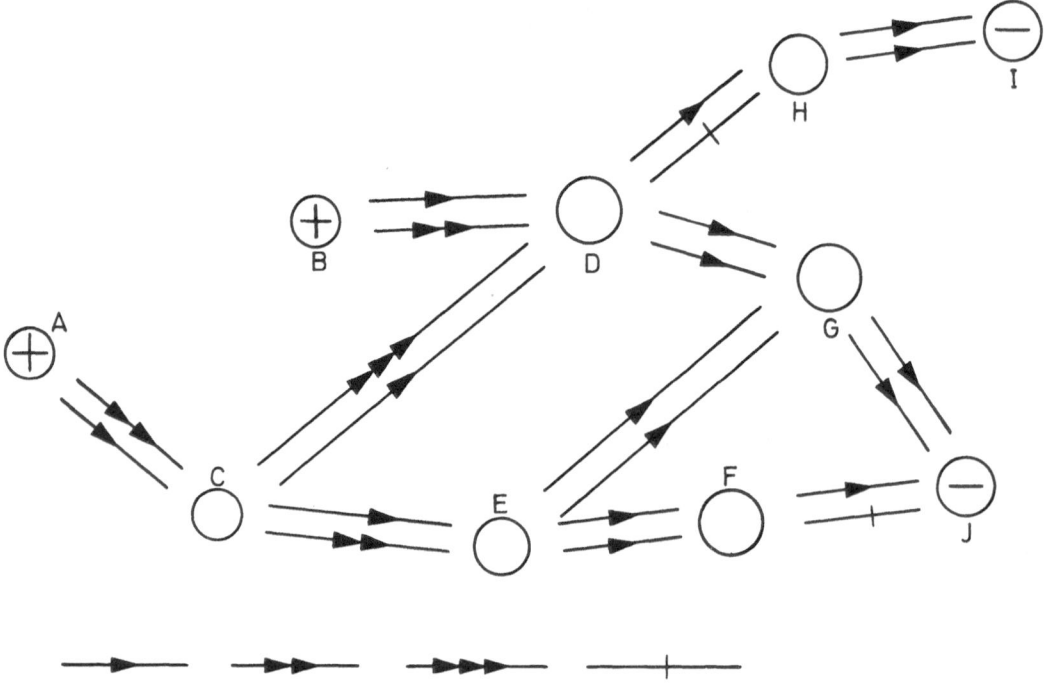

Figure 1. Simplified model of a metabolic map. Diagram showing relationship of genetic determinants (arrows) to cytoplasmic constituents (circles)

Firstly, anything which happens must be polygenic, which is why I personally dislike this word because to say a disease is polygenic is like saying it is unhealthy. It means nothing, because if it takes place in the cytoplasm, or if it takes place anywhere in the body, it must be under some sort of influence by the genes because everything is basically made from them. So it seems on simple grounds, one must say all things are polygenic, but, if one can relate things to some simple primary product, as in haemophilia or sickle cell disease, obviously one can relate it to a specific factor which one can infer and one can usefully talk about diseases which are related to specific genetic factors as genetic diseases. As you get further away from the primary genetic products, it gets more and more confused. The idea that there are two kinds of diseases, monogenic and polygenic, is a misunderstanding, and it is not possible to talk about a formal test for a polygenic system any more than it is possible to talk about a formal test for being alive. The mere fact that one is alive means one really must have a cytoplasm and it must be under some sort of control. The concept of a polygenic disease does not really get you any further than the concept of disease itself. The Hippocratic idea of a diathesis seems to me quite as scientific as heritability statements, and so on. The simplest situation is where you have some individuals and can take measurements and see if you have two sorts of humps, two differences rather than one. This may seem very simple, but the trouble with curves which are produced by real data is they nearly always have antimodes; if there is a true antimode, rather than a statistical one, this will only arise if the two constituent curves are over two standard deviations apart. This was known to Gauss and is the basis of his designing his voltmeters. This is very obvious when one thinks of it because it must be where the lines defining the normal curves are straight when they cross. As a true bimodality only arises if there is a basic differences of over two standard deviations, a little dip is statistically very unlikely to be related to this type of situation. One can make this very much more complicated by all sorts of statistical procedures, but there again one gets into difficulty because data can always be fitted by two measurements better than by one.

Secondly, one can try looking at the relatives. And there again this might seem simple to do but the difficulty is that one gets very much the same sort of association and intensities in the relatives in the one gene situation, as in the many gene situation. Indeed, these are extremely difficult to distinguish unless you get very large pedigrees, or unless you get a consistent clinical opinion on qualities as, for example, in the herditary xanthomatoses where there is a sufficient congruity of expert opinion to believe that there is a syndrome which runs in families in a predictable manner. This is not really a statistical matter. One can look at the correlation with relatives, which has sometimes been done under a misunderstanding that it is relevant; in fact it is not a discriminant because it gives the same results. Historically this was shown by Yule in 1904.

One can look at the parents, and this is of some importance because, in a dominant, of course, one parent has it and the other does not and, if it is rare, this is an almost invariable situation, while with the so-called many factor model there is obviously a parental tendency but it is very variable. This is extremely important because the only simple test you can do, which as far as I can see has almost never been done, is to look at the parental differences because one parent will have it and the other will not. The difficulty is that it is not known which; this rather entertaining statistical problem, which is similar to the linkage problem for two generations, has not yet been resolved although it is simple on computers.

Thirdly, one can look for association, which seems to me of some interest, particularly as an association has been found (and this seems to me one of the most important findings of the Seattle group) cholesterol level and ABO blood group.

Basically, I feel that one should get away from the idea that there are two separate mechanisms, a single gene mechanism and a multiple gene mechanism, and I think one should get away from these words, which are used variously. To talk about multifactorial is confusing because it is often used to include the environment, but no less a person than Mendel used the word factor to define the hereditary unit. It is used sometimes as synonymous with its Greek equivalent polygenic and by others as distinct from polygenic. Polygenic has even been related to polygenes, which are very interesting concepts, but there is no room for them, or, at least, nobody has found any yet, and so much is known about the genetic material, that I think we must doubt whether they exist as distinct from other genes.

Fourthly, there is yet another confusion; I had not heart of polyallelism being confused with polygenic, but I can see that could be yet a further reason for not using this word. How can one get one of this dilemma?

There are a lot of determinants of our variability, and we must accept that we do vary, and we must accept that our variation is largely determined by these heriditary units. If there is a large number of them, it seems that they will all be different, and, if they vary, some will be stronger than others. So one can formally ask the question "if we simplify the model and suppose that there really is just one very strong one, which has a relatively big effect, and that a proportion p of alleles have this, how strong is it and how common is it?" The gene frequency is p and it has an effect d, which is defined as half the distance between the two homozygotes, in terms of standard deviations. Now if you do that you then have an extremely simple system which is biologically plausible, but makes no demands on language or credulity, and allows one to eliminate many concepts, including significance tests, the splitting of variance, heritability, and polygenes.

Discussion

Dr. Fuhrmann: Dr. Edwards' paper emphasizes the importance of work like the fibroblast studies, getting close to the primary defect. The term ploygenic used in connection with these diseases has its problems. There is considerable confusion even between the terms "polygenic" and "multifactorial". Whereas "polygenic" originally has been reserved to define the additive action of many genes, each contributing a small fraction to some trait, it has been used by some authors in the broader sense implied by the term "multifactorial" meaning the combined action of several genes and environmental factors. Other authors restrict the term "multifactorial" to the original meaning of polygenic. Some models built on these concepts are very artificial. To me it seems that the finding of an apparently polygenic background of a disease always asks for a search for single major genes among the many contributing factors.

Dr. Motulsky: Relative to the argument, it is certainly quite clear that many genes are involved in the determination of a normal trait and we all accept it. We do not know how much each of these genes contributes to it. It may be very difficult for a normal trait like blood pressure or something like that, to all work it out. But if you take a disease trait, hypertension, or some of the things you are talking about, atherosclerosis, the number of factors entering into it probably is smaller and it is quite likely that major factors do play a role in these common diseases, and from the point of view of disease research strategy this really helps. If we grant that if he has let us say 10 factors, and one of these factors contributes 30 or 40% to the total variance, this is a major gene then by definition and this is one we can go after, by Dr. Edwards fibroblast or biochemistry or electronmicroscopy or what not, but that ultimately, to understand genetic disease etiology, we must try to search out for these major genes by methods other than statistics.

Dr. Edwards: The difficulty with the statistical model is it tells you of your families, 5% of them have a terribly interesting disease which then should have fibroblasts looked at, but it doesn't tell you which 5%. So it doesn't really help as a very good discriminant. Obviously, there are these multiple and in some cases preventable, and in some cases understandable, causes of hypercholesterolemia or anything else. The statistical approach doesn't tell you which places to investigate, which is why I can't see how its on the direct line of research in the seventies.

Dr. Slack: I would just like to ask Dr. Goldstein whether he has used his fibroblast cultures on heterozygotes from his monogenetically determined hypercholesterolemia which he did not select from families who first presented with tendinous xanthomata?

Dr. Goldstein: All the studies that we have done to date are with families that have clear-cut familial hypercholesterolemia with tendinous xanthomata. As I mentioned, of the 8 heterogytes two of them are overlapped into the normal range. The system needs to be refined considerably before one can begin to investigate all the forms of Type IIA and Type IIB hyperlipidemia, but I think the system does offer the promise of resolving some of these problems.

RELATIVE MOBILITY OF SERUM LIPOPROTEINS AND FAMILIAL HYPERLIPOPROTEINAEMIA TYPE III

J. Sobra, A. Heyrovský, M. Kvasilová, and R. Procházková

Some 15 years ago a special clinical and laboratory unit for active screening of patients with various forms of familial hyperlipidaemias has been established at the Third Medical Clinic of the Charles University in Prague. In the course of time over 3000 subjects with various forms of hyperlipidaemias and their affected and non-affected family members have been examined.

In our opinion any hyperlipoproteinaemia cannot be classified as secondary unless its genetically conditioned aetiology is excluded. This holds even for patients with another underlying disease; according to our experience there are in the population more familial than secondary hyperlipoproteinaemias.

Up to March 1972 we were able to detect various forms of familial hyperlipoproteinaemias in a total of 667 persons. The number of patients with individual types of hyperlipoproteinaemia and their relative proportion as compared with the findings of Fredrickson et al., 1973 is shown in Table 1. The frequency of various forms of xanthomatosis in our patients is presented in Table 2. A relatively high incidence of palpebral xanthomas in our patients with type IIA and IIB is due to the fact that they were screened in collaboration with dermatologists and ophthalmologists, who frequently encounter palpebral xanthomas in their consulting rooms.

Table 1. Frequency of individual types in our group of 667 patients with familial hyperlipoproteinaemia

Type	Fredrickson et al., 1971		Our findings, 1972	
	n	%	n	%
I	18	1.86	3	0.45
IIA			263	39.44
IIB	620	64.18	114	17.09
III	86	8.91	94	14.09
IV	171	17.70	148	22.18
V	71	7.35	45	6.75
Total	966	100.00	667	100.00

Table 2. Various forms of xanthoma and the percentage of their occurence in 667 patients with familial hyperlipoproteinaemias

Type	I	IIA	IIB	III	IV	V	Total
n	3	263	114	94	148	45	667
Xanthelasma palpebrarum	–	122 46.4%	40 35.1%	9 9.6%	14 9.5%	1 2.2%	186 27.9%
Xanthoma tendin.	–	61 23.1%	4 3.5%	12 12.7%	–	–	77 11.5%
Xanthoma tuberoerupt.	–	–	–	23 24.4%	–	–	23 3.4%
Xanth. str. palmare	–	–	–	17 18.0%	–	–	17 2.5%
Xanthoma eruptivum	–	–	–	–	–	13 28.8%	13 1.9%

Besides correlating the clinical and laboratory findings, our attention was drawn chiefly to a detailed qualitative analysis of serum lipoproteins after their separation by electrophoresis.

Material and Methods

Lipoprotein electrophoresis was performed in our laboratory in agarose gel according to Rapp and Kahlke (1968) with minor modifications (Sobra, 1972). Only fresh fasting sera, from 2 to 3 hours after blood collection were used for analysis. After staining with Sudan Black B, the glass plates were evaluated with the aid of an extinction densitometer ERI-65, Zeiss Jena.

The relative mobility of individual lipoprotein fractions was measured from the densitometric curves by projecting the peaks of the Gaussian curves into the distance between the start-line and the pre-albumin zone (Fig. 1).

During the last 4 years serum lipoprotein electrophoresis was performed on more than 1800 individuals. Other determinations included total cholesterol, triglycerides, total lipids and floating lipoproteins. Floating beta-lipoproteins were detected according to Fredrickson et al. (1968) in the preparative ultracentrifuge ICE model B-60 equipped with the swing-out rotor. The obtained supernatant was analysed by agarose gel electrophoresis and stained for lipids and for proteins.

Results and Discussion

Under well-standardized conditions it is possible to demonstrate by agarose gel electrophoresis in most fresh fasting blood sera 2 pre-beta-lipoprotein subfractions. The relative mobility (Rm) of the slower fraction is 0.50 and of the faster one 0.60. The fraction 0.60 prevails in most healthy control subjects, in

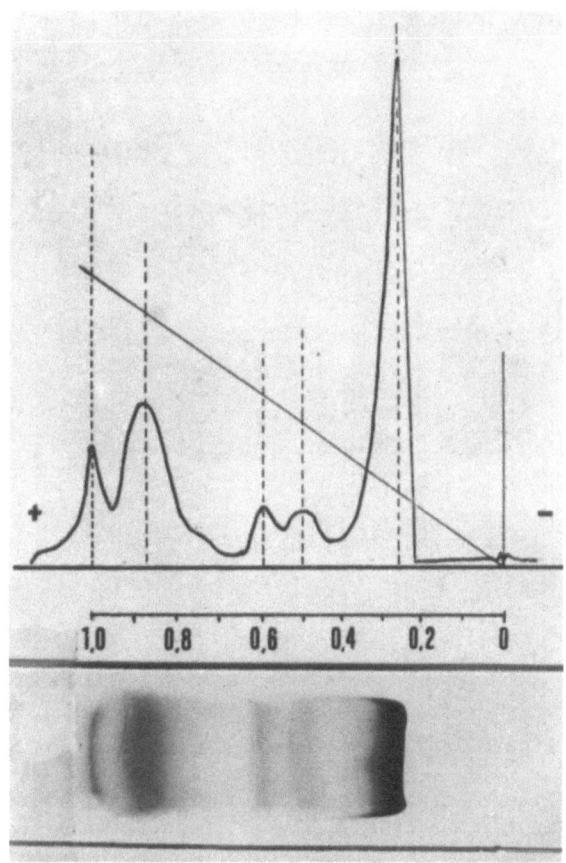

Figure 1. The measurement of the relative mobility (Rm) of individual lipoprotein fractions after agarose gel electrophoresis

most patients with type IIA (Fig. 2a) and in some patients with type III. An isolated occurrence of the fraction 0.50 without concomitant presence of the subfraction 0.60 could be established so far only in 6 individuals (1 woman with normal lipids and with a cancer of the stomach, 1 man with xanthoma disseminatum and 4 normal healthy subjects, 3 being members of the same family).

Both pre-beta-lipoproteins appear concomitantly in various relations in subjects with hyperlipoproteinaemias type IIB, IV and V, the fraction Rm 0.50 being dominant (Fig. 2b). Both subfractions are also present in some persons with type III and sporadically in type IIA.

In some patients with high triglyceride levels the two lipoprotein subfractions cannot be safely distinguished (Fig. 3). This is the case mainly in patients with alcohol-induced hyperlipoproteinaemia. Following 1-2 weeks of abstaining, the 2 subfractions became clearly separated.

Mutual relations of the two subfractions, their incidence in individual types of familial hyperlipoproteinaemias and their correlations with clinical manifestations are currently under study in our laboratory. The occurrence of two pre-beta-lipoproteins after separation by electrophoresis on cellulose acetate has been published recently by Dahlen et al. (1972).

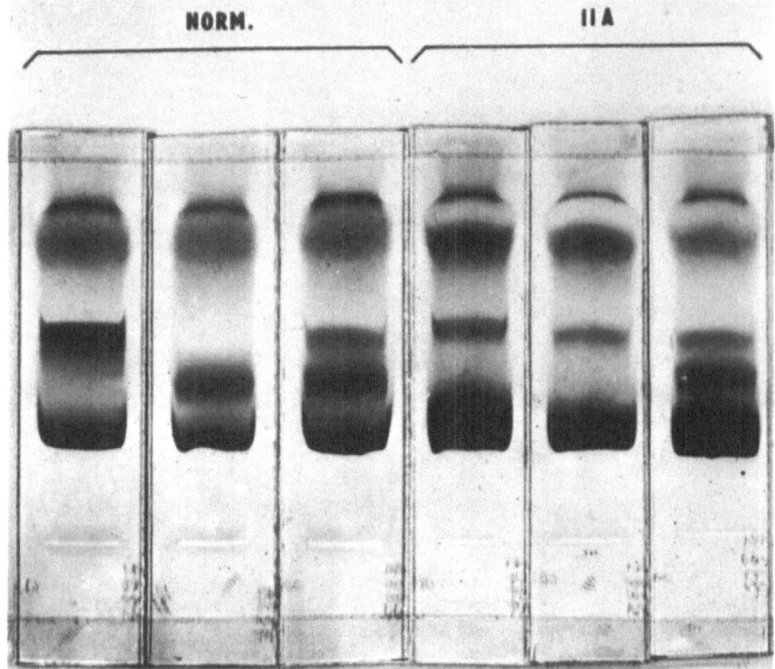

Figure 2a

Figure 2a/b. Separation of pre-beta-lipoprotein into two fractions in normals and in various types of hyperlipoproteinaemia.

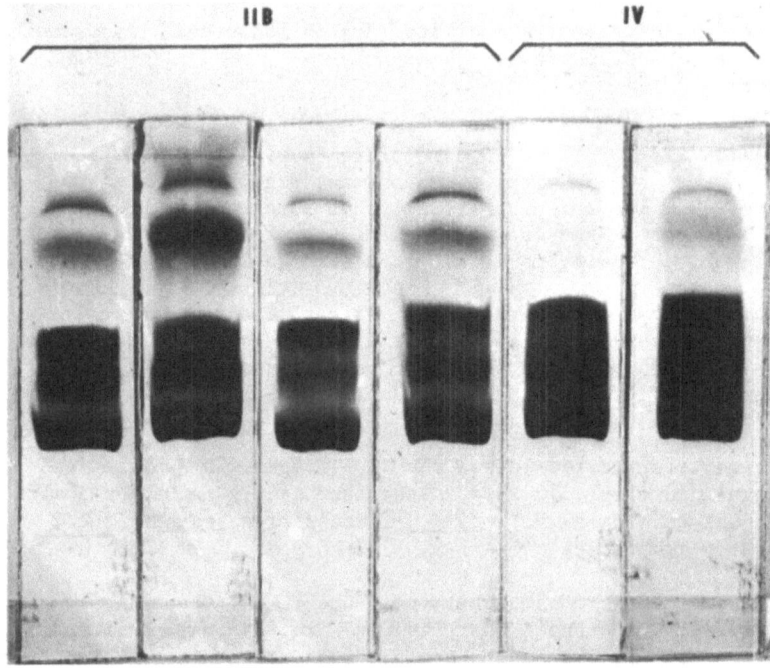

Figure 2b

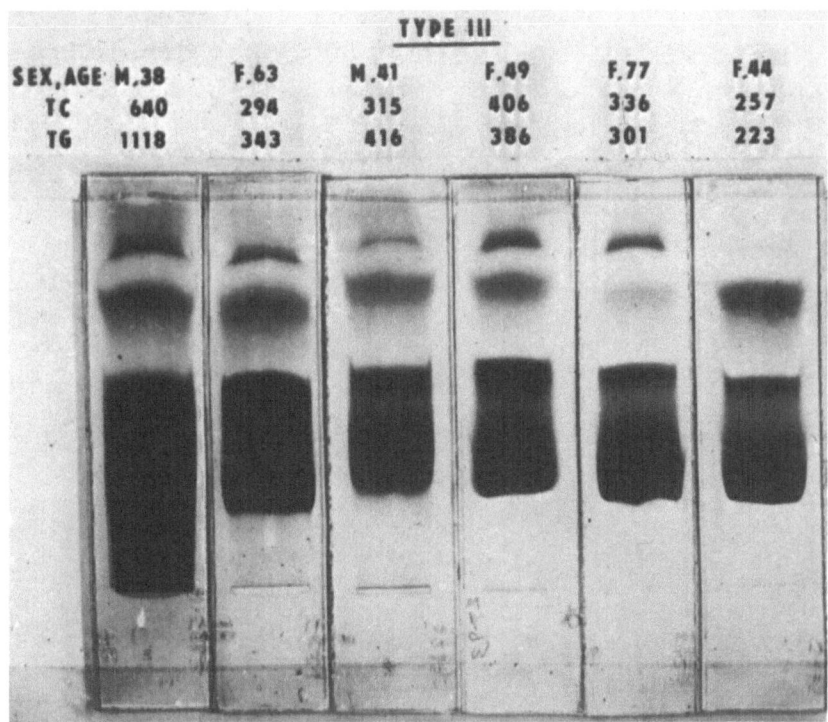

Figure 3. Agarose electrophoresis in type III hyperlipoproteinaemia showing the presence of the lipoprotein fraction with Rm 0.40

In type III hyperlipoproteinaemia, the densitometric curves reveal the presence of another lipoprotein fraction with Rm 0.40. Its presence may explain the occurrence of the well-known "broad band" in type III. From the pre-beta-lipoproteins the fraction Rm 0.60 is dominant in most persons with type III.

Fig. 4 shows 3 members of a family with type III hyperlipoproteinaemia. Both parents (father of 68, mother of 65) suffer from a mild form of hyperlipidaemia but their lipoprotein electrophoresis reveals a distinct rise of a lipoprotein with Rm 0.40. Their son (age 45) is the index patient; he has tuberoeruptive xanthomas in typical predilection localisations and xanthoma striatum palmare. The lipoprotein with Rm 0.40 is the dominant lipoprotein fraction in this subject. The parents are therefore thought to be heterozygotes and their son a homozygote of type III hyperlipoproteinaemia.

Another index patient with type III hyperlipoproteinaemia, a man of 39, has xanthoma striatum palmare and tuberoeruptive xanthomatosis with typical predilection localisation (elbows, knees, buttocks). The patient is a total albino and has suffered since childhood from ophthalmic migraines and horizontal nystagmus. He descends from a consanguinous marriage and is the first case described of coincidence of hyperlipoproteinaemia type III and albinism (5). Lipoprotein electrophoresis shows a typical "broad band" with a marked increase of the fraction 0.40. Floating beta-lipoproteins can be detected in the supernatant after ultracentrifugation at d 1.006.

The patient's brother, a man of 45, has suffered since the age of 42 from diabetes and has been treated with diet and insulin. He has shown normal serum lipid levels during repeated determinations. Agarose electrophoresis demonstrates however the presence of a lipoprotein component with Rm 0.40 and in the supernatant

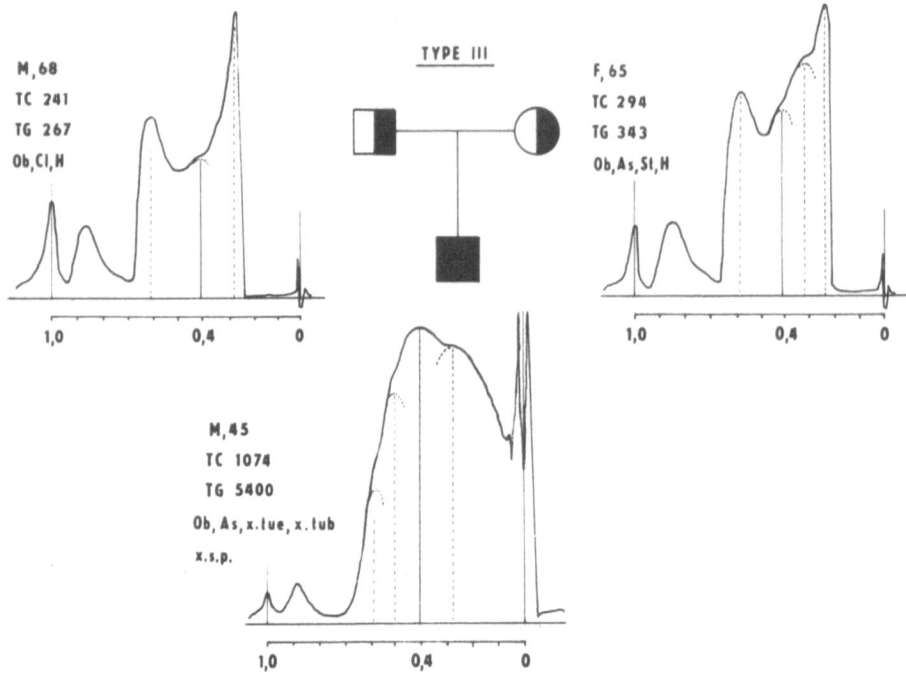

Figure 4. Densitometric curves of lipoproteins in parents showing the presence of fraction Rm 0.40 (heterozygotes) and with this fraction dominant in their son (homozygote)

obtained by ultracentrifugation at d 1.006, floating beta-lipoproteins are detected. We classify this normolipidaemic brother as a heterozygote of familial hyperlipoproteinaemia type III (Fig. 5).

Both the lipoprotein fraction with Rm 0.40 and floating beta-lipoproteins could be detected also in additional 7 normolipidaemic members from families of index patients with type III hyperlipoproteinaemia and this is the reason why even these subjects are thought to be heterozygotes of type III. It is interesting that in these normolipidaemic family members the cholesterol:triglycerides ratio is near 1.0.

In a total of 16 index patients with tuberoeruptive xanthomatosis and several other manifestations of type III hyperlipoproteinaemia and in 10 members of their families as well there was both a marked increase of the fraction with Rm 0.40 in agarose electrophoresis and the presence of floating beta-lipoproteins in the supernatant after ultracentrifugation at d 1.006.

The examination of the relative mobility of serum lipoproteins and the detection of the fraction with Rm 0.40 appear to provide a simple diagnostic method for normolipidaemic or borderline family members of type III index patients. We suggest that clinically non-affected family members having a lipoprotein fraction with Rm 0.40 on lipoprotein electrophoresis are type III heterozygotes.

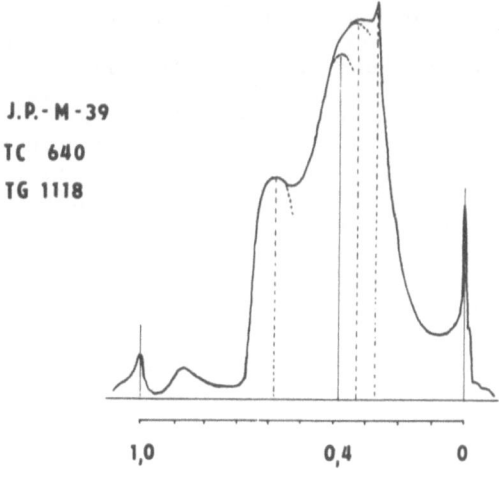

J.P.-M-39

TC 640

TG 1118

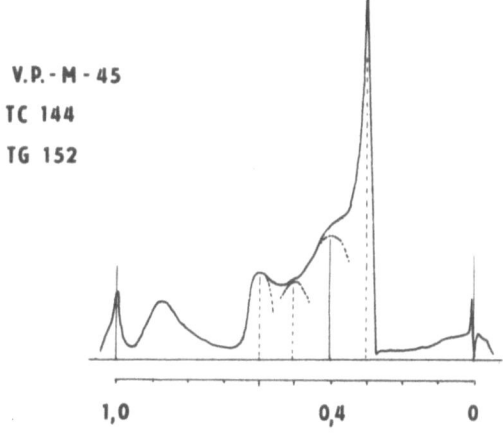

Figure 5. Densitometric curves of lipoproteins in an index patient with type
III hyperlipoproteinaemia (J.P., M,39 –
homozygote) and his brother (V.P., M,45
– heterozygote)

V.P.-M-45

TC 144

TG 152

Discussion

Dr. Holmes: An associate of Dr. Slack, Dr. Mosser is here with us; he also has
been very actively engaged in studies with the Type III hyperlipidemics.

Dr. Mosser: I think besides the exceptional pedigrees of Dr. Sobra which we have
seen and overlooking the pedigrees of Type III families, the presence or absence
of floating beta-lipoprotein or palmar xanthomata in families of these Type III
patients is not compatible with any simple Mendelian mode of inheritance. As Dr.
Slack has shown, the ratio of S_f 0-12 over S_f 12-20 obtained from Schlieren patterns by analytical ultracentrifugation of serum can be used to distinguish Type
III index patients from both controls and Type IV patients. These parameters may
therefore be suitable for quantitative genetic analysis in Type III families.

Comparing the Schlieren patterns obtained on 33 first degree relatives with the
mean of 24 index patients with Type III hyperlipoproteinemias and with the mean
plus or minus one standard deviation of 24 age and sex matched controls shows the
pattern of first degree relatives well between the index patients and the normal
range. As for the ratio of S_f 0-12 over S_f 12-20 the first degree relatives again
are found to be intermediate between the two groups. The number of first degree

relatives in this preliminary study is still small, but the distribution does not show any clear-cut bimodality but is skewed to the negative range, mainly due to the low range of four of the five first-degree relatives showing palmar xanthomata. If these are omitted, the mean value is still significantly different from the zero value of the control scores. The findings suggest that the phenotypic variations in both index patients with Type III and their first degree relatives are probably due to heterogeneity or to a multifactorial system of genetic and environmental factors, with a possible threshold effect for clinical manifestations and the presence of floating beta lipoprotein.

Dr. Hazzard: We studied a single large family from the Seattle area with clearcut Type III hyperlipoproteinemia in which the index case had tubero-eruptive xanthomas. In this large family of Irish extraction there were nine second generations and over fifty third-generation relatives. We were able to demonstrate vertical transmission of the Type III pattern in three of the nine second to third-generation branches of this family and we have chosen to interpret this as an autosomal dominant or in other words a simply inherited form of hyperlipoproteinemia. However, there are problems which exist in this. We see a coincidence of a Type IV pattern in numerous branches of this family, so an alternative hypothesis might be that the Type III and the Type IV represent two genetic disorders coinciding in a given individual to produce a severe Type III pattern. This obviously requires more analysis but to invoke more than two genes would seem very difficult in this particular family.

Dr. Heine, Oslo: I was interested in Dr. Sobra's point of a high mobility band, which is in our experience a normal band strongly related to the LPA lipoprotein of Professor Berg. The same was shown by Rider by using antisera to show lines of identity against this band and the LPA lipoprotein. I would be interested if your band is also the sinking pre-beta band. In families with Type IIA hyperlipoproteinemia with xanthomatosis we could also show that this was not associated with the hyperlipoproteinemia nor was it linked genetically to the gene for hyperlipoproteinemia.

Dr. Bierman: I would like to inject a word of caution about the interpretation of this lipoprotein associated with the Type III pattern with a 0.4 mobility as an abnormal lipoprotein. I think the best evidence to date suggests that it is a normally occurring lipoprotein increased in concentration, but it is not necessarily unique to this disorder, since there are other conditions which also will increase the concentration of this lipoprotein in other kinds of patients, therefore, increasing the ratio that Dr. Slack's colleague presented, such as in severe hypertriglyceridemia when all the fractions above flotation of S_f 12 will be elevated. Admittedly this is rare and probably would not confound genetic studies of families of patients with tubero-eruptive xanthomas too much, but it is just a note of caution.

Dr. Fuhrmann: I would like to support Dr. Hazzard's findings. We studied a large family of some 200 persons of which 121 belonging to 4 generations could be examined, with few exceptions including ultracentrifugation. Type III hyperlipoproteinemia was present in the proband, one of his sons and a grandson. A questionable floating pre-beta was found in other branches of this family showing vertical transmission. In addition, Type IV pattern was seen in numerous relatives.

I would like to ask Dr. Hazzard whether in his family there were children with a floating beta. Fredickson's group claimed that the youngest known case was 20 years old. Dr. Sobra has published a family, in which the 15 year old son of the index case showed a floating beta, and in our family we had suggestive evidence for the presence of floating beta-lipoprotein even in a two year old child, which had mildly elevated triglyceride levels.

Dr. Hazzard: We have not seen a floating beta in a child. I might say that two of the children, two and six years of age, of one of the branches of this family have persistent Type IV hyperlipoproteinemia. This again is consistent with either a Type III or IV pattern being contained in the individual, or Type III or Type IV disorder being primordial in the Type III development.

Dr. Little: For your information, Type III was reported in a child of age 11 by Dadolphen and Campbell in Canada. I think they reported it in the Lancet.

Dr. Lasser: We have reported a family from New Jersey, that we have interpreted up to now, that there may be two genes involved here, but there is a situation where we may see Type II in children as the premonitor of Type III or there is another gene because this particular patient on analytical ultracentrifugation shows an increased S_f 0-12 as well as S_f 12-100 and has 4 of his six sons affected with proven Type IIA. But it is my impression that with age their triglyceride is increasing although not into the abnormal range, but the older children seem to have more of a hint that their pre-beta will become increased.

Dr. Holmes: We have not had a chance to even consider the Type IV and/or Type V. Is there anybody here in the panel or among the participants who would like to make any very brief comments concerning these two groups?

Dr. Brunzell: We published recently some data in the Journal of Clinical Investigation suggesting that the presence of Type V lipoprotein pattern may simply represent saturation of removal capacity with elevations in very low density lipoproteins and thus a Type V pattern may be a Type IV individual with high triglyceride levels. Type IV's and Type V's seem to run in the same families, and an individual at different times will have either Type IV or Type V.

GENETICS AND ATHEROSCLEROSIS[*]

Arno G. Motulsky and Helge Boman

Evidence that genetic factors contribute to the development of atherosclerosis is not new (Adlersberg et al., 1949; Gertler and White, 1954; Thomas and Cohen, 1955; Russek and Zohman, 1958; Adlersberg and Schaefer, 1959; Shanoff et al., 1961; Rose, 1964; Walker, 1964; Slack and Evans, 1966; Suri et al., 1966). All writers on atherosclerosis and coronary heart disease usually refer to the role of heredity as an important etiologic factor, but hard data on the nature of the heredity unfortunately are lacking. Medical geneticists and public health specialists are attracted to genetic studies of atherosclerosis since genetically defined subpopulations at significantly higher risk might exist and elucidation of the pathophysiology of the defective metabolism could lead to possible prevention of premature coronary heart disease. The potential pay-off of genetic strategies in atherosclerosis research, therefore, is high.

Atherosclerosis as a Genetic Disease

Genetic diseases may be broadly classified in three categories: a) monogenic or Mendelian, b) polygenic, and c) chromosomal. Diseases inherited as Mendelian or monogenic traits individually are rare; as a group they are not uncommon (McKusick, 1971). Very few Mendelian diseases reach as high a frequency as atherosclerosis; sickle cell anemia and thalassemia major in some populations probably are the most common monogenic diseases, but very rarely exceed population frequencies of 1% (Weatherall and Clegg, 1972; Motulsky, 1973). Chromosomal aberrations individually are also uncommon. The nature of chromosomal defects makes them unlikely candidates to explain the genetics of atherosclerosis. Most common diseases are multifactorial and polygenic, i.e., multiple genetic factors interact with a variety of environmental and other unspecified nongenetic agents. A number of predisposing causes have already been identified in the etiology of coronary heart disease. Among such factors a genetic etiology is certain for diabetes (see Epstein, 1973 for references), hypertension (see Stamler et al., 1972, for references), and the hyperlipidemias (Kannel et al., 1971; Keys et al., 1970). Genetic factors might also play a role in tissue and blood vessel response to atherogenic stimuli, in arrangement of the collateral circulation of the coronary vasculature (see Bloor, 1972, for references), as well as in a variety of mostly unknown factors which lead to the final thrombotic events. Atherosclerosis as other common diseases, therefore, is likely to be an example of the interaction of genes with a variety of endogenous and environmental agents. Search for specific major genes comprising polygenic systems appears worthwhile.

Interaction of Heredity and Environment

It is useful to portray the pathogenesis of diseases as ranging over a spectrum from entirely genetic to entirely environmental causes. A few diseases such as Down's syndrome or hemophilia will manifest in practically all environments and such diseases are clearly mostly genetic in origin. Burns and trauma may be thought of as strictly environmental diseases. The remainder of illness presumably

[*]This investigation was supported in part by NIH Grant GM 15253 and by a Public Health Service International Research Fellowship (1 FO5 TWO 1905-2) to H.B.

occurs when gene-determined single or multiple factors interact with specific environmental factors. The exact contribution of genetic and environmental factors in most diseases remains unknown. However, whenever studies have been done on common diseases such as peptic ulcer (Cowan, 1973), hypertension (Platt, 1967; Pickering, 1967), diabetes (see Goldstein and Motulsky, 1974, for references), schizophrenia (Gottesman and Shields, 1973) and others, familial factors have been suggested. However, since the action of genes alone do not produce such diseases, enormous practical importance must be placed on environmental agents which may specifically interact with predisposing genetic factors. Identification of such genetic-environmental interaction may therefore be the key towards prevention and treatment. The marked increase of coronary heart disease in Western countries over the last decades (Stamler, 1973; Keys et al., 1966; Anderson, 1973) is an important example of the role of yet unidentified environmental factors in pathogenesis since genetic changes in the population could occur only over many generations or hundreds of years.

Genetic Approaches

1. Familial Concentrations. Many studies have been done on the frequency of coronary heart disease in relatives of patients with coronary heart disease as compared with controls (Gertler and White, 1954; Thomas and Cohen, 1955; Shanoff et al., 1961; Rose, 1964; Slack and Evans, 1966; Gertler et al., 1964; Deutscher et al., 1970; Hammond et al., 1971; Blacket et al., 1973). One difficulty with such studies is the exact criterion by which the diagnosis of coronary heart disease is made. Coronary heart disease may exist for many years before any symptoms are found. Different scoring criteria such as angina pectoris, certain electrocardiographic changes, coronary attacks, or death due to coronary heart disease proven by autopsy have been used in such studies. While the data differ slightly from study to study, there is general agreement that the frequency of coronary heart disease among first-degree relatives is increased between two to six times. Familial aggregation is particularly striking when examining the families of patients with early onset or of female patients (Slack and Evans, 1966). In this regard, coronary heart disease resembles other polygenic diseases where familial incidence is greatest among relatives of those affected at an earlier age and among relatives of the less commonly affected sex (Carter, 1969). Increased frequency of a disease in families does not necessarily prove that hereditary factors must be at play since a similar familial environment could make for familial aggregation. Other approaches, therefore, are required.

2. Twin Studies (see Fuhrmann, 1972). Twin studies on concordance of disease are performed on the rationale that twins are genetically identical and fraternal twins are genetically related such as sibs but that both types of twins share a similar environment. Concordance rates on unselected pairs of identical and fraternal twins, therefore, provide some hints about possible genetic etiology. Problems in scoring for coronary heart disease and in definition of concordance occur. How many years must twins be followed before assigning them to the concordant or discordant category? Studies which show lesser periods of follow-up show more modest increases in concordance between identical twins. A long-term Danish twin study (Harvald and Hauge, 1970) showed a concordance of 39% for identical male twin pairs as against 26% for nonidentical male twin pairs; 44% for female identical twins, and 14% for female nonidentical twins. The relatively high concordance (42%) in nonidentical twins of unlike sex when the female was the index case was of particular interest and is similar to that for identical twins of male sex. In this study patients were followed for a period of at least 10 years. Ideally, studies on the frequency of coronary heart diseases in identical twins reared apart would be helpful but sufficient data in this field are not available.

3. Migrant Studies. Several on-going investigations on the frequency of coronary heart disease with one sib remaining in the country of origin and the other sib moving to a geographic area of higher coronary heart disease frequency have not been fully reported yet. Such studies are being carried out with sibs in Ireland

and the United States (Trulson et al., 1964) as well as with sibs in Israel and the United States (Antonovsky, 1971). These and other investigations such as those reported on Oriental Jewish migrants to Israel (Toor et al., 1957) and Japanese migrants to Hawaii and America (Kagan et al., 1971) indicate a higher frequency of coronary heart disease among the sibs who moved to areas with higher coronary heart disease rates. These studies strongly suggest the importance of environmental factors but do not exclude the existence of genetically susceptible subpopulations.

4. Association with Genetic Markers. How could genetic studies be focused to get at more precise genetic markers than those provided by the clinical diagnosis of coronary atherosclerosis? Genetic studies on hyperlipidemia (Fredrickson and Levy, 1972), diabetes (see Goldstein and Motulsky, 1974, for references), and hypertension (Platt, 1967; Pickering, 1967) appear worthwhile. The role of heredity for other risk factors such as the putative driving and aggressive personality types (Rosenman et al., 1964) is more difficult to approach (Liljefors and Rahe, 1970). Specific single genetic markers can be studied. Thus, it has been shown that individuals with blood type A have a significantly increased chance of having thrombotic coronary heart disease (see Vogel and Kruger, 1968; Mourant, 1971). The reasons are unknown. Evidence is also mounting that individuals of blood group A have a somewhat higher cholesterol level than those of group B (Oliver et al., 1969; Langman et al., 1969; Mayo et al., 1969; Beckman and Olivecrona, 1970; Flatz, 1970; Wakely et al., 1973). In general, random testing of genetic markers which are not pathophysiologically related to coronary heart disease is not likely to be useful and more physiologic approaches have a higher priority in research design. Nevertheless, the availability of computers allows the sifting of large bodies of data by this approach. Spurious associations, however, might easily be established.

Genetic Analyses of Single Factors

Search for instances of rare Mendelian disorders which hide under the broad diagnostic umbrella of a common disease may be worthwhile. Such attempts have been useful for the separation of familial pheochromocytoma from hypertension (see Goldstein and Motulsky, 1974, for references), of partial HGPRT deficiency from gout (Greene, 1972), and of multiple endocrine adenomatosis from peptic ulcer (Schimke, 1973). Homocystinuria is associated with an increased tendency to thrombosis (McKusick, 1972). Could heterozygotes for homocystinuria who comprise approximately 1% of the population and have a partial enzyme defect have an increased frequency of coronary heart disease?

The familial hyperlipidemias are common and may be found in a significant proportion of patients with coronary disease. Elevated levels of plasma cholesterol (Adlersberg, 1951; Kannel et al., 1971) and probably triglycerides as well (Albrink and Man, 1959; Carlson, 1960; Albrink, 1962; Carlson and Böttiger, 1972) are known as significant risk factors for coronary heart disease. A genetic study directed at the hyperlipidemias has an a priori possibility of meaningful results. However, neither cholesterol nor triglycerides are primary gene products. It is therefore unlikely that unequivocal categorization of genetic classes will be possible by simple measurement of cholesterol and triglyceride levels in an individual case. Electrophoretic and ultracentrifugal phenotyping of lipids has been recommended and provide auxiliary tools (Fredrickson and Levy, 1972). However, the complexity of these procedures make population screening with such techniques difficult. In any case, those techniques do not aid in better genetic categorization (see below). Clear qualitative markers distinguishing affected from nonaffected patients would be ideal; such markers, however, have not been found yet.

Extensive evidence suggests that first-degree relatives in the normal population resemble each other in cholesterol levels (Schaefer et al., 1958; Mayo et al., 1969; Godfrey et al., 1972). Thus, many studies have shown significant parent-child and sib-sib correlation (Schaefer et al., 1958; Johnson et al., 1965) as well as high monozygote twin correlation of cholesterol levels (Osborne et al., 1959; Gedda and Poggi, 1960; McDonough et al., 1962; Jensen et al., 1965; Pikkarainen et al., 1966; Liljefors, 1970). The obtained correlations fall short of the expected theoretical values if cholesterol levels were entirely genetically determined and suggest that environmental factors interact with multiple genes in the determination of cholesterol levels. The unimodal pattern of cholesterol levels in the population is consistent with this interpretation. A Mendelian disorder such as familial hypercholesterolemia (see below) is too rare to affect the normal population distribution. It is particularly significant that correlations in cholesterol levels persist after sibs have lived in somewhat different environments for many years as shown in the Framingham study (Feinleib, 1972).

Studies of an Alaskan Kindred

In approaching the study of genetics of lipid levels we were encouraged by our finding that the gene for familial hypercholesterolemia as studied in a very large kindred in Alaska clearly behaved as an autosomal dominant trait (Schrott et al., 1972). In this kindred, we could differentiate between persons having normal and those with elevated plasma cholesterol levels with almost no overlap. This finding was interpreted to indicate that the gene causing the defect for familial hypercholesterolemia had shifted the normally polygenically distributed cholesterol levels to create a group of individuals with significantly higher mean levels of cholesterol. Against this background, consideration of the distribution of cholesterol or triglyceride levels in relatives of index cases with elevated lipid levels should allow distinction between polygenic and monogenic hyperlipidemia. If elevation of cholesterol levels, as an example, were due to multiple genes, the distribution of cholesterol levels among first-degree relatives would be unimodal but shifted to a higher mean, while if it were due to a single gene a bimodal population distribution (one similar to the normal curve, the other composed of the hypercholesterolemic relatives) would be obtained.

Seattle Myocardial Infarct Study (Goldstein et al., 1973a, 1973b)

1. Design and Frequency of Hyperlipidemia. During an eleven-month period, practically all patients with myocardial infarction in the Seattle metropolitan area were ascertained. Among 458 patients below the age of 60 years, 289 (85%) survived three months following the attack; among these, 366° (94%) were studied. Among 708 patients above the age of 60 years, 496 (70%) survived three months, every fourth patient was randomly selected and 134 patients were studied. Lipid levels in the 500 (366 and 134) study patients were determined and compared with those of controls. The control group was obtained by using the nonconsanguinous relatives of these patients. The 95th percentile of lipid levels was used as the cutoff limit and individuals whose levels were above the 95th percentile were arbitrarily considered as abnormal. Among the coronary population, 7.6% had cholesterol elevations alone, 15.6% triglyceride elevations alone, and 7.8% had elevations of both triglyceride and cholesterol. A total of 31%, almost a third of the coronary population, was affected with hyperlipidemia as compared to approximately 10% of the control population (5% hypercholesterolemia, 5% hypertriglyceridemia). Hyperlipidemia in the coronary cases was particularly striking in the young patients. In males, about 50% of the myocardial infarct survivors aged 50 years and below had hyperlipidemia.

2. Family Studies. 164 hyperlipidemic survivors were chosen as index cases for family investigations and first-, second-, and third-degree relatives were examined. There was no significant correlation in cholesterol or triglyceride levels between husbands and wives, arguing against a common environmental effect on lipid levels. Families were sorted into two groups according to whether their relatives had a significant elevation of lipid level. Those families where at least one relative had an elevation of lipid levels greater than the 99th percentile were further subdivided into those where the elevations were 1. in cholesterol alone,

2. in triglyceride alone, and 3. those where the elevation affected both cholesterol and triglyceride either together in the same individuals or separately.
When the data were thus sorted, three groups of disorders could be differentiated:
1. familial hypercholesterolemia, with cholesterol levels in the relatives distributed bimodally and triglyceride levels following a normal distribution; 2.
familial hypertriglyceridemia, with bimodal triglyceride distribution in relatives
and normal cholesterol distribution; and 3. "familial combined hyperlipidemia",
with bimodal triglyceride distributions in relatives while cholesterol distribution was shifted to a higher mean but was not bimodal. However, when the cholesterol levels of individuals with high triglyceride were considered separately in
this group, a bimodal distribution became apparent. We interpreted these findings
to suggest that the primary effect of this gene was "closer" to triglyceride metabolism than to cholesterol metabolism. When the frequency of hyperlipidemia among
the adult relatives of the three genetic groups was studied, about 50% of *adult*
sibs and about 25% of *adult* second-degree relatives were affected as expected with
autosomal dominant inheritance. These data are compatible with the concept that
three different genes, one affecting cholesterol metabolism alone, one affecting
triglyceride metabolism, and one affecting primarily triglyceride metabolism and
secondarily cholesterol metabolism were operative. In the combined hyperlipidemia,
many affected individuals had either an elevation of cholesterol alone or elevation of triglyceride alone. The reason for such variable expression is not apparent.

About 50% of children were affected in the hypercholesterolemic families suggesting that the gene had almost complete penetrance at a young age. The number of
affected children in familial hypertriglyceridemia and in combined hyperlipidemia
were only about 18% and 22%, respectively, of those expected. Full expression
seemed to occur only after the age of 25-30. Consistent with the clearer distribution of affected from normal adults by triglyceride rather than by cholesterol
levels in combined hyperlipidemia, elevated triglyceride levels were more frequently observed in children than elevated cholesterol levels. The low penetrance
of these disorders need to be kept in mind in evaluation of family studies and
limits seriously the use of lipid values in children, adolescents, and young
adults for genetic analysis.

Whereas familial hypercholesterolemia is generally recognized as a monogenic disorder by the medical and genetic community (for references see Fredrickson and
Levy, 1972), the recent studies by Glueck et al. (1971 and 1973) add additional
evidence to confirm single Mendelian inheritance in familial hypertriglyceridemia
and in combined hyperlipidemia. The manifestation rate or penetrance of the hypertriglyceridemic disorder in children appears higher in their data than in ours.
The reason for this discrepancy is not apparent.

Additional proof for the existence of these disorders as monogenic disorders
comes from apparently Mendelian segregation for all these disorders in *large* kindreds. If these disorders were polygenically inherited, monogenic inheritance
might be mimicked in small families but would be unlikely to simulate Mendelian
inheritance in a large kindred.

Miettinen et al. (1972) and Nikkilä and Aro (1973) have similarly reported on the
existence of the combined disorder particularly in patients with myocardial infarction. Unlike our group the bimodal distribution found in relatives could not
be demonstrated by the Finnish groups. These differences may relate to the significantly higher mean cholesterol levels in the Finnish population which may obscure possible bimodality. It is conceivable that demonstration of bimodality for
these disorders may not be possible in populations where mean cholesterols are
high. Patterson and Slack (1972) recently studied lipids in families of almost
200 survivors with myocardial infarction. A total of 127 first-degree relatives
of 18 male and 23 female index patients with hyperlipidemia were investigated. No
bimodality of lipids was detected among these relatives but the total numbers of
relatives were small. The need for a better genetic marker than lipid level alone
clearly is a real necessity.

Further analysis of our data revealed that 5.5% of our families had a slightly shifted unimodal distribution in cholesterol compatible with polygenic inheritance as would be expected from the familial correlation studies of cholesterol levels in normal families cited above. Our data demonstrated that more than half of our hyperlipidemic survivors (54%) suffered from a single-gene-determined hyperlipidemic disorder.

3. Age at Myocardial Infarction in Genetic Hyperlipidemia. The role of these genes in the determination of the onset of coronary heart disease was dramatic. Among males, the mean age of myocardial infarct in the group with familial hypercholesterolemia was 46 years; in the group with familial hypertriglyceridemia, 57 years; in the group with familial combined hyperlipidemia, 52 years. These values were significantly different from the mean observed age of 63 years for coronary attacks in our patients *without* hyperlipidemia (Table 1). These data also show that the presence of a familial disorder causes a much earlier onset of coronary heart disease in males as compared with females. The average mean age for the three monogenic categories was 52 years in males and 63 years in females. Males *without* hyperlipidemia had their heart attacks at a mean age of 63 years and females at 67 years. Thus, males with monogenic hyperlipidemia (all three types) had their infarct 11 years earlier than heart attack survivors without hyperlipidemias. Onset was 17 years earlier when the familial hypercholesterolemia group alone was considered.

Table 1. Average age[a] of patients with myocardial infarction by lipid characterization

Category	Males			Females		
	No.	Mean age ± SD (yrs)	Range (yrs)	No.	Mean age ± SD (yrs)	Range (yrs)
Familial hyper-cholesterolemia	13	46 ± 9	30–57	3	63 ± 12	46–71
Familial hyper-triglyceridemia	18	57 ± 12	33–74	5	65 ± 14	45–77
Familial combined hyperlipidemia	36	52 ± 9	34–65	11	62 ± 9	43–72
Polygenic hyper-cholesterolemia	22	58 ± 12	35–78	6	63 ± 6	48–70
Sporadic hyper-triglyceridemia	21	59 ± 11	39–69	10	68 ± 10	49–76
Patients without hyperlipidemia	267	63 ± 11	31–87	56	67 ± 11	35–86

[a]Corrected for ascertainment by multiplying the number of patients above 60 years by 4 since only 1 of 4 above this age was sampled. All patients aged 60 and below were studied for lipid categorization.

Significant differences were observed when the various subcategories were examined for the frequency of relatives dead of ischemic heart disease. Thus, almost twice the number of relatives of patients with hyperlipidemia died of ischemic heart disease (information from death certificates: 19% vs 35%). Similarly, death of myocardial infarction occurred at a younger age among relatives of the hyperlipidemic group.

4. Frequency of Genetic Hyperlipidemia in Myocardial Infarction. The incidence of monogenic hyperlipidemia among patients with myocardial infarction surviving three months or more was higher among younger patients. Below the age of 60 approximately 5% of all survivors had familial hypercholesterolemia, 5% had familial hypertriglyceridemia, and over 11% had the combined defect indicating that about 21% of all patients with myocardial infarct below the age of 60 had one of the monogenic defects. Above age 60, only 7% had one of the three disorders. Based on a frequency of 3% for coronary heart disease in the population aged 30-59 years, we calculated roughly that between 0.6% - 1% of the general population would carry any one of the three hyperlipidemic genes. These genes, therefore, would be among the most common disease-producing genes in our population. The high frequency of the combined disorder effectively rules out the possibility that this condition represents the interaction of familial hypercholesterolemia and hypertriglyceridemia.

Lipoprotein Phenotyping

Our studies did not indicate that lipoprotein phenotyping was of much help in delineating the familial genetic entities (Hazzard et al., 1973). In familial combined hyperlipidemia types IIa, IIb, IV, and V were found in different family members. While many family members with familial hypercholesterolemia were type IIa other types also were found. Similarly, while many family members with familial hypertriglyceridemia were type IV, other types were also observed. In a given family, all common types could be seen and occasionally patients changed from one type to another. Similar findings were obtained by Slack and Evans (1966) and Nikkilä and Aro (1973). We conclude that lipoprotein phenotyping in its present form is not a genetically determined phenotype and that determination of total cholesterol and triglyceride levels together with extensive family studies are of more help in pathophysiologic delineation than is lipoprotein phenotyping. Thus, the detection of type IIa in an individual could mean familial hypercholesterolemia, familial combined hyperlipidemia, or polygenic hypercholesterolemia. Similarly, type IV could mean nongenetic hypertriglyceridemia, familial hypertriglyceridemia, or familial combined hyperlipidemia.

Seattle Cord Blood Study

In another study, the significance of elevated triglyceride and cholesterol levels at birth as judged by cord blood screening was examined (Goldstein et al., 1973c). The upper 5% of 2000 consecutive samples of cord blood specimens were studied in detail. The cholesterol and triglyceride levels of parents and grandparents of these babies as well as of a control group of babies whose cholesterol and triglyceride levels fell in the middle of the total distribution were studied. No significant differences in cholesterol or triglyceride levels in parents or grandparents could be discerned in relatives of hyperlipidemic or normolipidemic babies. The frequency of grandparents who had died of myocardial infarction was 30% vs 31% among the normolipidemic and hyperlipidemic babies. Similarly, the frequency of living grandparents who had suffered a myocardial infarction was similar for normolipidemic and hyperlipidemic babies (5% vs 4.3%). These studies suggest that the determination of lipid levels of cord blood samples from neonates is not helpful in screening for the presence of hyperlipidemia as a risk factor for coronary heart disease. However, in these family studies, three families with familial hypercholesterolemia and one family with familial hypertriglyceridemia could be identified. The incidence of familial hypercholesterolemia is in keeping with our estimate of the population prevalence of this disease. These data are compatible with the findings of Kwiterowich (1973) that hypercholesterolemia can be detected at birth among the offspring in affected families. In such families the probability that a given child is affected is 50% and determination of cholesterol alone and particularly of LDL cholesterol is likely to detect affected infants. In mass screening, however, most elevated cholesterol levels will not indicate familial hypercholesterolemia and no single test is available to identify the few children affected with monogenic familial hypercholesterolemia. The lack of expression at birth in most cases of hypertriglyceridemia and combined hypertriglyceridemia makes it impossible to discover these disorders with existing markers.

Summary

Evidence is reviewed that the etiology of atherosclerosis is multi-factorial. Among etiologic agents a variety of genetic factors play a role. Atherosclerosis therefore behaves like most other common diseases. Strategy of genetic research in atherosclerosis involves search for major genes which affect risk facotrs. With these approaches, three major genes causing hyperlipidemia have been identified. These genes include one causing elevation of cholesterol - familial hypercholesterolemia, another causing elevation of triglyceride - familial hypertriglyceridemia, and a third causing elevation of both triglyceride and/or cholesterol levels in plasma - combined hyperlipidemia. Combined hyperlipidemia may manifest as hypercholesterolemia or hypertriglyceridemia alone. While children with hypercholesterolemia can be recognized already at birth, the other disorders rarely express in children. All three monogenic hyperlipidemias but particularly familial hypercholesterolemia and combined hyperlipidemia, are associated with premature coronary atherosclerosis in man. The mean age of patients with myocardial infarction associated with monogenic hyperlipidemia in our study was 52 years as compared with a mean age of 63 years in our normolipidemic patients with myocardial infarction. The most frequent monogenic disorder observed was familial combined hyperlipidemia affecting over 11% of patients with myocardial infarct 60 years and below.

Cord blood screening in a population-at-large cannot identify the familial hyperlipidemias, since most elevated cholesterol or triglyceride levels in cord blood have other causes. In affected families, only familial hypercholesterolemia can be identified at birth while the other disorders usually cannot.

PEDIATRIC ASPECTS OF ATHEROSCLEROSIS

Sidney Blumenthal

By virtue of the nature of coronary heart disease, only prevention can be expected to significantly reduce some of the absolute and most of the premature mortality, as well as the morbidity, of this disease. Preventive measures, to succeed,
must be instituted prior to the development of irreversible lesions. The atherosclerotic lesion first appears decades before the onset of any clinical manifestation (Strong et al., 1969; Lloyd et al., 1969; Holman et al., 1958). McMillan
indicates that the ultimate pathologic lesion may be the end result of several
possible pathologic reactions to a variety of noxious stimuli, and emphasizes
that for the general population, the critical time for atherogenesis and, thus,
prevention occurs in the third decade (McMillan, 1973). However, there exists a
group of individuals in whom the entire pathologic sequence of events is accelerated, so that, for them, the critical time is probably in childhood, perhaps in
the second decade. Roberts has demonstrated that the pathological appearance of
fixed lesions that develop early are identical to those that develop late (Roberts et al., 1973). The necessity for initiating preventive programs in all children may be debatable. There can be no disagreement, however, that such programs
should be initiated in childhood in those children identified as being at risk
for the premature development of coronary heart disease.

Fundamental to a scientific approach to prevention of disease is the identification of its cause(s) and pathogenesis. This information is not now available for
atherosclerosis. The desirability of elucidating the basic mechanisms and the
need for continuing research support to resolve these problems deserve the highest priority. However, programs of primary prevention need not and should not be
postponed. Sufficient information is available to allow us to proceed now, recognizing that any approach based upon present knowledge may need to be modified in
the future. The major unresolved question at this time is whether sufficient
knowledge is available to recommend such programs for the population at large, or
only for those at greatest risk.

Atherosclerotic plaques have been produced in experimental animals by feeding
high cholesterol, high saturated-fat diets. Arterial plaques have been shown to
regress in monkeys when a low cholesterol diet was introduced (Armstrong et al.,
1970; De Palma et al., 1970). Hypercholesterolemia has the highest association of
all risk factors with the development of atherosclerosis. Most agree that elevated serum lipids have a causal role in this disease. However, the "lipid hypothesis" is still not proven. Despite the publication of several studies of diet intervention, Cornfield and Mitchell[5] (1969) conclude that no evidence has yet been
produced to indicate that in man a cholesterol-lowering diet significantly reduces the mortality from coronary heart disease. Accordingly, the National Heart
and Lung Institute has recommended additional trials "to determine whether correction of the blood lipid abnormality by diets and drugs will modify morbidity and
mortality from coronary heart disease (Arteriosclerosis, NHLI Task Force, 1971).
The "lipid hypothesis" is now under investigation in a number of centers including a collaborative study by the Lipid Research Clinics supported by the Institute.

The best available evidence is that fatty streaks are precursors of fibrous
plaques and complicated lesions and that these processes follow a fairly predictable time sequence. Fatty streaks noted in early childhood increase in number
and in the extent of aortic intimal involvement during the second decade of life.

Progression to plaques and complicated lesions usually takes place in the third decade of life. Not all fatty streaks become plaques; they either regress, remain static or progress to the formation of plaques. Factors controlling these events have not been elucidated. In those individuals in whom the disease process is accelerated with the development of complicated lesions in childhood or adolescence, the reaction to environmental factors is hyper-responsive in character. One possible model of this phenomenon has been produced in sub-human primates by Clarkson and his colleagues (1971).

The preponderance of evidence indicates that atherosclerosis has many causes and that clinical manifestations make their appearance in varying degrees of severity, dependent in some measure upon the individuals' innnate susceptibility. This susceptibility is probably genetically determined. Responsible genes may regulate biochemical metabolism, structural differences in the arterial walls, end-organ response to stress and/or an hormonal regulating system. It is proposed that two groups of individuals can be identified from the general population, based upon the presence or absence of this innate susceptibility or hyper-responsiveness to environmental noxious factors. Design of prevention programs and optimal time of initiation of prevention in large measure is influenced by the belief of whether or not two populations exist. It is our contention that this is true, though further documentation is required.

Epidemiological studies in adults have established an association between certain individual characteristics and environmental factors with the premature development of atherosclerosis (Truett et al., 1967). The earlier in adult life these characteristics and factors are identifiable, the stronger their association. A profile can be developed reflecting the probability of occurrence of premature clinical events in an adult. Epidmiological studies have not established the causal relationship of these factors to the event, nor have they established the validity of these associations in children. There exists a strong assumption, but little published data, to indicate that adult risk factors are applicable to children. Jesse and her colleagues (in preparation) have been engaged in a study to determine whether premature myocardial infarction in fathers is associated with an identifiable pattern of risk factors among their progeny. Their data indicates that the progeny of cases had a significantly higher mean level of serum cholesterol as compared with progeny of controls (199.0 versus 176.2 mg per 100 ml) (p = .01). More important 11/70 progeny of cases were observed to have hyperlipidemia ($\geq$ 230 mg cholesterol per 100 ml), whereas 3.5/70 were expected. Among 54 families, the ability to identify children with hyperlipidemia was enchanced 3.5 fold (RR = $\frac{11 \times 66.5}{59 \times 3.5}$ = 3.54) if the male parent had experienced a myocardial infarction prior to the age of 50 years. Among 78 families, the ability to identify children with hyperlipidemia was comparable (3.8) and highly significant (p = .01). In addition, the weights of the progeny of cases exceeded that of progeny of controls. There was no difference between cases and controls in blood pressure determinations. The results of glucose tolerance tests will be presented elsewhere (Jesse et al., in preparation). It has been suggested that, inasmuch as alteration of environmental factors may require a changing of living habits in adult life, such habits are most easily established by training in childhood. There is a strong belief, but little evidence to prove, that children are more amenable than adults to the development of good health habits and that, once developed, these habits will persist throughout adult life. Success or failure in the training of a child so that he will do what is good for him depends upon a complex set of behavioral characteristics involving biological and social factors. Leventhal (1973) notes that "There is no evidence that children are more likely than adults to learn, believe and do what is good for health". In addition, factors affecting the stability of health habits developed in childhood are complex. All would agree with the virtue of attempting to instill good habits in early life. However, this must be a continuing educational process extending into adult life. The process of developing good health habits is as complex as that of changing poor health habits in adult life (Leventhal, 1973).

Those risk factors considered to be of major significance for a childhood population include hypercholesterolemia, hypertension, cigarette smoking, diabetes mellitus and obesity.

The most reliable predictor, in the adult, for the development of premature atherosclerosis is hypercholesterolemia. Normal values for plasma lipids and lipoprotein cholesterol concentrations for infants and children are not well standardized. Data now being collected via a variety of sources will shortly provide statistically valid information obtained from a large population base. Serum cholesterol levels rise rapidly from birth to two years of age (Levy et al., 1973). Conflicting values are reported for later childhood and adolescence (McGandy, 1971). Additional data for this age group is being analyzed (Jesse, 1973). Longitudinal studies reported by McGandy (1971) indicate that for high school children those at the upper end of the frequency distribution, remain at the upper end of the new and rising distribution one to three years later. After 13 years of age, mean annual increments are similar to that noted in the third decade of life (2-5 mg% per year) (McGandy, 1971). At the present time, there is still uncertainty in whether adult cholesterol levels can be predicted by the level obtained in early childhood (Kannel et al., 1972). The problem is confounded by the definition of "abnormality" in a situation in which mean values represent a continuous variable (Mitchell, 1973).

Major advances have been made in an understanding of the hyperlipidemias and a useful classification proposed by Fredrickson et al. (1967). Despite disagreements concerning some of the details of this classification, its introduction has clarified many issues. It recognizes that lipid disorders may be primary or secondary; that some primary disorders are common in childhood and are associated with premature coronary heart disease (Type II), some cause symptoms in infants, but are not associated with vascular disease (Type I); some seen in late childhood, are associated with some increased risk of coronary heart disease and of hypertension (Type IV). Exquisite genetic studies of primary hyperlipidemias have recently been reported by Goldstein, Motulsky and their colleagues (1973) and will be discussed in greater detail by Dr. Motulsky elsewhere in this volume. Their elucidation of the nature of the inheritance, and the significance of the type of hyperlipidemia, including that of a combined hyperlipidemia, is an index of the rapid progress being made in this field.

Primary Type II hyperlipoproteinemia is clearly associated with a high risk of premature myocardial infarction. Identification is possible in early childhood. The prevalence of this abnormality for different racial groups needs to be established. Some have suggested that the abnormality can be detected by analysis of cord blood plasma, while others have disputed this claim (Glueck et al., 1971; Lloyd et al., 1969). Identification by screening of cord blood would be highly desirable. The mean cord blood cholesterol has been reported to be 64 ± 18 mg/100 ml (Glueck et al., 1971). Type II hyperlipoproteinemia is defined by an increase in LDL with normal or slightly increased VLDL. Cord blood contains a relatively large amount of HDL. It does not contain chylomicrons and very little VLDL. Estimation of cord blood cholesterol without measuring LDL may be misleading. Furthermore, the presence of bilirubin or of hemolysis in the sample collected may affect the cord plasma cholesterol level (1-2 mg/100 ml) (Levy et al., 1973). Other factors apt to affect cord blood lipids include prematurity and intrauterine factors influenced by the maternal status. Hypercholesterolemia in cord plasma due to causes other than primary type II hyperlipoproteinemia require clarification as does the prevalence of normal cord plasma cholesterols in infants who are subsequently identified as having the disease. Although the problem of identification by analysis of cord blood has not been completely resolved, the opportunities are clear and solution of the problem appears to be imminent. Routine screening of cord blood is not advocated at this time. Plasma cholesterol levels during the first year of life vary markedly depending upon the type of formula and additional foods being consumed (Fomon et al., 1970), so that routine screening during the first year of life is not advocated.

448

The need to elucidate the problems still to be resolved should in no way reflect a pessimistic point of view. Rather the opportunities for early identification of an abnormality associated with a high risk of coronary heart disease in early adult life presents a stimulating challenge to effective preventive cardiology. This high risk population of children is the best model upon which dietary intervention is evaluated.

Recommended dietary changes in the infant seem innocuous. Schubert has reviewed the reasons for applying caution (Schubert, 1973). A potential deleterious effect upon the developing brain and nervous system may result from relative hypocholesterolemia. The total fat requirement for the infant is not known. A potential danger to the premature and young infant exists if total fat intake is less than 20% of caloric intake; the resulting increased protein intake may result in an excessive solute load to the infant kidney causing hypernatremia (Schubert, 1973). Linoleic acid is an essential fatty acid; the infant's minimal dietary requirement is approximately 1% of total calories and optimally 4.5% as found in human milk. Deficient dietary intake has been reported to result in dermatalogic problems in infants with development of eczematous changes. Furthermore, essential fatty acids have been identified as precursors of certain prostaglandins (Bergstrom et al., 1968). Other than those requirements established for linoleic acid in infants, additional data is available only from animal studies. The potential risks identified should caution those recommending restrictive dietary changes for the young infant. The need for such restrictions in the infant are difficult to justify. The potential risk must be weighed against the potential benefit for each infant; those with Type II hyperlipidemia as well as the normal infant.

Dietary fat requirements for the growing child are less critical than for the infant. Linoleic acid intake should approximate 2% of caloric intake. In the child, body stores are sufficient to prevent essential fatty acid deficiency except in very severe fat deprivation. Furthermore, it is well recognized that fat in food provides palatability to the diet of a rapidly growing child. Manipulation of the diet of "high risk" older children is accompanied by little risk to health. Manipulation of the diet of all children has its major impact psychologically. The fundamental question for the older child is not as much the risk, as the need for such dietary manipulation in the population at large.

Hypertension in the adult is a well-established risk factor for premature atherosclerosis. A prognostic relationship exists between arterial pressure and life expectancy at all levels of pressure, low as well as high, systolic and diastolic. The hypertensive risk is aggravated when it is associated with hyperlipidemia, especially in the young adult.

Arterial pressure is a continuously variable characteristic so that the accepted definition of an abnormal pressure of necessity utilizes some arbitrary point. "Abnormal" blood pressure in children requires better definition. Some have suggested that 2 SD above the mean for sex, age and weight be utilized. This has been useful for investigational purposes, but has not been accepted in clinical practice. Ongoing longitudinal studies should provide more generally acceptable values for children.

Treatment of adults with hypertension has shown a decrease in cerebrovascular accidents without a comparable decrease in coronary artery events (Freis, 1969). These studies have been performed on middle-aged individuals who probably have irreversible atherosclerosis. The possibility that therapy, initiated earlier in the process, might have more beneficial results is an intriguing suggestion. For those experiencing unanticipated signs and symptoms of the complications of hypertension in early adult life, detection and therapy in childhood is mandatory. How to identify these children is a pressing problem requiring clarification.

There are many gaps in our understanding of the natural history of essential hypertension, particularly its early stages. In contrast to the situation in adults, recognizable hypertension in children is usually secondary to an identifiable cause. Essential hypertension is rarely identified in early childhood. Hypertension develops over time and there is evidence that the processes which initiate elevations in arterial pressure are probably not the same as those which sustain it. Students of essential hypertension recognize the existance of familial aggregation and most believe that an hereditary factor is operational (Platt, 1947; Winkelstein et al., 1965). A highly significant relationship between casual blood pressure in adults and in their first degree relatives was reported by Miall more than twenty years ago (Miall et al., 1967). Recently, it has been shown that familial aggregation which occurs at all levels of pressure is measurable in children 2-14 years of age (Kass et al., 1969). Utilizing cross-sectional data supported by a limited number of longitudinal observations, it has been proposed that those children with blood pressures higher than the mean for their age will have the greatest rises in pressure in later life (Zinner et al., 1970). This imples that children are in a blood pressure "track" and that essential hypertension has its roots in early childhood. This is an important hypothesis requiring verification. If proven to be correct, it in no way indicates whether the influencing factors are genetic or environmental in nature. The role of inheritance of essential hypertension needs further documentation utilizing records of single families, family histories, twin studies, and measurements in relatives of patients with hypertension. Studies performed in twins reveal a higher correlation between monozygotic than dizygotic twins and between dizygotic twins than ordinary siblings (Stocks, 1930). Most agree that the evidence for inheritance is impressive, but that the mode of inheritance remains debatable (Pickering, 1967). Studies of the hemodynamics of essential hypertension reveal an heterogenic pattern (Frohlich et al., 1967). In fixed hypertension in the adult, total peripheral resistance is increased and cardiac output is normal or somewhat decreased depending upon the severity of the hypertension. In some adolescents with hypertension a syndrome has been described characterized by normal total peripheral resistance, increased cardiac output and decreased systolic ejection time. Hyperkinetic or hyperbeta adrenergic hypertension is usually labile in nature (Snyder et al., 1965). Some believe labile hypertension to be a precursor of fixed essential hypertension. A high incidence of a family history of at least one parent with essential hypertension in patients with labile hypertension has been reported (Snyder et al., 1965). Certainly labile hypertension deserves increasing attention, particularly when associated with a positive family history of essential hypertension, hyperlipidemia or an abnormal glucose tolerance test.

There is evidence that age, inheritance and environment are factors that determine arterial pressure. At least some adolescent patients with labile hypertension progress to fixed hypertension while others do not. The reasons are not clear; nor do we have any method of identifying those who will develop fixed hypertension. Is there a genetic defect in some? Answers to some of the remaining riddles of the natural history of essential hypertension require studies in infants and children (Kannel, 1972), preferably longitudinal rather than cross-sectional in nature. Failure thus far to explore the vagaries of arterial blood pressure in infants and children has resulted from the misconception that such pressures are difficult to obtain and are not reproducible. The experience of Kass and co-workers (1969) and Zinner and co-workers (1971) indicates that reliable blood pressures can be as readily obtained by specially trained nurses in children as in adults. The introduction of the Doppler sphygmomanometer in 1968 (Stegall et al., 1968; Uirby et al., 1969) has facilitated studies of blood pressure in neonates. Jesse, Hennekins, Spellacy and colleagues (in preparation) have documented the reliability of determinations obtained in infants and are engaged in a longitudinal prospective study to determine whether there is an association between levels of blood pressure in newborns and their families (Jesse et al., 1973). Pregnant women with essential hypertension (BP> 160/95) are the index cases. Their antepartum lipid profile, carbohydrate tolerance and blood pressure status are being obtained; the father and all children in the family are similarly evaluated during the mother's third trimester and annually thereafter. Blood pressures are obtained on the newborn infant on the day of delivery and daily for four days.

They are then repeated at one month, 3 months, 6 months and 1 year of age and annually thereafter. Information available at this time indicates that blood pressure determinations in the neonate are reproducible, systolic pressure variable during the first 2 days of life, stabilizes during the subsequent 3 days. It is significantly higher at 1 month, but does not rise from 1 to 3 months. The diastolic blood pressure is highly variable during the neonatal period and has no predictive value, possibly a manifestation of the marked changes in peripheral resistance during this period. The difference in systolic blood pressures between the mean neonatal level (80.4 mm Hg) and the mean infant level (108.1 mm Hg) is significant ($p < .001$).

The upper bound of the 95% two-sided confidence limit for a) newborn systolic blood pressure is 100 mm Hg (Day 0 - 1), b) neonatal systolic blood pressure is 100 mm Hg (Day 2 - 4), c) infant systolic blood pressure is 130 mm Hg (Month 1 - 3).

The intent in presenting this data, at this time, is to document the reproducibility of blood pressure determinations obtained by trained nurses, in the newborn, neonate and infant, and to urge other investigators to engage in studies in this age group. The results of association between levels of blood pressure in newborns and in their parents, to familial aggregation, to the relationship of such pressures comparing full and half-siblings, to that of "tracking", as well as any association with abnormal lipid levels will be presented in a subsequent publication.

I would like to conclude these comments concerning the pediatric aspects of the problem of essential hypertension by emphasizing that blood pressure is a graded variable and that "normality" needs to be redefined in terms of the relation of a child's blood pressure to the mean for age and sex and perhaps other characteristics as well. We know that in the adult pressure elevated above some arbitrary cut-off point, systolic or diastolic, casually or basally obtained, in either sex is potentially harmful. It becomes of greater importance if associated with a positive family history, elevated lipids, or an impaired glucose tolerance test. In addition, we know that an elevated pressure can be reduced by long-term medical therapy.

The greatest need is the ability to identify which child will show progressive elevations of blood pressure with advancing years. It is possible that these children can be identified by a positive family history of essential hypertension supported by tests (not yet elucidated) which may document hyper-reactivity of the vascular tree. We need to know whether effective treatment initiated before vascular changes become irreversible will alter prognosis. Longitudinal studies are necessary to provide opportunities to unravel some of these problems.

Cigarette smoking is a significant risk factor for coronary heart disease. The greatest risk occurs among young men who smoke heavily (Doyle et al., 1964). Cigarette smoking is increasing among adolescents in the United States, while it is declining among adults. The highest level of smoking among adolescents occurs in broken homes, in homes in which one or both parents smoke, or in which an older sibling smokes (Kahn et al., 1970). Smoking often becomes associated with a large number of satisfactions and may become psychologically addictive (Leventhal, 1973). Additional psycho-social factors require elaboration. Programs designed for the adolescent require the cooperation, by example, of all members of the household, as well as by teachers. Methodology needs to be developed and programs implemented to make cigarette smoking socially unacceptable by peer groups.

Obesity is another identified risk factor in adults. Obesity and hypertension are interrelated and obesity is often associated with abnormalities of glucose tolerance, insulin metabolism and hyperlipidemia (Karam et al., 1965; Jackson et al., 1971; Sims et al., 1971). It is difficult to establish the association of obesity alone as a risk factor for atherosclerosis. Furthermore, obesity is associated with serious aberrations in physical activity, as well as behavioral and sociological attitudes. Few would question the difficulty in achieving weight reduction in the obese adolescent or adult. A unique opportunity is available to those entrusted with the care of children.

Significant differences have been described in management of subjects in whom obesity developed in infancy as compared with late onset obesity. Obesity does not cause any recognizable health hazard to the infant or child, other than psychological. However, the obese infant is likely to become the obese adolescent or adult. Children who developed their obesity in infancy or early childhood have high fasting serum insulin and low circulating growth hormone levels. Adipose tissue cells are increased in size and number. Cheek has suggested that excessive weight gain in infancy results in an increased production of insulin affecting cell number and size (Cheek et al., 1970a, 1970b). The amount of food necessary to maintain obesity is then not excessive and a vicious cycle inititated (Cheek et al., 1970a). An appreciation of events taking place in the fetus is desirable for understanding changes in the neonate. Data is available concerning carbohydrate metabolism in the pregnancy triad: mother - fetus - amniotic fluid. Blood glucose homeostasis is maintained during pregnancy at a slightly lower level than during the non-pregnant state. Glucose freely passes the placental barrier. Insulin does not cross the placenta and insulin levels are low in the normal fetus. Spellacy (1967) has shown that insulin is slowly released by the fetus in response to a glucose load (Parra et al., 1971). The normal neonate requiring about 4-5 days before pancreatic beta cells release sufficient insulin to control the blood glucose pattern. Fetal insulin is recognized as an important growth factor (Pellacy, 1973). Human growth hormone, which does not cross the human placenta, is produced in relatively large amounts by the fetus. The significance of this observation is poorly understood.

Control of obesity in the infant and pre-school child will make prevention and treatment of the obese adult a more feasible objective. Physicians, parents and grandparents need re-education so that they do not utilize weight gain as an index of optimal health in the infant and pre-school child.

A major complication of diabetes is premature vascular disease. Amongst patients with atherosclerosis there exists a very high incidence of diabetes or of evidence of abnormal carbohydrate metabolism (Epstein, 1967). The mechanism for this association remains unsolved.

It seems clear that the nature of the atherosclerotic process is the same in the diabetic and non-diabetic, but that in the diabetic it occurs earlier, more often and with greater severity. Diabetes is frequently associated with hyperlipidemia; however, some diabetics develop vascular disease despite normal serum lipid levels. Insulin is an important controlling factor in both carbohydrate and lipid metabolism (Gertler et al., 1972). Unfortunately, present methods of treatment of diabetes (diet, insulin, oral agents) have not prevented the development of premature atherosclerosis. Nevertheless, there remains a strong belief among students of the subject that abnormal hormonal secretion and abnormal intermediary metabolism are related to the development of the vascular disease. Studies directed to resolving the question of whether or not the atherosclerotic process can be influenced by normalization of blood glucose in maturity-onset diabetes have been inconclusive (University Group Diabetes Program, 1970). Fajans (1971) emphasizes that present methods of treatment do not achieve normalization of blood glucose over a 24-hour period. Attempts to achieve this goal by transplantation of the pancreas in the juvenile diabetic are preliminary and encouraging (Lillehel et al., 1972).

Widespread involvement of smaller blood vessels (in addition to that of major arteries) has been described during the pre-diabetic stage of the disease (Fajans, 1971; Gunn et al., 1965). The direct effects of hormones upon vessel walls need investigation. It has been suggested that hyperinsulinemia may be more characteristic of chemical diabetes than hyperglycemia (Reaven et al., 1972). Inter-related factors other than hyperglycemia, hyperinsulinemia and hyperlipidemia are undoubtedly at work in the diabetic including obesity and hypertension.

The soundest advice at this time would be to encourage management attempting to achieve the optimal hormonal and biochemical control as soon as abnormal carbohydrate metabolism is detected (Fajans, 1972). In some this may consist only of dietary manipulation which prevents obesity predisposing to hyperinsulinemia. In others, insulin or drug therapy may be indicated. The desirability of identifying diabetes-prone children before overt disease becomes manifest seems self-evident.

In the existing social climate, problems related to contraceptive measures are of concern to pediatricians. Wynn notes that some women taking oral contraceptive preparations have elevated triglyceride levels noted within 6 weeks from the onset of medication (Wynn et al., 1966). Following discontinuation of the drug, blood concentrations usually return toward normal with six months (Aurell et al., 1966). Triglyceride elevations are related to the estrogen contained and are dose related (Spellacy, 1973). Women with hypertriglyceridemia prior to treatment demonstrate the highest concentrations when taking estrogen-containing drugs. Severe complications have been reported including vascular accidents (Zorilla, 1968; de Gennes, 1967) and pancreatitis (Davidoff, 1973). In the reported women with pancreatitis, Davidoff noted a frequent occurrence of moderate obesity, abnormal glucose tolerance curves in patients and their families, and evidence of familial hyperlipidemia (Davidoff, 1973). Spellacy believes that in order to minimize these metabolic effects, steroid contraceptives should contain small amounts or no estrogens and the progestogen dose should be low (Spellacy, 1973). Caution is indicated when prescribing steroid contraceptive agents or estrogens for other purposes in girls or in women with a family history of hyperlipidemia, diabetes or premature atherosclerosis and in those in whom serum triglyceride levels are abnormal.

We believe that it is possible to identify a group of children who are predisposed to the premature development of the clinical manifestations of atherosclerosis (Blumenthal, 1973). This presupposes that adult risk factors are applicable to children and utilizes the knowledge that most adult risk factors exhibit familial

Table 1.   Identification of "high risk" children

I. Children with

    A. Hyperlipidemia

        1. Primary
            Familial
            Nonfamilial
        2. Secondary
            Nephrosis
            Hypothyroidism

    B. Hypertension

    C. Diabetes

    D. Obesity

II. Progeny of adults with

    A. Hyperlipidemia

    B. Essential hypertension

    C. Diabetes

    D. Premature myocardial infarction

---

aggregation. Children are identified as outlined in Table 1. Once identified, the children and their siblings should have a physical examination, including a blood pressure determination with special attention directed to the minor technical problems required for this age group. Blood should be drawn for determination of lipids, and glucose and a glucose loading test performed. Appropriate advice and counselling should be given concerning diet, exercise habits, and cigarette smoking. Treatment of identified biochemical disorders should be individualized after consideration of the hazards (if any) of treatment versus procrastination. All such children and their families with or without identifiable abnormalities should be re-evaluated at one-year intervals.

In conclusion, we feel strongly that efforts aimed at prevention of the atherosclerotic process is the only method which will achieve a significant alteration in the excessive mortality and morbidity from this disease. The only means of prevention available at this time is that directed toward the reduction of risk factors, despite the lack of definitive evidence that this will in fact prevent the development or retard the progress of the disease. Prevention should be instituted prior to the critical time in which complicated, irreversible lesions develop. The debatable question is "Should preventive measures be directed at this time: to an identifiable 'high-risk' group of children, the childhood population at large or to the young adult?" Our position is that the main thrust should be directed at those children and young adults with an increased risk of premature atherosclerosis and its sequelae. To do otherwise presupposes greater knowledge of the causes of atherosclerosis than we now have. Others have suggested that dietary changes should be instituted in the general pediatric population (De Haas, 1973). There is a belief that habits of exercise and diet instituted in childhood will persist into adult life. This is a belief rather than a fact. The processes of behavioral influence are too complex for over-simplified conclusions.

Furthermore, we do not know whether modifying blood lipid levels by diet or drugs does actually retard the atherosclerotic process nor do we have information concerning possible toxicity in children. The potential ill-effects upon the fetus and infant are of even greater concern. Intervention upon children at increased risk should supply necessary additional data. As more information is accumulated, involving the entire population along similar lines may appear more justified.

Early identification of abnormalities in members of afflicted families provides the means for early treatment. When studies fail to produce any abnormal findings reassurance of the child and of the parents provide a major contribution to good mental health.

HERITABILITY OF SERUM LIPIDS AND LIPOPROTEINS

Arvid Heiberg

The factors which control the amounts of lipoproteins and lipids in plasma are only partly known. The importance of genetic factors are strongly established in primary hypercholesterolemia and other hyperlipoproteinemias and for normal cholesterol levels in mice and cows. Several investigators have shown a varying degree of genetic influence on serum cholesterol and phospholipids in man, but data on triglycerides and plasma lipoproteins are scarce.

Densitometric evaluation of lipoprotein electrophoresis can be used as a measure of plasma lipoprotein levels and it was found of interest to use this method in a twin study for evaluation of the genetic component in the control of serum lipoproteins and lipids.

Methods

Fifty pairs of twins, were randomly selected from the twin register of the Institute of Medical Genetics, University of Oslo, in such a way that 10 pairs of twins were sampled in each of the possible 5 groups: that is monozygous males, monozygous females, dizygous males, dizygous females and dizygous twins of unlike sex. The twins were between 18 and 24 years and in good health. They lived in most instances together or had recently separated.

Twin Zygosity. Confirmation of twin zygosity was achieved by testing at least 18 genetic marker systems. The probability for a pair classified as monozygous to be dizygous was determined to be less than 1 per mille for most of twin pairs, and for no pair did this probability exceed 0.5%, by marker system analysis in the 20 pairs. The dizygous pairs were different in from 1 to 7 marker systems.

There was no discrepancy between the results of the marker system analysis and morphologic inspection.

Total serum cholesterol and triglycerides were determined simultaneously after isopropanol extraction by standard auto-analyzer techniques. Phospholipids were determined as lipid phosphorus and total lipid computed from these results by the technique of Chandler and Wease. Lipoprotein lipids were determined by densitometry of the agarose gel electrophoretograms and the results were calculated as lipoprotein lipids by multiplication of the total lipid value by the percent dye uptake of each lipoprotein fraction.

Statistical analysis was performed following the instructions of Osborne and deGeorge, by comparing the mean intrapair variance, that is the difference within each pair with the interpair variance, that is the difference between pair, for the whole sample.

Results

Table 1 shows the intrapair and interpair variances for the different serum lipids and lipoproteins. As could be expected if there is a genetic influence on serum lipids there is a rise in the difference within pairs from monozygous to dizygous twins. The intrapair variance was smaller in monozygous twins than dizygous twins for all serum lipids and lipoproteins. The greater the magnitude of

these differences the greater should the genetic influence be. If there is a genetic influence the intrapair variance in twins should also be expected to be less
than the interpair variance as can also be seen from the table. These differences
are still apparent when the interpair variance is divided by the intrapair variance to obtain the value called F-ratio. This was highly significant for most lipids. Exceptions were seen for phospholipids and total lipids; in these instances
the difference between the intra- and interpair variance was not significant
(Table 2).

Table 1. Serum lipids and lipoproteins. Mean intrapair and interpair variance

	Choles-terol	Trigly-cerides	Phospho-lipids	Total lipids	ß-lipo-proteins	Pre-ß-lipo-proteins	α-lipo-proteins
Intrapair variance							
MM + MF	127	311	326	1308	1040	396	656
DM + DF	427	582	976	5375	1363	910	1629
DM + DF + DU	445	617	742	4735	1555	863	1301
Interpair variance							
All twins	2432	1855	1057	8681	6862	1549	1908

Table 2. Serum lipids. F-ratio for interpair/intrapair variance

	Choles-terol	Trigly-cerides	Phospho-lipids	Total lipids	ß-lipo-proteins	Pre-ß-lipo-proteins	α-lipo-proteins
MM + MF	19.20[a]	5.94[a]	3.24[a]	6.64[a]	6.60[a]	3.81[a]	2.91[b]
DM + DF	4.99[a]	3.19[a]	1.08	1.62	5.03[a]	1.70	1.16
DM + DF + DU	5.46[a]	3.00[a]	1.42	1.83[c]	4.41[a]	1.80[c]	1.47

[a] $p < 0.005$ [b] $p < 0.01$ [c] $p < 0.05$

The F-ratio for these variances, that is between interpair and intrapair for
lipoproteins are significant in a similar way in all monozygous twins, but not
for all dizygous twins. To calculate a meaningful estimate of the magnitude of
genetic influence is difficult, but the H-statistics is calculated in this way.

"H" is the variance within monozygous pairs subtracted from that of dizygous
pairs, divided by the dizygous pair variance. The larger the H-value, the greater
the genetic influence, or expressed differently the larger the difference between
the variance in monozygous and dizygous twins the larger the genetic influence.
Table 3 shows that the genetic control of serum cholesterol concentration seems

Table 3. H-values for serum lipid and lipoproteins

	Choles-terol	Trigly-cerides	Phospho-lipids	Total lipids	ß-lipo-proteins	Pre-ß-lipo-proteins	α-lipo-proteins
MM/DM	0.84[a]	0.24	0.14	0.66[b]	0.50	0.47	0
MF/DF	0.56	0.65	0.83[a]	0.82[a]	0	0.65	0.77
MM+MF/ DM+DF	0.74[a]	0.47	0.67[a]	0.76[a]	0.24	0.57	0.60
MM+MF/DM+ DF+DU	0.72[a]	0.50	0.56[b]	0.72[a]	0.33	0.54	0.50

[a] p <0.005 for F-ratio variance DZ/MZ.   [b] p <0.05 for F-ratio variance DZ/MZ.
[c] p <0.01 for F-ratio variance DZ/MZ.

to be more pronounced in males than in females, as judged from the H-value. There was no formal evidence for genetic control of serum triglyceride values, although the H-values were compatible with half of the variation being due to genetic variation. Phospho- and total lipid concentrations are also genetically influenced, phospholipids less so in the males.

For lipoproteins, H-values around 50% was found, but with considerable differences between males and females. Although not shown here, no greater variance was generally found in the lipoprotein and lipid parameters in the twins living apart than together, except in a few instances, but the differences were not significant and the groups have therefore been treated together.

In conclusion it can be stated that in this study cholesterol values are genetically influenced and the H-statistics suggest that between 56-84% of this variation is genetically determined. A substantial genetic influence was also apparent on other serum lipoproteins and lipids in this series of young, healthy twins. Thus this study further emphasises the importance of genetic factors in determining the concentration of serum lipids and lipoproteins.

THE INHERITANCE OF LIPOPROTEIN DISORDERS AND THE RISKS OF CORONARY DEATH IN FIRST-DEGREE RELATIVES OF 193 SURVIVORS OF MYOCARDIAL INFARCTION

David Patterson and Joan Slack

An unselected series of 108 and 85 female survivors of myocardial infarction have been investigated. Cholesterol and triglyceride levels, lipoproteins electrophoresis on cellulose acetate, and analytical ultracentrifugation have been used to determine their lipid status, compared with age and sex matched controls.

To allow comparison of lipid levels at different ages and between sexes, scores have been calculated for cholesterol and triglyceride levels (Patterson and Slack, 1972). All index patients and controls with cholesterol or triglyceride scores in excess of two standard deviations above the expected mean were designated hyperlipidaemic. This corresponds with the 96th percentile for cholesterol scores and the 93rd percentile for the triglyceride scores; the difference being due to the skewed distribution of cholesterol and triglyceride scores.

The distribution of cholesterol and triglyceride scores in the controls and index patients around the level expected for their age and sex is shown in Fig. 1. 2 standard deviations (2 S.D.) above the mean cholesterol score would correspond to a cholesterol level of 325 mg/100 ml. in a man aged 40 and 311 mg/100 ml. in a woman of the same age. 2 standard deviations above the mean triglyceride score would correspond to a triglyceride level of 212 mg/100 ml. in a man aged 40 and to a level of 130 mg/100 ml. for a woman aged 40. The lipoprotein electrophoresis in conjunction with the lipid levels enabled an assessment of the lipoprotein distribution to be made.

5% of the male controls were hyperlipidaemic compared with 22% of the male index patients. Only one male had Type II hyperbetalipoproteinaemia, 3 male controls had Type IV hyperprebetalipoproteinaemia, and one had the Type V abnormality. 13 male index patients had Type II hyperbetalipoproteinaemia and 11 had Type IV hyperprebetalipoproteinaemia.

14% of the younger female controls had hyperlipidaemia equally divided between the Type II and Type IV abnormalities. There were no older female controls. 33% of the female index patients had hyperlipidaemia, 17 of whom had Type II, and 11 Type IV abnormalities.

The lipoprotein distribution of the patients with hyperbetalipoproteinaemia diagnosed on the basis of the lipid levels and electrophoretic strip, was compared with the analytical ultracentrifuge data. 85% of the male index patients with Type II hyperlipoproteinaemia and 88% of the female index patients with Type II hyperlipoproteinaemia had the concentration of lipoproteins in Sf 0-20 elevated more than 2 S.D. above the expected mean. None of the 11 male nor 11 female index patients with hyperprebetalipoproteinaemia had the concentration of lipoproteins in Sf 0-20 elevated more than 2 S.D. above the expected mean. The correlation of serum cholesterol levels and the concentration of lipoprotein in Sf 0-20 was 0.81 and the correlation of triglyceride levels and the concentration of lipoprotein in Sf 20-400 was 0.80. It is therefore concluded that an estimation of the fasting cholesterol and triglyceride levels in conjunction with lipoprotein electrophoresis enables the classification of the distribution of lipoproteins to be made with confidence in accord with the W.H.O. classification (W.H.O., 1970).

234 first-degree relatives of index patients with lipoprotein abnormalities were contacted and fasting blood samples were obtained in 58% and their lipoprotein status assessed. The distribution of cholesterol scores in all the first-degree

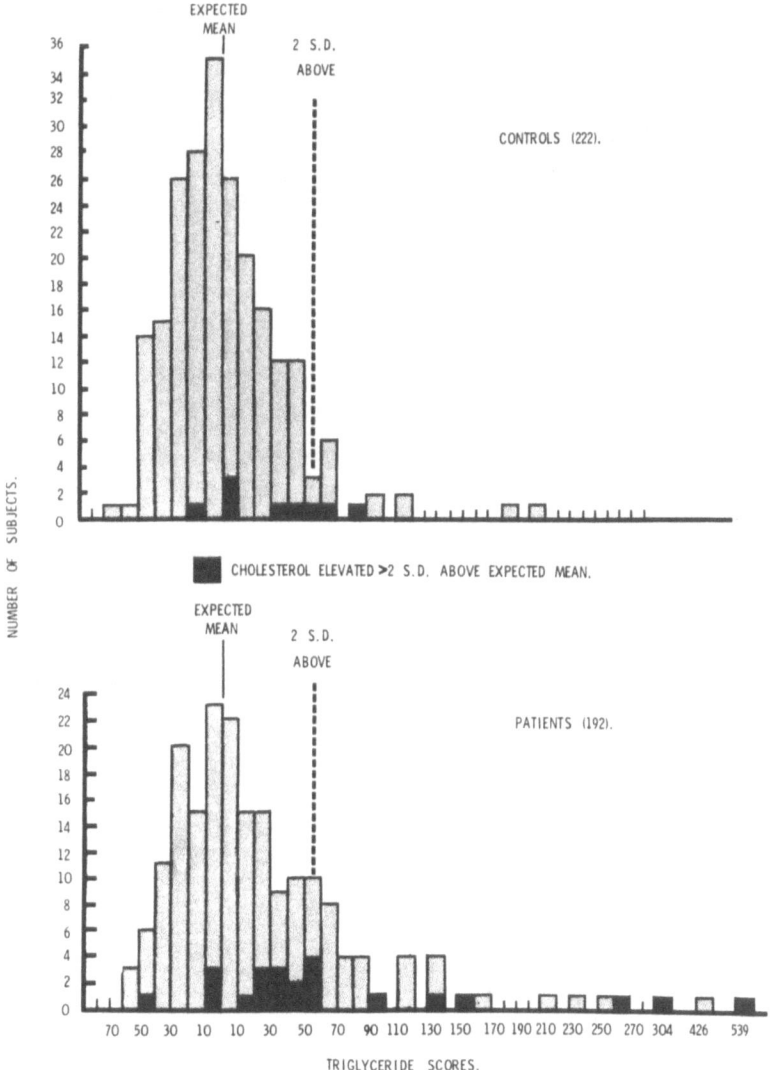

Figure 1(a). Distribution of triglyceride scores around the expected mean in controls and survivors of myocardial infarction

relatives of index patients with Type II hyperbetalipoproteinaemia is shown in Fig. 2. The index patients are not included in the distribution. The distribution is shifted to the right of the expected distribution, with 9 instead of the expected 2 subjects with cholesterol scores elevated more than 2 S.D. The mean cholesterol score is significantly different from the expected mean and even if the 9 frankly hyperlipidaemic relatives from 5 families are removed from the distribution, the mean of the main distribution is still significantly shifted to the right of the control distribution.

The distribution of cholesterol scores within these 5 families is compatible with the inheritance of hypercholesterolaemia in these families as a single gene effect when allowance is made for the number of first-degree relatives who were dead.

The distribution of the triglyceride scores of all the first-degree relatives is not shifted to the right but the mean score is significantly higher than expected and 8 relatives instead of the expected 2 have scores more than 2 S.D. above the

459

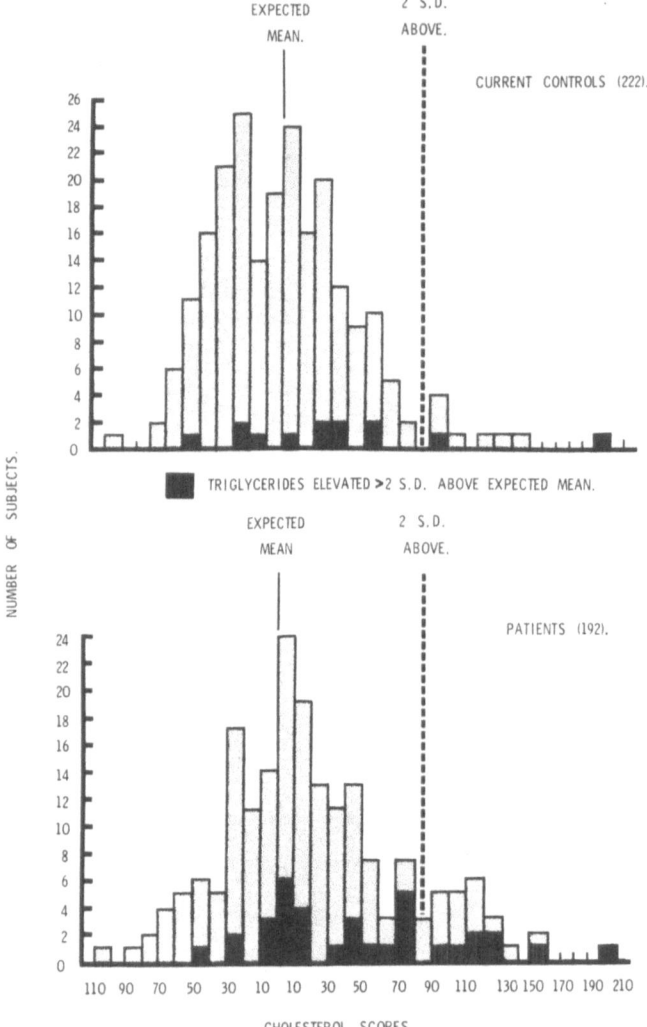

Figure 1(b). Distribution of cholesterol scores around the expected mean in controls and survivors of myocardial infarction

expected mean. 5 of the 8 outliers to the right of the distribution were found to be subjects with Type IIB hyperlipoproteinaemia.

If hyperbetalipoproteinaemia in the index patients were invariably due to the well recognised dominantly inherited condition, then with a 50% chance of an individual first-degree relative being affected, the number of families expected to have at least one affected member can be calculated from the distribution of family sizes. 19 families would be expected to have at least one affected and only 5 were found. The index patients in 4 of these 5 families was female. There results suggest that only one quarter of survivors with hyperbetalipoproteinaemia have the form that is inherited as an autosomal dominant and the remainder have an elevated level on the basis of polygenic inheritance.

The distribution of cholesterol and triglyceride scores in first-degree relatives of the index patients with hyperprebetalipoproteinaemia is shown in Fig. 3. No shift can be detected in either distribution. The mean triglyceride score is

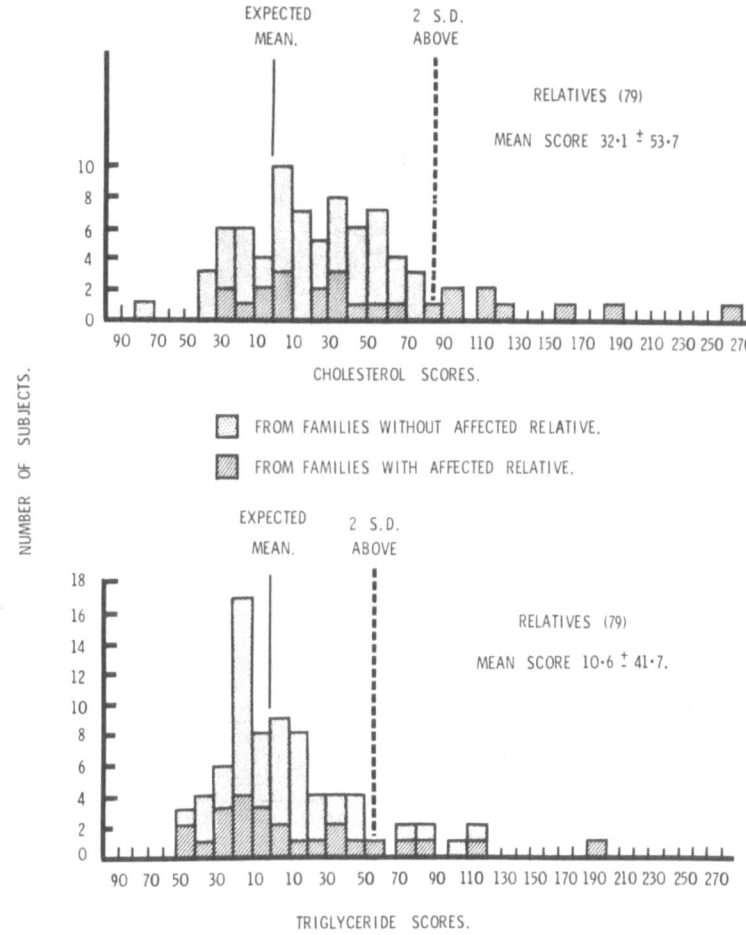

Figure 2. Distribution of cholesterol and triglyceride scores in first-degree relatives of hyperlipidaemic patients with Type II lipoproteinaemia on electrophoresis

significantly higher than expected while the mean cholesterol score is normal. If hyperprebetalipoproteinaemia were inherited as a dominant characteristic then 13 families of the index patients would be expected to have at least one affected member. Only 5 were observed. The numbers of subjects are too small to draw firm conclusions as to the mode of inheritance of Type IV hyperprebetalipoproteinaemia encountered in survivors of myocardial infarction but it is possible that not more than 1/3 of index patients with Type IV hyperprebetalipoproteinaemia have the form inherited as an autosomal dominant.

The raw data obtained in this study is strikingly similar to that of Goldstein et al. (1973). They studied 95% of the living first-degree relatives of index patients. However, it is unfortunate that their findings are reported to include unrepresentative proportions of second and third degree relatives whose ascertainment has led to a disproportionate incidence of lipoprotein abnormalities in those investigated. Further by excluding from their main analysis all families without an affected first-degree relative, they have excluded an unknown number of families on account of the affected sibling never being born or having died.

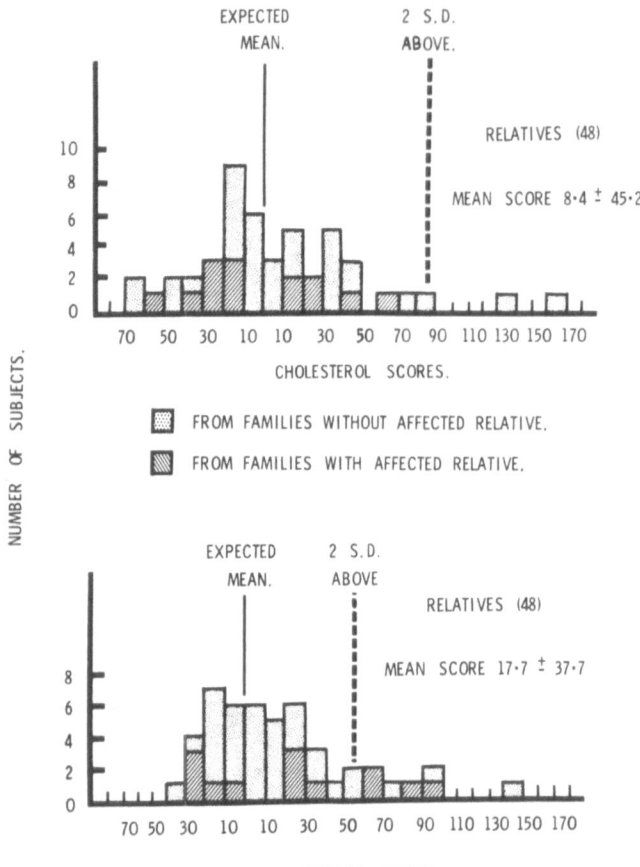

Figure 3. Distribution of cholesterol and triglyceride scores in first-degree relatives of hyperlipidaemic patients with Type IV lipoproteinaemia on electrophoresis

Life tables were constructed according to the method of Bradford Hill (1961), on all index patients and the cause of deaths of decreased relatives documented by reference to death certificates. Only certificates with a special mention of coronary artery disease were included. A comparison can then be made of the risks of coronary deaths in the general population with the risks to the first-degree relatives of male and female index patients have been considered in two groups: fathers, brothers, and sons in one group and mothers, sisters, and daughters in the other. The Registrar General's tables for England and Wales were used to calculate the risks of dying from coronary heart disease in the general population. The observed number of deaths was compared with the expected and expressed as a ratio.

When all the relatives of the index patients were considered together (Table 1) they had a 1-1/2 fold increased risk of a coronary death which is of the same magnitude as that found by Doll and Hill (1964) for cigarette smokers. The "younger" relatives had a 2-1/2 fold increased risk. The risks to the male relatives was approximately the same as to the female relatives.

The relatives of "younger" index patients with "normal" lipids also had an increased risk of a coronary death. This is suggestive that other genetically determined risk factors such as hypertension or coagulation problems are involved or else it reflects lipoprotein abnormalities in the first-degree relatives in spite of the index patients having normal lipids (Nikkilä and Aro, 1973). This increased risk was most marked amongst the younger relatives.

The risks to the relatives of index patients with Type II hyperlipoproteinaemia were significantly increased over the risks to the general population with the younger relatives having a five fold increase. These risks were considerably lower than described by Slack (1969) and Jensen et al. (1967) for subjects with familial hypercholesterolaemic xanthomatosis. The reason for this difference almost certainly lies in the low proportion of monogenic to polygenic modes of inheritance.

Table 1. Increased risk of a coronary death to first-degree relatives

Index patients	First-degree relatives	
	All relatives	"Younger" relatives
Whole group	x 1.5[a]	x 2.5[b]
"Younger" with "normal" lipids	x 1.9[a]	x 2.4[b]
Type II hyperlipoproteinaemia	x 2.5[b]	x 4.9[b]
Type IV hyperlipoproteinaemia	x 1.9	x 4.4[b]
Spouses with "normal" lipids	x 0.9	x 0.9

[a] $<0.05, >0.01$.   [b] $<0.01, >0.001$.   [c] <0.001.

The risks to the younger relatives with Type IV hyperlipoproteinaemia was of the same magnitude as that experienced by relatives of Type II patients. This suggests that Type IV hyperlipoproteinaemia may be an important and potentially dangerous risk factor. First-degree relatives of the spouses with normal lipids were found to have the same risk of a coronary death as that of the general population over the same period of time.

HYPERLIPIDEMIA IN SURVIVORS OF MYOCARDIAL INFARCTION: RELATIONSHIP BETWEEN GENETIC CLASSIFICATION AND LIPOPROTEIN PHENOTYPE[*]

William R. Hazzard, Joseph L. Goldstein, Helmut G. Schrott, Arno G. Motulsky, and Edwin L. Bierman

From the Departments of Medicine (Division of Metabolism and Gerontology, Veterans Administration Hospital, and Division of Medical Genetics, University Hospital) and Genetics, University of Washington, Seattle, Washington 98195.

The hyperlipidemic disorders have been classified according to several schemes (Ahrens et al., 1961; Beaumont et al., 1970; Fredrickson et al., 1967; Gofman et al., 1954; Havel, 1970; Thannhauser, 1958) but the system of assigning lipoprotein phenotypes introduced by Fredrickson, Levy, and Lees (Fredrickson et al., 1967) and subsequently endorsed in modified form by the World Health Organization (Beaumont et al., 1970) enjoys the widest current usage. Under the present system six lipoprotein patterns are recognized, based upon the whole plasma triglyceride (TG) and isolated low density lipoprotein (LDL), cholesterol concentrations, the presence or absence of chylomicrons in an overnight fasting plasma specimen, and the mobility of isolated very low density lipoproteins (VLDL).

Since many cases of hyperlipidemia are familial in occurrence, it might be assumed that lipoprotein phenotypes should be similar in hyperlipidemic members of a single family. The present study, proceeding from an investigation of the prevalence and genetic forms of hyperlipidemia among survivors of myocardial infarction, was designed to test this assumption.

In the parent study (Goldstein et al., 1973), age- and sex-adjusted fasting plasma TG and cholesterol levels from 500 three-month survivors of myocardial infarction were compared with similarly adjusted lipid levels in 950 non-related control subjects. Of the survivors, 164 (31%) were judged hyperlipidemic by virtue of an adjusted TG and/or cholesterol level exceeding the 95th percentile among controls. These 164 survivors in turn served as index cases for detailed family studies (Goldstein et al., 1973) which allowed their assignment to one of five genetically-defined categories: 1. Familial hypercholesterolemia; 2. Familial hypertriglyceridemia; 3. Familial combined hyperlipidemia (these three being separate, simply-inherited (i.e. monogenic) disorders); 4. Polygenic hypercholesterolemia; or 5. Sporadic (i.e., non-familial) hypertriglyceridemia.

The present study (Hazzard et al., 1973) determined the lipoprotein phenotype of 133 of these 164 survivors in a repeat fasting plasma speciment collected an average of 117 days after the initial sampling. In this manner we assessed the

[*]This work was presented in part at the 8th Session of the Association of American Physicians, Atlantic City, N.J., 2-3 May 1972, and published in the transactions.

Dr. Goldstein was supported by Special National Institutes of Health Fellowship GM 4784-01 and is now a Research Career Development Awardee (1-K4-GM 70, 277-01) from the National Institute of General Medical Sciences. His present address is the Division of Medical Genetics, Department of Internal Medicine, University of Texas Southwestern Medical School, Dallas, Texas 75235. Dr. Hazzard was the recipient of a Clinical Investigatorship of the Veterans Administration and is now an Investigator of the Howard Hughes Medical Institute. Dr. Schrott was supported by Special National Institutes of Health Fellowship HE-48 695. His present address is the Department of Medicine, University of Iowa, Iowa City, Iowa.

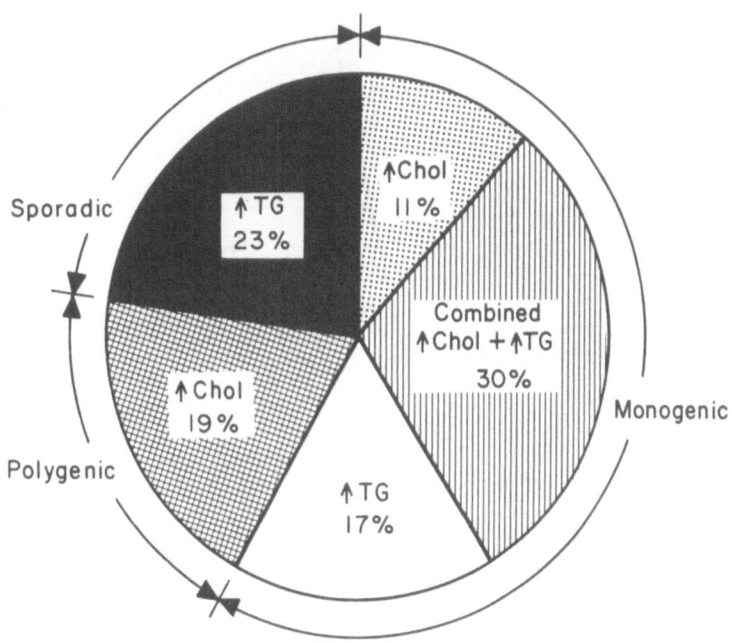

Figure 1. Genetic classification of 133 hyperlipidemic myocardial infarction survivors as determined from analysis of plasma lipid levels in their relatives

relationship of the lipoprotein phenotype of the survivor in this second specimen to his genetic classification, based upon the lipid levels of his relatives.

Among the survivors who were thus resampled (Fig. 1), 11% had familial hypercholesterolemia, 17% familial hypertriglyceridemia, 30% had familial combined hyperlipidemia, 19% polygenic hypercholesterolemia, and 23% sporadic hypertriglyceridemia. Among the same group, lipoprotein phenotypes were distributed as (Fig. 2): 26% normal; 25% IIa; 15% IIb; 32% IV; and 2% V. If a given lipoprotein phenotype were synonymous with the presence of a specific genetic lipid disorder, one might have predicted a close association of the IIa pattern with familial hypercholesterolemia, IIb with familial combined hyperlipidemia, and IV with familial hypertriglyceridemia. Indeed, in a general sense this proved to be true, since the mean LDL-cholesterol level discriminated statistically (P <.005) among the three monogenic disorders (Fig. 3): it was highest in survivors with familial hypercholesterolemia (261 ± 61 mg/100 ml [mean ± S.D.]); intermediate in those with familial combined hyperlipidemia (197 ± 50); and lowest in those with familial hypertriglyceridemia (155 ± 36). However, the LDL-cholesterol level did not distinguish polygenic hypercholesterolemia from familial combined hyperlipidemia nor sporadic from familial hypertriglyceridemia.

Most importantly, on an individual basis no lipoprotein pattern proved specific to any particular genetic lipid disorder; conversely, no genetic disorder was specified by a single lipoprotein pattern (Fig. 4). This lack of correlation occurred for several reasons: 1. lipid levels in some survivors fell below the 95th percentile(s) in the repeat sample (often as a result of clofibrate therapy in those with monogenic disorders), resulting in a normal lipoprotein phenotype; 2. lipid levels and lipoprotein phenotypes were similar in survivors with monogenic and non-monogenic (i.e. polygenic and sporadic) forms of hyperlipidemia; 3. despite the statistically significant differences in mean LDL-cholesterol levels among the 3 monogenic disorders, the degree of overlap made the LDL-cholesterol level an unreliable index of the genetic basis of the hyperlipidemia in the indi-

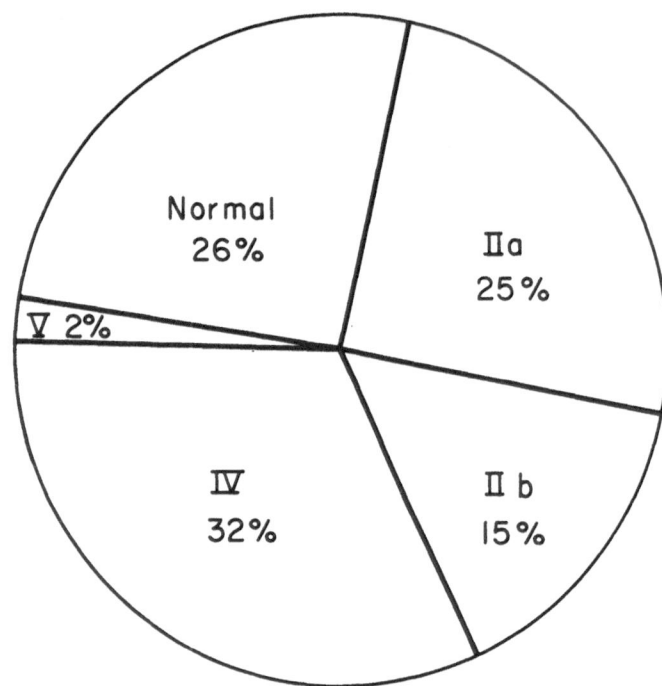

Figure 2. Lipoprotein phenotypes of 133 myocardial infarction survivors in a repeat fasting plasma specimen. All subjects were hyperlipidemic at the time of their original sampling. Four subjects with Type III have not been included

vidual survivor. It was of particular note that the mean LDL-cholesterol level among survivors in the largest group, with familial combined hyperlipidemia, very nearly coincided with the 95th percentile cut-point in the WHO classification scheme. As a result, approximately half the survivors with this disorder lay above this value (with IIa or IIb lipoprotein phenotype [depending upon the TG level]), while the remainder lay below it (with a normal or IV phenotype). Finally, although numerically uncommon, even the 4 subjects with ß-migrating VLDL (and a lipoprotein phenotype III) demonstrated lipoprotein and genetic heterogeneity, only one of the 4 having unequivocal broad-ß disease.

These studies thus suggest that lipoprotein phenotypes are not qualitative genetic markers but instead represent quantitative functions which may differ among individuals with a single genetic lipid disorder or be similar among persons with different genetic disorders. It remains to be seen whether the genetic classification of lipid disorders will prove more useful than the lipoprotein classification in its prognostic or therapeutic implications. However, from these studies it appears certain that the two are not synonymous among hyperlipidemic survivors of myocardial infarction.

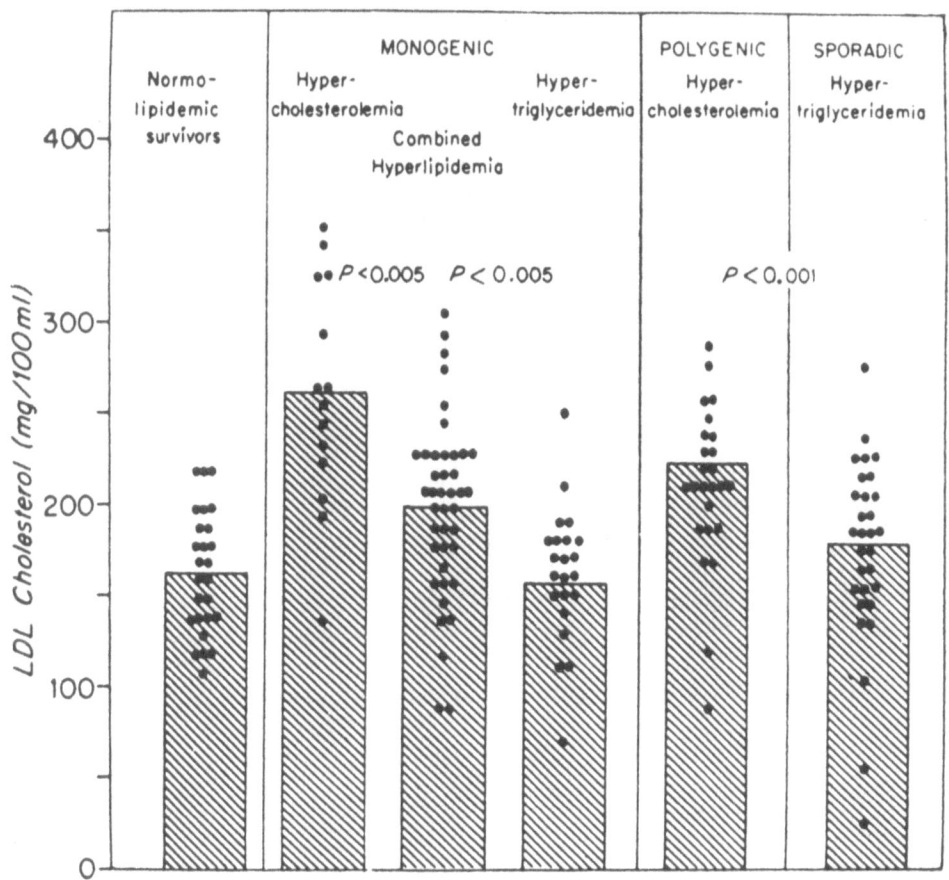

Figure 3. Low density lipoprotein (LDL) cholesterol levels of 133 hyperlipidemic myocardial infarction survivors upon repeat plasma sampling, grouped according to genetic classification. The normolipidemic survivors are 26 other survivors who had normal lipid levels in their original plasma samples and in whom family studies confirmed the absence of a genetic form of hyperlipidemia

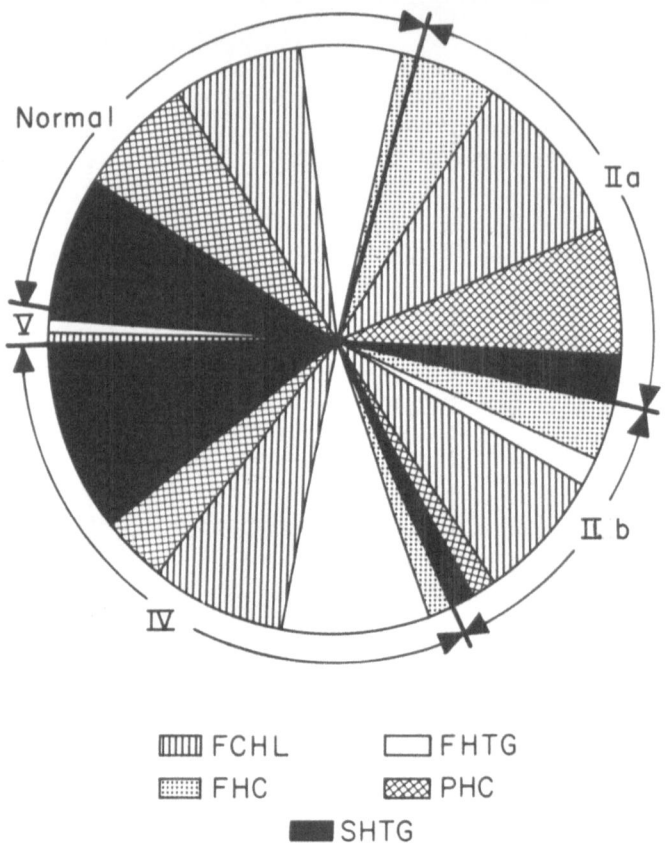

Figure 4. Genetic classification of hyperlipidemic myocardial infarction survivors grouped according to lipoprotein phenotype. FCHL = familial combined hyperlipidemia; FHC = familial hypercholesterolemia; FHTG = familial hypertriglyceridemia; PHC = polygenic hypercholesterolemia; SHTG = sporadic hypertriglyceridemia

QUANTITATIVE GENETIC STUDIES OF THE HUMAN PLASMA LP(A) LIPOPROTEIN

John J. Albers and William R. Hazzard

The Lp(a) lipoprotein has been suggested to be a qualitative autosomal dominant genetic marker in 30-45% of humans (Berg, 1968) but this has been challenged in later studies (Harvie and Schultz, 1970). Utilizing a sensitive radial immunodiffusion method (Albers and Hazzard, 1973), the present study was undertaken to characterize the mechanism of inheritance of the Lp(a) lipoprotein by quantification and genetic analysis of Lp(a) levels in 1251 adults, including 300 mother-father - offspring triplets.

1. Materials and Methods

a) Population. The population consisted of 1251 parents and grandparents of 133 non-hyperlipidemic and 126 hyperlipidemic newborn probands.

b) Blood Samples. Venous blood was drawn from overnight (12-14 hrs.) fasting human volunteers and the disordium EDTA plasma promptly separated at 4° and stored at -20°.

c) Lipid Analysis. Samples were extracted with zeolite and isopropanol and analyzed for cholesterol and triglyceride with the Technicon AutoAnalyzer I.

d) Quantitative Immunochemical Analysis. Quantitative immunochemical analysis were performed by single radial immunodiffusion (Albers and Hazzard, 1973).

2. Results

a) Relation of Lp(a) Levels to Age, Sex and Lipid Levels. Prior to genetic analysis, it was important to determine whether any relationship existed between Lp(a) levels and the sex or age of the individual. Lp(a) levels were found to be independent of age ($r=.036$; $.2>p>.5$). At the 5% level there was no statistically significant correlation of Lp(a) with either cholesterol or triglyceride levels in any of the groups of unrelated individuals ($n>244$).

b) Distribution of Lp(a) Levels Among Adult Subjects. The distribution of Lp(a) concentrations for the 1251 adult fasting subjects is shown in Fig. 1. The distribution was highly skewed (mean 9.7 mg/100ml, median 6.0). Seventy-eight percent of the subjects had detectable Lp(a) lipoprotein in whole plasma. Males and females had similiar distributions. There was no significant sex difference in either the mean or median Lp(a) levels: males, mean 9.3, median 5.8 mg/100ml; females mean 10.1, median 6.2 mg/100ml. Nine males (1.5%) and nine females (1.4%) had concentrations exceeding 50 mg/100ml with a maximum value among males of 125 mg/100ml and among females of 126 mg/100ml.

c) Relationship of Lp(a) Levels Among Family Members. The correlation of Lp(a) values among family members is shown in Table 1. Significant correlations between parents and offspring were found regardless of the sex of parent or offspring, contrasting with the lack of significant correlation between members of the husband-wife pairs ($r=0.023$). It was of note that the father-son correlation was comparable to the father-daughter and the mother-son comparable to the mother-daughter, indicating that the Lp(a) trait is not sex-linked. These data indicated that

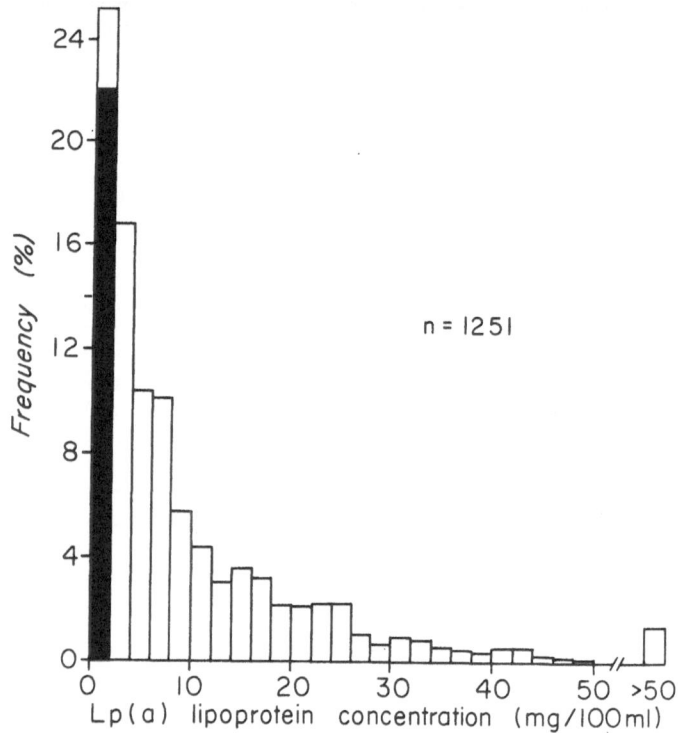

Figure 1. Frequency distributions of Lp(a) lipoprotein concentrations (mg/100ml) in 1251 adults. Solid bar represents the percentage of subjects with undetectable (<1.5 mg/100ml) Lp(a) lipoprotein concentrations in whole plasma

Table 1. Correlations of Lp(a) values between family members

Relationship	Sample Size	Pearson's Correlation Coefficient	Probability	Spearman's Correlation Coefficient
Offspring-Mother	300	.292	p<.01	.337
Daughter-Mother	163	.277	p<.01	.391
Son-Mother	137	.324	p<.01	.254
Offspring-Father	300	.458	p<.01	.398
Daughter-Father	163	.351	p<.01	.438
Son-Father	137	.556	p<.01	.367
Offspring-Parent	600	.370	p<.01	.375
Offspring-Midparent	300	.507	p<.01	.517
Husband-Wife (Grandparents)	300	.023	.5<p<.7	.038
Husband-Wife	246	-.021	.5<p<.7 .8<p< 1 [a]	-.004

[a]Probability value for Spearman's statistic.

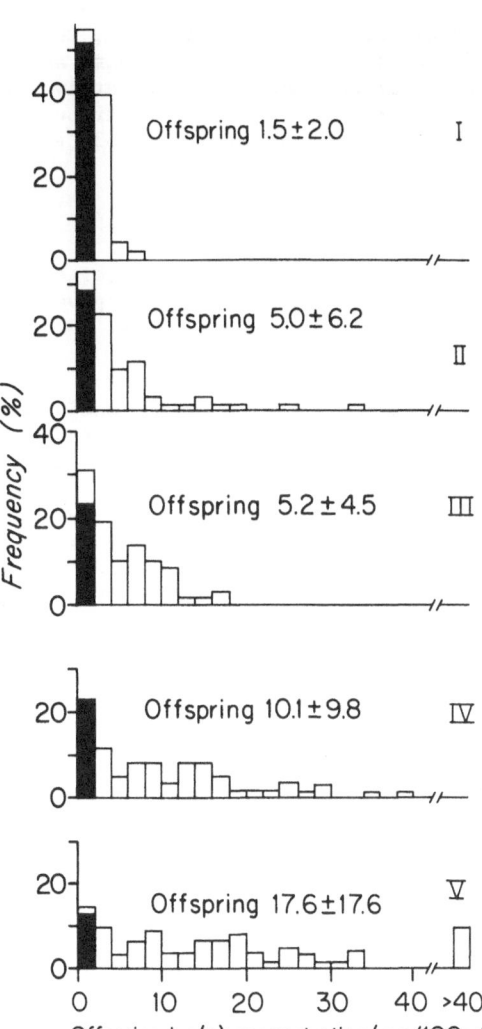

Figure 2. The frequency distributions of the Lp(a) lipoprotein concentrations of adult offspring derived from 5 groups of parents, quintiles I-V, having mean midparent concentrations of 1.3, 4.2, 7.7, 12.6, and 24.8 mg/100ml respectively. The mean ± S.D. offspring values for each quintile indicated

familial factors play an important role in the determination of Lp(a) lipoprotein levels. The absence of correlations in Lp(a) levels in husband-wife pairs suggest that these familial factors were primarily genetic in origin.

An estimate of heritability, that is, the proportion of the total phenotypic variance due to additive genetic variation, is equal to twice the parent-offspring correlation coefficient (Falconer, 1965). According to this formula, the heritability of Lp(a) using Pearson's correlation coefficient was 0.74. Using Spearman's rank correlation test, essentially the same estimate was obtained, i.e., 0.75.

In order to study the quantitative relationship of Lp(a) levels between parents and their offspring and specifically to look for evidence of bimodality consistent with a dominant mode of transmission, the 300 parent-offspring triplets were arbitrarily divided into quintiles of 60 families each with respect to midparent Lp(a) lipoprotein concentrations. The distribution of offspring and mean ± S.D. Lp(a) offspring concentrations from each of the five respective quintiles is shown in Fig. 2. As the midparent concentration increased, the offspring concentration increased correspondingly and the skewness and variance of the offspring frequency distribution increased, but there was no evidence of bimodality. In a further effort to detect bimodality and to study further the quantitative relationship of parent to offspring, those triplets in which one parent had an Lp(a) value of greater than 12 mg/100ml and the other had an Lp(a) value of less than 6 mg/100ml were analyzed separately. Even though the parental Lp(a) values were dissimilar and their Lp(a) distribution was clearly not unimodal, the Lp(a) distribution in the offspring (n=63) gave no evidence of bimodality.

3. Conclusions

Families could not be readily sorted for genetic heterogeneity in the present study because only one offspring was ascertained per family, necessitating pooling of family data. Thus a lack of completed ascertainment of all members was the major limitation in the study.

We can summarize our overall conclusions as follows. The Lp(a) lipoprotein is present in all or nearly all individuals in widely varying amounts. Lp(a) levels are not correlated with age, sex, or cholesterol or glyceride levels. The observed quantitative Lp(a) variation is determined by a multi-factorial mechanism with approximately 75% of the total variation genetically determined. Further analysis supports a polygenic model of inheritance, but does not rule out major gene effects. Furthermore, it is quite plausable that additional genetic herterogenity in the determination of plasma Lp(a) levels may be discovered upon a more detailed and extensive genetic study.

CORONARY ARTERY DISEASE RISK IN FAMILIAL TYPE II HYPERLIPOPROTEINEMIA

Neil J. Stone, Robert I. Levy, Donald S. Fredrickson, and Joel Verter

Prospective and retrospective analyses of coronary artery disease (CAD) risk for affected and non-affected members of kindred with familial hypercholesterolemia, (Type II hyperlipoproteinemia), vary considerably. Slack found that by age 60, the risk of CAD and CAD death in first degree male relatives of Type II propositi was 85.4% and 54.1% respectively (Slack, 1969). Furthermore, Jensen, Blankenhorn and Kornerup's 20 year follow-up study of 11 Danish kindred with familial hypercholesterolemia showed that CAD was diagnosed in almost one-third of affected subjects, but only in 1.3% of those not affected with hypercholesterolemia (Jensen et al., 1967). Harlan et al., however, report no apparent effect of hypercholesterolemia on longevity when they compared affected and non-affected individuals from one large American kindred. (Harlan et al., 1966). Although the authors felt that CAD at an "unusually early age was not epidemic in their kindred", symptomatic CAD occurred at mean age of 42 years among males and 50 years among females with hypercholesterolemia.

This report presents data from a systematic analysis of cardiovascular and lipoprotein status in 547 first degree relatives from 116 kindred with Type II hyperlipoproteinemia. The risk of CAD in adults with Type II has been compared with other family members with normal lipoproteins. Utilizing standardized cardiovascular study methods, comparisons were made between both sexes and over five decades to permit comparisons of CAD risk between subjects with other types of familial hyperlipoproteinemia and subjects in the general population.

The 116 propositi were among the first 118 consecutive patients seen at the National Institutes of Health Clinical Center with 1. a primary increase in low density lipoprotein cholesterol concentration which exceeded age-corrected upper 5% limits; and 2. either a similarly affected first degree relative or tendon xanthomas. The adult relatives of the propositi could be divided into three groups. The Group consisted of 380 living and 167 deceased first degree relatives of the propositi. This included 179 with Type II (II's) and 169 normolipidemic relatives (N's). The report of a larger cohort (1403 relatives) is in press (Stone et al., 1974). In that report, in addition to the first degree relatives of the propositi (Group I), two other groups are reported. In Group II were the first degree relatives of any Group I relative with Type II; similarly, in Group III were the first degree relatives of any member of Group II and Type II. This method of selection included all second and third generation Type II relatives and resulted in approximately as many normolipidemic relatives for study as those with Type II.

Lipid and lipoprotein studies utilizing paper electrophoresis and preparative ultracentrifugation were carried out as previously described. (Fredrickson et al., 1972). Subjects were instructed to maintain their weight and customary diet and to take no hypolipidemic medications for at least two weeks prior to sampling. Sampling was not performed until three months after an acute myocardial infarction.

Cardiovascular information was obtained from standardized interview, 12 lead ECG, and physician, hospital, and death records. CAD was designated by any of the following: 1. Angina pectoris according to Rose questionnaire; (Rose et al., 1968). 2. Q and QSI,1 items of the Minnesota Code on resting ECG; (Rose et al., 1968). 3. Coronary insufficiency occurring when chest discomfort was associated with either downsloping or flat ST segments depression of at least 1.0 mm or T wave inversion or both, but not associated with an elevation of heart enzymes or non-

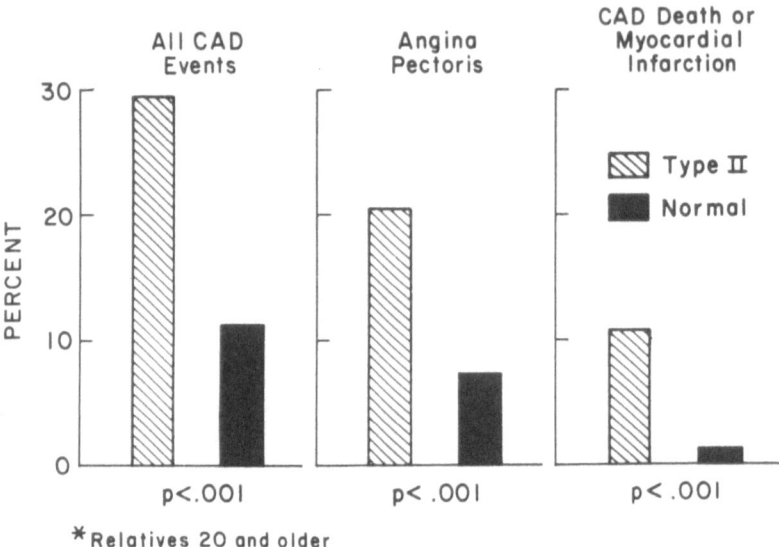

Figure 1. Prevalence of CAD endpoints in Type II and normolipidemic relatives

ischemic cause of chest pain; 4. Myocardial infarction documented with either cardiac muscle enzymes elevated in temporal profile consistent with acute cardiac muscle necrosis or ECG changes including the appearance of new Q waves, or both; 5. CAD death defined as occurring within two hours from the onset of symptoms as documented by a witness and occurring in the absence of chronic, debilitating diseases such as cancer.

Lipoprotein status was a decisive factor in assessing coronary risk. There was no significant difference between II's and N's with regard to age distribution, sex, hypertension, smoking habits, or body mass index. Yet CAD was three times more prevalent among II's than among N's (Fig. 1). Myocardial infarction was particularly evident in II's; 9.2% of Type II males and 5.8% of Type II females. Interestingly, the prevalence of abnormal Q waves on resting ECG's was similar among II's and N's.

Life table analysis demonstrated that in addition to the excessive CAD risk associated with the Type II trait, there was the additional hazard of early CAD onset. By age 40, the cumulative probability of fatal or nonfatal CAD was almost 19% for male Type II relatives vis-a-vis less than 1% for normolipidemic male relatives. By age 60, the risk had climbed to 65% (2 in 3) for male II's compared with only 16% (1 in 6) for male N's. In essence, the CAD risk for normolipidemic relatives lagged 20 years behind their Type II counterparts (Fig. 2).

Among females the results were less striking, but nonetheless significant by age 60. At that age, the risk of fatal or nonfatal CAD had reached almost 36% (1 in 3) for female II's contrasted with about 14% (1 in 7) for female N's (Fig. 3).

Thus, in this the largest study of CAD risk in kindreds with Type II hyperlipoproteinemia, affected male relatives were shown to have developed an early and excessive risk of a CAD event as compared with their otherwise similar normolipidemic relatives. Females with Type II presented with CAD at a later age, but still had far more CAD events than their normolipidemic counterparts. Family screening should be initiated when Type II hyperlipoproteinemia is diagnosed to identify individuals at high risk for CAD. This will be especially important if studies now underway can prove that treatment of Type II can cause regression or decreased progression of existing coronary lesions.

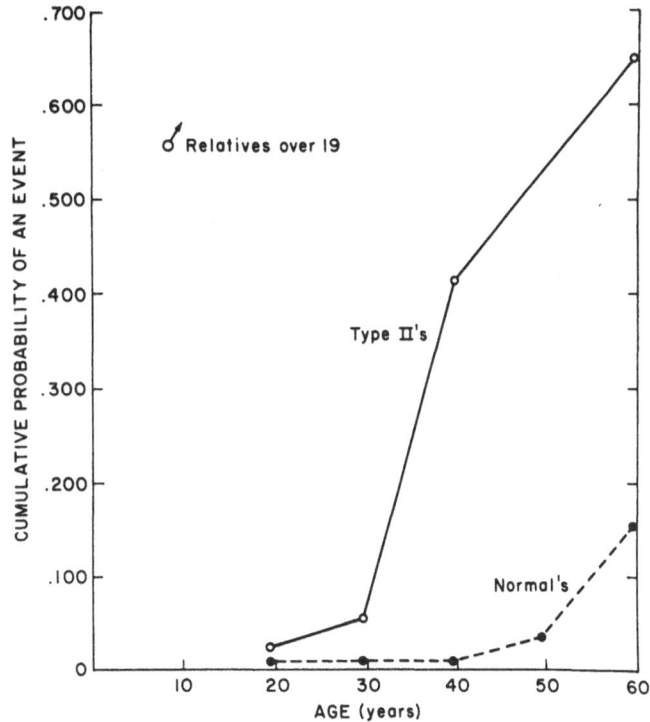

Figure 2. Cumulative probability by decade of fatal or nonfatal CAD events in male Type II and normolipidemic relatives

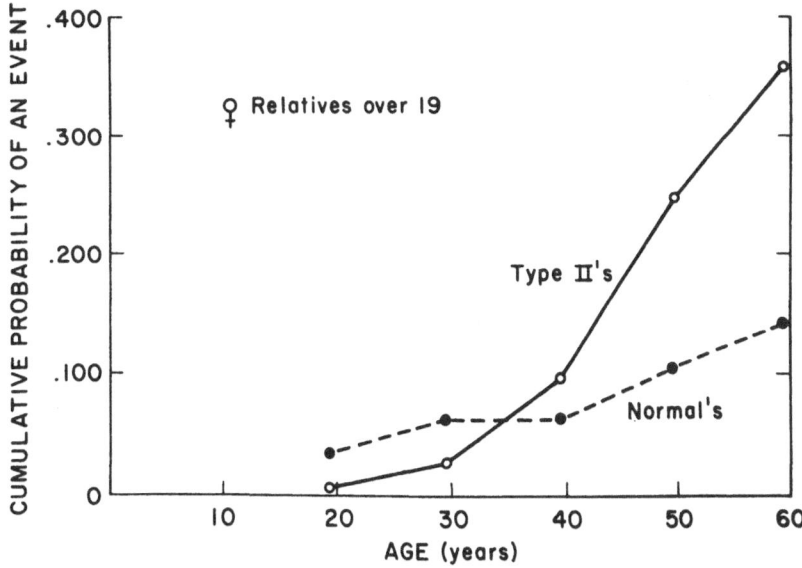

Figure 3. Cumulative probability by decade of fatal or nonfatal CAD events in female Type II and normolipidemic relatives

PROSPECTIVE STUDY OF CORD BLOOD CHOLESTEROL TO PREDICT LEVEL OF
CHOLESTEROL AND TYPE II HYPERLIPOPROTEINEMIA IN ADOLESCENCE

Iqbal Krishan, Curtis G. Hames, Herman A. Tyroler, and Caroline
Becker

Between January 1958 and July 1960, maternal and cord blood was obtained from 571
consecutive live births in a biracial rural general practice in Georgia, USA.
Following delivery of the infant, blood was obtained from a clean cut of the umbilical cord. Maternal blood was obtained at the same time.

In 1972, prospective study was conducted. Using the 1958-60 cord blood cholesterol levels, a stratified random sample was identified; 100% of those cord blood
cholesterols of $\geq$100 mg/100 ml were included in the sampling design.

Recall of the adolescents was accomplished between September and November 1972.
Fasting levels of total cholesterol, triglycerides and serum lipoproteins were
done.

The cumulative frequency of material cholesterol showed: Blacks have a mean cholesterol level lower than whites, both black and white women show a rise in cholesterol level during pregnancy, but the racial difference persists. The mean
cholesterol value of 196 blacks in this study was 245 mg/100 ml, and for 281
whites, 268 mg/100 ml. These means are highly significantly different with a p
value of less than .001. Additionally, when controlled for maternal age, this difference persists.

The mean cord blood cholesterol is 80 mg/100 ml, and the means for each of the
four race-sex groups are not different. Maternal serum cholesterol levels were
stratified in 50 ml increments (from: $\leq$149, 150-199, 200-249, 250-299, $\geq$300 ml/
100 ml). The means of all race-sex groups for each stratum of maternal cholesterol
are not different and indicate the total maternal cholesterol values do not predict the level of cord blood cholesterol in any of the four race-sex groups.

Using the three strata of cord blood cholesterol previously described ($\leq$68, 69-89,
$\geq$90 mg/100 ml), the mean 1972 adolescent cholesterol levels are not significantly
different; and, therefore, total cord blood cholesterol does not predict adolescent cholesterol level.

The correlation coefficient between cord blood and adolescent serum cholesterol
values for each of the race-sex groups did not show any statistically significant
differences. A total of 192 adolescents were recalled for studies in 1972 in the
approximate distribution of blacks and whites in the original 571 live births.

Turning now to the usefulness of total cord blood cholesterol levels to predict
presence of adolescent Type II hyperlipoproteinemia, it is apparent that the eleven adolescents with Type II are widely distributed across the cord blood cholesterol levels; they range from 58 to 109 mg/100 ml. The frequency of Type II hyperlipoproteinemia is not statistically different in the three strata. There were
three Type II's with cord blood cholesterol <68, three in the 69-89 cord blood
cholesterol level, and five in the >90 mg/100 ml, or 4.8, 4.4, and 8.1% respectively. Due to the small numbers, these percentages are not statistically significant, and 2 of the 5 Type II's had cord blood cholesterol levels of 90 mg/100 ml,
the value used as a cut-point. If the cut-point had been shifted to $\geq$91 mg/100 ml,
these two would have been included in the middle strata.

The frequency distribution of cord blood cholesterol of the adolescents who have
Type II hyperlipoproteinemia: two adolescents, one white female and one white

male, had cord blood cholesterol values of 90 mg/100 ml; and only one, a white female, had a cord blood cholesterol value over 100 mg/100 ml.

Glueck et al. (1971) presented data for 1800 consecutive unselected live births in a general hospital. The mean cholesterol was 63.8 $\pm$ 18.7; cord blood cholesterol levels greater than 100 mg/100 ml were arbitrarily defined as elevated based on the fact this was the mean cord blood cholesterol plus two standard deviations. In Glueck's study 3.6% of unselected live births had a blood cholesterol >100. In the Evans County study 8.3% of cord blood cholesterols were >100; however, since the mean cholesterol level was 80.3, almost 20 mg higher than the Glueck study, the value of the mean plus two standard deviations (80.3 + 2 (18,4)) would be 117 mg/ml. This represents only 1.6% of the population of Evans County.

It is unfortunate that there was no opportunity to measure the cord blood plasma concentration of low-density lipoprotein (LDL) cholesterol as reported by Kwiterovich et al. (1973). LDL cholesterol may well be a more sensitive indicator of Type II hyperlipoproteinemia in later life. Kwiterovich reported that three of twelve children re-examined one to two years after birth would have been considered normal at birth had the upper 5% for cholesterol concentration been used for diagnosis rather than LDL cholesterol. Only one observation, the white female with a cord blood cholesterol of 109 mg/100 ml, falls into upper 5% for cholesterol concentration in this Evans County study.

In summary, in a community-based study, maternal serum cholesterol did not predict cord blood cholesterol levels; in turn, cord blood cholesterol levels did not predict adolescent cholesterol of Type II hyperlipoproteinemia.

DETECTION OF FAMILIAL HYPERLIPOPROTEINEMIA BY CORD BLOOD ANALYSIS

Evan A. Stein, Dennis Mendelsohn and Israel Bersohn

In South Africa there exists a large difference in the incidence of coronary
artery disease (CAD) between the younger members, age 25-44, of the various ethnic groups. The most striking difference occurs between the Caucasian group,
which has the highest incidence in the world, and the Negroes, in whom the disease is rare. Furthermore, within the Caucasian group the Jewish and Afrikaans
sectors experience a higher incidence of CAD than the other Caucasian groups
(Schrire, 1971). In the present study an attempt was made to assess the contribution of genetically determined lipoprotein abnormalities towards CAD in South
Africa by cord blood analysis.

Methods

Neonatal serum was taken from the placental end of the umbilical cord before the
third stage of labour. Follow-up measurements were carried out on patients after
a 12-14 hour overnight fast. Total cholesterol (TC) and triglycerides (TG) were
measured on the Technicon AA II. Low density lipoprotein cholesterol (LDLC) was
calculated from the formula (Friedewald et al., 1972) LDLC = TC - (TG/5 + HDLC),
where high density lipoprotein cholesterol (HDLC) was measured in the supernatant
serum after precipitation with magnesium chloride and sodium phosphotungstate
(Burstein et al., 1971). Lipoprotein electrophoresis was carried out on Cellogel
membranes (Chemitron - Milano) which were stained with Fat Red 7B and then scanned on a Beckman Microzone densitometer.

Results

Four hundred and ninety-four Caucasian and 427 Negro neonates were screened.
Cord blood levels greater than the mean $\pm$ 2 SD were arbitarily defined as elevated. These levels were based on those found in the Caucasian group. Twenty-nine
neonates (25 Caucasian, 4 Negro) had cord blood TC levels greater than 117 mg%.
In 18 of these neonates, all Caucasian, the LDLC was greater than 66 mg%. Fifty-
five neonates (18 Caucasian, 37 Negro) had cord blood TG levels greater than 81
mg%. A highly significant difference (p <0.001) was found between the two groups
with regard to levels of TC, LDLC and TG (Fig. 1).

To data follow-up studies have been carried out on the Caucasian group. Sixteen
neonates with elevated cord blood TC and LDLC levels and 17 neonates with normal
cord blood TC and LDLC levels were re-examined at 1 and 2 years of age. Of these
33 infants both parents were studied at the time of the first yearly follow-up.
In 8 families, one of the parents - all under the age of 30 years - was diagnosed
as having hyperbetalipoproteinaemia (HBLP) (Group 1). The diagnosis of HBLP was
based on a TC greater than 250 mg%, LDLC greater than 180 mg%; elevation of the
beta-lipoprotein band on electrophoresis. In the other 8 families neither parent
had HBLP, (Group 2) and their mean TC and LDLC levels were similar to that of the
parents from the control group in which no case of HBLP was found (Fig. 2). The
infants from Group 1 showed, at one year, a mean TC level slightly higher than
the mean level of those infants from Group 2, and the control group. At the age
of 2 years, the 8 infants comprising Group 1 had a significantly (p <0.01) higher
TC than the other two groups (Fig. 2). This difference was highly significant
(p <0.001) when the LDLC levels were compared. An infant and similarly affected

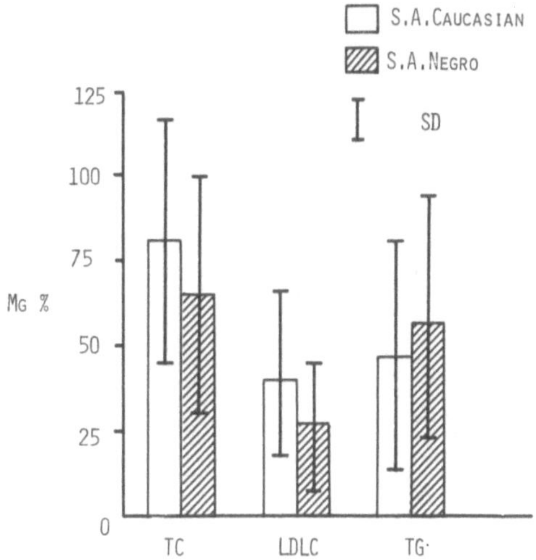

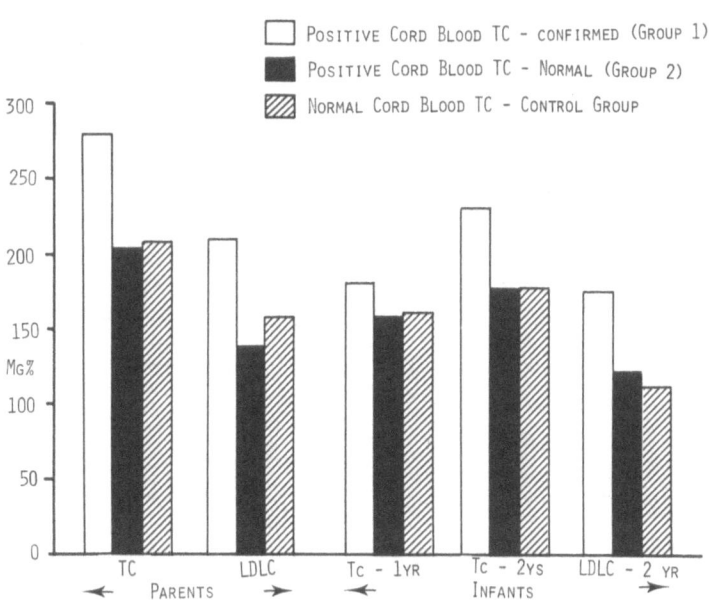

Figure 1. Mean values ± 2 SD for total cholesterol (TC) low density lipoprotein cholesterol (LDLC) and triglyceride (TG) in South African neonatal cord blood

Figure 2. Follow-up of the S.A. Caucasian group for hyperbetalipoproteinaemia – infants and parents

mother or father with HBLP was therefore identified in 8 of 494 consecutive un-selected live Caucasian births.

Fourteen infants, with elevated cord blood TG levels and 20 infants with normal cord blood levels were traced at 1 year of age. At this time both parents in all 34 cases were tested for hyperlipoproteinaemia. Six parents, from 5 families, were found to have hyperprebetalipoproteinaemia (HPHBLP) (Group 3). This was con-firmed on at least one other occasion. In all cases the fasting TG level was above 150 mg%, and the pre-beta-lipoprotein band was elevated on electrophoresis. In 9 families, were the neonates had elevated cord blood TG, (Group 4) and in parents of the 22 controls, where the cord blood TG was normal, no cases of HPBLP were found (Fig. 3). The mean TG levels in Group 4 and the control group was

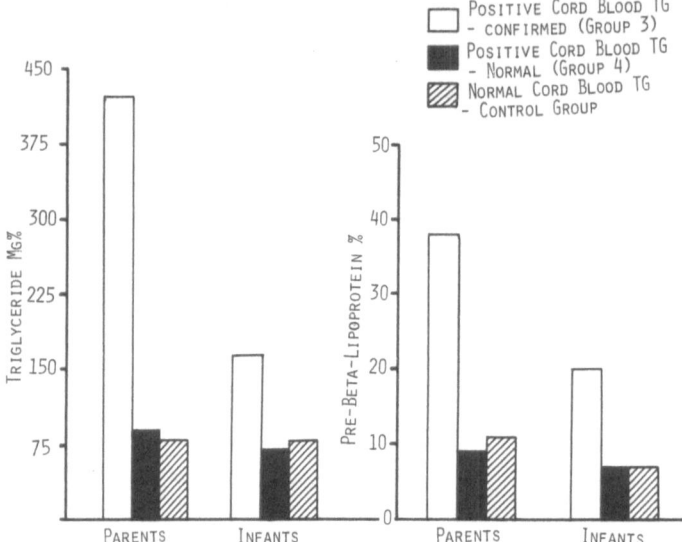

Figure 3. One year follow-up of the S.A. Caucasian group for hyperprebeta-lipo-
proteinaemia - infants and parents

66 mg% and 77 mg% respectively, with no increase in the pre-beta-lipoprotein band
on electrophoresis. At 1 year of age the infants from Group 3 were found to have
a significantly (p <0.001) higher TG level and pre-beta-lipoprotein band on electrophoresis, when compared to with those from Group 4. This difference also
existed between the infants of Group 3 and the control group (Fig. 3). A TG level
repeatedly above 220 mg% was found in the one infant whose parents both had HPBLP.
An infant and similarly affected parent with HPBLP was therefore identified in 5
of 494 consecutive unselected live Caucasian births.

Summary

This study shows that:

a) There is a significant difference in the concentrations of TC, LDLC and TG in
cord blood at birth between the South African Caucasian and Negro groups.

b) Familial HBLP and HPBLP can be identified by cord blood screening in unselected live births, although the incidence of false positives is high. The mean TC,
LDLC and TG levels ± 2 SD indicates an arbitary level above which a population at
risk can be said to exist. Confirmation of HBLP in the infant should be carried
out after 1 year, whereas HPBLP may be confirmed at a younger age.

c) The South African Caucasian group exhibits a high incidence of familial lipoprotein disorders as detected by cord blood screening (8 cases of HBLP and 5
cases of HPBLP in 494 births).

d) The incidence of familial HBLP, as found by cord blood screening, in the South
African Negro is very low.

PRE-BETA$_1$-LIPOPROTEIN: RELATIONSHIP TO ANGIOGRAPHICALLY PROVEN CORONARY HEART DISEASE AND TO Lp(a) LIPOPROTEIN

Kåre Berg, Gøsta Dahlén, Curt Erikson, Heikki Frick, Curt Furberg, and Mauri Wiljasalo

The Lp(a) antigen is a normal, genetically controlled, serum lipoprotein component demonstrable by immunological techniques. It is present in the sera of approximately 35% of healthy people of Western European extraction.

An atypical electrophoretic lipoprotein zone in the area between the ß-lipoprotein and pre-ß-lipoprotein zones was observed with a certain proportion of sera from healthy people when cellulose acetate electrophoresis was employed in a populations survey in Northern Sweden. The term pre-ß$_1$-lipoprotein was introduced for this lipoprotein component which, as judged from limited family data appeared to be governed by autosomal dominant inheritance. Comparisons between healthy people and patients with coronary heart disease with respect to presence or absence of this lipoprotein fraction suggested that it might be more frequent in people with coronary heart disease.

Certain properties of the pre-ß$_1$-lipoprotein suggested that it could be closely related, if not identical, to the lipoprotein carrying the Lp(a) antigen: the Lp(a) lipoprotein, and consequently also to the "sinking pre-ß-lipoprotein" of Rider, Levy and Fredrickson.

We wish to report the results of studying, blindly and independently, sera of 46 Finnish patients with suspected or angiographically proven coronary heart disease, with respect to Lp phenotype and presence or absence of pre-ß$_1$-lipoprotein. The purpose of this study was to investigate the possible correlation between Lp(a) antigen and pre-ß$_1$-lipoprotein and to find out if these serum lipoprotein phenomena were correlated with coronary heart disease.

Table 1. Lp(a) antigen and pre-ß$_1$-lipoprotein in 46 patients

	Number of individuals		
	Lp(a+)	Lp(a-)	Total
Pre-ß$_1$-lipoprotein present	16	1	17
Pre-ß$_1$-lipoprotein absent	11	18	29
Total	27	19	46

$x^2 = 11.73$, 1 D.F., $0.0005 < P < 0.001$.

The distribution of the 46 patients with respect to Lp(a) antigen and presence or absence of the pre-ß$_1$-lipoprotein is shown in Table 1. With the exception of one sample, all samples which exhibited the pre-ß$_1$-lipoprotein, were Lp(a+). In addition, 11 samples not exhibiting pre-ß$_1$-lipoprotein were Lp(a+). The atypical pre-ß-lipoprotein in the one exceptional sample may be distinct from pre-ß$_1$-lipoprotein as observed in most of the positive samples because it migrated distinctly slower than did pre-ß$_1$-lipoprotein in the remaining samples. Therefore, the results are compatible with the view that the immunological Lp test had revealed all samples containing true pre-ß$_1$-lipoprotein and several additional samples.

This study shows beyond any reasonable doubt that Lp(a) antigen and pre-ß$_1$-lipoprotein are indeed very closely related, and the data are compatible with the notion that pre-ß$_1$-lipoprotein is identical to the lipoprotein which carries the Lp(a) antigen: Lp(a) lipoprotein. Therefore, if pre-ß$_1$-lipoprotein occurs more frequently in patients with coronary heart disease than in healthy people, as was suggested by the studies in Northern Sweden, Lp(a) lipoprotein as revealed by antisera to the Lp(a) antigen should also occur more frequently in such patients.

Unfortunately, no extensive population study of healthy people in Finland has been conducted, with respect to Lp(a) antigen or pre-ß$_1$-lipoprotein. However, such studies have been conducted in neighboring Scandinavian countries and we have utilized the results of these studies for comparative analyses.

Table 2. Distribution of Lp phenotypes in 46 Finnish patients and in healthy Norwegians

| | Number of individuals | | |
	Lp(a+)	Lp(a-)	Total
Finnish patients	27 (59%)	19 (41%)	46
Healthy Norwegians	390 (35%)	719 (65%)	1109
Total	417	738	1155

x^2 = 9.60, 1 D.F., 0.002<P<0.005.

Table 2 shows the distribution of the Lp phenotypes in the 46 Finnish patients and in more than 1100 healthy Norwegians. There is a significant difference in the distribution of the phenotypes between the patients and the controls, the frequency of the phenotype Lp(a+) being 59% in the patients as opposed to only 35% among healthy persons.

Table 3. Occurrence of pre-ß$_1$-lipoprotein in 46 Finnish patients and in a population sample from Northern Sweden

| | Number of individuals | | |
	Pre-ß$_1$-lipoprotein present	Pre-ß$_1$-lipoprotein absent	Total
Finnish patients	17 (37%)	29 (63%)	46
Population sample from Northern Sweden	278 (23%)	951 (77%)	1229
Total	295	980	1275

x^2 = 4.35, 1 D.F., 0.03<P<0.05.

Table 3 shows a comparison between the patient group and a population sample from Northern Sweden, with respect to presence or absence of pre-ß₁-lipoprotein. The difference in distribution between the two samples is significant, 37% being positive in the patient series as opposed to only 23% in the population sample.

Thus, both Lp(a) antigen and pre-ß₁-lipoprotein occurred significantly more frequently in patients with coronary heart disease than in the healthy people.

There appeared to be a trend towards higher frequency of positives with respect to pre-ß₁-lipoprotein in the patients who had angiographically demonstrable coronary artery abnormalities: however, this trend was not statistically significant. There was, for both traits a tendency towards a higher frequency of positives in those with a positive family history with respect to coronary heart disease. However, these differences were not statistically significant. Among the patients with angiographically proven coronary artery disease, there was a statistically significant, positive correlation between smoking and presence of pre-ß₁-lipoprotein/Lp(a) antigen.

The mean plasma cholesterol value in people exhibiting pre-ß₁-lipoprotein (252 mg%) was higher than in those not possessing this component (221 mg%).

There was a tendency (not statistically significant) towards a higher cholesterol value in Lp(a+) than in Lp(a-) individuals. Those who were Lp(a+) without having the pre-ß₁-lipoprotein phenomenon had a mean cholesterol value which was practically the same as the one for Lp(a-) individuals.

From the data presented, we conclude that a strong, positive association exists between presence of Lp(a) antigen and of pre-ß₁-lipoprotein. The association suggests that the lipoprotein carrying the Lp(a) antigen: the Lp(a) lipoprotein, is closely related, if not identical, to the pre-ß₁-lipoprotein. However, lipoprotein components other than "true" pre-ß₁-lipoprotein may occasionally occur upon electrophoresis, in the area between ß-lipoprotein and regular pre-ß-lipoprotein.

Both Lp(a) antigen and pre-ß₁-lipoprotein occurred significantly more frequent in the group of patients analysed than in presumably comparable healthy populations studied previously. Thus, Lp(a) antigen/pre-ß₁-lipoprotein may represent a genetic risk factor with respect to coronary heart disease. If this is the case, the genetic background for this type of coronary heart disease may be different from that of the classical Type II hyperlipoproteinemia of Fredrickson and his coworkers, since it has been shown in other studies that no relationship exists between on the one hand Lp(a) antigen, pre-ß₁-lipoprotein and "sinking pre-ß-lipoprotein" and on the other hand hyperlipoproteinemia of Type II.

The positive association between Lp(a) antigen/pre-ß₁-lipoprotein and smoking in the most severely affected patients warrants further studies since it suggests the possibility of identifying a genetically distinct sub-population in whom smoking is particularly harmful.

Since Lp(a) antigen/pre-ß₁-lipoprotein can be determined early in life, the implications of the present results, if confirmed, for the attempts to prevent or delay manifestations of coronary heart disease are obvious.

PREVALENCE AND DISTRIBUTION OF FEMORAL ATHEROMAS IN HUMAN HYPERLIPO-PROTEINEMIA, TYPE II AND IV[*]

David H. Blankenhorn, Robert Barndt, Donald W. Crawford, Robert H. Selzer, and Edwin S. Beckenbach

The prevalence of femoral atherosclerotic lesions in Type II and Type IV hyperlipoproteinemia has been determined by performing Limited Femoral Angiography in 18 Type II and 10 Type IV patients attending a clinic for therapy of hyperlipoproteinemia. Patients studied were those willing to volunteer for femoral angiography as an experimental procedure for determination of lesion prevalence and possible guide to evaluation of their therapy. Written informed consent was obtained from all prior to angiography.

Lesion prevalence was determined from the angiograms in two ways: 1. The films were inspected visually and measurements made with a magnifying glass and micrometer caliper. 2. Films were scanned with an image dissector coupled to a digital computer. Suitable algorithms were employed to evaluate the digital data.

Limited Femoral Angiography

The patient, lightly premedicated, lay supine on the x-ray table with thigh externally rotated 45° and fixed in soft restraints. A No. 18 needle was inserted in one femoral artery below Poupart's ligament and a bolus of 20 cc 65% hypaque and 1.5 cc of 1% lidocaine was injected by hand. Fifteen films were exposed at two second intervals. Additional details of this procedure will be published.

Visual Lesion Measurement

Measurements were made on the superficial femoral artery immediately proximal to the point at which artery crosses behind the femur. Only films showing adequate filling of 20 cm of vessel and absence of motion were measured. A modification of the postmortem angiographic grading technique of Dejedar was employed (Dejedar et al., 1967). This modification provides atheroma grades equivalent to lesion grading in the International Atherosclerosis Project (early atheromas, raised lesions, complicated lesions, complicated lesions with calcification) (Guzman et al., 1968). Additional details will be published elsewhere (Crawford et al., in press).

Computer Measurements

Films were placed in an electronic image dissector. Ten centimeters of femoral artery, just proximal to the femoral crossing, were scanned perpendicular to the vessel at 25 micron intervals in steps of 25 microns. Digital data was obtained from these measurements and processed by computer. The vessel edge point in each scan line was located by determining maximum slope of film density. Edge irregularity was calculated from located edge points by comparing the results of two weighted smoothing operations, a 10 point fit and a 200 point fit. These procedures have been described previously in detail (Crawford et al., in press).

---

[*]Supported by PHS grants HL 14138 and RR-00443.

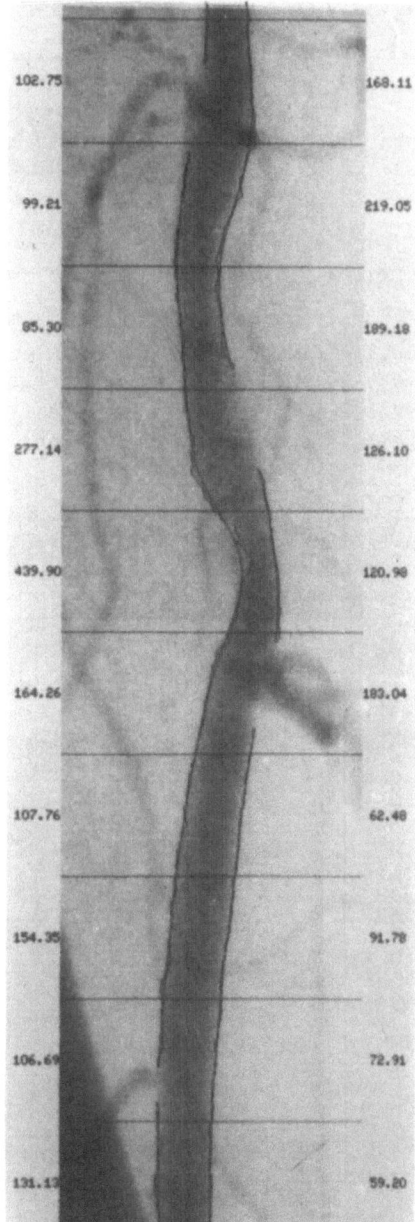

Figure 1. Femoral angiograms with computer generated edge irregularity measurements. Two curves have been fitted to each edge of the vessel and are reproduced on the figure by the computer. Edges are not drawn in areas where branches or other background shadow do not allow edge measurements to be made. The heavy non-vascular shadow at the lower left is the edge of the femur. See text for additional details

Fig. 1 illustrates edge irregularity measured by image dissector-computer for a 10 cm. segment of the angiogram of a 50-year-old man with Type IV hyperlipoproteinemia. The image shown was generated by computer following film scanning. The vessel is divided into centimeter segments and numbers at each side are average values for each segment of edge expressed as microns per scan line per centimeter. Edge irregularity exceeding 90 microns/scan line/cm. is currently considered evidence for presence of atheroma. This degree of edge irregularity can be consistently recognized by visual inspection of films. When visual inspection is compared with computer measurement of edge irregularity, the two parameters are highly correlated, r = .96; P <.001.

Table 1. Atheroma prevalence in Type II and Type IV hyperlipoproteinemia

Phenotype	Age	Previous MI	Atheroma	Advanced Atheroma (IAP III and IV)
II	20-51	11/18	17/18	6/18
IV	24-50	7/10	10/10	4/10

Table 1 presents lesion prevalence in Type II and Type IV. It should be noted that the age of patients is significantly lower than those generally studied by angiography for symptomatic peripheral vascular disease. In addition, the high prevalence of previous myocardial infarction (MI) reflects the population attracted to this clinic for hyperlipoproteinemia where emphasis is placed on therapy of cardiovascular disease. Fig. 2 shows that significant atherosclerosis was found in almost all patients (17 of 18 Type II; 10 of 10 Type IV). Significant atherosclerosis is defined for present purposes as any visible evidence of atheroma and/or vessel edge irregularity greater than 90 microns/scan line/cm. It is also noteworthy that advanced atheromas were found by visual grading in 6 of 18 Type II patients; 4 of 10 Type IV patients. Although advanced, these lesions did not cause symptoms of peripheral vascular insufficiency.

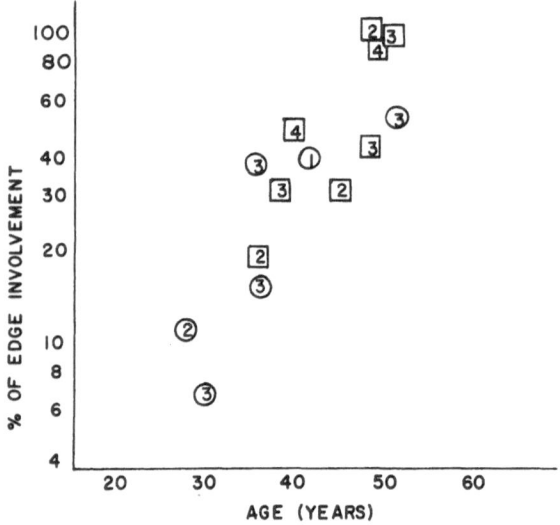

Figure 2. Relationship of age to lesion prevalence in Type II hyperlipoproteinemia. For details of figure consult text

Fig. 2 shows prevalence of lesions in Type II hyperlipoproteinemia patients as a function of age. The percent of vessel edge involved by significant atheromatosis (as previously defined) is shown on a logarithmic scale on the ordinate. Age is indicated on the abscissa. Patients indicated by squares are those with previous myocardial infarction. Patients indicated by circles had no previous infarction. The number in each patient's symbol indicates the prevalence of risk factors in addition to hyperlipoproteinemia, e.g., hypertension, smoking, diabetes, etc. A log linear increase in the percent of vessel involved by atheromatosis is shown to be a function of age little influenced by the occurrence of other additional risk factors.

These findings indicate that visible atheromas are common in the superficial femoral artery of young hyperlipoproteinemics, both those with and without previous infarction. Symptomatic peripheral vascular disease is not a prerequisite to diagnosis of femoral artery atherosclerosis in such patients. The technique for assessing atherosclerosis described here can be used for serial measurement of lesions and should be useful in evaluation of therapy.

PRIMARY HYPERLIPOPROTEINEMIAS AND OTHER RISK FACTORS IN PATIENTS WITH OCCLUSIVE ARTERIAL DISEASE OF THE LOWER LIMB

K.H. Vogelberg, H. Berger, F.A. Gries, Th. Koschinsky, W. Kübler, E. Schütz and Th. Stolze

During the past years the improved methods in discerning the disorders of lipid metabolism have shown that, besides beta lipoproteins, prebeta lipoproteins are also risk factors in the development of peripheral vascular disease (PVD)(Greenhagen et al., 1971; Kremer et al., 1973; Wollenweber et al., 1971). In order to get detailed informations of the relation between severity and localization of sclerotic lesions in PVD and lipid disorders we studied hyperlipoproteinemias (HLP) in 74 patients in whom angiography had been performed because of PVD of the lower limbs.

Methods

The concentration of triglycerides and cholesterol in the serum was determined by standard methods (Vogelberg et al., 1973). Lipoproteins were analyzed electrophoretically in agarose and by preparative ultracentrifugation (Vogelberg et al., 1973).

Glucose tolerance was tested by an oral load of 100 g glucose (Mehnert et al., 1972). Hypertension was defined as blood pressure >150 (systolic) and >90 mmHg (diastolic), obesity as overweight of >10% (Broca index). Habitual smoking was considered >5 cigarettes/d for >5 years. The sclerotic lesions were determined only by translumbal or retrograde transfemoral aortographies. The angiographies were evaluated by a point system which is demonstrated in Fig. 1: The sclerotic

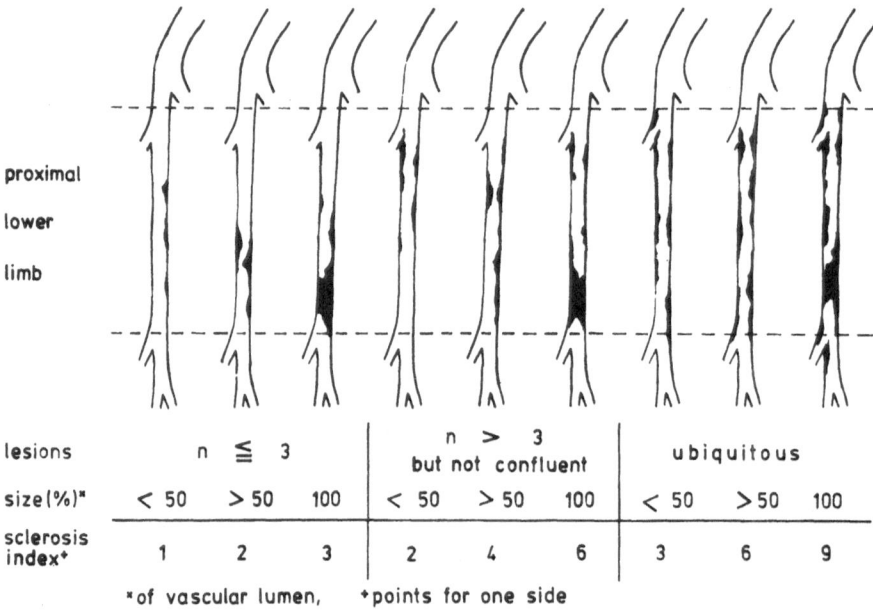

lesions	n $\leq$ 3			n > 3 but not confluent			ubiquitous		
size (%)*	< 50	> 50	100	< 50	> 50	100	< 50	> 50	100
sclerosis index+	1	2	3	2	4	6	3	6	9

*of vascular lumen,   +points for one side

Figure 1. Scheme for calculation of the sclerosis index shown for the proximal lower limb of one side

lesions of different localization could yield 1-18 points according to their severity. The points were summarized to form a sclerosis index for every vascular district (pelvis, proximal or distal lower limb).

Patients and Controls

The patients (60 men, 14 women) were admitted to the hospital for diagnosis or treatment of intermittent claudication. We selected 51 patients with primary HLP (21 of type IV, 4 of type II, 26 of type III), 9 patients with manifest diabetes mellitus, and 14 habitual smokers. Complications of atherosclerosis (gangrene, myocardial infarction) occurred above all in patients with diabetes and type IV. 86% of the patients with type IV simultaneously had two additional risk factors and at least 48% had five of them. Among smokers without any metabolic disorder the most frequent risk factor in addition was hypertension. Among patients with diabetes or HLP, except type III, at least every second person used to smoke.

The average age of the patients was between 55 (type II7 and 62 years (type IV). The age of the patients with HLP type IIa was generally lower (50 years), in diabetics without habitual smoking and without HLP it was significantly higher (68 years). Smokers who were diabetics or suffered from type IV HLP were 5 years younger than patients with the same disease who did not smoke.

The control group included 25 patients in the hospital with no intermittent claudication or other complications or atherosclerosis and were matched for age (18 men, 7 women). A disorder of glucose or lipid metabolism was not known. An angiographical examination was not carried out.

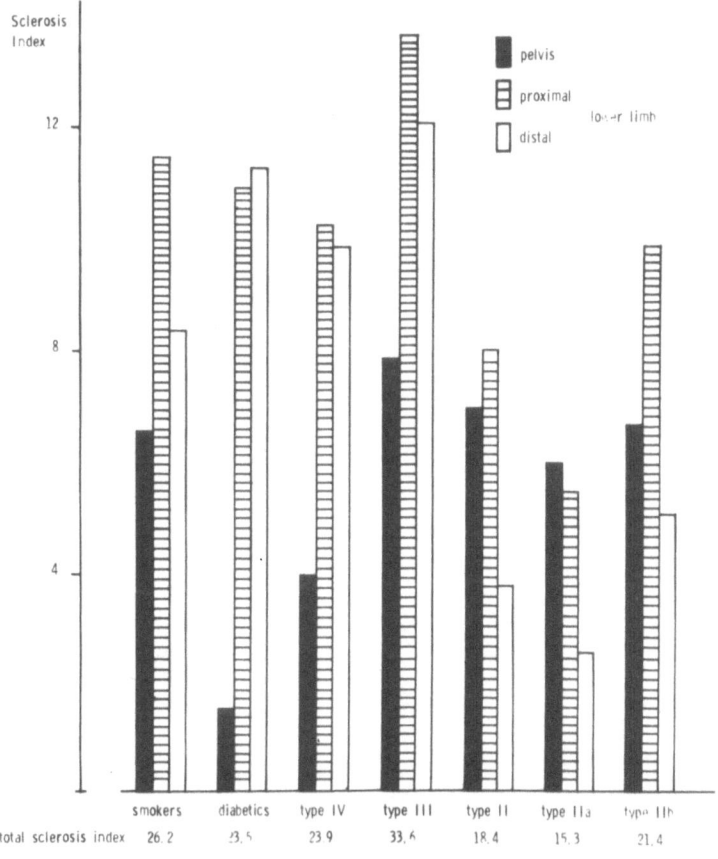

Figure 2. Severity and localization of atherosclerosis with peripheral occlusive disease according to different risk factors

489

Results

The evaluation of angiographies showed that the sclerotic lesions of PVD were more advanced among patients with hypertriglyceridemia than without an increase of triglycerides (Fig. 2). Total occlusions occurred in type IV nearly twice as often (76%) as in type II (42%). The severity of the sclerotic lesions decreased from type III to type IV and further to type IIb and finally type IIa. The sclerosis index was highest in type III, followed by smokers. It was higher in type IV than in diabetics. The gradual differences in the severity of sclerosis between type IV and III and between type IIb and IIa were similar.

Regarding the localization of the lesions it was found that arteries of the proximal lower limb were attacked preferentially in all groups except diabetics and type IV. The distribution pattern varied from group to group. A characteristic of diabetes and type IV was the minor involvement of the pelvic district.

The differences of the sclerosis pattern were more distinct when comparing type II and type IV among nonsmokers (Fig. 3). In type IV the arteries of the distal lower limb and in type IIa those of the pelvis were found to be even more sclerotic than of the proximal lower limb. It was shown that the sclerosis was worse among smokers than nonsmokers in type IV. In contrast to type IIa, habitual smokers were 5 years younger in type IV.

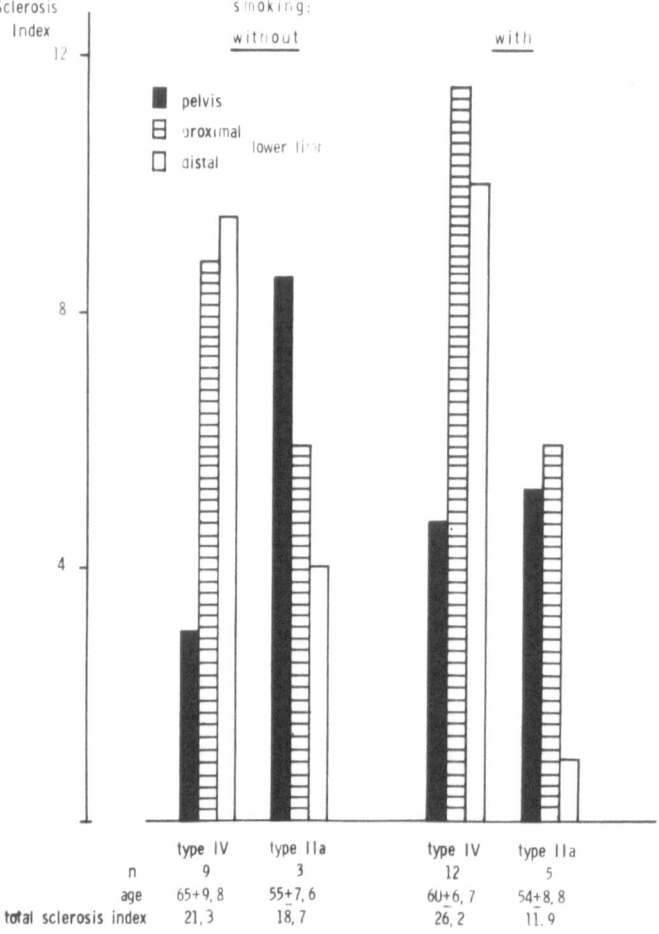

Figure 3. Influence of habitual smoking upon severity and localization of peripheral occlusive disease in primary hyperlipoproteinemia of type IV and IIa

As compared with type IV (and other HLP with raised prebeta lipoproteins), the angiographies of type IIa frequently showed a characteristic feature contrary to S-like windings of the great arteries (Schlosser et al., 1973), which could be seen mostly among older patients, constrictions like a string of pearls were only observed in type IIa.

Discussion

If we consider that the severest sclerotic lesions were seen in type III, as described by others (Zellis et al., 1970), it seems that the risk of atherosclerosis in PVD is greatest when both beta and prebeta lipoproteins are increased. Although the sclerosis index is higher in type IV than in type IIa and IIb, this does not necessarily imply a greater risk in type IV. Patients with this disease are 5-10 years older (Greenhalg et al., 1971; Slack, 1969) and most of them are suffering from additional diseases associated with sclerosis risks. Diabetes is very often seen among these patients (Knick et al., 1968; Righetti et al., 1973) and smoking seems to be a greater risk in this group than in patients with type II. In type II additional risk factors were only insignificantly higher than in controls. The frequent occurrence of type IV in PVD may be due to the fact that this disorder is less threatened by lethal complications than type II. From a functional point of view it should also be taken into account that a more proximal localization of sclerosis implies a greater risk than more distal sclerosis.

It is not known whether there is a relationship between type IIa and the morphological structure (vascular xanthomatosis) of medial sclerosis (Mönckeberg). In our opinion, the results presented as well as other information (Kannel et al., 1970; Leeren and Haarbrekke, 1971; Slack, 1969) show that in further investigations special attention should be paid to type II and III.

Summary

Angiographical examination of PVD of the lower limb of 51 patients with primary hyperlipoproteinemia, 9 patients with diabetes mellitus, and 14 habitual smokers indicated that the sclerotic risk of these factors varied. The severity of PVD of type IIa patients showed a characteristic feature of vascular atheroma, prefer ring the pelvic district, whereas in type IV patients and in diabetics the distal lower limb is preferred. Patients with type IIa and PVD were 5-10 years younger than those with type IV. Type IV was generally associated with 3 or more additional risk factors.

ATHEROSCLEROTIC LESIONS OF THE CEREBRAL ARTERIES IN YOUNG PERSONS[*]

Minoru Suzuki

Atherosclerosis in the cerebral arteries is generally believed to have a late onset. Fatty streak, or accumulation of lipid-laden cells (foam cells) and extracellular lipids in arterial intima, is usually interpreted as an early manifestation of atherosclerosis regardless of the location of major musculoelastic
arteries. However, our experimental studies on the cerebral arteries suggest that
accumulation of foam cells in the intima is a late change in advanced atherosclerotic lesions rather than an early event of intracranial atherosclerosis. Therefore, this study was undertaken in an attempt to elucidate the initiating mechanism of human intracranial atherosclerosis by investigating morphologic changes
of the cerebral arteries of young persons.

Materials and Methods

The brains removed at autopsy from 10 patients ranging from 3 months to 29 years
of age were perfused with buffered 3% glutaraldehyde through the internal carotid
and vertebral arteries within 3 to 8 hours after death. Glutaraldehyde-fixed specimens of the cerebral arteries were used for both light and electron microscopy.
Histologic sections were obtained from the anterior cerebral, middle cerebral,
posterior cerebral and basilar arteries; embedded in paraffin; cut 7 micra thick;
and stained with the hematoxylin-eosin, trichrome, aldehyde fuchsin van Gieson,
PAS and colloidal iron methods. Selected specimens were frozen-sectioned and
stained with Oil Red O solution. For electron microscopy, the samples were obtained from the anterior cerebral, middle cerebral and basilar arteries, postfixed in
buffered 1% osmium tetroxide, dehydrated through a series of ethanol-propylene
oxide, and embedded in Maraglas resin. Thin sections were doubly stained with 1%
lead citrate and 1% uranyl acetate solutions.

Results

The intracranial arteries of the patients of the *first decade* (4 cases ranging
from 3 months to 3 years of age) were normal. Normal intima of the arteries consisted of endothelium, PAS-positive thick basement membrane under the endothelium,
and internal elastic lamina (Fig. 1). However, musculoelastic intimal thickening
(intimal cushion lesion) was frequently noted at bifurcation sites of the arteries even in the youngest patient at the age of 3 months.

The intracranial arteries of the *second decade* group (3 cases at 17, 17 and 19
years of age) showed occasional foci of accumulation of small numbers of myointimal cells between the endothelial basement membrane and the internal elastic lamina (Fig. 2). Electron microscopically, the myointimal cells proved to be smooth
muscle accompanied by proliferation of collagen and appeared to have entered the
subendothelial space from the arterial media through apertures of the internal
elastic lamina (Fig. 3). Fragments of elastic fibrils, apparently newly formed
elastica, were frequently found in the region of the endothelial basement membrane.

---

[*]The postmortem materials used in this study were obtained by courtesy of Ethel
Erickson, M.D. and Sheldon Green, M.D. The study was supported by research grants
from the National Institutes of Health, USPHS (HL-05435) and from the American
Heart Association, Inc.

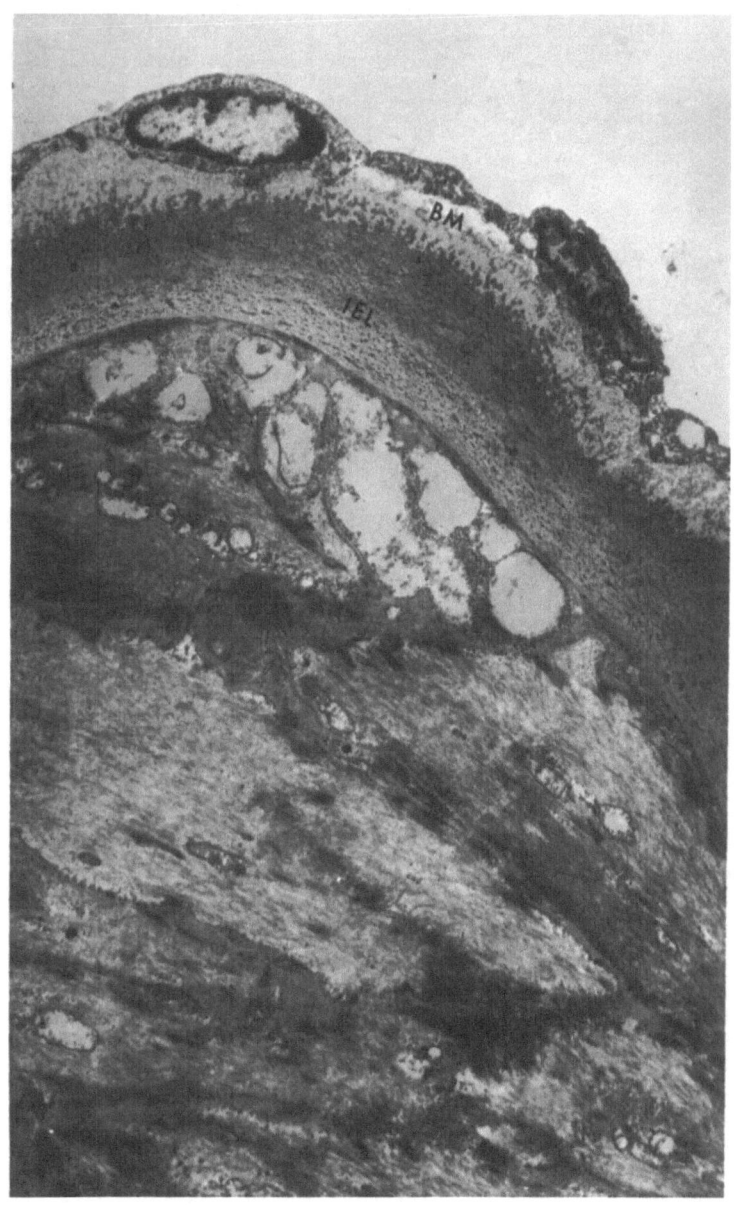

Figure 1. The anterior cerebral artery from a 19-month-old girl, showing normal intima. Normal intima of the intracranial artery consists of endothelium, thick basement membrane (BM) and internal elastic lamina (IEL)

Frozen sections of the arteries stained with Oil Red O failed to demonstrate either intracellular or extracellular lipids in the arterial intima. At the ultrastructural level, however, occasional osmiophilic intracellular and extracellular globules consistent with lipids were present in the intima, but foam cells were not found.

The intracranial arteries of the *third decade* group (3 cases at 20, 27 and 29 years of age) showed widened intimal lesions characterized by accumulation of smooth muscle cells, abundant collagen and amorphous material stainable by the

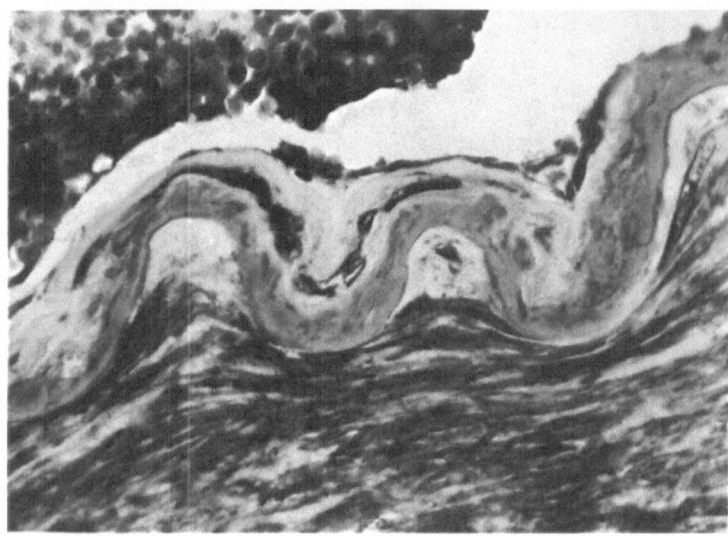

Figure 2. The middle cerebral artery of a 17-year-old woman, showing myointimal cells in the basement membrane between the endothelium and the internal elastic lamina. Masson trichrome stain (X 525)

colloidal iron method (acid mucopolysaccharide). Both intracellular and extracellular lipids were frequently found at electron microscopic level, but foam cells were uncommon.

Discussion

It is commonly held among the investigators of atherosclerosis research that fatty streaks observed in the intima of major musculoelastic arteries are an early manifestation of atherosclerosis that may progress to raised fibrous plaques or to complicated lesions. Atherosclerosis in the brain is believed by many pathologists to have a later onset (10 to 20 years) than in the coronary arteries and the aorta (Moossy, 1966). However, the results of this study indicate that early atherosclerotic changes of the cerebral arteries characterized by accumulation of smooth muscle cells in the intima occur during the second decade of life without formation of fatty streak. The emergence of smooth muscle cells accompanied by collagen between the endothelial basement membrane and the internal elastic lamina was a consistent finding in persons of the second and third decades. An observation made in this study that the smooth muscle entered the subendothelial space from the arterial media through apertures of the internal elastic lamina is consistent with similar findings in the experimental studies of the intracranial arteries (Suzuki et al., 1973) and of the non-cranial arteries (Ross et al., 1973). Intimal fatty streaks of the cerebral arteries were observed in the late third decade (Moossy, 1959), were noted later in life than those of the extracranial carotid arteries (Solberg et al., 1968), and were demonstrated in advanced atherosclerotic lesions (Hoff, 1972). In the present study, foam cells were also found in the arteries of the third decade, but minute lipid particles were recognizable both intracellularly and extracellularly in the second decade.

Conclusion

1. Intimal changes characterized by accumulation of smooth muscle cells and collagen (excluding intimal cushion lesion) develop in the intracranial arteries during

the second decade of life; 2. the smooth muscle in the arterial intima appeared to have derived from the media; and 3. fatty streak is a relatively late manifestation of the disease.

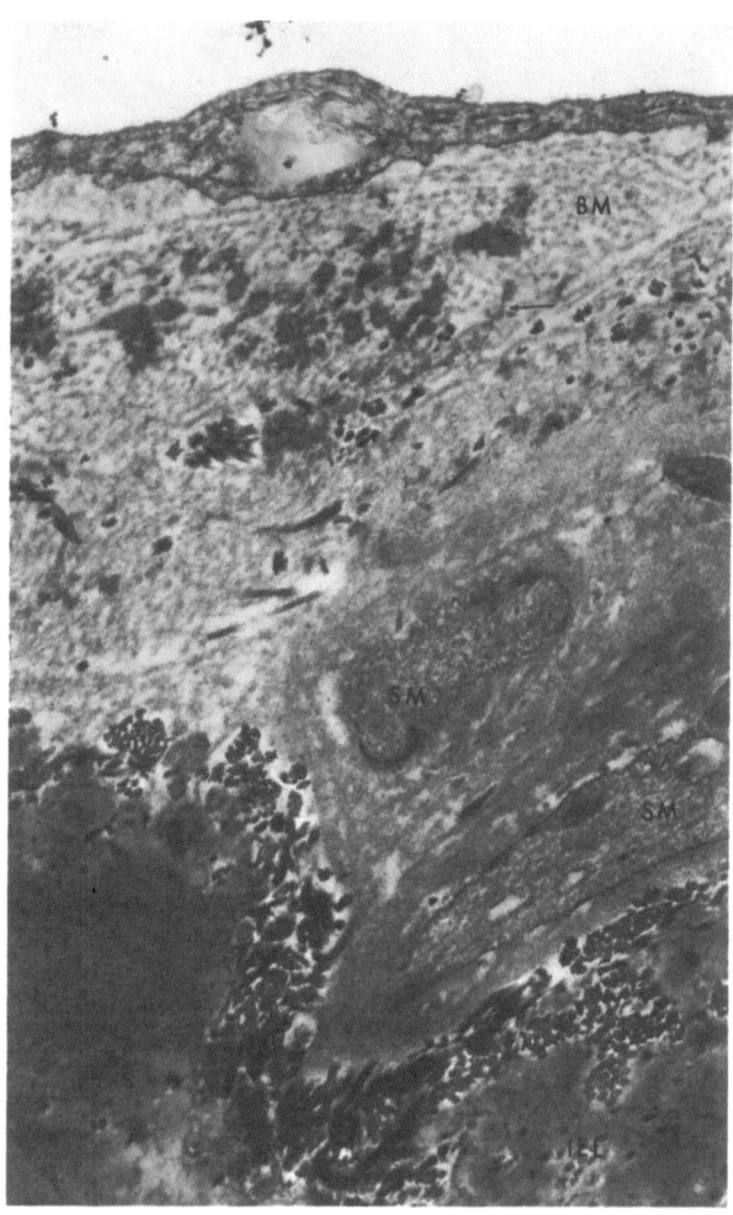

Figure 3. Intima of the middle cerebral artery from a 19-year-old woman. Smooth muscle cells (SM) appear to have entered the intima through an aperture of the internal elastic lamina (IEL). Small fragments of elastica (arrow) are recognizable in the basement membrane (BM) region under the endothelium (X 13,695)

XI

Plasma Lipids

WORKSHOP: Cholesterol and Triglyceride Metabolism in Man

Chairmen: R.J. Havel, USA
           E. Nikkilä, Finland

Participants: J. Boberg, Sweden
               G.S. Boyd, Great Britain
               H.S. Sodhi, Canada
               P.J. Nestel, Australia
               J. Glomset, USA
               A.N. Klimov, USSR

This workshop was concerned primarily with relationships between the transport of triglycerides and cholesterol in plasma lipoproteins and with their metabolism. This general topic is of increasing importance because of emerging evidence for interdependence between the transport of these two lipids and also because of the recognition that combined elevation of triglycerides (VLDL) and cholesterol (LDL) in blood plasma may be a major risk factor for atherosclerotic disease.

The session began with six presentations. J. Boberg (Uppsala) first reviewed his studies which indicate the dependence of VLDL-triglyceride secretion upon uptake of FFA in the liver in the postabsorptive state; lipogenesis in the liver and hepatic triglyceride stores may also contribute to this process. Removal of TG from the blood depends upon triglyceride hydrolysis catalyzed by lipoprotein lipase and (at least in adipose tissue) upon the capacity to esterify the resulting fatty acids. He indicated that high levels of VLDL may reflect disturbances of any of the processes that influence triglyceride secretion or removal.

G.S. Boyd (Edinburgh) followed with a review of the pathway for hepatic catabolism of cholesterol. He emphasized that the rate-limiting step in this process is the initial 7-a-hydroxylation of the ring. His studies show clear evidence for feedback inhibition of this step by bile acids and less by cholesterol -- this differs from regulation of hydroxymethyl-glutaryl-CoA reductase. He suggested that cholesterol in hepatic membranes remains in *situ* unless: 1. it is converted to cholesteryl esters; 2. it is attacked by 7-a-hydroxylase and converted to bile acids; 3. it is incorporated into lipoproteins secreted into the blood where it is subject to the lecithin-cholesterol acyltransferase (LCAT) reaction. The factors that control the utilization of hepatic cholesterol for the last of these processes are largely unknown.

H.S. Sodhi (Saskatoon) summarized his studies that indicate that catabolism of cholesterol to bile acids and excretion of neutral sterols are increased in primary hypertriglyceridemias. His work has led him to suggest that dietary cholesterol entering the liver or cholesterol newly synthesized in liver is first incorporated into plasma lipoproteins before catabolism, whereas cholesterol taken up in the liver from plasma lipoproteins is preferentially converted to bile acids. He hypothesized that catabolism of cholesterol is coupled to plasma triglyceride turnover.

P.J. Nestel (Canberra) reviewed his studies which show that increases in hepatic cholesterol synthesis, produced by treatment with bile acid-binding resins or phenobarbitone, are accompanied by increased VLDL-triglyceride and cholesterol levels. He suggested that hepatic synthesis of VLDL is a function of hepatic cholesterol synthesis.

J. Glomset (Seattle) briefly summarized his observations on patients with LCAT deficiency which support the concept that esterification of cholesterol in plasma is promoted by generation of excess polar cholesterol and lecithin associated with C-apoproteins when triglycerides are removed from chylomicrons and VLDL. Consistent with this hypothesis, abnormal VLDL and LDL rich in these lipids accumulate in the blood when patients with LCAT deficiency are fed fat-rich diets.

A.N. Klimov (Leningrad) described his studies which show that the major lipoprotein classes (VLDL, LDL and HDL) are present in the extracellular compartment of the arterial wall in man. VLDL and LDL accumulate with age and in uninvolved regions of atherosclerotic arteries, but this does not occur in veins.

The discussion following these presentations first focussed on the relationship between the formation of plasma cholesterol and cholesteryl esters on the one hand and of triglycerides on the other. Havel pointed out that, whereas nascent VLDL secreted from the Golgi apparatus of rat liver have the same content and composition of cholesteryl esters as do plasma VLDL, this may not be the case in man. K.T. Stokke (Oslo) reported that he had found no cholesterol-fatty acyl CoA transferase in human liver. Thus, in the post-absorptive state all plasma cholesteryl esters may be derived from the LCAT reaction. The amount of unesterified cholesterol entering the blood in chylomicrons and VLDL is uncertain because the content of cholesterol in newly secreted triglyceride-rich lipoproteins in man is unknown. In the rat, nascent VLDL have only about one-half as much unesterified cholesterol as plasma VLDL. The proportion of unesterified cholesterol that enter the blood in chylomicrons as opposed to VLDL is also uncertain. Whereas VLDL contain much more surface-cholesterol per unit weight of triglyceride than chylomicrons, considerably more triglyceride is usually transported in chylomicrons than in VLDL. Another uncertainty relates to the pathway of removal of chylomicron- and VLDL-cholesteryl esters in man although T. Redgrave (Melbourne) pointed out that chylomicron-cholesteryl esters are rapidly taken up in the liver of four mammalian species. Havel reported that O. Faergeman (San Francisco) has found that in the rat VLDL-cholesteryl esters are also rapidly taken up in the liver.

The discussion next turned to consideration of possible mechanisms for the increased rate of plasma cholesterol esterification and of cholesterol turnover in patients with hypertriglyceridemia. Some workers (Boberg, Havel) have found that many hypertriglyceridemic individuals do not have increased triglyceride turnover whereas others who use different methods (Reaven, Nikkilä) believe that triglyceride turnover is usually increased. One possibility for coupling of plasma cholesterol esterification to concentration of triglycerides was suggested by Havel: transfer of cholesteryl esters from HDL to the "core" of VLDL may facilitate the action of LCAT on HDL. If so, the reaction may be "pulled" by increased availability of VLDL-oil phase in hypertriglyceridemia rather than "pushed" by increased generation of surface lipids related to increased triglyceride turnover. Glomset and others have obtained evidence that is consistent with the "pull" mechanism. C. Fielding (San Francisco) pointed out that the bulk of plasma HDL may be far from an optimal substrate for LCAT since they contain a large amount of cholesteryl esters which are known to inhibit the reaction. Thus, rate of esterification *in vitro* may not reflect the dynamic situation *in vivo*.

If the action of LCAT is primarily to "scavenge" surface lipids related to triglyceride-transport, its action should be reduced in abetalipoproteinemia. Glomset observed that this appears to be the case. Ordinarily, LCAT-derived cholesteryl esters, largely transferred from HDL to LDL and VLDL, eventually enter the liver. The relationship of the extent of this transport to cholesterol catabolism and excretion was next discussed. The magnitude of these two processes appears to be similar; however, it was pointed out by several participants that the situation is very complex and no firm conclusions can presently be drawn.

Finally, the relationship between the lipoprotein vehicles for cholesterol and triglyceride to the accumulation of lipids in the arterial wall was discussed briefly. O. Stein (Jerusalem) stated that the pinocytotic pathway across arterial endothelial cells should transport particles up to 500-700 A diameter. In accord with this proposition, Klimov reported that he had been unable to produce arterial lesions by repeated intravenous injections of chylomicrons in rabbits.

A number of unsolved problems discussed in this workshop are susceptible to experimental attack. Elucidation of the complex relationships between cholesterol and triglyceride transport and metabolism should substantially increase our understanding of the regulation of plasma lipoprotein levels and the interrelationships among them.

METABOLIC STUDIES IN HYPERLIPIDAEMIA

Paul J. Nestel

Hypercholesterolaemia

Primary Hypercholesterolaemia. Several groups have published data based on common techniques and their findings may therefore be pooled. The sterol balance techniques provide information on the synthesis, absorption and turnover of cholesterol and on the turnover of bile acids. One finding that has emerged clearly is that metabolic hypercholesterolaemia occurring alone, and hypercholesterolaemia in association with hypertriglyceridaemia, are quite distinct. In most other respects, we are not close to understanding primary hypercholesterolaemia. I will now examine the various possibilities: 1. increased absorption; 2. increased synthesis; 3. diminished excretion; 4. inadequate feedback of endogenous synthesis by dietary cholesterol; 5. diminished clearance of the plasma pool of cholesterol implying a mal-distribution between the plasma and tissue pools of cholesterol.

The importance of dietary cholesterol as a determinant of the serum cholesterol level has become firmly re-established. Furthermore, it now seems unlikely that the absorption in man is limited to a few hundred milligrams. Recent long-term studies by Quintao et al. (1971) and by Kudchodkar et al. (1973) show that much greater amounts can be absorbed if the intake is high enough. At intakes of up to a 1g per day, about half may be absorbed; at higher intakes the fractional absorption becomes less. Dr. Sodhi has recently collated the data from his own and other workers' studies, notably from the Rockefeller University group: the relationship between intake and absorption was similar for most subjects irrespective of the type of hyperlipoproteinaemia. Allowing for the error of the methodology, hypercholesterolaemic subjects do not absorb excessive cholesterol provided they do not eat more than others and there is no evidence to suggest the latter. This implies that the reabsorption of the endogenous biliary cholesterol (about 1g/day) is also normal.

It has been suggested that the total synthesis of cholesterol and in particular that of bile acids is reduced in primary hypercholesterolaemia. I have compared the faecal excretion of these sterols in groups of subjects whose dietary intake was less than 100 mg per day: excretion therefore virtually equalled synthesis. Fig. 1 shows that 48 subjects with hypercholesterolaemia (in excess of 280 mg/100 ml) but normal serum triglyceride levels had values that were of the same order as 23 normocholesterolaemic subjects, when expressed per unit body weight. Only Miettinen's patients appeared to excrete less bile acids (Miettinen, 1971; Grundy and Ahrens, 1969; Grundy et al., 1969; Connor et al., 1969; Nestel, unpublished observations). The values in 11 New Guinea males, whose habitual intake of cholesterol is virtually zero, are of a similar order (Whyte and Nestel, unpublished observations). By contrast, in 22 subjects who were primarily hypertriglyceridaemic and in whom the raised serum cholesterol was attributable solely to an increase in very low density lipoproteins, bile acid production was clearly raised. Neutral sterol synthesis has not been plotted, because this is influenced by dietary cholesterol, which was greater than 100 mg per day in these subjects (Grundy and Ahrens, 1969; Miettinen, 1971; Sodhi et al., 1973; Nestel, unpublished observations).

Since dietary cholesterol has at most only a minimal effect on bile acid excretion in man, the production of bile acids in hypercholesterolaemia has been re-examined in a larger group consuming varying amounts of cholesterol. Fig. 2 shows that there is indeed a trend for patients with primary hypercholesterolaemia to

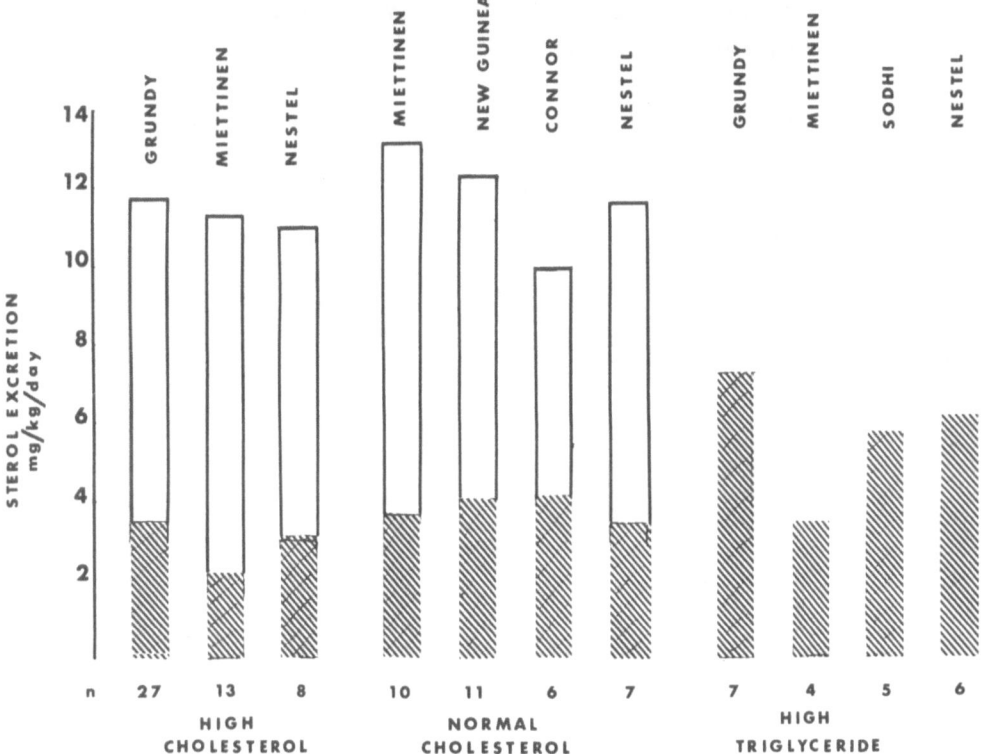

Figure 1. Sterol excretion in subjects with hypercholesterolaemia (>280 mg/100 ml) and normocholesterolaemia (<250 mg/100 ml), eating diets containing less than 100 mg cholesterol/day. (Bile acids = shaded area; total sterols = total area.) Bile acid excretion only is shown in hypertriglyceridaemia subjects (normal LDL cholesterol levels)

excrete less bile acid. The Figure also shows that the enhanced production in hypertriglyceridaemic subjects does not merely reflect overweight: 13 very obese subjects with normal plasma lipids, showed bile acid excretion which though increased (Nestel et al., 1973; Hunter and Nestel, unpublished), was nevertheless less than in the hypertriglyceridaemic subjects.

This difference in bile acid production was demonstrated initially by Kottke (1969) and more recently confirmed by Einarsson and Hellstrom (1972) who showed that hypercholesterolaemic subjects secreted less than normal amounts of biliary bile acids whereas this was raised in hypertriglyceridaemic subjects.

Despite their reduced production of bile acid (about which opinion is certainly not unanimous), hypercholesterolaemic subjects have a normal turnover of exchangeable body cholesterol. Fig. 3 shows data obtained from multicompartmental analysis by Samuel et al. (1973) using a 3-pool model, and by Nestel et al. (1969), Grundy and Ahrens (1969) and Sandhofer et al. (1972) whose 2-pool analyses have been reduced by 10% to make them comparable with Samuel's data. The values in 36 moderate to severe hypercholesterolaemic subjects resemble those in 32 normocholesterolaemic subjects. This may imply lesser conversion of cholesterol to bile acids as proposed by Miettinen, although the ratio of endogenous neutral sterol to bile acid excretion has been reported to be normal by others.

There is little evidence to suggest that feedback inhibition of synthesis is deficient in primary hypercholesterolaemia. Firstly, cholesterol turnover is not

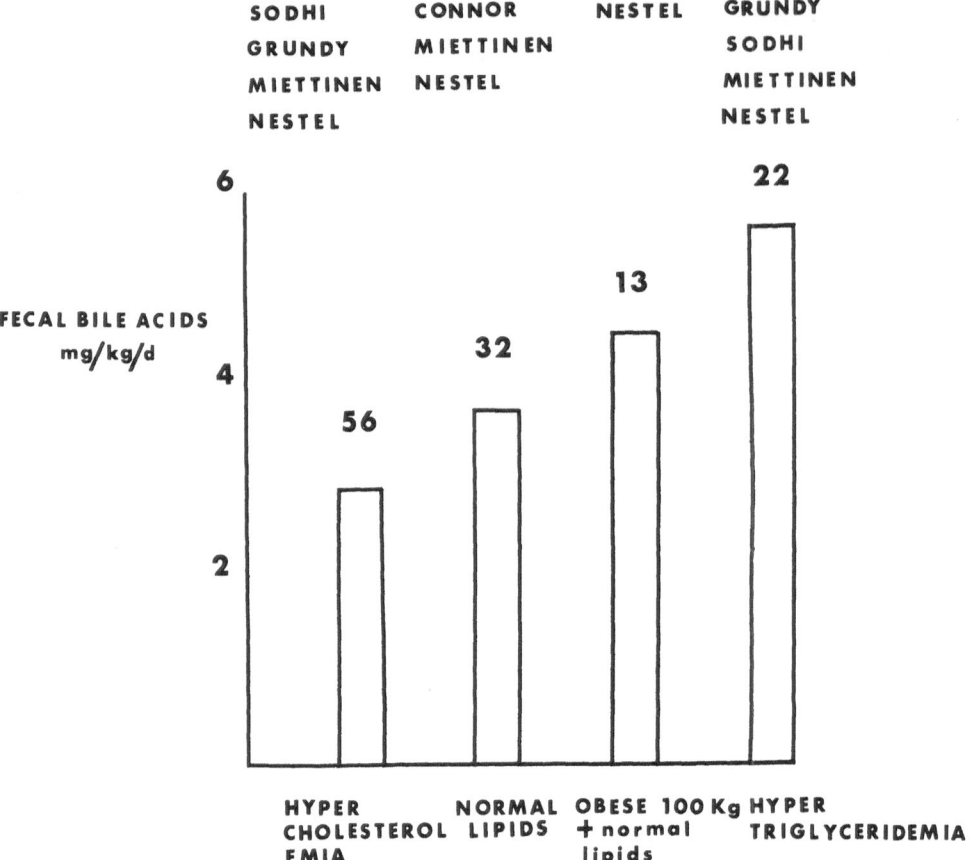

Figure 2. Faecal bile acid excretion in hyperlipidaemia and in obesity

raised and secondly, subjects in whom this problem has been specifically examined, show an appropriate degree of feedback inhibition, when reasonable amounts of cholesterol are eaten. We have shown that these patients respond sensitively to the relatively small increase of 216 mg/day (from 94 to 310) (Fig. 4). In the studies of Quintao et al. (1971) feedback inhibition and other compensatory mechanisms were overwhelmed in some subjects by 2-3g of dietary cholesterol. Interestingly, however, the retention of large amounts of dietary cholesterol was not reflected in marked increases in the serum levels. If inhibition of synthesis is appropriate for the change in absorption, then why does the serum concentration remain elevated? Does the initial expansion in the plasma pool alter the equilibrium between plasma and tissues?

Hypercholesterolaemia, defined as an increase in low density lipoprotein cholesterol is more likely to occur when cholesterol turnover is low than when it is high. It is low in hypothyroidism (Miettinen, 1970) and in the hypercholesterolaemia of anorexia nervosa (Nestel, unpublished observation). By contrast, serum cholesterol levels are not raised and may be low with resin therapy (Grundy et al., 1971; Goodman and Noble, 1968; Miller et al., 1973) even though the increase in synthesis appears to compensate for the increased loss. Other conditions with normal LDL cholesterol levels despite increased cholesterol turnover include Type 4 hyperlipoproteinaemia (Sodhi and Kudchodkar, 1973), and obesity (Nestel et al., 1973).

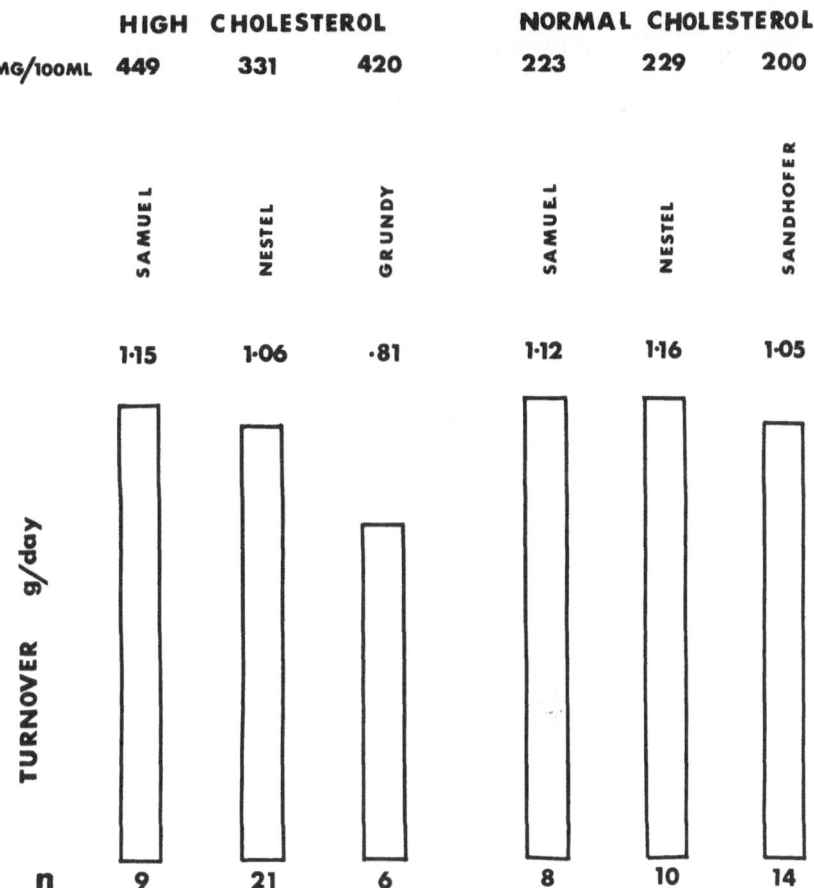

	HIGH CHOLESTEROL			NORMAL CHOLESTEROL		
MG/100ML	449	331	420	223	229	200
	SAMUEL	NESTEL	GRUNDY	SAMUEL	NESTEL	SANDHOFER
	1·15	1·06	·81	1·12	1·16	1·05
n	9	21	6	8	10	14

Figure 3. Comparison of cholesterol turnover in normocholesterolaemic and hyper-cholesterolaemic subjects (measured by isotope kinetics)

The amount of exchangeable cholesterol in the body does not appear to be increased even in severely hypercholesterolaemic subjects. This has been shown clearly for the rapidly exchanging pool A when the amount in the plasma is excluded (Nestel et al., 1969; Goodman and Noble, 1968). In the only study in which the slowly exchanging pools have also been adequately quantified, there is no relation between pool size and serum cholesterol concentration (Samuel et al., 1973).

This suggests that, in hypercholesterolaemia, a disproportionate fraction of the body's cholesterol is retained in the plasma, that is, the clearance of plasma cholesterol is inappropriately low in relation to the concentration. Research is therefore being directed at the regulation of the influx and efflux of cholesterol from plasma, the affinity of cholesterol for lipoproteins, the enzymes in the plasma that participate in cholesterol transport. Only a few points will be examined.

The metabolic fate of the protein component of low density lipoprotein resembles that of the cholesterol: the total turnover is normal though the fraction removed from plasma per unit time is decreased (Langer et al., 1972).

The influx of newly synthesized cholesterol believed to occur within very low density lipoprotein, can be studied in circumstances such as when turnover is stimulated by a bile acid-binding resin. Fig. 5 shows that this influx is not

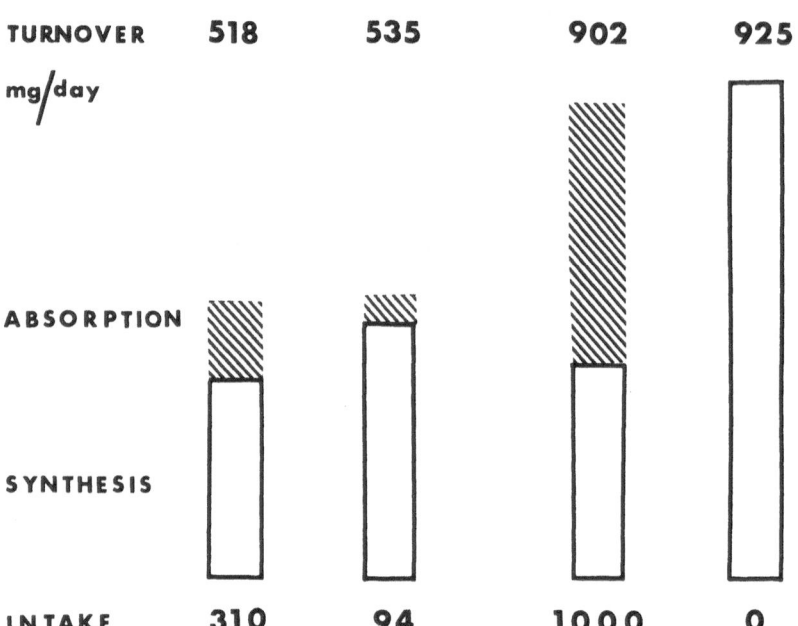

Figure 4. Cholesterol synthesis and absorption measured at 2 levels of cholesterol intakes in 4 hypercholesterolaemic patients and in 3 New Guinea males who habitually eat no cholesterol

significantly different from normal in primary hypercholesterolaemia. Nor is the efflux from low density lipoproteins diminished. On the other hand the influx is greatly increased in hypertriglycerideaemia (Miller, Clifton-Bligh and Nestel, unpublished observations). This is in accord with the previous observation that the turnover of plasma esterified cholesterol, measured by an in vivo technique, is significantly greater in hypertriglyceridaemic than in either normal or hypercholesterolaemic subjects (Nestel, 1970). Since this transport is mediated by the enzyme lecithin cholesterol acyl transferase, it is interesting to note the recent findings of Akanuma et al. (1973) that LCAT activity was also increased in hypertriglyceridaemic, overweight subjects.

Finally, hypercholesterolaemia is only the common manifestation of probably several genetically determined disorders. The non-uniformity in the responses to dietary cholesterol among the subjects studied by Quintao et al. (1971) illustrate the variety of metabolic disturbances that might characterize hypercholesterolaemia.

In summary then, primary hypercholesterolaemia is characterized by diminished clearance of cholesterol from an expanded plasma pool, possibly reflected in reduced bile acid excretion. Total cholesterol turnover and the amount of exchangeable body cholesterol are probably not increased. Dietary cholesterol leads to normal suppression of cholesterol synthesis. However, where hypercholesterolaemia

occurs together with hypertriglyceridaemia, then cholesterol synthesis and turnover, as well as bile acid production, are increased. In general, stimulating
cholesterol turnover lowers the plasma cholesterol concentration.

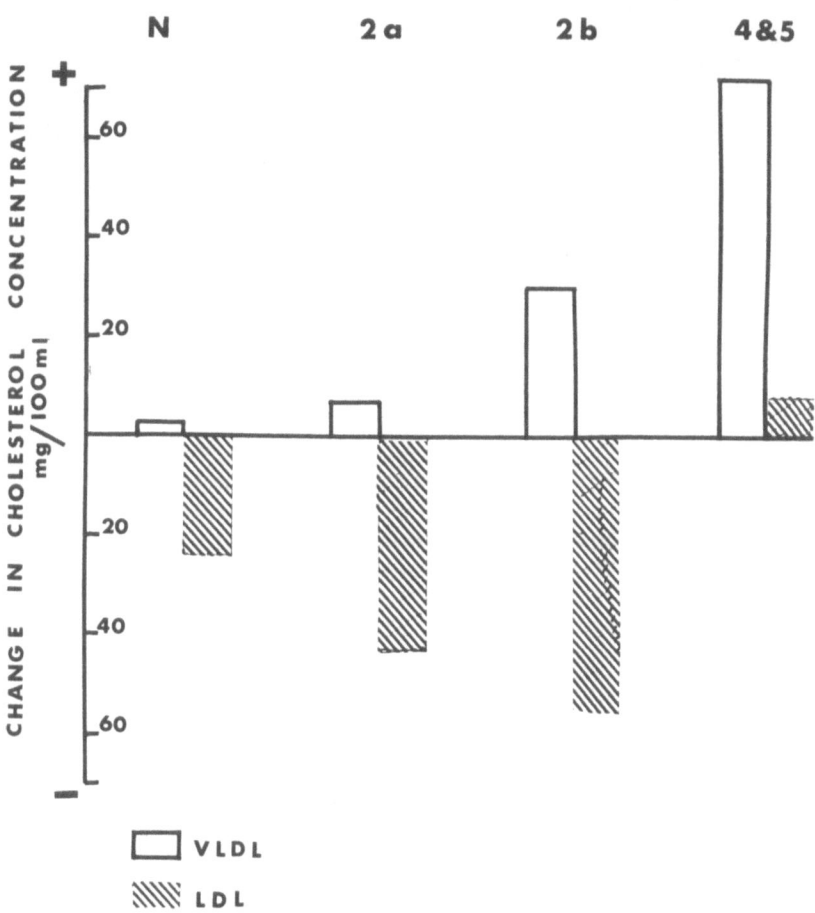

Figure 5. Influx of cholesterol into VLDL and efflux from LDL during colestipol
therapy - differences in the hyperlipoproteinaemias

Hypertriglyceridaemia

I will confine myself to several aspects of endogenous hypertriglyceridaemia. In
contrast to measurements of cholesterol turnover, the validity of the several
models of triglyceride turnover remains doubtful.

Since the rise in the plasma triglyceride concentration reflects changes in inflow or in outflow, one could establish the relative importance of overproduction
and deficient removal if the turnover of plasma triglyceride could be measured.
Both overproduction and inefficient removal might operate simultaneously especially since changes in inflow probably vary throughout the day, even with fat-free
diets, since the triglyceride concentration fluctuates appreciably during the day
and night even when carbohydrate-rich, fat-free diets are eaten. This suggests
that inflow and outflow of plasma triglyceride are not in balance throughout the
24 h and a measure of triglyceride turnover taken during only one phase of the
diurnal flux will only partly describe the basis for the hypertriglyceridaemia.

Most studies have hitherto been carried out during the fasting state, generally some 16 h after the last meal; findings from such studies may give incomplete information about the events that initiate the rise in the plasma triglycerides.

Without doubt, the most direct and accurate quantification of hepatic triglyceride production by isotopic means has been provided by the studies of Havel et al. (1970) and Boberg et al. (1972). By infusing radiopalmitate at a constant rate and measuring hepatic blood flow and the appearance of label in TGFA, the rate of secretion of labelled TGFA was obtained from the difference between the hepatic venous and arterial values and TGFA production was calculated from this value and the specific activity of hepatic venous FFA. In Havel's studies, the turnover of TGFA in a small group of hypertriglyceridaemic subjects was about 30% higher than among normotriglyceridaemic subjects, due to a greater hepatic uptake of FFA among the former. In this small group no correlation was found between TGFA production and triglyceride concentration. The studies were carried out for only 4 h, which was not sufficiently long to establish clear isotopic equilibration between VLDL-TGFA and plasma FFA among the hypertriglyceridaemic subjects, and so a possible underestimate of TGFA inflow was not excluded. At least 3 of their subjects were clearly overweight and, as has been suggested by Barter and Nestel (1973), hepatic fatty acids may be an additional source of VLDL-TGFA in obese subjects.

The studies of Boberg et al. (1972) also suggest that this technique may underestimate TGFA inflow especially in hypertriglyceridaemia. They base this on a comparison with two other methods that they had carried out in a large number of normal and in 14 hypertriglyceridaemic subjects. The first of these additional measurements is the chemical determination of the venous-arterial difference in the triglyceride concentration across the liver: the 'chemical triglyceride secretion', for which an analytical error of less than 2% is being claimed.

Since the isotopic secretion method appeared to give similar results to the chemically measured rates only at lower TGFA turnovers, it seems likely that the turnover was underestimated in Havel's hypertriglyceridaemic subjects. In the studies by Boberg et al. (1972), several of the hypertriglyceridaemic subjects clearly secreted more triglyceride as calculated by the direct chemical and the clearance methods. Overall, there was a significant correlation between the concentration and inflow transport of triglyceride among the hypertriglyceridaemic but not the normotriglyceridaemic subjects. Thus, the hypertriglyceridaemic subjects, although few in number, appeared to fall into a group with normal and another with raised triglyceride production. Since, in the majority of subjects, a very high correlation was found between TGFA inflow and the splanchnic extraction of FFA, it seemed likely that among that small group of hypertriglyceridaemic 'overproducers' in whom this correlation did not hold, the additional TGFA was derived from a hepatic source of fatty acids. Whether this alone implies a heterogeneous aetiology for endogenous hypertriglyceridaemia, a very likely possibility for a variety of other reasons, is uncertain. The preceding dietary intake of carbohydrate and the amount of stored hepatic fatty acid might account for such findings. The hypertriglyceridaemic group as a whole was homogeneous in one respect: the fractional turnover rate was low in all, indicating some degree of impairment of removal mechanisms.

To summarize the data derived from the studies of Havel et al. and Boberg et al., in terms of triglyceride kinetics, endogeneous hypertriglyceridaemia represents a heterogeneous disorder. Whereas the fractional removal of the expanded triglyceride pool is reduced in most hypertriglyceridaemic subjects in the fasting state, increased production of triglyceride has also been reported in a proportion of these subjects. This results from an increased hepatic uptake of FFA and from an additional source of hepatic fatty acids that may reflect increased lipogenesis from carbohydrate.

An older and much simpler technique is based on the rate of removal of triglyceride radioactivity from the plasma following the injection of a radioactive precursor such as glycerol or FFA. The problems of interpretation have been widely discussed but probably deserve restating since several very interesting studies utilizing this technique have been reported quite recently.

Studies in man by Carlson (1960) and Havel (1961) showed that following the injection of radiopalmitic acid, the initial portion of the specific radioactivity-time curve of plasma TGFA was exponential; from the area below the TGFA specific activity curve they calculated the fractional conversion of plasma FFA to TGFA. This was extended by Farquhar et al. (1965) and Reaven et al. (1965) who substituted radiolabelled glycerol for palmitic acid as precursor, calculating the fractional turnover rate from the half-time of removal of radioactivity in VLDL.

The crucial assumption in Farquhar's model is that the labelled precursor, glycerol, becomes incorporated into hepatic triglyceride and discharged into the plasma at a rate that is very much faster than the rate of removal of triglyceride from the plasma. However, this does not now appear to be true from the later studies of Quarfordt et al. (1970) which suggest that the turnover characteristics of the VLDL triglyceride pool are very similar to those of the immediate precursor pool in the liver. Significant amounts of labelled triglyceride would therefore continue to be discharged from the liver into the plasma VLDL during the period when measurements of the disappearance rate of VLDL radioactivity are being carried out. The specific radioactivity curve of the VLDL triglyceride would therefore represent both continuing inflow of label from the liver and outflow of label from the plasma whereas the assumption of Farquhar et al. was that it reflected outflow alone. Values for triglyceride turnover obtained by this method are appreciably less than the probable true values as discussed by Shames et al. (1970).

Furthermore, in studies carried out during high carbohydrate diets, the labelled precursor would not constitute the sole precursor, which would further underestimate the turnover.

This approach has been extended by Eaton et al. (1969) and Quarfordt et al. (1970) who used the method of multicompartmental analysis developed by Berman. Several models that appeared to be consistent with possible physiological pathways in the metabolism of FFA and TGFA, were constructed from the correspondence of the observed data with calculated data obtained with a digital computer.

These prolonged studies took into account the late curvilinear portion of VLDL-TGFA specific activity curves that could be explained only on the basis of several pools of fatty acids along the pathway of TGFA formation or some recycling of label. The inflow transport of TGFA was consistently higher with the high-carbohydrate diets which appeared to occur by way of a postulated slow conversion pathway. These studies also suggested that this increased conversion was brought about by greater diversion of FFA from pathways of oxidation and ketone-formation to production of TGFA. A similar mechanism has been put forward to account for the increased production of VLDL-TGFA in response to ethanol (Nestel and Hirsch, 1965; Wolfe et al., 1973).

Quarfordt et al. also observed a reduction in the fractional removal rate of VLDL-TGFA although they concluded that an increase in glyceride production from plasma FFA was the likeliest single prime pertubation brought about by high carbohydrate consumption.

Another important aspect of the studies of Quarfordt et al. was the finding that subjects with normotriglyceridaemia and those with endogenous hypertriglyceridaemia responded to carbohydrate diets with similar increments in triglyceride inflow. When studied in the fasting state after habitual diets both groups produced similar amounts of triglyceride but the subjects with endogenous hypertriglyceridaemia had significantly lower fractional removal rates.

Nikkila and Kekki (1971) who have used the Farquhar model extensively have also recognized the problems of deviation from the single exponential in the specific radioactivity curve of plasma triglyceride after injecting radioglycerol (though they did not analyze VLDL separately). They believed this to reflect the presence of a slow hepatic 'storage or non-secreting' pool with delayed secretion of label-led triglyceride, and to early recycling of label, especially when clearance of triglyceride was rapid. In contrast to the conclusions of Reaven et al. (1965) who concluded that in a normolipidaemic population the plasma triglyceride concentration was determined only by triglyceride inflow and not by clearance mechanisms, Nikkila and Kekki have observed variability in both inflow and clearance.

They have reported reduced fractional removal of triglyceride in hypothyroidism (Nikkila and Kekki, 1972). Among diabetics, they observed increased triglyceride turnover in non-ketotic adults and juveniles, though the fractional removal was low in severely hypertriglyceridaemic subjects (Nikkila and Kekki, 1973). Some reservations must be held about data derived with this technique and there is also a strong possibility that in diabetics, hepatic triglyceride stores might also contribute significantly to circulating TGFA (Basso and Havel, 1970).

Since many of the models that describe triglyceride transport are based on the relationship between plasma FFA and TGFA, changes in FFA transport must alter TGFA kinetics.

In the studies of Havel et al. (1970) and of Boberg et al. (1972) splanchnic up-take was highly correlated with FFA turnover, especially that fraction of the turnover that originated in splanchnic adipose tissue.

The magnitude of FFA transport might, therefore, be expected to determine the amount of FFA incorporated into plasma triglyceride and possibly the triglyceride concentrations. Studies by both Havel et al. (1970) and Boberg et al. (1972) do show significant correlations between the plasma FFA turnover and the secretion of TGFA from the liver as calculated from the appearance of radioactivity in the hepatic vein during constant infusions of radiopalmitate. In other studies by Sailer et al. (1966) and by Nestel (1967) in which the appearance of radioactivity in TGFA has been measured in peripheral and not hepatic veins during radio-palmitate infusions, similar correlations with FFA turnover have also been shown.

A correlation between plasma FFA turnover and the plasma triglyceride concentration has been reported by Nestel et al. (1970) among subjects with endogenous hypertriglyceridaemia on carbohydrate-rich diets. Recently, Boberg et al. (1972) have also observed a significant correlation between plasma FFA turnover and the plasma triglyceride concentration among hypertriglyceridaemic but not among nor-motriglyceridaemic subjects. Sailer et al. (1966) had previously reported signi-ficantly elevated concentrations of plasma FFA in patients with essential hyper-lipaemia.

Bolzano et al. (1972) have noted in hypertriglyceridaemic subjects a less effec-tive suppression of plasma FFA levels with sucrose than in normal subjects; hence, the esterification rate of FFA to TGFA was raised in hypertriglyceridaemia.

The relative importance of plasma FFA, in contra-distinction to glucose, as the substrate for plasma TGFA during high-carbohydrate diets, has recently been stud-ied in man by Barter and Nestel (1972). The proportion of VLDL-TGFA derived from circulating FFA was obtained from the ratio of specific radioactivities of VLDL-TGFA:FFA during prolonged constant infusions of radiopalmitic acid. This can be calculated as soon as the product (VLDL-TGFA) has reached isotopic equilibrium with its precursors, when its specific radioactivity also becomes constant. Fol-lowing 3 days of sustained carbohydrate feeding and while glucose was being con-sumed, plasma FFA accounted for as little as 10% of VLDL-TGFA. This contribution increased in the postabsorptive state, but even 20 h later reached only 70%. Con-versely up to 80% of TGFA was derived from glucose as measured from the incorpora-tion of ^{14}C-glucose (Barter et al., 1972). Since the labelling of VLDL-TGFA pre-ceded that of plasma FFA, it was concluded that liver was the site of lipogenesis.

The interrelationship of plasma FFA and triglyceride has also been studied by Barter et al. (1971) during alternating periods of sucrose consumption during the day and fasting by night. During the course of these pure sucrose diets, both the plasma triglyceride and FFA concentrations fell during the day and rose markedly only during the night; these diurnal fluctuations in triglyceride levels have also been reported by Schlierf and Dorow (1973). The significant correlations between the changes in FFA and triglyceride concentration suggest that part of the nocturnal rise in triglycerides is mediated by the flux of FFA.

The nocturnal increments of both lipids could be suppressed by infusions of insulin, although these findings may be equally related to enhanced clearance of triglyceride. Schlierf and Dorow were also able to suppress the nocturnal rise in triglyceride by giving nicotinic acid. The hypertriglyceridaemia during carbohydrate-rich diets may therefore be related to several factors: a) removal may diminish during the night as the plasma insulin level falls; b) production from plasma FFA may rise during the night when FFA turnover rises, and c) production from lipogenesis continues through the night with very high carbohydrate diets, though probably at a slower rate than during the day.

Wolfe (1972) has recently shown enhanced secretion of newly synthesized TGFA from the liver in obese subjects eating carbohydrate diets.

Finally, there is recent evidence other than from turnover studies for impaired clearance mechanisms in endogenous hypertriglyceridaemia. Human chylomicrons, infused intravenously, are removed at a rate that is inversely related to the endogenous triglyceride concentration (Nestel, 1964). Persson et al. (1972) have reported a significant inverse correlation between the plasma triglyceride concentration and the activity of lipoprotein lipase in adipose tissue. A preliminary report by Brunzell et al. (1972) suggests that plasma post-heparin lipolytic activity may become more readily depleted in those subjects with endogenous hypertriglyceridaemia in whom deficient removal of triglyceride can also be demonstrated by turnover techniques.

In this section I have stressed the importance of plasma FFA in determining the plasma TG level and have suggested that this may be more significant than lipogenesis from glucose. I have emphasized that periods of increased production alternate with periods of diminished removal and that until this distinction can be clearly identified it will not be possible to be certain which of these two mechanisms initiates a particular form of hypertriglyceridaemia.

CORRELATION OF KINETIC PARAMETERS OF CHOLESTEROL METABOLISM WITH SERUM CHOLESTEROL LEVELS[*]

Kurt Biss, Kang-Jey Ho, and C. Bruce Taylor

The factors affecting individuals' serum cholesterol levels are multiple and complicated. The present study was designed to determine a possible correlation of the individual serum cholesterol levels with various kinetic parameters of cholesterol metabolism in 15 healthy, white male subjects.

Materials and Methods

Fifteen healthy, ambulatory U.S. white males, age 30 to 62, with various serum cholesterol levels, ranging from 113 to 325 mg/100 ml, were maintained on their own regular diets which contained different amounts of cholesterol from person to person (300 to 1250 mg/day) during a 100 day metabolic study. Each subject received a single dose of 25 μci of cholesterol-4-^{14}C intravenously. A 5 ml blood sample was taken from each subject every day during the first week of the experiment, twice a week during the second and third weeks and once a week thereafter, up to a total period of 14 weeks. The serum cholesterol, triglyceride, phospholipid and total lipid levels were determined together with the radioactivity of serum cholesterol. Compartmental analysis of the disappearance curve of serum cholesterol specific activity was carried out by a computerized program based on the combination of the kinetic analyses reported by Gurpide et al. (1964) and the input-output analysis shown by Perl and Samuel (1969). The curves of all cases uniformly fit best a two-pool system.

Three 4-day stool samples were collected from each subject during 30 to 34, 60 to 64, and 90 to 94 days after the administration of cholesterol-4-^{14}C. The extraction and quantitation of fecal neutral sterols and bile acids, and also the fecal cholesterol and its specific activity were done by the methods described previously (Feldman et al., 1972). Such additional analysis of fecal specimen made it possible to calculate the rates of cholesterol absorption and synthesis. Regression analyses were done between serum cholesterol levels and all the kinetic parameters of cholesterol metabolism.

Results and Discussion

The fluctuation of individual body weights of all 15 subjects during the 100 day experimental period was minimal. The means and standard deviations of their serum total and free cholesterol, phospholipid, triglyceride, and total lipid concentrations are shown in Table 1. Among these 15 subjects the individual mean serum total cholesterol levels ranged from 113 to 325 mg/100 ml. For the same subject, this value was quite constant.

The individual values of various kinetic parameters of cholesterol metabolism are listed in Table 2. The rates of cholesterol absorption, synthesis, and excretion of each of 15 subjects are displayed in Table 3. The regression analyses revealed the following interrelationships among these kinetic parameters and their relationships to the serum cholesterol levels:

[*]This investigation was supported by Public Health Service Grant HL-13612-04 from the National Heart and Lung Institute and by a research grant from the Veterans Administration Hospital, Albany, New York (MRIS No. 8332-01).

Table 1. Changes of serum cholesterol, triglyceride, phospholipid and total lipid concentrations of the 15 subjects during the cholesterol metabolic study

Subject	Serum cholesterol (mg/100 ml)		Serum triglyceride (mg/100 ml)	Serum phospholipid (mg/100 ml)	Serum total lipid (mg/100 ml)
	Total	Free			
1	113 ± 7[a]	31 ± 3	119 ± 56	160 ± 17	382 ± 44
2	150 ± 13	38 ± 5	185 ± 65	190 ± 20	515 ± 69
3	158 ± 11	44 ± 5	239 ± 91	199 ± 18	595 ± 94
4	165 ± 17	47 ± 5	229 ± 64	198 ± 16	593 ± 77
5	202 ± 23	59 ± 6	384 ± 134	223 ± 22	802 ± 158
6	211 ± 12	65 ± 7	193 ± 51	226 ± 18	631 ± 66
7	212 ± 12	59 ± 5	190 ± 48	218 ± 19	594 ± 110
8	264 ± 26	74 ± 9	281 ± 72	311 ± 33	860 ± 93
9	267 ± 21	81 ± 9	444 ± 165	264 ± 31	972 ± 178
10	275 ± 28	73 ± 5	267 ± 64	267 ± 16	805 ± 78
11	288 ± 17	84 ± 5	387 ± 66	288 ± 19	957 ± 74
12	298 ± 35	84 ± 12	326 ± 81	300 ± 40	928 ± 103
13	300 ± 53	81 ± 6	349 ± 115	270 ± 32	907 ± 123
14	317 ± 26	88 ± 11	297 ± 88	297 ± 34	911 ± 96
15	325 ± 29	88 ± 9	470 ± 93	327 ± 29	1111 ± 110

[a] Mean $\pm$ SD of 22 determinations throughout the experimental period.

1. The rate of absorption of dietary cholesterol was directly proportional to the daily cholesterol intake with a theoretical mean maximal absorption capacity of 345 ± 73 mg/day (95% confidence intervals). The absorption efficiency was fixed at an average of 37%.
2. The rate of absorption or the input of the dietary cholesterol into the system resulted in a mean 16.6% suppression of endogenous cholesterol synthesis. The maximal suppression was only 25% of the total body cholesterol synthesis in this group of subjects.
3. The turnover rate of body exchangeable cholesterol was proportional to the rate of synthesis but not to the rate of absorption, suggesting no increase of fecal output of sterols as a compensatory mechanism for the influx of dietary cholesterol.
4. The elevation of serum cholesterol levels was accompanied by proportional increase in serum phospholipid and triglyceride levels. This was true even for the random unfasted sera.
5. The serum cholesterol levels, however, were not correlated with any of the kinetic parameters of the cholesterol metabolism except for a weak negative

Table 2. Various kinetic parameters of a two compartment model of cholesterol metabolism obtained from the 15 U.S. white males in this study

Subject	M_A gm	M_B gm	M_T gm	$\bar{t}$ (days)	I_T mg/day	K_{AB}	K_{BA}	K_A	$\frac{1}{\alpha}$ (days)	$\frac{1}{\beta}$ (days)
1	26.48	47.57	74.05	44.60	1660	0.05960	0.03317	0.06271	7.11	67.57
2	25.84	58.49	84.33	47.28	1784	0.11410	0.05039	0.06903	4.60	62.50
3	19.51	16.86	36.37	32.39	1123	0.06130	0.7091	0.05756	6.06	40.48
4	21.88	66.13	88.01	50.89	1729	0.10460	0.03462	0.07904	4.88	74.63
5	34.89	72.36	107.25	65.81	1629	0.06324	0.03049	0.04671	7.72	90.90
6	26.41	36.45	62.86	59.56	1055	0.04250	0.03080	0.03996	9.89	81.97
7	37.51	58.48	95.99	101.00	951	0.03720	0.02386	0.02534	12.71	129.87
8	25.11	33.45	58.56	61.59	951	0.08750	0.06569	0.03786	5.65	70.92
9	28.27	39.96	68.23	48.76	1399	0.14210	0.01006	0.04949	3.65	54.95
10	22.78	42.54	65.32	38.64	1691	0.06420	0.03438	0.07420	6.39	61.35
11	33.39	56.75	90.14	61.52	1465	0.06742	0.03966	0.04389	7.22	79.37
12	30.96	21.33	52.29	34.83	1501	0.09108	0.13220	0.04850	4.07	38.31
13	23.36	43.68	67.04	51.82	1294	0.11640	0.06228	0.05538	4.58	63.29
14	26.34	46.72	73.06	50.05	1460	0.11910	0.06713	0.05542	4.44	60.61
15	32.49	87.27	119.76	80.39	1490	0.06634	0.02470	0.04585	7.81	113.64
Mean	26.68	48.67	76.22	55.28	1412	0.08710	0.0473	0.05273	6.45	72.69
SD	4.99	18.36	20.95	17.18	270	0.03000	0.0282	0.01341	2.36	23.72
SE	1.29	4.74	5.41	4.43	70	0.00770	0.0072	0.00346	0.61	6.12

M_A, M_B, and M_T: Pool sizes of compartments A, B and their sum respectively.

$\bar{t}$: Mean transit time of the tracer cholesterol.

I_T: Daily total input of cholesterol into the system from outside the system.

K_{AB}, K_{BA} and K_A: Rate constants for cholesterol transport from pool A to B, from pool B to A, and from pool A to outside the system, respectively.

α, β: The slopes of the first and second exponential curves, respectively.

correlation with the turnover rate. Such "independence" of the serum cholesterol levels strongly suggests that there are probably some genetic, dietary,
and other yet undertermined factors which may specifically affect the structure and metabolism of circulating lipoproteins and consequently affect the
serum cholesterol levels.

Table 3. The rates of absorption, synthesis, and excretion of cholesterol in the
15 U.S. white males during the experiment while on their own regular daily diets

Subject	Rate of absorption			Rate of synthesis	Rate of excretion
	mg/day	% of $\dot{Q}$ diet	% of I_T	mg/day	mg/day
1	175	31.81	10.54	1485	1660
2	380	44.70	21.30	1404	1784
3	193	32.16	17.18	930	1123
4	135	24.54	7.80	1594	1729
5	319	37.52	19.58	1310	1629
6	229	36.64	21.70	826	1055
7	124	38.15	13.03	827	951
8	340	42.50	35.75	611	951
9	427	34.16	30.66	972	1399
10	190	33.04	11.23	1501	1691
11	174	34.16	11.87	1291	1465
12	141	35.25	9.39	1360	1501
13	177	41.64	13.67	1117	1294
14	105	35.00	7.19	1355	1460
15	171	38.00	11.47	1329	1490
Mean	219	36.25	16.16	1193	1412
SD	99	4.96	8.05	294	270
SE	26	1.33	2.08	76	70

$\dot{Q}$ diet: Daily intake of cholesterol in the diet (mg/day).
I_T: Daily total input of cholesterol into the system = Rate of absorption + Rate
of synthesis.

THE RELATIONSHIP OF ESTERIFICATION OF PLASMA CHOLESTEROL TO HYPERTRIGLYCERIDEMIA

Harbhajan Singh Sodhi and Bhalchandra Kudchodkar

It was shown by us recently that hepatic synthesis of cholesterol was related to plasma levels of triglycerides in hyperlipemic patients (Sodhi and Kudchodkar, 1973a); and it was postulated that hepatic synthesis of plasma lipoproteins, especially very low density lipoproteins (VLDL), is a major determinant of cholesterol synthesis in man (Sodhi and Kudchodkar, 1973b). We now present evidence to suggest that the rate of esterification of plasma free cholesterol is also related to cholesterol synthesis and turnover of plasma lipoproteins.

The rate of esterification of plasma free cholesterol were determined by in vivo and in vitro methods. The turnover rates of plasma cholesterol esters were calculated from the specific activity slopes of plasma free and esterified cholesterol after an intravenous injection of radioactive mevalonate (Nestel and Monger, 1967). In vitro activity of lecithin cholesterol acyltransferase (LCAT) was determined

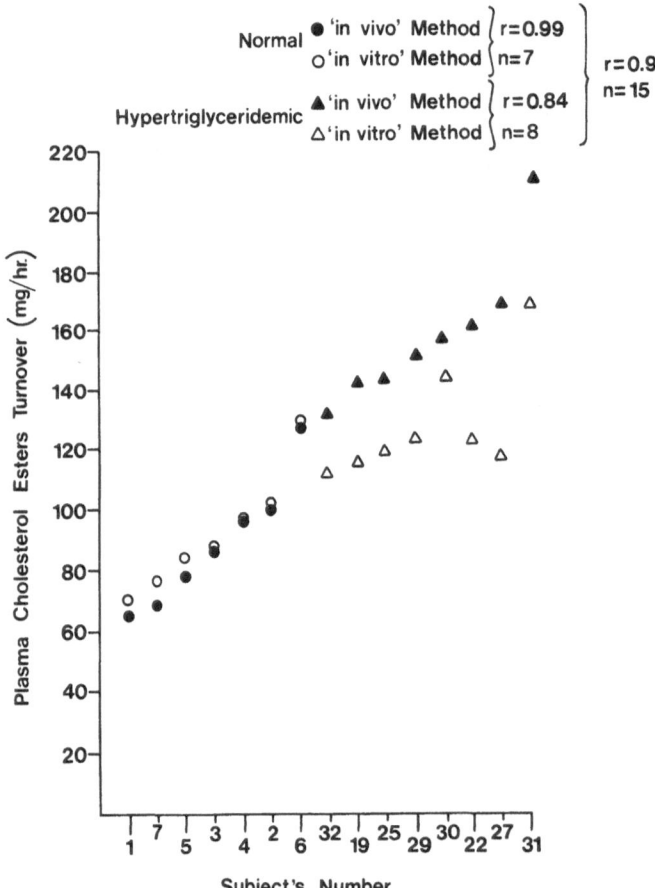

Figure 1. Results of in vitro and in vivo esterification of plasma free cholesterol in normo- and hypertriglyceridemic subjects

by incubating the patient's own plasma at 37°C in a Dubnoff's incubator. The patient's plasma was labelled by intravenous injection of radioactive mevalonate, so that the radioactive cholesterol was in the physiological state. From the changes in the amounts and specific activity of plasma free and esterified cholesterol during one hour of incubation, the rates of esterification of plasma free cholesterol were calculated.

In normotriglyceridemic subjects, the results obtained by in vivo and in vitro methods gave almost identical values (Fig. 1), thus validating the thesis that plasma LCAT is responsible for the esterification of plasma free cholesterol in man. However, in hypertriglyceridemic patients the results obtained by the in vitro method were consistently lower than those obtained by the in vivo method (Fig. 1).

In order to study the effect of hypertriglyceridemia on the in vitro activity of LCAT, different amounts of VLDL triglycerides were added to aliquots of plasma, and the LCAT activity was determined. The control aliquots of plasma contained 1.03 mg of triglycerides in each ml, and the activity in this sample was assumed to be 100. Addition of VLDL triglycerides up to about 1 mg showed a modest increment in the LCAT activity, but further increment in the concentrations of VLDL triglycerides decreased the activity of LCAT as determined in vitro (Fig. 2). Despite this effect, the values obtained by even the in vitro method were significantly greater in hypertriglyceridemic than in normo-triglyceridemic subjects (Fig. 1).

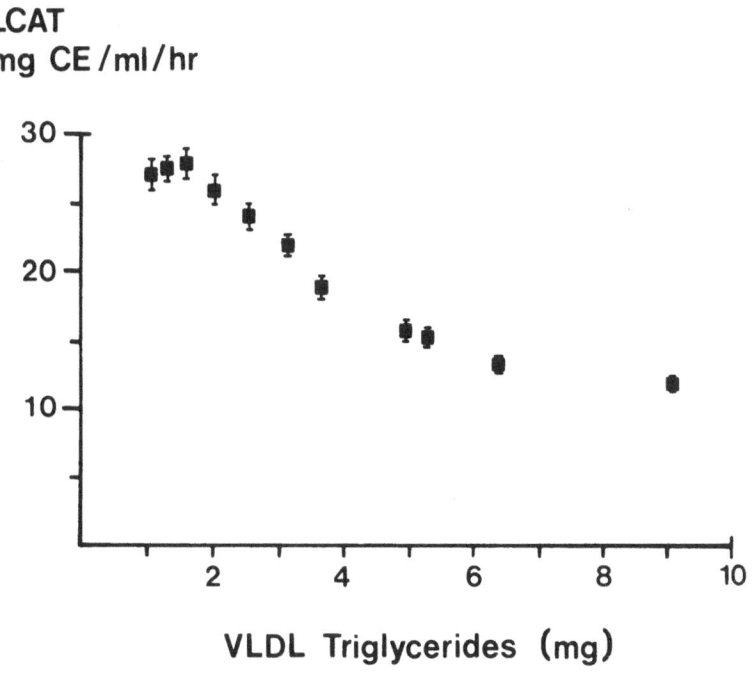

Figure 2. Effect of plasma very low density lipoprotein triglycerides on the activity of LCAT determined in vitro

Net turnover rates of plasma cholesterol esters determined in vivo were 188 ± 26 mg/hour in the hypertriglyceridemic group and 116 ± 18 mg/hour in the normotriglyceridemic subjects. Their correlation coefficient with plasma triglyceride concentrations was 0.87, and statistically it was highly significant (p <0.001).

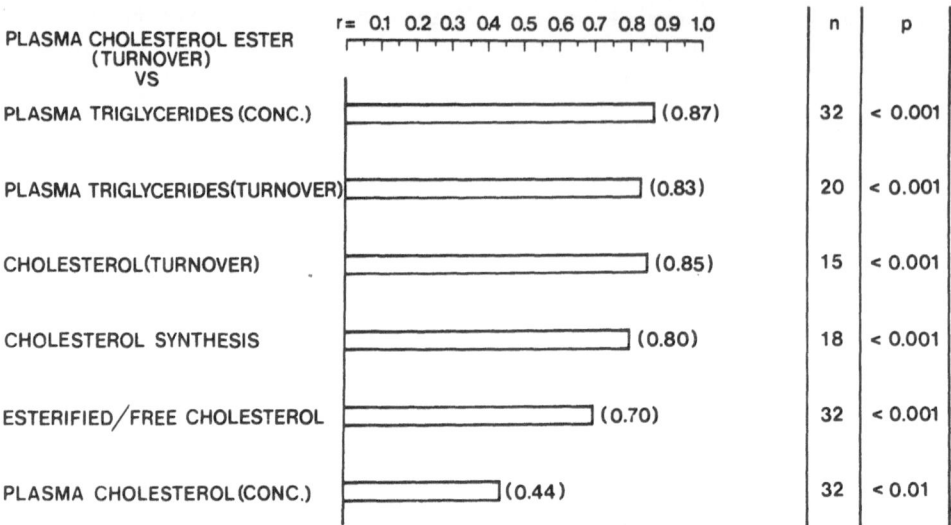

Figure 3. Correlations of turnover rates of plasma cholesterol esters with some parameters of plasma cholesterol and triglycerides

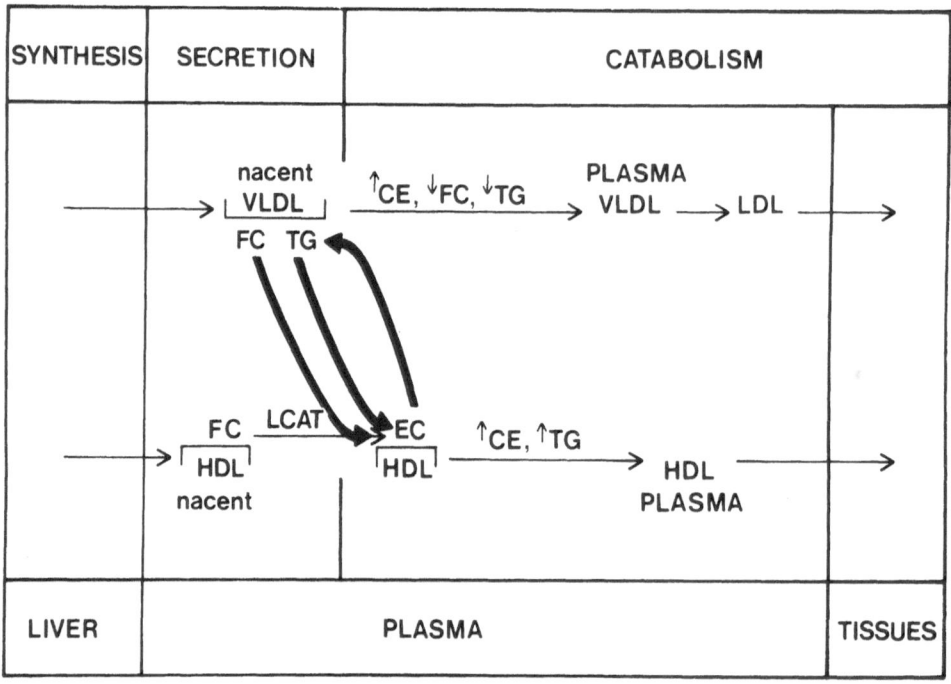

Figure 4. Role of LCAT in catabolism of plasma lipoproteins

Turnover of plasma cholesterol esters had only a poor correlation with levels of plasma cholesterol (Fig. 3), but its correlations with values of cholesterol turnover (derived from kinetic analysis of plasma cholesterol specific activity) and with absolute rates of cholesterol synthesis (determined by cholesterol balance) were excellent (Fig. 3). Its correlation with the relative rates of cholesterol synthesis (determined from the incorporation of acetate and mevalonate into plasma free cholesterol) was also excellent ($r=0.79$). These data indicated that esterification of plasma free cholesterol was related on one hand to cholesterol turnover and on the other to plasma triglycerides. Since the increase in plasma triglycerides (or VLDL) per se cannot explain the increased activity of LCAT in hypertriglyceridemic subjects, the latter may well be related to increased turnover of plasma VLDL seen in patients with moderate hypertriglyceridemia (Reaven et al., 1965).

It is suggested that the free cholesterol is incorporated into plasma lipoproteins as a structural component, and any loss of free cholesterol through its esterification must be associated with other metabolic changes in the structure of plasma lipoproteins. In this sense, esterification of plasma free cholesterol may represent only one aspect of complex and interrelated metabolic reactions involving peptides and other lipids in the turnover of plasma lipoproteins (Fig. 4).

The ratio of esterified cholesterol (EC)/free cholesterol (FC) in plasma VLDL is significantly lower than that in plasma low density lipoproteins (LDL) or high density lipoproteins (HDL) (Rose, 1972). Since elevations of plasma triglycerides above normal are primarily due to increases in plasma VLDL, one would expect that EC/FC ratios in hypertriglyceridemic subjects would be lower than in those with normal plasma triglycerides. Experimental observations, however, indicated that EC/FC ratio was, in fact, significantly ($p < 0.05$) greater in hypertriglyceridemic patients (2.48) than that in normotriglyceridemic subjects (2.06). The ratios showed a significant correlation with the turnover rate of plasma cholesterol esters (Fig. 3). suggesting that the greater the activity of LCAT, the greater the esterified fraction of total plasma cholesterol. The ratios also had significant correlations with relative rates of cholesterol synthesis. We investigated three different groups of subjects made up of 11, 16, and 19 volunteers on ordinary diets. The EC/FC ratio in each case showed a significant correlation with the endogenous synthesis of cholesterol ($r=0.72$, 0.43, and 0.55). This suggests that the EC/FC ratio may be a rough index of the relative rates of cholesterol synthesis in man.

ROLE OF A LIPID CARRIER PROTEIN IN THE CONTROL OF LIPID SYNTHESIS, METABOLISM, AND TRANSPORT

Mary E. Dempsey, Kim E. McCoy, Thelma D. Calimbas, and John P. Carlson

In previous studies, we showed that squalene and sterol carrier protein (SCP), a soluble liver protein, is essential for conversion of water-insoluble precursors to cholesterol by liver microsomal enzymes (e.g. Ritter and Dempsey, 1970, 1971, 1973; Dempsey, 1974a, b, c; and Fig. 1). Our initial reports were confirmed by several laboratories (e.g. Scallen et al., 1971; Rilling, 1972; and Johnson and Shah, 1973).

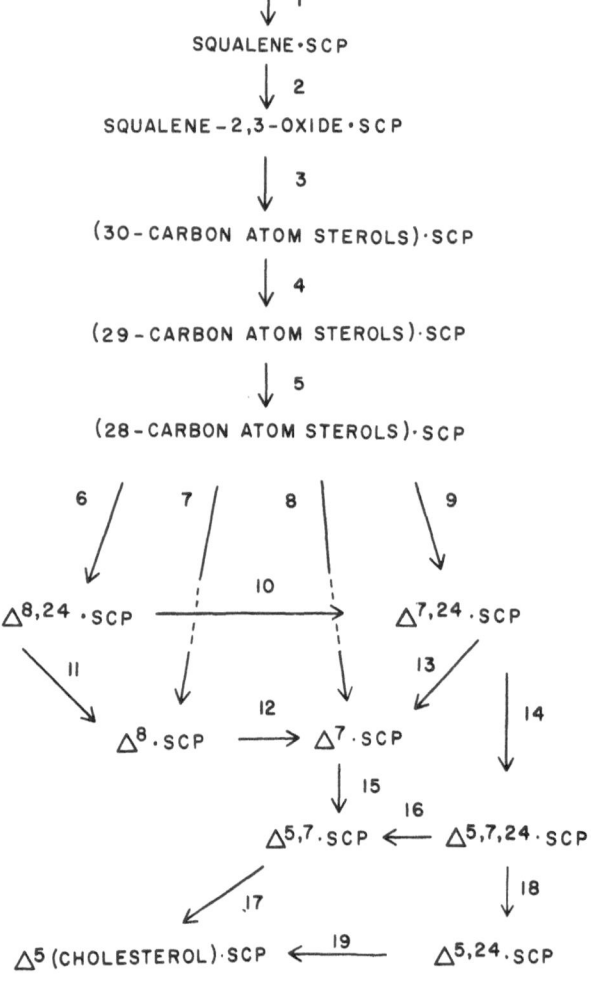

Figure 1. Outline of pathways and intermediate compounds in the later stages of cholesterol biosynthesis; role of SCP. Intermediates are shown as SCP complexes and position of unsaturation is indicated by the delta (Δ) symbol

The purpose of this article is to summarize some of our recent findings on the structural, functional and regulatory properties of SCP, as well as the ubiquitous presence in nature of SCP or an SCP-like protein.

Structural Properties of SCP and Lipid Binding. We have developed two techniques for purifying SCP from the soluble fraction of homogenates; one involves heat treatment of the soluble fraction at high ionic strength (Ritter and Dempsey, 1970, 1971, 1973); the other avoids the heat step (McCoy et al., 1973; and Dempsey, 1974a). These methods yield a partially purified preparation of the sterol-free or protomer form of SCP (pro-SCP), (M.W. 16,000 daltons). Homogeneous pro-SCP (as determined by polyacrylamide gel electrophoresis at several pH values) is obtained by ion exchange chromatography of the partially purified preparation (Dempsey, 1974a, c). Studies with various lipids have shown that SCP has a high affinity for squalene, sterol precursors of cholesterol, phospholipids, long chain fatty acids, and water-insoluble precursors of steroid hormones and bile acids (Dempsey, 1974c). SCP thus appears to be a lipid carrier protein (Dempsey, 1971; Ritter and Dempsey, 1973).

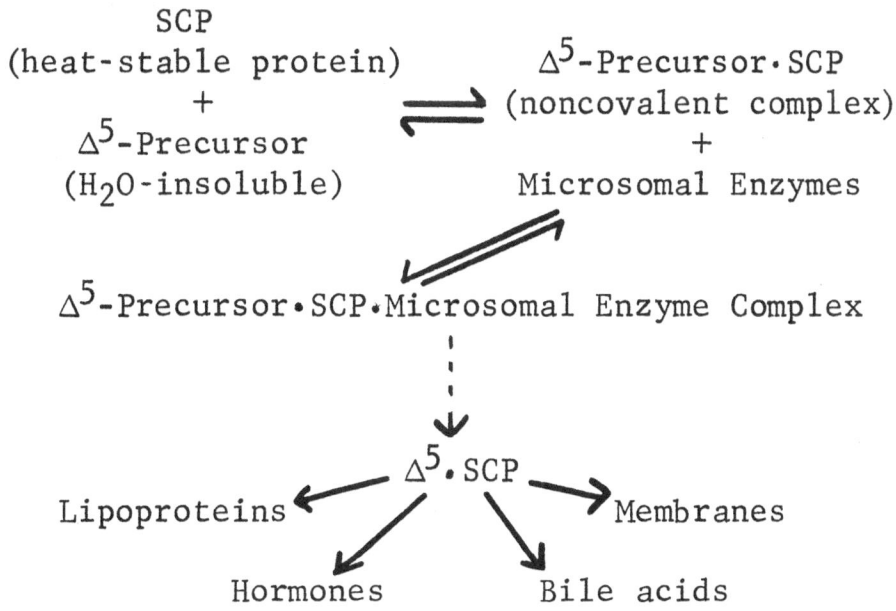

Figure 2. Proposed mechanism of SCP function and biological roles

With regard to cholesterol synthesis, our data indicate that pro-SCP forms a non-covalent, high molecular weight (>150,000 daltons) complex with a cholesterol precursor (Fig. 2) (Carlson et al., 1973). This complex combines with a specific microsomal enzyme. The precursor-SCP is converted to its product, the following precursor-SCP, which then combines with the microsomal enzyme next in the sequence of cholesterol synthesis. Finally, cholesterol-SCP results (Fig. 2; cf. also Fig. 1).

Functional Similarity of SCP to a Plasma Lipoprotein. The high density lipoprotein (HDL) fraction of human plasma contains SCP-like activity (Ritter and Dempsey, 1971; Koehler and Dempsey, 1973). This activity is associated predominately with one of the major HDL apo-polypeptides, apo-Gln-II (also designated apo-A-II), (Dempsey et al., 1972). The latter observation suggests certain structural similarities between apo-Gln-II (Brewer et al., 1972) and SCP, e.g. apo-Gln-II has a molecular weight of 16,000 daltons, as does pro-SCP (Dempsey, 1974c).

Participation of SCP in Cholesterol Metabolism. Regarding the initial stages of steroid hormone synthesis, a cholesterol·liver-SCP complex is metabolized by adrenal mitochondrial enzymes to pregnenolone (Kan et al., 1972). Steroids formed from pregnenolone are progressively more water-soluble and not bound by SCP (Ritter and Dempsey, 1971). In addition, Kan and Ungar, (1973) isolated a heat-stable protein from adrenal tissue which is structurally similar to liver-SCP and functions with the adrenal mitochondrial enzymes catalyzing cholesterol side-chain cleavage yielding pregnenolone.

With regard to bile acid formation (Fig. 3), bile acids themselves (e.g. cholic acid and chenodeoxycholic acid) are water-soluble and not bound by SCP (Ritter and Dempsey, 1971; Grawbowski et al., 1973). However, early products of cholesterol metabolism to bile acids (e.g. 7a-hydroxycholesterol; cf. also Fig. 3) are bound by SCP and liver microsomal 12a-hydroxylase has a specific requirement for SCP (Grawbowski et al., 1973). It appears that other enzymes in the initial stages of bile acid synthesis (cf. Fig. 3) may also require SCP for maximum activity.

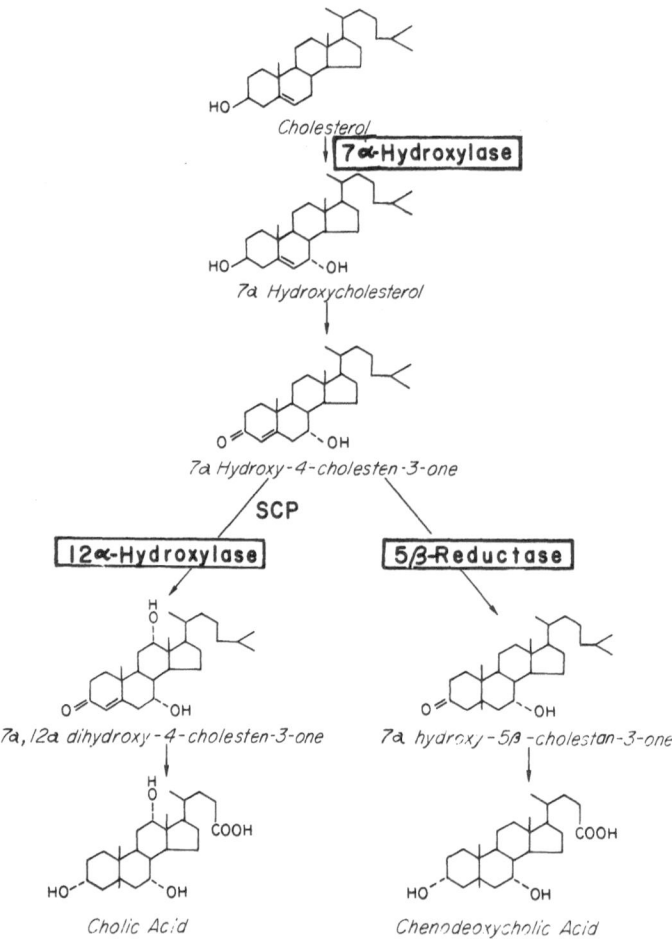

Figure 3. Pathways of conversion of cholesterol to bile acids

Ubiquitous Occurrence of SCP or an SCP-Like Protein. SCP was first discovered in rat liver (Dempsey, 1974c); more recently, a structurally and functionally similar protein was purified from human liver (Dempsey et al., 1972; and from various mammalian tissues (e.g. heart, kidney, adrenal, intestine, lung, spleen, brain, muscle) (Kan et al., 1972; McCoy et al., 1973). An intriguing finding is that SCP is present in protozoa (Calimbas, 1972, 1973; and Dempsey, 1974b, c). Protozoan SCP has the same molecular weight and similar functional properties as liver SCP, e.g. protozoan SCP will substitute for liver SCP in reactions catalyzed by liver enzymes and liver SCP will substitute in the same manner for protozoan SCP. SCP or an SCP-like protein is also present in yeast (Rilling, 1972). The ubiquitous occurrence of SCP in mammalian tissues as well as lower forms of life suggest that a requirement for SCP or an SCP-like protein may be a general biological requirement for water-insoluble steroid synthesis, metabolism, and transport – plus regulation of these processes (Dempsey, 1974b, c).

Possible Role of SCP in Regulation of Lipid Synthesis, Metabolism, and Transport.
The various functions of SCP in sterol synthesis, metabolism and transport alluded to in the preceeding sections suggest that a cholesterol·SCP or lipid·SCP complex could participate in the regulation of these interrelated processes (cf. Fig. 2 and Dempsey, 1974b). Indeed, preliminary findings by Carlson et al. (1973) indicate that SCP is capable of modifying the activity of a major regulatory enzyme in cholesterol synthesis (ß-hydroxy-ß-methylglutaryl-CoA reductase), possibly by an allosteric mechanism. Ritter et al. (1972) also noted that the level of cellular SCP could regulate the pathways by which cholesterol is synthesized, i.e. at high levels of SCP the pathway involving saturated side-chain sterol intermediates would predominate.

It is apparent that further extensive studies are needed for complete elucidation of the various physiological roles of this versatile protein, SCP.

IMPAIRED FATTY ACID INCORPORATION INTO ADIPOSE TISSUE (FIAT) IN HYPERTRIGLYCERIDEMIA. EFFECT OF INTRAVENOUS FAT INFUSION ON FIAT[*]

Göran Walldius, Lars A. Carlson, Hans Lithell, Anders G. Olsson, Paolo Rubba, and Bengt Vessby

In the development of hypertriglyceridemia (HTG) two general mechanisms may be operating: 1. *Increased production* of triglycerides (TG) from the liver, 2. *Decreased removal* of TG from the blood to peripheral tissues (adipose tissue, muscles). A *combined* defect of increased production and decreased removal of TG may also give rise to HTG. Many studies have shown that low removal of TG from blood is the most important mechanism underlying HTG (for review, Carlson, Olsson, 1973).

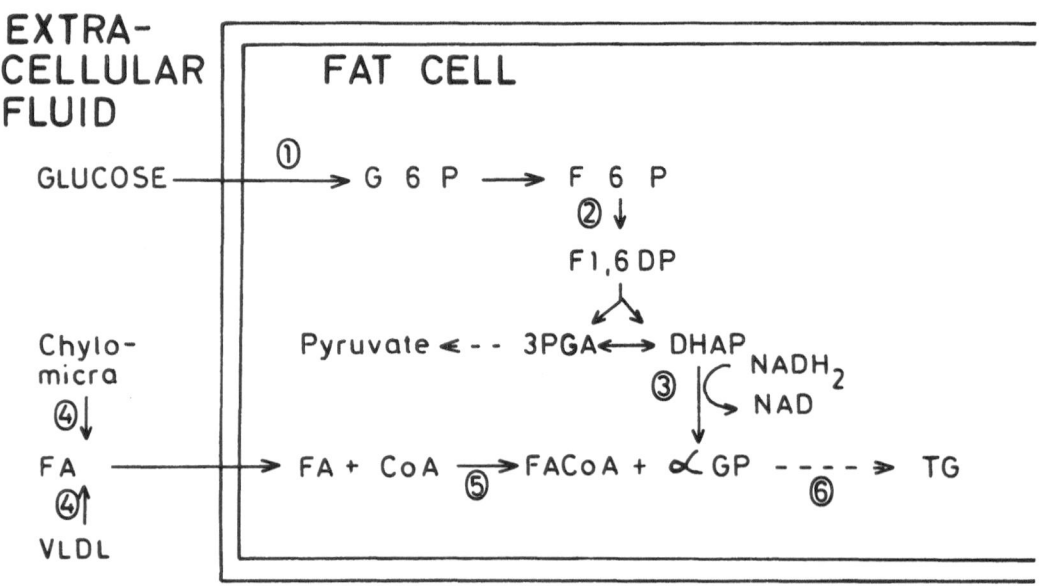

Figure 1. Regulation of plasma triglyceride (TG) uptake by adipose tissue

In the *removal* process TG-rich chylomicrons and TG in very low density lipoproteins (VLDL) are (a) hydrolyzed probably by the same enzyme system(s) lipoprotein lipase (LLA) in the capillary wall (Fig. 1). Fatty acids (FA) and glycerol are formed in this process. FA are then either (b) *taken up* by the tissue or (c) re-entering blood as free fatty acids (FFA). Subnormal adipose tissue LLA has been found in some subjects with moderate GTG, but no difference was obtained when LLA was expressed per "total body fat" (Persson, 1973). Different results have been obtained for postheparin lipoprotein lipase activity (PHLA) in HTG. However, the interpretation of PHLA values as reflecting adipose tissue (AT) LLA is complex. The role of AT-LLA in other types of HTG than type I is as yet not conclusive.

---

[*]Supported by a grant from Swedish Medical Research Council (19x-204).

During the last two years we have focussed our interest on mechanism (b). We have named this process FIAT (Fatty acid Incorporation into Adipose Tissue). The results obtained show that low FIAT is often found in HTG. FIAT values in different types of HL as well as the effect of acute elevation of plasma TG in vivo on FIAT will be presented.

Materials and Methods

Young healthy male and female students, mean age 24 years, as well as men and women, mean age 53 years, not suffering from acute or malignant disease, overt endocrine disorder or given any therapy directed towards HL, participated in the study (Table 1). After an overnight fast, blood was taken for lipid determination, ultracentrifugation and classification of type of HL (Walldius et al., 1973). A needle biopsy from lower abdominal subcutaneous fat was taken. 25-75 mg of adipose tissue was then incubated in triplicate in a buffer medium containing labelled fatty acids (^{3}H-FA) and labelled glucose (^{14}C-glucose). After two hours of incubation lipids were extracted, FIAT and GLIAT were determined. Lipolysis was determined as glycerol release into incubation medium (Walldius et al., 1973). Total body fat was calculated from height and weight (Persson, 1973). Blood sugar and insulin were determined as described (Carlson et al., 1973) and exogenous TG as described (Carlson, Rössner, 1972).

Table 1. Fasting concentration of plasma triglycerides (mmol/1) and cholesterol (mg/100 ml), age (years), FIAT ($\frac{nmol}{3}$/g/hr), GLIAT (nmol/g/hr) and glycerol (nmol/g/hr). m ± SEM

| | Type of hyperlipidemia | | | | | |
	YN	NTG	II B	III	IV	V
N	22	24	13	4	39	3
TG	1.05 ±.05	1.55 ±.09	3.29 ±.37	6.07±1.79	4.44 ±.44	11.6 ±3.2
CHOL	179 ± 5	221 ± 6	346 ± 9	361 ± 50	279 ± 11	260 ± 56
AGE	25 ± 1	51 ± 2	55 ± 2	61 ± 6	51 ± 1	52 ± 11
FIAT	201 ± 27	156 ± 11	74 ± 9[c]	82 ± 4[b]	88 ± 6[c]	59 ± 23
GLIAT	161 ± 10	199 ± 12	141 ± 19[a]	89 ± 10[b]	135 ± 13[b]	83 ± 60
GLYCEROL	634 ± 40	468 ± 35	413 ± 42	542 ±110	655 ± 51[b]	578 ± 332

[a]p <.05, [b]p <.01, [c]p <.001 indicates degree of significance versus NTG.

In part of the study, 11 subjects with normal lipid values and 13 subjects with HTG were given 10% Intralipid®-S (IL) as a constant infusion (5.4 ml/kg/min) from 8 o'clock in the morning to 11 o'clock. TG, FIAT, GLIAT and lipolysis were determined before and after the infusion.

Results

Young male and female subjects with normal TG and cholesterol values (YN) had high FIAT and GLIAT values compared with the other groups of subjects (Table 1).

No sex difference was found. In all groups of subjects with HTG low values for
FIAT and GLIAT were found. Subjects with HTG were somewhat more obese than normals. If FIAT values were multiplied by total body fat (assuming that the obtained FIAT value was representative for all body fat) subjects with HTG still had
lower FIAT values than normals (NTG). The FIAT values (nmol/body/hr) for NTG was
2.16, type II B 1.17 (p <.01), type III 1.42, type IV 1.42 (p <.01) and for type
V 0.54. In type IV, HTG glycerol release was higher than in the other groups.

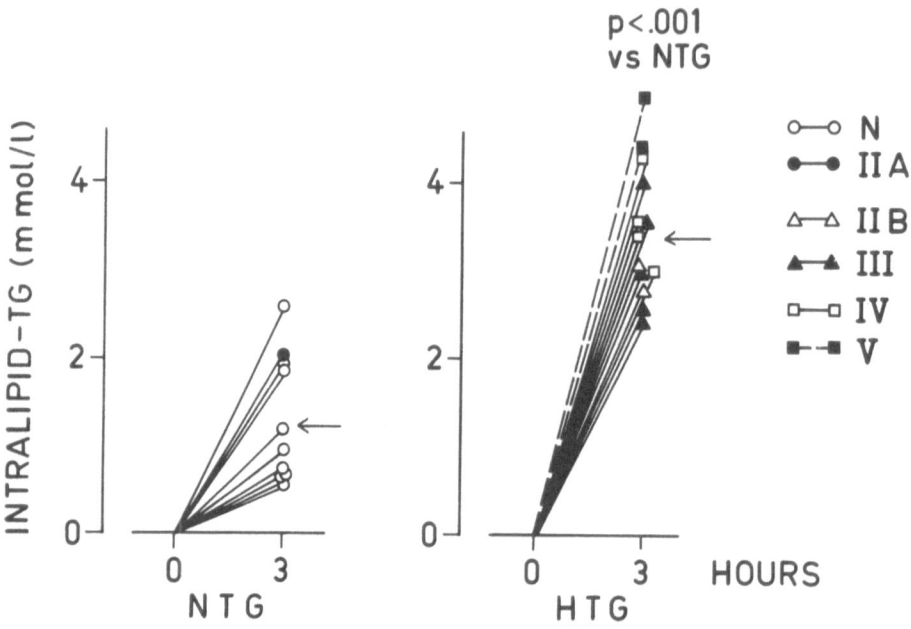

Figure 2a. Increase in intralipid-triglycerides (TG) after infusion of intra-
lipid®-S

When IL was given to subjects with different types of HTG (Fig. 2a), ILTG values
for normals increased to 1.15 mmol/1 and for subjects with HTG to 3.60 mmol/1
(determined by nephelometry). This acute elevation of chylomicron like TG rich
particles did not influence blood sugar or insulin after 3 hours of infusion. As
shown in Fig. 2b, FIAT was not influenced by the acute increase in TG. The only
difference between normals and subjects with HTG were FIAT and GLIAT values which
were significantly lower in subjects with HTG. FIAT was negatively correlated to
TG in all subjects (r = −.56, p = <.01).

There was a high correlation (r = .72, p <.001) between fasting plasma TG and
ILTG after three hours IL infusion (ILTG3). ILTG3 was negatively correlated to
FIAT before and after IL infusion (r = .69 and r = .65, both p <.001) (Fig. 2c)
as well as to GLIAT before and after IL infusion (r = .61, p <.005 and r = −.70,
p <.001). There was no relation between ILTG3 and AT glycerol release before and
after IL infusion.

Discussion

In studies on the pathogenesis of HTG, interest has as yet not been focussed on
the metabolic step *after* the action of LLA, i.e. FIAT. Our studies demonstrate
that *adipose tissue in HTG has a decreased capacity to incorporate externally sup-*
plied fatty acids and glucose. FIAT values were corrected for isotopic dilution

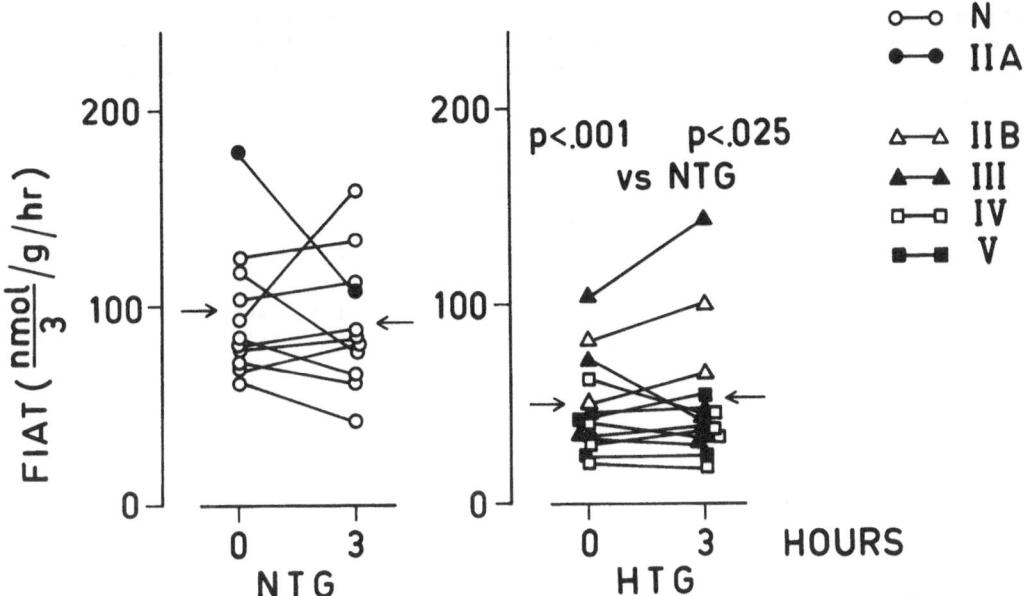

Figure 2b. Fatty acid incorporation into adipose tissue (FIAT) before and after infusion of intralipid®-S

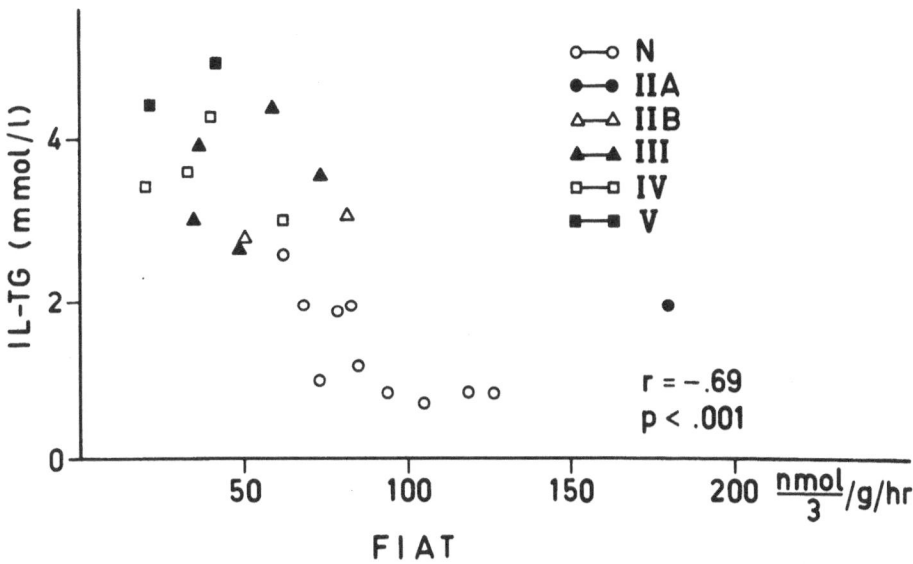

Figure 2c. Correlation between intralipid®-triglycerides (IL-TG) after infusion of IL and fatty acid incorporation into adipose tissue (FIAT)

(from AT non-labelled FA) in the incubation medium (Walldius et al., 1973). In type IV, HL high AT lipolysis might contribute to HTG.

Acute elevation of plasma TG by Intralipid®-S infusion did neither inhibit nor stimulate FIAT, GLIAT or glycerol release from AT. Apparently AT is insensitive to short-term elevation of TG both in normal subjects and in subjects with HTG.

Subjects with high ILTG3 and low FIAT had high plasma TG values. The inverse relationship between ILTG3 and FIAT and GLIAT might indicate that AT is rate-limiting in the removal of exogenous TG. From these results we put forward the hypothesis that *low FIAT function may cause HTG by reducing TG removal.*

Summary

Subcutaneous adipose tissue was obtained by a needle biopsy technique from subjects with different types of hypertriglyceridemia (HTG). Specimens were incubated in an isotopic medium and incorporation of fatty acids (FIAT) and glucose (GLIAT) was determined. FIAT and GLIAT were significantly lower in HTG than in normolipidemia. Three hours infusion of fat (IL) did not alter FIAT or GLIAT. Low FIAT and low removal values were found in HTG. The results suggest that low FIAT function may cause HTG by reducing TG removal.

INTERRELATIONSHIP OF PLASMA FREE FATTY ACIDS AND BLOOD BETA-HYDROXYBUTYRATE CONCENTRATION IN CORONARY ARTERY DISEASE

P. Gosh and C.N. Hales

The incidence of coronary artery disease (CAD) has increased during the latter half of this century and accounts for 33 per cent of male deaths between the ages of 45-54 years and 25 per cent of male deaths between the ages of 35-44 years (Oliver, 1969). The aetiology is multifactorial and hyperlipidaemia has been found to be an important factor. This includes elevations of both cholesterol and triglyceride concentrations in the blood. In addition, increased concentrations of insulin have been found in CAD (Peters and Hales, 1965; Nikkila et al., 1965). It is possible that insulin plays a role in atherogenesis by increasing the production of triglyceride. The purpose of this study was to find out whether insulin might regulate the metabolism of free fatty acids (FFA) to triglycerides in liver. The pathway of metabolism of FFA is shown in Fig. 1. If insulin modifies the metabolism of FFA by liver, it may affect the proportion of FFA converted to triglycerides as opposed to ketone bodies.

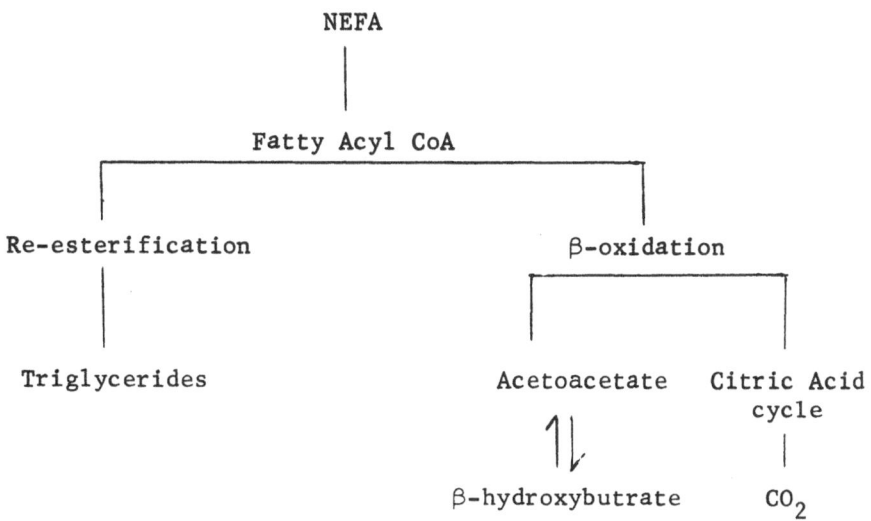

Figure 1. Pathway of free fatty acids or nonesterified fatty acids in liver

In order to investigate this possibility we studied 12 controls, 12 subjects with hyperlipidaemia without clinical artery disease (non-ischaemic hyperlipidaemia), and 30 subjects with coronary artery disease. The age, relative weight and the average blood pressures of these groups were similar. Each subject was studied with a 50 g oral glucose tolerance test after a 12 hour fast. In addition to measurements of FFA and ß-OHB, glucose, insulin and triglycerides, various other parameters were measured. The results showed a closely similar pattern in plasma FFA and blood ß-OHB concentrations in all three groups, although there were significant differences in the actual concentrations. When the fasting plasma FFA and blood ß-OHB concentrations were plotted together, there was a highly significant positive linear correlation between the two in fasting controls (r = 0.82). This was not however significant in CAD patients under similar conditions (r = 0.062).

When the plasma FFA and blood ß-OHB during every point of the glucose tolerance
test were plotted together, there was a positive correlation in all three groups.
The angle of the regression lines, however, was different. The regression lines
were parallel and similar in the two abnormal groups, indicating less ß-OHB formation whether the circulating FFA was similar or higher than the values in controls (Fig. 2).

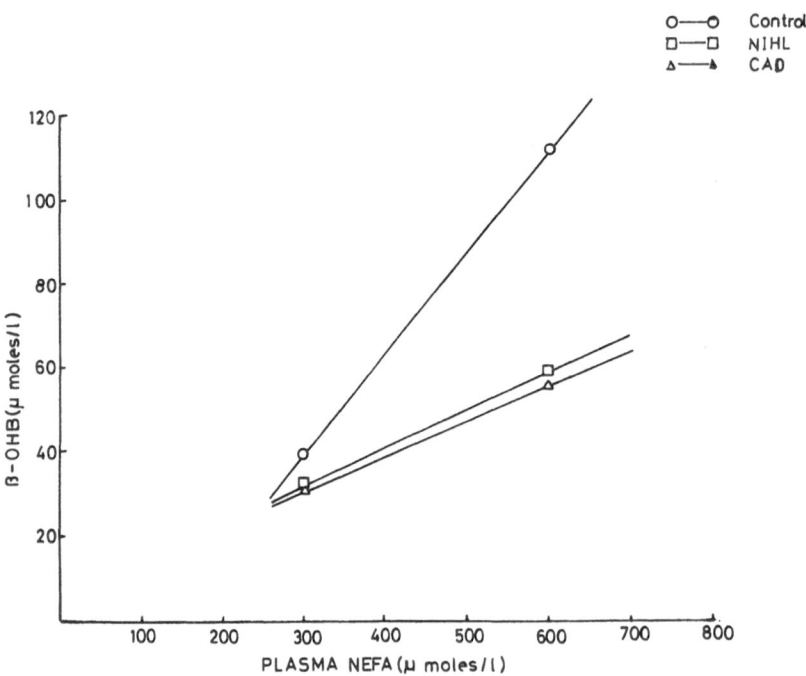

Figure 2. Correlation between plasma NEFA (or FFA) and blood ß-OHB concentrations

The ß-OHB concentration may be reduced as a result of increased utilization of
ketone bodies or increased amount of fatty acids entering the citric acid cycle
or a change in the ratio of acetoacetic to ß-hydroxybutrate. It is unlikely that
ketone bodies were utilized in excess or more fatty acids entered the citric acid
cycle, although no direct evidence was obtained in this study. A separate study
involving six controls and six subjects with CAD did not show any significant difference in the ratio of ß-OHB/AC-Ac between two groups. The results of the glucose
tolerance tests were then analysed to find out whether changes in insulin and triglyceride concentrations were associated with the changes observed in the relationship between FFA to ß-OHB. A 95 per cent confidence limit on both variables
(FFA and ß-OHB) was drawn from the 12 pairs of observations in fasting controls
(Fig. 3). About two-thirds of the subjects in the CAD group had their results outside the confidence limit and one-third of the same group had their results within the 95 per cent confidence limits. The analyses of the results of glucose and
insulin concentration in these two sub-groups showed that those who were outside
the confidence limits had lower glucose and higher insulin concentrations compared to those who were inside the limit. The insulin/glucose ratio illustrates
this point (Fig. 4). In addition, 11 out of 19 patients in the sub-group outside
the limit had abnormally elevated triglyceride concentrations whereas only two
out of 11 patients in the other sub-group had similar results.

This work suggests that insulin may be an important factor in the control of ketogenesis and triglyceride synthesis in liver. Raised insulin concentration may

direct fatty acids towards re-esterification. As increased insulin concentration occur in CAD, an agent which reduces the concentration of insulin may lower the triglyceride concentration and reduce the incidence of CAD.

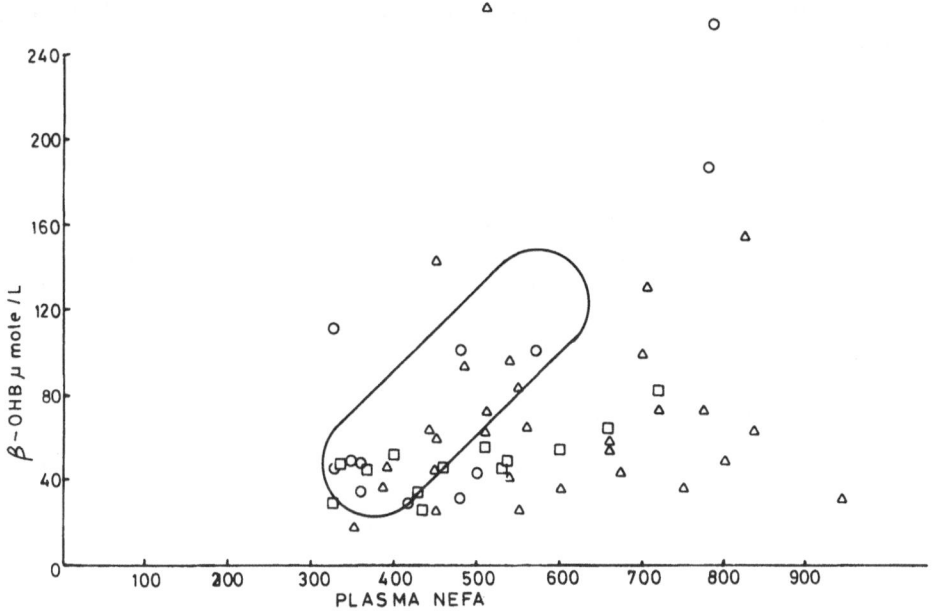

Figure 3. 95 per cent confidence limits of both plasma NEFA (or FFA) and blood ß-OHB concentrations in fasting controls

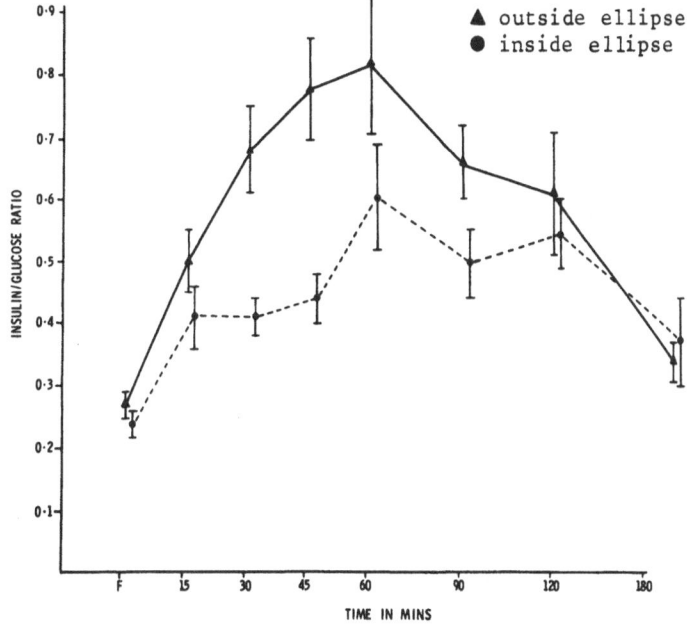

Figure 4. Insulin/glucose ratio following oral glucose in 2 sub-groups in CAD

ELIMINATION OF CHOLESTEROL AS BILE ACIDS IN HYPERLIPOPROTEINEMIAS TYPE II AND IV

Kjell Hellström, Kurt Einarsson, and Mora Kallner

Several studies indicate that cholesterol metabolism is regulated differently in hyperlipoproteinaemia type II and type IV (cf. Miettinen, 1973). Data on the turn-over of the two bile acids synthesized in the liver (cholic acid and chenodeoxy-cholic acid) show that the formation of bile acids in patients with a type II lipoprotein pattern is lower than in those with type IV (Kottke, 1969; Einarsson and Hellström, 1972; Wollenweber and Stiehl, 1972). This difference is mainly due to a subnormal synthesis of cholic acid in type II and an abnormally high forma-tion of this bile acid in most subjects with type IV (Einarsson and Hellström, 1972). Further evidence that these two types of hyperlipoproteinaemia represent different entities of diseases affecting bile acid metabolism was obtained by studying the effect of hypolipemic drugs.

Material and Methods

The controls were healthy subjects, 6 females (F) and 4 males (M). Their means ($\pm$ SEM) for age, serum cholesterol (C) and triglycerides (Tg) were 53 ± 3 yrs, 228 ± 9 and 123 ± 12 mg%, respectively. Of the hyperlipemic patients, 9 (all F) showed a type IIa (age 56 ± 2 yrs, C 391 ± 11 mg%, Tg 126 ± 8 mg%) and 6 (3 F, 3M) a type IIb (58 ± 3 yrs, C 328 ± 11 mg%, Tg 281 ± 23 mg%) lipoprotein pattern; hyperlipoproteinaemia type IV was encountered in 22 (4 F, 18 M) patients (age 52 ± 2 yrs, C 239 ± 11 mg%, Tg 388 ± 31 mg%) and hyperlipoproteinaemia type V in 5 (2 F, 3 M) (age 50 ± 3 yrs, C 285 ± 33 mg% and Tg 1922 ± 159 mg%).

Many of the patients suffered from coronary heart disease. None showed evidence of hypo- or hyperthyroidism, alcoholism or liver disease. During the months before and during the study they were not taking antibiotics or drugs known to have hepa-totoxic effects. When re-examined during treatment with clofibrate (2 g/day) or cholestyramine (10-14 g/day), the patients had already been prescribed the drugs for more than one month.

Experimental Procedure. All patients were hospitalized and maintained on a stan-dardized diet of natural type. About 40 per cent of the calories were supplied as fat.

[14]C-cholic acid (5 µCi) and ^{3}H-chenodeoxycholic acid (15 µCi) were given orally in the morning before breakfast. At least 4 specimens of duodenal bile (5-10 ml) were collected at 1-3 day intervals. The specific radioactivities of cholic and chenodeoxycholic acid were determined in each sample. The half-life, pool size and turnover of the compounds were calculated as described by Lindstedt (1957). Further details of the methods used have been published earlier (Einarsson and Hellström, 1972).

Results

Basal Condition. In the control subjects the half-life, pool size and daily syn-thesis of cholic acid averaged 2.6 days, 823 mg and 281 mg/day, respectively (Table 1). The half-life of this acid was almost the same in all groups of

Table 1. Bile acid turnover (means ± SEM) under basal conditions in the whole series of patients and in the sub-groups studied before (B) and during (D) treatment with clofibrate or cholestyramine. Number of patients in parenthesis

Lipoprotein	Treatment	Cholic acid			Chenodeoxycholic acid			Combined	
		$t_{1/2}$	Pool size	Turnover	$t_{1/2}$	Pool size	Turnover	Pool size	Turnover
		days	mg	mg/day	days	mg	mg/day	mg	mg/day
Control (10)	–	2.6±0.7	823±133	281±44	4.1±1.1	602±75	138±24	1424±186	419±62
IIa (9)	–	2.5±0.4	447±112[a]	120±15[b]	3.0±0.5	696±118	169±17	1144±210	289±27
IIb (6)	–	2.9±0.8	629±143	164±30	4.7±1.0	947±102[a]	176±36	1576±227	340±56
IV (22)	–	1.8±0.2	1669±234[a]	764±102[b]	2.4±0.2[a]	733±90	221±22	2402±273[a]	985±104[b]
V (5)	–	2.5±0.8	2088±750[a]	587±128[a]	3.2±0.8	873±129	235±57	2961±800[a]	822±172[a]
II (6) B.	clofibrate	2.7±0.7	676±201	195±59	3.4±0.6	838±99	192±31	1514±270	387±70
D.	"	2.7±0.6	623±153	172±20	3.6±0.7	631±107	132±20	1255±233	304±36
IV (6) B.	"	0.9±0.1	1552±486	1076±333	1.5±0.1	636±109	293±51	2188±420	1379±221
D.	"	1.6±0.5	809±298	243±85[c]	2.1±0.4	588±184	216±53	1396±303[c]	549±97[d]
II (4) B.	cholestyramine	2.6±1.2	360±268	89±29	3.2±1.7	776±517	163±19	1136±782	253±46
D.	"	1.2±0.5	1058±263[d]	815±423[c]	0.7±0.3	364±98	398±142[c]	1423±327	1213±561[c]
IV (5) B.	"	1.1±0.5	1166±441	804±308	1.6±0.3	513±193	240±119	1670±180	1044±90
D.	"	0.7±0.2	906±497	987±578	0.7±0.4	630±372	650±229[d]	1530±160	1637±170

[a] $0.01 < p < 0.05$, [b] $0.001 < p < 0.01$ (comparisons with controls),
[c] $0.01 < p < 0.05$, [d] $0.001 < p < 0.01$ (comparisons with pretreatment values).

patients. Lower values were recorded for the pool size (447 ± 112 mg) and turn-over (120 ± 15 mg/day) of cholic acid in the patients with a type IIa lipoprotein pattern. Although not significant on a statistical basis, both parameters tended to be subnormal in the patients with type IIb. In the patients with types IV and V, the values for the pool size and turnover of cholic acid were 2-3 times higher than those of the controls (Table 1).

In the controls the half-life of chenodeocycholic acid exceeded that of cholic acid by about one day; the pool size (mean 602 mg) and turnover (144 mg/day) were lower than for cholic acid (Table 1). A different pattern was encountered in the patients with a type II lipoprotein pattern, characterized by chenodeocycholic acid as the dominant bile acid. In the controls the quotient for the pool size of cholic acid in relation to chenodeocycholic acid averaged 1.4, whereas in types IIa and IIb it was 0.6 and 0.7, respectively. The mean quotient for the turnovers of the two bile acids was 2.0 in the controls, 0.7 in type IIa and 0.9 in type IIb. In type IV, the pool size and daily synthesis of chenodeocycholic acid did not differ significantly from the control values. Due to the large pool size and turnover of cholic acid, their quotients for cholic acid in relation to chenode-ocycholic acid synthesis averaged 2.4 (pool size) and 3.4 (turnover).

Treatment with Clofibrate. In 4 out of 6 patients with hyperlipoproteinaemia type II the concentrations of cholesterol and triglycerides decreased during treatment with clofibrate (Einarsson et al., 1973); the other two patients displayed a simi-lar tendency in the case of triglycerides. These effects were not accompanied by consistent changes in half-life, pool size and turnover of the bile acids (Table 1, Fig. 1).

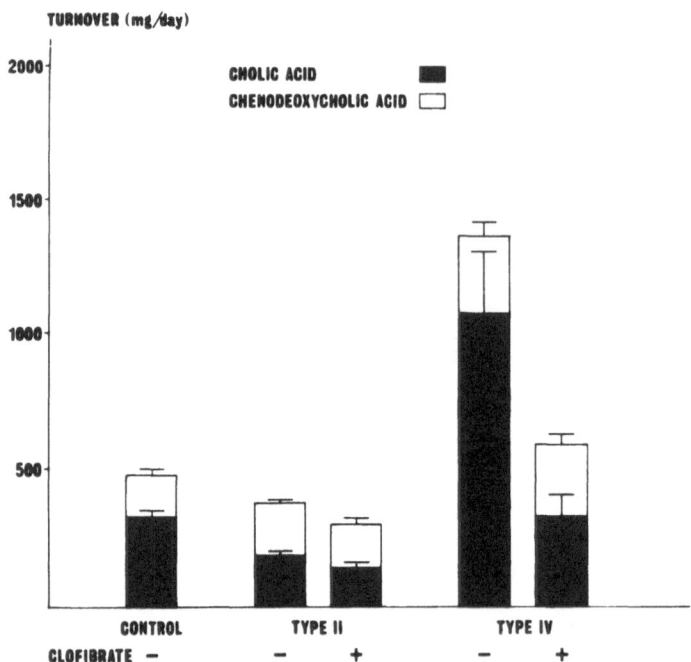

Figure 1

During treatment with clofibrate the serum triglycerides and pre-β-lipoproteins decreased markedly in 5 of the 6 patients with hyperlipoproteinaemia type IV. Ad-ministration of the drug had no significant effect on the half-life and pool size of cholic acid but the turnover decreased in all subjects, on the average from

1076 ± 243 to 333 ± 85 mg/day (p<0.025). Mainly due to the marked change in cholic acid formation, the total synthesis of the primary bile acids was much lower
while the patients were on clofibrate (Fig. 1).

Treatment with Cholestyramine. In 3 out of 4 patients with hyperlipoproteinaemia
type II, serum cholesterol decreased significantly during treatment with cholestyramine. At the same time the pool size and turnover of cholic acid increased in
all subjects, on the average 3 and 10 times, respectively (Table 1, Fig. 2). The
synthesis of chenodeoxycholic acid was also somewhat elevated. The total formation
of bile acids rose by a mean of about 1 g/day.

Quite a different reaction pattern was encountered in the patients with type IV.
Treatment with cholestyramine did not accentuate the high cholic acid formation
recorded during basal conditions but the turnover of chenodeoxycholic acid increased moderately in all subjects (Table 1, Fig. 2). Total bile acid formation
tended to be higher during treatment but the difference was not statistically
significant.

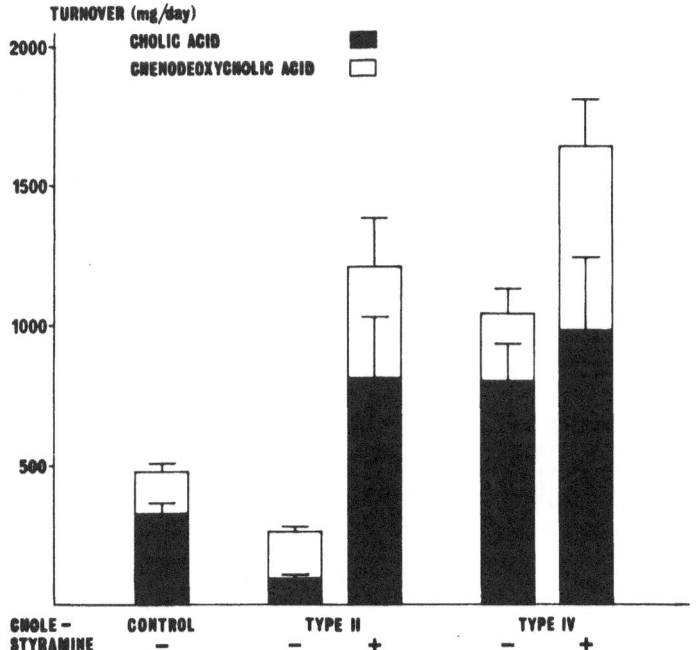

Figure 2

Discussion

In relation to the normolipemic controls, the patients with hyperlipoproteinaemia
type IIa had a subnormal and those with type IV an elevated cholic acid synthesis.
These changes were not conditioned by differences in body size since the daily
synthesis of cholic acid per kg body weight in the controls (4.0 ± 0.6 mg/kg) was
higher than in type IIa (1.9 ± 0.2 mg/kg, p<0.01) but lower than in type IV (9.7
± 0.3 mg/kg, p<0.01). Due to the relatively high formation of chenodeoxycholic
acid in patients with type IIa, their total bile acid synthesis was however, within the normal range. In type IV the combined formation of cholic and chenodeoxycholic acid exceeded that of the controls even when calculated per kg body weight.

The patients participating in these studies had been admitted consecutively to the ward because of hyperlipoproteinaemia. Most of those with a type II lipoprotein pattern turned out to be women, whereas most of those with type IV were men. Bile acid turnover in relation to both type of hyperlipoproteinaemia and sex consequently had to be evaluated from a small number of subjects. Even so, the turnover of cholic acid in patients with hyperlipoproteinaemia type II was significantly lower than in the controls of the same sex. Furthermore, the men with type IV had a higher bile acid formation than the male controls. No such difference was obtained for the women. Although not significant on a statistical basis, the formation of bile acids (in absolute amounts or calculated per kg body weight) tended to be higher in the males than the females, a tendency which applied to the controls as well as to the hyperlipemic subjects.

The present studies demonstrate that it is the cholic acid rather than the chenodeocycholic acid metabolism which is abnormal in hyperlipoproteinaemia. The low quotient for the turnover of the two bile acids in type II changed to normal during treatment with cholestyramine. This effect was achieved mainly by a stimulated formation of cholic acid, thus indicating that the low formation under basal conditions is due to homeostatic factors rather than to an inability of the liver to produce cholic acid.

BILE ACID KINETICS IN HYPERLIPOPROTEINEMIA[*]

Bruce A. Kottke, Connie L. Stamnes, Nancy E. Tyler, and Mary A. Carey

On the basis of lipoprotein composition and structure, the hyperlipoproteinemias have been classified into six major types, and it is generally conceded that these types represent distinct disease entities. Hence, they might be expected to be associated with concurrent abnormalities of lipoprotein metabolism and possibly also with alterations of cholesterol metabolism. Langer et al. (1972) showed that the catabolism of low density lipoproteins is slowed in type II_a hyperlipoproteinemia compared to normal. A distinct metabolic defect in lipoprotein metabolism has also been shown in type III hyperlipoproteinemia (Quarfordt et al., 1971). Miettinen et al. (1967) reported that patients with familial type II_a hyperlipoproteinemia have a lower rate of excretion of fecal bile acids than do normals.

In 1969, we (Kottke, 1969) reported that rates of cholic and chenodeoxycholic acid synthesis were significantly lower in patients with type II_a hyperlipoproteinemia than in patients with type IV or V hyperlipoproteinemia; this has been confirmed by Einarsson and Hellström (1972). Herein we report an expansion of our previous series of patients, with data from 34 patients with hyperlipoproteinemia and three normal controls. Because of the possibility (Vlahcevic et al., 1972) of alterations in bile acid pool sizes in patients with cholelithiasis, we have considered the presence of gallbladder disease as a factor in the analysis of our data. In addition, we calculated our data on the basis of both body weight and body surface area.

Methods

During the studies, the patients ate ordinary foods on a dietary regimen similar to what they had been following for months prior to the study. Cholesterol content of the diets ranged from 150 to 275 mg/day and fat content was 50 to 60 g/day, except in four studies cholesterol was 500 to 650 mg/day and fat content was 60 to 90 g/day. Patients were maintained in a steady state throughout the study. The synthesis rates and pool sizes of the two primary bile acids, cholic acid and chenodeoxycholic acid, were measured by the Lindstedt (1957) technique using [carboxyl-^{14}C]cholic acid and randomly labeled [^{3}H]chenodeoxycholic acid.

Results

Synthesis Rates. The present data (Table 1) confirm our previous observation (Kottke, 1969) that the synthesis rates of cholic and chenodeoxycholic acids are significantly lower in patients with type II_a hyperlipoproteinemia than in patients with other forms of hyperlipoproteinemia including type II_b or in normals. Although the synthesis rates of these two bile acids were high in type IV and V hyperlipoproteinemia, this increase was not significant compared to our small number of normal controls.

All of these differences persisted after patients with a previous cholecystectomy, known cholelithiasis, or the subsequent development of cholelithiasis were excluded. The ratio of cholic acid synthesis to chenodeoxycholic acid synthesis was

[*]Supported in part by NIH Grant HL-14196.

not clearly altered by the type of hyperlipoproteinemia present. In all groups of patients, the fractional turnover rate of cholic acid was greater than that of chenodeocycholic acid. The fractional turnover rates of both primary bile acids were significantly lower in patients with type II_a than in patients with type IV or V. The fractional turnover rate of chenodeoxycholic acid was increased in type IV as compared to normal controls.

Pool Sizes. Type II_a hyperlipoproteinemia was characterized by low pools of both cholic and chenodeoxycholic acids (Table 1), whether the pool sizes were calculated as absolute values or on the basis of body weight or body surface area. Type IV was characterized by a significant decrease in the size of the chenodeoxycholic acid pool, regardless of how the data were calculated. In both instances, elimination of patients with a previous cholecystectomy or known gallbladder disease did not change these differences.

Table 1. Mean pool sizes and synthesis rates

Acid	Type II_a (N = 11)	Type II_b (N = 4)	Type IV (N = 14)	Type V (N = 5)	Normal (N = 3)
			Pool size (mg/m^2)		
Cholic	305^a	544	471	689	654^a
Chenodeoxycholic	416^a	843	534^f	763	$980^{a,f}$
			Synthesis rate (mg/m^2)		
Cholic	$85^{a,b,e,f}$	127^e	311^f	295^b	161^a
Chenodeoxycholic	$74^{a,b,c,d}$	121^a	231^b	227^c	145^d
Total	$159^{a,b,c,d}$	248^a	542^b	522^c	306^d

^{a,b,c,d} $P < 0.01$. ^{e} $P < 0.02$. ^{f} $P < 0.05$. Comparisons are between same letters.

Conclusion

Although these data are of a preliminary nature because of the small number of normal controls, our findings strongly suggest that types II_a, II_b, and IV hyperlipoproteinemia are characterized by distinctive abnormalities of bile acid kinetics. These observations suggest that either specific lipoproteins may regulate bile acid metabolism or the lipoprotein defect of the hyperlipoproteinemia may be secondary to a primary defect in bile acid synthesis. In addition, our findings suggest that investigations of the relationship of bile acid metabolism to cholelithiasis will need to consider the lipid status of the patients with cholelithiasis.

Miscellaneous

INFLUENCE OF DIETARY CHOLESTEROL ON SKIN LIPÍD SYNTHESIS IN MAN. EVIDENCE FOR A POSITIVE FEEDBACK MECHANISM

Dennis Mendelsohn and Harold C. Seftel

Elucidation of the mechanisms of abnormal lipid metabolism in man have been hampered mainly by the difficultires in obtaining representative tissues for biochemical scrutiny. Concerning cholesterol metabolism, the most easily available human tissue, blood (either whole or its separate components), is unable to synthesise this sterol to any significant extent. Human skin however, is capable of a wide variety of biosynthetic functions and is also an active site with regard to cholesterol and fatty acid synthesis. Employing the relatively painless skin punch biopsy technique, Mendelsohn and Mendelsohn (1972) demonstrated that patients with Type II hyperlipoproteinemia had approximately three times the concentration of cholesterol in their skin together with a significantly increased rate of dermal cholesterogenesis when compared with normal subjects. Also, by incubating skin slices of Type II patients with both acetate and mevalonate, evidence was obtained that the increased enzymatic activity occurred before the stage of mevalonate formation, indicating the possibility that 3-hydroxy-3-methylglutaryl coenzyme A reductase was the enzyme affected. These findings supported the contention that the skin was very active as far as cholesterol biosynthesis was concerned and also suggested that other body tissues (e.g. arterial) might behave similarly in Type II patients who have a known predilection for atherosclerosis and its complications. We have also shown in unpublished experiments that gross dietary manipulation in humans can produce marked changes in skin lipid metabolism. The present report describes the effect of alteration of one dietary constituent only, i.e. cholesterol, on the metabolism of fatty acids and cholesterol in the skin of man.

The dietary cholesterol intake of two adult volunteers (one male – age 42 years and one female – age 36 years) was adjusted to less than 200 mg daily for three weeks. After this period, 1g cholesterol per day dissolved in about 30 ml mixed vegetable oil was added to the diet for four weeks. Thirty millilitres of mixed vegetable oil alone was then given with the diet for two weeks and the experiment continued for a further two weeks on the original diet. Full thickness, skin punch biopsies (4mm diameter) were taken from the scapular region at weekly intervals. These were immediately trimmed of excess subcutaneous tissue, weighed and then incubated at 37° for 2 hours in air in 1 ml Krebs-Ringer phosphate buffer, pH 7.4, containing 25 µCi sodium-acetate-1-^{14}C (50mCi/mmol). After digestion and extraction of lipids from the skin slices by the usual procedures, radioactivity was determined in total fatty acids and cholesterol (as the digitonide). Previous experiments had shown that over 90% of human skin digitonide-precipitable sterols consisted of cholesterol. Total cholesterol in each biopsy specimen was also measured employing o-phthalaldehyde.

During the period of cholesterol feeding, the biosynthesis of skin cholesterol increased by 15.3% in the male and 14.8% in the female; i.e. from 32-49 and 23-34 nmoles acetate incorporated into cholesterol/g skin respectively. Total skin cholesterol (mg/g skin) rose from 1.1-2.2 in the male and 1.6-2.4 in the female. In both cases, upon removal of cholesterol from the diet, dermal sterol synthesis dropped markedly before returning to basal levels while total cholesterol fell slowly. Incorporation of radioactivity from acetate into total fatty acids followed that of cholesterol. Changes in serum cholesterol for the duration of the experiment were unremarkable in each subject.

Dietschy and Wilson (1970) found that in the rat and squirrel monkey dietary supplementation with cholesterol produced no significant alteration of sterol synthesis in the skin. A possible explanation for the discrepancy in our results might
be due to the fact that whereas in the above mentioned species cholesterol accounts for less than 50% of skin digitonide-precipitable sterols, in man this
figure is well over 90%. However, it is of interest in this regard that Ho and
Taylor (1968) demonstrated in some mammalian species, e.g. rabbit and prairie dog
but not rat, increased feeding of cholesterol led to a raised cholesterol content
of most tissues but especially so in aorta and skin. Our findings indicate that
probably in contrast to the liver, a positive feedback for cholesterol and fatty
acid synthesis exists in the skin of man with accumulation of the former therein
during high dietary intake of this sterol. Upon removal of excess cholesterol
from the diet, its concentration in the skin fell slowly and still had not returned to basal levels after four weeks. Furthermore, the level of serum cholesterol
gave no indication of the metabolic changes taking place in the skin. If a similar train of events as described above occurs in the human arterial wall *in vivo*,
then dietary cholesterol may be of greater importance in the pathogenesis of
atherosclerosis than has hitherto been assumed.

Due acknowledgement is made to the South African Medical Research Council and the
Atomic Energy Board for the assistance and support enabling the research concerned
to be undertaken, and for permission to publish the results of the work.

XII
Lipolytic Enzymes

Chairmen: W.V. Brown, USA
          H. Greten, West Germany

Participants: Th. Olivecrona
              Ch.J. Fielding, USA
              E.L. Bierman, USA
              J.A. Glomset, USA
              D. Steinberg, USA

Transport in the plasma of dietary and endogenously produced lipid provides for internal balance of caloric supply between the various organs and tissues. The normal metabolism of the lipoproteins responsible for this transport is dependent on the proper functioning of a group of lipolytic enzymes. Lipoprotein lipase is felt to be primarily responsible for hydrolysis of the triglycerides on chylomicra and the very low density lipoproteins (VLDL) before their uptake as fatty acids (or partial glycerides) by extra-hepatic tissues. The purification and characterization of lipoprotein lipases from several sources has progressed rapidly during the past four years. The first two papers in this workshop will discuss the lipoprotein lipase of bovine milk (Dr. Olivecrona) and that from plasma after heparin injection (Dr. Fielding).

The metabolism of lipoproteins also involves the so-called surface components or polar lipids, which include phospholipids and free cholesterol. At least two plasma enzymes have been characterized which may play important roles in this area. The properties of post-heparin phospholipase will be reviewed by Dr. Bierman and those of lecithin cholesterol acyl transferase (LCAT) by Dr. Glomset. Finally, the release of stored lipid for its return to the plasma pool as fatty acids will be reviewed by Dr. Steinberg.

LIPOPROTEIN LIPASE OF BOVINE MILK

Thomas Olivecrona, Olle Hernell, and Torbjörn Egelrud

About 2 years ago we described a method for the purification of a lipoprotein lipase (LPL) (Egelrud and Olivecrona, 1972) from bovine milk. This is an advantageous starting material since there is as much enzyme activity in 1 liter milk as there is in 2 liters of rat post-heparin plasma or in 60 kg of hen adipose tissue. The main purification was obtained by affinity chromatography on agarose with covalently linked heparin. Similar procedures have since been used successfully with lipoprotein lipases of other origins (Greten and Walter, 1973; Bensadoun et al., 1973).

The affinity chromatography demonstrated that the enzyme forms a strong, reversible, ionic bond with heparin. Thus, if enzyme and heparin are present together at physiological pH, ionic strength etc., they will form a complex.

The physiological lipid substrate for the enzyme is long chain triacylglycerols. The milk LPL hydrolyses the two primary ester bonds (Nilsson-Elle, et al., 1973), but may act initially mainly on the 1-ester bond (Moorley and Kuskis, 1972). The initial products of the lipolysis are fatty acids and 2-monoacylglycerols. The monoacylglycerols are probably split only after isomerization. These products are not water soluble and the reaction is dependent on an efficient fatty acid acceptor, e.g. serum albumin.

Efficient hydrolysis of long chain triacylglycerols is promoted by the apolipoprotein R-Glu (C II) (Havel et al., 1973). However, the enzyme has catalytic activity also in the absence of the activator peptide (Egelrud and Olivecrona, 1973). With long chain triacylglycerols the basal activity is about 5% of the optimal, activator stimulated activity. With tributyrylglycerol the activity is about half of the optimal activity against long-chain triacylglycerols, and the activity against tributyrylglycerol is not much stimulated by activator. The enzyme also has activity against the water soluble substrate paranitrophenyl acetate and in this system no effect of activator can be demonstrated. Thus, the activator is not necessary for catalysis to occur, but modifies the substrate, or the enzyme, to promote activity against the physiological substrate, long chain triacylglycerols.

We have recently adapted our method to the purification of a lipoprotein lipase from human milk (Hernell and Olivecrona, unpublished). In bovine milk, most of the enzyme is in the skim milk, bound to the casein micelles, whereas in human milk, most of the LPL is bound to the milk fat droplets, and one must first make a lipid free, soluble enzyme preparation. Therefore, the initial steps of the purification were quite different from those used with the bovine milk, However, also with the enzyme from human milk, the main purification was obtained by affinity chromatography on heparin-Sepharose. This gave us a preparation with a specific activity of 140 µeq fatty acid released per min and mg protein at 25°C, which is about half of that for the enzyme from bovine milk, but about 5 times higher than that previously reported for enzyme purified from post-heparin plasma (Fielding, 1970). Our preparation contained several proteins, as judged by SDS-acrylamide gel electrophoresis. One of the bands, accounting for about half the staining intensity, appeared to coincide in its distribution in the fractions with the enzyme activity. It was the only band on the gel that stained also with the PAS reaction. The bovine milk LPL also gives this reaction, and the LPL from swine adipose tissue (Bensadoun et al., 1973) and from human post-heparin plasma are also glycoproteins, since they bind to concanavalin-A. The molecular weight of the peptide chain was about 63.000. Our data thus suggest that the enzyme in human milk may have a molecular weight and specific activity similar to that in bovine milk.

We have raised a rabbit antibody to the bovine milk LPL. This antibody also precipitates the human milk LPL, further suggesting a similarity between the two enzymes. Human post-heparin plasma contains at least two separate lipases (LaRosa et al., 1972). One has the classical characteristics of a lipoprotein lipase. Thus, it is stimulated by serum and is inhibited by high salt concentration. The other lipase probably originates in the liver and is inhibited by serum but not by high salt concentration (Krauss et al., 1973). When human post-heparin plasma was incubated with the rabbit antiserum to bovine milk LPL, the enzyme activity measured in a "lipoprotein lipase assay" decreased by more than three fourths, whereas the lipase activity measured with 0.75 M sodium chloride but no serum present was essentially unchanged. These results suggest that the antiserum precipitated the lipoprotein lipase but not the liver lipase and show that the human post-heparin plasma lipoprotein lipase also has immunological determinants in common with the bovine milk lipase.

The bovine milk enzyme is probably the only lipoprotein lipase that can be obtained at sufficient purity in adequate quantities (milligrams or tens of milligrams) to permit a chemical and physical chemical characterization. Our studies suggest that this enzyme has many properties in common with the human lipoprotein lipases, which should encourage us to embark on a more detailed study of the molecular properties of the bovine milk lipoprotein lipase.

Finally we would like to point out that there are two lipases present in human milk (Hernell and Olivecrona, unpublished). One is the lipoprotein lipase, with properties very similar to the lipase in cow's milk. The other enzyme which is not present in cow's milk, differs in several respects. It is stimulated by bile salts and is present in much higher activity than the lipoprotein lipase. Therefore human milk should *not* be used without fractionation for studies on lipoprotein lipase, as has been successfully done with bovine milk.

HEPARIN-RELEASED LIPOPROTEIN LIPASE

C.J. Fielding

Circulating lipoprotein triglyceride fatty acid (TGFA) is cleared in extrahepatic tissues by a pathway which requires hydrolysis prior to uptake and utilisation. Physiological studies indicate that the bulk of TGFA is removed by these tissues, and only a small fraction (about 15%) by the liver (Bergman et al., 1971). It is well known that heparin releases a triglyceride hydrolase into the plasma from a superficial, probably extracellular binding site that is highly reactive with triglyceride-rich lipoproteins (chylomicrons and very low density lipoproteins, VLDL). Release of the enzyme can also be demonstrated by perfusion of isolated organs such as the heart (Fielding, 1972). After passage of heparin through the tissue, ability of the tissue to catabolise TGFA is virtually abolished (Borenzstayn and Robinson, 1970). On these grounds, heparin-released lipoprotein lipase (LPL) is believed to represent the major or only enzyme system involved in the catabolism of TGFA in peripheral tissues. LPL activity is virtually undetectable in the plasma prior to the injection of heparin. Other lipoprotein lipase activities are present intracellularly in many tissues and in milk.

The heparin-released LPL has been highly purified in a number of laboratories and characterised in terms of its substrate specificity, molecular properties, and the dependence of activity on the presence of a protein cofactor which is a component of the natural lipoprotein substrates. A second, heparin-released lipase of hepatic origin has been purified and characterised by Greten and co-workers (Greten et al., 1972). Space permits the discussion here only of research in which LPL was distinguished from post-heparin hepatic lipase, either by purification or by the use of appropriate differential inhibitors.

Distribution of Heparin-Released LPL. Only a fraction of total tissue LPL appears to play a direct role in the clearance of circulating lipoprotein triglyceride. In adipose tissue, where adipocyte and stroma-vascular fractions can be readily dissociated with collagenase, most of the recovered enzyme activity is associated with the adipocyte fraction (Rodbell, 1964). Similarly, only a small proportion of heart LPL is released by perfusion with heparin (Borenzstayn and Robinson, 1970). The proportion of the total lipase activity of postheparin plasma which represents LPL has also been the subject of a number of studies, which have presented conflicting conclusions. In general terms, studies which used natural lipoprotein substrates or triglyceride-lecithin dispersions in the assay of post-heparin lipolytic activity have found that the major part of activity showed the properties of LPL, in terms of substrate specificity and reaction with inhibitors of LPL or hepatic lipase (Fielding, 1972; Boberg and Carlson, 1964). On the other hand, in studies using triglyceride-Triton X100 substrate the major part of activity assayed had the properties of hepatic post-heparin lipase (Krauss et al., 1973). It has to be borne in mind that both lipases are physiologically supported at cellular binding sites and therefore not present in free solution. Nevertheless, the differences in "proportions" of post-heparin lipases reported by different laboratories may be due in large part to differences in assay technique, as is shown by our recent studies in which the same sample of human post-heparin plasma was assayed by each procedure, under saturating conditions with respect to each substrate. As shown in Table 1, with M-NaCl as inhibitor of LPL, the extent of

inhibition obtained with the two assays is quite different, indicating the expected greater "proportion" of hepatic lipase obtained when using triglyceride-Triton
X100 substrate. Similar results have been obtained using protamine as inhibitor
of LPL. As discussed above, in animal post-heparin plasma, the proportion of LPL
assayed with triglyceride-lecithin does appear to approximate to the proportional
clearing of TGFA by the extrahepatic tissues in the intact animal. Triglyceride-
Triton X100 substrate clearly gives a quite different estimate. There are no adequate data at present to determine whether this is also the case in man and in
pathological conditions of lipoprotein metabolism.

Table 1. Inhibition of human post-heparin plasma by M-NaCl, assayed with triglyceride-lecithin and triglyceride-Triton X-100 substrates. Plasma was assayed at
timed intervals following the administration of 0.2 mg heparin/kg body wt. *Conditions:* pH 8.6, 37°C. Assays were for 30 min in the presence of saturating concentrations of substrates

Interval post-heparin (mins)	Triglyceride-lecithin		% inhib.	Triglyceride-Triton X-100		% inhib.
	-NaCl[a]	M-NaCl		-NaCl	M-NaCl	
5	6.8	1.6	76	10.5	7.2	32
10	6.9	1.2	83	10.4	8.1	22
30	3.7	0.8	78	6.7	6.2	8
60	0.9	0.5	45	2.2	3.6	-[b]

[a]Assays -NaCl: assayed at ionic strength I = 0.15; (O. Faergeman and C.J. Fielding, unpublished results).
[b]Hepatic post-heparin lipase in post-heparin plasma is stimulated to about 150%
of control values in the presence of M-NaCl (ref. 2). Correction has not been
made in the values presented.

Purification and Properties of Heparin Released LPL. LPL purified to at least
95% homogeneity, as determined by polyacrylamide gel electrophoresis, has been
obtained by several laboratories using procedures based on affinity-flotation of
lipase triglyceride complex, fractionation with detergents, and subsequent chromatography of the solubilised active fraction by ion exchange chromatography (Fielding, 1969; Fielding 1970). The relative activity of purified LPL with emulsified,
micellar and soluble ester substrates is shown in Table 2. In contrast to other
triglyceride lipases such as pancreatic lipase (Sarda and Desnuelle, 1958) or the
lipoprotein lipase of bovine milk (Egelrud and Olivecrona, 1973), heparin-released LPL shows a high degree of specificity for reaction with long-chain neutral
glycerides. Purified LPL also shows minor activity with phospholipid substrates
(lecithin, phosphatidyl ethanolamine) but only at high pH (>10) (C.J. Fielding,
unpublished experiments).

Whilst a number of studies have been made of the cofactor dependence of LPL species from tissue cell homogenates and from milk, less attention has been paid to
this property with the heparin-released lipase species. Ganesan and co-workers
(Ganesan et al., 1971) reported studies on the cofactor activity of the major
human VLDL polypeptides with purified heparin-released LPL from man and several
animal species. Evidence was obtained for the existence of two LPL components.

Table 2. Substrate specificity of heparin-released LPL from rat plasma. *Reaction conditions:* pH 7.0, 37°C. Assays were for 10 minutes in the presence of saturating concentrations of substrate and of VLDL protein where applicable

Substrate	Maximal reaction velocity	
	−apoVLDL	+apoVLDL
Triolein-lecithin 10%	2.1	3.6
1,2-diolein	2.4	3.3
2-monolein (emulsion)	0.8	0.8
2-monolein (micellar)	0.2	0.2
Tributyrin	0.2	0.2
nitrophenyl acetate[a]	<0.01	<0.01

[a]Assayed spectrophotometrically.
[b]Mole $^{-7}$.mg protein·sec^{-1}.

One, activated by apolipoprotein C-1 (C-terminal serine)[*], was released from the liver; the second, activated by apolipoprotein C-2 (C-terminal glutamic acid) was derived from the extrahepatic tissues. In this laboratory we have sought and failed to find evidence for lipase activated by C-1 apolipoprotein in our purified preparations of human or rat post-heparin LPL (Havel et al., 1973), which were activated only by apolipoprotein C-2.

Kinetic studies of the mechanism of cofactor activation of the LPL reaction have shown the following features: 1. cofactor protein increases the catalytic rate for LPL, but is not a prerequisite for activity; 2. cofactor activity is pH dependent and is more marked at the lipase pH optimum (8.0-8.5) than under physiological conditions; 3. cofactor dependence is limited to reactions at a lipid-water interface; 4. cofactor-induced increase in the rate of lipolysis probably results from the appoximation of a positively charged amino acid residue of the cofactor to the lipase active site (Fielding, 1973).

LPL-mediated catabolism of triglyceride represents a key reaction in plasma lipid metabolism and is now receiving increased attention from investigators in spite of operational difficulties associated with instability of the enzyme protein and the very small amounts released into the plasma by heparin. Future progress will depend on the distinction of this lipase from the several other similar activities present in the tissues and in post-heparin plasma.

POST-HEPARIN PHOSPHOLIPASE

F.L. Bierman

After intravenous injection of heparin to man, enzymatic activities appear in plasma active on a variety of lipid substrates including phospholipids (phosphatidyl ethanolamine and phosphatidyl choline) (Vogel and Zieve, 1964). Post-heparin

---

[*]Terminology of human VLDL polypeptides is that used by Ganesan et al. (1971) to describe the species isolated by Brown et al. (1969).

phospholipase appears to release fatty acids from the C-1 position (Vogel and Bierman, 1967); the kinetics of appearance and disappearance of the activity from the circulation is similar to that observed for other substrates (triglyceride emulsions, monoglycerides and diglycerides). Phospholipase activity appears to be active *in vivo*, since during constant heparin infusion and sampling of plasma with paraoxan inhibitor to block *in vitro* lipolysis, VLDL lecithin decreases in parallel with reduction in triglyceride (Vogel and Bierman, 1968; 1970). This suggests a multi-enzyme lipolytic system physiologically acting on both coat and core of triglyceride-rich lipoproteins to produce a triglyceride-poor, lecithin-poor, cholesterol-rich remnant (Vogel et al., 1971).

Thus far, attempts at physical-chemical separation and purification have failed to separate triglyceridase from phospholipase activities (Vogel et al., 1971) consistent with the possibility that a similar enzyme is acting on both substrates. Studies on tissue sites of origin thus far have suggested that phospholipase is derived predominantly from the liver and not adipose tissue. Dose-response curves with heparin have failed to differentially release various enzyme activities. In normal subjects there is a high correlation among levels of triglyceridase, monoglyceridase and phospholipase activities. In subjects with deficiency of post-heparin lipolytic activity secondary to other diseases (e.g. insulin deficiency, thyroid deficiency), all post-heparin activities decrease in parallel and respond in parallel to treatment (Bierman, 1972; Baum et al., 1973). With estrogen-induced inhibition of release of lipolytic enzymes by heparin, all activities decrease in parallel (Hazzard et al., 1972). In some subjects with reduced PHLA, however, normal monoglyceridase activity is maintained in the face of reduced phospholipase and triglyceridase activities.

Thus, there is a close physiological association between post-heparin triglyceridase and phospholipase activities, which suggests a combined action in the catabolism of VLDL to produce cholesterol-rich remnants. Hydrolysis of the phospholipid coat of a lipoprotein may be essential to allow enzyme access to core triglyceride. Whether phospholipase is a completely separate enzyme or is part of an enzyme aggregate coming from one or more tissue sources is still an open question.

LECITHIN: CHOLESTEROL ACYLTRANSFERASE

John A. Glomset

Lecithin:cholesterol acyltransferase (LCAT) is a plasma enzyme that catalyzes the transfer of fatty acids from the lecithin to the cholesterol of circulating lipoproteins. Although not strictly a lipolytic enzyme, it does catalyze the conversion of lecithin to lysolecithin; and discussion of its function seems appropriate for a symposium on lipolytic enzymes because its physiologic role appears to be closely related to that of lipoprotein lipase (Schumacher and Adams, 1970; Glomset and Norum, 1973). According to the available evidence (Glomset, 1968; 1972), LCAT is synthesized in the liver, but acts in the plasma in close association with high density lipoproteins (HDL). By catalysing the transfer of fatty acids from the lecithin to the cholesterol of HDL, the enzyme directly forms HDL cholesteryl esters and lysolecithin. In addition, the LCAT reaction has important indirect effects: 1. It indirectly diminishes the unesterified cholesterol and lecithin of plasma lipoproteins such as low density lipoproteins (LDL) and very low density lipoproteins (VLDL). These polar lipids exchange readily among lipoproteins, and this in effect creates a pool of substrate for the LCAT reaction from which HDL unesterified cholesterol and lecithin can be replenished. 2. The LCAT reaction tends to increase the lysolecithin content of other plasma proteins (especially albumin), since lysolecithin also redistributes following the LCAT reaction. 3. The LCAT reaction increases the cholesteryl ester content of LDL and VLDL, apparently by promoting the transfer of newly formed cholesteryl esters from HDL. These direct and indirect effects can be readily demonstrated by incubating normal plasma lipoproteins with LCAT. However, the relative changes obtained are small; and until recently their significance was unclear. Fortunately, the discovery of familial LCAT deficiency (Norum and Gjone, 1967; Norum et al., 1972) has provided an entirely new perspective. Patients with this disease have plasma lipoproteins that are abnormal by many criteria (Glomset and Norum, 1973). All of the lipoproteins contain abnormally high proportions of unesterified cholesterol and lecithin relative to cholesteryl ester, and in addition some are abnormal in appearance upon electron microscopy, some migrate abnormally upon electrophoresis, and some bear no resemblance at all to normal lipoproteins. Studies of the effects of the LCAT reaction on these lipoproteins (Glomset and Norum, 1973; Norum et al., unpublished) have yielded striking results that can be summarized as follows. Incubation of the patients' unfractionated plasma with partially purified LCAT: 1. decreases the plasma unesterified cholesterol and lecithin, primarily by affecting large aggregates of these lipids that have the same density as LDL; 2. increases the plasma cholesteryl ester, primarily by increasing the content of cholesteryl ester in normal-sized LDL and VLDL; 3. increases the total concentration of normal-sized LDL in the plasma and increases their rate of flotation; 4. increases the concentration of apolipoprotein A-I in the HDL class; 5. alters the appearance of the HDL upon electron microscopy from that of stacked discs and small particles to that of normal HDL; and 6. increases by 2- to 3-fold the relative content in the patients' VLDL of material similar to the Shores' "arginine-rich" peptide.

The fact that incubation with LCAT markedly alters the patients' lipoproteins is consistent with the concept that normal lipoproteins, freshly isolated from plasma, have already reacted extensively with LCAT in vivo. This would explain why little further change occurs upon incubation of normal plasma in vitro and why more than two thirds of the cholesterol of freshly obtained normal plasma is already esterified. The effects of incubating the patients' plasma with LCAT are also consistent with the concept that the LCAT reaction markedly alters the distribution of lipids and peptides among plasma lipoproteins, and that the source of the unesterified cholesterol and lecithin for the reaction, the site of the reaction, and the ultimate carriers of most of the cholesteryl esters formed by the reaction may be entirely different lipoproteins.

A major problem that remains to be clarified concerns the physiological role of the reaction. Schumacher and Adams (1970) have suggested that the LCAT reaction removes the surface lipids of chylomicrons and VLDL following degradation of the latter by lipoprotein lipase. Our results support this suggestion, especially since the large aggregates of unesterified cholesterol and lecithin in the patients' plasma decrease markedly in concentration when the patients consume fat-free diets (Glomset et al., unpublished). These aggregates may be derived from chylomicron surfaces; and since they serve as a major source of unesterified cholesterol and lecithin when the patients' plasma is incubated with LCAT in vitro, it is possible that they accumulate abnormally in the patients' plasma because of the absence of LCAT activity. The role of the LCAT reaction may be to prevent these aggregates from accumulating by converting excess surface lipid from chylomicron "remnants" (Redgrave, 1973) to a form that can be cleared by alternate pathways since the cholesteryl esters formed when the patients' plasma is incubated with LCAT largely become associated with relatively normal VLDL and LDL. This might free apolipoprotein-C components that would ordinarily be associated with the unesterified cholesterol and lecithin to take part in the activation of newly secreted chylomicrons, as proposed by Havel et al. (1973).

REGULATION OF HORMONE-SENSITIVE LIPASE AND LIPOPROTEIN LIPASE IN ADIPOSE TISSUE

Daniel Steinberg and John C. Khoo

My remarks will be limited to some comments on the relationship between hormone-sensitive lipase and lipoprotein lipase in adipose tissue and their response to hormones. It has been recognized for some time that the rates of fat mobilization from adipose tissue tend to vary inversely with the levels of lipoprotein lipase in the tissue. For example, during starvation there is a marked decrease in lipo-protein lipase concentration and an increase in the rate of free fatty acid (FFA) release. On refeeding, lipoprotein lipase levels increase and rates of FFA release decrease. Exposure of adipose tissue *in vitro* to lipolytic hormones (or to dibu-tyryl cyclic AMP) increases the rate of FFA release and the tissue concentration of hormone-sensitive lipase activity while decreasing the tissue concentration of lipoprotein lipase activity. This reciprocality between the two enzymes has led to several hypotheses. It has been suggested, for example, that both lipase activ-ities might be referable to a single enzyme protein, its activity toward lipopro-tein substrate being favored under some circumstances (possibly due to structural modification of the enzyme protein) while its activity toward stored triglycer-ides might be favored under other circumstances. This possibility seems unlikely since lipoprotein lipase and hormone-sensitive lipase have been at least partially resolved from each other (Huttunen et al., 1970). Another hypothesis to explain the reciprocal relationship is that the same system that leads to activation of hormone-sensitive lipase simultaneously leads to a *de*activation of lipoprotein lipase (Robinson and Wing, 1970). This hypothesis is attractive because of its analogy to metabolic control in other systems. For example, epinephrine activates phosphorylase in the liver and at the same time converts glycogen synthase to the relatively inactive D form (Rall et al., 1956; DeWulf and Hers, 1968). Thus, there is a "push-pull" regulation of glycogen breakdown and synthesis. Studies in our laboratory over the past few years have led to an elucidation of the mechan-isms involved in the conversion of hormone-sensitive lipase to its activated form (Huttunen et al., 1970; Huttunen and Steinberg, 1971). This has allowed us to put the latter hypothesis to a critical test and it is the results of those experi-ments that I want to report today. First, let me quickly review our current under-standing of the regulation of hormone-sensitive lipase.

It has been known for a number of years that the action of lipolytic hormones in adipose tissue is associated with an increase in cyclic AMP concentrations (But-cher et al., 1968; Manganiello et al., 1971; Butcher et al., 1965) and that inhi-bitors of phosphodiesterase can mimic or amplify the action of the lipolytic hor-mones (Vaughan and Steinberg, 1963). It has now been established that the link between cyclic AMP and the actual activation process is cyclic AMP-dependent pro-tein kinase (Huttunen et al., 1970; Soderling et al., 1973; Khoo et al., 1973). Partially purified hormone-sensitive lipase, free of endogenous protein kinase activity, can be activated 50 to 100% by brief incubation with protein kinase, ATP, Mg^{2+} and cyclic AMP (Huttunen et al., 1970). All of these cofactors are ab-solute requirements for the activation process. Furthermore, it has been shown that there is a transfer of phosphate from ATP to the enzyme protein during the activation and that this parallels the activation process very closely (Huttunen et al., 1970). It appears that the protein kinase acts directly on the lipase i.e. that there is no other enzyme involved. (In the case of the phosphorylase system, phosphorylase kinase is the immediate target of activated protein kinase, the active phosphorylase kinase then in turn converting phosphorylase to its active, phosphorylated form (Walsh et al., 1968).

Dr. John C. Khoo in our laboratory has examined the possibility that the same pro-tein kinase system that activates hormone-sensitive lipase might deactivate lipo-protein lipase. Lipoprotein lipase prepared from various sources was treated with protein kinase, ATP, Mg^{2+} and cyclic AMP under exactly the conditions used for activation of hormone-sensitive lipase (Khoo et al., 1973). Preparations used included: 1. acetone powder extracts of human adipose tissue prepared by the method of Korn (1955); 2. lipoprotein lipase released from rat epididymal fat pads into a heparin-containing medium; 3. lipoprotein lipase from an acetone powder of human milk; 4. lipoprotein lipase in crude extracts of human and chicken adipose tissue (not treated with acetone). The latter preparations included a significant level of hormone-sensitive lipase activity (assayed at pH 7.0 in the absence of added lipoprotein activators) but total activity was markedly enhanced by the addition of serum or of apoLp-Glu (Brown and Baginsky, 1972), indicating the presence of high levels of lipoprotein lipase activity. Incubation with the cyclic AMP-dependent protein kinase system led to significant increases in lipase activity assayed at pH 7.0 in the absence of lipoprotein activators, as expected. The percentage increase in activity under conditions optimal for lipoprotein lipase assay, on the other hand, was much smaller. In absolute terms, it was essentially equal to the increments observed in the absence of lipoprotein activators (Table 1). In other words, the results suggest that the hormone-sensitive

Table 1. Lack of effect of protein kinase on lipoprotein lipase activity in human and chicken adipose tissue fractions[a]

Additions	Lipolytic activity		Absolute change	Percentage change
	−cAMP and MgATP	+cAMP and MgATP		
	nmoles FFA/mg protein/hour			%
Human[b]				
None	120	200	80	+67
Human serum (50 µl)	486	532	56	+9.5
ApoLp-Glu peptide (10 µg)	470	520	50	+10.6
Chicken[c]				
None	584	1482	898	+154
Chicken serum (25 µl)	2473	3365	892	+36

[a] The large increment in lipase activity in the presence of added serum or apoLp-Glu peptide is taken to indicate that assay under those conditions measures predominantly lipoprotein lipase. The fact that the absolute increment in total lipase activity was similar in the presence or absence of serum or apoLp-Glu implies that all of the activation is referable to the hormone-sensitive lipase in the fractions.

[b] pH 5.2 precipitate fraction prepared from 100,000 x g supernatant of human subcutaneous adipose tissue.

[c] pH 5.2 precipitate fraction prepared from abdominal adipose tissue of laying hen.

lipase remaining in this preparation was activated but that nothing happened to the absolute level of lipoprotein lipase activity. The latter acted essentially as a "diluent", reducing the percentage activation observed but not decreasing the absolute increment in activity, presumed to be referable to the hormone-sensitive lipase content. It was felt important to carry out this somewhat more difficult experiment to rule out the possibility that the other preparations might contain only an already deactivated form of lipoprotein lipase. Finally, we have also looked for a protein kinase effect on the triglyceride lipase of hepatic origin purified by Greten et al. (1972) from post-heparin human plasma. Results were again negative.

None of the several additional preparations of lipoprotein lipase tested showed any effect at all of preincubation with the protein kinase activation system. Thus, while the "push-pull" hypothesis is theoretically attractive, we can find no evidence to support it. Nikkila and Pykallisto have pointed out that there is also a close reciprocal relationship between elevation of FFA levels in adipose tissue and decreases in lipoprotein lipase activity. They suggest that the fall in lipoprotein lipase activity seen under conditions associated with rapid fat mobilization simply reflects an inhibitory effect of high FFA concentrations on lipoprotein lipase activity or lipoprotein lipase biosynthesis (Nikkila and Pykallisto, 1968). Still another hypothesis is that of Patten, who suggests that a decrease in the ATP concentration during conditions of fat mobilization may account for the decreases in lipoprotein lipase activity (Patten, 1970). However, it should be noted that ither investigators have demonstrated increased fat mobilization *without* significant changes in ATP concentration (Jarret et al., 1972).

Returning to hormone-sensitive lipase for a moment, let me briefly report our recent results in human adipose tissue. Human adipose tissue is much less active metabolically than rat tissue and appears to be less sensitive to hormonal stimulation. However, hormone-sensitive lipase from human tissue has been partially purified by Dr. John C. Khoo and shown to have properties very similar to those of the enzyme in rat adipose tissue. The response of the enzyme to cyclic AMP-dependent protein kinase is similar in magnitude to that previously observed with rat enzyme and, except for some minor quantitative differences in optimal cofactor concentrations, the two systems seem to be in every way similar (Khoo et al., 1974). Thus, the marked difference in hormonal responsiveness is most likely attributable to differences in receptors and/or their interaction with adenylate cyclase in the membrane rather than to differences in the hormone-sensitive lipase enzyme itself or the relationship between protein kinase and hormone-sensitive lipase. It will be of interest to explore adipose tissue of other species in view of the marked differences that have been reported in hormonal responsiveness, both qualitative and quantitative. Certainly some of the differences must be based on differences in receptor systems in the cell membrane since adipose tissue from some species responds perfectly well to one hormone that is effective in rat adipose tissue while not responding at all to other such hormones (Rudman and di Girolamo, 1967). The question of interest is whether all of the species differences reside in the cell membrane-adenylate cyclase system or whether there are some species in which the basic mechanism of lipase activation is qualitatively or at least quantitatively different.

OBSERVATION IMPLICATING THAT FAMILIAL TYPE I HYPERLIPOPROTEINEMIA IS NOT A POST-HEPARIN-LIPASE DEFICIENT CONDITION

Finn Damgaard-Pedersen and Jørn Dyerberg

Familial type I hyperlipoproteinemia or familial hyperchylomicronemia is defined as a condition with:

1. Type I lipoprotein pattern as shown by serum lipoprotein electrophoresis.
2. Low PHLA (Post-Heparin-Lipase-Activity).
3. Clearing of the chylomicronemia within a few days on a fat-free diet.

Besides these major criteria the patients present: abdominal pain attacks and eruptive xanthomatas related to fat intake, hepato-splenic enlargement and sometimes acute pancreatitis.

In spite of the very high triglyceride and moderately elevated cholesterol concentration in the blood, the patients do not seem to develop atherosclerotic vascular diseases more frequently than normal persons. (The oldest type I patient we have investigated is now 45 years old). Reduction of plasma triglyceride concentration in type III, IV and V hyperlipoproteinemia by steroids such as norethindrone acetate (Glueck et a., 1969; 1971) or oxandroline (Glueck, 1971) has been reported to be accompanied by an increase of PHLA, and it has been accepted that PHLA reflects, at least partly, the activity of the lipoprotein lipase, the enzyme responsible for removal of chylomicrons and very-low-density lipoproteins from the blood. We have treated five type I patients by giving oxandrolone, and observed a normalisation of PHLA but no change in serum-triglyceride concentration.

Materials and Methods

Six type I patients are presented in Table 1. Of the six patients 3 children, BSP, SSN, and DSN, aged 13, 14 and 10 years, and 2 adults HVJ and GH, aged 45 and 34 years, were treated for 7 days with oxandrolone (17-ß-hydroxy-17-α-methyl-2-oxo-5-α-androstan-3-one). The children got 5 mg/day and the adults 7.5 mg/day. PHLA was measured as described earlier (Faergeman and Damgaard-Pedersen, 1973) using a modification of the Intralipid method of Boberg and Carlson. Quantitative lipoprotein electrophoresis was carried out as described by Dyerberg and Hjorne (1970). Serum triglycerides, cholesterol, phospholipids, and total lipids were analysed using conventional methods. Adipose tissue lipase activity was measured by using the "direct incubation" method described by Persson et al. (1972). Inhibition studies using 1M sodium chloride and protamine sulfate were performed as described by Faergeman & Damgaard-Pedersen (1973).

Results

As shown in Fig. 1 oxandrolone treatment increased PHLA in all patients to normal or higher than normal level.

Fig. 2 shows that no change occurred in serum triglyceride concentration during the study. Lipoprotein electrophoresis revealed that all the triglycerides were found in the chylomicron fraction before as well as after oxandrolone treatment.

Inhibition study showed that the increased PHLA was inhibited 74 per cent and 57 per cent by 1M sodium chloride and protamine sulfate respectively.

Table 1. Typical plasma lipid and lipoprotein values in six patients with type I hyperlipoproteinaemia

Pt.	Total lipids g/l	Triglycerides mmol/l	Cholesterol (tot.) mmol/l	Phospholipids mmol/l	Lipoproteins g/l (9)				max. PHLA (percent of normal (13))[a]
					Chylomicr.	β-lipopr.	pre-β lipopr.	α-lipopr.	
A { ♂ 250960 BSP	41.22	39.95	12.96	–	31.20	5.50	3.05	1.45	–
–"– b	8.92	5.20	5.46	4.21	0.15	2.95	4.45	0.65	49%
♀ 181159 SSN	32.70	35.44	5.26	5.33	21.09	4.33	7.65	3.18	55%
♀ 050562 DSN	35.00	39.46	9.91	5.36	23.78	3.24	7.80	3.96	51%
B { ♂ 240428 HVJ	–	52.20	15.40	–	Type I hyperlipoproteinaemia pattern, qualitatively evaluated.				51%
♀ 240639 GH	–	20.20	8.16	–					32%
♀ 280936 IS	–	20.60	6.88	–					32%

A: Family 1. B: Family 2.

[a]Normal value: 100 per cent corresponding to 228 μmoles of fatty acids deliberated/liter plasma/minute (S.D. 26 μmoles of fatty acids deliberated/liter plasma/minute).

[b]After 3 days on a total fat-free diet.

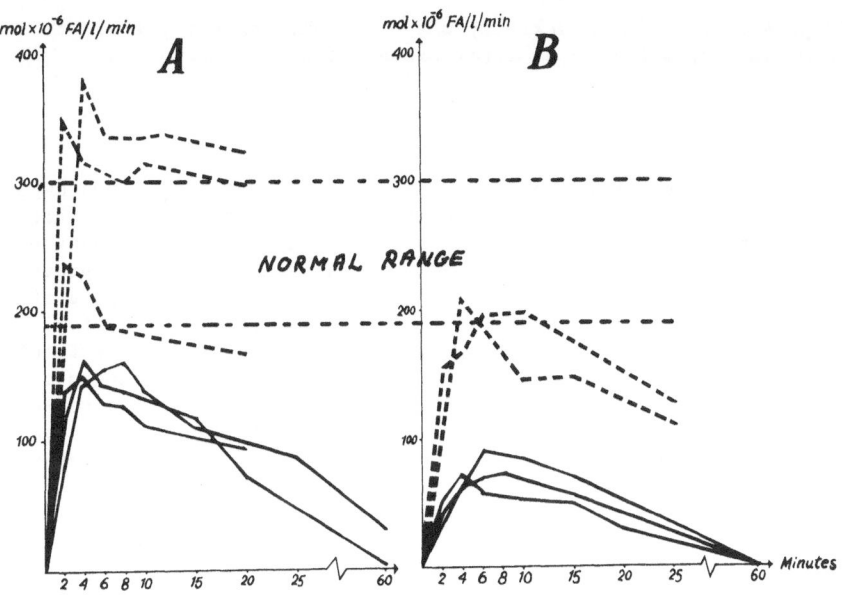

Figure 1. PHLA measured in venous blood after a single i.v. dose of heparin (20 I.U. per kilogram body weight).
A: Family 1, three members, treated with oxandrolone 5 mg/day for 7 days,
B: Family 2, three members, two treated with oxandrolone 7.5 mg/day for 7 days,
——————— PHLA before treatment,
-------- PHLA after treatment

Figure 2. Serum-triglycerides concentrations in 5 patients with familial type I hyperlipoproteinemia.
A: Before oxandrolone treatment,
B: After oxandrolone treatment (7 days)

Adipose tissue lipase activity was not significantly different from zero either in measurements before or after oxandrolone treatment.

Discussion

It is well known that the lipolytic activity measured in postheparin plasma (PHLA) is due to several enzymes. The quantitatively most important are lipoprotein lipase, hepatic triglyceride lipase, and monoglyceride lipase. During inhibition studies using 1M sodium chloride it is shown that only lipoprotein lipase is almost totally inhibited (95%) whereas triglyceride lipase is stimulated and mono-glyceride lipase only inhibited to a minor degree (Greten et al., 1970). Our results indicate that the increase in PHLA by oxandrolone-treatment is caused mostly by an increase in lipoprotein lipase activity, because of the 74 per cent inhibition of PHLA in vitro by 1M sodium chloride in the assay medium. This increase, however, is not related to an increased lipoprotein lipase activity in adipose tissue, as lipoprotein lipase activity in fat biopsies was zero during the whole study.

The increased release of lipoprotein lipase from non-adipose tissue like muscle, heart, kidney, or long may be responsible for the normalised PHLA.

This normal PHLA, however, did not correct the hyperchylomicronemia. This fact can be explained by assuming that oxandrolone increases the activity of an abnormal lipoprotein lipase, which acts on an artificial substrate like Intralipid, but does not attack chylomicrons. Such a lipase has been described by Schriebman et al. (1973). The existence of such an abnormal lipoprotein lipase will be in agreement with the finding of enormous accumulation of chylomicrons in type I patients in spite of a relatively moderate decrease in PHLA (several type I patients have PHLA of more than 50 per cent of normal level). The possibility of different metabolic defects, resulting in the same lipoprotein abnormality must strongly be considered in this type of hyperlipoproteinemia.

Conclusion

It is possible to normalise the PHLA in type I patients by oxandrolone treatment, but the hyperchylomicronemia persists. PHLA normalization may be due to an abnormal lipoprotein lipase released from non-adipose tissue.

The results of these investigations indicate that PHLA measurements should not be used as a major criteria in establishment of the diagnosis Familial type I hyperlipoproteinemia. Instead we suggest measurements of lipoprotein lipase activity in fat biopsies.

Acknowledgement. Oxandrolone was kindly supplied by G. D. Searle A/S, Copenhagen, Denmark.

SEPARATION AND CHARACTERIZATION OF TWO TRIGLYCERIDE LIPASE ACTIVITIES FROM HUMAN POST-HEPARIN PLASMA

Christian Ehnholm, Walter Shaw, Heiner Greten, Wolfgang Lengfelder, and W. Virgil Brown

Introduction

The lipase activities of post-heparin plasma have been shown to hydrolyze many classes of lipids, including: a) triglycerides (TG), diglycerides (DG) and monoglycerides (MG) (Shore and Shore, 1960; Greten et al., 1969; Fielding, 1972; Greten, 1972), b) phospholipids (Vogel and Zieve, 1964; Vogel and Bierman, 1967) and c) long-chain fatty acyl coenzyme A derivatives (Jansen and Hulsman, 1973). Attempts to physically separate enzymes specific for the hydrolysis of each of these lipid classes have been unsuccessful. Recent studies have shown that at least two triglyceride lipase activities exist in post-heparin plasma (LaRosa et al., 1972; Greten et al., 1972; Fielding, 1970). They have been characterized after partial purification from swine post-heparin plasma (Ehnholm et al., 1972). One of these was similar in its characteristics to the lipoprotein lipase of adipose tissue (Bensadouw et al., unpublished) and the other differed from lipoprotein lipase in its lack of activation by plasma cofactor and in being stimulated rather than inhibited by exposure to solutions high in ionic strength. This hydrolase was also active against phospholipids. The techniques used successfully in the separation of swine triglyceride lipase have now been applied to the study of human post-heparin plasma.

Materials and Methods

Blood was collected from normal subjects 10 min after intravenous injection of sodium heparin (Riker Laboratories), 60 U/kg body weight. The blood was centrifuged immediately at 4°, the plasma decanted and stored frozen at -20° until used.

Enzyme Assays

Triglyceride Lipase Assay. In a total volume of 1 ml, each vial contained: 2.8 umole triolein (0.044 μC/μmole), 3.75 mg gum arabic, 10 mg bovine serum albumin and 5 μl of post-heparin plasma or variable volumes (50-200 μl) of enzyme solutions. Final buffer concentration was 0.2 M Tris-HCl. With regard to ionic strength and pH, two standard sets of conditions were chosen to provide maximum activity of the hepatic lipase or lipoprotein lipase — 0.75 M NaCl and pH 8.8 for hepatic lipase and 0.075 M NaCl, pH 8.2 and 20 μg per ml of apoLp-Glu for lipoprotein lipase. The incubations were performed for 30 min at 28° and terminated as described earlier (Ehnholm et al., 1972).

Phospholipase A_1 Assay. Phospholipase A_1 activity was determined using $1-(1-{}^{14}C)$ acyl-2-acyl phosphatidylethanolamine as substrate (Ehnholm et al., unpublished).

Separation of Plasma Triglyceride Lipase. Aliquots of 10 ml of post-heparin plasma were added to 250 ml centrifuge tubes containing 200 ml of acetone. After 10 min the tubes were centrifuged at 2000 x g for 10 min and the supernatant discarded. The precipitate was then sequentially washed with 200 ml portions of acetone (x1), heptane (x2), ethanol-ether (1:1, v/v)(x2) and ether (x1). All solvents were at $0-4^{\circ}$. After drying under nitrogen the remaining ether was evaporated in a vacuum dessicator. The powder was dissolved in 10 ml of 0.005 M Nabarbital buffer (pH 7.4) and centrifuged for 10 min at 12,000 x g. The extract was then applied to a column of Sepharose 4B (2.5 x 10 cm) containing covalently linked heparin (Olivecrona, 1971). The column had previously been equilibrated with a 0.005 M Na-barbital buffer containing 0.15 M NaCl. After application of 200 ml of 0.4 M NaCl the column was eluted with a linear gradient of NaCl from 0.4 to 1.5 M in the same barbital buffer.

Concanavalin A Chromatography. Preparations of hepatic lipase obtained by gradient elution from the heparin-Sepharose were further purified by Concanavalin A-Sepharose chromatography. A column of Con-A Sepharose (Pharmacia Fine Chemicals) (1x 10 cm) was initially washed with 100 ml of 1.0 M NaCl-0.005 M Na-veronal buffer, pH 7.4. The enzyme sample in 0.75 M NaCl-0.005 M Na-veronal was applied to the column. It was then washed with 100 ml of 1.0 M NaCl-Na-veronal. The lipolytic activity was eluted with 0.005 M Na-barbital buffer containing 1.0 M NaCl and 1.0 M α-methyl-D-glucopyranoside (CalBiochem).

Other Methods

Protein was determined by the method of Lowry et al. (1951) using bovine serum albumin as standard. Polyacrylamide gel electrophoresis (10% acrylamide) was performed in the presence of sodium dodecyl sulfate by the method of Weber and Osborn (1969).

Isoelectric focusing: Enzyme solutions were dialyzed against 1% glycine and applied in a 0-55% (w/v) sucrose gradient on a 110 ml focusing column (LKB Instruments). Final concentration of carrier ampholyte (pH 3-6) was 1% (w/v). Electrofocusing was conducted for 36 hours at 500 volts.

Results

Heparin-Sepharose chromatography of delipidated post-heparin plasma gave one peak of triglyceride lipase activity (Peak I) eluting with 0.6 to 0.75 M NaCl (Fig. 1) when assayed with no activator apolipoprotein added. When apoLp-Glu was present in the assay, a second peak of activity (Peak II) eluted between 1.0 - 1.4 M NaCl. The enzyme in Peak I did not require a serum cofactor and was most active when assayed in solutions of 0.5 to 1.0 M NaCl. The second lipase, Peak II, required apoLp-Glu for activity and only apoLp-Glu produced activation. This activity was inhibited when assayed in the presence of 0.5 to 1.0 M NaCl (60%) or protamine sulfate, 1.0 mg/ml (40-80%). Thus the second peak had the characteristics of lipoprotein lipase.

The triglyceride lipase eluting first from the heparin-Sepharose column also had phospholipase A_1 activity (Fig. 2). In previous studies the release of triglyceride lipase and phospholipase has been shown to occur simultaneously (Jansen and Hulsman, 1973). However, there are conflicting data in the literature as to whether these two activities can be related to a single enzyme. Peak I was therefore further purified on Con-A Sepharose. As can be seen in Table I the two enzymes co-chromatograph and the ratio of triglyceride lipase activity to phospholipase activity of the purified enzyme was very similar to that obtained in the original post-heparin plasma. On polyacrylamide gel electrophoresis in the presence of sodium dodecyl sulfate one major band was obtained with an apparent molecular weight of 64,000. Isoelectric focusing of the preparation after Con-A Sepharose chromatography gave a major peak of activity with a pI of 4.1. The ratio of triglyceride lipase to phosphatidylethanolamine lipase activity across this peak ranged from 1.0 to 1.2. The identical recoveries and similar chromatographic properties suggested that a single enzyme was the major source of the phospholipase and triglyceride lipase activities monitored during the purification. Further evidence was provided by thermal inactivation studies. During incubation at both 30° and 37° the percentage of the original triglyceride lipase and of the phospholipase activity remaining were identical when plotted versus time.

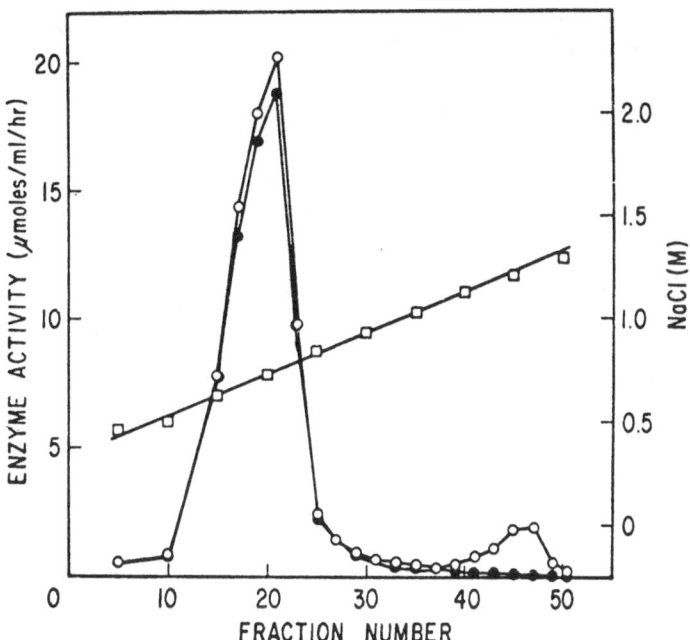

Figure 1. Heparin–Sepharose affinity chromatography of delipidated human post-heparin plasma.
Triglyceride lipase activity was measured in each fraction (13.5 ml) indicated by addition of 0.1 ml of eluate to the standard assay system. The NaCl in the final assay mixture was contributed entirely by the column eluate. One series of assays (o – o) contained 20 µg of apoLp-Glu per assay the other one (•–•) no apoLp-Glu. Starting material 460 ml post-heparin plasma. ☐ – ☐ NaCl molarity of eluting buffer

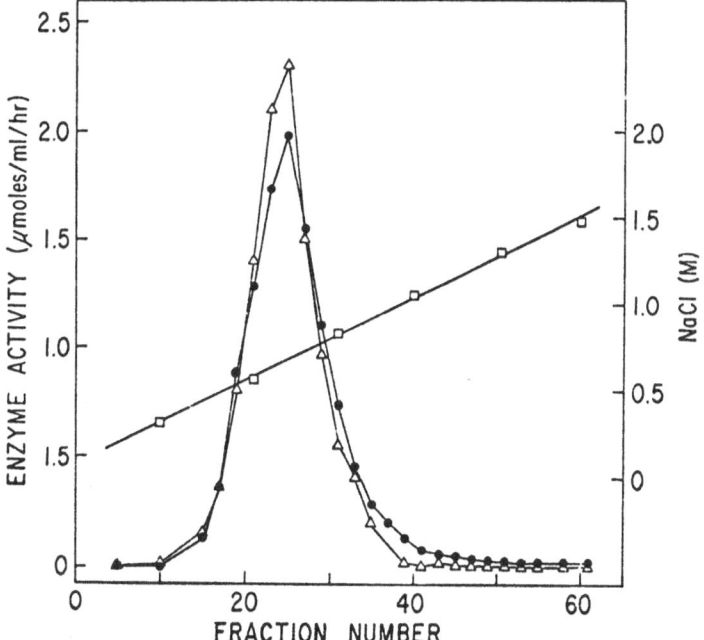

Figure 2. Heparin–Sepharose affinity chromatography of delipidated human post-heparin plasma.
Triglyceride lipase (o-o) and phosphtidylethanolamine lipase (Δ-Δ) activities were measured from the fractions indicated using the standard assay system. ☐ – ☐ NaCl molarity of eluting buffer

Table 1. Purification of triglyceride lipase and phospholipase from human post-heparin plasma

Fraction	Total TG activity	Yield	Total PE activity	Yield	Ratio of TG/PE
	(μmoles free fatty acid per hour)	%	(μmoles free fatty acid per hour)	%	
Post-heparin plasma	1320	100	1088	100	1.21
Delipidated post-heparin plasma	360	27	883	81	0.41
Heparin affinity column	404	31	612	56	0.66
Con-A affinity column	323	25	268	25	1.21

Discussion

In the present study two different triglyceride lipase activities have been separated from human post-heparin plasma. The designation lipoprotein lipase seems appropriate for the activity eluting at higher ionic strength since it is virtually identical in its characteristics to lipoprotein lipases previously purified from porcine adipose tissue (Bensadoun et al., unpublished) and post-heparin plasma (Ehnholm et al., 1972), bovine milk (Egelrud and Olivecrona, 1972) and chicken adipose tissue (Egelrud, 1973). The properties of the second post-heparin plasma triglyceride lipase resembled those of an enzyme obtained from liver perfusates (Spitzer and Spitzer, 1956; Hamilton, 1964) and that partially purified from hepatocyte membranes (Assmann et al., 1972). Recently this form of triglyceride lipase has also been purified from human (Greten et al., 1972) and porcine (Ehnholm et al., 1972) post-heparin plasma. The absence of this lipase activity in post-heparin plasma of hepatectomized swine indicates that the liver plays a major role in the generation of this enzyme activity. We therefore suggest this triglyceride lipase be referred to as "hepatic lipase". The presence of at least two different triglyceride lipases in human post-heparin plasma helps to explain the conflicting data in the literature on the effect of high ionic strength in the assay of lipase activity in post-heparin plasma.

In addition to triglyceride lipase activity, the hepatic lipase also showed phospholipase A_1 activity. The experiments reported strongly suggest that a single enzyme has ester hydrolase activity against both phospholipid and triglyceride and thus confirm and extend earlier findings. Whether this enzyme in vivo acts as a phospholipase or a triglyceride lipase or both needs further study.

SELECTIVE MEASUREMENT OF LIPOPROTEIN LIPASE AND HEPATIC LIPASE IN POST-HEPARIN PLASMA

Ronald M. Krauss, Robert I. Levy, and Donald S. Fredrickson

Two triglyceride lipase activities are released into plasma by heparin injection (LaRosa et al., 1972; Fielding, 1972; Krauss et al., 1973). One is derived from the liver (LaRosa et al., 1972; Fielding, 1972; Krauss et al., 1973; Assmann et al., 1973; Greten et al., 1972); the other originates from extrahepatic tissues and is commonly termed "lipoprotein lipase" (Korn, 1959). We recently have reported that both enzymes in post-heparin plasma in the rat are capable of hydrolyzing very low density lipoproteins (Krauss et al., 1973; Krauss et al., in press), but the capacity of the hepatic enzyme to hydrolyze chylomicron lipids is relatively limited (Krauss et al., in press). A second distinction is that the extrahepatic lipase is more sensitive to inactivation by salt and protamine sulfate (LaRosa et al., 1972; Fielding, 1972; Krauss et al., 1973). This feature has served as a means for the selective measurement of the two lipase activities in rat post-heparin plasma (Krauss et al., 1973). Plasma is incubated with a ^{14}C-triolein emulsion at substrate saturation (8.5mM) at pH 8.6. Prior incubation of the plasma with protamine, 3 mg per 0.05 ml, for ten minutes at 27°C results in greater than 90% inactivation of extrahepatic lipase ("protamine-inactivated activity") and retention of more than 90% of the hepatic enzyme activity ("protamine-resistant activity").

The purpose of the present study was to adapt this selective assay to the measurement of post-heparin lipolytic activity (PHLA) in humans. If hepatic lipase contributes significantly to human PHLA, as it does in the rat (Krauss et al., 1973), a number of previous observations made on the basis of total activity may require re-evaluation. Of particular interest is familial hyperchylomicronemia (Type I hyperlipoproteinemia), a disorder characterized by impaired clearance of dietary fat. While the primary defect in this disease is generally believed to be a deficiency of lipoprotein lipase (Fredrickson et al., 1963; Harlan et al., 1967), there have been reports of normal or only slight depressed levels of PHLA in some patients (Fredrickson and Levy, 1972).

The validity of the selective assay procedure in humans was assessed using enzyme extracted from samples of normal adipose tissue and liver obtained at laparotomy. As in the rat, the adipose tissue enzyme was protamine-inactivated, and the hepatic enzyme was protamine-resistant. Both activities were measured in plasma, and attained maximal levels ten minutes after intravenous heparin (10 u/kg). Each exhibited a broad pH optimum between 8.0 and 9.6, and was linear for 90 minutes at 27°C with up to 0.06 ml plasma per ml assay. Measurement of the two lipases in 89 normal subjects revealed significant age and sex variation (Table 1). Protamine-resistant activity was highest in adult males; protamine-inactivated activity was greatest in young males (18 years and under). In females the level of protamine-inactivated lipase activity was directly correlated with age. The mean level doubled between the second and sixth decades and then approached the value found in the young males.

Lipid and lipoprotein analyses were used to categorize 51 patients with familial hyperlipoproteinemia by the system of Fredrickson and Levy (1972). Plasma from hyperlipemic patients was diluted for use in the lipase assay so that endogenous triglyceride contributed less than 5% of the total substrate. In the group of 14 patients with Type I hyperlipoproteinemia, the mean protamine-inactivated lipase activity was less than one-tenth normal in each age and sex group (Fig. 1). The protamine-resistant activities were normal except in adult males, in whom the mean was reduced by about one-third. 90% tolerance limits were established for

Table 1. Heparin-released plasma lipase activities in normals

Sex	Age	N	Triglyceride lipase activity μmoles FFA/ml/hr	
			Protamine resistant	Protamine inactivated
Males	5 - 18	10	11.0 ± 3.1[a]	6.7 ± 1.6[a,b]
	19 - 65	33	15.0 ± 5.3[a,b]	4.1 ± 1.7[a]
Females	0 - 18	11	11.1 ± 3.8	3.8 ± 1.1[b,c]
	19 - 65	35	10.8 ± 3.3[b]	4.6 ± 1.8[c]

[a]Difference between younger and older males,
Significant $p < 0.01$.

[b]Difference between males and females,
Significant $p < 0.001$.

[c]Significant correlation with age, $p < 0.001$.

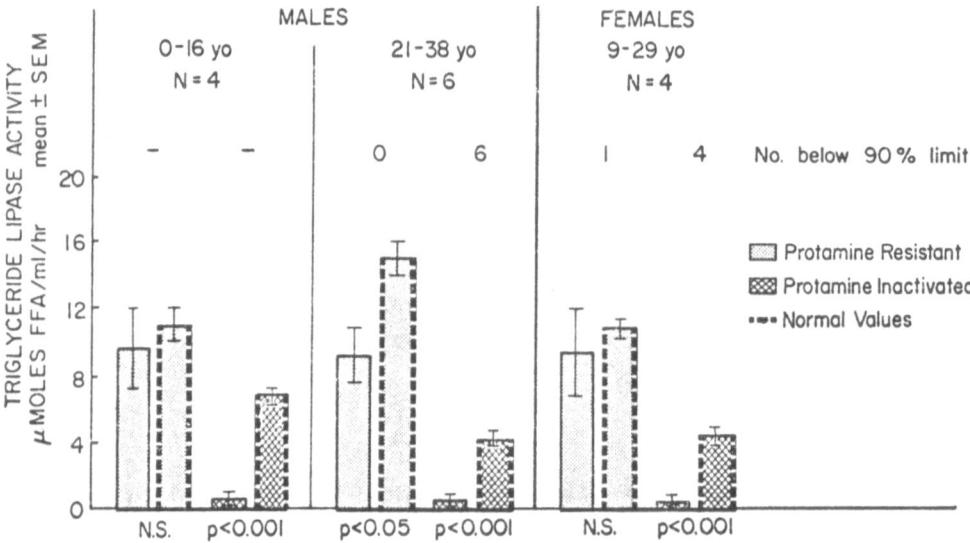

Figure 1. Plasma post-heparin lipase activities in patients with Type 1 hyperlipoproteinemia. The 90% tolerance limits were not calculated for normal males under
age 19 since the number of subjects was too small

normal females and adult males; each of the ten Type 1 patients in these categories fell below the limits for protamine-inactivated lipase, while only one
was below the limit for protamine-resistant lipase (Fig. 1). Mean values for both
activities were normal in the group of 37 patients with Types 3, 4, and 5 hyperlipoproteinemia. Two patients with "Type 5", however, were found to have protamine-
inactivated lipase values well below normal, and within the range observed in
Type 1 patients.

Since a number of patients with hyperlipoproteinemia were on diets restricted in
fat content, the effects of altering diet composition were studied (Table 2).
When fat intake was reduced to below ten grams per day and carbohydrates corre-

Table 2. Effect of diet composition on lipase activities in normals

Diet	Sex	N	Lipase activity umoles FFA/ml/hr ± S.D.	
			Protamine resistant	Protamine inactivated
Basal (2 weeks)	Males	4	12.5 ± 3.4	4.1 ± 1.8
	Females	4	12.8 ± 3.0	3.8 ± 1.0
	All	8	12.6 ± 3.0	3.9 ± 1.3[a]
Low Fat (2 weeks)	Males	4	13.4 ± 1.6	2.0 ± 1.0
	Females	4	14.5 ± 4.8	1.6 ± 0.3
	All	8	13.9 ± 3.8	1.7 ± 0.7[a]
High Fat (1 week)	Females	3	11.8 ± 2.7	2.6 ± 0.2

[a]Difference between basal and low fat,
Significant p <0.001.
All individual values were the means of at least 3 determinations
for each patient on each diet.
Basal diet contained 20% of calories as protein, 40% as carbohy-
drate, and 40% as fat.
Low fat diet contained less than 10 grams fat per day, with iso-
caloric substitution of carbohydrate.
High fat diet contained greater than 150 grams fat per day, with
isocaloric reduction of carbohydrate.

spondingly increased for a period of two weeks the protamine-resistant lipase
activity in normals was reduced by more than 50%. Even at this level, however,
the activities remained three to five times higher than in the Type 1 patients.
An isocaloric diet high in fat (greater than 150 grams per day) had no significant effect on activity of either enzyme (Table 2).

Among other clinical conditions in which selective measurement of lipase activities is of interest is hypothyroidism. Low levels of PHLA have been reported
in this disorder (Porter et al., 1966), but the features of the Type 1 syndrome
are not ordinarily observed. In three adult female patients with clinical and
biochemical evidence of hypothyroidism, protamine-inactivated lipase was normal
(4.7 ± 1.4 u) while mean protamine-resistant lipase was significantly reduced
(6.2 ± 0.8 u, < p 0.001).

Administration of norethindrone acetate, a progestin, has been shown to increase
PHLA and to reduce lipid levels in patients with Type 5 hyperlipoproteinemia, but
not in those with Type 1 (Glueck et al., 1971). In each of three normal subjects,
a ten day course of this drug at a dose of 5 mg/day resulted in a significant increase (p <0.01) in protamine-resistant lipase (mean increase 30%) whereas
protamine-inactivated lipase activity was reduced (mean reduction 25%, N.S.).

A three week episode of infectious mononucleosis with hepatic involvement in a
normal subject afforded the opportunity to observe serial changes in the two
lipase activities. Protamine-inactivated lipase was unaffected, while protamine-

resistant lipase activity was depressed by up to 75%, returning towards baseline with resolution of hepatic dysfunction.

The selective assay of plasma post-heparin lipase activities thus has been shown to be of clinical value. A specific enzyme defect has been defined which offers a useful criterion for classifying patients with familial hyperchylomicronemia. In addition, selective changes in lipase activities may now be detected in other conditions affecting lipid levels, such as hypothyroidism, hepatic disease, dietary fat restriction, and drug therapy. Further studies may help to clarify the respective roles of hepatic and extrahepatic enzyme activities in lipoprotein catabolism.

EFFECT OF UNSATURATED PHOSPHATIDYLCHOLINE ON THE LIPOPROTEIN LIPASE ACTIVITY IN VITRO *

B. Blaton and H. Peeters

Lipoprotein lipase (LPL) from cow's milk is only active in the presence of a plasma lipoprotein cofactor (Korn, 1955) and of phospholipids (Scanu, 1967). The temperature, presence of ions, source of triglycerides, and the LPL activators must be well controlled (Greten, 1972). Plasma cofactor peptides from lipo-proteins have been intensively studied as enzyme activators (Bier and Havel, 1970; Havel et al., 1970; La Rosa et al., 1970). The possible relationship of the source of the enzyme with the polypeptide specificity was suggested by the data of Gannesan et al. (1971). More attention was given to the role of phospholipids in the hydrolysis of triglyceride emulsions by Chung et al. (1973). They showed that the lipoprotein lipase activity decreased remarkably when the chain length of the saturated acyl chains in the phosphatidylcholine increased. However the influence of the double bonds in PU-PC was not investigated.

It is known that intravenous injection of polyunsaturated phosphatidylcholine (PU-PC) increases the enzymatic activity of cholesterase and phospholipase in the arterial wall (Patelski et al., 1970). Studies on the treatment of human hyper-lipoproteinemia with PU-PC showed a significant decrease of cholesterol and phospholipid but not of plasma triglycerides (Blaton et al., 1972; Peeters et al., 1971; 1973). In view of the uncertainties of the effect of PU-PC on the hypertri-glyceridemia we investigated the effect of different PC-species on the lipo-protein lipase activity in vitro, using a well-defined artificial triglyceride emulsion and cow milk lipase.

Materials

Enzyme Preparation. The enzyme preparation was carried out essentially according to Bier and Havel (1970). Acetone butanol powders were prepared by extraction of 1 g crude LPL with 40 ml precooled acetone. The procedure was repeated twice, respectively with 25 ml butanol and 25 ml acetone. The powder was air-dried and stored at -20°C, in portions of 200 mg. The working sample with a concentration of about 4% in 0.1 M NaCl was kept at 4°C and used within 4 h.

Preparation of Cofactor Lipoprotein and LPL-Activators. Human plasma lipoproteins were prepared by ultracentrifugation from overnight-fasted, normal male donors (Blaton et al., 1973). Apo-VLDL, prepared according to Koga et al., (1970) was used as a cofactor lipoprotein. Purified soybean phosphatidylcholine (EPL - pure) and samples of essential phospholipids (EPL - Lipostabil) were provided by Nattermann (Köln). Egg-yolk phosphatidylcholine purified on Al_2O_3 was also used (Vandamme et al., 1968). Saturated PC was prepared by hydrogenation of the un-saturated form from egg-yolk and EPL samples. Bovine serum albumin (Poviet) was used as free fatty acid acceptor.

Substrates. 100 mg of triolein (applied Sciences) or 100 mg corn oil were mixed with PC in chloroform in ratios described under results. After evaporation of the organic solvent, the lipids were dispersed in 3 ml 0.15 M NaCl by sonification with a Branson Sonifier B-12 for three 30 sec periods at 50 Watt.

* This work was supported by Grant no. 1206 from the Nationaal Fonds Geneeskundig Wetenschappelijk Onderzoek, Belgium.

Analytical Methods

Biochemical Methods. Proteins were determined according to the method of Lowry et al. (1951). PC was extracted from EPL (Lipostabil) by the method of Folch (1951). Free fatty acids were determined by titrimetry (Dole, 1956) and by colorimetry (Novak, 1965). The fatty acid spectra were determined by GLC as described by Blaton et al. (1970).

Assay Procedure for LPL. A solution of 0.1 ml albumin (20 mg %), 0.1 ml apo-VLDL (20 mg %), 1.2 ml LPL (4%), and 0.8 ml NaCl (0.8%) was adjusted to pH 8.8 in the titration vessel of a pH-stat TTT-2 (Radiometer). After mixing the solution with 0.6 ml substrate adjusted to pH 8.8, the enzymatic hydrolysis was followed continuously by pH titration with 0.1 M NaOH during 45 minutes at 37°C in N_2-atmosphere. A comparison between the results obtained by pH-stat titration and those of several free fatty acid determination methods always indicated slightly higher results with the first procedure.

Results

Effect of the Substrate and of Cofactor Lipoprotein on the LPL Activity. The hydrolysis of a purified triolein substrate and of a corn-oil substrate were activated to the same extent by phosphatidylcholine from egg-yolk. Thus corn oil was selected as the triglyceride substrate for further studies.

The rate of hydrolysis is increased in the presence of apo-VLDL, but much more when PC is present. From the activation curve we extrapolated optimal concentration of the cofactor pipoprotein.

Phospholipase as a Contaminant of LPL. Based on three different arguments, practically no phospholipase is present in the milk-LPL preparations. There was no lipoprotein lipase activity on a specific PC-choline substrate. A second argument is the fact that phospholipase is thermostable, whereas after heat denaturation the milk LPL is no longer active. Finally the GLC patterns of the liberated free fatty acids are not influenced by the presence of PC in the substrate (Table 1).

Table 1. Fatty acid composition of different substrates and of LPL activators

| % FA | Substrate | | Activators | | | |
| | Triolein | Corn Oil | EPL - PC | | Egg-yolk PC | |
			Native	Hydrogenated	Native	Hydrogenated
16:0	–	11	15	14	33	35
16:1	–	tr.	tr.	–	2	–
18:0	–	4	3	86	14	61
18:1	100	23	11	–	32	tr.
18:2	–	54	65	–	15	–
18:3	–	8	6	–	1	–
20:0	–	–	–	–	–	4
20:4	–	–	–	–	3	–

Influence of PC-Species on LPL Activity. FA-spectra of the substrate and of the activators are given in Table 2. We studied different molar ratios of PC to TG and observed a different activation of the lipoprotein lipase (Fig. 1). There are

Table 2. Influence of PC on the hydrolysis of corn-oil triglycerides by LPL

% FFA	Substrate		
	Corn oil	Corn oil + EPL pure 0.1 mol PC/mol TG	Corn oil + egg-yolk PC 0.135 mol PC/mol TG
16:0	16	15	16
16:1	1	1	1
18:0	6	6	6
18:1	21	21	22
18:2	47	48	46
18:3	9	9	9

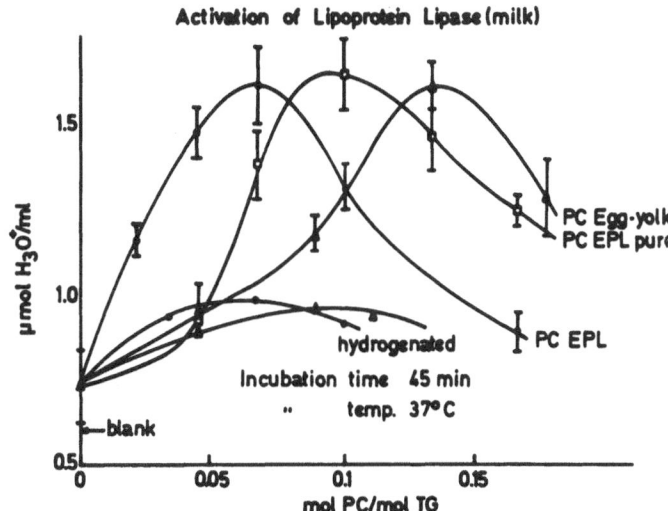

Figure 1. Proton liberation from corn-oil substrate after addition of EPL or egg-yolk PC as LPL activators

three zones in each activation curve: a zone of increasing activity due to molar increase of PC, a zone of optimal LPL activity at an optimal molar ratio of PC/TG, followed by an inhibition zone at higher PC concentration. It seems that the activation properties of phospholipids on LPL are not only dependent upon the nature of the phospholipids employed or upon the chain length and hydrophobic quality of the acid, but also upon the contribution of their double bonds. An experimental proof was given by hydrogenation of unsaturated egg-yolk and EPL PC-species. After saturation to 16:0 and 18:0 as predominant fatty acids, these lecithins showed only little LPL activation, corresponding to the results obtained by Chung et al. (1973) in his study with pure dipalmitoyl PC. The differences observed between PC from EPL and EPL-pure must be ascribed to the presence of the deoxycholate in EPL which is extracted together with PC.

Conclusion

The results demonstrated that cow-milk LPL contains little or no phospholipase activity and that apo-VLDL as well as phospholipids act as LPL activators. Differences between polyunsaturated phosphatidylcholine species demonstrate the importance of the chain length of the fatty acids but especially of their double bonds. From this it appears that the phospholipid molecule has detergent properties which cannot be disregarded.

It is also possible that the phospholipid molecule plays a role by promoting a better interaction between enzyme and substrate, possibly by charging the surface structure of the substrate or affecting the structure of the enzyme of the apo-protein activator or of both. We believe that the phospholipids, as compared with the apolipoprotein activator, interact rather with the substrate than with the enzyme. From these experiments it appears that essential phospholipids can play a role in triglyceride metabolism.

LIPOLYTIC ACTIVITIES OF HEPATIC PLASMA MEMBRANE ORIGIN IN POST-HEPARIN PLASMA

Gerd Assmann, Ronald M. Krauss, Donald S. Fredrickson, and Robert I. Levy

Following the intravenous injection of heparin, lipolytic activities against long-chain tri- di- and monoglycerides, short chain triglycerides and phospholipids are released into plasma (Shore et al., 1953; Shore and Shore, 1961; Fielding, 1970; Levy and Swank, 1954; Meyers et al., 1955; De Meis and Maroja, 1967; Yasuoka and Fujii, 1971; Vogel and Bierman, 1967; Vogel and Zieve, 1964). It has been demonstrated from our laboratory and others that, in addition to lipoprotein lipase of extrahepatic origin, post-heparin plasma contains a triglyceride hydrolase released from the liver (LaRosa et al., 1972; Krauss et al., 1973; Assmann et al., 1973; Fielding, 1972; Greten et al., 1972).

In an attempt to define the subcellular localization of lipolytic activities released by heparin from the liver, rat liver homogenate, cytosol, microsomal, lysosomal, mitochondrial and plasma membrane fractions were prepared. The purity of the cell fractions was monitored by both enzymatic measurement and electron microscopy (Assmann et al., 1973). The plasma membrane and endoplasmic reticulum fractions appeared to be about 10% cross-contaminated according to their content of glucose-6-phosphatase and 5' nucleotidase, respectively. Lysosomes prepared by continuous sucrose gradient were free of mitochondria. The mitochondrial fraction contained acid phosphatase and cytochrome C oxidase activities, suggesting less than 2% contamination with lysosomes. The specific activity of the marker enzyme 5'-nucleotidase in the plasma membrane preparations was enriched 16.3 fold over that in whole homogenate. In electron micrographs the plasma membranes were vesicular and contained junctional complexes; only an occasional patch of rough endoplasmic reticulum was seen.

Triglyceride hydrolase activity was determined as triolein-triton X-100-albumin emulsions, monoglyceride hydrolase activity as monoolein-sodium taurodeoxycholate-micellar solution and phospholipase activity with sonified triton X-100-sodium taurodeoxycholate-phosphatidylethanolamine emulsions. Assays were carried out at substrate saturation and pH optima.

Triglyceride hydrolase activity in post-heparin plasma from the isolated perfused rat liver had a pH optimum of 9.5 and a Km of 1.28 mM (Assmann et al., 1973). When assay conditions optimized for the post-heparin perfusate were employed for individual subcellular fractions, plasma membrane preparations showed the highest specific triglyceride hydrolase activity (Assmann et al., 1973a). When corrected for contamination with other subcellular fractions, the specific activity was more than 7 times higher than in any other cell fraction.

Monoglyceride hydrolase activity in the post-heparin perfusate had a pH optimum of 8.6 and a Km of 3 mM (Assmann et al., 1973b). Specific activities in plasma membrane fractions and microsomal fractions were about equally high. High specific activities of both phospholipase A_1 and A_2 have also been found in liver plasma membranes, as previously reported by others (Torquebiau-Colard et al., 1970; Victoria et al., 1971; Newkirk and Waite, 1971; Nachbaur et al., 1972; Newkirk and Waite, 1973).

Triglyceride lipase activity, monoglyceride-hydrolase activity and phospholipase activity could be released from plasma membranes by heparin. Small amounts of heparin were enough to release more than 90% of the lipolytic activities from plasma membranes. The effects of protamine and sodium chloride, as well as pH optima and Km values, were identical for enzymes released from plasma membranes and from the isolated perfused liver.

Further purification of the plasma membrane released lipolytic activities was achieved by heparin affinity chromatography. Five protein fractions were collected from the column, the first and second one containing more than 92% of protein initially applicated to the column (Fig. 1). In several experiments, essentially all triglyceride hydrolase and phospholipase activity was bound to column;

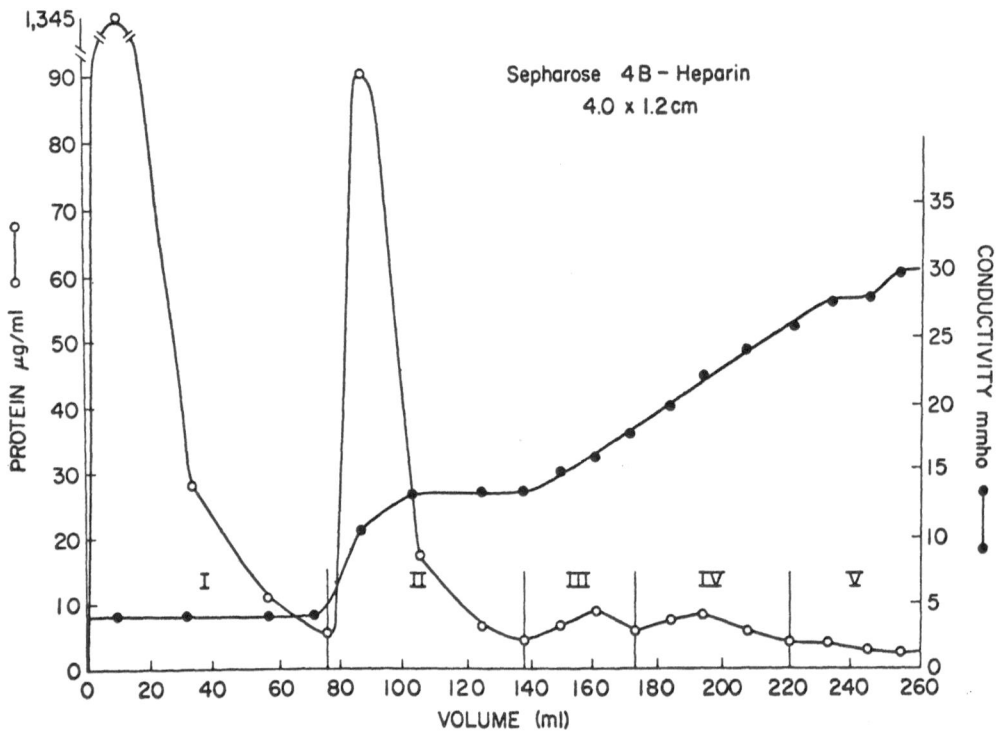

Figure 1. Plasma membranes were prepared from 25 Osborn-Mendel male rats (250-300 gm) as described (12), and enzyme ectivities eluted by incubation of plasma membranes in glycine buffer, pH 9.6, I = 0.1 for 60 min at 27°C. The eluant (12.6 ml) was applied to a column of heparin-sepharose (12 x 40 mm) previously equilibrated with the glycine buffer. Protein was determined according to Lowry (22). Peak I eluted with the original buffer; peak II eluted with 0.16M NaCl in glycine buffer, and peaks III-V eluted with an NaCl gradient (0.16M - 0.52M) in glycine buffer

whereas, consistently about 60% of the monoglyceride hydrolase eluted in the void volumn peak (Table 1). Using an NaCl gradient, triglyceride hydrolase and phospholipase activity were reproducibly released from the column between conductivities 16-26 mMho (peak IV, Fig. 1), their specific activities being 200-400 fold increased over those in plasma membranes. The activities were recovered from the affinity column with 17% and 32% yield, respectively (Table 1). The relatively low recovery is most likely attributable to the instability of lipolytic activities in their purified form.

Enzymatic activity could be partly restored by the presence of 1.25 M salt. Addition of serum caused no increase in activity of the triglyceride hydrolase after its partial purification (Assmann et al., 1973a).

Table 1. Heparin sepharose chromatography hepatic plasma membrane eluant

| | | % Recovery | | | |
Fraction:	I	II	III	IV	V
Protein	92.3	4.8	0.9	1.0	0.5
Lipase activities:					
Triolein	17.7	2.1	6.6	17.3	2.2
Monoolein	59.0	0.7	2.0	4.2	0.4
Phosphatidyl-Ethanolamine	12.3	2.7	6.0	32.1	3.3

Enzyme activities were measured in aliquots of the indicated column fractions (Fig. 1) as follows:

1. Triglyceride hydrolase. Per ml of assay:

   Tri[1-^{14}C]olein   9 µmoles (2.1 µC/µmole)
   1% Triton X-100: 45 µl
   Fatty acid free albumin: 15 mg
   glycine buffer pH 9.6, I = 0.1 to volume.

2. Monoglyceride hydrolase. Per 0.3 ml of assay:

   [2-^{3}H]monoolein: 1.7 µmoles (8.8 µC/µmole)
   sodium taurodeoxycholate: 3 mg
   Tris-HCl buffer, pH 8.6, 0.05M NaCl.

3. Phospholipase. Per 30 µl assay:

   Phosphatidyl [1,2-^{14}C]ethanolamine (24 µC/µmole): 167 nmoles
   Tris-HCl buffer pH 8.6, I = 0.1 to volume, containing 0.18%
   Triton X-100 and 0.24% sodium taurodeoxycholate.

Reaction products were separated by thin layer chromatography and counted by standard techniques.

In an attempt to define the stereospecificity of the triglyceride hydrolase released from liver plasma membranes into the plasma we used several specifically labeled substrates (Assmann et al., 1973b). Triolein was randomly labeled in the carboxyl fatty acid carbons, with ^{14}C, as well as selectively with [1-^{14}C] oleic acid in either position sn-1, sn-2, or sn-3.

The stereochemical specificity of the heparin released triglyceride hydrolase was also investigated using specifically labeled glyceryl diether monoesters, the ester being in either position 1, 2 or 3.

With both triolein and dioctadecenyl-glycerylether-monoesters it was established that the triglyceride lipase specifically attacks the two primary ester positions with the same reaction rate, producing primarily a secondary ester (2-monoglyceride) as reaction product (Assmann et al., 1973)(Fig. 2). We did not obtain conclusive evidence bearing on the possibility that isomerization of 1, 2 (2, 3) diglyceride to 1,3 diglyceride or 2-monoglyceride to 1-monoglyceride is an obligatory step in enzymatic breakdown of triglycerides to glycerol.

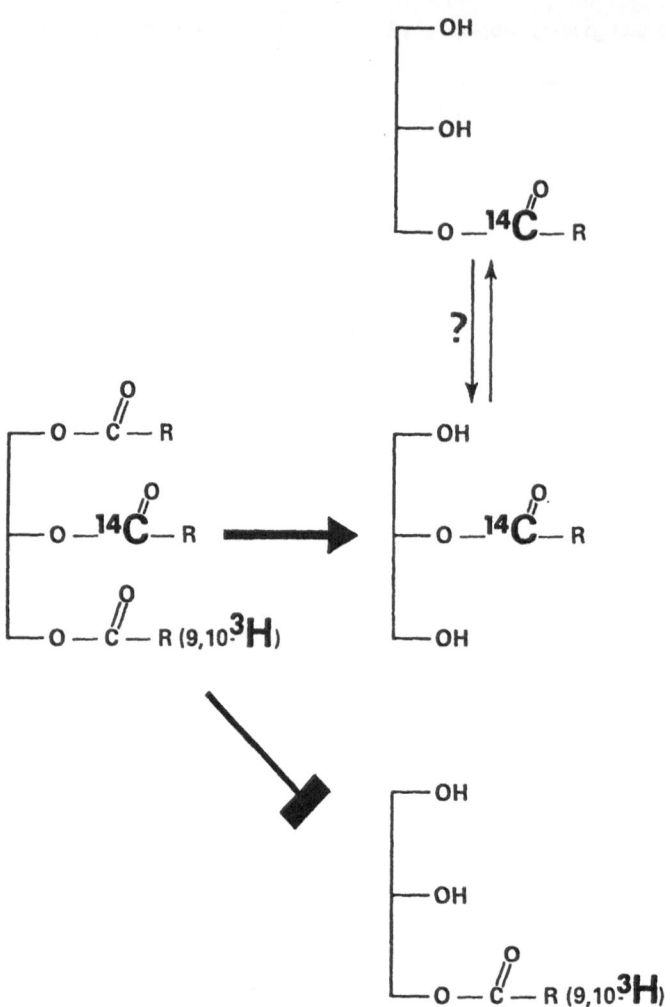

Figure 2. Formation of 2-monoglyceride from triglyceride

ASSAY OF ACTIVATORS FOR SERUM LIPOPROTEIN LIPASE

Peter Chu, A. L. Miller, and G. L. Mills

The measurement of the serum level of most of the apo-lipoproteins is a tedious operation, unsuited to routine use. But two of these proteins, namely those designated as CI and CII, are known to stimulate the activity of lipoprotein lipase, and are thus open to estimation *via* a sensitive enzymic reaction. The purpose of this report is to describe some results which have been obtained with an assay based on the observation by Whayne and Felts (1970) that guinea pig post-heparin plasma does not hydrolyse Intralipid unless it is activated by the addition of human or rat serum.

The assay is carried out by incubating the substance to be tested, at 37°, with the buffered Intralipid mixture shown in Table 1. At zero time, and again after 60 min, two samples, each of 1 ml, are withdrawn and extracted with 5 ml of Dole's mixture (isopropanol, 200 ml; heptane, 50 ml; 1 N H_2SO_4, 5 ml; Brij 35, 3.7 gm).

Table 1. Medium for the assay of lipoprotein lipase activator. This mixture will accommodate up to 2 ml of the solution to be tested. A standard curve is prepared, using the reference serum, for each batch of assays

10% Intralipid	1.5 ml
TRIS Buffer (1.35M; pH8.4)	0.75
15% Bovine Albumin soln. (pH8.4)	2.25
Ammonia solution (0.025M)	1.0
Post-heparin guinea pig plasma	1.0
Test solution	x ml
NaCl solution (0.15M)	(2-x) ml

The fatty acids liberated by hydrolysis of the Intralipid are determined by titrating aliquots of the resulting heptane extract with 0.01M NaOH using Thymol Blue indicator. Since pure activator was not available to us, a large sample of normal serum has been used as a source of an arbitrary standard. This was divided into samples of 2.5 ml and kept frozen, a procedure which has proved to be more reliable than freeze-drying. The activating capacity of this serum has been defined as 100 units/ml.

The response of the system is shown in Fig. 1, which demonstrates that the amount of fatty acid liberated during the digestion is a linear function of the activator level up to 0.8 ml of standard serum (80 units). It is therefore important to assay highly active specimens at more than one level to ensure that the linear part of the response is not exceeded. Incubation periods of 60 and 90 min produce response curves of essentially the same shape, and the shorter time has been adopted for routine purposes.

The average activating capacity of sera from healthy subjects with normal lipoprotein patterns is 75 ± 6.25 units/ml, of which virtually all is in the lipoprotein fractions. Thus, the HDL fraction contains 67 ± 11% of the total serum activity, while the VLDL and LDL contribute 16 ± 8.5% and 13 ± 10% respectively. Only 3% remains in the residual infranatant after centrifugation at 1.21 g/ml.

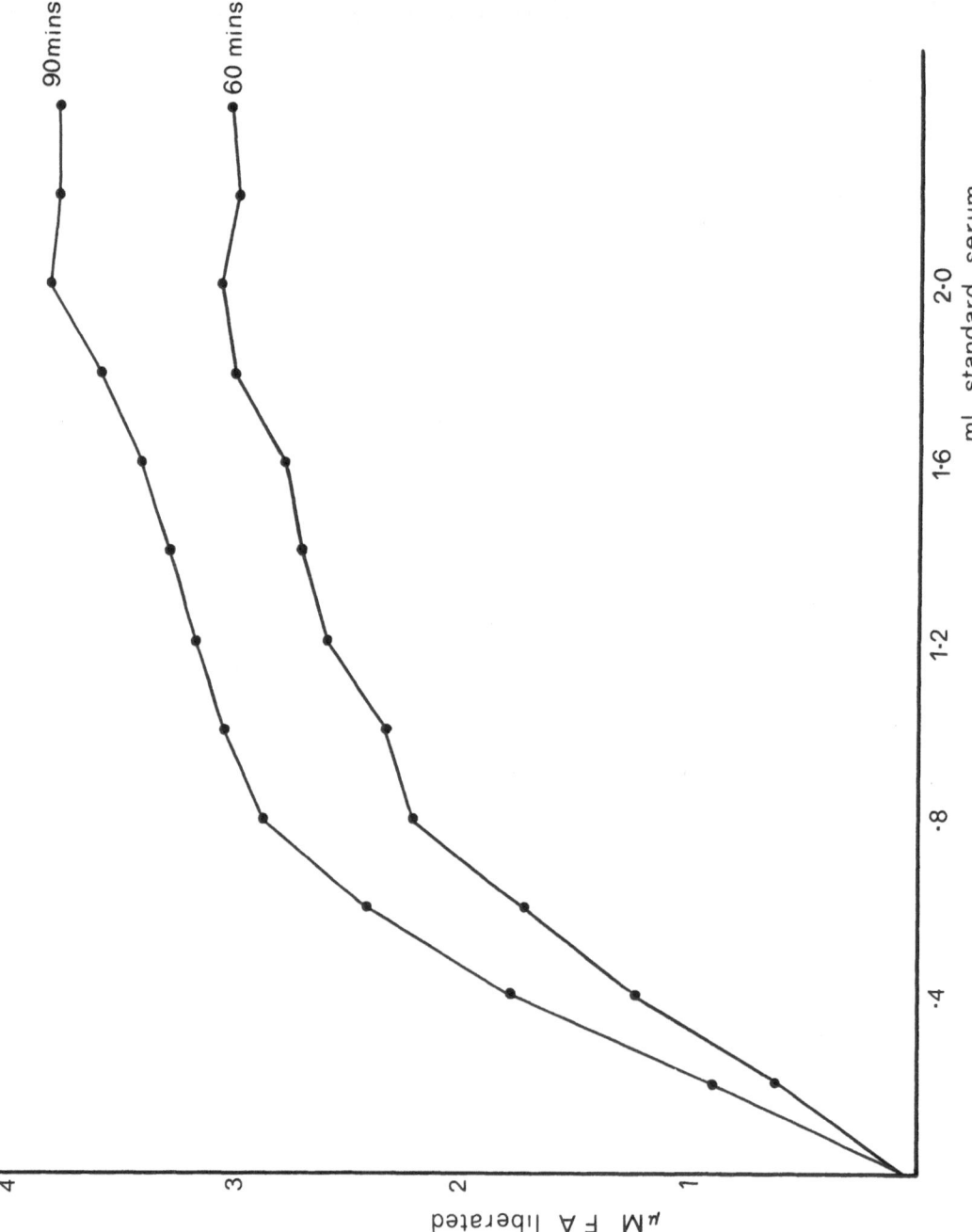

Figure 1. The amount of fatty acid liberated (μmoles) by guinea pig post-heparin lipase from buffered Intralipid substrate after incubation at 37° for (a) 60 min and (b) 90 min, in the presence of different volumes of the same human serum

Table 2. The level of lipoprotein lipase activator in normal subjects and in representative examples of different hyper-lipoproteinaemias. Also shown is the proportion of the total found in the major lipoprotein fractions after isolation by sequential ultracentrifugation. The specific activity of the VLDL and LDL was determined from their concentrations estimated by analytical ultracentrifugation

Lipoprotein Pattern	Serum activator level (units/ml)	Proportion in lipoprotein fraction:				Specific activity	
		VLDL %	LDL %	HDL %	Residue %	VLDL units/mg	LDL units/mg
Normal	75±6.25	13±10	16±8.5	67±11	3±3.8	57	3.6
Type II	127	31	22	36	10	29	2.3
	85	36	18	33	12	35	5.9
Type III	127	44	11	44	0	17	6.4
Type IV	93	54	14	27	5	15	3.2
	110	52	16	30	2	19	5.9
	105	52	19	29	0	19	6.4
Type V	135	48	18	33	0	-	-
	223	61	9	31	0	5.6	18.5
	154	71	11	12	6	9.8	9.0
Obstructive jaundice	105	38	62	0	0	-	-
	188	21	75	4	0	33	17

In hyperlipoproteinaemics, the absolute level of activator is elevated in the VLDL fraction, but is little changed in the LDL (even in hypercholesterolaemics) and is usually depressed in the HDL (Table 2). The HDL and VLDL are approximately equal in activating capacity in hyperlipoproteinaemias of Types II and III, but the progressively increasing average contribution of the VLDL to the serum lipoprotein levels in Types IV and V leads to this fraction becoming the principal reservoir of activator. By contrast, the most active fraction in cases of obstructive jaundice is the LDL, which in these subjects contains the abnormal lipoprotein-X. The level of HDL is often depressed in this disease and this must, at least in part, explain the low activating capacity of this fraction.

It is interesting to find (Table 2) that the specific activating capacity of the LDL (units/mg lipoprotein) varies comparatively little, whereas that of the VLDL falls as the serum level of these lipoproteins rises, reflecting the low protein content of the large particles. Only in obstructive jaundice and perhaps in some patients with Type V hyperlipoproteinaemia is the specific activity of the LDL much increased.

The observations of the preceeding paragraphs suggest that the activator may be one of the apo-lipoproteins that are more commonly found in the VLDL and HDL than in the LDL, i.e. the so-called A and C apo-lipoproteins. The fact that a highly purified specimen of LP-X has been found to activate the assay system is consistent with the activator being one of the C-proteins, and this conjecture is supported by the observation that highly purified lipoprotein-A and lipoprotein-B, donated by Dr. P. Alaupovic, were totally inactive. By contrast, a specimen of purified lipoprotein-C prepared in our laboratory from the VLDL of a hypertriglyceridaemic patient had a powerful stimulating action, which was also the case with the pure peptides CI and CII (also provided by Dr. Alaupovic), at a concentration of 35 μg/ml. It seems highly probable therefore that the activating substance which is being determined by this assay is the peptide which stimulates the lipoprotein lipase of man.

XIII

Factors Contributing to Genesis
of Hyperlipoproteinemia and/or
Atherosclerosis

Immunological Factors

IMMUNOLOGICAL FACTORS OF ATHEROSCLEROSIS

J. L. Beaumont and V. Beaumont

Introduction

In the field of vascular diseases, there is one variety of vascular lesion in
which the role of immunological factors is well documented. This immune vascular
disease, secondary to hetero- or autoimmunization, induces widespread lesions in
the small arteries and capillaries, frequent glomerulonephritis, but no cardiovascular ischemic complications.

Atherosclerosis appears in a different light to the pathologist, the clinician,
and the immunologist. In atherosclerosis, two fundamental lesions are associated
to form, in the intima and media of large arteries, the specific atheromatous
plaque: an intimal deposit of lipids, mainly cholesterol, and fibrous thickening
(Lenegre et al., 1959). This widespread and early basic lesion reduces the
caliber of the arterial lumen, but with generally no dramatic clinical consequence for a long time. Later on, modifications of the atheromatous plaque and
secondary thrombosis may occur, leading to clinical ischemic disease of the heart,
brain, and lower limbs. In this evolutive disease, several risk or associated
factors, differently combined, are known to interfere, but their proper responsibility as direct or indirect atherogenic factors is not easy to assess. Similarly,
immunological factors may also be buried in this long silent period, and some
recent data suggest that they may play a role in the constitution of the atherosclerotic lesion.

This report will examine:
the facts suggestive of a relationship between immunology and atherosclerosis;
the role of these immunological factors in the mechanism of atherosclerosis, the
question being: Is atherosclerosis an immunological disease? or are immunological
factors, alone or in association, implicated in the genesis of the atheromatous
disease?

At present, there is evidence that immunoglobulin-mediated mechanisms may be involved in the process of atherosclerosis in at least two conditions: autoimmune
hyperlipidemia with subsequent ischemic disease in man; arteriopathies induced in
animals by hetero-immunization. These two conditions are the result of the antibody activity of immunoglobulins.

Autoimmune Hyperlipidemia (AIH)

1. Background

In rare IgA or IgG myelomas, a major hyperlipidemia is associated (see review by
Dixon et al., 1965), and in some of these cases it was found that the myeloma
immunoglobulin forms complexes with the circulating lipoproteins (Heremans, 1960;
Lewis and Page, 1965; Cohen et al., 1966; Beaumont et al., 1965a).

The AIH concept appeared in 1964-65 (Beaumont and Lorenzelli, 1967), when after
finding antibody-like antilipoprotein activity of the myeloma protein in one
IgA K myeloma associated with hyperlipidemia, a similar activity was found for
non-myeloma immunoglobulins in a case of hyperlipidemia without myeloma. In this

AIH induced by antilipoproteins, hyperlipidemia was the result of the accumulation of circulating complexes.

Since then it was demonstrated that:
binding to lipoproteins was the result of the activity of the antibody site of the immunoglobulins (Fab fragment)(Beaumont et al., 1970a); several types of AIH may occur, which differ by the site involved reacting on lipoproteins and by the corresponding antibody (Beaumont et al., 1970a; Beaumont, 1969a).

AIH may also be induced by antienzyme antibodies which inhibit heparin (Glueck et al., 1969; Beaumont and Lemort, 1970). This allowed to widen the initial concept of AIH to all hyperlipidemias induced by an antibody able to inhibit lipolysis of lipids carried in the blood; so that AIH may be induced either by antilipoprotein or by antienzyme or any other antibody activity related to the lipolytic process (Beaumont, 1970).

Experimental hyperlipidemias were inducible in rabbits by immunization (Beaumont and Beaumont, 1968) and an antilipoprotein autoantibody was demonstrated in this experiment (Beaumont et al., 1969).

The occurrence of atherosclerosis in AIH was suggested by the high frequency of associated ischemic diseases in non-myeloma as well as in myeloma cases (Beaumont, 1965; Beaumont et al., 1967b). It seems now definitely established, by finding in two myeloma cases studied at autopsy, typical and severe atherosclerotic lesions containing Ig-LDL complexes (Lewis and Lazzarini-Robertson, 1973).

2. Definition and General Mechanism

AIH is a metabolic disease of immune origin. In AIH, lipoproteins accumulate in the circulating blood as a result of an inhibition of the lipolysis of the lipids they carry. This inhibition may be induced either by antilipoprotein antibodies reacting with the surface of lipoproteins at sites which are necessary for a correct lipolytic enzyme attack or by antienzyme antibodies which inhibit directly the enzyme before its reaction with the lipoprotein sites.

This general mechanism is suggested by finding slowed clearing of circulating lipoproteins in AIH, which is illustrated by vitamin A tolerance test (Beaumont et al., 1968) and by low postheparin lipase activity in AIH induced by antiheparin antibody (Glueck et al.,1972; Beaumont and Lemort,1970). We have recently studied in vitro the inhibitory activity of pure immunoglobulins from AIH cases in test systems, including postheparin lipase or adipose-tissue lipase and purified lipoprotein-activated substrates. AIH antilipoproteins as well as AIH antienzyme antibodies were able to inhibit fatty acid release in these conditions (Beaumont, unpublished observation).

According to its definition, AIH includes at a molecular level many possible forms which differ by the reacting site involved and by the corresponding antibody. By the one study of myeloma cases, several of them were evidenced and it is obvious that several and probably many other sites do exist.

This molecular diversity is in good accordance with Burnet's hypothesis (Burnet, 1959), which allows to expect that there would not be two exactly similar cases of an autoimmune disease.

The molecular diversity, which does not exclude in each case highly specific antigen-antibody specificity, allows a large scale of variation from one case to another for the biopathological and clinical expressions of the resulting metabolic impairment. For this reason, it is not surprising that AIH was found in hyperlipoproteinemias of almost all types referred to in the presently used classification.

3. Detection and Diagnosis

Why AIH was not brought to light till recent years may be explained. First, research in the field of lipid and lipoprotein was moving along lines where interference of an immune mechanism was not expected; second, at first sight, hyperlipidemias and hyperlipoproteinemias of immune origin do not differ from the types already classified in the albumin electrophoretic system (WHO Bulletin, 1970); third, in AIH, with the exception of myeloma cases in which there may be an antibody excess, circulating antibodies are inhibited by the antigens which are usually in great excess in blood. Usually little or no free antibody activity can be demonstrated in whole serum and plasma, and special purification procedures are needed to free the antibodies from their blocking antigens; fourth, AIH antibodies are usually not precipitating, so that specially sensitive procedures are necessary; fifth, a test useful for one type of AIH may be negative in other types, in which different antigen antibody reactions are involved.

However, the following list of presumptive signs and of tests useful for diagnosis at present may be given.

a) Presumptive Signs. Hyperlipidemia in myeloma or macroglobulinemia. Although such cases are rare, their study is worthwhile and will surely give more information on the diversity of AIH.

All signs of blood lipoprotein "instability" : cryoprecipitation, which was seen with IgM antilipoprotein (Lewis et al., 1966); precipitation by simple dilution in saline, which was seen with IgA anti-Lp Pg (Beaumont et al., 1970); impaired electrophoretic characteristics in cases of antilipoprotein form of AIH : no lipoprotein migration into starch gel (Cohen et al., 1966); lipoprotein precipitation or trailing in agarose gels, especially when albumin is omitted; abnormal β and α arcs in serum immunoelectrophoresis (Beaumont et al., 1970a).

Spontaneous agglutination of lipid particles (Beaumont, 1970; Beaumont and Lorenzelli, 1972) : in non-myeloma as well as in myeloma cases, spontaneous agglutination of circulating lipid particles, especially chylomicra and VLDL, may be seen by examining the plasma and serum with the naked eye and under the microscope. The agglutinates may be found in fresh plasma or serum and also in the creamy layer which floats in some cases after one night in the refrigerator at +4oC. Such agglutinates may be solubilized by the addition of an excess of the corresponding antigen and contain antilipoprotein antibody which after appropriate purification may be added to lipid particles to reproduce in vitro agglutination.

The phenomenon of spontaneous lipid-particle agglutination is positive only in some cases of the antilipoprotein form of AIH. It is negative in the antienzyme form of the disease. A negative result does not exclude the presence of antilipoprotein antibodies.

b) Diagnostic Tests. These tests are meant to detect antigen-antibody reactions in vitro between serum immunoglobulins and specific molecules related to lipoprotein metabolism. Except for myeloma cases with an antibody excess, the tests are usually not positive with whole serum and, as said above, reactive immunoglobulins need to be separated from their blocking antigens by different methods (Beaumont and Lorenzelli, 1967; Beaumont and Delplanque, 1969), combining pH variations, chromatography, ultracentrifugation, and detergents. The possible use of affinity chromatography with activated CNBr Sepharose is under investigation.

Four tests have been used to detect antigen-antibody reactions in AIH:

Three of them are available to clinical and epidemiological work : immunodiffusion tests by Ouchterlony's method (Beaumont et al., 1970); passive hemagglutination tests (HAP) using benzidine- (Beaumont, 1965) or chromium chloride- (Beaumont et al., 1969a) sensitized red cells; passive agglutination of synthetic, activated lipid emulsion (ALEA) tests (Beaumont and Lorenzelli, 1972). The results of these tests depend on the nature of the antibody and the antigen involved in the reaction. First, the valence of the antibody is important : for instance (Beaumont et al., 1970a) HAP and immunoprecipitation tests were highly positive in the first anti-Lp Pg myeloma case studied, in which the IgA antibody was for a large part highly polymerized. On the other hand, immunoprecipitation was negative and HAP was only weakly positive in a second IgA anti-Lp Pg myeloma in which the IgA was not polymerized, although this antibody had the same activity when its interaction with purified lipoproteins was studied in gel-filtration experiments (Beaumont et al., 1970a)(see later). Second, the nature of the antigen is also important : for example, antiheparin antibodies may be detected by ALEA test using lipoprotein-heparin or albumin-heparin activated emulsions and are not detected by HAP experiments; some antilipoprotein antibodies may react better in ALEA than in HAP tests and vice versa. Third, it is very important, while performing these tests, that no antibody inhibitors are present in the test system : for this reason, we perform HAP and ALEA tests without any macromolecular diluent (Beaumont et al., 1969a; Beaumont and Lorenzelli, 1972). HAP and ALEA tests may be sensitized by the use of an antiimmunoglobulin antiserum, as in Coombs' method. However, many positive reactions are seen with this method and it is sometimes difficult to make sure of their specificity. Work is going on at present in our laboratory on this problem.

The fourth test, which may be called the gel-filtration test (GFT)(Beaumont et al., 1970), is the most sensitive and has the great advantage to evidence direct intermolecular interaction of purified IgG with purified antigen (such as beta-lipoprotein (Beaumont et al., 1970), alpha-lipoprotein (Beaumont et al., 1970), or heparin (Beaumont and Lemort, 1970).

Unfortunately, this test is time-consuming, needs purification steps, and is not yet convenient for systematic detection studies. However, it is important to point out that this test may be the only positive one, even in myeloma cases.

4. Types of Antibodies Involved in AIH

a) Antilipoprotein Antibodies. In this form of AIH, there is a mixed hyper-lipidemia with cholesterol and triglyceride increase. The hyperlipoproteinemia type may look like types III or V as well as, sometimes, types I, IIb, or IV. The hyperlipidemia is partly sensitive to dietary changes, but a low fat or a low carbohydrate diet does not normalize it. The vitamin A tolerance test elicits an abnormally high and prolonged hypervitaminemia. Plasma postheparin lipase activity is variable. The serum contains soluble lipoprotein-Ig complexes which may be seen by the above described methods.

In the antilipoprotein antibody AIH, cutaneous, tuberous, and simple xanthomatosis may be seen especially in myeloma cases in which the lipidemia reaches very high levels.

At present, several myeloma and non-myeloma cases were studied:

Myeloma Antilipoprotein AIH. Two types have been fully described today : the IgA anti-Lp Pg and IgG anti-Lp A.S. myelomas.

In the IgA anti-Lp Pg myeloma, the active M protein is an IgA K which reacts with alpha- and beta-lipoproteins of all human beings and all animals studied (rabbit, rat, guinea pig, chicken). There are about 60 sites on the human beta-Lp and 20 on the alpha-Lp molecules. Part of the antigen can be extracted by ether and contains a phospholipid (Beaumont et al., 1970). Two cases were studied which differ by the degree of polymerization of the IgA molecule : in the two cases there was a combined hyperlipidemia of very high degree, xanthomata and severe ischemic disease of heart and lower limbs.

In the IgG anti-Lp A.S. myeloma, the active M protein is an IgG K which reacts with the alpha- and beta-lipoproteins of the patient's plasma, in 3 of 50 human sera studied. It does not react with rabbit Lp. In one of the 3 reactive human sera all, in the two others only some (about 30%), of the alpha- and beta-Lp molecules reacted. In this case there were no xanthomata and no clinical signs of ischemic disease.

Other Cases. Through the courtesy of Mrs Lewis, we were able to study the activity of her two very completely studied cases. One of them is an IgA K myeloma, which was first described in 1965 (Lewis and Page, 1965). In HAP and ALEA tests, the serum of this patient (Serum GOD...) behaved like anti-Lp Pg myeloma serum, but a more complete study would be necessary to confirm complete identity. The second was an IgG K myeloma (Lewis et al., 1973)(Serum HOP...) which proved different from anti-Lp Pg. The specificity in this case, in which there were circulating Lp-Ig complexes, remains to be determined.

It is likely that several of the other cases of myeloma with hyperlipidemia, which were studied by others, were AIH. Recently we had the opportunity to study completely four new cases (Beaumont, unpublished): one IgG K in which the IgM component reacted with alpha-Lp and albumin : in this case there were simple xanthomas and ischemic heart disease; one IgG K which reacted with beta- and alpha-lipoproteins : the complexes in this case were cryoprecipitable; there were simple xanthomas and no clinical ischemic disease; one IgA K which seemed to react only with VLDL; and one IgM K which seemed to react with both alpha- and beta-lipoproteins.

Non-Myeloma Antilipoprotein AIH. At present, we have studied 15 patients. In these cases, there was spontaneous agglutination of lipid particles.

Whole serum gave usually no or only weak positive agglutination reactions in HAP or ALEA tests. The purified antibodies were precipitating in vitro in one case (Beaumont et al., 1965) and not precipitating in the others, but gave positive tests in HAP and ALEA.

In many cases, the reacting sites seemed to be common to alpha- and beta-lipoproteins. However, in the two last cases studied, only beta-lipoprotein and, in one case, only albumin reacted. The exact type of the Ig antibody and of the reacting antigen site were not determined in the first cases studied, because there is much less circulating antibody in non-myeloma than in myeloma AIH. However, in the two last cases which we have been studying for five years in one, and two years in the other, the reacting system involves, in the first: IgG and chylomicra and VLDL as the reacting antigen, in the second: a more complex combination in which there is an IgG which reacts with beta-lipoproteins, and IgM which reacts with the IgG.

Ischemic disease is frequent and often precocious in the non-myeloma AIH we have studied (Beaumont et al., 1967a; Beaumont et al., 1968).

5. Antienzyme Antibody AIH

All the myeloma and non-myeloma cases actually known are antiheparin and antiheparin-lipase AIH.

a) Myeloma Antiheparin AIH. Two types have been fully described today: the IgA λ SAb and the IgG K ED.

In the IgA Λ Sab (Beaumont and Lemort, 1970; Beaumont and Lemort, unpublished), the hyperlipidemia was of the mixed type with predominant hypertriglyceridemia. Although there were no typical signs of myeloma, there was in the serum a monoclonal IgA Λ which reacted with heparin and heparin fragments, as demonstrated by direct gel filtration tests as well as by the ALEA tests described above, and also by the inhibition of antithrombin activity of heparin. Each IgA Λ molecule reacted with two heparin molecules. Fragments of hydrolyzed heparin, which had no more antithrombin activity and no sulfate, were potent inhibitors, thus demonstrating that the binding was independent of the polyanionic properties of heparin.

In the IgG Κ ED (Glueck et al., 1972), a very well-studied crystallizable immunoglobulin, it was demonstrated, using isotopic-labeled heparin, that the purified IgG and its Fab fragment bound heparin. In this case, it was demonstrated that the IgG inhibited, in vivo as well as in vitro, the anticoagulant activity of heparin and the postheparin lipase activity. There were diffuse atherosclerotic lesions at autopsy.

In IgA Λ Sab and IgG Κ ED myelomas, there was a hyperlipidemia with predominant hypertriglyceridemia, which varied widely from one test to another. The lipoprotein pattern was of type IV or V.

b) Non-myeloma Antiheparin AIH. Antiheparin immunoglobulins have been detected in several cases of dysgammaglobulinemias, associated with lupus erythematosus (Glueck et al., 1969) and also in two cases in which there was no detectable dysglobulinemia (Beaumont and Lemort, unpublished). In these cases, the hyperlipidemia is usually a predominant hypertriglyceridemia but it may be absent, and it seems likely that there are different types.

c) Thrombosis and especially recurring venous thrombosis were present in several of the patients in which antiheparin antibodies were found.

No epidemiological study is available so far for a frequency estimation of AIH in the population. However, among 270 hyperlipidemic patients with a milky or turbid plasma, 2% large agglutinates and 20% small agglutinates suggestive of anti-Lp AIH were found.

6. Experimental AIH (Beaumont and Beaumont, 1968; Beaumont et al., 1969b)

In animals, immunization procedures often produce hyperlipidemia with sometimes a milky serum, especially in rabbits and chickens. This hyperlipidemia may occur early, during the 4th to 6th week of the immunization course and then it is usually transient. Sometimes it begins later, 12 weeks or more after the end of the immunization course and may be permanent (Beaumont and Beaumont, 1968). The proof of experimentally produced AIH was made in a rabbit which became highly hyperlipidemic 16 weeks after several injections of complete Freund's adjuvant. In this case, an Ig which behaved like an anti-Lp autoantibody linked to the circulating Lp could be extracted (Beaumont et al., 1969b). This antibody reacted with a Lp site which is not present in all rabbits and is probably allotypic.

To experimental AIH may probably be attributed some hyperlipidemias associated with cancers, especially Walker rat carcinoma (Posner, 1960) and hamster Greene lymphoma (Albrink and Albrink, 1969; Beaumont and Beaumont, unpublished). This possibility is actually under study in our laboratory.

7. Atherosclerosis in AIH

Although there are no statistical figures to assess it, atherosclerosis is very likely one of the possible tissue complications of AIH for the following reasons: Clinically defined ischemic diseases are frequently associated with myeloma AIH although they are rather infrequent in the usual myeloma; ischemic diseases were usually associated to non-myeloma AIH and sometimes in rather young patients in which AIH was the only obvious factor (Beaumont et al., 1967a); atherosclerosis was found at autopsy (Lewis and Lazzarini-Robertson, 1973). Moreover, in a recent work, complexes made of LDL-Ig were found in the vessel wall of two cases of myeloma-antilipoprotein AIH (Lewis and Lazzarini-Robertson, 1973).

Clinical ischemic disease and atherosclerosis at autopsy were present both in antilipoprotein and antiheparin AIH.

The mechanism by which AIH induces atherosclerosis may be different for antilipoprotein and antoheparin types. In either, there is hyperlipidemia which is an already known factor of atherosclerosis. Additionally, in the antilipoprotein type, the circulating Ig-Lp complexes may be harmful by themselves. Some of them move through the arterial wall like other circulating macromolecules and, as they are rather instable, they may precipitate in the intima and yield subsequent accumulation of lipids and cholesterol. It is noteworthy here that the complexes we have studied until now do not fix complement, since it is understandable that the tissue of the vessel is not immediately and dramatically damaged like in other immune-complex diseases, for example serum sickness. By this hypothesis, atherosclerosis in antilipoprotein AIH would be an "autoimmune cholesterol-rich complex disease". In antiheparin AIH, there are no circulating lipoprotein-Ig complexes, but a thrombotic tendency seems to be associated to the antienzyme hyperlipidemia. This factor may contribute to the atherosclerotic lesions and its thrombotic complications.

8. The Origin of the Antibody Production which induces AIH is not known

Available data suggest that several mechanisms may be responsible. In myeloma cases it seems likely that the producing clones develop without any specific stimulation. In non-myeloma cases it is the general problem of tolerance failure in autoimmune disease, and genetic as well as acquired factors may be expected.

9. Treatment

In our experience, AIH may be influenced by a low caloric diet and also by antilipemic drugs like clofibrate or nicotinic acid. However, the improvement is usually only partial and the lipidemia does not return to normal. This was also the case in one of the myeloma AIH studied by Lewis and Page (1973).

We have made a few nonconclusive assays with corticosteroids, penicillamine (Beaumont et al., 1967b), and chlorambucil. However, recently it was demonstrated in a myeloma case that an immunosuppressive therapy was able to reduce both the antibody level and hyperlipidemia (Lewis et al., 1973). This is an encouraging result which suggests new lines for hypolipidemic drug research. But a very careful approach will be necessary to apply immunosuppressive treatment to non-myeloma cases, because the risk of treating may be higher than the risk of hyperlipidemia itself, which may be well tolerated for years. The ideal treatment to look for would be blocking specifically the AIH antibodies and only them.

10. Related Conditions

Other autoimmune disorders may be encountered in autoimmune hyperlipidemia : several antiheparin cases were found in lupus erythematosus (Glueck et al., 1969). However in the cases we have studied, there was no evidence of an associated lupus or immune arthritis, or thyroid or kidney disease. A mild anemia was rather frequent. No systemic study of the serological immune reactions was done for the present.

As was stated above, the frequency of AIH was not determined but it is felt that it may be the cause of many "primary" hyperlipidemias. On the other hand, some "secondary" hyperlipidemias are likely to be AIH : especially in nephrotic syndromes, in viral hepatitis, and in some cases of cirrhosis of the liver.

Autoimmune hypolipidemia was also described (Noseda et al., 1969) as a result of the antilipoprotein antibody activity of immunoglobulins: In these cases the reacting lipoprotein sites seem different from those involved in AIH : they are localized on the protein moiety of the LDL molecule (Riesen et al., 1972).

Immunization-Induced Arteriopathies

I. The Facts

1. Immunological injuries to arterial tissue are well known to result from repeated injections of antigens in appropriate experimental conditions related to serum sickness (Dixon et al., 1965; Cochrane, 1971; Germuth et al., 1967). It was demonstrated that, in these conditions, the histological lesions were due to the trapping of large circulating antigen-antibody complexes by a filtering membrane in the vessel wall (Cochrane, 1963). The subsequent segmental arteritis involves mainly small arteries and capillaries, with secondary tissue damage, especially in the kidneys. But deposit of immune complexes in coronary arteries and aortic wall, was also visible under the microscope, and hydrodynamic conditions proved to play an important part in their localization (Kniker and Cochrane, 1968).

2. Major lesions of large and medium arteries can also be induced by immunological procedures (Schmitt, 1942; Brochs, 1945; Saphir et al., 1968; Scebat et al., 1967a; Minick et al., 1966; Levy, 1967; Beaumont and Beaumont, 1968). Some of them, especially in rabbits, may lead to histological lesions which, in time, look much like human atherosclerosis.

a) The Inducing Antigens. Repeated injections and usually large doses of immunizing material are needed. Several kinds of antigens may induce arterial lesions:

Vascular wall antigens: Active immunization with homologous or heterologous aorta homogenates in toto (Scebat et al., 1967a; Beaumont and Beaumont, 1968) or with purified vascular wall antigens, such as structural glycoproteins and elastin (Robert et al., 1971) in Freund's complete adjuvant, induces a high ratio of arterial lesions in rabbits. There is no difference in the incidence and severity of the lesions when intimal or medial aortic tissue is used (Scebat et al., 1967a), but it seems that elastin injection, though less antigenic, leads to much more severe injury.

Other antigens: Anyway, the arterial lesions are not specific to the injected antigen. The same lesions have been induced by several different antigens : liver and kidney tissue homogenates, purified plasma proteins (albumin, gamma-globulins, beta-lipoproteins), and even Freund's adjuvant alone (Beaumont and Beaumont, 1968).

b) The Immunological Features. The occurrence of the vascular lesions is related to the immunizing process : the stronger the sensitization, the wider the lesions; when Freund's adjuvant is omitted, lesions can be obtained, but of a much lesser degree; the use of immunosuppressive agents, though not quite conclusive, seems to reduce their spreading.

Delayed hypersensitivity tests were found to be positive (Renais et al., 1973).

Circulating antiartery antibodies have been demonstrated in passive hemagglutination and double diffusion tests. But it must be said that no parallelism was found between production and level of antiartery antibodies and the arterial lesion. Major lesions may occur without any detectable antiartery antibody (Renais et al., 1973).

c) Associated Conditions. Hyperlipidemia beginning in the course of immunization, is quite common (Beaumont and Beaumont, 1968; Renais et al., 1973; Minick et al., 1966; Scebat et al., 1967b; Crocket et al., 1968). Transient or permanent, it may be of immune origin (see above). However, no correlation can be found between the degree of hyperlipidemia and the incidence of arterial lesions.

A moderate arterial hypertension develops in 20% of immunized rabbits (Renais et al., 1973).

d) Nature of the Induced Lesions. The early lesions are not characteristic of atherosclerosis. They develop in large arteries, but contain less or no lipid and cholesterol, and are much more destructive, with early and severe alterations of the elastic structures of the vessel.

However, when rabbits can be kept alive for several months after the end of immunization, the lesions become more atherosclerotic and lipid deposits can be seen in degenerative foci (Renais et al., 1973). The influence of aging in transforming a fresh experimental lesion into an atheromatous-like lesion was already demonstrated in cholesterol-fed rabbits (Constantinides, 1965).

Lesions of coronary arteries following cardiac transplantation in man and dog can also be attributed to an immunological mechanism (Glueck et al., 1969). The lesions consist essentially of fibrous intimal thickening with perivascular and parietal infiltration. It is noteworthy that this first lesion, characteristic of an immunological reaction, can be modified by associated conditions in the recipient : the lesions are much more severe in hypertensive patients, and hyperlipidemia leads to an extensive atheroma (Thomsen, 1969).

II. Mechanisms of Immunization-Induced Arteriopathies

Although the facts are obvious, the mechanism by which lesions are induced remains open to discussion:

1. According to the hypothesis of many authors, autoantibodies reacting with components of the arterial wall stimulate the lesions.If this hypothesis turns out to be correct, the resulting atherosclerosis, which would develop with aging, would be the result of a direct alteration in the vessel wall. However, there is no absolute proof available yet of this mechanism.

2. On the other hand, the pathogenic role of circulating immune complexes is clearly established by two possible main types:

a) In the first, which respond to the now classical immune complex disease, the complexes are produced with a heterologous antigen. In this type, the complexes usually contain no lipids but often react with complement and might yield rather destructive lesions containing little cholesterol, when they are fresh. These lesions could be at the root of a secondary atherosclerotic lesion when cholesterol deposit would develop.

b) In the second type, which responds to one of the patterns of AIH, the complexes are produced with autologous lipoproteins, contain lipids and cholesterol and do not react with complement. These complexes might induce directly a lipid-rich lesion resembling the atherosclerotic one with, at the beginning, little damage to the elastic and muscular structures of the artery.

The Mechanism of Atherosclerosis — an Attempt at Synthesis Including Immunological Factors

Some of the above-mentioned facts, especially the preferential possibility of eliciting arterial lesions by elastin immunization, and the inverse relation between the antigenicity of elastin and the lesions produced, seem to support an immunological theory of atherosclerosis as part of the general mechanism of aging (Robert, 1971). For these authors, atherosclerosis could be the consequence of an autodestruction of the artery by an immunological process, where structural constituents of the arterial wall are implicated; the sequence being : localized degradation of elastin tissue; autoantibody formation; reaction of antibodies, especially antielastin, with the arterial wall; selfmaintenance of the process, the origin of which is due either to activated sensitization to altered tissue constituents, or activation of a forbidden clone.

We feel that this theory has the disadvantage of not including all the factors concerned in atherosclerosis and its etiological factors.

For instance:
The correlation between atherosclerosis and some inherited disorders of lipid metabolism, such as familial type II hyperlipoproteinemia, is not easily explained, and no immunological mechanism was found up to now.

Medium and large arteries, the elective site of atherosclerosis, have no antigenic properties, and elastin can be found in many other places.

On the contrary, all possible immunological factors listed above easily take place with the numerous other known factors of atherosclerosis, if the atherosclerotic lesion is considered as *the result of a disturbance of the physiological flow of molecules through the wall of large arteries.*

Some of the main arguments supporting this view must be recalled:

1. There are no capillary vessels in the intima and the inner part of the media of large and medium arteries.
1. The cholesterol molecule is not synthesized in significant amounts in the vessel wall; is not catabolized by the cell which cannot open the sterol ring; is almost insoluble unless it is included in lipoproteins.
3. There is a permanent flow from the blood through arterial intima and media of macromolecules including lipoproteins.
4. Most of the molecules which flow through the intima of the arteries are easily metabolized even when their carrier is degraded, because they are soluble or degradable in soluble pieces. For the cholesterol molecule, which is not synthetized or degraded in the arterial wall, an outflow must be postulated to equilibrate the inflow and a "maximum capacity" of this outflow or excretion (MCE chol) may be also postulated and should be rather low.
5. The volume of the flow, the stability of the lipoproteins which carry cholesterol, their reactivity with the arterial tissue, and the ability of macrophages to synthesize new lipoproteins in the arterial wall may be the main limiting factors of cholesterol transfers from the circulating blood to the artery and from the artery to the blood.

The preceding assumptions may be summarized in the following equations: In normal conditions, cholesterol leaving the artery (excreted cholesterol : E chol), in a period of time, is equal to the amount of cholesterol entering it (blood cholesterol : B chol) and no cholesterol is deposited (D chol):

$$E\ chol = B\ chol\ ;\quad D\ chol = 0$$

A deposit of cholesterol and atheroma will arise when:

$$E\ chol < B\ chol$$

so that

$$D\ chol = B\ chol - E\ chol$$

Two different conditions may then lead to a cholesterol deposit : if the flow of B chol entering the artery is abnormally high and exceeds the capacity of excretion of a normal artery:

here

B chol > MCE chol

B chol > E chol

if maximum capacity of excretion of a "diseased" artery is abnormally reduced and falls under the normal flow of B chol:

here

MCE chol < normal

MCE chol < B chol

In this theory, the factors of atherosclerosis may be classified with regard to their influence on the physiological flow of molecules through the intima of arteries. Some of them can be briefly listed:

1. *Among Factors Increasing Blood Cholesterol Flow*, hyperlipidemia, and specially type II hyperlipoproteinemia, predominates. The general increase in circulating beta-lipoprotein transfer into tissues result in cholesterol deposition not only in arteries, but also in skin, cornea, cardiac valves, and tendons. Most of the other types of hyperlipidemia are also atherogenic, except pure hypertriglyceridemia type I and IV.
Arterial hypertension which increases the gradient between vascular lumen and tissues, may increase the transfer of all molecules, including lipoproteins, into the intima, so that the MCE chol may be overcome without hyperlipidemia. Pulmonary atherosclerosis secondary to pulmonary hypertension is a good example.

2. *Among Factors Reducing the Arterial Maximum Capacity of Excretion*, all factors modifying the structure and metabolic activity of the arterial wall may lead to a MCE chol reduction and subsequent atherosclerosis : for instance, atherosclerosis in graft vein segments which have no vasa vasorum.

3. The association of these two types of mechanism is probably the most usual condition of atherosclerosis in man, in which several risk factors are implicated.

4. Furthermore, some of those risk factors proceed by a different mechanism, but may act in complicating the basic lesion : for instance, thrombosis and its factors; tobacco smoking which induces modification of vasomotoricity and hence circulatory disturbance.

Although this theory may seem rather too simple and is still hypothetical in many aspects, it has several advantages:
The two classical theories of atherosclerosis need no longer to be opposed because in this new view the lesion may be induced either by an overload of the artery by molecules coming from the blood or by a primary alteration of the arterial tissue itself.

The statistical correlations between risk factors and atherosclerosis are taken into account with the possibility, in individual cases, of the predominance of one factor like hyperlipoproteinemia as well as of associations.

The existence of atherosclerosis with and without hyperlipidemia is easily understood and, in general, the fact that no risk factor seems absolutely necessary.

The central role of cholesterol remains clear even in the absence of a hyperlipidemia. Indeed, the accumulation of cholesterol in the lesions is the passive result of any disturbance in the flow of molecules through the avascular zone of the artery. The same accumulation of cholesterol occurs when similar conditions are realized in other tissues.

The role of the arterial structure is obvious.

In this general mechanism, the immunological factors easily fall into place without making of atherosclerosis a new "directly immunological disease":

1. Autoimmune hyperlipidemia may act in two ways : by increasing the flow of B cholesterol in all cases;
by a combined increased flow and some kind of direct damage to the vessel wall which may induce a diminished E chol excretion capacity in the antilipoprotein type of AIH in which unstable lipid-rich complexes enter the vessel wall. By this hypothesis, the atherosclerotic lesion would be the result of a variety of immune-complex diseases which differ from other immune-complex arteritides by three fundamental properties : the autoimmune origin of the complexes, their high lipid and cholesterol content, their noninteraction with complement.

2. Immunization-induced arterial lesions may result:
from an increase of B cholesterol when autoimmune hyperlipidemia is associated;
from an alteration of the vessel wall, and hence a decreased MCE and E chol when one of the two following conditions is realized:

Flow into the arterial wall of immune complexes rich or not in lipids : in the second case, the accumulation of lipids will be a secondary result of the arterial wall alteration;

Direct alteration of the vessel wall by "anti-artery" antibodies, with the result of secondary accumulation of cholesterol coming from the blood.

Conclusions

The fact that immunological factors are involved in the production of atherosclerosis in man should be considered in all studies on the mechanism and treatment of this disease including prevention. Immunological factors may act as a cause of a known atherogenic condition like hyperlipidemia in autoimmune hyperlipidemia. They may also have a more direct action on the arteries in heteroimmunization-induced lesions.

From a molecular point of view, the role of immunological factors in atherosclerosis seems to result from an antibody activity of circulating immunoglobulins rather than from cellular attached antibodies:

In autoimmune hyperlipidemia the arterial lesions may be secondary to the increase in circulating lipoprotein blood level and, when the antibodies show anti-lipoprotein activity, to the antigen antibody complexes which circulate in the blood and may infiltrate the artery. In the latter case, atherosclerosis appears like a variety of autoimmune complex disease.

In the heteroimmunization experimental model, the lesions may be due either to associated autoimmune hyperlipidemia with or without circulating complexes or to other sorts of complexes made of immunoglobulins and hetero-antigens. In the latter case, the arterial lesions are a consequence of the classic form of immune-complex disease.

Other mechanisms are possible, such as direct action of "antiartery" antibodies of an immunological origin or other atherogenic factors.

The different immunological factors, which are already known or may be expected, are easily placed in a general theory of atherogenesis in which the atherosclerotic lesion is the result of a disturbance of the physiological flow of molecules, and especially of cholesterol, through the arterial wall. In this view, the disease may be correlated with immunologic factors in many different ways.

There is room for extended research along these lines and perhaps for new therapeutic and preventive approaches.

ANTIBODIES AGAINST VASCULAR ANTIGENS

S. Gerö, Judit Székely, Magdolna Bihari-Varga, and Éva Szondy

1. It is generally accepted that arteriosclerosis is a polyaetiologic and presumably polypathogenetic disease caused by a combination of individually different factors. From the considerable amount of information obtained in the last
10 years, it seems likely that allergic and autoimmune processes may also play a
role in the chain of events leading to the atheromatous vascular changes (Gerö,
1969).

The presence of autoantibodies against arterial tissue in the sera of sclerotic
patients has been demonstrated by several authors (Stein et al., 1965; Jezkova
and Pokorny, 1967; Szigeti et al., 1968).

In our department, the frequency of occurrence of antibodies against homologous
aortic tissue was previously examined by the thrombocyte immune adhesion (TIAT)
test (Gerö, 1972).

As shown in Table 1 positive results were obtained in 60% of cases with various
clinical manifestations of arteriosclerosis and negative results in all the control subjects. No notable difference could be demonstrated between the lipid contents of the serologically reactive and nonreactive sera.

Table 1. Autoantibodies in arteriosclerosis (TIAT test)

Diagnosis	Number of patients	Pos.	Neg.
Coronary sclerosis	18	11	7
Myocardial infarction	20	14	6
Cerebral sclerosis	9	4	5
Arterioscler. obliterans	3	1	2
Total	50	30	20
Control	50	0	50

Next, to throw more light on the antigenic properties of the human arterial wall,
an extraction-fractionation procedure, basically that of Robert et al. (1968),
was applied to the aortic tissue.

The obtained fractions : calcium-chloride-tris-citrate (CTC) extract consisting
mainly of proteoglycans, water-soluble tropocollagen, TCA-soluble collagen,
structural glycoproteins (SGP) and elastin were characterized by immunochemical and thermoanalytical methods and their antigenic properties were investigated individually.

The aortic fractions were not homogenous : by disc electrophoresis, performed
according to the method of Ornstein and Davies, 1964, at least two bands could
be established in all fractions. These findings are in accordance with those of

Robert et al. (1971) who also established the heterogeneity of the same aortic fractions by the method of Ouchterlony. They found cross-reactions between the vascular antigen fractions and their antisera, indicating the presence of a water-soluble form of SGP and of elastin in the CTC extract and the presence of a small amount of SGP in purified elastin.

Table 2 summarizes the results of the assays for the demonstration of antibodies against the four main antigenic fractions isolated from macroscopically intact human aortas. It can be seen that the presence of autoantibodies against the CTC extract of human aorta was established by both the linear immunodiffusion and passive hemagglutination test in the sera of about 50% of the patients with coronary sclerosis, myocardial infarction and cerebral sclerosis. In 11 cases with arteriosclerosis obliterans negative results were found. Again, both tests were negative in the 22 control subjects.

Table 2. Immunological tests with aortic fractions

Methods	CTC extr. (Sol.prot.)				TCA-sol. collagen		Struct. GP		elastin	
	linear[a] immunodiff.		passive[b] hemaggl.		linear[a] immunodiff.		linear[a] immunodiff.		linear[a] immunodiff.	
Diagnosis	n[c]	pos.	n[c]	pos.	n[c]	pos.	n[c]	pos.	n[c]	pos.
Coronary scler.	31	15	17	14	24	0	32	0	24	0
Myocardial inf.	18	4	16	12	17	0	11	0	17	0
Cerebral scler.	22	10	29	21	19	0	24	0	19	0
Arterioscler. oblit.	11	0	–	–	12	0	12	0	11	0
Phlebothrombosis	12	1	15	2	10	0	8	0	12	0
Control	22	0	22	0	22	0	22	0	22	0

[a]Positive reaction: 1:16 - 1:32 serum dilution.

[b]Positive reaction: 1:32 - 1:128 serum dilution.

[c]n = number of cases.

But no antibodies could be demonstrated by the linear immunodiffusion test against SGP, elastin, and collagen-containing fractions in the cases investigated until now. Here we have to mention that Stein et al. (1965), by the use of the passive hemagglutination test, succeeded in demonstrating antibodies directed against elastin in the sera of apparently healthy and atherosclerotic individuals as well.

Next we used CTC extracts of atheromatous aortas. Here also, about 50% of the patients with various clinical manifestations of arteriosclerosis and in patients with arteriosclerosis obliterans, positive precipitation could be demonstrated by Oudin's method. The sera of healthy controls gave negative reactions.

The CTC extracts prepared from normal and pathological aortas were analyzed by a complex thermoanalytical method, derivatography (Paulik et al., 1958). Fig. 1 shows the differential thermal gradient (DTG) curves. The peak at 240°C indicates the thermal decomposition of the glucosaminoglycan components of the proteoglycans, while the 560°C peak is characteristic for that of their protein components (Bihari-Varga, 1971). According to the data obtained by quantitative evaluation of the decomposition curves, the amount of glucosaminoglycans in the CTC extract of intact and of calcified lesions containing aortas is rather similar, while in the aortas with lipid plaques the GAG-concentration is twice as high.

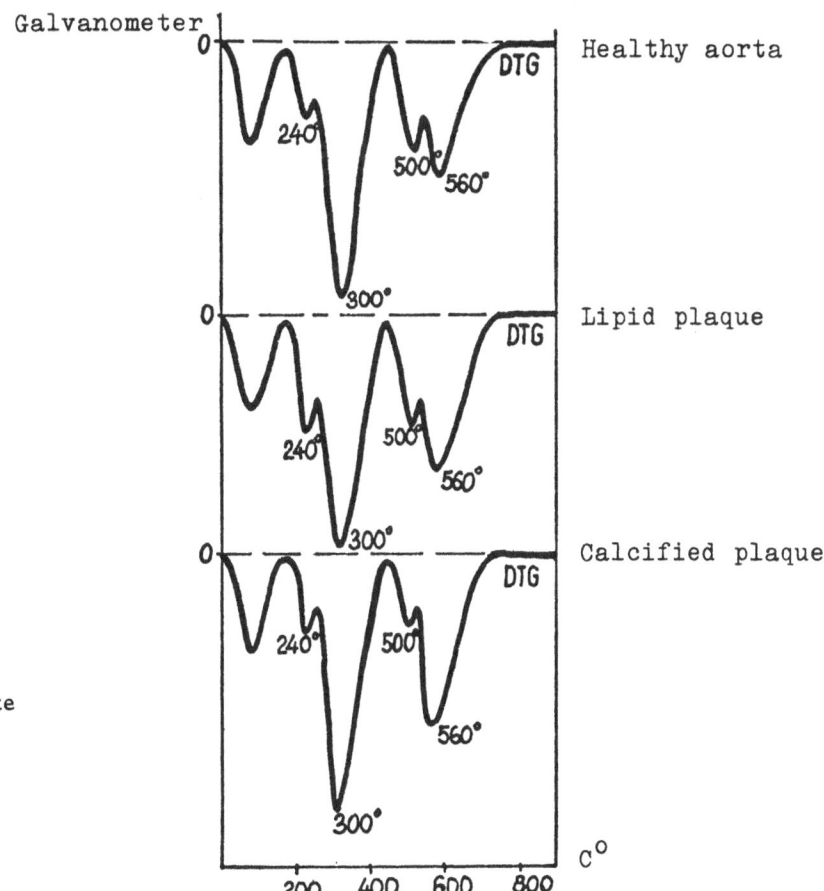

Figure 1.
CaCl$_2$-TRIS-citrate
extract

2. The increasing number of surgical interventions using homologous venous grafts in the arterial system suggested the significance of studies on the antigenicity of venous tissue. Again, in a certain number of cases, phlebothrombosis is a chronic disease of a cyclic course, characterized by the alternation of active and inactive phases. This course exhibits similarity with allergic events. Based on the assumption that autoimmune mechanisms may take part also in the pathology of phlebothrombosis, we attempted to demonstrate antibodies against venous tissue in the sera of patients with phlebothrombosis.

To this end, antigens were prepared from human vena cava tissue according to the method reported before.

Table 3. Immunological tests with vein CTC extract

Methods	Linear[a] immunodiffusion			Passive[b] hemagglutination		
Diagnosis	n[c]	pos.	neg.	n[c]	pos.	neg.
Phlebothrombosis	53	40	13	11	7	4
Control	22	0	22	22	0	22

[a] Positive reaction: 1:16 - 1:32 serum dilution.

[b] Positive reaction: 1:31 - 1:128 serum dilution.

[c] n = number of cases.

It was shown by disc electrophoresis of the CTC extracts of human aortic and venous tissue that there was a difference in the pattern of the two extracts the number of the fast-moving bands was higher in the venous than in the aortic extract.

Table 3 shows that the assays for antivenous antibodies were positive with the linear immunodiffusion test in 75% and with the passive hemagglutination test in more than 60% of the cases investigated until now.

The immunological properties of the other macromolecular venous tissue components are the subject of our current investigations.

HYPERIMMUNO-GLOBULINEMIA-LIPOPROTEINEMIA AND ATHEROGENESIS[*]

Lena A. Lewis and A. Lazzarini-Robertson, Jr.

The role of immuno-globulin bound lipoproteins in atherogenesis is not clear. While such an association of immuno-globulins and lipoproteins has been recognized as a possible etiologic factor for some hyperlipoproteinemias (Beaumont, 1969) the number of cases with this type of hyperlipidemia which have been available for detailed study of the atherosclerotic disease is limited. This report presents studies on two patients who were known to have hyperimmuno-globulin-hyperlipoproteinemia for 21 and for five years respectively.

Patients and Materials

Patient G had tuberous xanthomas and greatly elevated serum lipid, very low density, VLDL, (i.e. -S70-400) and low density, LDL, (i.e. -S25-70) lipoprotein levels when first examined at the Cleveland Clinic. His serum cholesterol and triglyceride levels, initially and usually throughout the 21 year study have been above 800 and 1000 mg per dl, respectively, despite attempts to regulate them with diet or diet plus drugs. An earlies report (Lewis and Page, 1965) summarized the first ten years of study on this patient. Fifteen years after his initial examination he was found to have bilateral popliteal aneurysms. Angiograms showed diffuse aneurysmal disease involving aorta, iliac arteries, superficial femoral arteries and the popliteal arteries. An aorta bilateral common iliac aneurysm-ectomy with replacement with a dacron graft was done. A year and a half later a thrombosis of the left popliteal necessitated a bypass graft from the common femoral to the popliteal artery. During the five years since vascular surgery he has done very well. Repeated coronary angiograms have shown only minimal coronary artery changes. The xanthomatous lesions have decreased in size since clofibrate treatment in addition to diet was started in 1968. His serum lipoproteins when studied by ultracentrifugation have consistently shown greatly elevated levels of VLDL, LDL and low levels of HDL. The ultracentrifugally concentrated lipoprotein fractions have contained IgA globulin in addition to lipoproteins. The IgA globulin snd lipoproteins migrate on paper electrophoresis as a single very concentrated fraction with trailing edge with "saw-tooth" appearance, with mobility of pre β-lipoprotein.

Patient H when first examined at the Cleveland Clinic in 1967 was 67 years of age and was found to have multiple myeloma and diffuse xanthomatosis. Her serum triglyceride and cholesterol levels were greatly elevated and all of her lipoproteins migrated electrophoretically to the γ-globulin position. She had greatly elevated concentration of IgG type K. She responded well to therapy which included initial plasmapheresis and melphalan (L-phenylalanine mustard) therapy. Her serum IgG concentration decreased from 4.0 to 1.0 g per dl and serum cholesterol and triglycerides became normal and the serum lipoproteins showed the electrophoretic mobility of normal β and α-lipoproteins. The improved serum protein and lipoprotein patterns were maintained for nearly five years. She then had a relapse, and infections developed. Autopsy showed diffuse aortic atherosclerosis, but absence of gross coronary lesions.

---

[*]These studies were supported in part by Grant HE 6835 from the National Heart and Lung Institute.

Methods

Lipids (Sperry and Webb, 1950; Technicon Autoanalyzer Methodology, 1962; Van Handel and Zilversmit, 1957), lipoproteins (Lewis et al., 1952) and protein electrophoretic patterns (Meites and Faulkner, 1961) were determined on serum taken when the patients were fasting and before initiation of any treatment. During the period of treatment the levels of these serum constituents were determined when the patients returned for clinical evaluation. After techniques for immuno-globulin quantifications were developed they were also measured (Fahey and Lawrence, 1963). Tissue cultures (Robertson, 1967) were made of tissue obtained at operation or at autopsy.

Results

1. Patient G

A. *Studies of Serum and Bone Marrow*. The serum of patient G has consistently shown increased levels of VLDL, 600-1000 mg per dl, LDL, 800-1200 mg per dl, IgA, 1500-3400 mg per dl, and low LDL, <150 mg per dl. (Table 1). The supernant fraction after ultracentrifugation at d 1.21 contained IgA in addition to lipoproteins. The complexing of IgA with lipoproteins has been observed throughout the 21 years of study. It is a very firm association which is not broken by ultracentrifugation at high salt concentration or by electrophoresis at pH 8.6. Dissociation was achieved by ultracentrifugation of the lipoprotein - IgA complex in a sucrose gradient of low ionic concentration and low pH.

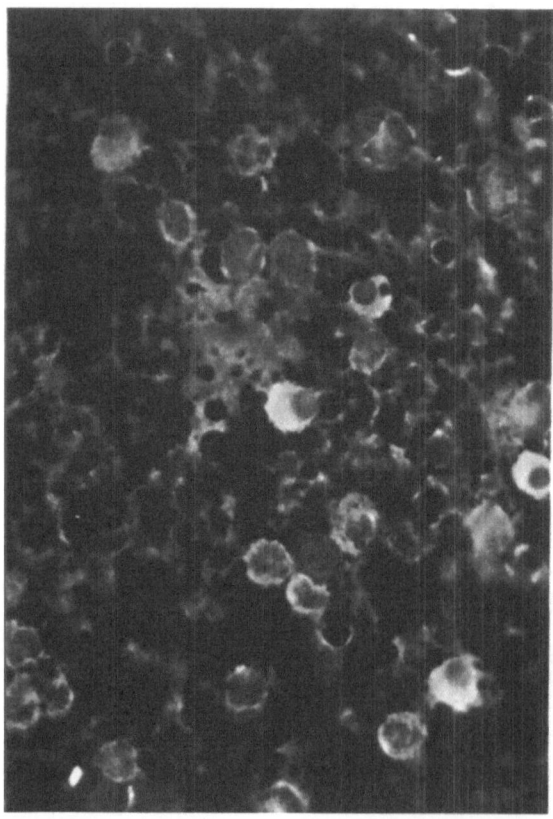

Figure 1. Bone marrow of patient G showing fluorescence of plasma cells when reacted with anti β-lipoprotein antisera

Until 1971 examinations of serum for type of light chain present in IgA showed both K and λ chains, but since then only λ chains have been demonstrated. Studies of the patient's bone marrow up to 1971 showed increased percentage of plasma cells, 8 to 20% most of which were mature cells. Since then increased numbers of plasma cells, some of which were immature and atypical in form have been present. Immuno-fluorescent studies of the bone marrow have shown immuno-fluorescence of plasma cells both for IgA and LDL antibody (Fig. 1).

B. *Special Histologic and Tissue Culture Studies.* Histologic examination of a biopsy specimen of patient G's skin was made. Areas of grossly normal skin showed presence of intracellular lipids in the dermin as well as in the keratinized epidermis (Fig. 2). The xanthomatous skin showed extensive lipid infiltrate surrounding hair follicles in dermis as well as large accumulation of lipids in the keratinized epidermal surface.

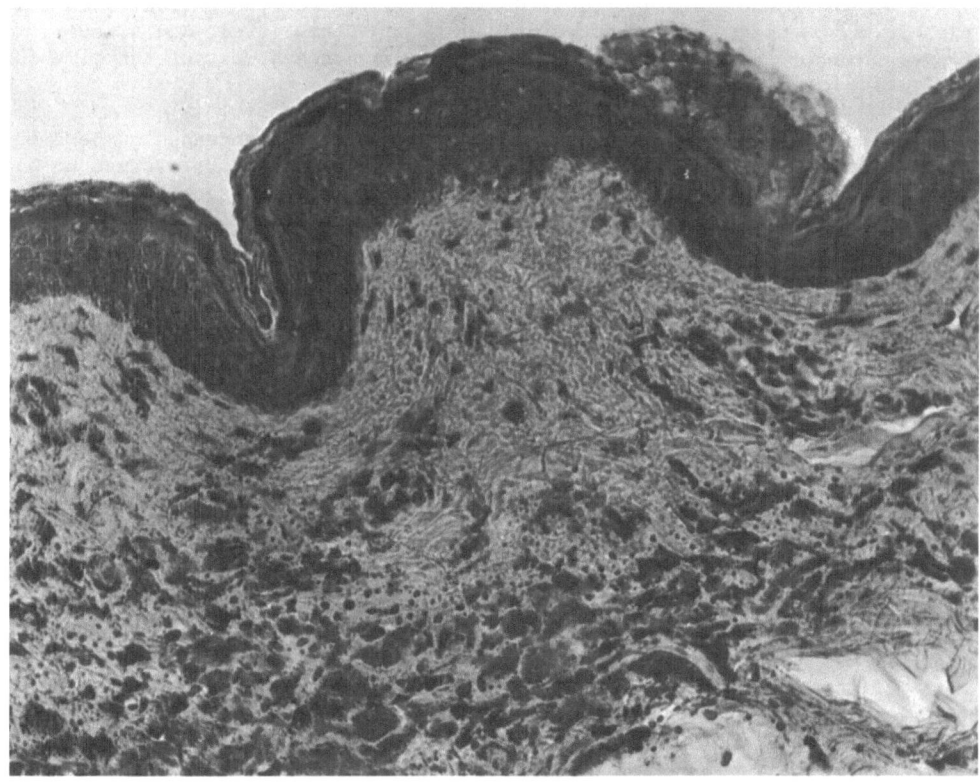

Figure 2. Cross section of epidermis and subdermis of grossly normal skin in patient G showing abundance of intracellular lipids in all layers including keratinized epidermal cells. Frozen section Sudan hematoxylin stain (121 X)

In dermal giant Touton cells developed in cell culture from resected xanthomatous lesions, an abundance of membrane-bound intracellular lipid is present. These cells also showed positive immuno-fluorescence both against IgA and LDL antibody. Xanthomatous skin from patients with hyperlipidemia but normal immuno-globulin levels showed fluorescence only against LDL antibody.

Bone marrow cells were cultured and after ten passages in semisynthetic media containing 10% autologous serum, the cells showed presence of intracellular lipid vacuoles.

Cultures of the femoral artery intimacytes showed marked differences in the intracellular accumulation of lipid droplets between contigous cells of vascular
smooth muscle. These intracellular vacuoles showed positive immuno-fluorescence
with both IgA and LDL antibody.

2. Patient H

A. *Studies of Serum and Bone Marrow*. Initial studies of serum proteins, lipids
and lipoproteins on Patient H showed greatly elevated levels of IgG, cholesterol,
triglyceride and lipoproteins. The lipoproteins were bound to the IgG and migrated in the position of IgG during electrophoresis at pH 8.6 (Fig. 3). The
serum had a high viscosity and contained cryoglobulin. As noted above, the association of lipoprotein with immunoglobulin was not broken by electrophoresis
but when the serum was subjected to ultracentrifugation at d 1.063 and d 1.21
lipoproteins free of IgG were concentrated in the top fraction and IgG in the
bottom of the ultracentrifuge tube. During treatment of the patient with immunosuppressive drugs her serum IgG, lipid and lipoprotein levels and viscosity decreased to near normal levels where they were maintained most of the time for
nearly five years (Lewis et al., 1973).

Examination of the patient's bone marrow showed greatly increased numbers of
plasma cells many of which were immature. Positive immuno-fluorescence of plasma
cells was observed both for IgA and LDL antibody. The diffuse xanthomatoses persisted despite improvement in serum lipid and lipoprotein levels.

B. *Special Histologic and Tissue Cultures Studies*. Autopsy examination showed
diffuse atherosclerosis of the aorta, but there was absence of gross coronary
lesions. Tissues were studied by immuno-fluorescent techniques for qualitative

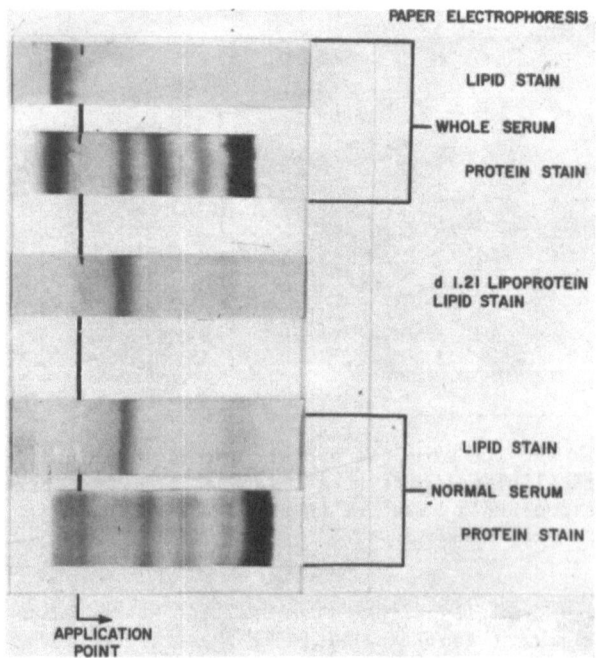

Figure 3. Serum lipoproteins and protein patterns of patient H with hyperlipidemia
and multiple myeloma. Note that lipoproteins migrate with identical mobility to
that of IgG. After removal of immunoglobulins, the lipoproteins show a characteristically normal mobility (Barbitol buffer, pH 8.6)

Table 1. Serum immunoglobulin and lipid levels 1965-73

	IgA mg/dl	T.C. mg/dl	T.G. mg/dl	-S. density 1.21, mg/dl				
				70-400	40-70	25-40	20-25	1-10
May 26, 1965	Very con.	1105		940	1180	705	750	<54
May 3, 1966	Very con.	1143		1060	1180	920	700	<54
December 18, 1966	Very con.	1108	1200	840	760	705		<90
March 28, 1968	1700	558	750	168	470	700		<145
January 10, 1969	2000	615	765					
April 15, 1969	2000			82	196	450		56
August 18, 1969	1600	632	784					
February 23, 1970	1400	742	780	196	570	980	40	135
August 11, 1970	3400	575	750	376	420	705		trace
November 30, 1970	2000	664	872	370	750	840		trace
May 12, 1971	2600	655	850	122	1055	540	890	
June 29, 1971	2700	485	1150	270	1055	- 1150 -		120
February 23, 1972	1875	675	900					
May 24, 1972		725	1100					
May 3, 1973		725	2325	590	240	700		0

Table 2. Immunoglobulin-lipoproteins at cell level

   Diagnosis = Multiple Myeloma Xanthomatosis. For 5 years - Chemotherapy.

Tissue Cells at Autopsy	IgG	IgA	Fibrin	LDL	HDL
Skin (Xanthoma)	+++	+	+	+++	-
Thoracic Aorta	+++	+	++	+++	+
Myocardium	+++	±	+	+++	-
Coronary Artery	++	-	+	-	-
Spleen[a]	+++	+	++	+	-
Liver	+++	+	+++	+++	+++
Kidney	+++	+	++	++	+
Bone Marrow	++	+	+	++	-

[a]Spleen Cells in culture continued high rate of IgG synthesis after ten passages.

Table 3. Some of studies reported showing association of lipoproteins, immunoglobulins and notes on incidence of atherosclerosis

Author	Journal	Patient Age & Sex	Immuno-globulin	Atherosclerosis	Other Notes
Beaumont, J-L.	Progr. Biochem. Pharmacol, 1968 4:110	59 M	Type IgA	Angina pectoris myocardial. infarct. ASO	multiple myeloma
Beaumont, J-L., Lemort, N., Halpern, B.	C.R. Acad. Sc. Paris (1970)1:271:2452	38 M	IgA IgAλ antiheparin antibody	Angina pectoris	
Beaumont, J-L., Antonnucci, M., Lemort, N.	Annal. Biol. Chem. (1970) 28:387	47 M / 62 M / 52 F	IgA IgA IgG	ASO with angina pectoris Angina pectoris; died of M.I. Not mentioned	
Lewis, L.A., Page, I.H.	Am. J. Med. (1964) 38:286	48 M	IgA	ASO	
Lewis, L.A., Van Ommen, R.A., Page, I.H.	Am. J. Med. (1966) 40:783	57 F	IgM	0	
Lewis, L.A., Page, I.H., Battle, J.D. deWolfe, V.G.	IRCS (1973)1:40	68 F	IgG	Atheroscl. aorta	(multiple myeloma)
Perrault, M., Dupperat, B., Dry, J., et al.	Ann. Med. Interne (1971)122:799	53 F	IgG λ	Some decrease in peripheral circulation systolic bruit over rt. carotid	(multiple myeloma) 5 yrs. after plane xanthoma manifest.
Feiwell, M.	Brit. J. Derm. (1968) 80:719		Cryoglob.	Gross atheroma in aorta, femoral & popliteal vessels	Xanthomatosis
Kodama, H., Nakagama, S., Tonioku, K.	Arch. Derm. (1972) 105:722	48 F	IgG K	Not mentioned	Plane xanthomatosis "other physical findings not remark-able

Table 3 (continued)

Author	Journal	Patient Age & Sex	Immuno-globulin	Atherosclerosis	Other Notes
Levin, W.C., Abqumrad, M.H., Ritzmann, S.E. et al.	Arch. Int. Med. (1964) 114:688	58 M	IgG K	Acute myocardial infarct.	xanthomatosis Precipitin lines on immunoelectrophoresis suggested association of IgG with lipoprotein.
Cohen, L., Blasdell, R.K., Djordjewichy, J. et al.	Am. J. Med. (1966) 40:299	55 F	IgG (? assoc. of IgG with lipo-protein)		Familial xanthomatosis, lipidemia, multiple myeloma
Kayden, H.J., Franklin, E.C.	Circulation	40 M	Υ = glob. binds LDL lipoprotein	Not mentioned	xanthoma; increased plasma cells in bone marrow
Noseda, G., Bütler, R., Schlumpf, E. et al.	Schweiz Med. Wchsch (1971) 101:893	68 F	IgA		multiple myeloma peripher. pulse OK Heart Normal
Noseda, G., Riesen, W., Bütler, R.	Schweiz Med. Wchsch (1971) 101:1787	Sera of 23 myeloma patients showed multiple myeloma, binding activity against ß-lipo. Cardiopulmonary findings not remarkable.			

demonstration of immunoglobulin, fibrin-fibrinogen, LDL and HDL. Tissues thus studied included skin, thoracic aorta, myocardium, coronary artery, spleen, liver, kidney and bone marrow. Table 2 summarizes the results and shows that IgG and LDL were both found in all tissues examined except the coronary arteries which showed neither component.

Examination of grossly normal abdominal skin showed presence of abundant intra and extracellular stainable lipids in the dermal layers as well as in the keratinized epidermis. Skin cells were cultured in autologous media and rapidly dividing dermal cells showed intracellular lipid vacuoles. Such vacuoles also showed positive immunofluorescence after incubation for 60 minutes with IgG antibody.

The thoracic aorta showed intra and extracellular lipids in inner intima, in contrast to the anterior descending coronary artery which showed extensive intimal fibroplasia without extensive lipid deposits. The coronary lesions did not show positive immunofluorescence for IgG or LDL antibody, while intracellular accumulation of LDL apoprotein and of IgG in aortic cells of inner intima was demonstrated (Table 2). The intracellular localization in the aorta of the immunoglobulin and of the LDL were very similar. Significant localization of fibrin-fibrinogen was noted in the atherosclerotic areas of the aorta.

Discussion

The present study of two patients with hyperlipoproteinemia-hyperimmuno-globulinemia has shown that association of lipoprotein with immunoglobulins does not prevent the deposition of lipids and lipoproteins in arterial tissue. In both patients, one with greatly elevated levels of IgA globulin, the other with high IgG globulin, advanced atherosclerotic lesions were demonstrated in the aorta. During the period of study, 21 and five years respectively, both lipids and immunoglobulins were elevated. From study of the families of both patients, there was no evidence to suggest that the hyperlipidemia was familial. The exact duration of the elevation of lipid-lipoprotein immunoglobulin levels could not be determined, but they were established to be present for 21 and five years, respectively. Whether the association of immunoglobulin-lipoproteins in the serum retarded the development of atherosclerosis from the speed that would have been operative had only the greatly elevated serum lipid-lipoprotein levels been present without elevated immunoglobulin levels is impossible to answer. It may be pertinent that the distribution of atherosclerotic involvement, being greatest in the aorta, was similar in the two patients.

At the time that atherosclerosis was demonstrated in our two patients, they were at the age where atherosclerosis is most common. Patient G had had consistently excessive elevated lipid and lipoprotein levels for 13 years when he had arterial surgery.

Studies by others of patients showing association of lipoproteins and immunoglobulins, and notes concerning incidence and nature of their atherosclerotic lesions if given are summarized in Table 3.

Many of the patients in whom serum lipoprotein-immunoglobulin association has been observed have had as the primary disease, multiple myeloma, in which it is generally recognized that serum lipid and lipoprotein levels are low (Lewis and Page, 1954) and atherosclerosis is not a usual complication (Beaumont, 1969). While information is not always given concerning atherosclerosis in the patients it was a major finding in many of the patients on whom clinical notes were given.

In a patient with possible association of lipoprotein with IgG reported by Levin et al. (1964) xanthomatosis of coronary arteries involving all three vascular coats with predilection for the advantial tissue and perivascular fat was noted. No lipid stained material either in or adjacent to plasma cells was found in frozen sections of spleen, which would suggest that lipoproteins were not present in the plasma cells as whole intact molecules. Whether the Lp of the lipoprotein was present was not determined. In our studies presence of the protein of the lipoprotein was demonstrated.

Localization of lipoprotein and immunoglobulins in other tissues, and celles besides arterial tissue suggests the generalized nature of the lipoprotein-immunoglobulin distribution.

Summary

The role of immunoglobulin-bound lipoproteins in atherogenesis is not clear. We have studied two patients with immunohyperlipidemia and severe atherosclerosis. Patient G has a 21 year history of tuberous xanthomas and greatly elevated serum lipids. Firmly bound circulating IgA-lipoprotein complexes were demonstrated by ultracentrifugation. Symptomatic, atherosclerotic aortoiliac and popliteal aneurysms required surgical repair while repeated cineangiographic studies showed minimal coronary artery lesions. Cell culture studies demonstrated reversibility of intracellular lipids by xanthoma cells but not by aortic intimacytes in which intracellular IgA-LDL complexes were found. Clinical diagnosis in Patient H was multiple myeloma and diffuse xanthomatosis. Serum lipoproteins migrated with IgG type K. With chemotherapy, lipoprotein and globulin levels were reduced to normal for almost five years. Autopsy showed diffuse aortic atherosclerosis but absence of gross coronary lesions. IgG-LDL complexes were shown in the aorta, kidney, liver, and skin but were absent in coronary arteries. High rate synthesis of IgG by spleen cell cultures continued after several passages.

These studies suggest that the binding of serum lipoproteins to abnormal immuno-globulins does not prevent their deposition in aortic atheroma.

We thank Drs., J. D. Battle, Jr., I. H. Page, and V. G. deWolfe who gave us the opportunity to study these patients and collaborated with us in the investigations.

WORKSHOP: Atherosclerosis-Hypertension Interrelationships

Chairmen: R. R. H. Lovell, Australia
           A. G. Shaper, England

Participants: C. G. Caro, England
               W. Hollander, USA
               S. Renaud, France
               S. L. Skinner, Australia
               Dr. Hood, Sweden

The participants were specifically asked to address themselves to the question: "What indications are there of a relationship between blood pressure and the development of arterial lesions?" The background was set by Dr. C. G. Caro (London) who considered that there was considerable evidence that the transport of certain macromolecules (albumin, cholesterol associated with lipoprotein) between blood and the arterial wall depended on the level of the shear rate or shear stress at the wall (Caro, 1973). (The shear rate represents the velocity gradient in the blood immediately adjacent to the wall; the shear stress is the tangential force, i.e. product of shear rate and blood viscosity). Dr. Caro considered that the transport of matter to the wall was primarily brought about by molecular diffusion and that hydrodynamic (bulk) flow had a negligible role. He emphasised that his comments related to the movement of macromolecules within a thin layer of plasma immediately adjacent to the artery wall and that he could at present make no comment on the uptake process, or transport within the artery wall. In his view vessel wall permeability is not altered by pressure changes and the concept of pressure-driven insudation of plasma constituents was not acceptable. The uptake process at the blood-wall interface is the rate controlling step in this total transport process and this shows a substantial temperature dependence.

With reference to Dr. Caro's expressed view that the concept of insudation of plasma constituents was not acceptable as a factor in promoting atherosclerosis in hypertension because the permeability was not altered by pressure changes, Dr. Haust (London, Ontario) pointed out the following: If one considers rightfully that the process of insudation is *not* merely a passive process, but rather a consequence of an active focal reaction of the vascular wall to injury operational at a given site, indeed, there is no basic disagreement between that school of thought and the interpretation of Dr. Caro's statement.

Dr. W. Hollander (Boston) described new pharmacological approaches to hypertensive and atherosclerotic disease based on animal studies. Hypertensive and atherosclerotic vascular disease are characterised by lipid deposition and proliferation of smooth muscle cells and connective tissue proteins in the arteries. The aorta and heart of animals (rat, rabbit) in which hypertensive and atherosclerotic disease had been produced, were examined for DNA, lipids, collagen, esastin and protein. Antiproliferative drugs such as colchicine, penicillamine, cortisone and aspirin all suppressed fibrous plaque formation. Colchicine and cortisone inhibited both the lipid deposition and the proliferation of connective tissue and smooth muscle cells in the diseased arteries while penicillamine and aspirin inhibited only the fibrotic changes in the artery. Dr. Hollander suggested that the use of antihypertensive drugs in combination with colchicine appeared to be maximally effective in preventing hypertensive vascular disease and complicating atherosclerosis.

Dr. S. Renaud (Lyon) discussed the influence of hypertension on dietary-induced atherosclerosis in rats (Renaud and Allard, 1963; DuPont et al., 1973). In both spontaneous and metacorticoid hypertensive rats, the hyperlipemia (cholesterol and triglycerides) resulting from the high fat diet feeding was considerably higher than in the normotensive. This serum lipid elevation might contribute to the acceleration of atherosclerosis by hypertension. Concerning the lesions observed in the aorta, in hypertension alone there was subendothelial deposition of fibrin and proteinaceous material, in addition to reduplication of endothelial basement lamina. In hyperlipemic normotensive animals, there was intimal deposition of fat droplets and numerous lipid laden cells. In hypertensive-hyperlipemic animals, the subendothelial space was occupied by smooth muscle cells, pools of osmiophilic bodies, proteinaceous material and cholesterol clefts. This type of lesion was particularly striking in the mesenteric arteries, leading to a considerable thickening of the intima. In the rat, hypertension might enhance the development of hyperlipemia-induced atherosclerosis by several mechanisms. One way appears to be by increasing the transport of blood elements through the arterial wall.

The concept that the renin-angiotension system might be involved in the development of hypertensive vascular disease was discussed by Dr. S. L. Skinner (Melbourne and Copenhagen) in relation to experimental atherosclerosis and hypertension. When rabbits are fed an atherogenic diet, renin secretion is suppressed without change in the diastolic blood pressure (Ampbell et al., 1973a). The effect occurs at the level of serum cholesterol found in man and cannot readily be accounted for by commonly recognised influences. When rabbits are made hypertensive by cellophane perinephritis, renin secretion is also suppressed and returns to normal in the chronic phase of hypertension. Feeding cholesterol to such animals accelerates the atherosclerotic process but again suppresses renin levels (Campbell et al.,1973b). These findings show that, as with essential hypertension, experimental renal hypertension can develop with suppression of renin levels and further, that acceleration of the atherosclerotic process in such hypertension is unlikely to be due to changes in the renin-angiotensin system. Dr. Skinner emphasised that these findings were not relevant to fibrinoid hypertensive vascular disease, in which the association with elevated renin and angiotensin is more convincing. In response to a question from Dr. Caro, Dr. Skinner pointed out that in order to answer the specific question "Does an elevated level of circulating angiotensin accelerate the deposition of lipid in the arterial wall more than can be accounted for by the associated hypertension alone", it would be necessary to use a model for hypertension in which renin and angiotensin were persistently elevated. This might be achieved with the unilateral renal artery clip model with contralateral kidney intact.

Dr. Hood (Malmö) pointed out the striking differences to be found within an individual at necropsy in the severe hyperbetalipoproteinaemias. There could be an advanced ulcerating atherosclerosis covering the whole aorta, and at the same time, moderately elevated non-ulcerating atheroma in the pulmonary artery and thin milky deposits in the femoral vein. He considered that this showed the influence of blood pressure from a normal mean pressure to very low pressure, as the physio-chemical state of the blood was identical for the three vascular areas.

Dr. Hood also described his clinical and epidemiological studies (Hood et al., 1973; Hood, 1972). A large group of survivors of myocardial infarction (MI) with first attacks below the age of 50 years, were studied and comparisons made with individuals from a randomised population group of 50 year old males. The ratio of MI survivors to the population study group was always far below 1.0 when the serum cholesterol was low, whether or not blood pressure or serum triglycerides were high. There were indeed very few MI survivors with low diastolic blood pressure and serum triglycerides and even fewer with low diastolic blood pressure and low serum cholesterol.

Dr. Hood then presented data on successive cohorts of actively treated severe hypertensives, analysed for 5 and 10 year mortality. There was a striking decrease in 5 year mortality as regards cerebrovascular lesions, congestive failure and uraemia. Analysis of 10 year mortality showed improvement in cerebrovascular lesions but myocardial infarction remained stable. When the material was subdivided according to age at start of treatment, there was a suggestive decline in the 5 year mortality from MI among those of 50 years of age or less at the start of treatment. Dr. Hood argued for the active tracing of asymptomatic hypertensives and their early treatment.

Dr. E. G. J. Olsen (London) described the International Atherosclerosis Project (IAP) (Robertson and Strong, 1968) in which 23,000 aortas and sets of coronary arteries were studied, including some 2,000 hypertensive subjects. These hypertensive subjects were compared with normotensives with regard to the extent of fatty streaks and raised lesions (fibrous plaques, complicated and calcified lesions) separately and combined in the aorta and the three coronary arteries. There were significant differences in the extent of fatty streaks in the abdominal aorta between hypertensives and normotensives, particularly in the younger men (25-44 years). At all ages there were differences in raised lesions between the two groups. In the coronary arteries, both fatty streaks and raised lesions were significantly more frequent in the hypertensives at ages 25-54 years in men and women. Some anomalous findings suggested that as raised lesions increased in extent, they encroached on the area previously occupied by fatty streaks.

Raised lesions tended to increase with increasing age in hypertensive and normotensive subjects, but in some location-race groups, particularly those with high levels of atherosclerosis, there was no evident increase with age. This suggested that hypertensive subjects had a higher mortality rate at younger ages than normotensives and that this was proportional to the severity of the hypertension. Overall, the IAP showed that hypertension accelerated the progression of atherosclerosis, particularly with regard to the raised lesions.

Dr. A. Trillo (London, Ontario) pointed out that while there was general acceptance that hypertension precipitates or aggravates the development of atherosclerosis, there was no agreement at present as to what hypertension per se actually does to the arterial wall. Data from experimental metacorticoid hypertension in rats suggested that hypertension without other factors being present, produced intimal lesions comparable to those described as gelatinous elevations, and considered by many to represent early atherosclerotic lesions (Trillo et al., 1970; Trillo et al., 1971).

When hypertensive animals were rendered hyperlipemic, the aortic lesions represented a combination of processes of insudation of blood components, lipid accumulation, cellular necrosis and presence of cholesterol in both, intima and media. These lesions were similar to the early atherosclerotic lesions but were more diffuse. He presented a series of slides to illustrate the early and advanced lesions showing a morphologic sequence of insudative lesions to early atherosclerotic plaques.

Dr. E. B. Smith (Aberdeen, Scotland) and her colleagues had developed a method for the quantitative measurement of electrophoretically and immunologically intact plasma constituents in intima (Smith and Slater, 1972). In 24 normotensive and 6 hypertensive subjects coming to autopsy, blood samples have been obtained during the week before death, thus allowing direct quantitative comparison of the concentrations of plasma constituents in the artery wall and in the circulating plasma. The diffusely thickened intima which is "normal" in human aorta in the third decade and upwards contains large amounts of most plasma constituents. On a volumetric basis the concentration of LD-lipoprotein in the intima is approximately the same as in the plasma and is highly correlated with it, but the 'volume of the patient's plasma' from which the lipoprotein is derived remains rather constant. This suggests the concept that a rather constant amount of "whole plasma" enters the intima, carrying with it an amount of LD-lipoprotein which is proportional to the plasma lipoprotein concentration.

In the 24 normotensive subjects the normal intima contained LD-lipoprotein equivalent to 1349 ± 95 µl of the patient's own plasma/100 mg dry tissue, whereas in the 6 hypertensives it was significantly higher at 2166 ± 154 µl (p <0.001). Thus it appears that in hypertension more plasma enters or is retained in the intima, and combined hypertension and hypercholesterolaemia have an additive effect on the amount of LD-lipoprotein in the intima.

LD-lipoprotein has a molecular weight of 2 million, so it is difficult to visualize it diffusing across the cell membrane. Relative to their concentrations in plasma, LD-lipoprotein has the highest concentration in intima and albumin (M.W. 68,000) the lowest. From several experimental studies it appears that large molecules rapidly cross the intact aortic endothelium in pinocytotic vesicles, and this may be the mechanism involved, but it is also possible that in the middle-aged human the endothelium is not intact and plasma can "leak" between damaged cells (Smith and Slater, 1973).

WORKSHOP: Hormones and Atherosclerosis

Chairman: M. F. Oliver, Great Britain

Participants: A. M. Barrett, Great Britain
              P. A. Bastenie, Belgium
              H. A. Eder, USA
              R. F. Mahler, Great Britain
              I Shkhvatsabaja, USSR

One of the more neglected subjects related to the pathogenesis of atherosclerosis is the influence of hormones. The effects which hormones may have on the development of arterial lesions are, in many respects, quite different from those which initiate the syndrome of ischaemic heart disease. For example, lack of thyroid and insulin can lead to atherosclerosis while a sudden increase in the plasma and tissue concentration of catecholamines is a major cause of the onset of symptoms of ischaemic heart disease. Again, the extent and type of arterial lesions show little difference in young women compared with young men, while there is a striking sex difference in the incidence of ischaemic heart disease under the age of 50. There are many areas in the field of atherosclerosis where scant attention has been paid to the influence of hormones and these include their effects on plasma low density (LDL) and very low density (VLDL) lipoprotein concentrations, on the lipoprotein structure itself, on platelet aggregation, on fibrinogen and on fibrinolysis and, most important of all, arterial wall metabolism. This Workshop was designed to elucidate some of these problems.

A. M. Barrett (Leeds) reviewed the field of *catecholamines and atherosclerosis*. Some of the relevant acute effects of catecholamines are a) vasoconstriction outside skeletal muscle b) lipolysis with elevation of free fatty acids (FFA) c) increased platelet adhesiveness d) cardiac acceleration with a tendency for dysrhythmias. It is important to distinguish between those actions which might be implicated in the genesis of atheroma from those which may precipitate clinical features in the presence of established ischaemic heart disease. Two major classes of compound, which have interested most pharmacologists and are currently under widespread investigation, are hyperlipidaemic agents and specific adrenoceptor antagonists. The original clear distinction between these two types of therapy have become blunted recently. There is evidence, for example, that the hypolipidaemic agent, clofibrate, may reduce the incidence of sudden death in anginal patients and that the antianginal beta-adrenoceptor antagonists can reduce lipid response to "stress" conditions.

All four of the accepted risk factors associated with the development of ischaemic heart disease - hyperlipidaemia, hypertension, cigarette smoking and physical inactivity - have a connexion with sympathetic activity. Acute elevation of FFA by infusion, or by subcutaneous administration of catecholamines, is followed by a delayed increase in other serum lipids. Some forms of hypertension are associated with elevated plasma catecholamine values. Nicotine will raise circulating levels of catecholamines, and cigarette smoking raised plasma FFA and increases platelet stickiness in man. Heavy smokers have higher levels of plasma LDL and VLDL than non-smokers. Physical training programmes may lead to an increase in vagal dominance, inferring a previous state of sympathetic dominance.

There are general theoretical objections to the useful interpretation of blood catecholamine levels as a true index of sympathetic activity, mostly because of the extraordinary capacity of adrenergic nerve terminals to recapture (uptake 1 process) released nor-adrenaline. This results in the fact that only 25% of the total amount of transmittor released is likely to appear in the general circulation. Many drugs, especially tricyclic antidepressants, depress the uptake process for nor-adrenaline but we do not know if their widespread use has a significant effect on the development effect of atheroma and associated complications. A correlation has been shown, however, between the administration of amitriptyline and the incidence of sudden and unexpected death in patients with a diagnosis of ischaemic heart disease. Attention has also been given to the findings that "emotional stress", such as associated with public speaking, leads to elevation of plasma nor-adrenaline, a rise in free fatty acids and in triglycerides. Beta-adrenoceptor antagonists do not effect catecholamine secretion but do prevent the elevation in plasma FFA and VLDL. Does this have any potential therapeutic importance? Is the benefit of beta-adrenoceptor blockade measured solely in terms of direct reduction in the cardiac action sympathetic neurohormones or is the inhibition of emotion-based fluctuations in serum lipids important?

Adrenaline and nor-adrenaline increase platelet coupling in vitro and acute exercise has been shown to raise the level of platelet adhesiveness. Whether this is due to catecholamines or a secondary consequence of increased FFA is not clear. Additional effects of FFA are the increased deposition of triglyceride in human tissue culture cells, and perhaps their accumulation in ischaemic myocardial cells leading to ventricular arrhythmias and impaired myocardial contractility.

There is ample evidence to show that catecholamine-induced mobilisation of FFA is sensitive to beta-adrenergic receptor blockade but there is no evidence at present that such drugs would decrease the incidence of cardiac arrhythmias or the overall death rate in patients presenting with symptoms of myocardial infarction. We do not yet know whether it is of benefit to prevent FFA mobilisation during the first hours after infarction, as the appropriate studies have not been made.

Finally, the drug Clofibrate is of interest. It is mainly bound to plasma albumin and might impede the access of FFA to albumin and thereby diminish FFA transport. This in its turn might be expected to reduce the supply of long chain fatty acids for hepatic lipid synthesis. It is possible that the drug could exert an indirect anti-sympathetic action in limiting changes in FFA liberation.

P. A. Bastenie (Brussels) gave an account of atherosclerosis in association with *clinical and pre-clinical hypothyroidism*. The time-honoured concept that myxoedema leads to severe atherosclerosis has been questioned in recent years. This is mostly because patients rendered severely hypothyroid with radio-iodine do not show more severe atherosclerosis than would have been expected. Although there are other reasons for doubting the atherogenetic effect of thyroid insufficiency, the evidence in its favour is strong. Most cases of spontaneous myxoedema in the adult are due to almost complete destruction of the thyroid by a process of auto-immune thyroiditis. Consequently, the pituitary shows increased thyrotropic cells which are the source of high levels of serum TSH. There is an increase in plasma cholesterol, LDL, plasma triglyceride and VLDL: the lipoprotein pattern of hypothyroidism is similar to that observed in type II and type III genetic hyperlipoproteinaemias.

Latent lymphocytic thyroiditis has been observed with high frequency at the autopsy of patients dying from miscellaneous diseases and is especially common in hypothyroidism. The same auto-immune reactions have been observed in these miscellaneous diseases with an increased amount of thyrotropic cells in the pituitary and of THS in the serum. Whereas in the past asymptomatic thyroiditis was undetectable during life, it can now be diagnosed by the presence of specific serological or cellular immune reactions against thyroid extracts or thyroid cells. It is characterised by changes in iodine metabolism and the presence in the serum raised TSH levels.

In many of these asymptomatic cases blood cholesterol levels are also raised. When carefully matched paired controls are studied, a significant increase is found in serum cholesterol concentrations in patients with thyroiditis compared with normal subjects. Asymptomatic thyroiditis, as detected by significant auto-immune reactions, may thus be considered as a condition of pre-myxoedema and is characterised by increased levels of TSH and serum cholesterol.

An association has repeatedly been found between latent thyroiditis and myo-cardial infarction in female patients, although the correlation is not signifi-cant for males. Other associations which have been seen are with obesity, hyper-tension and diabetes. In a recent enquiry into the presence of latent thyroiditis in 406 women, the prevalence of myocardial infarction was four times in excess of that found in those without thyroiditis. Similar results have been found in routine autopsy material in men as well as in women. These findings suggest that asymptomatic thyroiditis is a risk factor for coronary disease, particularly in women over the age of 50.

Thyroiditis or its underlying metabolic defect is only one factor among many others. Its part may be relatively unimportant when other more potent risk fac-tors are at work. In their absence, the thyroid factor may well prove to be of aetiological significance and only prospective studies will ascertain its im-portance.

H. A. Eder (New York) spoke on the subject of *oestrogens and atherosclerosis*. Data from the USA on differences in the incidence of ischaemic heart disease showed a fivefold excess under the age of 55 in males compared with females. In the black population in the USA the difference is not so great and in areas of low incidence of atherosclerosis the sex difference does not exist. The sex dif-ference has been thought by many to be due to the difference in the level of sex hormone secretion, and the high incidence in older women related to the menopause. An alternative explanation is the selective removal from the population of males at high risk and this is an interesting point which deserves further investi-gation. The administration of oestrogens to males raises the level of cholesterol in HDL and lowers cholesterol in LDL and VLDL. This is probably due to altered composition of LDL rather than an absolute decrease in the amount. Androgens have an opposite effect with lowering of cholesterol in HDL and raising of cholesterol in LDL and VLDL. This is not, however, a constant finding and in some individuals androgen actually lowers the cholesterol in LDL. The side effects of feminisation together with a mean rise of serum triglyceride recently shown by the Seattle group, suggest that this approach to the problem of ischaemic heart disease may be unacceptable and incorrect. Occasionally marked hypertriglyceridaemia can occur and, once the oestrogen is withdrawn, reduction of high serum triglyceride levels. The rationale for the use of oestrogens has now been eliminated as a re-sult of the finding within the Coronary Drug Study of an excess incidence of pulmonary embolism, thrombophlebitis and also of new events of myocardial infarc-tion in individuals receiving premarin, conjugated equine oestrogens.

Another effect of oestrogens is on elastin and collagen. In the thoracic aorta of rats made hypertensive by renal clips, there is an increase in the concentrations of these proteins compared with controlled animals. When rats are pre-treated with oestrogens, these effects of hypertension on aortic smooth muscle proteins disappear. Furthermore, oestrogens suppress the increase in alkaline phosphatase seen in the same tissue samples of hypertensive rats. Oestrogens also appear to suppress lyzosomal activity.

There are a great many opinions about the effect of insulin on lipid synthesis in the arterial wall with evidence for and against a positive action. R. F. Mahler (Cardiff), considered the influence of *insulin on the arterial wall* and reported evidence from rats made diabetic with alloxan. The incorporation of lino-leic acid, particularly into neutral lipids was appreciably reduced, although there was no change in the incorporation rate into phospholipids. When these rats were treated with insulin, there was no statistical increase in the incorporation

rate. In human arteries, obtained from autopsy, incubated with linoleate and
insulin, there was some incorporation of linoleate into neutral lipids, although
no change in phospholipids. The incubation of arterial intimal cells in culture,
obtained from the pig showed an increase in glucose incorporation in the presence
of insulin.

Studies of a cyclic-AMP dependent lipase in arterial tissue show different sensi-
tivities. Human arterial tissue is sensitive to nor-adrenaline; and the coronary
artery is a good deal more sensitive than the femoral artery and the aorta does
not show much response at all. Insulin is well known to restrain the stimulating
effect that adrenaline has on hormone sensitive lipase and adipose tissue. In the
coronary artery, the stimulation produced by nor-adrenaline was significantly
suppressed by 10 u.units/ml of insulin and with five times that concentration
complete suppression of nor-adrenaline stimulated lipolysis was achieved. This
degree of suppression was most marked for the coronary artery.

There has been much interest in the effect of hypoglycaemic drugs recently and
Mahler reported that the incorporation of acetate into lipid, which is slightly
increased by insulin, was equally stimulated by tolbutamide but, significantly,
suppressed by phenformin.

Finally, there is more plasma lipolytic activity in women than in men. Once women
reach the menopause this difference is lost. The same applies to rats - male rats
when young have less lipolytic activity than females.

II. A. Eder (New York) commented on *lipoproteins in diabetes*. Rats made diabetic
by the administration of streptozoazine have high levels of serum lipid. These
are higher than in sucrose fed rats. They also have elevated levels of blood
glucose and low levels of serum insulin. VLDL is markedly elevated and so also
are LDL. There are differences in the apoproteins of these lipoproteins. In a
sucrose fed rat the C2-peptide, analogous to human C2, is increased relative to
the C3-peptide. In a diabetic rat, the ratio is reversed. These changes are most
likely to be seen in VLDL. In the diabetic VLDL, the C3-peptide is the most
rapidly moving protein. These findings might be relevant to the changes in lipoprotein lipase activity that are seen in these diabetic rats, since the C-pep-
tides are in the high density lipoprotein fraction. The diabetic rats have increased amounts of lipoprotein lipase and the C-protein is probably the activator of this system.

I. Shkhvatsabaja (Moscow) described the effect of *steroid hormones on types of
hyperlipoproteinaemia in atherosclerosis*. A correlation exists between the level
of serum cholesterol and the concentrations in the urine of 17-oxycortico-
steriodism (17-OCS), free cortisol, 17-ketosteroids and free andosterones.
Marked hypercholesterolaemia was accompanied by marked reduction in the excretion
of these hormones.

A study was carried out in 138 patients with coronary disease between the ages of
30 and 59 years. The types of hyperlipoproteinaemia were defined according to the
Frederickson classification and data analysed according to polyacrilamide gel
electrophoresis or the analytical ultracentrifuge. Thin layer chromatography was
used for estimating the steroid hormones in the urine.

In Type IIA, when only serum cholesterol concentrations are increased, there is a
decrease in the total quantity of 17-OCS in the urine. In Type IIB, in which the
increase of concentration of lipoprotein is associated with a rise in triglycerides as well as cholesterol, there is an increase in the content of 17-OCS in the
urine and in cortisol. The excretion of 17-OCS was most marked in patients with
Type IV hyperlipoproteinaemia - that is in those with the largest increase in
serum triglycerides. In patients with abnormal tolerance to glucose, there was
an increase in total 17-OCS as well as in biologically-active cortisone compared
with coronary patients without abnormal tolerance to carbohydrate. In patients

with Type IIB hyperlipoproteinaemia and a disturbance of tolerance to carbohydrate, the urinary content of 17-OCS and free cortisol was very similar to
that in corresponding patients with Type IV hyperlipoproteinaemia.

It is known that in adipose tissue, cortisol activates cyclic AMP and thence lipolysis of stored triglyceride. Increase in the content of glucocorticoid could increase adipose tissue lipolysis with a release of free fatty acids into plasma,
leading in its turn to an increase in serum triglycerides and VLDL. These studies
may explain the increased triglyceride concentration which has been observed in
patients during the first day following myocardial infarction where there is a
sharp increase in the activity in the pituitary-adrenal axis.

N. M. Gerasimova (Moscow) spoke on the *effect of cortisol on plasma lipoproteins*.
In rabbits and rats with experimental atherosclerosis, cortisol was given at a
level of 5 mg/100 g weight and analysis was made of plasma lipoproteins. This
led to an increase in beta-lipoproteins and particularly pre-beta-lipoproteins.
VLDL increased in the majority of normal rabbits and at the same time there was
an increase in the content of 3'5' AMP in the urine of these animals. Cortisol
may increase the synthesis of 3'5' AMP, and therefore of adipose tissue lipolysis
resulting in increased plasma FFA and leading to increased synthesis of triglyceride and VLDL. In rabbits resistant to the development of atherosclerosis,
cortisol led to a decrease in the concentration of VLDL and LDL.

The *discussion* which followed raised several problems. Are oestrogens less harmful for women than for men? Is it the joint oestrogen-progesterone preparations
which are the most conducive to thrombosis? Is the depression of TSH levels in
an acute heart attack catecholamine-induced? Carotenoid pigments, which are the
precursors of vitamin A, are carried by LDL and in hypothyroid patients can be
very high with reduced conversion to Vitamin A: does this influence connective
tissue metabolism adversely? Growth hormone is elevated after myocardial infarction: does it increase VLDL though increased adipose tissue lipolysis?
Can cholesterol inhibit the uptake 2 mechanism of nor-adrenaline round an
atherosclerotic plaque increased by the presence of cholesterol in the plaque?

INFLUENCE OF LIPIDS ON THE PROGESTERONE-BINDING AFFINITY OF SERUM ALBUMIN AND α_1-ACID GLYCOPROTEIN

Ulrich Westphal and W. B. Owen Edelen

If a highly purified commercial HSA* preparation is delipidated by extraction with chloroform-methanol at 4°, its binding affinity for progesterone increases about 2 1/2 fold. This was determined by equilibrium dialysis and evaluated by the method of Scatchard (Westphal, 1971; Fig. VI-4). Since pure albumin preparations contain small amounts of firmly bound fatty acids that are removed by organic solvents, addition of fatty acids to delipidated HSA should inhibit interaction with progesterone. This was found when 5 moles of lauric acid were added per mole of nondelipidated or delipidated HSA; in either case, the nK value was reduced to less than half (Westphal, 1971: Fig. VI-4).
The presentation of the binding data as straight lines, and their extrapolation to the abscissa, is an oversimplification; the experimental points would better fit to a concave curve, indicating more than one type of binding sites (Westphal and Harding, 1973). However, the low water solubility of progesterone does not permit complete evaluation of the binding system at higher progesterone concentrations. The influence of the fatty acid on the number of progesterone-binding sites is, therefore, uncertain.
Addition of myristic and palmitic acid to delipidated HSA reduced the affinity for progesterone in a similar way as shown for lauric acid.
Binding of ligands to serum albumin is a very non-specific phenomenon. Because of our interest in the interaction of steroid hormones with high-affinity binders in serum and hormone target tissues, we investigated the influence of lipids on the binding of progesterone to α_1-acid glycoprotein, a serum protein with properties similar to those of the highly specific steroid-binding proteins found in blood serum.

AAG binds Δ_4-3-ketosteroid hormones according to the polarity rule, i.e., mainly by hydrophobic forces (Westphal, 1971: Chapter XIII). The binding affinity decreases with increasing number of polar groups in the steroid molecule. Delipidation of chromatographically pure AAG results in about 2 1/2 fold enhancement of binding affinity for progesterone; the number of binding sites increases from a fractional value to about 1 (Ganguly et al., 1967: Fig. 2). Re-addition of the lipid extracted during delipidation essentially restores the lower binding affinity and capacity characteristic of the AAG before delipidation.

I would like to comment here on a practical point concerning the equilibrium dialysis experiments. We had much difficulty over the years with inconsistency of the affinity constants determined for the progesterone-AAG complex. In spite of all precautions, scrupulous cleanliness of vessels, solutions, etc., the values were not well reproducible - until we found that manipulation of the dialysis bags with (well-scrubbed) hands causes a marked decrease of binding affinity.

This is shown in Table 1. The nk values increase 2 1/2 to 3 times by using surgical gloves when handling the bags. The effect is smaller, but definite also for progesterone interaction with HSA. Similar results were obtained by different investigators.

---

*Abbreviations used: HSA, human serum albumin; AAG, α_1-acid glycoprotein or orosomucoid.

Table 1. Influence of skin secretions on progesterone binding affinity of α_1-acid glycoprotein and human serum albumin

Progesterone complex with	nK values obtained		Increase by factor of	Investigator
	without gloves M^{-1} x 10^{-5}	with gloves M^{-1} x 10^{-5}		
AAG Prep. 1	4.9	12.9	2.6	OE
2	4.7	13.1	2.8	OE
3	5.1	13.9	2.7	OE
2	5.4	14.9	2.8	TK
3	6.1	17.7	2.9	TK
HSA Prep. 1	4.3	4.9	1.1	GH
2	3.2	4.3	1.3	GH
3	1.8	2.5	1.4	GH

Working under lipid-free conditions, we than investigated the influence of various lipids on progesterone binding to AAG. Fig. 1 shows the inhibition by the presence of 0.5 mole palmitic acid per mole AAG. The nK value is reduced; there is no decrease of n. A similar inhibition was observed when a small amount (0.2 mole per mole AAG) of cholesterol was added to the progesterone-AAG system. The results obtained with these and some other lipids are compiled in Table 2. In all these cases, the n value was not significantly affected by the inhibiting lipids.

Table 2. Inhibition of progesterone - AAG interaction by lipids. Equilibrium dialysis, 50 mM phosphate pH 7.4, 4°

Inhibitor	Mole inhibitor per mole AAG	K M^{-1} x 10^{-5}	% Inhibition
None (control)	-	10.3	-
Lauric acid	1	4.9	44
Mystric acid	1	3.2	69
Palmitic acid	0.5	3.4	67
Cholesterol	0.2	4.3	58

The influence of phospholipids on the affinity of the progesterone - AAG complex was investigated in a similar way. Fig. 2 documents the inhibition effected by the presence of 8 moles phosphatidyl ethanolamine per mole AAG, and indicates some reduction of the n-value. Table 3 summarizes the effects of the phospholipids. Binding inhibition was obtained in all cases; the n values were slightly reduced.

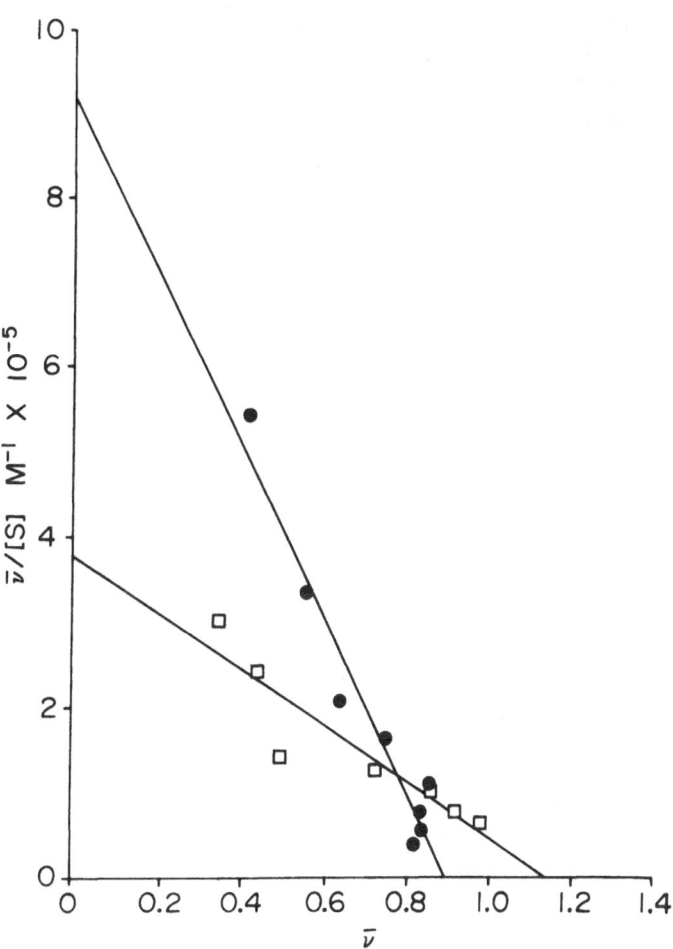

Figure 1. Binding of progesterone to AAG. Inside solutions (2 ml), containing
1 mg AAG/ml, in the absence (circles) and presence (squares) of 0.5 mole sodium
palmitate per mole AAG; outside solutions (4 ml), containing 2, 3, 4, 6, 8, 10,
12, and 18 µg ^{3}H-progesterone per ml. Equilibrium dialysis in 50 mM phosphate
buffer, pH 7.4, 4°, 72 hrs. The buffer contained 50 moles EDTA per mole AAG. The
data are presented according to Scatchard, by plotting $\bar{\nu}$/[S] vs. $\bar{\nu}$, where $\bar{\nu}$ indicates moles of bound progesterone per total protein, and [S] the molar concen-
tration of unbound progesterone. The slope of the lines yields nK, and the inter-
sect with the abscissa gives n

Table 3. Inhibition of progesterone – AAG interaction by phospholipids.
Equilibrium dialysis, 50 mM phosphate pH 7.4, 4°

Inhibitor	Mole inhibitor per mole AAG	nK M^{-1} x 10^{-5}	% Inhibition
None (control)	–	16	–
Phosphatidyl serine	8	8	50
Phosphatidyl ethanolamine	8	7	56
Phosphatidyl inositol	8	6	63
Phosphatidyl choline	8	10	38

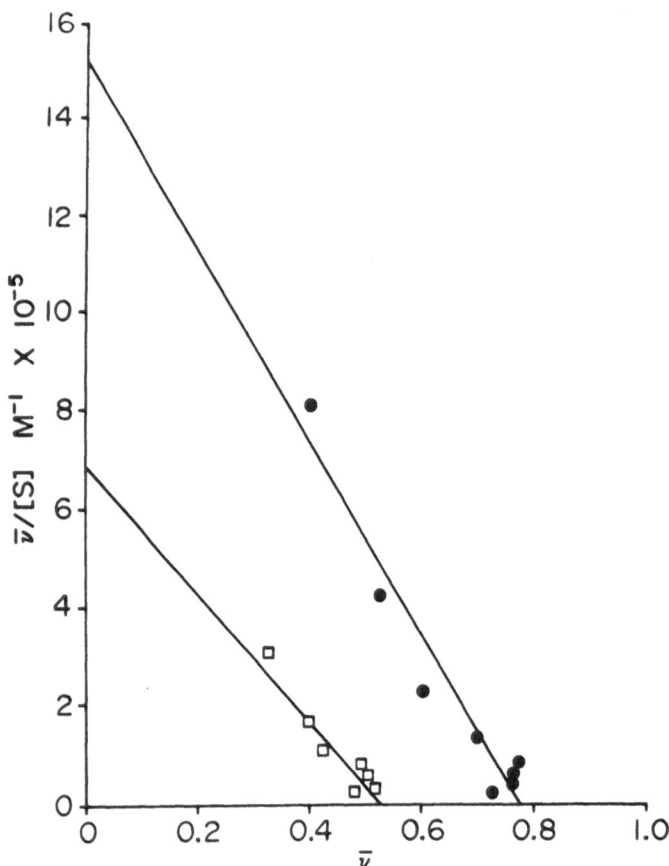

Figure 2. Binding of progesterone to AAG, in the absence (circles) and presence (squares) of 8 mole phosphatidyl ethanolamine per mole AAG. Equilibrium dialysis for 12 hrs at 22°, followed by 36 hrs at 4°. Other conditions as in Fig. 1

The following conclusions are drawn from our studies:

Various lipids (fatty acids; phospholipids; cholesterol) and secretions of the human skin inhibit the binding of progesterone to AAG in a similar way as fatty acids reduce progesterone interaction with serum albumin. The inhibition appears to be noncompetitive. We assume that the inhibiting lipids occupy hydrophobic areas neighboring the binding site, thus causing decreased binding affinity, but no definite influence on the n value.

THE INFLUENCE OF EXERCISE ON GROWTH HORMONE (STH) - SECRETION IN MALES WITH ATHEROSCLEROTIC LESIONS

H. Ditschuneit, H. H. Ditschuneit, E. Küter, D. Rakow, H. U. Klör, and J.-D. Faulhaber

The best known physiologic significance of growth hormone (GH) is induction and maintenance of longitudinal growth. An isolated GH deficiency does not induce fatal metabolic disturbances but it severely retards skeletal development. As GH secretion persists in adulthood, it remains questionable whether the only function of GH is stimulation of growth. Several clinical and experimental observations indicate that GH may increase fat catabolism which can be recognised by a lowering of respiratory quotient and increased ketogenesis (Prader et al., 1967; Rabinowitz, Klassen and Ziegler, 1965; Tanner and Whitehouse, 1967; Gaebler, 1930; Bennett et al., 1948).

In addition, the following facts seem to indicate that GH plays an important role in the development of atherosclerotic processes.

1. In ateliotic dwarfs with isolated GH deficiency no signs of atherosclerosis were found up to an age of 80 years, though most of them suffered from hyperlipoproteinaemias Type IIa and IIb and from subclinical diabetes (Merimee, 1972).

2. The ultimate fate of 80% of diabetic patients is determined by vascular disease. Besides a hyperlipidemia, which surely contributes to the development of atherosclerosis, elevated GH levels are observed in diabetes, too (Hansen, 1970; Pfeiffer, 1965).

3. Moreover, in many acromegalics exhibiting severe vascular disease without elevated plasma lipids, the plasma GH concentrations are consistently elevated (Friedberg, 1959; Hurst and Loque, 1966; Wright et al., 1970).

These observations stimulated us to investigate the relation of GH to several parameters of lipid metabolism in patients with myocardial infarction.

Methods

3 months after recovery from myocardial infarction documented by clinical, electrocardiographical and laboratory evidence, 32 patients were subjected to manual ergometric exercise over 20 minutes. At zero time, and at 10 and 20 minutes of exercise pulse rate, FFA, glycerol, ß-hydroxybutyrate, triglyceride (TG), total cholesterol (TC), plasma insulin and GH were measured. The mean age of the patients was 53.2 ± 2 years, body weight averaged 73.0 ± 2.1 kg. The levels of TG and TC were 184 ± 30 mg% and 223 ± 10 mg%, respectively. The hyperlipoproteinaemias observed could be classified as Type IIa, IIb and IV by lipoprotein electrophoresis. 25 subjects who had normal plasma lipids and who showed no signs of vascular disease as judged by oscillography, ECG and ophthalmoscopy were chosen as controls. The means of age and weight were 38.6 ± 2 years and 74.8 ± 1.8 kg, respectively. The TG values averaged 109 ± 8 mg%, TC was 191 ± 7 mg%. The experimental conditions were the same as stated above.

Results and discussion

During physical exercise there is an increase of plasma GH. As Fig. 1 shows, a strong correlation exists between the intensity of physical strain as expressed

by the pulse rate and the GH concentration. In order to guarentee the same stimulus of GH secretion in both groups we only chose those of the controls who had
the same pulse rates under exercise as the atherosclerotic patients.

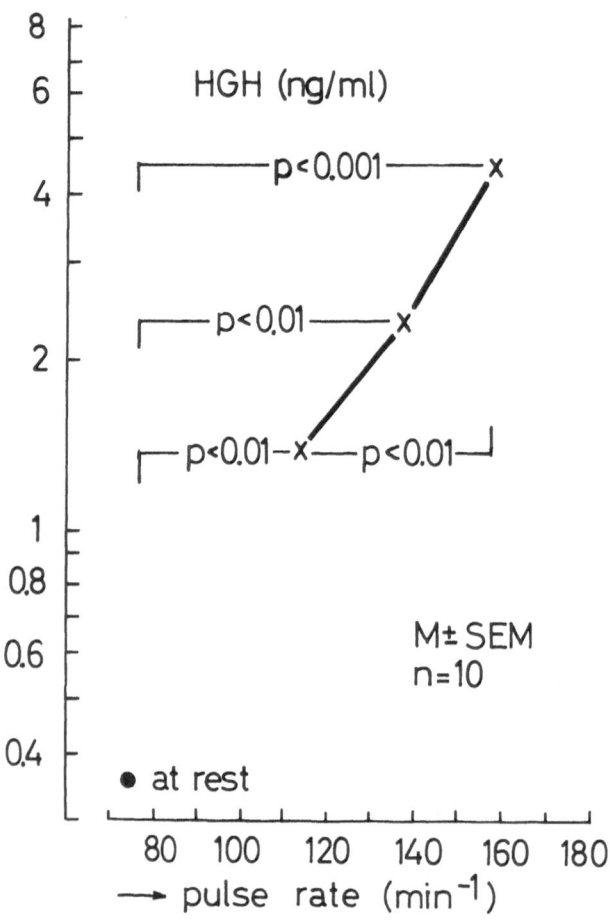

Figure 1. Increase of human growth hormone (HGH) in relation to pulse rate under
ergometric exercise

The patients with infarction already showed elevated GH concentrations of 1.7 ±
0.3 ng/ml at rest. The exercise induced a further increase of high significance
after 10 and after 20 minutes (Fig. 2). While the GH levels in normals only
reached 3.8 ± 1.0 ng/ml the patients with ischaemic heart disease showed a level
of 9.1 ± 1.9 ng/ml which exceeded that of normals nearly thrice.

The higher levels of GH in atherosclerotics both at rest and during physical
strain caused a higher increase in ß-hydroxybutyrate than in normals. The elevation of free glycerol was more pronounced in ischaemic heart disease, too. The
FFA slightly decreased under the working load in both groups while the plasma
insulin remained unchanged. To our great surprise both plasma triglycerides and
total cholesterol rose significantly during exercise in both groups. The increase
was still greater in myocardial infarction than in controls. Actually, we don't
have a reasonable explanation for these findings.

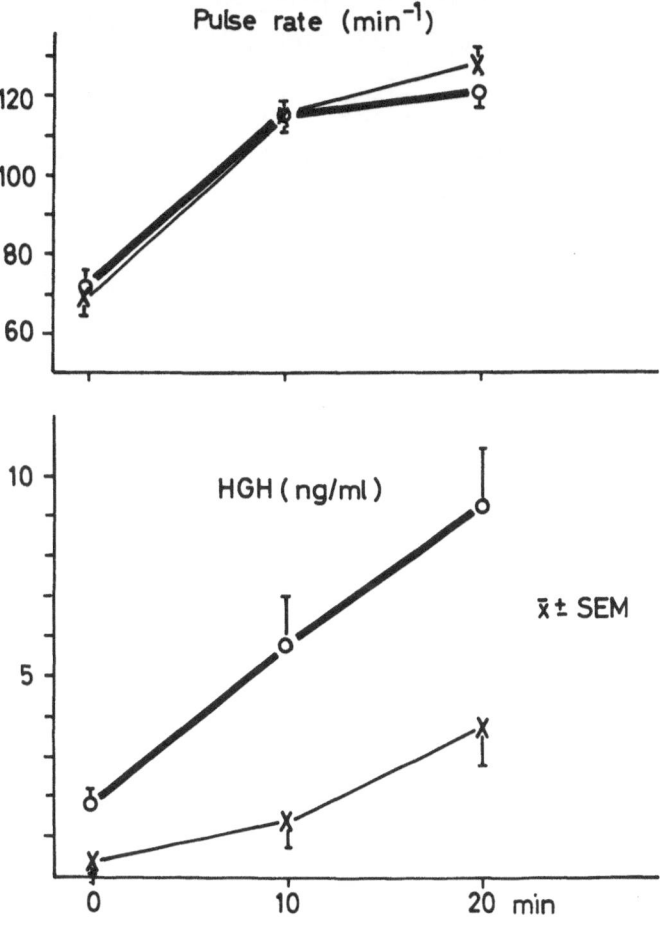

Figure 2. Increase of human growth hormone (HGH) and pulse rate under ergometric exercise over 20 minutes in 32 atherosclerotic patients and 10 normals

These results together with the clinical evidence cited at the beginning indicate that GH may be of great importance for the development of atherosclerotic processes. Under these aspects the GH mediated oxidation of FFA may play an important role.

As Fig. 3 shows, an infusion of GH over several hours greatly enhances the formation of ß-hydroxybutrate, which is a sensitive indicator for the extent of fatty acid oxidation.

Though the FFA level raises considerably under the GH infusion, this increase per se does not enhance ketogenesis, since a similar rise in plasma FFA caused by heparin infusion does not induce a comparable elevation of ß-hydroxybutyrate (Fig. 3).

We may summarize our results by saying that hyperlipidemia alone might not suffice to induce atherosclerotic changes. In addition, an increased level of GH which promotes fatty acid oxidation may be necessary for the development of vascular disease.

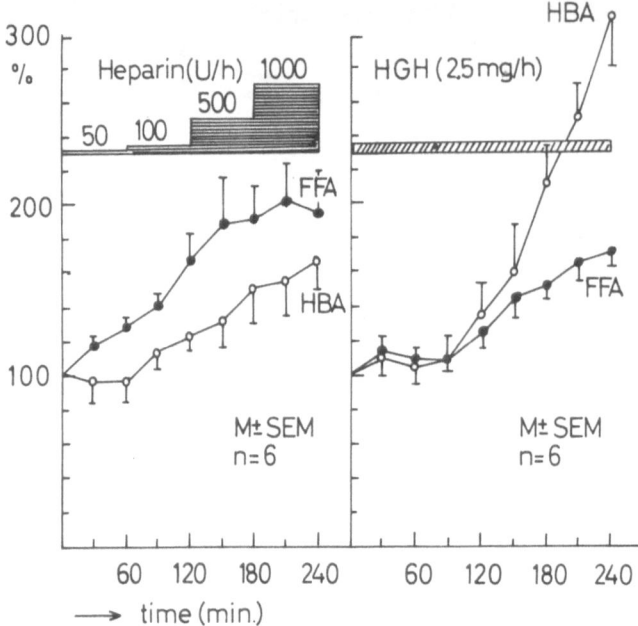

Figure 3. Effect of infusion of heparin and of human growth hormone (HGH) on free fatty acids (FFA) and ß-hydroxybutyric acid (HBA) in healthy volunteers

TYPE III HYPERLIPOPROTEINEMIA SECONDARY TO HYPOTHYROIDISM

Norman L. Lasser, John Burns, and Susan Solar

Type III hyperlipoproteinemia is an uncommon form of human hyperlipidemia characterized by accumulation of abnormal very low density lipoproteins (VLDL) with beta, rather than pre-beta, electrophoretic mobility. Although it is usually considered a primary disorder, it has been reported to occur secondary to systemic lupus erythematosus and diabetic ketoacidosis (Fredrickson and Levy, 1972; Stern et al., a972). It has also been described, without documentation, as occurring secondary to hypothyroidism (Fredrickson and Levy, 1972; Koppers and Palumbo, 1972; Wieland and Seidel,1973), which is usually associated with the type II disorder (Fredrickson and Levy, 1972). A case has also been described in which type III hyperlipoproteinemia is greatly aggravated by hypothyroidism (Hazzard and Bierman, 1972).
We have had the opportunity to study a case in which the type III pattern is clearly secondary to hypothyroidism, which, in this case, converts the pattern observed in a patient with familial hyperlipoproteinemia from type IV to type III.

Methods

Plasma cholesterol and triglycerides were determined simultaneously in the Technicon Auto Analyzer (Kessler and Lederer, 1965; Rush et al., 1970). Electrophoresis was carried out in agarose as described by Noble (1968), utilizing Bio Rad slides and Fat Red 7B staining. Preparative ultracentrifugation was carried out by the method of Havel, Eder, and Bragdon (Havel et al., 1955), and analytical ultracentrifugation was kindly performed by Dr. Frank T. Lindgren by methods previously described (Lindgren et al., 1972).

Results

Case Report. The propositus, a 49-year old female, was referred because of grossly elevated serum lipids. She had a long history of hypertension and angina. Seven years prior to her referral she had been told she had an underactive thyroid and given medication which was discontinued 1 1/2 years prior to her visit, precipitating increased fatigability. The patient was menopausal at the time of her visit and had a family history of hypothyroidism and diabetes. Her physical examination was consistent with typical hypothyroidism. At the time of her first visit she had a hematocrit of 35, a blood sugar of 272 mg/dl, uric acid of 9.1 mg/dl, and creatinine of 1.5 mg/dl. Nine months later, after she had been treated for hypothyroidism, her anemia had improved and her uric acid and creatinine were in the normal range. Her initial thyroid function tests were all markedly below normal, with a thyroxine of 2.0 mg/dl (normal 5.4-13) and a radioactive iodine uptake of only 3%. Her initial cholesterol values were about 800 mg/dl, with serum triglycerides of approximately 2,000. Lipoprotein electrophoresis after ultracentrifugation was consistent with the type III pattern, with a narrow band of beta-migrating material visible in the d<1.006 fraction and a broad beta band in the whole plasma. This initial electrophoresis pattern is shown in Fig. 1, as are those of succeeding samples taken after therapy with triiodothyronine (T3). After she had been treated for approximately a week and T3 dosage was up to 10 micrograms per day, her plasma still had the appearance of that of a type III, but was beginning to have a small amount of pre-beta material which merged with beta in the 1.006 top. By the time she was up to 25

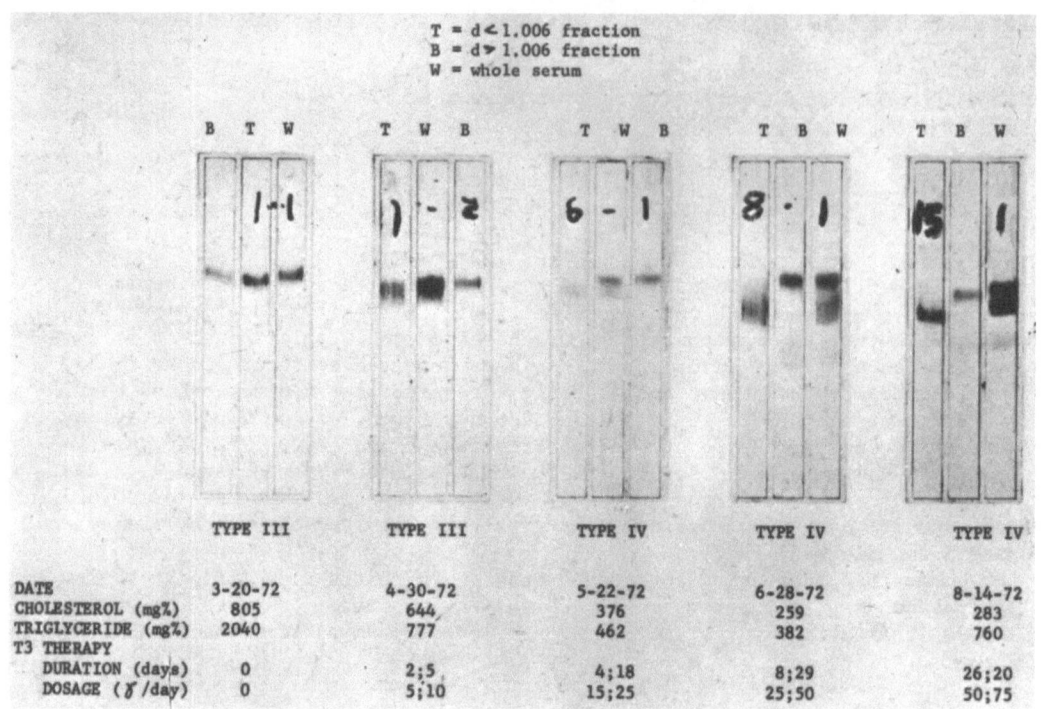

T = d<1.006 fraction					
B = d>1.006 fraction					
W = whole serum					

Figure 1. Electrophoretic patterns and plasma lipids with triiodothyronine

	TYPE III	TYPE III	TYPE IV	TYPE IV	TYPE IV
DATE	3-20-72	4-30-72	5-22-72	6-28-72	8-14-72
CHOLESTEROL (mg%)	805	644	376	259	283
TRIGLYCERIDE (mg%)	2040	777	462	382	760
T3 THERAPY					
DURATION (days)	0	2;5	4;18	8;29	26;20
DOSAGE (γ/day)	0	5;10	15;25	25;50	50;75

micrograms per day three weeks later, her pattern had the appearance of a typical type IV, with floating beta no longer detectible. The patient was given as
much as 75 micrograms of T3 per day, her pattern retaining the typical appearance
of a type IV. Note the multiple pre-beta bands to be seen in the fourth microscope slide.

Lipoproteins During Course of Therapy. As seen in Fig. 1 the patient's lipids
fell precipitously after she was started on T3, the cholesterol reaching a low
of 259, with the triglycerides 382 at this time, when the patient was on 50 micrograms of T3 per day. At the time patient had also lost 25 pounds, which she
gradually regained.

During the next period her lipid values remained the same, but the patient
noticed an increased frequency of angina compared to the period prior to the in-
stitution of therapy. After eleven months of T3 therapy varying from 25 to 75 mcg
per day, a sample was obtained for analytical ultracentrifugation, and the ultracentrifuge pattern obtained is shown in Fig. 2. The pattern, taken while the
patient was on 50 micrograms per day, has the appearance of that of a typical
type IV, with a VLDL peak at about $S_f 100$.

After a year of therapy the patient's thyroid medication was discontinued for a
period of 4 days. At the end of this period electrophoresis pattern had reverted
back to one resembling that of a type III, and there was an elevation of her
serum lipids. Her d<1.006 fraction demonstrated material which migrated on
electrophoresis only slightly faster than the beta in the bottom fraction or the
whole serum. After two days 5 micrograms per day, she again demonstrated two pre-
beta bands in her top fraction, as well as in the whole serum. While the double
pre-beta remained apparent in samples taken over the next month, the whole serum
again had the appearance of that of a typical type IV patient. Her cholesterol
reached a peak of only about 450 during the period of no therapy, and the chol-

esterol/triglyceride ratio in her VLDL increased from 0.27 to 0.33, but not into the usual type III range. During this period, samples were obtained for analytical ultracentrifugation, which showed a VLDL fraction which had shifted slightly to a lower S_f value, with the suggestion of a double peak around S_f100. Two days later the peak had broadened and showed a plateau between S_f40 and S_f70.

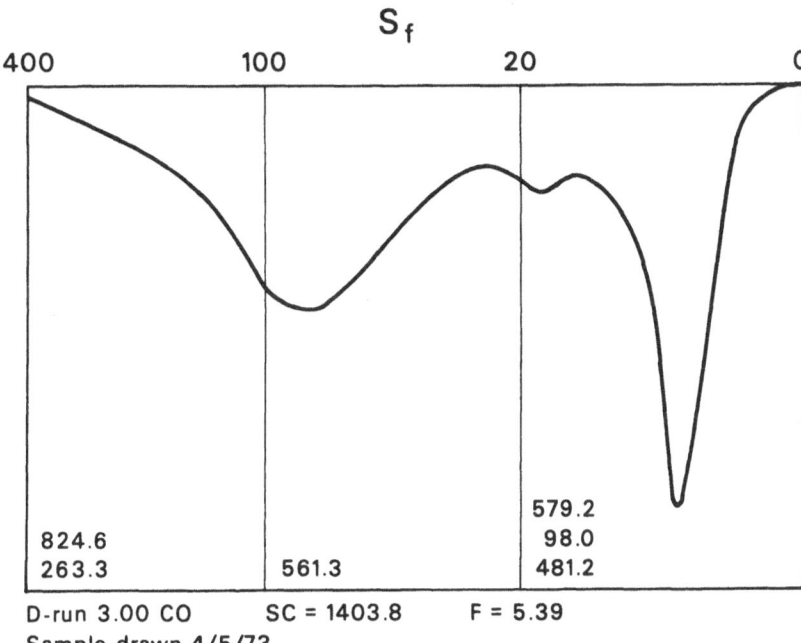

S_f

| 400 | 100 | 20 | 0 |

824.6
263.3

561.3

579.2
98.0
481.2

D-run 3.00 CO   SC = 1403.8   F = 5.39
Sample drawn 4/5/73
Analytical ultracentrifugation courtesy of F.T.Lindgren

Figure 2. Analytical ultracentrifuge pattern of serum after one year's therapy with triiodothyronine

As T3 was gradually reinstituted, the patient's lipid levels returned toward their prior values, but the patient noted that her increased frequency of angina was related to any T3 dosage exceeding 25 micrograms per day, at which level she has been maintained.

Family Studies. A major question which arose was whether the type III pattern seen in this patient had been present prior to the hypothyroidism, which simply aggravated the hyperlipidemia, or the pattern was secondary to hypothyroidism, either through production of a secondary hyperlipidemia or conversion of a previously existing one to the type III form. In order to answer this question it was desirable to study as many relatives of the propositus as possible for hyperlipidemia. Plasma cholesterol and fasting triglycerides were measured in forty-three of her relatives, and the results are shown in Fig. 3. It can be seen that hyperlipidemia is present in every generation of this family which was examined and that the disorder was apparently transmitted by the patient's father. The patient (after T3 therapy), both her siblings, and their affected children were all found to have a type IV pattern, there being a combined hyperlipidemia in the parents and only a hypertriglyceridemia in the children. Among the family members of the patient's paternal aunts there are cases of combined hyperlipidemia, hypercholesterolemia, and hypertriglyceridemia. Note that the husband of one of the aunts is presumed to have had hyperlipoproteinemia, possibly familial hypercholesterolemia, since he died in his forties of a myocardial infarction, as did one of his sons.

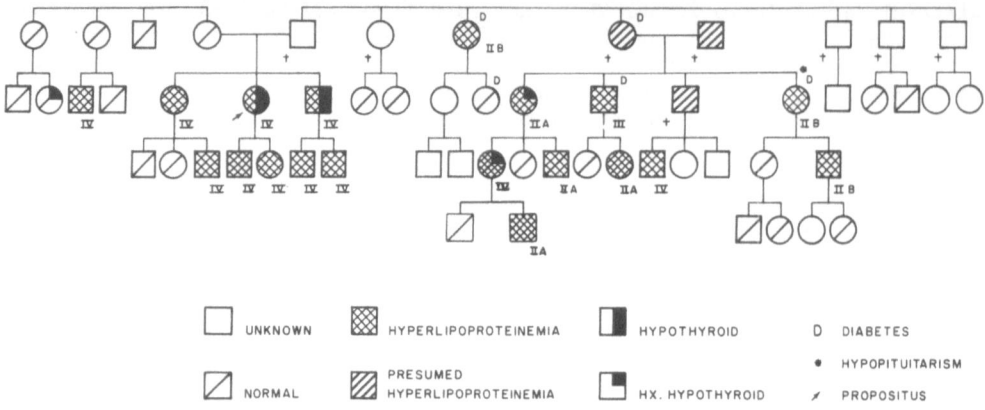

Figure 3. Hyperlipidemia in relatives of propositus. Roman numerals refer to types according to WHO classification

The plasma of all the relatives was ultracentrifuged and the VLDL examined for floating beta lipoprotein. As can be seen in Fig. 3, this material was found in only one relative, a first cousin, but it is not known at this time whether or not he was hypothyroid. Note that the propositus' brother (M.O.) was hypothyroid. The cholesterol/triglyceride ratio in VLDL was measured in 17 of the relatives, both normal and hyperlipidemic, and it was abnormal (0.75) only in the brother (M.O.).

Discussion

We have concluded that both the analytical data and the results of the family study are most consistent with the interpretation that this is an example of a familial combined hyperlipidemia with dominant inheritance, in which the lipoprotein pattern becomes that of a type III patient in the presence of hypothyroidism. The electrophoretic patterns in Fig. 1 clearly demonstrate that the patient had a type III pattern when she was hypothyroid, and that this was converted to the type IV pattern when the hypothyroidism was treated. That this latter pattern was indeed type IV is clear from the analytical ultracentrifuge pattern shown in Fig. 2. No abnormal intermediate/density lipoprotein is present when the patient is receiving thyroid medication, eliminating the possibility that the patient remained a type III in whom the floating beta lipoprotein was simply not visible by conventional means.

Familial combined hyperlipoproteinemia and its inheritance pattern has recently been described by Rose and Goldstein and their collaborators (Goldstein et al., 1973; Rose et al., 1972), and the pattern demonstrated in Fig. 3 would seem to be consistent with their descriptions. Thus, most of the subjects who are affected demonstrate the type IIB or type IV pattern, although IIA and III are also found. As discussed earlier, it is possible that the husband of one of the propositus' aunts had familial hypercholesterolemia, since he and one of his sons died at such an early age. This may explain why the type IIA pattern is found in his descendents, although his grandson, whose father also died in his forties, demonstrated a type IV pattern, and not type II. Thus the propositus does not represent someone in which type III was produced as a secondary hyperlipoproteinemia, but rather a familial combined hyperlipidemia which was transformed in the presence of hypothyroidism. The one relative who also demonstrated the type III pattern may have hypothyroidism when he is examined for this possibility, but the type III pattern has been described in combined hyperlipidemia, as has the type

IIA pattern (Goldstein et al., 1973). It is also possible that hypothyroidism itself is inherited in this family. It is interesting that the one relative in whom the VLDL cholesterol/triglyceride ratio was abnormal also had hypothyroidism, although no floating beta was visible in his VLDL.

The finding in this patient that hypothyroidism can cause the appearance of beta-VLDL when only alpha-VLDL was present without hypothyroidism, is consistent with results previously described both in humans and in animals. Hazzard and Bierman have concluded, on the basis of the case they have described (Hazzard and Bierman, 1972), that secondary factors may interact with the primary metabolic defect causing type III hyperlipoproteinemia to influence the expression of this disorder. They have clearly demonstrated that hypothyroidism is one of these secondary factors. Moreover, Shore et al. (1973) have shown that hypothyroidism in animals causes the accumulation of the abnormal intermediate density lipoprotein found in type III, and that this lipoprotein is rich in the arginine-rich peptide found in the C family of VLDL lipoproteins. An increased proportion of this arginine-rich peptide has also been demonstrated in humans with the type III disorder (Havel and Kane, 1973), so that it is possible that this peptide is transferred to the surface of VLDL as C-proteins are lost during the conversion of VLDL to low-density lipoproteins. Although the mechanism underlying these findings and the conversion of the type IV to the type III pattern in the patient described is unclear, all of the results emphasize the possible role of hypothyroidism in the mechanism of the production of hyperlipoproteinemia, particularly when it is the type associated with the presence of beta-VLDL. It seems quite likely that the mechanism involved an effect of thyroid hormone on the rate of metabolism of the short-lived intermediate density lipoprotein which normally appears during conversion of VLDL to LDL, but which has been shown to accumulate in patients with the type III disorder (Bilheimer et al., 1971; 1972).

It has been suggested by some investigators that hypothyroidism in the form of subclinical myxedema may be implicated in a surprisingly large proportion of cases of hypercholesterolemia (Fouler et al., 1970; Calay et al., 1971).

The possibility that hypothyroidism plays a surprisingly large role in the production of hyperlipoproteinemia is an intriguing one, and is worthy of further investigation, particularly in view of the findings presented here.

XIV
Plasma Lipoproteins

WORKSHOP: Plasma Lipoproteins

Chairmen: P. Alaupovic, USA
          D. Seidel, West Germany

Participants: A. M. Gotto Jr., USA
              G. K. Kostner, Austria
              R. I. Levy, USA
              L. A. Lewis, USA
              A. V. Nichols, USA
              H. Peeters, Belgium

The main purpose of the workshop on lipoproteins was to sort our the available
information, to summarize some of the more important achievements and to indicate, whenever possible, the future trends. With the primary focus on the chemistry of human plasma lipoproteins, the program of the workshop included the
following topics and presentations: 1. Isolation and characterization of apolipoproteins, 2. Isolation and characterization of normal lipoprotein species,
3. Isolation and characterization of abnormal lipoprotein species, 4. Lipid-
binding properties of apolipoproteins, 5. Structure of lipoproteins, 6. New developments in analysis of apolipoproteins and lipoproteins, and 7. Nomenclature
of apolipoproteins and lipoproteins.

It was indeed very appropriate to begin the lipoprotein workshop with a presentation on recent advances in *the isolation and characterization of apolipoproteins*. In discussing this topic, Dr. Levy appropriately pointed out that progress in this area of lipoprotein chemistry can only be described as phenomenal.
In 1966, at the First International Symposium on Atherosclerosis, only apolipoproteins A and B* were recognized as identifiable protein moieties, while the

---

*Abbreviations and nomenclature: VLDL, very low density lipoproteins (d <1.006
g/ml); LDL, low density lipoproteins (d 1.006-1.063 g/ml); LDL_1, subclass of
low density lipoproteins (d 1.006-1.019 g/ml); LDL_2, subclass of low density
lipoproteins (d 1.019-1.063 g/ml); HDL, high density lipoproteins (d 1.063-1.21
g/ml); HDL_2, subclass of high density lipoproteins (d 1.063-1.125 g/ml); HDL_3,
subclass of high density lipoproteins (d 1.125-1.21 g/ml); VHDL, very high density lipoproteins (d >1.21 g/ml); α-LP, α-lipoproteins, lipoproteins with an
electrophoretic mobility of α-globulins; ß-LP, ß-lipoproteins, lipoproteins
with an electrophoretic mobility of ß-globulins; pre-ß-LP, pre-ß-lipoproteins,
lipoproteins with an electrophoretic mobility of $α_2$-globulins. In this report
the apolipoproteins were designated according to the ABC-nomenclature (Alaupovic, 1971). ApoA, apolipoprotein A consisting of two nonidentical polypeptides A-I and A-II; A-I polypeptide contains glutamine as the C-terminal and
aspartic acid as the N-terminal amino acid; A-II contains glutamine as the C-
terminal and pyrrolidone carboxylic acid as the N-terminal amino acid. In other
systems of nomenclature (Scanu et al., 1969; Lux et al., 1972) A-I is designated as Fraction III or apolipoprotein Gln-I (apoLP-Gln-I) and A-II as Fraction IV or apolipoprotein Gln-II (apoLP-Gln-II). ApoB, apolipoprotein B; ApoC,
apolipoprotein B; ApoC, apolipoprotein C consisting of three nonidentical polypeptides C-I, C-II and C-III; C-I polypeptide is characterized by N-threonine
and C-serine, C-I by N-threonine and C-glutamic acid and C-III by N-serine and
C-alanine. In other systems of nomenclature, C-I is designated apolipoprotein
Ser (apoLP-Ser) or Fraction V, C-II as apolipoprotein Glu (apoLP-Glu) or Fraction V, and C-III as apolipoprotein Ala (apoLP-Ala) or Fraction V. LP-A, lipoprotein A, lipoprotein family characterized by the presence of ApoA (A-I and
A-II); LP-B, lipoprotein B, lipoprotein family characterized by ApoB; LP-C,
lipoprotein C, lipoprotein family characterized by ApoC (C-I, C-II and C-III);
Lp(a), polymorphic form of lipoprotein B or LDL; LP-X, lipoprotein X, low density lipoprotein characteristic of obstructive jaundice.

entry of apolipoprotein C (Gustafson et al., 1964) was looked upon with skepticism. In 1973, there were at least seven or eight recognized apolipoproteins or polypeptides. One of the most significant achievements during this time period was the recognition that ApoA or the major protein of HDL consists actually of two nonidentical polypeptides designated as A-I and A-II (Shore and Shore, 1968). This was followed by the confirmation of ApoC and its resolution into three non-identical polypeptides referred to as C-I, C-II and C-III (Brown et al., 1969). Studies on the physical, chemical and immunological properties of these polypeptides culminated in the first successful determination of the amino acid sequence of C-III polypeptide (Brewer et al., 1972b). Brewer et al. (1972a) also determined the amino acid sequence of A-II polypeptide, and Shulman et al. (1972) elucidated the sequence of C-I polypeptide. At a regular session preceding the lipoprotein workshop, McConathy and Alaupovic (1973) announced the isolation and partial characterization of a minor polypeptide found mainly in HDL and designated previously as "thin-line" polypeptide. On the basis of immunological properties, electrophoretic mobility in 7% polyacrylamide gel and characteristic amino acid and carbohydrate composition, these authors concluded that "thin-line" polypeptide is the apolipoprotein of a distinct lipoprotein family present mainly, although not exclusively, in HDL_3. According to the ABC nomenclature (Alaupovic, 1971) this protein moiety is designated as apolipoprotein D (ApoD) and its corresponding lipoprotein(s) as lipoprotein family D (LP-D). Another minor apolipoprotein was identified by Shore and Shore (1973) in VLDL.

It exists apparently in three polymorphic forms and has been designated, due to its relatively high content of arginine, as the arginine-rich polypeptide. A polypeptide of similar properties and amino acid composition was also isolated from VLDL by Shelburne and Quarfordt (1973). From the available information it is not yet possible to establish whether this polypeptide is a part of the ApoC complex or a separate protein moiety capable of forming its own family of lipoproteins. Such forthcoming information is expected with great interest.

Dr. Levy cautioned investigators that the finding of a protein in a lipoprotein complex after delipidation does not necessarily prove that it is an apolipoprotein. Many plasma proteins may adsorb to lipoprotein complexes and may therefore be isolated with them. He also cautioned that the apolipoproteins may undergo changes during isolation and delipidation (Herbert et al., 1973) and that therefore the finding of multiple protein forms may be misleading.

The recognition of at least eight polypeptides as specific lipid carriers indicates that the plasma lipoprotein system may consist of a greater number and types of lipoproteins than previously suspected. The effect that this development has already had on the existing views regarding the definition and classification of lipoproteins was discussed by Dr. Kostner in his presentation on *the isolation and characterization of normal lipoprotein species*. Immunological characterization of intact and delipidized lipoproteins showed clearly that each major density class was heterogeneous with respect to its apolipoproteins; in this respect, VLDL represented the most heterogeneous group of lipid-protein complexes. Recent studies in the author's and other laboratories suggested that zonal ultracentrifugation (Wilcox et al., 1969) was the most accurate and reliable method for the isolation of lipoprotein density classes. Utilizing this procedure, LDL_2 preparations contained almost exclusively ApoB. Similar preparations isolated by ultracentrifugation in fixed-angle rotors contained, however, ApoB and ApoA polypeptides. The HDL could be separated by zonal ultracentrifugation into HDL_2 and HDL_3 subclasses. The region between these two classes contained a negligible amount of a lipoprotein characterized by the exclusive presence of A-I polypeptide. Immunological testing of isolated VHDL also revealed the exclusive presence of the A-I-containing lipoprotein. On the other hand, VLDL, LDL_1, HDL_2 and HDL_3 displayed the same degree of apolipoprotein heterogeneity whether isolated by zonal or standard ultracentrifugal techniques. Attempts to separate individual lipoproteins from these density classes were based on the postulate that the plasma lipoprotein system consists of a mixture of lipoprotein families, each of which is characterized by a single, distinct apolipoprotein (Alaupovic, 1968).

The HDL$_2$ preparations gave positive reaction with antibodies to LP-A, LP-B, Lp(a) and LP-C. By utilizing a procedure including immunoadsorption, column chromatography on Sepharose 4B and hydroxyapatite, and precipitation with 33% polyethylene glycol (Kostner and Alaupovic, 1972) the HDL$_2$ subclass was fractionated into four or five lipoprotein species. The LP-B and Lp(a) were separated from other HDL$_2$ lipoproteins by immunoadsorption with antibodies to LP-B. Further separation of LP-B and Lp(a) could be achieved by fractionation on Sepharose 4B (Ehnholm et al., 1971). Hydroxyapatite column chromatography of the remaining lipoproteins resulted in partial separation of LP-A and LP-C families. However, a clearcut separation of these two lipoprotein species required precipitation of LP-A by 33% polyethylene glycol. The LP-A family was subfractioned into LP-A and LP-A-I by chromatography on columns containing monospecific antibodies to A-II polypeptide. HDL$_3$ was fractionated by similar procedures into LP-A and LP-C. Application of these separation procedures to VLDL or LDL$_1$ resulted in isolation of products still containing several individual lipoprotein families. These results in conjunction with immunological testing (Alaupovic et al., 1972) have demonstrated that VLDL and LDL$_1$ consist of an association complex(es) of lipoprotein families and triglyceride. The lipoprotein density fractions of d >1.025 g/ml are mainly mixtures of distinct, separable lipoprotein families, whereas density fractions of d <1.025 g/ml consist of lipoprotein families complexed with triglycerides. The concept that density classes of lipoprotein contain several separable lipoprotein species has been supported by a number of recent studies. For example, Albers et al. (1972) have established that lipoprotein with S$_f$ 0-2 consist of a mixture of separate LP-A, LP-B and Lp(a). It has also been established by use of either immunological (Pearlstein and Aladjem, 1972) or chromatographic (Shore and Shore, 1973) techniques that VLDL represent a mixture of distinct lipoprotein subpopulations or species differing in protein components. These new experimental findings argue strongly against the prevailing concept according to which the polydisperse density classes of lipoproteins are considered as the basic physical-chemical entities of the plasma lipoprotein system. This concept ignores the marked heterogeneity of major classes and obscures the significance of apolipoproteins as the essential determinants of the compositional and structural stability of lipoproteins. In contrast to this operational concept, the chemical concept emphasizes the significance of apolipoproteins or their constitutive polypeptides for the formation of lipoproteins, and incorporates within its framework all other physical, chemical and immunological properties of lipoprotein families. Thus, it extends rather than negates a concept based on strictly physical characteristics of plasma lipoproteins.

Recent advances in the chemistry of apolipoproteins have already dramatically influenced our views and concepts about the lipid transport system. By disclosing an unsuspected chemical and metabolic complexity of lipoproteins, these findings have stimulated intensive efforts to redefine and/or identify the fundamental physical-chemical entities of the plasma lipoprotein system, to develop methods for their isolation, and to search for their specific roles in transport of lipids. These efforts should dominate the lipoprotein field in the foreseeable future, because identification of basic lipoprotein units is an essential requirement for any meaningful probe into their structure and metabolism.

In his presentation on *isolation and characterization of abnormal lipoprotein species* Dr. Seidel strongly pointed out that the importance of such efforts has already proved useful for a better understanding of abnormal plasma lipid concentrations in some forms of dyslipoproteinemia. The careful analysis of the lipoproteins revealed abnormalities of their protein moieties in many cases.

One form of hyperlipoproteinemia well known for many years, is the hyperlipoproteinemia accompanying obstructive jaundice. Recent studies have well documented that the characteristic elevation of unesterified cholesterol and phospholipids in patients with obstructive jaundice are due to the presence of a low density lipoprotein of abnormal composition and properties (lipoprotein X) (Seidel et al., 1969). The protein lipid composition of the isolated LP-X is unique and consists of 6 per cent protein, 65 per cent phospholipids, 23 per cent unesterified cholesterol, 2 per cent cholesterolesters and 3 per cent triglycerides. The protein moiety of LP-X consists of a combination of 40 per cent albumin and 60 per cent apo C (Seidel et al., 1970). In the electro-micrograph LP-X appears as a spherical particle, larger than normal LDL with a diameter ranging from 300 to 700 A, and in contrast to normal lipoproteins with a strong tendency to aggregate and to form discs. It consists of a phospholipid, cholesterol, apo C wall. The albumin portion of LP-X seems to be masked in the core of the native particle (Hamilton et al., 1971; Seidel et al., 1972a). It has been proposed that the specific combination of apo C and albumin may play an important role in maintaining the structural integrity of this lipoprotein particle characterized by the high phospholipid-protein ratio of 11. Other liver disorders are often associated with decreased concentration of serum α- and pre-ß-lipoproteins, when lipoprotein electrophoresis is applied as criterion. Further characterization of these two classes of plasma lipoproteins, however, demonstrated that the decreased concentration of HDL is primarily due to an impaired lipid binding capacity of apo A resulting in an abnormally high protein lipid ratio and in severe cases a lack of neutral lipids. In contrast to normal α-lipoproteins, this fraction does not stain for lipids, but shows two distinct and non identical precipitin bands on immunoelectrophoresis and immunodiffusion. The isolated VLDL from patients with liver disorders revealed a regular particle size and a protein-lipid ratio close to normal, but develop ß-mobility on electrophoresis. Analysis of the protein moieties of this fraction indicated a lack of apo A. It therefore was suggested that disturbed liver function leads to the synthesis of an altered apo A resulting in α-lipoproteins with dissociated apo A peptides and in very low density lipoproteins devoid of apo A. Both findings may be explained by an impaired capacity of this apolipoprotein A to bind neutral lipids (Seidel et al., 1972b).

Abnormalities of the apolipoprotein composition were also found in patients with familial lecithin: cholesterol acyltransferase deficiency, which is most pronounced in the LDL fraction. Immuno-chemically, this fraction shows apo A, apo B as well as apo C. Three different lipoprotein subfractions can be isolated from this density class. The normal ß-lipoproteins showing only apo B as apolipoprotein, a second, triglyceride rich, lipoprotein with normal ß-mobility but consisting of apo B and apo C and a third lipoprotein very similar the lipoprotein X (Seidel et al., 1972c; Torsvik et al., 1972). The HDL fraction of these patients contains significantly less lipoproteins than normals with a reduced capacity to take up lipid stain and shows thereby some similarity with the HDL fraction of patients with severe liver disease.

Disturbances of the thyroid gland are also known to influence the plasma lipid values. Hypothyroidism leads to an increase of ß-lipoproteins and hypercholesterolemia. Hyperthyroidism is followed by hypocholesterolemia but not by a decrease of the ß-lipoproteins when lipoprotein electrophoresis is applied as criterion. This discrepancy has recently been solved by the detection and isolation of a ß-lipoprotein with an abnormally low cholesterol content and in contrast to normal ß-lipoproteins within the HDL fraction. It therefore has been designated ß-HDL (Wieland und Seidel, 1972). The protein portion of ß-HDL consists of apo B and a second protein moiety not yet identified, but different to the known apo-peptides. Since it is not possible to enrich the ß-HDL with lipids it was concluded that it is the specific combination of apo B with the second protein compound rather than the availability of lipids which determines the protein lipid composition of this abnormal plasma lipoprotein.

Among the familial types of hyperlipoproteinemia up to now only one form (type III) broad-ß disease is known to show an abnormal lipoprotein designated floating-ß. This lipoprotein is believed to be an intermediate between normal VLDL (pre ß-lipoproteins) and normal LDL (ß-lipoproteins). It develops ß-mobility but consists in contrast to normal ß-lipoproteins of apo B and apo C. Because of its relatively high triglyceride content it appears within the VLDL fraction (Quarfordt et al., 1971).

Since all of the abnormal lipoprotein compounds share common physio-chemical and chemical properties with normal plasma lipoproteins specific techniques combining various methods are necessary for their isolation. Only the analysis of homogenous and intact particles should be considered in the evaluation of the biodynamics of lipid metabolism.

In his discussion of *lipid-binding properties of apolipoproteins*, Dr. Gotto briefly reviewed the progress achieved in this area of lipoprotein chemistry and then presented in more detail some of the most recent results obtained in his laboratory. These studies (Jackson et al., 1973a; Jackson et al., 1973b; Morrisett et al., 1973) were based on the assumption that binding of phospholipids by plasma apolipoproteins is a prerequisite for their association with cholesterol, cholesterol esters and triglyceride. Several methods have been employed for assessing the interaction between plasma apolipoproteins and phospholipids. The first method suitable for assay of small quantities of apolipoproteins or peptide fragments employed defatted ß-hydroxybutyrate dehydrogenase (apodehydrogenase) from mitochondria; this enzyme has an absolute requirement for phosphatidyl choline. The relative affinity of the apolipoprotein or its fragment for phosphatidyl choline was tested by inhibition of the reactivation of the apodehydrogenase.

A second method utilized ultracentrifugation to isolate stable complexes formed by the association of lipids and proteins at densities intermediate between those of lipid and those of protein. By careful selection of conditions for ultracentrifugation and use of a salt-sucrose gradient spanning an appropriate density range, the complex of reconstituted apoprotein and phospholipid could be obtained free of excess unbound lipid or protein. Spectroscopic measurements of fluorescence and circular dichroism could be used to assess changes in the conformation of the protein as a consequence of the binding of phospholipid. The fluorescence spectrum of an apoprotein or fragment containing tryptophan would be expected to undergo a blue-shift if the binding of phospholipid resulted in the change of the environment around a tryptophan residue from a more hydrophilic to a more hydrophobic character. All apoproteins and fragments which bind phospholipid thus far have been found to exhibit this property and to show an accompanying increase in the α-helical structure as assessed by circular dichroism.

A final method utilized electron microscopy with negative staining to detect the effects of an apoprotein on the structure of bilaminar vesicles of phospholipid. When a soluble, detergent-free apoprotein or its fragment which was capable of interaction with phospholipid was added to a preparation of phospholipid vesicles, the vesicles became aligned as linear arrays of stacked discs.

These methods have been used to show that the carboxyl cyanogen bromide fragment of A-II polypeptide (apoLP-Gln-II) binds phosphatidyl choline, while the amino terminal fragment does not and that synthetic fragments of C-III polypeptide (apoLP-Ala), 41-49 and 48-79, bind phospholipid while the shorter fragments, 55-79 and 69-79, do not exhibit binding.

Further discussion of the *lipid-binding properties of apolipoproteins* by Dr. Peeters focused on the thermodynamics of binding. The lipid-protein bond is a key problem in the study of lipoproteins, as it is responsible for the stability of the molecules and for the variations in composition found in disease. To elucidate this binding, the most straightforward approach is to recombine apolipoprotein with various lipid components. By means of several techniques, such as ultracentrifugal flotation, circular dichroism, and fluorescence spectroscopy, important information has been obtained concerning the composition and structure of relipidated apo-HDL (Scanu et al., 1970; Lux et al., 1972). None of these techniques, however, provides information about the thermodynamics of such a system, and therefore microcalorimetry is a useful tool to follow complex formation at the very moment when components are mixed. From measurements of the heat a binding curve can be drawn, and from this a direct determination of the binding enthalpy and the composition of the complex can be obtained.

We first applied this technique to a model study of the binding of fatty acid and phospholipid to bovine serum albumin (BSA), using an LKB batch calorimeter. The heat of binding of lysolecithin to delipidated BSA and to BSA relipidated with oleic acid was measured in the microcalorimeter at 25°C, in order to check whether there is any competition between fatty acid and phospholipid for binding sites on BSA. This reaction is highly exothermal and takes place immediately. In Fig. 1 the binding enthalpy is plotted as a function of the molar lysolecithin/BSA ratio. From this it appears that the binding enthalpy for lysolecithin steadily decreases with increasing fatty acid relipidation (14 Kcal/mole BSA for delipidated BSA down to 2 Kcal/mole BSA for a protein containing 5 moles oleic acid). Moreover, a least-square fitting of the curve to a Klotz equation shows that there is always *one* binding site available to lysolecithin, and the binding constant remains of the order of 3×10^4. Thus, fatty acid binding does not compete with phospholipid binding, which takes place at another specific site. This strongly contrasts with the results obtained with binding of a dye, where the nonspecific interactions are completely displaced by fatty acid binding (Peeters et al., 1972).

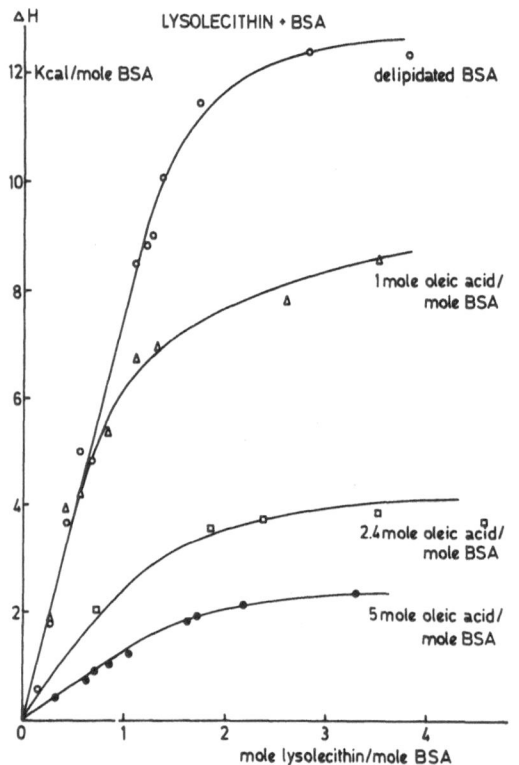

Figure 1. Binding of lysolecithin to delipidated and relipidated BSA

The study of lysolecithin binding was extended to human apoHDL, and the results are shown in Fig. 2. The binding reaction is more strongly exothermal (28 Kcal/mole apo HDL); and the complex composition is completely different, as the binding involves 78 moles lysolecithin/mole apoprotein (Rosseneu-Motreff et al., 1973).

The binding enthalpy is derived not only from complex formation, but also from the rupture of the phospholipid micellar structure and probably from a rearrangement of the lipoprotein itself. This complex formation is affected by ionic strength, as the presence of 1 M NaCl decreases the binding enthalpy (20 Kcal/mole apoprotein) and affects the complex composition. This is in agreement with recombination experiments performed in the untracentrifuge (Morrisett et al., 1973).

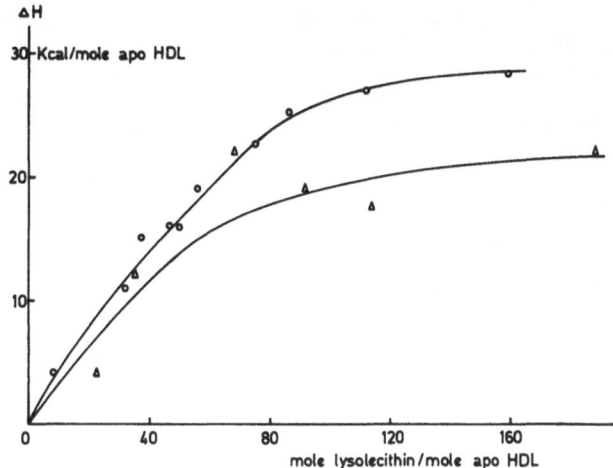

Figure 2. Binding of lysolecithin to human apo-HDL
(o) Binding curve measured in a carbonate-bicarbonate buffer pH 9.6, μ = 0.05
(Δ) Binding curve measured in the same buffer in presence of 1 M NaCl

A second set of experiments on apoHDL relipidation, performed with synthetic
dicaproyl and dilauroyl lecithins, demonstrates the influence of fatty acyl chain
length on phospholipid binding. Fig. 3 shows that an increase of the fatty acyl
chain length increases the binding enthalpy and also the molar ratio of phospholipid to apoprotein in the complex.

This approach should be suitable for further studies with isolated polypeptides
and other lipids. It should provide information of use in the evaluation of the
modalities of lipid binding during the formation and degradation of lipoproteins.

Closely related to the problems of lipid binding are questions of the overall
structure of lipoproteins, which was discussed by Dr. Nichols. Productive approaches to the determination of the overall size, shape and internal organization of lipoproteins currently include electron microscopy and X-ray scattering.

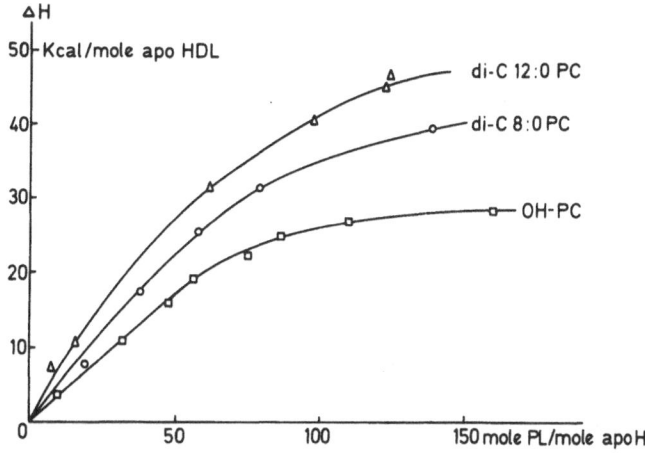

Figure 3. Influence of the fatty acid chain length on the binding of phospholipids to apo-HDL
□ Lysolecithin, O Synthetic di-Caproyl lecithin, Δ Synthetic di-Lauroyl lecithin

Aspects of internal structure, such as conformation of the constituent components, interactions among components and molecular motion of the components are now accessible to evaluation in many instances. Methodological approaches used in evaluation of the latter properties include: nuclear magnetic resonance, electron spin resonance, optical rotatory dispersion, circular dichroism, infrared and fluorescence spectroscopy.

Based on data from electron microscopy and X-ray scattering, models have been proposed for the major classes of serum lipoproteins, particularly the HDL and the LDL. Significant differences in these models are apparent and elucidation of actual structure is currently a most challenging and actively pursued problem. This discussion will focus primarily on the problem of the overall structure of HDL and LDL.

Under electron microscopy using negative staining (Forte and Nichols, 1972) HDL appear as particles with diameters of 95-100 Å for HDL_2 and 70-75 Å for HDL_3. When observed in hexagonally packed arrays, the HDL appear essentially as spherical particles with granular surface features. When observed as separate particles, the images frequently suggest substructural organization.

X-ray scattering data for HDL_2 (Shipley et al., 1972) have been interpreted as consistent with a spherical model having an electron-dense shell of 11 Å thickness, made up of protein and the polar ends of the phospholipid molecules. This shell surrounds an electron-deficient inner lipid core of 86 Å diameter which consists of apolar moieties (cholesteryl esters, triglycerides and acyl chains of the phospholipids). When the X-ray data are compared with theoretical scattering curves for models of uniform electron density there is little indication that HDL structure consists of an aggregate of lipoprotein subunits. The X-ray data, however, indicate small deviations from spherical symmetry and show need for further analytical work. From the standpoint of possible introduction of artifacts, the X-ray method maintains lipoproteins in an aqueous environment and avoids potential structural alterations which may occur during dehydration in the negative staining procedure of electron microscopy.

Electron microscopy data for LDL (Forte and Nichols, 1972; Gotto et al., 1968b; Pollard et al., 1969) have provided consistent information on the overall size (190-250 Å diameter) and shape (essentially spherical) of this lipoprotein species. Interpretation of micrographs with respect to surface organization has differed. One interpretation (Forte and Nichols, 1972) proposes a spherical structure with serrated edges and a strandlike surface network; another interpretation (Gotto et al., 1968b) proposes a structure with a surface consisting of 20 globular protein subunits (50 Å diameter) arranged in dodecahedral pattern with icosahedral symmetry. The detailed nature of the latter model derives from apparent resolution gained by dense staining of the LDL preparations and from three-dimensional isodensity maps constructed from the electron micrographs (Pollard and Devi, 1971). In both of the above models the interior of the LDL is considered to consist of an apolar core, primarily cholesteryl esters and triglycerides.

X-ray scattering studies of LDL (Mateu et al., 1972) have provided data compatible with a spherical particle of 220 Å diameter. The surface organization proposed is essentially in accord with the electron microscopic dodecahedral model except that each of the 20 globular units is considered to be a trimer composed of subunits of 8000 daltons each. The above models provide both a description of the possible organization of the surface protein subunits as well as an estimate of expected subunit molecular weight. Available physical-chemical data on the LDL protein moiety show considerable variation in subunit molecular weight values, ranging from 27,000 to 246,000 daltons (Pollard et al., 1969; Smith et al., 1972). Confirmation of the surface subunit organization of LDL awaits further definition of the molecular properties of its protein moiety.

An extraordinary aspect of the x-ray scattering model is the requirement that the bulk of the LDL lipid be organized into a spherical bilayer shell of 65 Å average radius. Such a model of LDL would have an inner aqueous region surrounded by a protein-stabilized lipid bilayer. A bilayer organization is not incompatible with lipoprotein morphology since single-bilayer structures in both LDL and HDL fractions have been well documented in specific disease states. In LDL of LCAT-deficient plasma (Glomset et al., 1973) and of cholestasis plasma (Hamilton et al., 1971; Seidel et al., 1972a) single-bilayer vesicular structures have been demonstrated, with diameters ranging from 400-600 Å. Discoidal lipoprotein structures of single-bilayer thickness (40 Å) have been described in HDL of LCAT-deficient (Forte et al., 1971) and of cholestasis (Utermann et al., 1972) plasma. Specific aspects, however, of the proposed bilayer model of LDL are indeed novel. Such aspects include the high content of cholesteryl esters in a bilayer structure and the mode of interaction of the protein moiety with the bilayer; these and other points require further experimental information. The bilayer model also raises questions relating to lipoprotein metabolism. In particular, there is the question of how such an LDL structure may arise from the proposed metabolic degradation (Levy et al., 1971) of precursor VLDL to product LDL.

Finally, the data for the overall size and shape of VLDL indicate a spherical morphology with particle sizes ranging from 300-900 Å (Forte and Nichols, 1972). The general view of the internal structure of VLDL is that it consists of an apolar lipid core (triglycerides and cholesteryl esters) stabilized by a surface coat of protein, phospholipid and unesterified cholesterol.

With this brief overview we see that the investigation of lipoprotein structure still poses fascinating problems and that there are clear signs of exciting developments and insights in the foreseeable future.

Dr. Lewis discussed *new developments in analysis of lipoproteins and apolipoproteins.* Separation of lipoprotein classes by ultracentrifugation has been recently refined (Lindgren and Jensen, 1972), and isolation of fractions by precipitation techniques, including the use of heparin-Mn^{++} (Gotto et al., 1968a), sulfated dextrans (Peeters, 1971), and heparin-Ca^{++} (Lopez-S. et al., 1971), has been reported. Precipitation techniques have recently also been described for making lipoproteins visible in gels after electrophoresis (Seidel et al., 1973; Wieland and Seidel, 1973). Isolation of the LP-A, LP-B, and LP-C families from human high density lipoproteins has also been accomplished (Kostner and Alaupovic, 1972). Several chromatographic techniques are now available for the preparation of individual apolipoprotein polypeptides (Shore and Shore, 1969; Scanu et al., 1969; Brown et al., 1969).

With the availability of pure lipoproteins and apolipoproteins, specific antisera have been prepared, and immunochemical techniques for the identification and quantitation of lipoproteins have been developed. The methods include immunodiffusion in 1% agarose for LP-B quantification (Lees, 1970), double antibody radioimmunoassay (Schoenfield et al., 1972), radioimmunoassay for assay of two circulating high density apolipoproteins (Starr et al., 1973) and electroimmunoassay (Laurell, 1972). Utilizing "crossed electrophoresis" and specific antisera, superimposed components that form the LP-B can be demonstrated (Wilkenson and Mills, 1972). Identification and quantitation of LP-X may be achieved by electrophoresis in agar gel, in which LP-X has a distinctive anodal mobility (Seidel, 1971; Magnani and Alaupovic, 1972).

Isoelectric focusing was found by Scanu et al., 1973 to give good separation of soluble forms of VLDL apolipoproteins and to be useful as a check of purity of lipoprotein fractions. Isoelectric focusing has also been used by Sodhi et al., 1973 for the study of lipoproteins.

Quantitation of individual apolipoproteins has been accomplished recently by scanning of polyacrylamide gel electrophoretic patterns of tetramethyl urea-delipidized lipoproteins (Kane, 1973) and by gravimetric analysis of apolipoprotein fractions dried to constant weight (Lee and Alaupovic, 1973).

In the last presentation of the workshop, Dr. Alaupovic discussed briefly the most commonly used systems of *nomenclature of apolipoproteins and lipoproteins*. As expected, these systems have reflected very closely the changing conceptual views about lipoproteins as a unique physical-chemical and physiological system of macromolecules. In general, there are two types of apolipoprotein and lipoprotein nomenclatures: one is based on the operational and the other on the chemical classifications of lipoproteins. In the former, hydrated densities and electrophoretic mobilities have been utilized as the main criteria for defining and classifying the basic lipoprotein components of the system. In the latter type, the apolipoproteins or their constitutive polypeptides have been recognized as the specific and distinct markers of the lipoproteins forming individual constituents of the lipid-transport system.

Historically, the first operational nomenclature was based on the migration of lipoproteins during free-boundary electrophoresis into the α_1- and ß-globulin positions. The protein moiety of α-lipoproteins was referred to as α-protein or α-P and that of ß-lipoproteins as ß-P. With the advent of electrophoresis on various supporting media, the resolution of low-density lipoproteins into pre-ß- and ß-lipoprotein classes introduced a third protein moiety, the pre-ß-protein or pre-ß-P. The second operational nomenclature, presented in Figure 4, evolved from the concept maintaining that the lipoprotein density classes represent the basic chemical and metabolic components. The protein moieties were designated as apolipoproteins of a particular major or minor density class: in the abbreviated forms, they were called apoVLDL, apoLDL, apoHDL, etc. The operational nomenclature has culminated in recent proposals to designate apolipoproteins or polypeptides by their chromatographic elution patterns. The major protein moieties of HDL separated by Sephadex gel filtration were called fractions III and IV and the minor polypeptides fraction V (Scanu et al., 1969). The water-soluble polypeptides of apoVLDL separated by DEAE-cellulose column chromatography were designated as D_1, D_2, D_3 and D_4 in order of their elution (Brown et al., 1969). Although simple and useful in the developmental stages of lipoprotein chemistry and metabolism, the operational nomenclatures are either inaccurate or have limited potential for development into general systems of lipoprotein nomenclature. Designations such as apoVLDL, apoLDL, apoHDL, etc., refer to several rather than single apolipoproteins or polypeptides, because each density class is heterogeneous with respect to the protein moieties. The same is true for terms such as pre-ß-P, α_1-P or fraction V. On the other hand, designations such as D_1, D_2 or fraction III refer to single polypeptides, but are not a part of, or cannot be developed into, a system encompassing all polypeptides, apolipoproteins and lipoproteins.

The two chemical systems of nomenclature, however, possess the capability for expansion into comprehensive classification schemes. Development of both systems was prompted by the recently recognized complexity of the apolipoproteins and the inadequacy of operational classification systems to provide a sound theoretical basis for new experimental facts. One of these employs the C-terminal amino acids as the markers and names for individual polypeptides (Shore and Shore, 1969; Brown et al., 1969), whereas the other utilizes letters and numbers as designations for apolipoproteins, polypeptides and polymorphic forms (Alaupovic, 1968; 1971). Nomenclature based on determination of C-terminal amino acids is limitless in its applicability to individual polypeptides and their corresponding lipoprotein species. For example, R-Gln-I or apoLP-Gln-I refers to a distinct polypeptide. In the form of LP-Gln-I, it can be used as a designation for the lipoprotein species that is characterized, irrespective of its hydrated density or electro-phoretic mobility, by the exclusive presence of this polypeptide. Unfortunately, several shortcomings limit severely the potential usefulness of this system. Some polypeptides have identical terminal amino acids (Table 1). This problem can be further complicated by possible microheterogeneity at the C-terminus. However, as pointed out by Herbert and Fredrickson at the Conference on Serum Lipoproteins in Graz (October 21 and 22, 1973), probably the most serious disadvantage of this nomenclature is its failure to permit recognition of the fundamental kinship between homologous proteins from different species if their

Table 1. Nomenclature of Apolipoproteins

Apolipo-proteins	"ABC"		Carboxyl-terminal amino acids		Column chromatographic fractions		Density classes
	Constitutive polypeptides	Polymorphic forms			DEAE-cellulose	Sephadex	
ApoA	A-I	A-I-1 A-I-2, etc.	R-Gln-I	apoLP-Gln-I	-	III	ApoHDL-I
	A-II		R-Gln-II	apoLP-Gln-II	-	IV	ApoHDL-II
ApoB	NK	NK	R-Ser	apoLP-Ser	-	-	ApoLDL
ApoC	C-I	C-I-1 C-I-2 C-I-3	R-Ser	apoLP-Ser	D_1 - -	V	ApoVLDL-I
	C-II	NK	R-Glu	apoLP-Glu	D_2	V	ApoVLDL-II
	C-III	C-III-0 C-III-1 C-III-2 C-III-3 C-III-4	R-Ala	apoLP-Ala$_0$ apoLP-Ala$_1$ apoLP-Ala$_2$	- D_3 D_4 - -	V	ApoVLDL-III
ApoD	NK	NK	NK		-	-	

C-termini differ. These shortcomings are not inherent in the ABC nomenclature. This system is an expression of the theory of lipoprotein families (Alaupovic, 1968; 1971). According to this concept, the plasma lipoprotein system consists of free or associated forms of lipoprotein families or species each of which is characterized by the presence of a single, distinct apolipoprotein or its constitutive polypeptides. At the present time, there are four recognized apolipoproteins, designated by letters as apoA, apoB, apoC and apoD. If an apolipoprotein contains nonidentical polypeptides, these are designated by Roman numerals in addition to the letter indicating its parent protein. For example, ApoA consists of A-I and A-II, and ApoC of C-I, C-II and C-III polypeptides. Arabic numerals denote the possible polymorphic forms of each polypeptide, such as C-III-0, C-III-1 and C-III-2. The designation of corresponding lipoprotein species utilizes the same system of letters and numerals preceded, however, by the abbreviation LP for lipoprotein. Thus, the lipoprotein species characterized by the presence of ApoA is called LP-A, the one by ApoB the LP-B, and so on. If additional evidence shows that some or all of the polypeptides form their own lipoprotein species, they can be designated as LP-A-I, LP-C-III-2, etc. The entire system is, of course, applicable to homologous proteins or polypeptides of all other animal species. Among the presently available systems, the ABC nomenclature has the greatest potential and flexibility for accomodating existing as well as new information about the highly complex chemistry of plasma lipoproteins. Its main shortcomings may arise either from improper groupings of polypeptides into apolipoprotein clusters or an inherent limitation to describe specific function or origin of individual polypeptides or their lipoprotein species.

FUNCTION AND STRUCTURE OF PLASMA LIPOPROTEINS

Gerd Assmann and Donald S. Fredrickson

It is appropriate that a session devoted to the plasma lipoproteins begin with a
lecture concerned with structural aspects of lipoproteins even though there is
still much about this subject that is unknown. In order to achieve a complete
understanding of how any biological system functions it is necessary to know the
detailed molecular composition and structure of that system. The ultimate model
of a lipoprotein must explain in detail how proteins and lipids are held together
in an organized three dimensional structure. While we are still a long way from
such knowledge about lipoproteins and membranes in general, progress at both the
theoretical and experimental levels in recent years has created a stage where at
least the gross aspects of the organization of the proteins and lipids in plasma
lipoproteins can be discerned.

Here we will first review some more general aspects of the appearance and composition of plasma lipoproteins and then progress to a description of experiments
conducted in Bethesda over the last year which provide some new insights into the
interaction of lipids with apolipoproteins. The results conclude with a considerably updated model of a plasma lipoprotein.

The plasma lipoproteins have developed in higher forms of life for the inter-
organ transportation of lipids, substances of little solubility in water (Nelson,
1972; Scanu, 1973; Fredrickson, 1973). The major lipids in transit are triglycerides. They are always accompanied by cholesterol and phospholipids in macromolecular complexes with specific proteins. The lipids and proteins are present
in relatively fixed proportions that differ greatly in different lipoprotein species. Their high content of lipid makes the lipoproteins lighter than the other
plasma proteins, a property which is the basis for the commonly used method of
isolation by flotation in the ultracentrifuge.

Classification of the plasma lipoproteins has been based mainly on differences in
the size and charge of the complexes. The major families of lipoproteins, which
are separated by ultracentrifugation (Fig. 1) are the chylomicrons, very low density lipoproteins (VLDL), low density lipoproteins (LDL), and high density lipoproteins (HDL). VLDL and chylomicrons range in particle diameter from 200-1000 Å;
LDL from 200-220 Å; HDL from 50-100 Å.

Chylomicrons are lipoproteins of $S_f > 400$ which arise from the gastrointestinal
tract and serve to transport glycerides of dietary origin from the intestine into
the lymph. The catabolism of chylomicron triglyceride is catalyzed by lipolytic
enzymes, mainly lipoprotein lipase. The latter enzyme acts principally in the
capillary endothelium of adipose tissue and skeletal muscle. Chylomicron "remnants", relatively enriched in protein, phospholipid and cholesterol, are then
thought to be cleared by the liver.

The chemical composition of a chylomicron particle varies with the size of the
particle and the conditions under which it is collected. On the average they contain 80 to 95% by weight of triglyceride and only one to two percent of protein.

VLDL comprise a family of macromolecules rich in endogenous triglyceride with a
broad S_f range of 20-400, isolated between density 0.95 and 1.006 gm/ml. VLDL
have been shown to arise from the liver and from the intestine. Evidence suggests
that VLDL are stored in the Golgi apparatus of hepatocytes and intestinal epithelial cells prior to secretion into plasma or lymph.

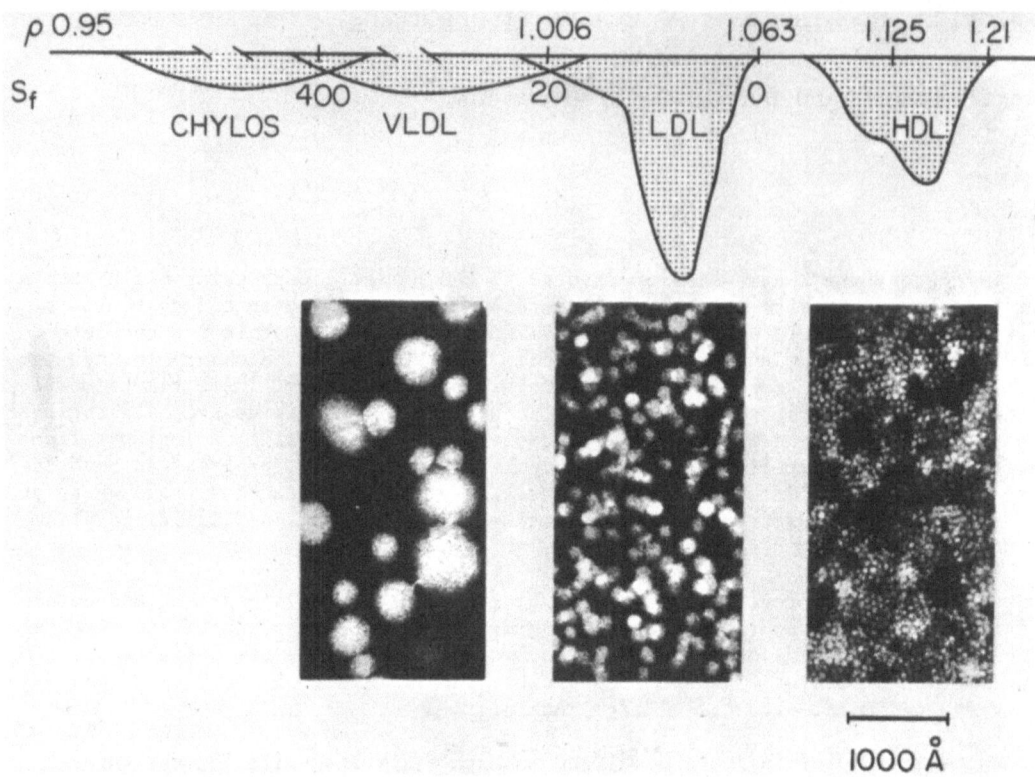

Figure 1. Three of the four major lipoprotein families in plasma represented by the Schlieren patterns generated by them in the analytical ultracentrifuge (top) and their appearance in the electron microscope under negative staining. Chylomicrons are not shown. The abbreviations and other details are explained in the text

The chemical composition of VLDL is shown in Fig. 2. VLDL are composed of 90% lipid and 10% protein. The major lipid component is triglyceride. The protein component consists of at least four major proteins. The major protein component is designated apoLDL and is shared with the low density lipoprotein family. Three other distinct proteins, designated as apoC-I, II and III are shared with the high density lipoprotein family. One of the C apoproteins, apoC-II, has been shown by a number of investigators to activate lipoprotein lipase (LaRosa et al., 1970; Havel et al., 1970).

The primary sequences of apoC-I and apoC-III have been determined in Bethesda and are shown in Fig. 3. ApoC-I contains 57 amino acid residues; apoC-III contains 79 amino acid residues. ApoC-III is a glycoprotein containing galactose, galactosamine and one or two moles of sialic acid.

The primary structures of proteins permit comparison that may shed light on their relationship and evolution. Barker and Dayoff have made a genetic comparison of the sequences of these two apolipoproteins (Barker and Dayoff, 1973). By their technique, C-I and the amino terminal portion of C-III, residues 1-59, appear to have arisen from a common ancestral gene. Possibly they began as proteins of similar length and during their divergent evolution C-III was elongated and acquired a glycosidyl side chain. The specific functions of apoC-I and C-III related to lipoprotein structure or metabolism are as yet unknown.

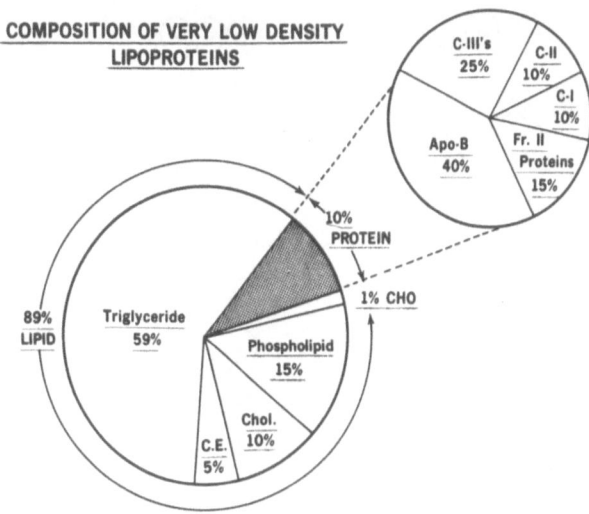

COMPOSITION OF VERY LOW DENSITY LIPOPROTEINS

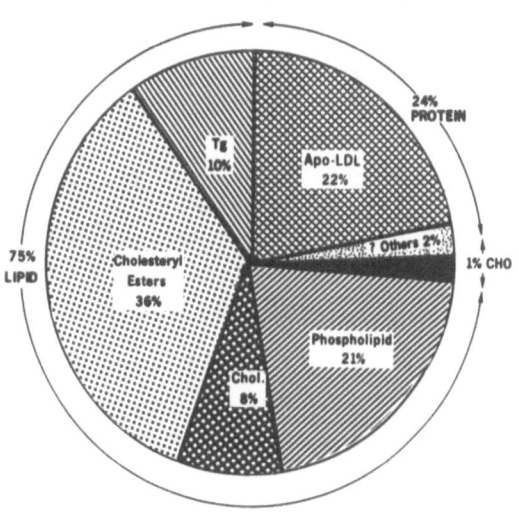

COMPOSITION OF LOW DENSITY LIPOPROTEINS

Figure 2. Protein and lipid composition of human very low, low, and high density lipoproteins

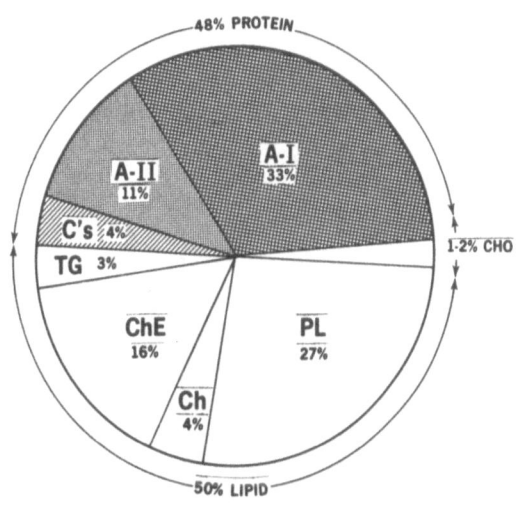

COMPOSITION OF HIGH DENSITY LIPOPROTEINS

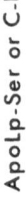
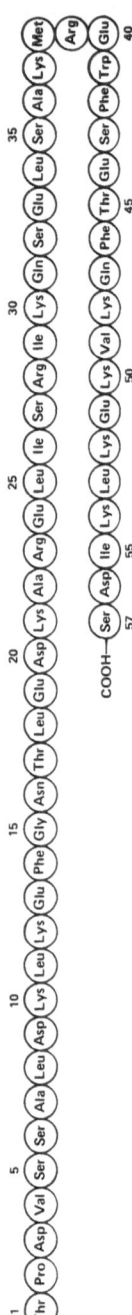
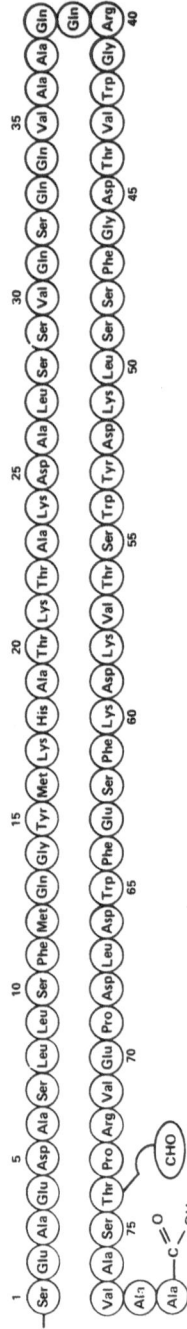
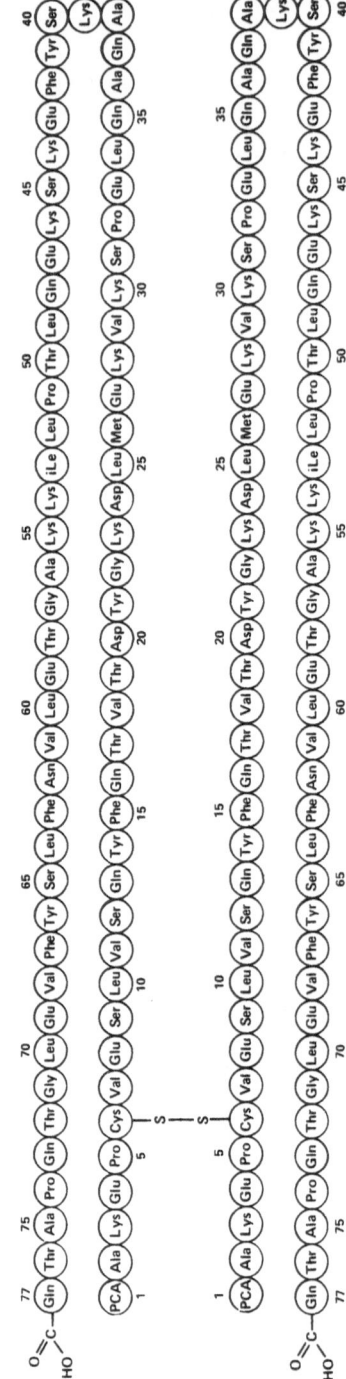

Figure 3. The amino acid sequences of apoC-I, apoC-III and apoA-II from human plasma lipoproteins

The protein moiety of VLDL is believed to be the principal precursor of the LDL protein. Studies in recent years have indicated that VLDL, after entering the plasma, are metabolized, at least in part, to LDL (Eisenberg et al., 1972). The conversion of VLDL to LDL in plasma appears to be a unidirectional process without any evidence for recycling of LDL into VLDL.

LDL transport the bulk of plasma cholesterol, and because hypercholesterolemia is often associated with atherosclerosis, the understanding of the metabolism of LDL has long been considered of major importance. The principle LDL apoprotein also appears to be one of the apoproteins of paramount importance in triglyceride transport as demonstrated by certain mutants (Fredrickson et al., 1972). The synthesis and degradation of LDL are currently being investigated in a number of laboratories.

The chemical composition of LDL is shown in Fig. 2. If we take a rough average for these particles, LDL are composed of 75% lipid, and 25% protein. The major lipid component is cholesteryl ester. The protein component of LDL (apo B) has been difficult to characterize due to its insolubility following delipidation. The molecular weight determined in various laboratories has ranged from approximately 28,000 (Pollard et al., 1969) to 275,000 (Smith et al., 1972). Whether it consists of one protein or an association of one or more monomers is not established. Further studies will be required to fully characterize the protein moiety of LDL.

For the remainder of this presentation we will concentrate on HDL in some considerable detail. In contrast to LDL, the proteins in HDL are soluble in aqueous solution and have been well-characterized. HDL float between density 1.063 and 1.210 gm/ml. From the early days of ultracentrifugal fractionation, it has been conventional to divide HDL into two major subclasses: HDL_2, isolated between densities 1.063 and 1.12, and HDL_3, isolated between densities 1.12 and 1.21 gm/ml. Since significant chemical differences are perceptible only at the outer extremes of the HDL distribution, studies on HDL have mainly been made with pools containing both HDL_2 and HDL_3.

An average chemical composition for HDL is given in Fig. 2. The lipid consists mainly of cholesteryl esters and phospholipid, there being about four moles of phosphatidylcholine per mole of sphingomyelin. About 90% of the protein moiety of HDL is composed of two major apoproteins which are designated as apoA-I and apoA-II, or by their COOH-terminal amino acids as apoGln-I and apoGln-II; the remaining 10% is mainly composed of apoC-I, apoC-II and apoC-III.

A wide variety of methods have been used in different laboratories for the isolation of apoproteins in HDL (Fredrickson et al., 1972). In our experience satisfactory preparations are achieved by delipidation of HDL with organic solvent, followed by gel filtration and ion exchange chromatography. With gel chromatography on Sephadex G-200, apoA-I elutes before apoA-II, while the pattern is reversed on ion exchange chromatography. Both apoA-I and apoA-II migrate in polyacrylamide electrophoresis as single bands. ApoA-I is a single chain protein with a molecular weight of approximately 28,000. The complete amino acid sequence of apoA-I has not yet been reported. The primary sequence of apoA-II, however, has been completed in this laboratory and is shown in Fig. 3.

The structure of apoA-II is unusual, perhaps unique, in that it contains two identical monomers which are linked through a disulfide bridge at residue 6. ApoA-II contains no carbohydrate; it also lacks histidine, arginine and tryptophan. The amino terminal residue is pyrrolidone carboxylic acid.

Although the lipid composition and protein structure of HDL are reasonably well-understood, the quarternary structure of the HDL particle and the molecular organization of the lipid and protein are as yet undefined. In general, the lipid moieties in the HDL particle are likely assembled in one of two different ways, illustrated in Fig. 4, in which only phospholipids are represented.

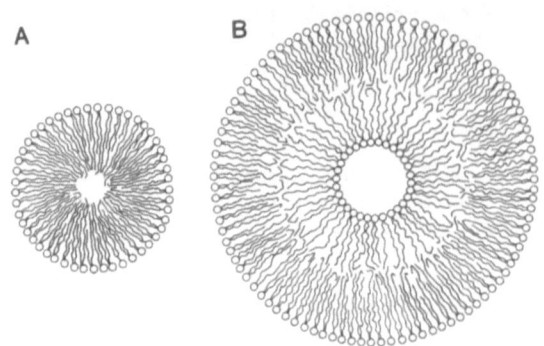

A B

Figure 4. Schematic representation
of a micelle (A) and lipid bilayer
(B)

A micellar-like structure with the polar phospholipid headgroups all oriented to
the outside, and the fatty acid hydrocarbon chains inside, is schematically shown
in A. A spherical bilayer structure with polar phospholipid headgroups both outside and inside is schematically shown in B.

Data derived from X-ray techniques by Shipley et al. (1972) have indicated that
HDL has an organized symmetrical structure with a relatively electron-poor, non-
polar, central region and a relatively electron-rich polar outer region. Trans-
lated in terms of the organization of lipids, the polar headgroups of phospholipids are thought to have a surface location in HDL, whereas the hydrocarbon
chains of the phospholipids and cholesteryl esters would be located in the interior of the particle. Various studies on the action of different phospholipases
upon intact HDL particles have led to a similar conclusion in that most of the
phospholipid headgroups in HDL are hydrolyzable by these enzymes and are therefore located on the surface.

Recently, collaboration between our laboratory and the NHLI Laboratory of Chemistry have permitted application of Fourier transform-coupled nuclear magnetic
resonance (NMR) techniques to the study of HDL structure (Assmann, unpublished
results). ^{31}P-NMR has been particularly useful for evaluating the location of the
phospholipid headgroups in the HDL particle. It has been previously demonstrated
that paramagnetic ions, like Eu^{+++}, permit differentiation of the internal and
external surfaces of lipid bilayers. In lecithin bilayers, Eu^{+++} will strongly
interact with the outer phosphorus groups. Eu^{+++} will not penetrate the bilayer
hydrophobic area and is thus not available to bind the inner phosphorus atoms.

The ^{31}P signal in NMR spectroscopy of lecithin molecules in the lipid bilayer
arrangement is composed of a single component consisting of both the inside and
outside phosphorus atoms. In the presence of Eu^{+++} there are two components. One
component corresponds to internal lecithin molecules which are in contact with
the ion free internal aqueous phase. The other component is shifted to a high
field and corresponds to molecules at the external surface in contact with the
bulk salt solution.

When HDL were titrated with Eu^{+++} we observed a gradual shift of both the lecithin and sphingomyelin ^{31}P resonance (unpublished results). No unshifted component, as in the case of a lipid bilayer, is left. We concluded that essentially
all phospholipid phosphorus is located at the outer surface of the HDL particle.
These combined results indicate that the HDL particle is a spherical micelle with
all the phospholipid headgroups located at the outer surface. The micellar arrangement of lipids does not necessarily apply for all other lipoproteins. Small-
angle X-ray scattering data of LDL obtained in Luzzati's laboratory by Mateu et
al. (1972) have been interpreted as consistent with a spherical lipid bilayer in
which the distribution of the two major lipid components, phospholipids and cholesteryl esters, is uniform on the two sides of the bilayer.

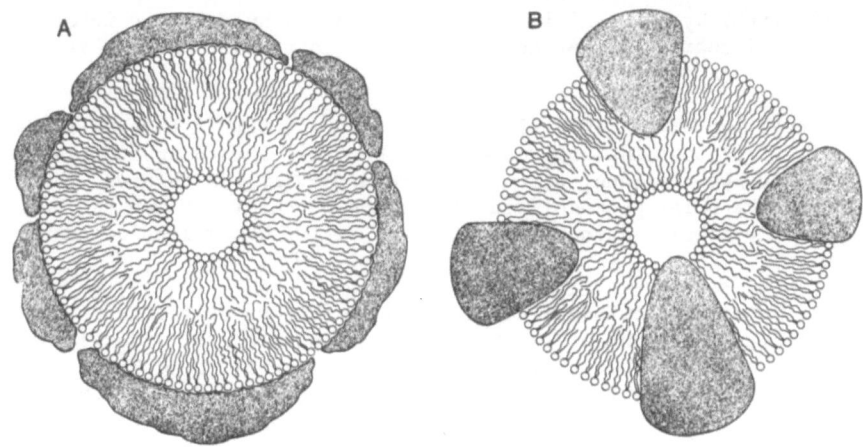

Figure 5. Two possible modes of interaction of lipids with proteins

The location of the protein in lipoproteins is currently a matter of debate.
There are two basic possibilities for the interaction of lipids and proteins
(Fig. 5). In the left hand model (A, Fig. 5), the protein surrounds the bilayer
or micelle. The major force of interaction between lipid and protein is hydro-
philic in nature. This model is similar to the membrane model proposed by
Danielli and Davson (1935).

The model on the right (B, Fig. 5) shows the protein arranged perpendicular to
the surface of the micelle or bilayer. The major force of interaction between the
lipid and protein in this model is hydrophobic in nature. The model is similar to
the membrane model of Singer, in which protein icebergs swim in a sea of lipid
(1971).

A model for HDL, proposed by Forte et al. (1968) and based primarily on electron
microscopic data, consists of four to five subunits packed together with an overall diameter of 70-100 Å. Electron dense regions in the center of the subunit
structure have been described, representing either protein or polar headgroups of
phospholipids. In this model, each subunit is thought to have its own complement
of lipid and protein, the lipid being in the center with each subunit surrounded
by protein (Gotto, 1969).

In order to determine whether the major forces involved in lipid-protein interactions in HDL are hydrophilic or hydrophobic or both, ^{13}C NMR spectroscopy has
been used (Assmann, unpublished results). This technique offers exciting possibilities for exploring structural questions related to lipoprotein research,
since it is possible by isotopic labeling of specific carbons with 90% ^{13}C (its
natural abundance is only 1%) to focus specifically on the mobility and the environment of individual carbon atoms in a lipid or protein. The techniques of
chemical enrichment of ^{13}C at specific locations in the phospholipid headgroups
of lecithin and sphingomyelin as well as specific carbon atoms of saturated and
unsaturated fatty acids in these and other lipids have been first developed in
the laboratory of Stoffel (Stoffel et al., 1972). The application to NMR-studies
of lipid-apoprotein interaction has proved the usefulness of this physical technique (Stoffel, personal communication).

Localized motion along an aliphatic chain, like a fatty acid or cholesterol side
chain, is reflected in NMR measurements. In lecithin, for instance, differences
in motional freedom of individual carbon atoms along the fatty acid chain and the
phosphorylcholine moiety, can be determined through the measurement of spin-
lattice relaxation times (Levine et al., 1972). Whether the apolipoprotein interacts with the phosphorylcholine moiety of phosphatidylcholine (PC) and sphingo-

myelin (SPM) by hydrophilic interaction, or by hydrophobic interaction with fatty acid alkyl chains, can be determined by a change in motional freedom of the respective groups.

The insertion of a ^{13}C label in the choline moiety in phospholipids permitted specific focus on the environment of the lecithin and sphingomyelin polar headgroups in HDL (Assmann, unpublished results). It was observed that the environment of the polar phospholipid headgroups of PC or SPM was the same for phospholipid in a simple lipid bilayer and the native HDL molecule (Assmann, unpublished results).

On the contrary, however, the presence of the HDL protein considerably influenced the magnetic environment in the neighborhood of the α-carboxyl carbon atom of lecithin and the cholesteryl ester carboxyl carbon atom. These results, taken together with data derived from P-NMR spectroscopy, suggested that the major force of interaction between HDL apoproteins and phospholipids is hydrophobic in character, although the importance of some hydrophilic bondings on certain sites cannot be entirely excluded.

Let us examine further the molecular basis of lipid-protein interactions in HDL as suggested by adapting the above findings to knowledge of apoprotein structure. The implications may be broader than for HDL alone. A major question that arises is: what is the specificity of the primary sequence of an apolipoprotein that permits binding or strong association with lipid? From membrane biochemistry it is known that some membrane proteins are amphipathic, that is, they possess one hydrophobic region which is embedded in the interior of a lipid bilayer and in contact with the hydrophobic lipid tails, and they possess one or two hydrophilic regions which project out into the aqueous medium outside or inside the membrane. Hydrophilic protein areas are made of ionic and highly polar amino acid residues; hydrophobic areas are made up of nonpolar residues. An example of a membrane protein with linear amphipathic properties is glycophorin isolated from red cell membranes by Marchesi and co-workers at the NIH (Marchesi et al., 1973). It consists of a protein chain of about 200 amino acid residues to which are attached a large number of oligosaccharide chains. Most remarkably, these sugar residues, which are, of course, highly polar, are all found on half the chain. This region is followed by a highly hydrophobic stretch of about 25 amino acid residues and finally by a hydrophilic region, which has no sugar residues, near the carboxyl end of the chain. It is believed that glycophorin spans the entire erythrocyte membrane. Its hydrophilic portions protrude from either surface of the membrane and its intervening hydrophobic portion is embedded in the membrane interior.

Inspection of the primary structure of apolipoproteins (Fig. 3) so far known reveals that there are no remarkable linear amphipathic areas or long, distinct hydrophobic areas that obviously account for hydrophobic interaction between protein and lipid. There are numerous hydrophobic amino acid residues but they are distributed over the entire length of the molecule. There are also a relatively small number of "acid-base pairs"; i.e., adjacent diamino and dicarboxylic acids scattered along the chains.

Although apolipoproteins apparently have no linear amphipathic properties, they may, nevertheless, have amphipathic properties that arise from their conformation; that is, their secondary and tertiary structure. On close inspection of the primary sequence of apoA-II, one can see that the distribution of hydrophilic and hydrophobic amino acid residues in certain areas is not random. There are certain regularities that are evident.

If one, for instance, constructs an α-helical area between residues 11 and 30 of apoA-II (Fig. 6), the nonrandom distribution of amino acids becomes apparent (Assmann and Brewer, unpublished). Polar residues such as lysine, glutamic acid, aspartic acid and tyrosine are totally located on one α-helical surface area. Hydrophobic amino acid residues like valine, methionine, phenylalanine and leucine are located on the opposite helical surface. We may predict, therefore, that

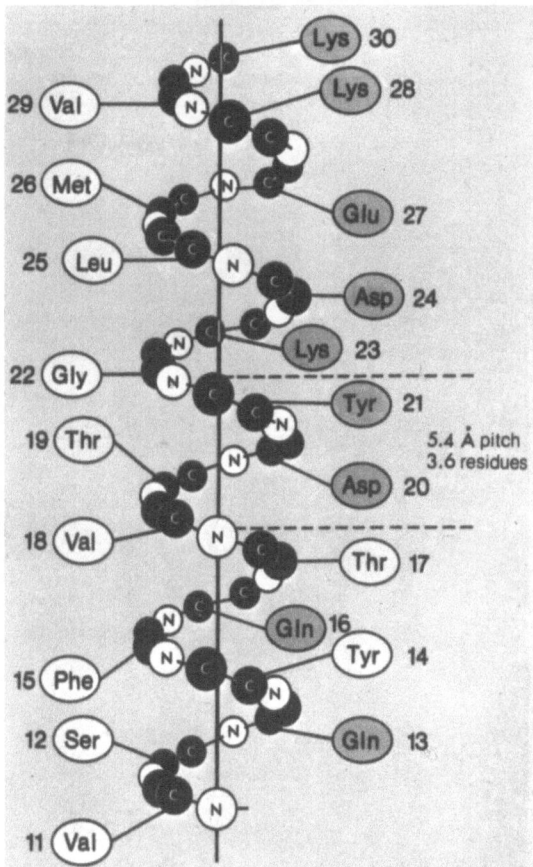

Figure 6. Theoretical construct of an α-helical area of apoA-II with amphipathic properties. A right-handed α-helix with 3.6 amino acid residues per turn and a periodicity of 5.4 Å between residues 11 and 30 of apoA-II reveals hydrophobic amino acids (Val, Phe, Leu, Met) on one helix surface area and charged (Lys, Glu, Asp) on the opposite helix surface area (Assmann and Brewer, unpublished results)

the primary sequence of lipid-binding apolipoproteins is so designed that it provides a hydrophobic surface of significant length when the protein assumes a helical conformation to bind lipid. Similar sequence areas in this and other apolipoproteins are present, thereby permitting the formation of "conformational amphipathic properties" that may be a prerequisite for lipid binding.

It has now been amply demonstrated in a number of laboratories that apoproteins usually contain a certain amount of α-helix, even when delipidated, and that this helical content invariably increases when the apoproteins, or major segments of them, are recombined with phospholipids (Fig. 7) (Assmann and Brewer, unpublished; Lux et al., 1972).

If the 15-20 amino acid residues in the area shown in Fig. 6 are arranged in a α-helix, a maximum length of approximately 20-25 Å would result. The resultant hydrophobic helix surface area would be equivalent to the dimension of a C_{18}-fatty acid chain in its fully extended form. Thus, apoA-II theoretically has at least one surface, dependent on its conformation, that would permit it to interact hydrophobically with phospholipid fatty acid chains.

The presence of an apolipoprotein in a lipoprotein macromolecule does not necessarily mean that it is a lipid-binding protein. In the experiments on HDL, apoA-I, in contrast to A-II, seems to be a poor phospholipid-binding protein (Assmann and Brewer, unpublished results). The incorporation of apoA-I into HDL appears to require the presence of apoA-II, indicating that protein-protein interactions are probably very important for the integration of apoA-I into the native HDL particle. Thus, apoA-II appears to be a phospholipid-binding protein, whereas the function of apoA-I in native HDL remains to be defined.

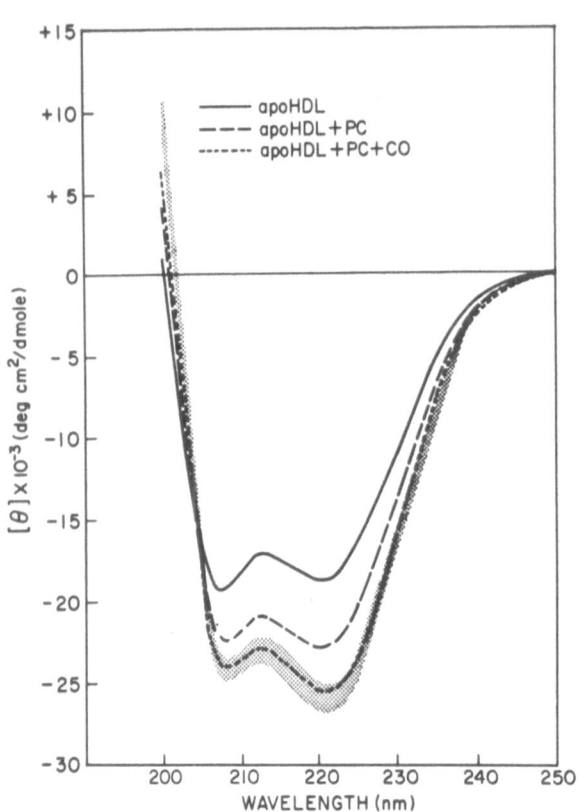

Figure 7. The far-ultraviolet
CD spectra of apoHDL, apoHDL
recombined with phosphatidylcholine alone (apoHDL + PC),
and apoHDL recombined with both
phosphatidylcholine and cholesteryl oleate (apoHDL + PC +
CO). The shaded area represents
the range of the CD spectra of
five separate HDL preparations
(Assmann and Brewer, unpublished;
Lux et al., 1972)

Based on these results, and the theoretical consideration outlined, Assmann and
Brewer have constructed a new model for HDL as shown in Fig. 8. This model of
HDL is still highly schematic and incomplete. For example, the steric arrangements of cholesteryl esters and cholesterol in the lipoprotein are not known.
Protein icebergs are shown half-submerged in micellar lipid. The distribution of
phosphatidylcholine and sphingomyelin is illustrated as though it were random,
but it may be that these phospholipids are arranged in a more specific way. The
apoproteins shown here are oriented perpendicular to the surface. ApoA-II is
arranged such that its amphipathic areas, derived from its conformation, are
in hydrophobic interaction with the alkyl chains of phospholipids. ApoA-I is
shown as principally having protein-protein interactions with apoA-II.

The full elucidation of the quarternary structure of a lipoprotein macromolecule
will not be possible for some time to come. It one considers, however, the extraordinary increase in detailed information about apolipoproteins alone that has
occurred in the last five years, it is easy to perceive the advances that will
come. There is no want of excitement in this particular section of the search
for more knowledge relevant to atherosclerosis.

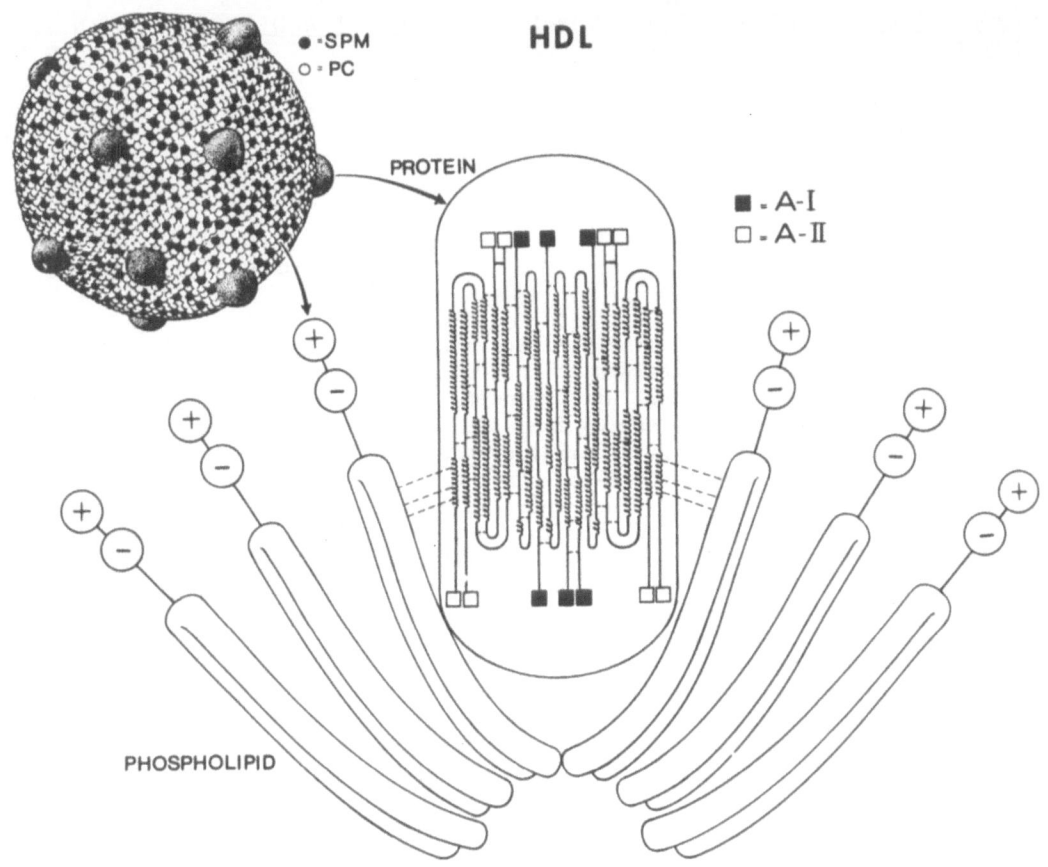

Figure 8. Hypothetical model for HDL (Assmann and Brewer, unpublished results)

LIPOPROTEIN SYNTHESIS, INTRACELLULAR TRANSPORT AND SECRETION IN LIVER*

Y. Stein and O. Stein

Introduction

Very low density lipoproteins (VLDL) of serum are considered to be the main carriers of "endogenous" triglycerides in contradistinction to chylomicrons, which
carry "exogenous" triglycerides. With respect to size, they form a rather heter-
obenous family of particles, ranging from 300 to 800 Å in diameter, and are
characterized by their high triglyceride content, 50-70% by weight, which is
responsible for their density of less than 1.006. The other components of VLDL
are cholesterol, phospholipids, carbohydrates and proteins. The protein moiety,
(which will be designated apolipoprotein) contributes 6-13% of weight and during
the last few years it has been shown to consist of several different protein
molecules. Low density lipoproteins (LDL) have an average particle size of 200 Å
and are considered the main carriers of serum cholesterol, which makes up 40-
45% of their weight. The other major component of LDL is protein (20-25% by
weight) which consists mainly of a single molecular species which is the same as
the major VLDL apolipoprotein. The two lipoprotein classes (VLDL and LDL) will
be considered together, since there exists between them a precursor-product
relationship. The source of origin of serum VLDL has been shown to be confined
mostly to the liver (Stein and Shapiro, 1959; Havel et al., 1962) and to a more
limited extent to the small intestine (Roheim et al., 1966a; Ockner et al.,
1969; Windmueller et al., 1970; Tytgat et al., 1971).

Intracellular Sites of Synthesis of VLDL Components

Lipid. Two approaches have been used to study the intracellular site of synthesis
of VLDL components, i.e., subcellular fractionation and radioautography. First
came the demonstration that the microsomal fraction derived from liver homogenates is the richest in enzymes active in esterification of fatty acids to triglycerides (Stein and Shapiro, 1958; Weiss and Kennedy, 1960). Next the role of
the microsomes in triglyceride synthesis was studied in rat liver perfused with
labeled fatty acid and it was shown that the triglyceride with the highest specific activity was first isolated from the microsomal fraction (Stein and Shapiro,
1959). Likewise, enzymes active in the various steps of phospholipid synthesis
are present mainly in the microsomal fraction of both liver (Stein and Shapiro,
1957; 1958; Weiss et al., 1956) and intestine (Brindley and Hubscher, 1965).
Improvements in isolation techniques permitted the subfractionation of the microsomes into rough (ribosome-bearing) and smooth microsomes. In the liver both
these subfractions have been shown to catalyze the synthesis of lecithin from
labeled glycerol (Glauman and Dallner, 1968) and of cholesterol from labeled
mevalonate (Chesterton, 1968). Autoradiography permitted for the first time to
localize in the intact cell the synthetic pathways studied hitherto in isolated
fractions. With the help of this method it became possible to demonstrate the
presence of labeled triglyceride in the endoplasmic reticulum of liver already
2 min after injection of labeled fatty acids or glycerol. This radioautographic
reaction was seen over both rough and smooth endoplasmic reticulum and often the
regions of transition between the two showed the presence of labeled triglyceride (Stein and Stein, 1966; 1967).

---

*This investigation was supported in part by a research grant from the Myra Kur-
land Heart Fund, Chicago, Ill., and by a grant from the Ministry of Health, the
Government of Israel.

Similarly, radioautography at the electron microscope level was instrumental in the intracellular localization of triglyceride synthesis to the elements of the endoplasmic reticulum in the cell of the small intestine (Jersild, 1966b; Strauss, 1968). One of the sites of cholesterol esterification might be present also in the endoplasmic reticulum, as VLDL isolated either from the Golgi apparatus of rat liver (Mahley et al., 1969) or from rat intestinal lymph (Ockner et al., 1969) contain two thirds of their cholesterol in esterified form. However, in the human, cholesterol esterification occurs predominantly in the circulation. This reaction is catalyzed by lecithin-cholesterol acyl transferase (LCAT) which transfers the fatty acid from the 2 position of lecithin to free cholesterol (Glomset, 1969). Indeed, familial deficiency of LCAT results in the absence of cholesterol ester from serum lipoproteins (Norum and Gjone, 1967).

Protein. Even though a minor component, the protein moiety of VLDL, of both liver and intestinal origin, plays a major role in the secretion of the particle into the circulation. Thus, interruption of protein synthesis by puromycin (Robinson and Seakins, 1962; Jones et al., 1967) ethionine (Robinson and Harris, 1961; Schlunk et al., 1968) or cycloheximide (Bar-on et al., 1973) results in a marked depression of serum lipoproteins. The proteins of the VLDL belong to the class of secretory proteins, the synthesis of which is usually effected on membrane-bound ribosomes (Redman, 1968). Synthesis of specific serum lipoproteins (Bungenberg de Jong and Marsh, 1968) has been also carried out in an in vitro system in the presence of rat liver ribosomes. The mechanism which controls the rate of apolipoprotein synthesis has not been elucidated so far. Under certain experimental conditions, such as partial hepatectomy followed by regeneration (Infante et al., 1968; Girard et al., 1971) or high concentrations of fatty acid (Ruderman et al., 1968; Alcindor et al., 1970) in a liver perfusion system, there seems to be stimulation of apolipoprotein synthesis. The origin of these apolipo-proteins has been studied by Windmueller et al. (1973) who have demonstrated that while synthesis of all apolipoproteins of VLDL does occur in the liver, the small intestine is able to synthesize little or none of the apolipoproteins charac-terized by a rapid mobility on polyacrylamide gel. These investigators postulated that VLDL of intestinal origin acquire the small "fast moving" apolipoproteins in the intestinal lymph and in the circulation (Windmueller and Spaeth, 1972; Wind-mueller et al., 1973).

Carbohydrate. The carbohydrate constituents which have been identified in human plasma lipoproteins are glucosamine, galactose, mannose and sialic acid, and are present in the form of glycoproteins (Marshall and Kummerow, 1962). During the formation of glycoproteins the various sugars are added in a stepwise manner to the protein moiety. Thus N-Acetyl glucosamine may be added to the nascent poly-peptide chain still at the polysomal level (Molnar, 1967). The addition of man-nose is catalyzed by enzymes present in the membranes of the rough endoplasmic reticulum, however, the addition of galactose, a presursor of glucosamine occurs mainly at the level of the Golgi apparatus (Whur et al., 1969; Wagner and Cynkin, 1971). The final step of glycosidation of serum lipoproteins in the liver occurs also in the Golgi apparatus, as the highest specific activity of the enzyme which transfers glucosamine to serum lipoproteins was found in that frac-tion (Lo and Marsh, 1970). More recently a high specific activity of galactosyl transferase has been found in a purified Golgi fraction derived from rat intes-tinal mucosa (Mahley et al., 1971).

Synthesis of High Density Lipoproteins

Serum high density lipoproteins (HDL) are composed of about 50% protein, 30% phospholipid and 20% cholesterol, the latter mostly in the form of cholesterol ester. Like the other lipoproteins described so far, they originate mostly from the liver (Windmueller and Spaeth, 1967) and to some extent also from the small intestine (Windmueller and Spaeth, 1972). Their independent origin from serum VLDL has been indicated by the presence of α protein in patients with a beta-lipoproteinemia (Gotto et al., 1971). In experimental animals use was made of

orotic acid, known to inhibit release of β lipoproteins from the liver, in order
to study the synthesis and release of HDL. Livers of orotic acid-fed rats were
shown to release labeled phospholipid and cholesterol into the perfusate, but
hardly any triclyceride (Windmueller and Levy, 1967). The synthesis of the protein moiety of serum HDL was studied with the help of labeled precursors and
incorporation of label into HDL protein was demonstrated both in a perfused
liver (Roheim et al., 1966b) and in vivo (Shiff et al., 1971; Faloona et al.,
1968). More recently HDL protein was shown to be released into the lymph and into
the perfusion medium by isolated rat intestine (Windmueller and Spaeth, 1972).
Analysis of the various HDL apolipoproteins following perfusion with radioactive
amino acids revealed that while all the apolipoproteins of HDL released by the
liver were labeled, in case of the intestine - "the fast moving components" were
not labeled. These findings may indicate that while the liver secretes apparently
a complete HDL particle, the HDL derived from the intestine obtains some of its
apolipoproteins from the serum (Windmueller et al., 1973).

Secretory Pathway of VLDL

Early studies with labeled fatty acids have shown that about 20 min elapse between the time of formation of labeled triglyceride in the liver and its appearance in the circulation (Stein and Shapiro, 1959; Havel et al., 1962). Since the
half-life of the fatty acid in the circulation is extremely brief, it was possible to consider the labeling of liver triglyceride as a pulse labeling and
follow the intracellular route of labeled triglyceride from the site of synthesis
to the site of secretion with the help of radioautography. These studies have
shown that the above mentioned lag period can be accounted for by the findings
that the VLDL particles, which originate in the endoplasmic reticulum are first
transported to the Golgi apparatus and subsequently reach the sinusoidal cell
border inside membrane-bound vacuoles (Stein and Stein, 1967). The final step
in the secretory process consists of the fusion of the membranes of secretory
vesicles with the plasma membrane and release of the lipoprotein particles into
the space of Disse. A similar sequence of events is envisaged also for the intracellular transport and secretion of VLDL in the small intestine in fasting
animals and in man (Tytgat et al., 1971; Jones and Ockner, 1971). Diversion of
bile or administration of cholestyramine resulted in the disappearance of VLDL
particles from the intestinal cells (Jones and Ockner, 1971). The question
whether intestinal VLDL should be considered as small chylomicrons (Windmueller
et al., 1970; Tytgat et al., 1971), or a distinct particle population (Mahley et
al., 1971) has not been resolved so far. In Golgi apparatus isolated from rat
intestinal mucosa, VLDL particles and chylomicrons were found in separate secretory vesicles; this was interpreted as an indication that they might be segregated in the Golgi apparatus (Mahley et al., 1971).

Even though the general route of the secretory pathway of VLDL has been outlined,
the site of the coupling between the lipid and protein moieties has yet to be
localized. Lipoprotein granules large enough to be distinguished from the
matrix are first noted at the regions of transition between rough and smooth
endoplasmic reticulum, and it is possible that the lipoprotein particle is
formed there. Recently, the transport of serum glycoproteins was studied in rat
liver microsomes and it was proposed that the polypeptide chain which is released from the ribosome may not reach the lumen of the cisterna, but travel
inside the membrane of the rough endoplasmic reticulum proper till it reaches
the smooth endoplasmic reticulum or the Golgi apparatus (Redman and Cherian,
1972). This is not true for albumin which reaches the lumen of the cisterna
directly after its release from the ribosome. Since serum lipoporteins are
complex proteins, one might envisage the possibility that the apolipoprotein
portion might be transported in a manner similar to that of the glycoprotein.
If such a mechanism were operative, one might consider the presence of a limited
apolipoprotein pool, from which the lipoprotein particles are formed during their
passage through the cisternae of the endoplasmic reticulum. The presence of a
pool of apolipoproteins and the site of lipid-protein attachment was studied

in the intact rat (Buckley et al., 1968) and in perfused rat liver (Bar-On et al., 1973). Cycloheximide introduced into the perfusion system inhibited incorporation of labeled amino acid in perfusate proteins, but esterification of newly added fatty acid into complex lipids proceeded at a normal rate. For about an hour after interruption of protein synthesis, secretion of VLDL proceeded at about 60% of the normal rate indicating that intracellular transport and release of VLDL are not dependent on concomitant protein synthesis. Thus it seems that there might be a small intracellular pool of apolipoproteins which may serve as acceptor of lipid synthesized after inhibition of protein synthesis (Bar-On et al., 1973).

Some circumstantial evidence suggests that the transfer of VLDL into the Golgi apparatus in the hepatocyte might require energy. This is based on the finding of accumulation of VLDL particles in the cisternae of the endoplasmic reticulum and their absence from the Golgi apparatus 3-5 hours after administration of ethionine, at a time when there is a significant fall in cellular ATP (Farber, 1967; Baglio and Farber, 1965).

The secretory of the HDL particle has not been elucidated so far and its presence in the secretory vesicles of the Golgi apparatus remains to be demonstrated.

Regulation of VLDL Synthesis

One approach to the study of the regulation of VLDL synthesis is through investigation of the various types of fatty liver. As mentioned previously, interference with protein synthesis by injection of puromycin, ethionine or carbon tetrachloride results in a decrease in lipoprotein secretion and in the development of fatty liver. It seems of interest to point out that the degree of lipid accumulation in the liver was not related only to the degree of inhibition of protein synthesis, but rather to a rise in serum free fatty acids (Glaser and Mager, 1972; Bar-On et al., 1972). Accumulation of triglyceride, in the face of normal protein synthetic activity might act as a trigger for the synthesis and secretion of serum VLDL, which has also found its intrastructural expression in the form of numerous VLDL particles in the Golgi apparatus of the hepatocyte (Roheim et al., 1971). Additional support for the role of high concentration of liver triglyceride in the stimulation of VLDL synthesis and secretion was derived from the finding that feeding of a high sucrose diet to rats results in a very marked increase of incorporation of amino acids into VLDL protein and a rise in serum VLDL levels (Shiff et al., 1971). It seems plausible that the trigger for the enhancement of the synthesis of VLDL protein described above is linked to the process of mobilization of the accumulated triglyceride which is stored in the liver in the form of large cytoplasmic droplets. The mobilization of triglyceride from the intracellular lipid droplet was investigated recently (Bar-On et al., 1971) and the question asked was whether the triglyceride is mobilized as a whole molecule or whether it has to undergo hydrolysis. To that end liver triglycerides were labeled with ^{3}H-glycerol and ^{14}C-palmitic acid and liver perfusion was started at a time when most of the labeled triglyceride was present in the intracellular lipid droplet. During three hours of perfusion secretion of labeled triglyceride occurred, and the ratio of ^{14}C-palmitate/^{3}H-glycerol in triglycerides of the perfusate and of liver microsomes were similar and different from that in the intracellular lipid droplet. This ratio rose also at later times of perfusion, indicating that the ^{14}C-palmitate moiety of the droplet triglyceride had been used for the newly synthesized lipoprotein molecules. Moreover, while the specific activity of the palmitic acid labeled triglyceride in the microsomes and in the lipid droplet was similar, the specific activity of glycerol labeled triglyceride in the microsomes was only half of the lipid droplet. Thus, when the triglyceride of the intracellular lipid droplet is mobilized for secretion, it has to undergo hydrolysis and it is the fatty acid portion which is mostly reutilized.

Another type of fatty liver which helped to elucidate an important aspect of
VLDL secretion was orotic acid. Incorporation of this drug into a synthetic
diet results in the accumulation of osmiophilic particles in the cisternae of
endoplasmic reticulum (Novikoff et al., 1966) and a failure to secret VLDL into
the circulation (Windmueller and Levy, 1967). The interference with VLDL secretion occurred in spite of no reduction in protein synthesis (Deamer et al.,
1965) and secretion of serum proteins of density greater than 1.21 (i.e. serum
albumin) (Roheim et al., 1966b). In a recent study the osmiophilic droplets
("liposomes")were isolated from orotic acid-treated livers, and their apolipoprotein composition examined on polyacrylamide gel electrophoresis (Pottenger
and Getz, 1971). It became evident that apolipoproteins derived from the "liposomes" had the same composition as normal serum VLDL, apart from one missing
band. This band has been shown to be immunologically identical with one just
preceding it, and the faster mobility of the latter was due to a different
sialic acid content (Brown et al., 1970). Thus it appears that interference with
the glycosidation process does affect the intracellular transport and secretion
of otherwise fully assembled VLDL particles.

The delivery of the VLDL from its intracellular site of formation is achieved
by a secretory vesicle which migrates from the Golgi apparatus and fuses with
the sinusoidal cell membrane. Recently several reports have appeared, which have
dealt with the participation of microtubules in the process of secretion in endocrine glands (Lacy et al., 1968; Williams and Wolff, 1970; Malaisse-Lagae et
al., 1971; Pelletier and Bornstein, 1972). In rats pretreated with colchicine
and injected with ^{14}C-palmitic acid or ^{3}H-leucine, there is a five-fold reduction
in the appearance of labeled triglyceride or labeled protein in the circulation.
The dose of colchicine employed caused no impairment in esterification of fatty
acids into triglycerides and caused only a slight (less than 15%) depression in
protein synthesis in the liver. By the use of Triton WR 1339 it was possible to
demonstrate that the fall in both labeled and total triglyceride in the serum
of colchicine-treated rats was due to impairment of VLDL release from the liver.
In addition, when lipoproteins were isolated from sera of rats injected with
leucine-^{3}H but not given Triton, it became evident that administration of
colchicine resulted in a reduction of serum VLDL by 80% of HDL by 20%, while the
d > 1.21 level remained unchanged. However, the specific activity of the proteins in all the fractions was reduced by 50%, thus indicating that colchicine
inhibited the secretion of all of them. The morphological counterpart of the
impaired release is the accumulation of large secretory vesicles, filled with
nascent VLDL in the hepatocyte (Fig.1)(Stein and Stein, 1973). Thus it seems
that the microtubular system might be operative also in the normal release of
lipoproteins into the circulation.

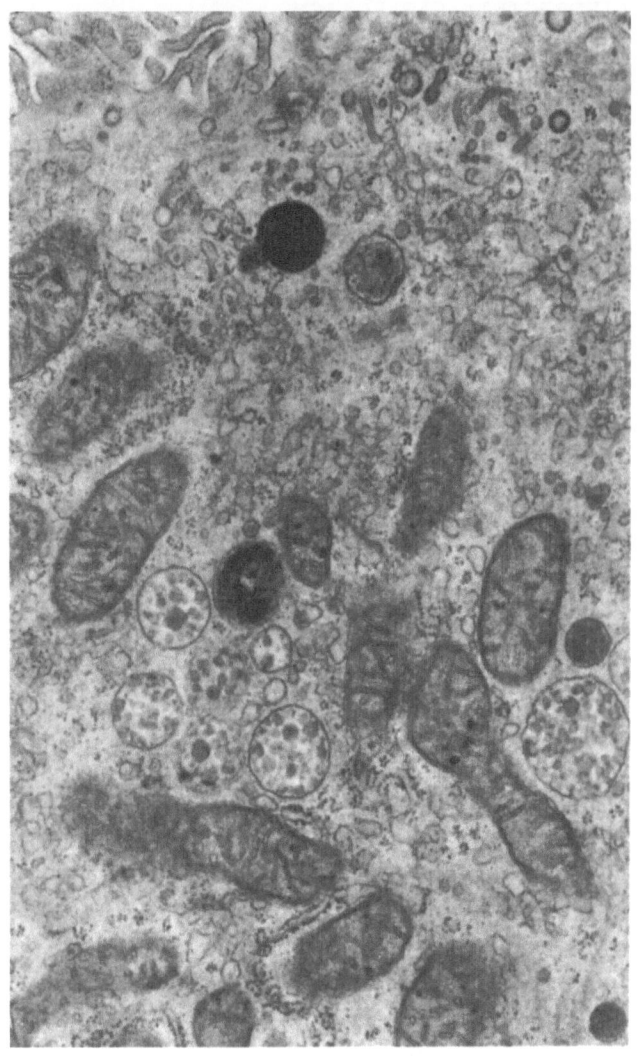

Figure 1. Electron micrograph of liver or rat 180 min after injection with colchicine. Secretory vesicles containing many VLDL particles are seen in the cytoplasm (X 21.910)

LIPOPROTEIN CATABOLISM

Daniel Steinberg

Introduction

The study of lipoprotein degradation poses certain very special problems. The lipoprotein molecule is something of a chimera. Unlike a well-behaved, covalently constructed molecule like DNA or a simple protein, it represents a less tightly bound complex of proteins and lipids - and they don't sit still. The ready exchange of free cholesterol between lipoprotein molecules is well recognized. The same is true for phospholipids. Thus, it is very difficult to interpret turnover studies based on labeling of these lipid components. As we shall discuss, at least some of the protein moieties also exchange rapidly between lipoprotein fractions. So the investigator is plagued by the vagaries of a system that has maddening, will-o'-the-wisp qualities about it. At least the cholesterol esters, some of the apoproteins, and the triglycerides exchange slowly enough so that kinetic studies can be meaningful and the studies I will review today deal primarily with the latter two moieties.

My charge from the Program Committee was to review advances since our last symposium in the area of lipoprotein catabolism. Such a discussion necessarily overlaps with and cannot be separated from advances in lipoprotein structure, where considerable progress has been made in the past four years. Nor can it be separated from a discussion of enzymes known to modify lipoprotein structure. Both of these topics are covered elsewhere in this Symposium and so I shall limit myself primarily to certain aspects that bear directly on the removal of lipoproteins from the plasma compartment.

Defective Catabolism in Hyperlipoproteinemic Patients

Interest in the mechanisms of lipoprotein removal from the plasma has been heightened in recent years as we have become aware that in many of our hyperlipoproteinemic patients the defect probably lies in removal mechanisms rather than in an overproduction of lipoproteins (Table 1). This is clearly the case in familial hyperchylomicronemia or Type I hyperlipoproteinemia. Production rates are not at issue here, that being solely a function of fat intake. The patients show no chylomicronemia on a fat-free diet, yet show massive chylomicronemia even on modest fat intake. Obviously, they have a defect in the rate of removal of chylomicrons and that has been correlated with a deficiency of lipoprotein lipase (Havel and Gordon, 1960; Fredrickson et al., 1963; Harlan et al., 1967; Bradford et al., 1968). The successful resolution during the past several years of post-heparin lipolytic activity derived from the liver and that derived from peripheral tissues, including adipose tissue has eliminated what seemed a paradox. Some of these patients, while they have very low levels of lipoprotein lipase in adipose tissue biopsies, show post-heparin plasma lipolytic activity that is far from zero. Now we know, as discussed below, that the lipolytic activity that they do show after heparin injection is mostly derived not from the adipose tissue or other peripheral tissues but from the liver.

In Type II disease, studies by Langer, Strober and Levy (1972) in ten patients have shown that the defect again is probably in removal rates. They found that the apparent half-life of LDL (low density lipoprotein) apoprotein was markedly reduced. However, total production (i.e. the product of the fractional catabolic rate and the LDL pool size) yielded values for daily flux within normal limits.

Table 1. Hyperlipoproteinemic states in which defective catabolism has been implicated

---

All familial hyperchylomicronemias (Type I; prob. Type V)

Many familial hyperbetalipoproteinemias (Type IIa)

Many familial hyperprebetalipoproteinemias (Type IV)

On the other hand, Walton, Scott and coworkers reported normal fractional catabolic rates for LDL in a small series of Type II patients (Walton et al., 1963). Whether the difference in findings is based on patient selection — indicating heterogeneity of mechanisms in patients with Type II disease — or in technique cannot be decided at this time.

Studies by Havel and his coworkers (1970) and studies by Quarfordt et al. (1970), show that at least some patients with Type IV hyperlipoproteinemia have predominantly a defect in removal of VLDL (very low density lipoprotein) triglyceride. In both studies, the fractional removal rate was markedly reduced, with almost no overlap between controls and patients with Type IV hyperlipemia. On the other hand, net production of VLDL triglyceride on diets containing the usual intake of carbohydrate (40% of total calories) was not statistically different. The mean value in the patients was very slightly higher than that in controls but this difference was felt to be too small to account for the degree of hypertriglyceridemia observed. Other investigators, on the other hand, have presented evidence for high production rates in some of their Type IV patients (e.g. Reaven et al., 1965). Again, the question of heterogeneity within the group we call "Type IV" must be considered a real possibility (see review by Nikkila, 1969).

What I would like to do now is to take the four major classes of plasma lipoproteins one by one and discuss our present understanding of their catabolism.

Chylomicron Catabolism

The removal of chylomicrons is a complex process. The cholesterol and triglyceride components have very different fates, as suggested first by Havel et al. (1963). They showed that when the liver was excluded from the circulation, the initial rate of triglyceride disappearance was relatively unimpaired while cholesterol disappearance rate was much slower. Redgrave (1970) isolated what he called chylomicron "remnants" shortly after injection into rats and also studied tissue distribution of the cleared cholesterol and triglycerides from the injected chylomicrons. As shown in Fig. 1, the "remnants" had a much smaller diameter, a higher density and much less triglyceride relative to cholesterol than the parent chylomicrons. Ten minutes after injection, 79% of the cleared cholesterol was in the liver but only 21% of the cleared triglyceride. This differential removal of chylomicron components has been demonstrated in sheep and in dogs also (Bergman et al., 1971). In sheep, almost none of the chylomicron cholesterol was taken up in the lower part of the body and fully 76% was taken up in the liver. Later, we shall have to ask if there is any similar complexity in the process of VLDL removal.

LaRosa and coworkers (1972) provided the first evidence for a second post-heparin triglyceride lipase. Its hepatic origin is now clearly established and its properties have been well-described (Krauss et al., 1973b; Greten et al., 1972; Ehnholm et al., 1973; Assman et al., 1973). The physical resolution of the two enzymes from post-heparin plasma by Ehnholm et al. (1973) opens the way to complete characterization of them and unambiguous assessment of the relative

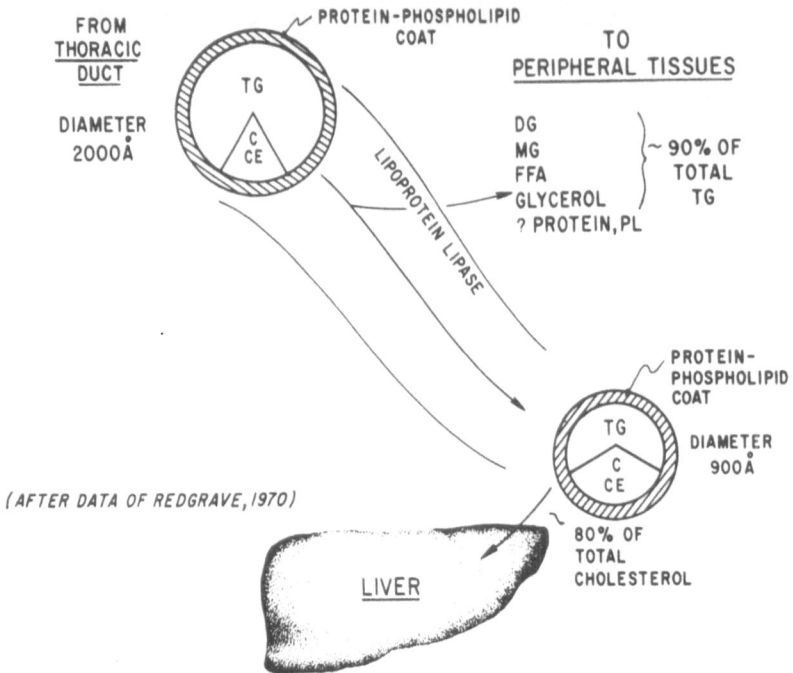

Figure 1. Scheme depicting the differential fate of cholesterol and of triglyceride (TG) during removal of chylomicrons from the plasma (Chylomicron ⟶
"Remnant"). Based on data of Redgrave (1970) and Bergman et al. (1971)

amounts of each in post-heparin plasma. It also should be possible now to develop
specific antibodies that will help in the quantification of them and in the
localization of these enzymes in tissue. At this meeting, Krauss et al. (1973b)
report a simple method for distinguishing the two activities in post-heparin
plasma. In fourteen patients with familial hyperchylomicronemia, the peripheral
lipoprotein lipase activity contributed only minimally to the total post-heparin
lipolytic activity. The absolute level of peripheral lipoprotein lipase activity
was only 10% of normal; in contrast, the level of the hepatic enzyme was only
slightly less than normal. One can conclude that the hepatic enzyme alone is
incapable of maintaining normal rates of chylomicron clearance. However, this
does not rule out a role for the hepatic lipase in the overall metabolism of
chylomicrons. Specifically, the hepatic lipase may be essential in the removal
of the "remnants" that are taken up by the liver.

Very Low Density Lipoprotein (VLDL) Catabolism

Since our last Symposium, we have lost our innocence regarding the complexity of
VLDL, thanks to the work of a number of investigators (Gustafson et al., 1966;
Brown et al., 1969, 1970; Shore and Shore, 1969; Scanu et al., 1969). Brown, Levy
and Fredrickson (1969) first clearly established the fact that VLDL contained, in
addition to apoLDL, three distinct low-molecular weight proteins — apoLp-Glu,
apoLp-Ser and apoLp-Ala (designated by their C-terminal amino acid residues).*

---

*These apoproteins as a group are also referred to as "apolipoprotein C" and the
 subfractions correspond as follows: apoLp-Ser = C-I; apoLp-Glu = C-II; apoLp-Ala
 = C-III (Alaupovic et al., 1972).

These three proteins represent 40 to 50% of the total protein, the bulk of the remainder being identical in all respects to the apoprotein found in LDL (Gotto et al., 1972). Now, since LDL under steady-state conditions contains little if any of the low-molecular weight proteins, these must be lost somehow during the conversion of VLDL to LDL. On the other hand, the HDL (high density lipoprotein) fraction *does* contain small but real concentrations of these same small apo-proteins. ApoLp-Glu and apoLp-Ala are in rapid equilibrium with their counter-parts in VLDL as shown by the *in vitro* mixing studies of Bilheimer, Eisenberg and Levy (Bilheimer et al., 1972; Eisenberg et al., 1972) and by Havel, Kane and Kashyap using lipoprotein lipase activator activity as a marker (Havel et al., 1973). So, as shown in Fig 2, one can draw a picture of VLDL, 60% or more tri-glyceride by weight, associated with at least 4 different apoproteins. Three of these can exchange reversibly and rapidly with HDL, as indicated on the left.

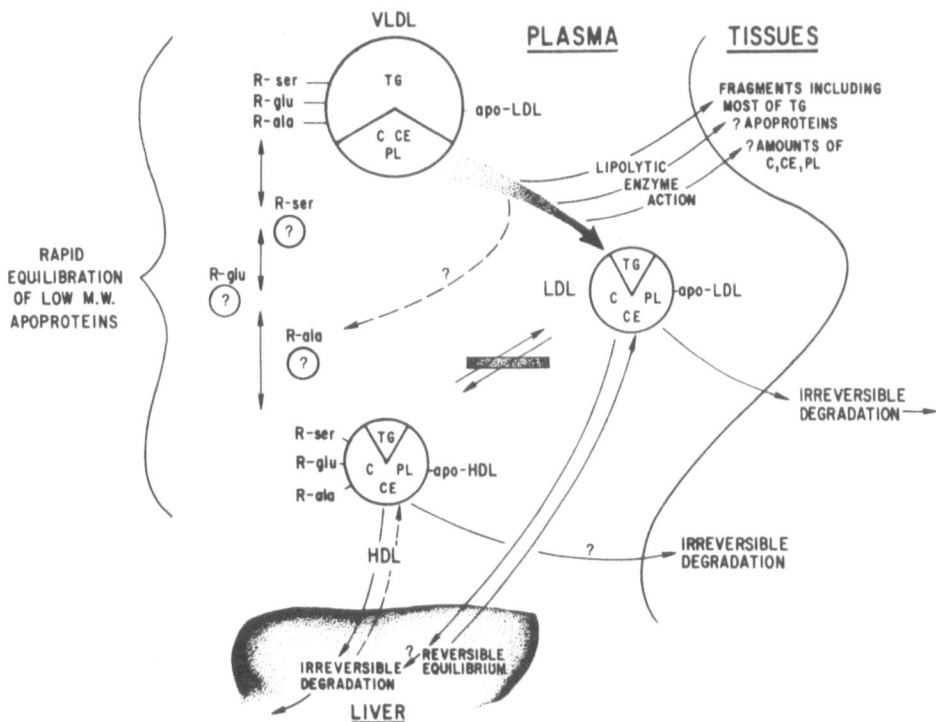

Figure 2. Lipoprotein-apoprotein exchanges and interconversions. Schematic rep-resentation of lipoprotein transformations within the plasma and removal from the plasma. The low-molecular weight apoproteins (R-ser, R-glu, R-ala corre-sponding to apoLp-Ser, apoLp-Glu and apoLp-Ala) are shown to be rapidly ex-changing between VLDL and HDL. Whether this occurs concurrently with transfer of some lipid or not is uncertain and the lipid moieties transferring with them are indicated by circles containing question marks. The ultimate fate of these apoproteins remains to be established. Note that interconversion of LDL and HDL does not apparently occur at all. Reversible equilibrium of LDL with a hepat-ic pool has been established as has irreversible degradation in the periphery, as discussed later in the text. Irreversible degradation of HDL in the liver has been demonstrated, as discussed later; the possibility of reversible equilibrium of HDL with a hepatic pool is not ruled out

During conversion of VLDL to LDL, almost all of the triglyceride is lost and so is much of the protein. Certainly, all of the small apoproteins are lost, as already mentioned. Is any of the apoLDL lost into tissues during VLDL breakdown or does all of it wind up in the LDL fraction? Recent isotopic and analytic studies by Eisenberg, Bilheimer, Lindgren and Levy (1973) suggest that the LDL is mostly or fully retained. VLDL subfractions of S_f 40 up to 500 were isolated from a hyperlipemic patient and after delipidation their apoprotein content was determined by chromatography on Sephadex G-150. As shown in Table 2, the amount of apoLDL per particle in the S_f 147, 82 and 41 fractions was about the same while the amounts of apoLP-Glu plus apoLp-Ala fell by 50%. The largest VLDL, S_f 500, seemed to contain more LDL than the smaller fractions. However, note that in going down from S_f 500 to S_f 41 the amounts of the small apoproteins dropped almost by a factor of 10 while apoLDL dropped only by a factor of 2. So we can conclude that much or all of apoLDL is carried right through to LDL while the other apoproteins are progressively stripped off (along with the triglycerides and some of the phospholipid and cholesterol).

Table 2. Composition of VLDL subfractions

Median S_f for fraction	Total	TG	apoLDL	apoLp-Glu + apoLp-Ala
	Mass per particle (Daltons x 10^{-6})			
500	176	123.2	0.81	3.77
147	30.9	19.7	0.30	0.97
82	16.0	8.8	0.33	0.76
41	8.2	3.6	0.44	0.47

(Data of Eisenberg, Bilheimer, Lindgren and Levy, BBA, in press)

How is this effected? Since heparin injection dramatically accelerates the process (*in vivo* only) it is assumed that lipoprotein lipase is responsible. However, in the absence of a heparin injection the levels of lipoprotein lipase in the plasma are low and hydrolysis is presumed to take place predominantly within the capillary bed. Robinson's early evidence that lipoprotein lipase must reside in part in the capillaries and electron microscopic evidence for margination of

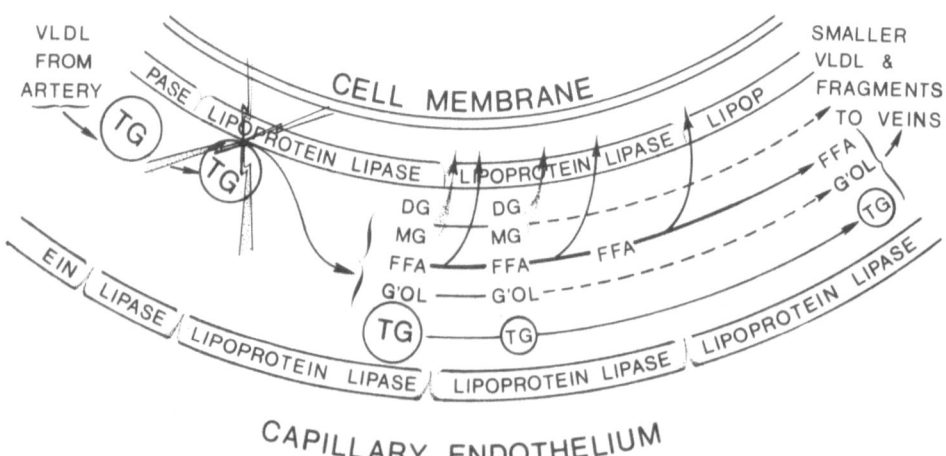

Figure 3. Schematic representation of the fate of VLDL in the capillary bed

chylomicrons and large lipoproteins (i.e. adherence to the endothelium) suggests a scheme (Fig.3) similar to that for chylomicron removal (Robinson and Harris, 1959; Wasserman and Mc Donald, 1963; Schoefl and French, 1968). On reaching the capillary, the lipoprotein (chylomicron or VLDL) interacts with lipoprotein lipase on or in the capillary endothelium leading to lipolysis. Some of the products move immediately across the capillary for uptake by tissue cells. However, not all of the products are taken up in a single passage. A fraction of the FFA (free fatty acid) and glycerol released, certainly escapes uptake and appears in the peripheral circulation. Human studies by Eaton, Berman and myself (1969) suggested that a large part of the VLDL triglyceride fatty acids mix with FFA in the periphery before being taken up. Bergman et al. (1971) have shown in sheep and dogs that as much as 40% of the triglyceride fatty acids in chylomicrons are released as FFA prior to ultimate removal from the plasma. The stripped down lipoprotein — stripped down to varying degrees presumably — then reappears in the peripheral circulation. The scheme shown in Fig. 3 addresses itself only to lipoprotein lipase, the original "clearing factor". Actually, we know that many enzymes are at least potentially involved in lipoprotein breakdown, some of which are listed in Table 3. Heparin injection increases plasma levels not only of lipoprotein lipase but also of the triglyceride lipase of hepatic origin, already discussed, phospholipase A and lower glyceridase activity or activities.

Table 3. Plasma enzymes possibly involved in lipoprotein catabolism

---

Lipoprotein lipase (from adipose tissue and other peripheral tissues)

Hepatic triglyceride lipase

Monoglyceride lipase

Phospholipase(s)

Lecithin-cholesterol acyltransferase

Others?

Although not heparin-dependent, LCAT (lecithin-cholesterol acyl transferase) is constantly present in plasma and also plays a role. The relative importance of these lipoprotein-degrading enzymes and the possible interactions among them remain to be determined.

LDL Catabolism

When we turn to LDL catabolism, we find ourselves in relatively unknown territory. In the case of VLDL, it was obvious that hydrolysis and removal of glycerides had to be a key to catabolism and that lipases must be involved. Does anything analogous happen with LDL? Are any of the same lipolytic enzymes involved? The LDL fraction contains very little triglyceride (less than 10% by weight) and in normal individuals it is a reasonably homogeneous preparation. On the other hand, there *are* several reports indicating both variability from subject to subject and microheterogeneity in given subjects (Adams and Schumaker, 1969, 1970; Fisher et al., 1972). Moreover, some patients with elevated VLDL (Type IV hyperlipoproteinemia) have significant concentrations of lower density LDL in their plasma, that is, molecules with S_f values between 10 and 20 (Fisher, 1970; Hammond and Fisher, 1971). The concentration of such molecules in normal individuals is extremely small and difficult to detect at all. Slack and Mills (1970) have reported small but statistically significant differences in lipid composition between LDL fractions from normal subjects and those from Type II patients. So, the possibility that within the LDL density range there is a metabolic "chain" analogous to that for VLDL catabolism has not been ruled out. Fisher, Berman and coworkers (unpublished results) have presented some preliminary evidence for just such transformations within the class of LDL molecules but the exact nature and the physiologic significance of such LDL transformations remains to be established. Since LDL is not convertible to HDL — the apoproteins are quite distinct and tracer studies indicate no conversion — the LDL is in a sense the end-of-the-line and we need to know where and how it exits from the plasma.

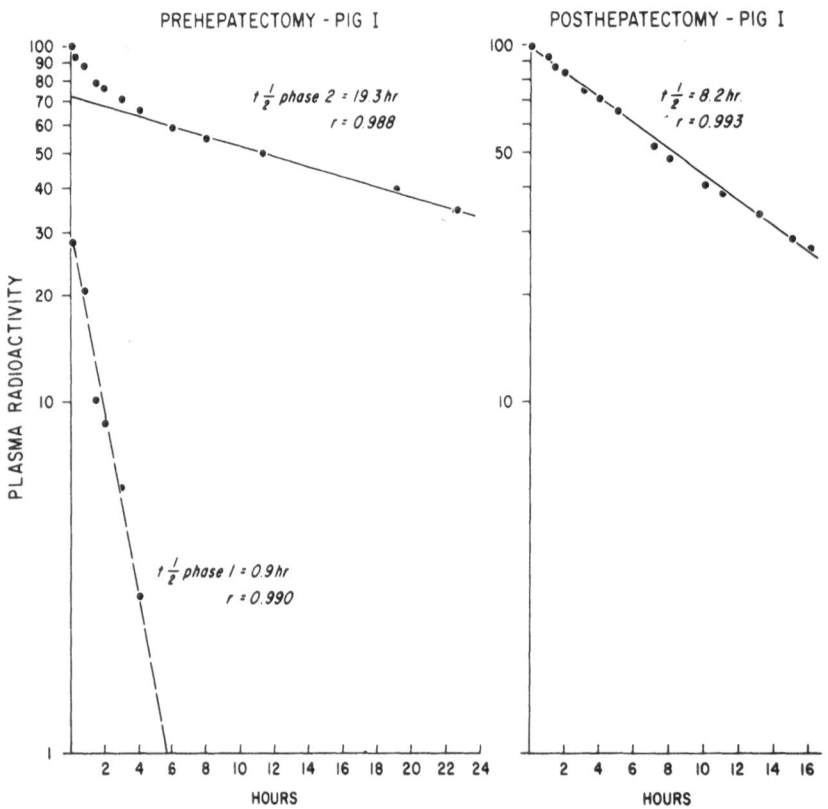

Figure 4. Results of a representative experiment in which ^{125}I-LDL (d 1.019 – 1.063) was injected intravenously into a pig. The left panel shows the experimental points for disappearance of plasma radioactivity as a function of time; the lower curve results from subtraction of the second exponential from the primary curve. The right panel shows the disappearance of plasma radioactivity in a later experiment on the same animal after complete removal of the liver, as discussed later in the text

Our group in La Jolla has been trying to learn something about LDL disposal (Sniderman et al., 1972, 1973a,b,c; Steinberg et al., 1973). We have used pigs because their lipoprotein pattern is close to that of man and they are of good size. When ^{125}I-labeled LDL (d 1.019 – 1.063) was injected into normal pigs it showed a biexponential decay from the plasma compartment (Fig.4). At all times after injection, over 95% of the label in plasma was recovered in the LDL fraction. The more rapid, initial disappearance (half-life about 50 minutes) does not merely reflect heterogeneity of the injected labeled molecules as shown by reinjection studies. When plasma was drawn from a primary recipient about four hours after the original injection, and this plasma was injected into a secondary recipient, a biexponential decay was seen that duplicated almost exactly the curve seen in the primary recipient. Thus, we conclude that the first phase of disappearance represents recycling between LDL in the plasma and an extravascular pool (or pools) of LDL. Table 4 summarizes kinetic data from 13 studies in intact swine. The mean half-life for the initial phase of disappearance was 0.83 hours and that for the second phase of disappearance was 22.5 hours. It can be seen that the results from animal to animal are included in a fairly narrow range. A more meaningful description of degradation is the fractional catabolic rate (FCR), calculated by analysis of the biexponential decay curve assuming a simple two-pool model according to Mathews (1957). The value for the intact animals was 0.042 per hour, that is a little over 4% of the plasma LDL pool being irreversibly degraded per hour.

Table 4. Kinetic parameters for ^{125}I-LDL disappearance in intact swine

	Phase I half-life (hour)	Phase II half-life (hour)	Fractional catabolic rate (hour^{-1})
Mean $\pm$ SEM (n = 13)	0.83 $\pm$ 0.06	22.5 $\pm$ 1.7	0.042 $\pm$ 0.003

(Data of Sniderman, Carew, Chandler and Steinberg, 1973; Steinberg, Carew, Chandler and Sniderman, 1973)

We then determined the tissue distribution of the labeled LDL in animals sacrificed at different intervals following its injection. Correction for trapped plasma in the tissues was made by injecting ^{14}C-labeled Dextran just prior to sacrifice. The only tissue found to contain very significant concentrations of label was the liver. It contained an amount of radioactivity, most of it precipitable by trichloroacetic acid that corresponded to 12 to 19% of that remaining in the plasma at the time of sacrifice (Table 5). The total radioactivity in the liver was relatively constant whether the animal was sacrificed at 8 hours or up to 122 hours after the original injection. Certainly, there was no apparent time trend. This suggests a hepatic pool in rapid equilibrium with the LDL in plasma. The *total* extravascular LDL pool size was calculated from analyses of the plasma decay curves in these experiments. As shown in Table 5, the *total* extravascular pool amounted to some 20% of the *plasma* LDL pool. Thus, the pool in the liver seems to account for about three quarters of the total extravascular pool and represents the *major* extravascular pool.

This finding was certainly compatible with the proposal that the liver might be taking up and destroying LDL. Liver has been implicated as the site of LDL catabolism in rats (Hay et al., 1971). We repeated our kinetic studies in pigs that had undergone complete extirpation of the liver. Circulation to the rest of the viscera was maintained by insertion of a porto-caval shunt. We fully expected the disappearance rate of labeled LDL to decrease after hepatectomy but found, to our surprise, that it was not decreased at all. A representative result is shown in Fig. 4. In fact, as can be seen, the LDL disappeared more rapidly after hepatectomy. The other notable finding was that the disappearance was now *mono-exponential*, that is, there was no sign of the initial, more rapid phase of disappearance seen in all of the intact animals. This is consonant with the conclusion, drawn from the tissue distribution studies, that the liver contains the major extravascular pool of LDL. The fact that disappearance was monoexponential also indicates kinetic homogeneity. This is relevant since pig LDL has been

Table 5. Comparison of the size of the intrahepatic LDL pool, determined directly, with the size of total extravascular LDL pool, calculated from disappearance curves

Time of sacrifice (hr)	Total ^{125}I liver/ total ^{125}I plasma x 100	Total extravascular ^{125}I-LDL pool/plasma ^{125}I-LDL pool x 100[a]	% of extravascular pool accounted for by liver pool
8	12	29	41
16.5	19	22	86
17	15	16	94
52	14	18	78
99	14	18	78
122	18	22	82
	15.3 ± 1.1	20.8 ± 1.9	76.5 ± 7.5

[a]Determined from plasma decay curve.

(Data of Sniderman, Carew, Chandler and Steinberg, 1973; Steinberg, Carew, Chandler and Sniderman, 1973)

reported to be separable into two components differing in density (Janado et al., 1966; Janado and Martin, 1968). The second component, isolated at d 1.060 – 1.090, was presumably not an important contribution in the present studies since we prepared and labeled the fraction d 1.019 – 1.063. Moreover, recent studies by Jackson et al. (1973) show that the protein moiety in the two pig LDL fractions are probably identical.

Results in 5 studies pre- and post-hepatectomy are summarized in Table 6. Each animal served as its own control. The fractional catabolic rate before hepatectomy averaged 0.046 per hour in these five animals and after hepatectomy averaged 0.076 per hour, an increase of well over 50%. At the bottom of the Table are data from three dog studies done in an analogous way. The results were the same in the sense that the post-hepatectomy disappearance curve was monoexponential and the calculated fractional catabolic rate was increased. The increase in fractional catabolic rate after hepatectomy was even more marked, over 100%.

During the hepatectomy studies in swine, we measured total LDL protein concentration as well as LDL protein radioactivity. As shown in Table 7, both the radioactivity of the injected labeled LDL and the total LDL protein concentration fell at the same rate. In other words, the specific radioactivity of the LDL did not change significantly even though as much as 50 to 75% of the total LDL had disappeared by the end of the study. Not shown here, LDL cholesterol levels fell comparably. This finding validates the use of the ^{125}I-labeled LDL as a suitable tracer for circulating LDL. Another conclusion is that fractional catabolic rate is not necessarily a function of LDL concentration. Even though total LDL concentration dropped by a factor of 2 or more, the fractional rate constant did not change. This tends to further validate the findings of Langer, Strober and Levy (1972) as reflecting a true defect in removal rate in Type II patients. They observed an *inverse* correlation between fractional catabolic rate and LDL concentration in different patients. The question arose as to which was cause and which was effect. The present results suggest that LDL concentration per se does *not* affect fractional catabolic rate.

Table 6. Comparison of **fractional** catabolic rates of LDL before and after hepatoectomy in swine

		FCR before	FCR after
		$(hour^{-1})$	$(hour^{-1})$
Swine		0.047	0.070
		0.044	0.063
		0.047	0.077
		0.047	0.070
		0.044	0.101
	Mean $\pm$ SEM (n=5)	0.046 $\pm$ 0.001	0.076 $\pm$ 0.006
Dogs	Mean $\pm$ SEM (n=3)	0.030 $\pm$ 0.001	0.062 $\pm$ 0.001

(Data of Sniderman, Carew, Chandler and Steinberg, 1973; Steinberg, Carew, Chandler and Sniderman, 1973)

Table 7. Comparison of rates of disappearance for ^{125}I-LDL and of total LDL protein in five hepatectomized swine

Half-life of plasma radioactivity	Half-life for decrease in LDL protein
(hours)	(hours)
9.9	9.6
11.0	11.4
9.0	9.3
9.8	10.2
6.9	7.2

(Data of Sniderman, Carew, Chandler and Steinberg, 1973; Steinberg, Carew, Chandler and Sniderman, 1973)

Another conclusion that can be drawn is that, at least under the conditions of our experiment, little or no LDL was being contributed to the plasma by any extrahepatic tissue. This is not necessarily in conflict with the evidence that the intestine *can* produce VLDL and, from it presumably, LDL under some circumstances. These animals were fasted overnight prior to the study and they, of course, had no biliary flow and therefore no fat absorption was going on.

What can we conclude about LDL catabolism from these findings? At the very least, we can conclude that extrahepatic tissues certainly have some capacity to remove LDL irreversibly from the plasma compartment. In other words, we can conclude that the liver is certainly not the *exclusive* site for LDL catabolism. In fact, the data suggest that LDL removal is primarily a peripheral process.

What does the unexpected *increase* in removal rate after hepatectomy mean? One must first ask whether it only reflects some aspect of the deterioration of an animal deprived of its liver. Every effort was made to maintain these animals in a physiologic state. Blood glucose was maintained by constant infusion, of course, and pO_2 and pCO_2 were held within normal limits as was total blood volume and hematocrit over the period of study. The animals survived up to 24 hours and no data were used beyond the point when blood pressure could not be maintained within normal limits. Nevertheless, the possibility that the derangement responsible for the increased catabolic rate is related to some nonphysiologic process remains. For example, is there accumulation of some plasma component that destabilizes lipoproteins? Speaking against this is the fact that the catabolic rate was constant from the very beginning of the study. If we were dealing with some progressive change following hepatectomy, one might have anticipated that the catabolic rate would start close to the normal value and progressively increase. This was not observed. Furthermore, when labeled plasma from a hepatectomized pig was injected into an intact pig, the Phase II half-life was normal, showing that the LDL was not irreversibly damaged in some way. Finally, our preliminary studies show that *H*DL protein and albumin do not fall acutely after hepatectomy.

If we accept for the moment the possibility that the increased catabolic rate is a reflection of the loss of a function normally carried out by the liver, we can speculate about the possible mechanisms involved. These speculations may be justified since they do in fact suggest experimental approaches. One is looking for some hepatic function that prolongs the lifetime of the LDL molecule. The scheme shown in Fig. 5 may help us discuss the possibilities. We can visualize two (or more) populations of LDL molecules — possibly a continuous spectrum of molecules — in which one category (LDL_1) has a half-life like that seen in intact animals and the other (LDL_2) has a much shorter half-life, like that seen in hepatectomized animals. Is it possible that LDL generated from VLDL (or directly secreted by the liver if that occurs) picks up lipid from the periphery and normally delivers that lipid back to the liver? If the liver were unavailable to serve as an unloading point, is it possible that this lipid-enriched LDL might have a shorter half-life in the plasma? For example, the mechanism by which sterol is mobilized from tissues and taken to the liver for ultimate disposal has not been identified. The work of Glomset and Norum (1973) on LCAT has let to a logical hypothesis on this score. While LCAT prefers *H*DL as a primary substrate, its action leads in turn to compositional changes in other lipoprotein fractions. LDL might be one such vehicle and the short half-life of LDL in the hepatectomized animals could be rationalized on such a basis. It is equally possible that phospholipid or triglyceride is being picked up as well as or in addition to cholesterol. Thus, the loss of the liver as the presumed ultimate source of LCAT or as the site for modification of circulating LDL may be important. Finally, the inverse hypothesis could also be entertained, namely, that LDL is constantly being recirculated throug the liver where it picks up lipids and that the absence of that recycling leads to the short half-life observed. Undoubtedly, other explanations can be put forward. The two that I have suggested are testable and we are testing them.

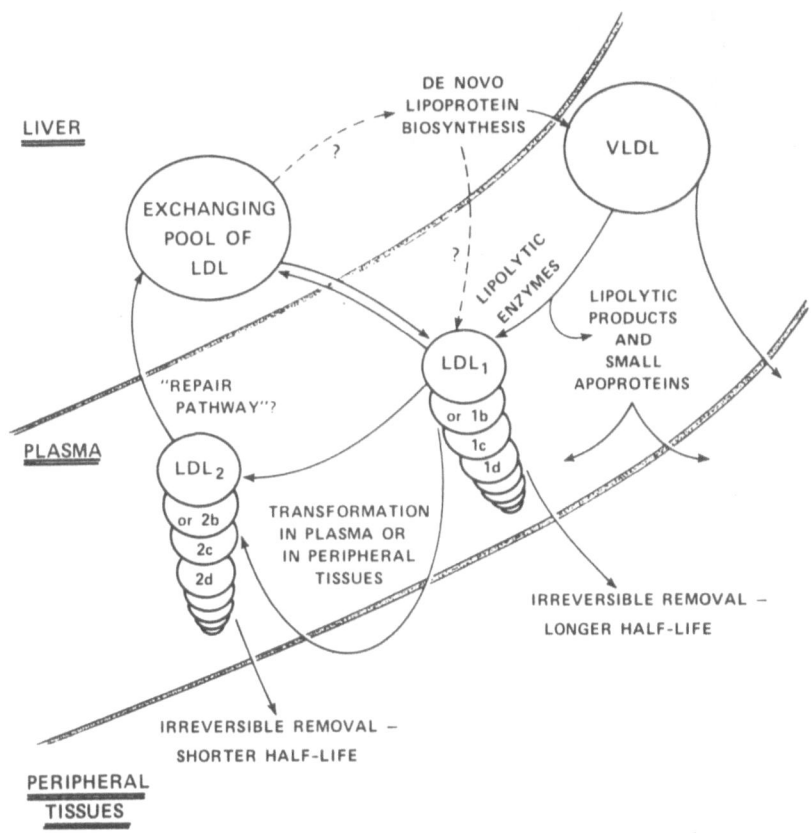

LIVER

DE NOVO
LIPOPROTEIN
BIOSYNTHESIS

VLDL

EXCHANGING
POOL OF
LDL

LIPOLYTIC
ENZYMES

LIPOLYTIC
PRODUCTS
AND
SMALL
APOPROTEINS

LDL₁

or 1b

1c

1d

"REPAIR
PATHWAY"?

PLASMA

LDL₂

or 2b

2c

2d

TRANSFORMATION
IN PLASMA OR
IN PERIPHERAL
TISSUES

IRREVERSIBLE REMOVAL –
LONGER HALF-LIFE

IRREVERSIBLE REMOVAL –
SHORTER HALF-LIFE

PERIPHERAL
TISSUES

Figure 5. Schematic representation of one possible hypothesis to explain the more
rapid disappearance of LDL in hepatectomized animals. LDL is considered to arise
primarily from breakdown of VLDL. The primary product (LDL₁) is shown undergoing
an unspecified transformation, possibly pick-up of cholesterol or other lipids
from peripheral tissues, that converts it to a molecule in the second population.
The second population under normal conditions reenters the liver and is modified
to the LDL₁ form once again. In the absence of the liver, the LDL that has been
modified in the periphery, being unable to traverse the "repair pathway" has a
shorter half-life in the plasma compartment

HDL Catabolism

Finally, let me review some recent work on HDL catabolism in the rat carried out
by Roheim, Rachmilewitz and the Steins in Jerusalem (Roheim et al., 1971; Rachmilewitz et al., 1972). They used ^{125}I-labeled HDL preparations screened biologically by passage through a primary recipient and then transfused into a second
recipient. As shown in Fig. 6, beyond 2 to 3 hours the disappearance was mono-
exponential. Whether there is some initial equilibration with extravascular
spaces during the first couple of hours is not entirely clear. The mean half-life
for the first-order disappearance was 10.5 hours. During the disappearance of
labeled HDL there was little or no change in the distribution of radioactivity
among serum fractions, over 90% remaining in the HDL, confirming that there is
no conversion of HDL to LDL and no sizable conversion to VLDL.

Their animals were sacrificed in groups at various time intervals after injection
and the results at 4 hours and at 12 hours are summarized in Table 8. The results
are expressed as percentage of injected dose recovered per gram of tissue. More

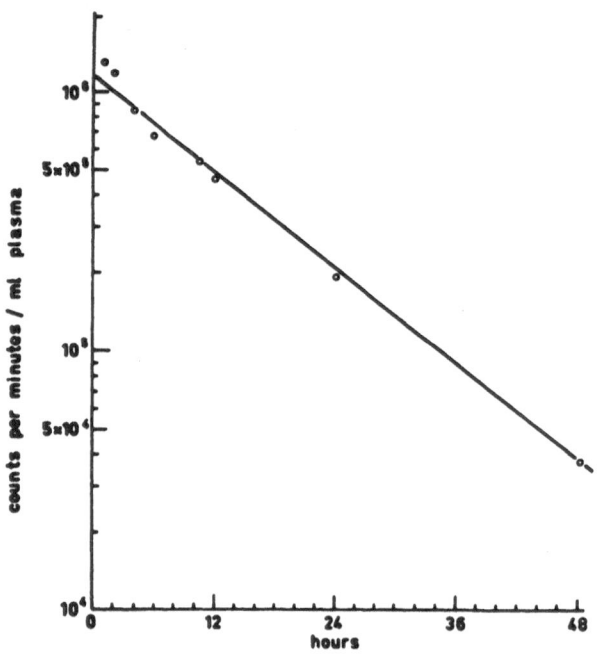

Figure 6. Time course of the disappearance of ^{125}I-HCL from the blood stream of rats (mean values for three studies) (Data of Roheim et al., 1971)

Table 8. Tissue distribution of [125]I[a] after injection of ^{125}I-HDL into rats

Tissue	Percentage of injected dose/gram tissue	
	at 4 hours	at 12 hours
Liver	2.1	1.5
Small intestine	0.6	0.7
Heart	0.9	0.8
Lung	0.9	0.8
Kidney	1.2	0.9
Spleen	2.1	2.0
Stomach	0.6	0.5
Muscle	0.3	0.2

[a]85-93% trichloroacetic acid-precipitable.

(Data of Roheim, Rachmilewitz, Stein and Stein, 1971)

than 85% of the recovered radioacitvity was still precipitable by trichloroacetic acid. The liver and the spleen showed the highest concentrations of radioactivity. In view of its size, the liver accounted for the largest amount in any organ although it is difficult to assess the importance of the muscle, its mass being so huge. The radioactivity in the liver, studied autoradiographically, was predominantly in parenchymal cells, almost none being found in the sinusoidal spaces and only a small percentage in Kupffer cells. Although most of the radioactivity was precipitable with trichloroacetic acid, only a third or less was recognized by antibody against HDL initially, and even less was immunochemically competent at later times, showing that protein degradation was proceeding.

These results demonstrate nicely that HDL catabolism is occurring in the liver. It is less certain what fraction of the *total* HDL catabolism is accounted for by the liver. Every tissue examined contained radioactivity although at lower concentrations than the liver. Of course, the steady-state concentration in a tissue need not be a reliable guide to the rate at which that tissue is degrading the protein in question, so the presence of label in other tissues need not reflect irreversible degradation there. Our preliminary studies in hepatectomized pigs at any rate would support their interpretation that liver is the major site of HDL breakdown.

Concluding Remarks

I have tried to veview some of the highlights of recent research on lipoprotein catabolism. Obviously, the review is incomplete. I should note particularly the omission of more than passing reference to LCAT. The role of this enzyme in lipoprotein metabolism is obviously of great importance. The work of Glomset and Norum and their coworkers on patients with LCAT deficiency makes this evident. Dr. Glomset and Dr. Norum have recently published an excellent and complete review of the subject (1973) and I have taken that as my justification for limiting discussion of LCAT since something had to be deleted.

The significant advances in lipoprotein structure and in characterization of enzymes modifying lipoprotein structure seem to be revealing an ever increasing complexity of the system in which we are interested. While this makes life difficult in some ways and is discouraging in some respects, one has the distinct feeling that a pattern is emerging and that the schemes we are able to draw four years from now will represent a much closer approximation to the true picture even if those we draw today are not. It is to be hoped that this basic information will be of vital importance in elucidating the defects in inherited hyperlipoproteinemias, in devising interventions designed to control plasma lipoprotein levels and in so doing control the development of atherosclerosis.

COMPARATIVE ELECTROPHORETIC PROFILES OF SERUM LIPOPROTEINS

Charles E. Day and Catherine Alexander

Reduction of hyperlipoproteinemias is accepted almost universally as one way to retard atherogenesis. An enormous research and development effort is expended each year in the search for hypolipidemic drugs. Rats or mice are generally used in the primary screening and subsequent follow-up testing for hypolipoproteinemic agents. But the lipoproteins of both rats and mice are quite different quantitatively and qualitatively from human lipoproteins. Clearly better animal models simulating the human lipoprotein spectrum are needed for atherosclerosis research, especially in the pharmaceutical industry. The primary requirement for such an animal model is an elevated low density lipoprotein (LDL) level and a high LDL/ HDL ratio. Secondary considerations include size, cost, and ease of handling and maintenance of the animal. Size and cost are major considerations for drug screening, since compounds are usually available in only very small quantities and large numbers of animals are required. The purpose of this investigation was to survey the electrophoretic profiles of serum lipoproteins of several animals in an effort to discover a better animal model for human serum lipoproteins suitable for drug evaluations.

Materials and Methods

Animals were obtained from colonies maintained at The Upjohn Company, from commercial suppliers of laboratory and/or exotic animals, or from the wild in Michigan. In a few cases serum was obtained from commercial suppliers of animal sera or the slaughterhouse. Agarose gel electrophoresis was performed on fresh animal sera by a method previously described (Hatch et al., 1973). Slides were stained overnight in Oil Red O. Serum cholesterol analyses were performed by an automated ferric chloride procedure (Block et al., 1966). Electrophoretic mobilities relative to a bromphenol blue albumin reference were measured to the nearest 0.01 mm with a microcomparator. Semi-quantitative densitometric scans were made with a Beckman Analytrol® equipped with a Microzone® attachment or a Quik-Scan® densitometer from Helena Laboratories.

Results and Discussion

Agarose gel electrophoresis with subsequent lipid staining was performed on the sera of 34 animal species (Table 1) with representatives from each of the major classes of vertebrates. Although it is not possible to be sure without subsequent isolation and electrophoresis, it was assumed that the slowest moving lipoprotein band (with a mobility comparable to human LDL) was LDL and that the fastest migrating lipoprotein was HDL. LDL/HDL ratios were calculated on this basis. The ratios are probably artificially high because of the more intense staining of lipoproteins in the LDL band with a higher proportion of non-polar lipids. Relative electrophoretic mobilities were not a suitable means to categorize lipoproteins.

Only five species had a LDL/HDL ratio of 1.0 or greater and a cholesterol greater than 100 mg/dl. These were the human, pig, opossum, garter snake and green snake (Fig. 1-3). The reptiles are especially interesting because the LDL/ HDL ratio in the more than one dozen individuals examined were always much greater than one. In the garter snake there is much individual variation (Fig. 3). This variation could be explained by possible differences in sex or dietary

Table 1. Serum cholesterol levels and lipoprotein ratios in thirty-four species of vertebrates

Common name	Scientific name	Sex	Serum cholesterol (mg/dl)	LDL/HDL Ratio
Mongolian gerbil	Meriones unguiculatus	M	104	0.58
Chinese hamster	Cricetulus griseus	M	180	0.23
Golden hamster	Mesocricetus auratus	M	112	0.60
White-tailed antelope squirrel	Ammospermophilus leucurns	–	182	0.59
Woodchuck	Marmota monax	–	108	0.54
Guinea pig	Cavis porcellus	M	27	1.86
Rat	Rattus norvegicus Upj:TUC(SD)spf	M	123	0.45
Mouse	Mus musculus Upj:TUC(ICR)spf	M	120	0.20
Goat	Capra hircus	–	80	0.82
Sheep	Ovic aries	–	60	0.72
Cow	Bos taurus	M	96	0.32
Human	Homo sapiens	M	216	1.88
Rhesus monkey	Macaca mulatta	M	136	0.59
Pig	Sus domesticus	F	–	2.57
Dog	Canis familiaris	M	114	0.26
Cat	Felis domesticus	–	108	0.60
Opossum	Didelphis virginiana	M	198	1.00
Rabbit NZW	Oryctolagus cuniculus	M	57	1.44
Black-tailed jack rabbit	Lepus californicus	–	19	<1
Salamander	Ambystoma tigrinum	–	47	>1
Frog	Rana pipiens	F	72	>1
Turtle	Chrysemys picta marginata	F	75	1.17
Common garter snake	Thamnophis sirtalis sirtalis	–	122	10.35
Keeled green snake	Ophreodrys aestivus aestivus	–	618	5.06
Trout	Salmo trutta	–	–	<1
Carp	Cyprinus carpio	–	176	0.14
Dogfish	Amia calva	F	77	0.47
Japanese quail	Coturnix coturnix japonica	M	216	0.45
White Carneau pigeon	Columba livia	M	362	0.50
Ringneck pheasant	Phasianus colchicus	M	155	0.48
White Leghorn chicken	Gallus domesticus	M	104	0.45
Goose	Anser anser	M	203	0.59
Turkey	Meleagris gallopavo	–	125	0.55
Duck	Anas platyrhynchos	M	144	0.26

history since both these factors were unknown for the individuals used from this species. Although the data is still preliminary, reptiles appear interesting enough to warrant more detailed studies on lipoprotein structure and metabolism and their suitability as models for human hyperlipoproteinemias. Our data on snakes is also in agreement with that of Mills and Taylaur (1971) who found very high levels of LDL in a water snake and grass snake with a composition not unlike human LDL! Porcine lipoproteins have been well characterized and are reasonably similar to human lipoproteins. However, the size, expense of maintaining, and difficulty of handling swine, even miniature ones, precluse their large scale use, especially for pre-clinical evaluation of new drugs. Lipoproteins of small marsupials have received practically no attention.

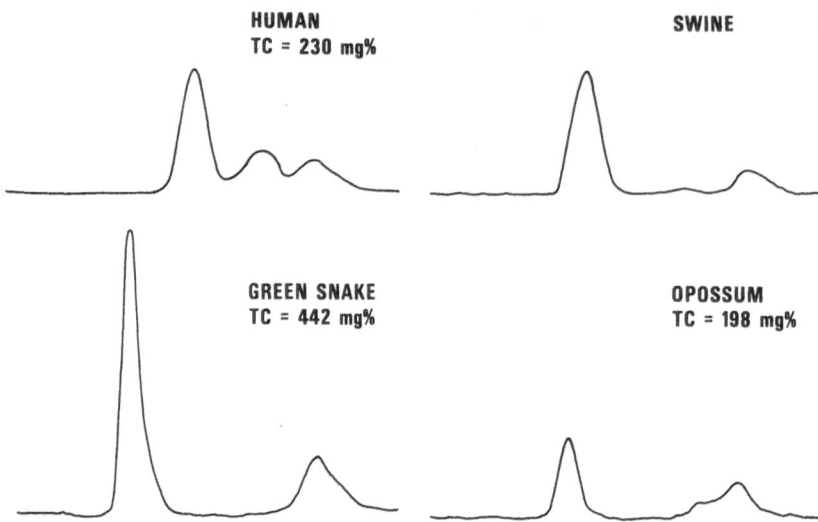

Figure 1. Lipoprotein electrophoretograms from the sera of three species most closely simulating the human pattern. TC = serum total cholesterol

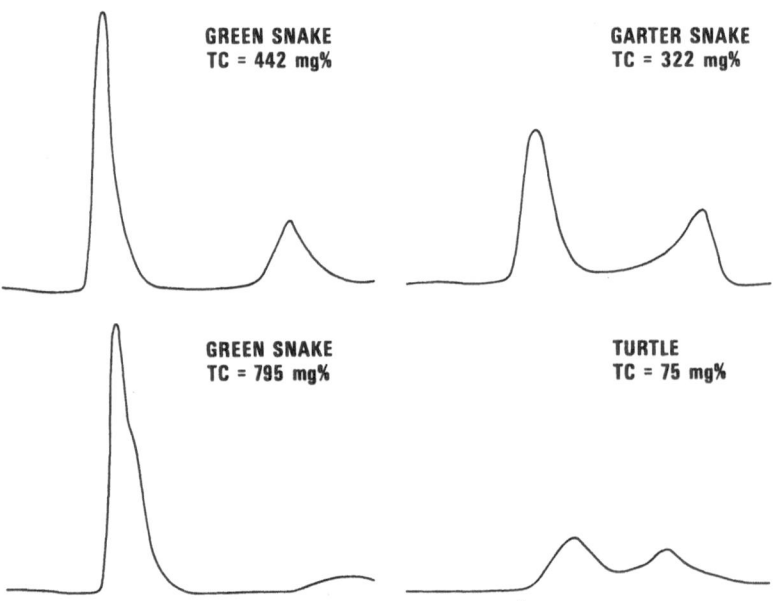

Figure 2. Serum lipoprotein patterns from three species of reptiles. TC = serum total cholesterol

Although a few species with high LDL levels were discovered, there is no evidence to indicate that these animals develop premature atherosclerosis. Even if they develop no spontaneous lesions their usefulness to atherosclerosis research should not be overlooked. It is quite possible to have an animal with a lipoprotein system identical in structure and metabolism to the human system, which still develops no atherosclerosis because of possible differences in the structure and metabolism of its arteries or differences in other factors such as hemodynamics. In the snake for example, there is a virtual absence of branching in the arterial tree, the aorta is not very muscular and is very thin walled, and the blood pressure is probably low because of the low resistance to flow. Factors such as these, and not the lipoproteins, will probably determine its susceptibility to atherosclerosis. However, if the lipoprotein system simulates that of humans, then these animals may be quite useful in the pre-clinical evaluation of hypolipoproteinemic agents.

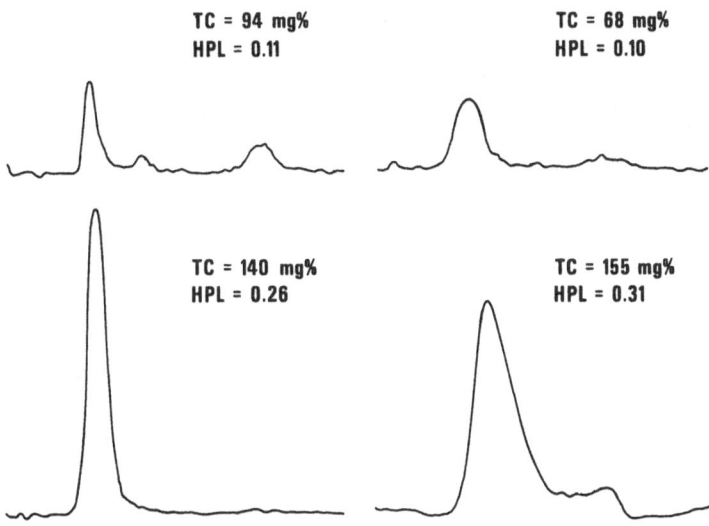

Figure 3. Variation in the serum lipoprotein patterns from several individuals common garter snakes. TC = serum total cholesterol, HPL = heparin precipitating lipoproteins

STUDIES ON APOLIPOPROTEIN D
A NEW PROTEIN MOIETY OF THE HUMAN PLASMA LIPOPROTEIN SYSTEM*

W. McConathy and P. Alaupovic

Studies on the human plasma lipoprotein system have demonstrated its antigenic heterogeneity (Aladjem et al., 1957). The basis for this heterogeneity has been clarified by the isolation and characterization of several antigenically distinct polypeptides: A-I, A-II, C-I, C-II, C-III and LP-B (Shore and Shore, 1968; Brown et al., 1969; Alaupovic et al., 1972). A previously uncharacterized determinant designated as "thin-line" polypeptide occurs primarily in HDL (Ayrault-Jarrier et al., 1963) but its presence has also been demonstrated in LDL (Lee and Alaupovic, 1970) and VHDL (Alaupovic et al., 1966). When tested by double diffusion analysis, HDL gives two precipitin lines with anti-HDL_3: a thin precipitin line nearer the antigen well due to the "thin-line" polypeptide and a broad precipitin line nearer the antibody well due to LP-A (Alaupovic et al., 1972). This report describes the isolation and partial characterization of the antigenic determinant previously designated as "thin-line" polypeptide.

One liter of pooled human plasma was utilized as starting material for each isolation. The HDL_3 (d = 1.12-1.27 g/ml) was isolated by standard ultracentrifugal procedures, dialyzed and totally delipidized with chloroform-methanol (2:1, v/v). The apoHDL was solubilized and applied to hydroxylapatite-cellulose column (2:1, v/v) in 0.001 M K_2HPO_4, pH 8.0, as previously described (McConathy and Alaupovic, 1973). The fraction eluted with 0.001 M K_2HPO_4, pH 8.0, was rechromatographed under identical conditions until a single band was obtained by polyacrylamide gel electrophoresis. The fraction from hydroxylapatite cellulose column was chromatographed on Sephadex G-100. A major symmetrical peak was eluted from the Sephadex column with 2 M acetic acid. Polyacrylamide gel electrophoresis of the isolated major fraction (Fig. 1) gave a single band with a mobility intermediate between the bands corresponding to A-II and C-II. This band did not correspond to any known apolipoprotein or polypeptide bands.

The major fraction from Sephadex column reacted only with antiserum to HDL_3 and antiserum to the isolated Sephadex fraction. This precipitin line was identical with that of the "thin-line" polypeptide in intact HDL_3 (Fig. 2). The antiserum to the isolated polypeptide reacted only with its corresponding antigen and not with A-I, A-II, C-I, C-II, C-III, LP-B or albumin. It was concluded that the isolated polypeptide corresponded to the antigenic determinant designated as "thin-line" polypeptide.

Amino acid analysis of the isolated "thin-line" polypeptide demonstrated the presence of all the common amino acids. The composition was different from all previously characterized apolipoprotein polypeptides (Shore and Shore, 1968; Brown et al., 1969). Carboxypeptidase A and B analyses of the isolated polypeptide indicated leucine as C-terminal amino acid. Preliminary carbohydrate analyses indicated the presence of mannose, galactose, glucose, glucosamine and sialic acids; they accounted for approximately 12-15% of the dry weight of the "thin-line" polypeptide.

---

*This study was supported in part by Grant HL-6221 and HL-7005 from the U.S. Public Health Service and by the resources of the Oklahoma Medical Research Foundation.

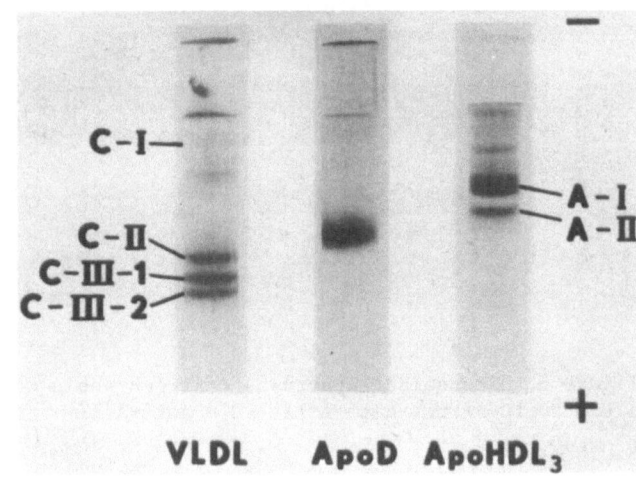

Figure 1. Basic polyacrylamide gel electrophoresis patterns of VLDL, ApoD ("thin-line" polypeptide) and ApoHDL₃

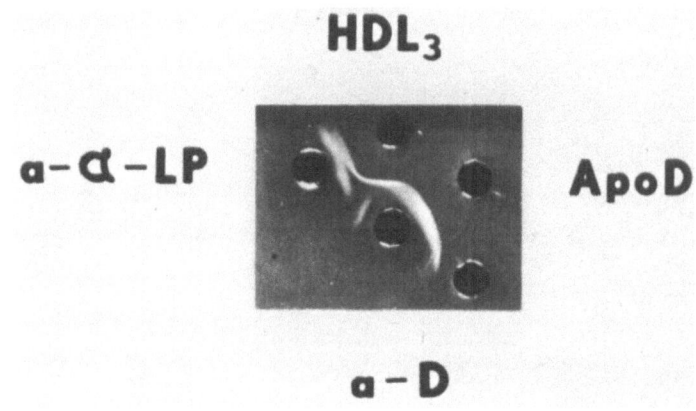

Figure 2. Double diffusion analyses in 1% agarose gel of antiserum to ApoD (a-D) and reactions of identity of antigens and antobodies to ApoD. a = anti

"Thin-line" polypeptide was detectable in fresh plasma or serum with anti HDL₃ or anti "thin-line", both in the presence or absence of 5,5'-dithiobis (2-nitro-benzoic acid), an inhibitor of lecithin:cholesterol acyltransferase (Stokke and Norum, 1971). Immunoelectrophoretic analysis of fresh plasma or serum demonstrated the non-identity of "thin-line" polypeptide and LP-A (Fig. 3). It was also shown that the mobilities of LP-A and "thin-line" polypeptide were different. The non-identity of LP-A and "thin-line" polypeptide has already been demonstrated by double diffusion (Lee and Alaupovic, 1970). Positive Oil Red-O staining of the "thin-line" immunoprecipitin line clearly indicated the lipoprotein nature of this polypeptide.

Fractionation of neuraminidase-treated HDL₃ on a Concanavalin A-Sepharose 4B column resulted in separation of "thin-line" polypeptide from LP-A and LP-C.

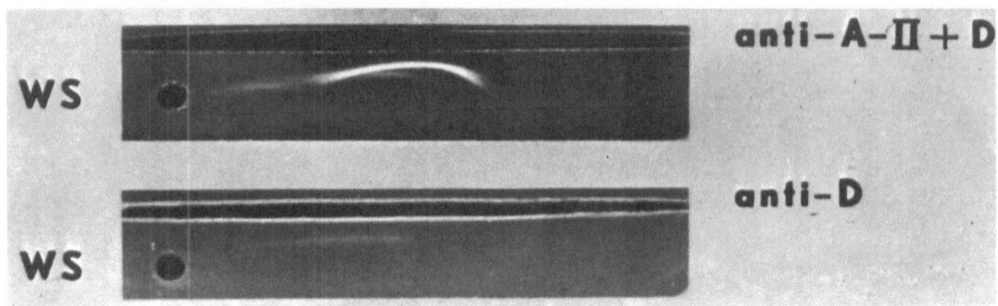

Figure 3. Immunoelectrophoresis of fresh whole serum in 1% agarose gel. WS = fresh whole serum, anti-A-II + D = anti-A-II + anti-ApoD, and anti-D = anti-ApoD

These results indicate the lipoprotein nature of "thin-line" polypeptide and its occurrence as a distinct lipoprotein species. According to the ABC nomenclature (Alaupovic, 1972), this protein is designated as apolipoprotein D (ApoD) and its corresponding lipoprotein(s) as lipoprotein family D (LP-D).

CHARACTERIZATION OF LOW DENSITY LIPOPROTEINS FROM PATIENTS HOMOZYGOUS FOR FAMILIAL HYPERBETALIPOPROTEINAEMIA

Gervase L. Mills and C. Emlyn Taylaur

At the last Atherosclerosis Symposium, Slack and Mills (1970) described the unusual composition of the LDL of patients suffering from familial hyperbetalipoproteinaemia (referred to below as LDL-H), the details of which are included in
Table 1. Attention was also drawn to the fact that this composition would be expected to result in a molecule of higher density than normal, whereas LDL-H
behaves like a substance with either an abnormally low density, or an abnormally
high molecular weight. We now propose to report the results of further physical
and chemical studies which habe been made on the LDL of subjects who are homozygous for this disease. These were of both sexes, in the age range from 10 to
20 years, and were classified by the criteria laid down by Nevin and Slack (1968).
Typical physical characteristics of the LDL from these patients are compared with
the corresponding fraction from control subjects in Table 1. From this it appears
that the molecules of LDL-H have a slightly higher average molecular weight, and
a somewhat lower hydrated density than those of the normal LDL. Moreover, this
combination approximates closely to the values calculated for a normal LDL of
the same flotation rate. The LDL-H are therefore not abnormally dense molecules
of high molecular weight, and their high flotation rate must be the consequence
of some structural or compositional change which counterbalances the effect to be
expected from their low content of triglyceride.

Evidence of an effect of this kind has been found in a study made in collaboration
with a group of physicists at Queen Elizabeth College in London, which suggests
that LDL-H may have a bigger dielectric decrement than normal (Grant et al., 1972).
This is illustrated by the values quoted in Table 1. Since the molecules of both
the normal and the anomalous LDL have been shown by electron microscopy to be
spherical, this finding can be interpreted as an indication that LDL-H binds an
unusually large amount of water, which tends to normalise the hydrated density of
these molecules.

In an attempt to detect any abnormality of composition which might offer an explanation for an increase in hydration, or some change in molecular structure,
we have subjected the LDL-H to more detailed chemical analyses, as follows.

When LDL-H is separated by sequential ultracentrifugation into fractions of
narrow density range, their subsequent analysis gives evidence of three components
of mean hydrated density of about 1.015, 1.03 and 1.045 g/ml respectively. By
comparison with the corresponding fractions from the LDL of healthy control subjects, the first two have an abnormally low proportion to triglyceride, with a
raised cholesteryl ester. By contrast, the third fraction, which accounts for only
about 9% of the total LDL, has a normal composition. In all the fractions of
LDL-H, the proportions of unesterified cholesterol, phospholipid and protein are
indistinguishable from those of the control fractions (Table 2). In the familial
hyperlipoproteinaemic therefore, it appears that 90% of the normal LDL may be
replaced by relatively low density components in which the triglyceride content
may be as low as 1 - 2%.

The investigation of the constituent parts of LDL-H has yielded the following
additional information:

1. the fatty acid patterns of the lipid esters in the LDL-H, as determined by gas
chromatography, do not differ significantly from those of controls. There is thus
no evidence to suggest that either the presence of an uncommon fatty acid, or an

Table 1. The composition and physical properties of LDL from patients homozygous for familial hyperbetalipoproteinaemia compared with the corresponding lipoproteins from control subjects. Five patients were studies, but not by all methods in each case

		LDL-II (Homozygous FH)	LDL (Control)
Cholesteryl ester		43.2[a]	39.5 ± 2.3[a]
Unesterified cholesterol		11.7	9.0 ± 0.4
Triglyceride		2.0	7.3 ± 1.4
Phospholipid		20.6	21.2 ± 1.0
Protein		22.6	22.4 ± 1.3
Hydrated density	(g/ml)	1.0250	1.0283
$S_{20,w}$	$(\times 10^{13})$	4.9	5.3
$D_{20,w}$	$(\times 10^{7})$	1.81	1.91
Molecular weight	$(\times 10^{-6})$	3.8	3.3
Dielectric decrement	(ml/g)	127.7	107.8 ± 1.73
Hydration	(g/g)	0.14	0.044 ± 0.024
Lecithin		61.3[b]	67.4[b]
Sphingomyelin		31.9	24.6
Lysolecithin		2.0	2.6
Phosphatidylethanolamine		4.0	3.2
Phosphatidylserine		1.0	2.2
Hexoses		2.4[c]	3.1[c]
Amino-sugars		1.2	1.6
Sialic acid		0.9	1.2

[a] Composition is expressed as a percentage of total lipoprotein.

[b] Lipid phosphorus expressed as a percentage of total phosphorus.

[c] Expressed as a weight percentage of apo-lipoprotein.

unusual proportion of polyunsaturated acids could be responsible for the structural modification of the lipoprotein.

2. the amino-acid composition of the protein moiety obtained by extraction of the LDL-H with ethanol/ether is almost identical with that of control LDL, and with that reported for LDL by Levy et al. (1967).
This confirms earlier immunological evidence that the normal and the abnormal LDL have a common protein.

3. it can be shown by two dimensional immunophoresis that the LDL-H contains both the B and C apo-lipoprotein in proportions which fall within the range observed for normal subjects. The properties of the LDL-H cannot therefore be ascribed to an unusually high proportion of the C component.

Table 2. Weight percentage of subfractions of LDL from a patient homozygous for familial hyperbetalipoproteinaemia and a control subject. The density ranges quoted for these fractions have not been corrected for re-distribution of salt in the ultracentrifuge

Density range of subfraction (g/ml)	LDL-H (Homozygous FH)					LDL (Control)				
	CE	UC	TG	PL	Pro	CE	UC	TG	PL	Pro
1.020 - 1.030	42.4	10.4	5.6	20.9	20.9	37.7	9.1	11.2	21.1	20.1
1.030 - 1.040	47.0	11.4	2.0	20.8	18.6	40.7	9.6	7.1	22.5	20.2
1.040 - 1.050	46.1	11.0	2.4	21.4	19.2	41.1	8.9	5.8	23.1	21.1
1.050 - 1.063	40.8	10.2	6.7	19.0	23.2	42.1	8.8	6.9	20.3	21.9

4. although the proportions of the minor phospholipids have been shown by thin-layer chromatography to be the same in LDL-H as in the normal lipoproteins, the proportion of lecithin may be somewhat less, and that of sphingomyelin correspondingly more than the average values for control subjects (Table 1). However, not only are the observations few in number, but they also fall within the range observed for normal LDL and cannot be regarded as definitely abnormal.

5. analysis of LDL-H from one subject disclosed a normal amount of amino-sugar and sialic acid in the apo-lipoprotein, whereas the hexose content was diminished by an amount equivalent to 1 residue per mole of protein of molecular weight 27000 (Table 1).

Although the significance of the two last studies needs to be established by additional observations, it is evident that the differences in chemical composition between LDL-H and normal LDL are very small and, at least when considered individually, do not provide a convincing explanation for the anomalous density of the former. Thus the available evidence appears to favour the hypothesis that LDL-H is an abnormal arrangement of chemically normal constituents.

LIPOPROTEIN ABNORMALITIES ASSOCIATED WITH TYPE III HYPERLIPO-PROTEINAEMIA

Joan Slack and G. L. Mills

The diagnosis of Type III hyperlipoproteinaemia presents little problem in patients with primary hyperlipoproteinaemia who are found to have beta migrating lipoprotein of density less than 1.006, especially if palmar xanthomata are present at the time of clinical examination. However, careful and repeated observation of 24 index patients, who have exhibited both these criteria on at least one occasion, has lead us to realise that "floating beta" lipoprotein is not always demonstrable in the serum.

Fredrickson et al. (1972) have suggested that total serum cholesterol/triglyceride ratios are helpful in distinguishing patients with Type III hyperlipoproteinaemia from normal, but Hazzard et al. (1973) finding a mean and standard deviation serum cholesterol/triglyceride ratio to be 2.4 ± 0.9 in normal serum, 0.83 ± 0.19 in patients with Type III and $0.85 - 0.37$ in patients with Type IV, concluded that the serum cholesterol/triglyceride ratio clearly distinguishes the Type III patient from the normal but fails to distinguish Type III from Type IV. They concluded that cholesterol/triglyceride ratio in isolated VLDL (Sf 0-20) distinguishes Type III from other types of primary hyperlipoproteinaemia, finding the mean in patients with Type III to be 0.60 ± 0.11 and in patients with Type IV to be 0.27 ± 0.06; however, in their series, the ratio VLDL cholesterol/triglyceride failed to distinguish all Type III patients from the range found in normal sera where the ratio was 0.35 ± 0.08.

The presence or absence of "floating beta" lipoprotein in first degree relatives of Type III index patients is not compatible with any simple Mendelian pattern and since Fredrickson et al. (1972) have found that Type IV hyperlipoproteinaemia may be found more frequently than expected among the relatives of index patients with Type III, it is necessary for further genetic investigation of the Type III abnormality to use quantitative measurements which might distinguish subclinically affected relatives from normal individuals and from those who may exhibit characteristics of other primary hyperlipoproteinaemia states.

We have, therefore, examined the results of repeated biochemical investigations of fasting serum, both during exacerbation and remission, from 24 index patients who have at some time exhibited both "floating beta" lipoprotein and palmar xanthomata in an attempt to determine the best quantitative measurement for use in genetic analysis of families of index patients with Type III hyperlipoproteinaemia.

The following methods have been used:- Measurement of serum cholesterol and triglyceride by the method of Sperry Webb (1950) and Van Handel and Zilversmit (1957) respectively, electrophoresis of lipoproteins on agarose gel by the method of Noble (1968) and analytical ultracentrifugation as described by De Lalla and Gofman (1954).

Fig. 1 shows the Schlieren patterns obtained by analytical ultracentrifugation of serum from a normal female and a female patient with Type III hyperlipoproteinaemia. We have noted the following major differences in the two patterns and have come to recognise these differences as important in distinguishing the Type III pattern from other primary lipoprotein abnormalities, and the normal.

1. There is a concave slope noticeable in the second frame which slopes downwards.

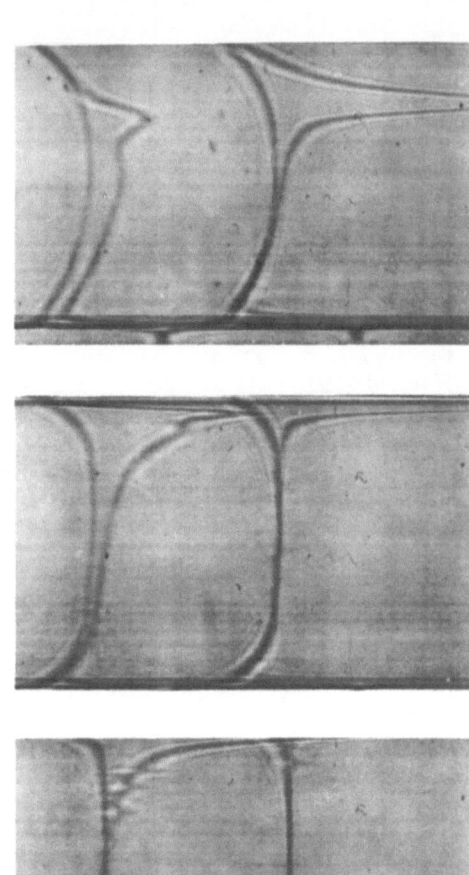

Figure 1. Schlieren patterns of low density lipoproteins taken after centrifugation in d = 1.063 Na Cl at 52,640 rev. per. min. at 0, 6 and 30 mins. after reaching full speed. Upper patterns from female index patient with Type III hyperlipoproteinaemia and lower patterns from female control

2. In the second frame, a small peak appears at the base of the cell.
3. In the third frame, two peaks of a biphasic curve appear.
4. Both these peaks are about the same height.

Fig. 2 shows diagramatically the characteristics of the Schlieren patterns obtained from the 24 controls carefully matched from a population sample with the 24 index patients with Type III hyperlipoproteinaemia.

For quantitative analysis it is necessary to find the best method of expressing the characteristic differences between index patients and other types of hyperlipoproteinaemia by a single quantitative measurement; and we have found by a process of inspection and trial and error that a good and convenient measurement is the ratio:- Sf 0-12/12-20.

As for other lipid measurements, there is a small but distinct advantage in using log. transformation of this value for statistical calculations requiring a normal

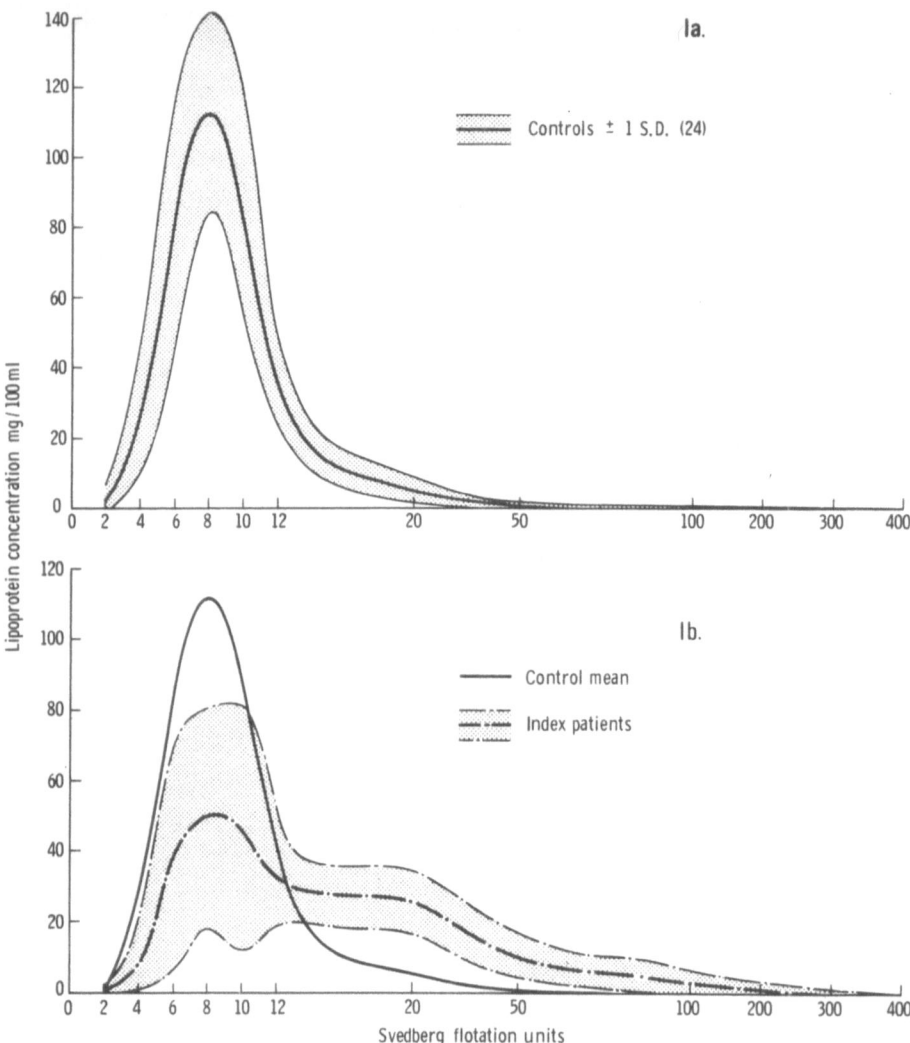

Figure 2. Schematic representation of patterns obtained from analytical ultra-centrifugation of low and very low density lipoproteins. The lipoprotein flota-tion rate in Svedberg units is shown on the horizontal axis. The height of the curve is proportional to the concentration of lipoproteins at each step along the flotation axis
a) from 24 CONTROLS, showing the mean and one standard deviation above and below the mean,
b) from 24 INDEX PATIENTS with Type III hyperlipoproteinaemia showing the mean and one standard deviation above and below the mean. The mean in 24 matched Controls is shown by the solid line

distribution and we have therefore, used the log. transformation of the ratios in order to make comparisons between the groups of patients and controls who are necessarily composed of individuals of variable ages and sex. Standard deviation scores are calculated from the formula:

$$\text{SD score} = \frac{x - \overline{X}_c}{SD_c} .$$

Where $\overline{X}_c$ and SD_c are the expected mean and standard deviation calculated from a large control population and x is the measured value in any individual. The standard deviation score of the large control series is thus 0 ± 1 and the individual standard deviation score is the proportion of one standard deviation above or below zero.

Table 1. Standard deviation scores $\pm$ 1 SD of serum lipid concentrations in Type III and IV hyperlipoproteinaemia

	Type III	Type IV
Numbers	24	15
Serum Cholesterol	2.14 ± 1.75[a,b]	0.66 ± 1.06
Serum Triglycerides	2.53 ± 1.37[a]	2.56 ± 1.25
Log. $\dfrac{\text{Cholesterol}}{\text{Triglycerides}}$	-1.59 ± 0.90[a]	-2.35 ± 1.41
Sf 0 - 12	-2.31 ± 1.71[a,c]	2.55 ± 0.13
Sf 12 - 20	1.50 ± 0.70[a]	1.76 ± 0.19
Log. $Sf \dfrac{0-12}{12-20}$	-3.28 ± 0.99[a,c]	-0.41 ± 0.83

Significance of difference from 0 ± 1.
Significance of difference from Type IV.

[a] $p < .001$ shown.
[b] $p < .01$ shown.
[c] $p < .001$ shown.

Table 1 shows a comparison of standard deviation scores calculated from log. transformation of serum cholesterol, triglycerides and the ratio serum cholesterol/triglycerides, lipoprotein concentrations and the ratio Sf 0-12/12-20 in patients with Types III and IV hyperlipoproteinaemia. Our results are in close agreement with Hazzard et al. (1973) in that for serum cholesterol/triglyceride ratios, there is a significant difference between controls and patients with Type III hyperlipoproteinaemia, but no significant difference between patients with Type III and patients with Type IV hyperlipoproteinaemia. When the standard deviation scores of the ratio log. Sf 0-12/12-20 is used there is a significant difference between the patients with Type III hyperlipoproteinaemia and both controls and patients with Type IV.

When the ratio log. Sf 0-12/12-20 was calculated repeatedly in one patient both in and out of remission, with and without "floating beta" lipoprotein and compared with the ratio log. serum cholesterol/triglycerides, the ratio log Sf 0-12/12-20 remained consistently more than 3 standard deviations below that expected for her age and sex, suggesting that this quantitative measurement was more consistently characteristic of the genetic abnormality associated with Type III hyperlipoproteinaemia and might prove suitable for genetic analysis of families of Tape III index patients.

FLOTATION CHARACTERISTICS OF THE LIPOPROTEIN ACCUMULATED IN THE PLASMA OF TYPE III PATIENTS

J. Patsch and S. Sailer

Lipoprotein typically accumulated in the plasma of type III patients (Lp-III) was isolated quantitatively by means of a rate-zonal ultracentrifugation procedure (Fig. 1).

In order to get information on the flotation properties of Lp-III in the angle-head rotor, sera of type III patients were collected in polyallomer tubes at nonprotein solvent densities (d 1.006, 1.019, 1.025, 1.035, 1.050, and 1.063 resp.). Ultracentrifugation was carried out in type 50 Ti anglehead rotor at 45,000 rpm, 15° C, for 18 hours (1.4×8^{10} g min.). After centrifugation, the top layers were separated from the infranatant by a tubeslicing technique, and separately centrifuged in the zonal rotor (Fig. 2).

Fig. 3 shows the flotation properties of Lp-III and LDL in the anglehead rotor. By these experiments, the proper density for the selective flotation of Lp-III proved to be 1.025.

Fig. 4 demonstrates lipoprotein electrophoresis in agarose gel of type III and type IV plasma, supranatant and infranatant at densities 1.006 and 1.025 respectively. In type III, after density adjustment of the plasma with KBr to a density d 1.025, the top layer revealed a band in the pre-ß position and a second one (Lp-III), with a mobility slower than pre-ß and somewhat faster than ß. This Lp-III band was not found in the top layer of type III plasma at d 1.006. Further, this band was never demonstrable in the top layer of plasmas other than type III at d 1.006 or 1.025.

These data show that the density d 1.025 is optimal for typing of hyperlipoproteinaemias using combined ultracentrifugation in anglehead rotors and agarose-gel electrophoresis.

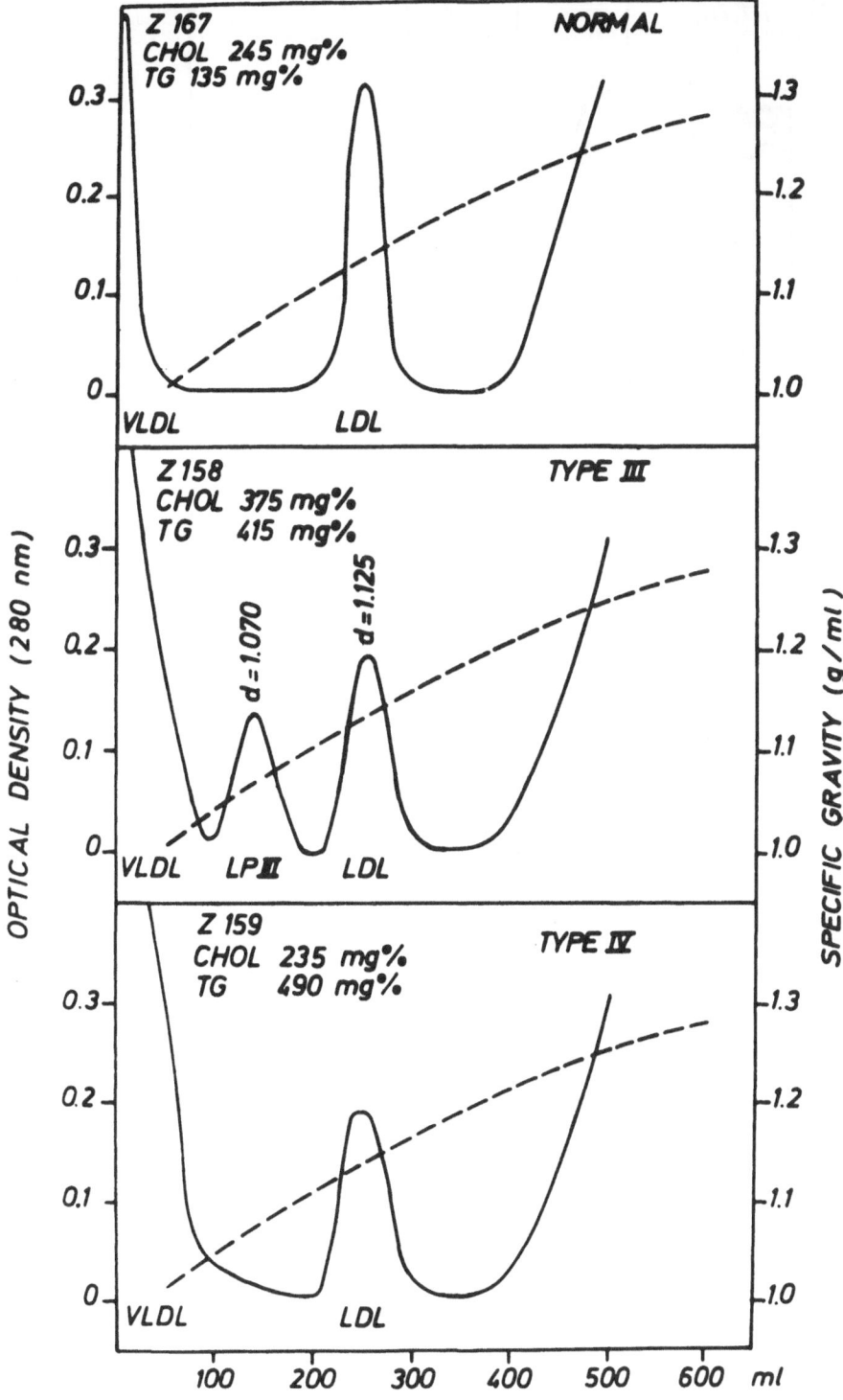

Figure 1. Isolation of LP III by zonal ultracentrifugation

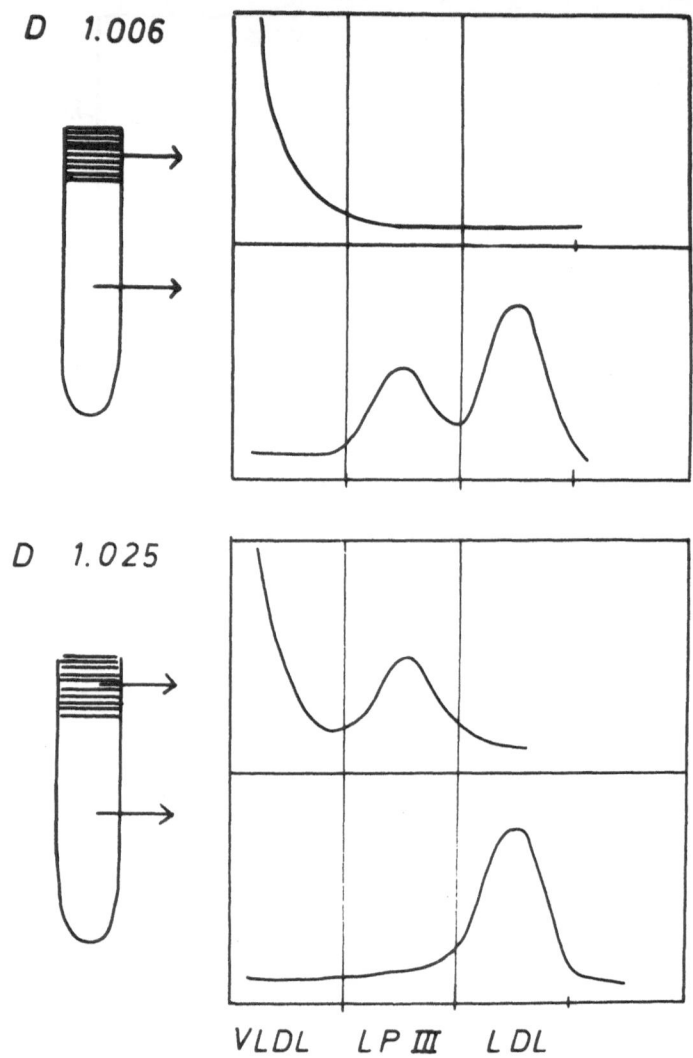

Figure 2. Type III plasma zonal rotor in anglehead T_i-14

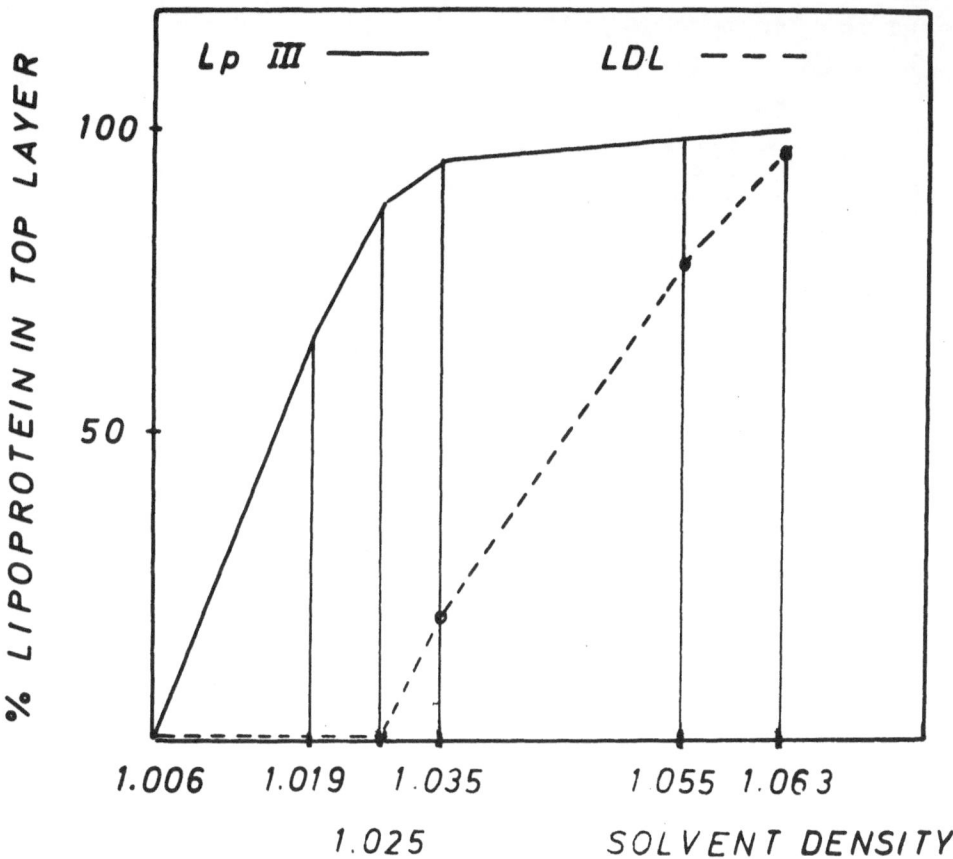

Figure 3. Ultracentrifugation of plasma in anglehead rotors Ti 50/65 (45.000 rpm, 18 hours, 1.4×10^8 $g \cdot min$)

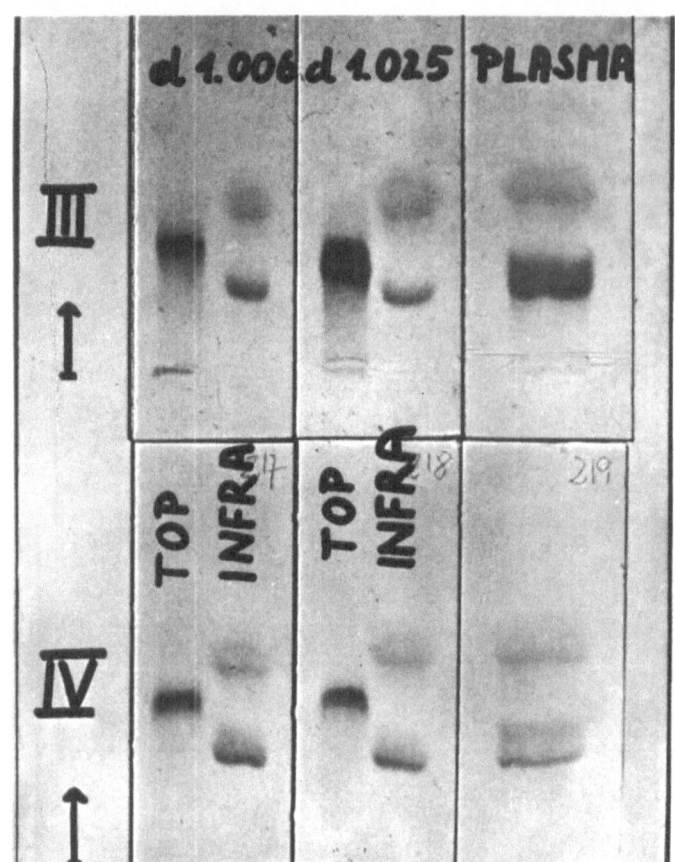

Figure 4. Lipoprotein electrophoresis (agarose gel) of Type III and Type IV plasma, supranatant and infranatant at densities 1.006 and 1.025

LIPOPROTEIN PATTERN IN TYPE III AND TYPE IV PATIENTS DURING PROLONGED FASTING

S. Sailer and J. Patsch

VLDL, "Lp-III", and LDL were isolated quantitatively by means of rate-zonal ultracentrifugation. Apolipoprotein proteins were detected by double immunodiffusion technique using mono-specific antisera to lipoprotein families. In VLDL of type IV and of type III patients, Apo-B and Apo-C were detectable in all instances. The same was true for Lp-III. In LDL before the fasting period only Apo-B was detectable.

Three patients of type III and three patients of type IV have been studied during a starvation period after a fast of 15 hours, 3, and 6 days respectively. Fig. 1 and 2 represent the typical behavior of the lipoprotein density classes d < 1.063. The figures give the concentration in mg/100 ml plasma.

In type IV patients, during starvation, the concentration of VLDL decreases rapidly, some new density classes between VLDL and LDL fractions became detectable, the concentration of LDL increased, Apo-C became detectable also in some LDL fractions (Fig. 1).

In contrast, the VLDL concentration of type III patients decreased slower, the concentration of Lp-III increased and the LDL concentration remained roughly unchanged. Apo-C was detectable during the whole starvation period only in the VLDL and Lp-III fractions (Fig. 2).

These findings support the hypothesis of a defect in conversion of VLDL to LDL in type III patients.

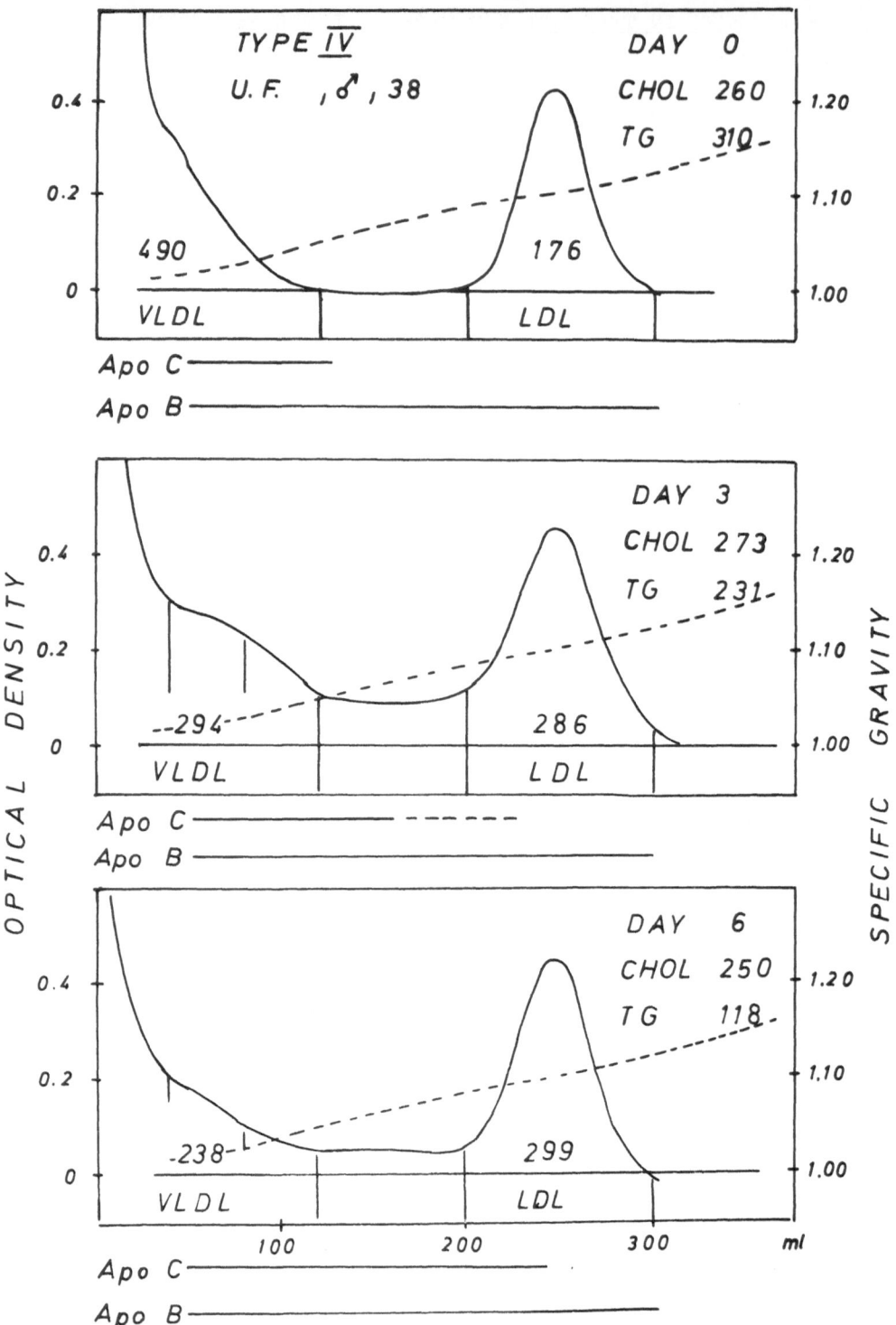

Figure 1. Zonal ultracentrifugation of plasma after fasting for 14 hours, 3 days, and 6 days (type IV patients)

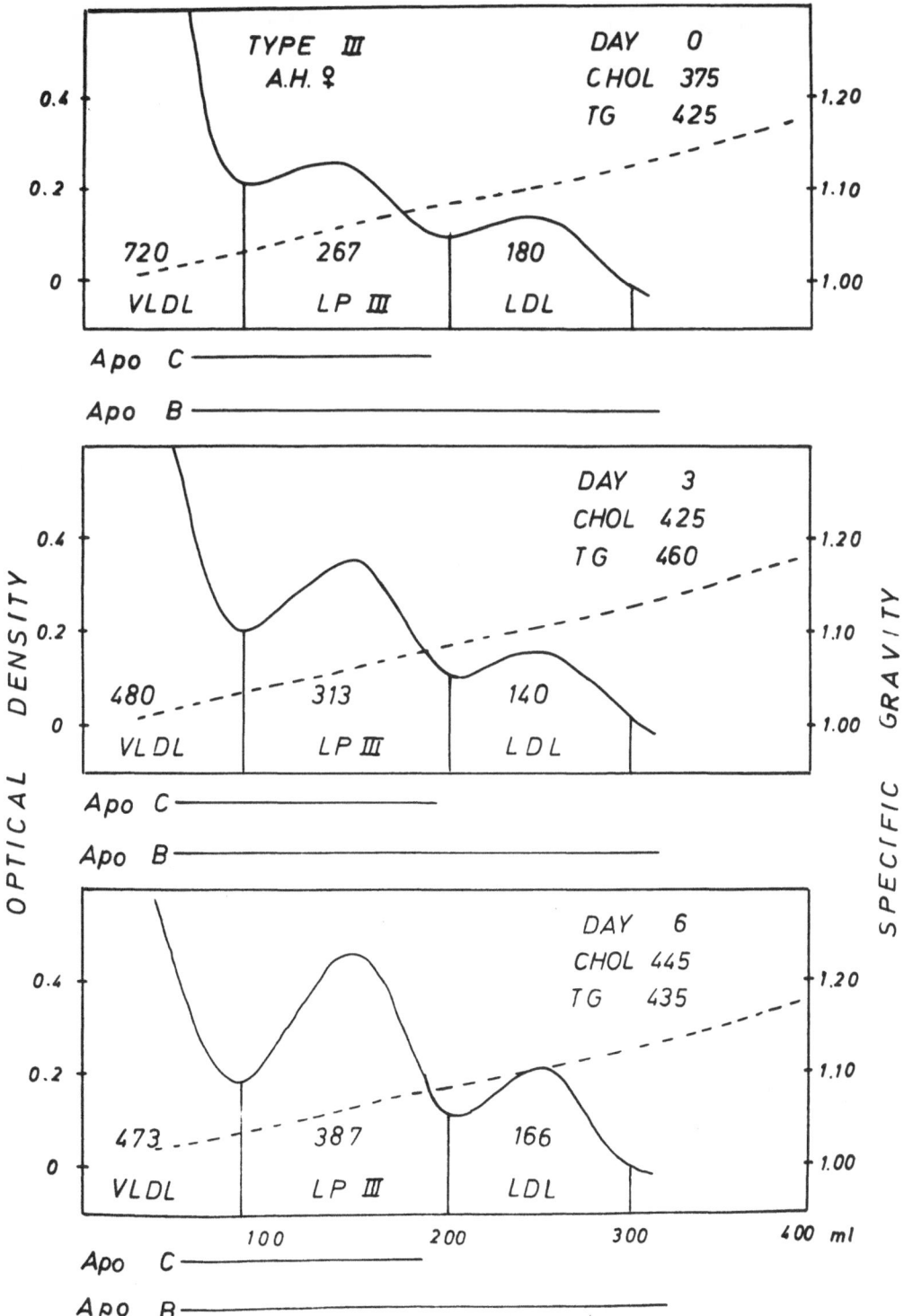

Figure 2. Zonal ultracentrifugation of plasma after fasting for 14 hours, 3 days, and 6 days (type III patients)

XV

Risk Factors

Chairmen: H. G. Rose, USA
         A. Little, USA

Participants: D. F. Brown, USA
             A. Menotti, Italy
             L. Wilhelmsen, Sweden
             D. E. Strandness, USA
             B. F. Rifkind

HYPERLIPOPROTEINEMIA AND ATHEROGENESIS

D. F. Brown

Since this Congress convened four years ago, lipoprotein typing has come into
widespread use and I will discuss whether or not this has provided us with more
useful information than earlier studies which confined themselves to serum cholesterol and triglyceride levels. From the public health standpoint, prevalence of
hyperlipoproteinemia is important. In the United States Wood (1972) has reported
prevalence in a California population and I have reported similar findings in
Albany, New York (Brown and Daudiss, 1973). These studies have demonstrated the
rarity of Type I hyperlipoproteinemia and that Types III and V are uncommon.
Types II and IV, however, are quite prevalent — the latter being predominantly
a disorder of young and middle-aged men. In 1300 apparently healthy blood donors
in Albany, New York, the prevalence of Type II hyperlipoproteinemia was about
equal in both sexes and increased with age. The overall prevalence in this population was approximately 100/1000. By contrast, Type IV hyperlipoproteinemia was
much more prevalent in men than in women at all ages — the overall prevalence
being 261/1000 for men and 82/1000 for women. In men aged 35-44 in this population, 35% exhibited the Type IV disorder according to the criteria of Fredrickson (1972).

What information have we on these two forms of hyperlipoproteinemia as risk factors and how do they relate to earlier findings on cholesterol and triglyceride
levels? Since time does not permit a detailed review of the literature, I will
dispense with the Type II disorder fairly quickly because I think evidence for
its atherogenicity is overwhelming. This has been evident on the basis of clinical experience (Jensen et al., 1967) and evidence that coronary artery disease
manifests itself at a significantly younger age in subjects with this disorder
than in normolipemic subjects (Slack, 1969). While very few prospective studies
have specifically identified Type II hyperlipoproteinemia on the basis of lipoprotein analyses, the disorder nevertheless is readily identified on the basis of
elevated serum cholesterol levels in subjects with normal triglycerides. As early
as 1966 we used this indirect method of lipoprotein typing (Brown et al., 1966)
and we and others, including Carlson (1972) in a recent communication, have demonstrated that elevated LDL are associated with premature atherosclerosis. I suspect that the very numerous studies reported in the literature correlating elevated cholesterol levels with atherosclerosis in general reflect this role of LDL
since it is the major cholesterol transporting fraction.

What about the role of elevated VLDL? The marked difference in the prevalence of
this disorder in men and women demonstrated in the American population suggests
the possibility that this may in part explain the much higher prevalence of
ischemic heart disease in the male. Moreover, since the major lipid component of
VLDL is triglyceride, one might also jump to the conclusion that the few studies

697

equating elevated triglyceride levels with an abnormal prevalence of coronary artery disease might have been the result of elevated VLDL levels. In 1969 I reported an increased incidence of ischemic heart disease with elevated triglyceride levels (Brown, 1969). Data from that report reproduced in Fig. 1 relates the 7-year incidence of ischemic heart disease to increased levels of cholesterol alone or triglyceride alone. In 205 subjects with very definitely elevated triglyceride levels of approximately 250 mg%, the incidence of ischemic heart disease was significantly higher than in subjects with lower triglyceride levels.

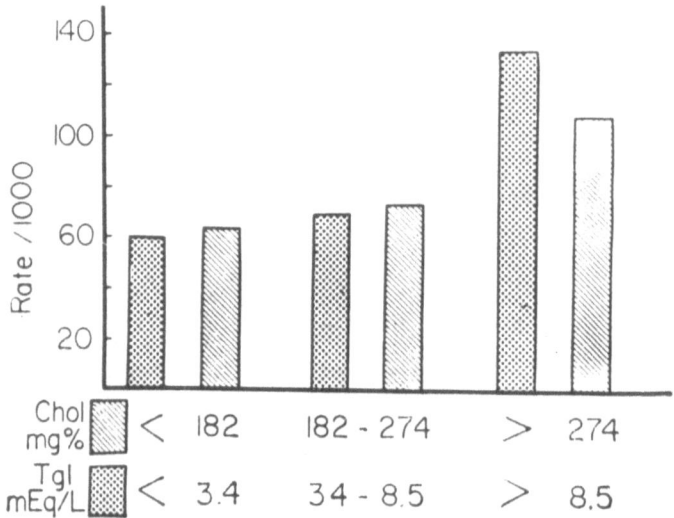

Figure 1. 7-year incidence of ischemic heart disease as related to serum cholesterol or triglyceride levels

In this report, however, I took some pains to point out then, as I will now, that not all patients with elevated triglyceride levels have isolated elevation of VLDL — that is, Type IV hyperlipoproteinemia. The Type IV label implies elevated VLDL with normal LDL. No prospective study to date has clearly identified fasting subjects with isolated VLDL elevation. Since VLDL contain substantial amounts of cholesterol as well as triglyceride, some subjects with VLDL elevation will exhibit coincident hypercholesterolemia especially if LDL and HDL levels in these subjects are near the upper limits of normal, since total cholesterol is the sum of LDL, VLDL and HDL cholesterol. A problem in interpreting studies on serum triglyceride levels is that many patients with this abnormality have coincident cholesterol elevation and it is not always possible to determine from the data whether this total cholesterol level represents coincident increase in LDL or is solely due to VLDL elevation. I am not confident that the risk attributable to elevated triglycerides has not in fact been due to coincident LDL elevation. Accordingly, I think future studies attempting to link triglyceride elevation to coronary artery disease must include measurement of LDL cholesterol to assess the independent contribution of VLDL elevation as a risk factor. LDL cholesterol can be approximated without elaborate studies as indicated below by assuming that VLDL cholesterol is equal to $\dfrac{\text{triglyceride concentration}}{5}$

and that HDL cholesterol approximates 45 mg%.

$$\text{Total cholesterol} = \text{LDL} + \text{VLDL} + \text{HDL cholesterol},$$

$$\text{VLDL cholesterol} = \frac{\text{triglyceride}}{5},$$

$$\text{HDL cholesterol} = 45 \text{ mg\%},$$

$$\text{LDL chol.} = \text{total chol.} - \frac{(\text{triglyceride} + 45)}{5}.$$

While this method is not as good as direct quantitation of lipoproteins, it is an improvement on analyses based solely on total cholesterol and triglyceride levels. This formula has recently been applied to data from the Albany Cardiovascular Health Center population to measure prevalence and 10 year incidence of ischemic heart disease in relation to LDL and VLDL levels. Ischemic heart disease was considered present if the patient exhibited unequivocal evidence of one or more of the following: myocardial infarction, angina pectoris, abnormal ECG response to exercise or sudden death. On the basis of lipoprotein levels, patients were assigned the label of normolipemic, Type II or Type IV hyperlipoproteinemia. The Type II label in this analysis includes subjects with Type IIa and Type IIb hyperlipoproteinemia. Unlike previous studies, typing was based not on a single annual measurement but on the type that the patient exhibited over a 10-year period. Since the majority of patients did not consistently demonstrate normolipemia or a particular type, the analysis was based on subjects who exhibited the abnormality 100% of the time or greater than 60% of the time. Prevalence data demonstrated in Fig. 2 was based on the type of hyperlipoproteinemia that the patient exhibited in 1963 and exhibited subsequently either until he died or until the time that this analysis was made in 1973. On this basis, ischemic heart disease was significantly more prevalent in Type II subjects and in those with the Type IV disorder than in normolipemic subjects. In subjects who were free of ischemic

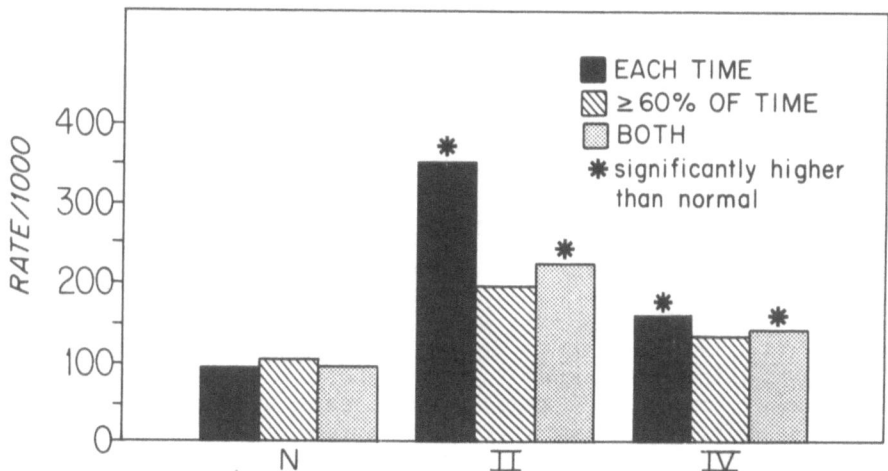

Figure 2. Prevalence of IHD in 1470 men according to lipoprotein types

heart disease in 1963, the 10-year incidence of this disease was calculated and again related to lipoprotein type. A rather surprising finding in this analysis (Fig. 3) was that the incidence of ischemic heart disease over this period of time was not significantly higher in Type II subjects than in normolipemic subjects but was significantly higher in subjects with Type IV hyperlipoproteinemia. A possible explanation for the absence of risk associated with the Type II disorder in the last 10 years may be that the Type II disorder has already exerted its deleterious effect on the coronary arteries prior to 1963 whereas the Type IV disorder requires a long period of time to exert this effect. It is known that subjects with Type II hyperlipoproteinemia exhibit clinical manifestations of coronary artery disease at a young age. A recent study by Klemens et al. (1972) in

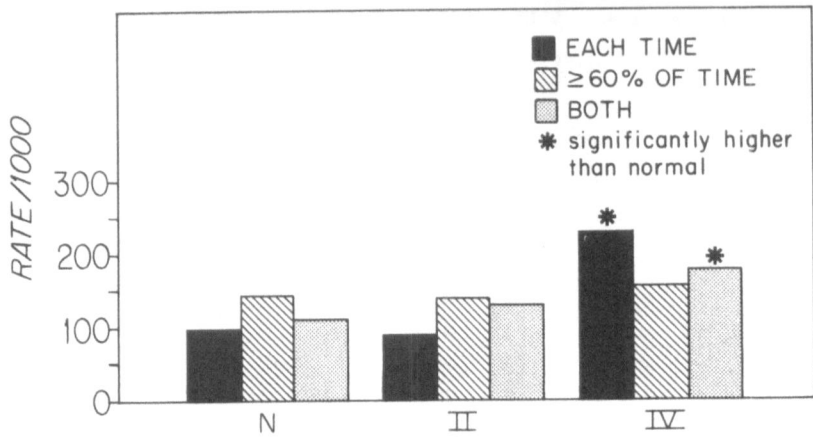

Figure 3. 10-year incidence of IHD in 1312 men according to lipoprotein type

patients with myocardial infarction, angina without infarction and patients with
no evident coronary artery disease has shown that Type II and Type IV hyperlipoproteinemia were correlated with the disease, that the Type II disorder
prodominated in younger people and that type IV predominated in the older age
group. In a study by Carlson (1972) LDL and VLDL elevation alone or in combination were considered as risk factors only in subjects under 60 years of age.
On the basis of currently available data, however, and until such time as more
accurate measurements of low density and very low density lipoproteins are made
in prospective epidemiologic studies, one cannot feel completely confident that
VLDL elevation plays an important role in atherogenesis.

Added to the limitations of lipid methodology in the epidemiologic studies has
been the difficulty in clearly defining subjects with coronary artery disease or,
stated in another way, in defining that apparently healthy subjects are free of
coronary atherosclerosis. In these studies, coronary artery disease has been
defined purely on clinical grounds. We now know on the basis of coronary angiographic and autopsy studies that significant coronary artery disease can exist
and remain undetected by any clinical means. In Albany, Dr. Sosa and I have carried out lipoprotein typing on over 1000 subjects undergoing selective coronary
angiography. Data have been analyzed in the first 733 of these subjects of whom
561 were men and 172 women. The prevalence of hyperlipoproteinemia in this group
of subjects is shown in Fig. 4. The findings indicate that the prevalence of
hyperlipoproteinemia is higher in subjects with diseased vessels than in those
with normal or minimally diseased vessels. It is also evident that this relationship of hyperlipoproteinemia to coronary artery disease is less marked in subjects
over age 44 than in subjects younger than 44. Accordingly, a more detailed analysis of the types of hyperlipoproteinemia is demonstrated in Fig. 5 for men and
women under 44. The left hand bar demonstrates subjects with normal vessels or
less than 20% luminal occlusion and the right hand bar subjects exhibiting greater
than 20% luminal occlusion of any coronary artery. The majority of subjects included in this right hand bar in fact exhibited greater than 80% occlusion. In
men with normal vessels or minimal disease, a significantly higher percentage
had normal lipids than did those with more severe disease. In this latter group,
Type IV and Type II hyperlipoproteinemia was more prevalent than in those with
healthy vessels or minimal disease but the differences were statistically significant only for the Type II disorder. The finding of note is the remarkably high
prevalence of the Type IV disorder, namely in 27% of subjects with healthy
vessels or minimal disease. In 26 young women with normal vessels or minimal
disease, 85% exhibited normal lipids, 12% Type IV and 4% Type II hyperlipoproteinemia. In 15 young women with more advanced disease, one-third had normal

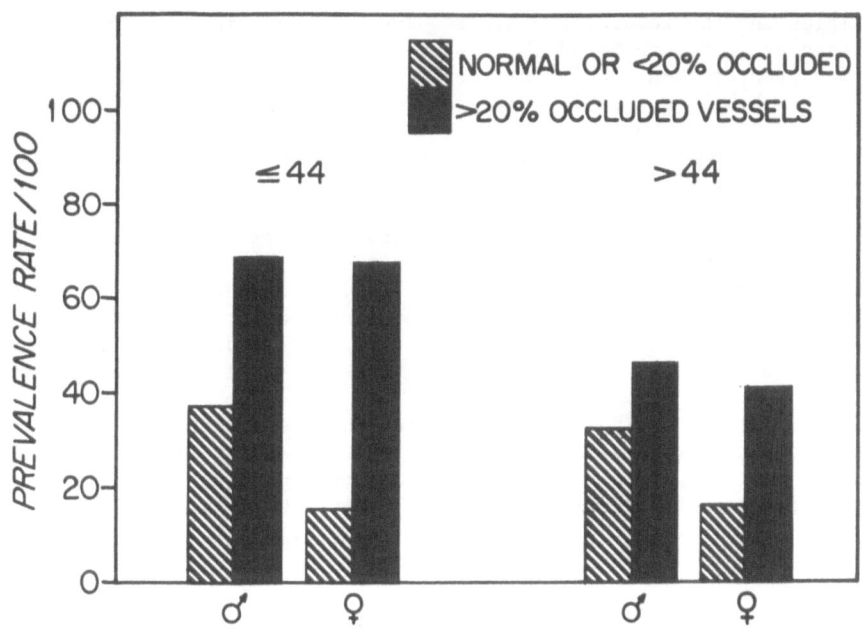

Figure 4. Prevalence of hyperlipoproteinemia in 561 men and 172 women according to age, and state of occlusion of coronary arteries

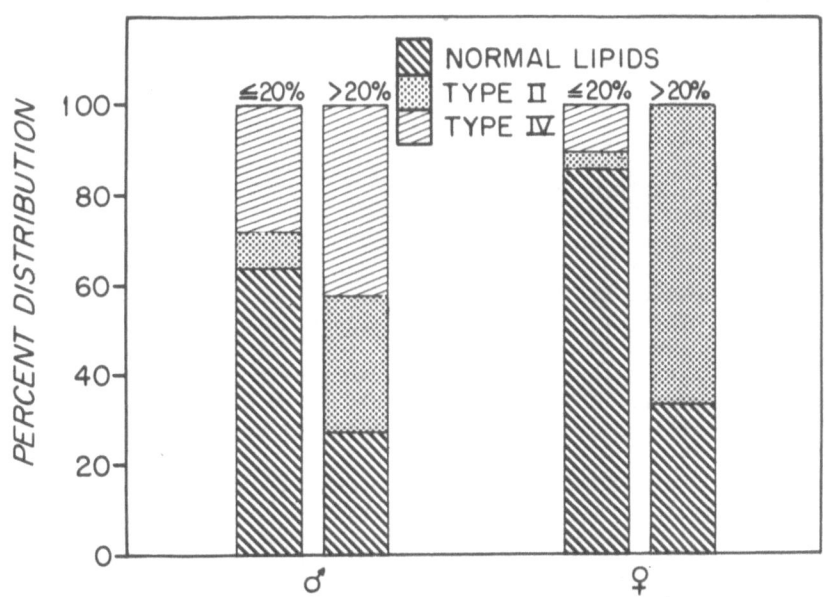

Figure 5. Distribution of blood lipid patterns in subjects aged under 45 years, according to state of occlusion of coronary arteries

lipids and the remainder exhibited Type II hyperlipoproteinemia and not one of
these subjects exhibited the Type IV disorder. Eleven of these 15 women exhibited greater than 80% luminal occlusion of one or more coronary arteries, 9 of
these exhibiting Type II hyperlipoproteinemia and 2 normal lipids. These data
convincingly demonstrate the role of elevated low density lipoprotein levels in
coronary atherosclerosis and fail to implicate the Type IV disorder in young
women with this disease. The high prevalence of the Type IV disorder in men with
apparently healthy vessels makes it difficult at this time to positively link
elevated VLDL with atherogenesis in the male sex but accumulation of a larger
series of patients may reveal a statistically higher prevalence of this disorder
in males with more advanced disease. In view of the remarkably high prevalence of
this disorder in the male sex and the fact that its dietary and drug management
is quite different from that of the Type II disorder, continuing work must be devoted to identify with certainty its possible role as a risk factor.

Acknowledgements. The studies reported in this presentation were carried out in
collaboration with J. A. Sosa, M.D., Chief of Adult Diagnostic Cardiology and
J. T. Doyle, M.D., Director of the Cardiovascular Health Center and Chairman of
the Division of Cardiology at Albany Medical College.

MULTIVARIATE PREDICTION

A. Menotti

Doctors in general and epidemiologists in particular usually mean by risk factors
those characteristics which, if measured in subjects free from clinical manifestations of a disease, make it possible to identify those who are at higher risk
of developing the disease within a given period of time, as compared to others
belonging to the same population group.

This concept has been mainly applied to coronary heart disease (CHD) and to coronary risk factors, whereas this is not the case for atherosclerosis *per se*,
which can be considered neither an end-point nor a condition that can be early
diagnosed by such measurements.

Even though the idea of risk factors can be and has been extended also to other
complications of atherosclerosis, the concept of multivariate prediction is
properly applied at the moment mainly to some well-defined manifestations of CHD
where risk factors are used as possible predictors of the disease.

It is well known that 40 or more factors have been identified or at least suspected (Strasser, 1972), but that only a few of them have been shown to be consistently reliable in predicting the excess coronary risk.

Some of the equivocal interpretations of many claimed risk factors have relied
for many years on the almost exclusively univariate approach in the analysis of
the material collected in longitudinal studies; that is, correlating classes of
single risk factors with the subsequent incidence of the disease. Obvious drawbacks of the univariate analysis soon became clear, since the possible predictors
of the disease were many and they were possibly correlating and interacting with
each other in many different and unknown ways.

Simple analysis of more than one factor at the same time, performed by the standardization of rates or by the use of cross-classifications, have readily shown
their limitations and inefficacy.

The multivariate approach has been attempted only in relatively recent years and
so far only in a few studies. The data presented here belong to the "Seven Coun-

tries Study" (Coronary heart disease in seven countries, 1970) which has been among the first to employ such techniques.

At the moment at least two valid models are available, together with many solutions, for the estimation of the coronary risk as a function of several risk factors measured some years in advance. The experience gained within some major prospective studies with the multiple regression linear function, and more especially with the multiple logistic function (MLF), has provided good evidence of their interest and value. The MLF ($y = 1/1 + e^{-(a+b,x, + b_2x_2....+ b_nx_n)}$), first applied to the Framingham data (Cornfield, 1967; Truett et al., 1967), resembles a flat S-shaped curve which has some other biological analogies. It estimates the probability (y) of developing CHD within a defined period of time as a function of several risk factors (the x's). The solution of the equation, by assigning to y the value of 1 or 0 (for cases and non-cases respectively) and the actual levels of risk factors to the x's, allows us to estimate the value of a (a constant) and of the b's, which are individual coefficients for the single risk factors (Table 1). Several means are available for evaluating a solution.

Table 1. Example of a solution of the multiple logistic function generated by pooling the European samples of the "Seven Countries Study". Incidence of "Hard-criteria CHD" predicted by five risk factors in five years

	Coefficients
Age (years)	0.078
Body mass index[a]	0.016
Systolic blood pressure (mm Hg)	0.020
Serum cholesterol (mg/dl)	0.010
Smoke[b]	0.104
Constant	−14.211

[a] $\dfrac{\text{weight (kg)}}{\text{height (m}^2)}$.

[b] Code: never smoked or ex-smoker = 3; less than 5 cigarettes per day = 4; 5-9 = 5; 10-19 = 6; 20-29 = 7; 30 or more = 8.

In non-technical terms the findings are as follows:

1. The solutions in general describe fairly well the material from which they have been generated, that is, they indicate that the material does fit well into the model. The back-application of constant and coefficients to the material yields individual estimates of y (probabilities) which can be arranged in rank order, allowing the computation of the correlation coefficient between observed and expected cases in arbitrary classes of risk, (Table 2), and this is usually above 0.90 (Keys, 1972).

2. The histograms representing the distribution of the observed cases in decile classes of risk show that a good discrimination is obtained, since usually 1/3 or more of all cases occur in the highest decile of risk, and about 1/2 in the upper two deciles (Keys, 1972).

3. The levels of the single coefficients are irrelevant to the independent predicting power of the single factors, but a rough guide to this is given by the ratio of the coefficient to its standard error (t test). Such an approach, and comparison of the discriminating power of different solutions which include or

exclude a specific factor (while others are kept fixed), have shown that major predicting power is attributable to age, serum cholesterol, blood pressure (either systolic or diastolic) and smoking habit, whereas little or no independent contribution is provided by body weight (and other indirect measurements of fatness), physical activity, body shape, pulse rate etc. Unfortunately little or no data are available on blood glucose and glucose tolerance test.

4. The four or five basic risk factors have substantially the same predicting power in different populations, even though the coefficients may vary in terms of different levels of significance.

5. The use of solutions for the estimation of risk in populations different from those which have generated them has indicated that the relative risk (tested by the correlation between predicted and observed cases in decile classes of risk) is rather good; whereas the absolute risk, that is the prediction of the number of incidence cases from one population to another has been less satisfactory. For example the U.S. solutions tend to overestimate incidence in European groups; while the European solutions tend to underestimate the U.S. incidence. This means that some factors not considered here are responsible for the excess of risk in the Americans as compared to European men, even when age, blood pressure, serum cholesterol and smoking habits are similar.

Table 2. Example of the correlation between observed and expected cases of CHD in decile classes of risk when the solution is applied back to the individuals of the same population. (Seven Countries Study; European samples; incidence in 5 years of "Any Criteria CHD" predicted by age, systolic blood pressure, serum cholesterol and smoking habit)

Decile of risk	Observed cases (x)	Expected cases (y)
1	9	9.31
2	19	14.28
3	16	18.49
4	22	22.67
5	27	27.50
6	37	33.22
7	34	40.79
8	53	50.65
9	78	67.73
10	110	125.70
Total	405	410.32

$y = -2.4152 + 1.0728 \, x$. $r = 0.9814$.

Altogether the MLF seems to be a powerful even though still imperfect tool; at the moment it is apparently able to explain a great part of the disease (but probably no more than 50 to 50% of it) when some few well-established risk factors are considered. Nevertheless this is to date the best tool we may use for some purposes. These include

a) the proper evaluation of "new" risk factors in prospective studies;
b) the identification of high risk individuals within a population, independently from the solution employed;
c) the estimation of the possible reduction of incidence as a result of interven-

tion on risk factor levels;
d) comparing the observed reduction of the estimated risk following a preventive treatment with the expected one.

On the other hand more work should be done on this model on the available prospective material, and possibly also on other models, in order to improve the present predictive possibilities.

EARLY DIAGNOSIS

A. Little

Introduction

Ideally, in the practice of medicine, it is better to prevent than to attempt to cure. However, atherosclerosis is never likely to be completely preventable. Therefore, physicians are continuing to develop methods for the earliest possible diagnosis of the disease. As new methods become available, they require comparison with older ones in order to determine their value. The earlier the diagnosis, the more likely is treatment to be effective in causing regression of lesions or in preventing ischemic tissue damage. The recent improvement in methods for eliminating atherosclerotic risk factors and the development of surgical techniques for correcting potentially serious arterial obstructive lesions makes the early diagnosis of atherosclerosis very important. The next three speakers will discuss methods for the early diagnosis of coronary and peripheral atherosclerosis and of screening for hyperlipidemia. They were selected to speak to us because of their experience and current research in these fields. They have been asked to consider the following points. Is it possible to diagnose "early atherosclerosis" or are we still only recognizing advanced, irreversible disease? Does earlier diagnosis with present methods improve prognosis? Are there practical methods for the diagnosis of early lesions? Will they help us to elucidate the cause of the disease and the effect of treatment on the lesions? Should screening for hyperlipidemia involve the entire population or only selected groups of subjects? Can we assure hyperlipidemic patients that we can decrease risk of atherosclerotic complications by lowering plasma lipids? Are these methods for early diagnosis of atherosclerosis and of screening for hyperlipidemia fully evaluated or is there much work still to be done?

EARLY DIAGNOSIS OF CORONARY HEART DISEASE

Lars Wilhelmsen

Pathogenetic Considerations

It is generally assumed that the presence of early clinical signs of coronary heart disease (CHD) represents advanced or late stages of coronary artery disease. According to Baroldi (1965, 1967), however, in 6 per cent of cases with recent myocardial infarction (AMI) a functionally important obstruction of a coronary artery was not demonstrable. In about half of the cases with recent AMI no acute occlusion of any type was observed, and in the residual cases a thrombus — possibly secondary to the infarct in several cases — was found (Baroldi, 1973). This is in conformity with many autopsy studies after sudden coronary death (SCD). The role played by the small vessels and collaterals is insufficiently known.

Disturbed function of either the contractile elements of the myocardium or the estimated 10 per cent of it having more purely electrical activity may be more important than is generally considered. Thus, cardiac dysrhythmias certainly play a key role.

Aims of Early Diagnosis

There are at least two aims of early diagnosis of CHD. Firstly, a clinical one; namely to be able to initiate *therapy* in an *individual* before a more serious event occurs. That is, to quote an example, what we are aiming at when we try to identify unstable or preinfarction angina and other symptoms and signs which may be immediate fore-runners of an AMI or SCD. These premonitory symptoms and signs will not be discussed in more detail in this presentation.

The second aim is exemplified by the *group* diagnosis with more strictly preventive aspects. The following presentation will be restricted to this second aspect and to methods which can be used in fairly large groups of people from the general population.

Methods for Early Diagnosis

a) *Coronary Angiography*. Coronary angiography is evidently an effective tool, but it is not applicable to large, healthy populations because of complicated and expensive methodology and some, though small, risks of complications. In selected series of patients published so far (Bruschke et al., 1973) and hitherto unpublished data from Göteborg it has been shown that extensive vascular changes carry a higher risk for a fatal outcome than more discrete ones. But several cases have been seen still alive in spite of severe three-vessel disease on the angiogram 10 years ago.

It is too early to form an opinion whether recently developed methods for non-invasive evaluation of myocardial blood flow (Zaret et al., 1973) will prove to be useful and sufficiently cheap for general use.

b) *Symptoms*. The presence of chest pain occurring during exercise has been associated with about three times higher risk than absence of this symptom (Rose, 1971; Punsar & Karvonen, 1973). It has not been consistently shown whether this increase of risk is unrelated to other risk factors for CHD. In a study of unselected patients surviving an AMI angina pectoris was found prior to the AMI in only 50 per cent of the patients (Elmfeldt & Wilhelmsen, 1972).

Dyspnea when walking uphill or dyspnea on even less exertion increased the risk of later AMI by about two times and was an independent predictor in multivariate logistic analysis (Wilhelmsen et al., 1973). The relationship was stronger between fatal IHD and dyspnea than between non-fatal AMI and dyspnea (unpubl. observ.). Dyspnea is also a predictor for death among those who have already experienced an AMI (Elmfeldt & Wilhelmsen, 1972). It is very probable that the rapid reversible increase of left atrial pressure occurring during a load in patients with CHD can cause a reversible increase in airway resistance and be responsible for the dyspnea (Pepine & Viener, 1972).

c) *Electrocardiogram*. The risk of later CHD events increases about three-fold by having ST and/or T-changes in the resting electrocardiogram (Rose, 1971). Blackburn et al. (1970) have shown that especially diphasic or flat T-waves, but also first degree AV block or minor prolongation of the PR interval and frequent ventricular premature beats, increase the risk of subsequent CHD independently of other risk factors present.

d) *Exercise Testing*. Many have hoped that it should be possible to improve the prediction of early CHD by applying graded exercise ECG in a prospective population study. Thus, it has been used by Rumbal and Acheson (1963), Astrand (1969) and Blackburn et al. (1970) and others.

We have collected data from a random population sample of men all aged 50 at entry to the study in 1963. An exercise test on a bicycle ergometer with increasing loads up to maximum was carried out in 790 subjects in 1967 (Grimby et al., 1970). To date a 6-year follow-up is available (Wilhelmsen et al., to be published). The end points have been fatal CHD and non-fatal AMI. ST- or T-changes (Minnesota Code 4:1-3 or 5:1-3) increased the risk of later CHD about three-fold. The ratio was, however, about the same for rest as for the different work loads up to maximum exercise. There was good correlation between ST-T changes and ventricular premature beats. In this study (Vedin et al., 1972) as well as in the Tecumseh Study (Chiang et al., 1969) there was a relationship between ventricular arrhythmias and CHD. Very few data of predictive importance appeared from the measurements of work capacity such as heart rate at different loads etc.

According to our results in an age- and sex-standardized population, exercise testing is a heavy undertaking which does not seem to offer a sufficient body of new information for prediction in the general middle-aged male population.

e) *Non-Invasive Methods*. The possibilities of using non-invasive methods for analysis of especially left ventricular function have not been sufficiently tested as yet. The left ventricular ejection time (LVET) is often, but not always, shortened and the pre-ejection period (PEP) often, but not always, prolonged in clinical CHD as after an AMI (Wikstrand et al., 1973).

It is possible that stress tests, for example static work loads, may increase the yield of these methods as well as other non-invasive techniques such as phonocardiography and measurement of the left atrial and ventricular volume by ultrasound technique. Less time-consuming methods which are adapted for use by technicians need to be developed and tested in normals and patients with varying degrees of CHD.

Finally, it has to be stressed that we know very little about the possible preventive effects of changes of risk factors and to what extent early CHD may be reversible.

EARLY DIAGNOSIS OF PERIPHERAL ATHEROSCLEROSIS*

D. E. Strandness, Jr.

The diagnosis of peripheral atherosclerosis can be objectively established and disease progression followed by a variety of simple, noninvasive methods. The fibrous and complicated plaques as they project into the lumen of the artery will reduce the pulse pressure distal to the lesion(s) by an amount proportional to the resistance offered by the lesion and the associated collateral arteries (Edholm et al., 1951; Strandness and Bell, 1965). This pressure drop can be enhanced by increasing limb blood flow either by exercise or reactive hyperemia (Keitzer at al., 1965; Schultz et al., 1967).

The simplest approach is to measure the systolic pressure at the ankle by plethysmographic methods or the ultrasonic velocity detector and express the value as a percentage of the arm systolic pressure (the ankle pressure index) (Carter, 1968, 1969; Strandness, 1971). Normally, the ankle pressure should be greater than 97% of the arm pressure (Carter, 1969). When exercise is added to the procedure and the ankle pressure is monitored after completion of the walking time,

*Supported in part by National Institutes of Health Grant HE 10502-05.

the pressure gradient is increased and the period of post-exercise hyperemia is prolonged (Strandness, 1970).

Normal subjects, when stressed maximally, will have a transient fall in ankle pressure but within one to two minutes, the pressure will return to within 10-20% of the baseline level (Fig. 1). Patients with peripheral atherosclerosis subjected to a much lower constant workload (2 mph on a 12% grade) will sustain a greater drop in pressure and, most importantly, a much delayed return to the baseline level (Fig. 2). As the disease progresses, both the resting ankle pressure will decrease and the post-exercise response will become increasingly abnormal.

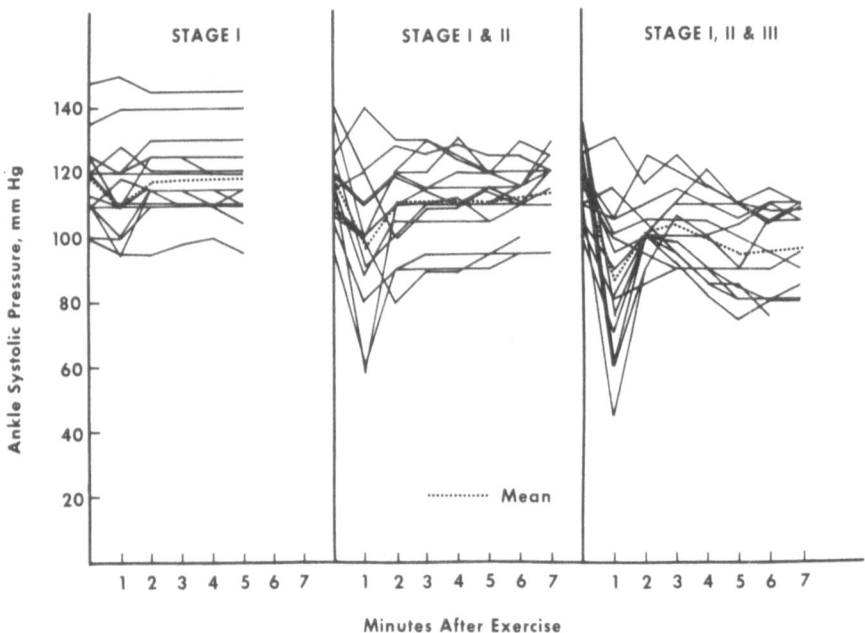

Figure 1. The changes in ankle systolic blood pressure that followed graded treadmill exercise. Stage I -- 1.7 mph on a 10% grade; Stage II -- 3.4 mph on a 14% grade; Stage III -- 5 mph on an 18% grade. Each stage was three minutes in duration. During the 30-second transition between stages, the subject stepped off the treadmill while the speed and elevation were adjusted for the next stage. (From Strandness, D.E., Jr. (Ed.) *Collateral Circulation in Clinical Surgery*. Philadelphia: W.B. Saunders Co., 1969

It is also possible to measure the calf blood flow before and after exercise to bring out the abnormalities produced by atherosclerosis. As noted in Fig. 3, there is an inverse relationship between the calf blood flow and the ankle blood pressure response (Summer and Strandness, 1969). For routine studies and mass screening, the ankle pressure measurement is preferred because the technique is much simpler to carry out and it provides essentially the same diagnostic information.

Another promising approach to the early diagnosis of peripheral atherosclerosis is that described by Zelis et al. (1970). These authors measured the *peak* reactive hyperemic blood flow in the calf after cuff occlusion of arterial inflow. It was found that two of 11 type II, nine of 12 type III and one of 10 type IV lipoprotein abnormalities had peak flows lower than normal. The impressive obser-

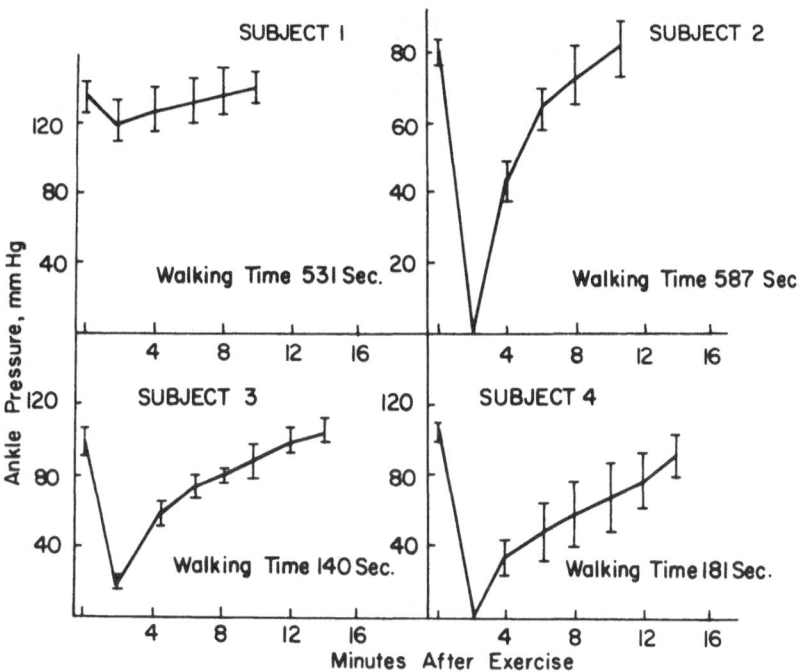

Figure 2. The mean ankle systolic pressure changes and one standard deviation are shown. The patients all walked the same duration on four successive days. The variation in response reflects the variation in the extent of the disease. The treadmill speed was 2 mph with a grade of 12%. (From Strandness, D.E., Jr.: *Peripheral Arterial Disease*. Boston: Little, Brown and Company, 1969

vation was that the flow abnormality was reversible in six patients with type III disorders who were studied before and after three-six months of treatment by diet and cliofibrate. These studies are difficult to perform well and do not lend themselves to large patient populations but certainly deserve verification by other investigators.

A key and yet unanswered question is the stage at which peripheral atherosclerosis can be detected. Evidence is accumulating that the process can be diagnosed well before symptoms appear. Advanced lesions, based upon morphological changes, will not be detectable unless a pressure-flow abnormality occurs either at rest or following a period of flow increase. Carter (1972) has shown that plaques compromising the arterial cross-section by 25% or more will produce a fall in the ankle pressure after exercise.

The recent development of the ultrasonic arteriogram may provide another noninvasive method of establishing the presence of the intimal irregularity produced by this disease (Hokanson et al., 1971; Mozersky et al., 1972). This technique which utilizes the Doppler effect can be used to generate images of the area of the artery where blood is flowing. Plaques can be observed as filling defects similar to those observed by conventional contrast arteriography. This technique has the advantage of being able to examine the lumen geometry in both the longitudinal and transverse planes at selected sites such as the carotid bifurcation, the common femoral, superficial femoral and popliteal arteries. The method remains in the development stage but does hold great promise as some of the technical problems are overcome.

Even considering some of the limitations of the current technology, it is both feasible and reasonable to apply the physiologic study methods to this important problem. First of all, it is possible to assess the incidence of this disease in patients considered at risk and establish the true incidence of the problem. Secondly, it will be possible to establish the relationship between peripheral atherosclerosis and involvement in the coronary, cranial and extracranial arteries. Thirdly, it is now established that disease progression can be objectively determined by these study methods (Strandness and Stahler, 1966; Mozersky et al., 1972a,b). This latter factor is extremely important in establishing the efficacy of current, or proposed, methods of treatment. This is an important consideration because it is essential that we have objective data available to support the role of intervention in not only preventing the disease but stopping disease progression once it is detected.

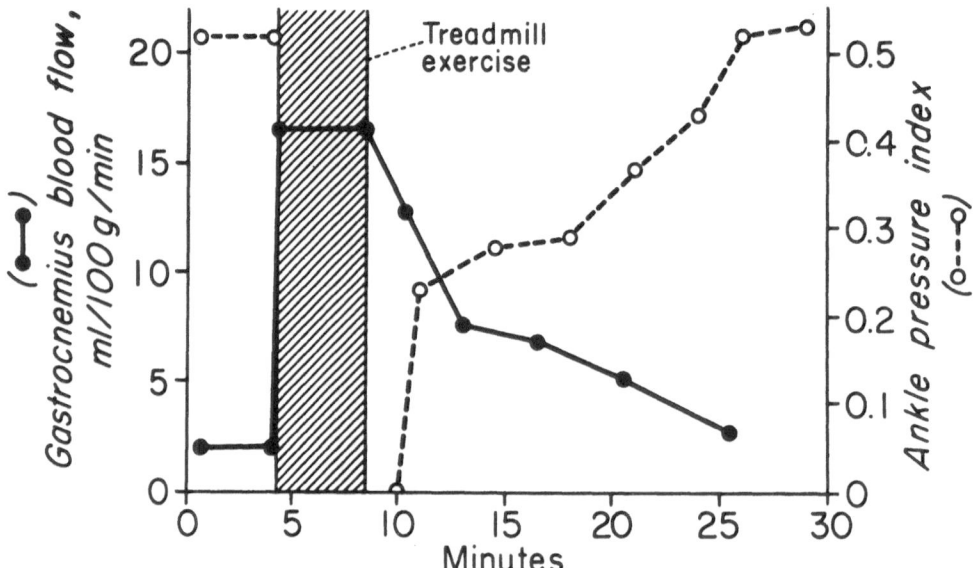

Figure 3. The inverse relationship between the calf blood flow (measured plethysmographically) and the ankle pressure index. This patient had peripheral atherosclerosis and intermittent claudication. The patient walked to the point of developing calf pain which forced him to stop

SCREENING FOR HYPERLIPIDEMIA IN RELATION TO ATHEROSCLEROSIS

B. F. Rifkind

Several major criteria should be considered before screening for a disorder can be advocated on a large scale (Sharp, 1968). They include that the disorder should be both severe in its consequences and prevalent, tests should be available for its ready diagnosis, and treatment should be available for the abnormal subjects identified by the screening process. I shall evaluate screening for hyperlipidemia in these terms with the purpose of demonstrating that its current status fulfills some, but not all, of these requirements. I shall not consider screening for other coronary heart disease (CHD) risk factors though these may be simultaneously screened for in certain types of population surveys.

Severity. The severe consequences of CHD hardly needs to be dwelt upon except to emphasize the high mortality of the first attack of myocardial infarction and that a frequent initial manifestation is sudden death, stressing the need for identifying subjects at risk by screening programs before symptoms emerge.

Prevalence. The prevalence of CHD also hardly needs restating. In the United States, cardiovascular disease is responsible for a high proportion of all death, and of these cardiac deaths, arteriosclerotic disease accounts for the majority. Many studies have demonstrated that hyperlipidemia is prevalent in CHD subjects, especially in younger age groups. Nevertheless, by no means do all CHD subjects have hyperlipidemia, and indeed many subjects lack any of the major risk factors. The definition of hyperlipidemia is, in fact, somewhat arbitrary, lipid levels throughout the range that operates in most advanced societies being associated with CHD risk. The aim of detecting hyperlipidemic subjects is to identify a group whose CHD risk considerably exceeds that of subjects with so-called normal lipid levels.

Test Availability. The advent of automated analytical systems now permits large numbers of lipid (cholesterol and triglyceride) determinations to be performed. There are, however, several problems still associated with the mass determination of lipids. The variation in accuracy amongst the many methods which are currently used to determine cholesterol is insufficiently appreciated. Using the Abell-Kendall method for cholesterol determination as the gold standard, many common methods produce results considerably in excess. Failure to allow for such variation can be a major source of error. Levels of precision and accuracy between or within laboratories employing a given method also leaves much to be desired. There is an urgent need for international standardization of lipid determinations, both to serve the individual patient and to permit comparisons of data collected in different laboratories.

A rule of thumb which can be used in screening is to regard subjects whose total cholesterol exceeds the 90% cutoff and/or whose triglyceride exceeds the 95% cutoff as potentially hyperlipoproteinemic. The selection of the 90% instead of the 95% cutoff for cholesterol is based on observations that in about 10% of Type II subjects, although the LDL cholesterol exceeds the 95% cutoff, the total plasma cholesterol lies within the 90-95% range.

Available Treatment. Perhaps the most difficult problems that flow from population screening relate to treatment of abnormal subjects. A useful group of lipid lowering diets and drugs are now available. However, no categorical evidence exists to show that correction of hyperlipidemia will prevent vascular disease although much circumstantial evidence and several encouraging recent clinical trials point in that direction. The number of hyperlipidemic subjects generated by screening programs is daunting; using popular definitions of hyperlipidemia about 8% of the population will be so defined. Proper management of these subjects, after demonstration of hyperlipidemia, involves further evaluation by a clinician, including the exclusion of secondary causes of hyperlipidemia. Subsequent management also requires the input of physicians and nutritionists and followup of the patient. The conduct of large-scale population screening therefore involves laboratory personnel, physicians, nutritionists, administrators, blood drawers, interviewers, etc.

Bearing in mind that treatment has not yet been demonstrated to be effective, the time cannot yet be held to have arrived when large-scale screening programs should be routinely undertaken. Rather, limited, well conducted pilot programs with defined objectives should be instituted.

Whom to Screen. General principles which underly selection of populations for screening include potential access to the whole population and the recognition of hyperlipidemia at as early an age as possible so that therapy can, at least theoretically, be introduced before atherosclerotic disease becomes irreversibly established, and so that behavioral modes leading to aggravation of CHD risk factors can be corrected, though very little is known about the latter.

Tables 1 and 2 summarize some of the groups that may be considered for general population screening. The use of umbilical cord blood screening is attracting much attention as a means of potentially obtaining easy access to the whole population. While cases of familial Type II hyperlipoproteinemia can be detected, rather little is known about its overall sensitivity and specificity. Umbilical cord blood screening, or screening of school children, is also limited by the probability that only certain forms of hyperlipoproteinemia can be detected at this stage. The main problem in screening in adult life is to obtain and organize access to the population. An alternative high yield approach is to screen the asymptomatic relatives of hyperlipidemic subjects.

Table 1. Population screening

Possibilities	Comments
Cord blood	Allows early diagnosis Familial Type II only Measure LDL cholesterol Further evaluation required
High school children	Allows early diagnosis Familial Type II and some Type IV Screen for other risk factors
Young and middle- aged adults	More difficult to organize ? need to obtain repeat determinations Screen for other risk factors

Table 2. Selected group for screening

Subjects with
    premature vascular disease, xanthomas, early corneal arcus,
    family history of premature vascular disease, xanthomas, hyperlipidemia.

First degree relatives of   hyperlipoproteinemic index cases

XVI
Prevention

Chairman: M. F. Oliver, Great Britain

Participants: A. G. Shaper, Great Britain
               M. Steinbach, Romania
               G. Tibblin, Sweden
               O. Turpeinen, Finland
               R. J. Jones, USA
               R. W. Wissler, USA

HARD AND SOFT WATER IN RELATION TO THE INCIDENCE OF CARDIOVASCULAR DISEASE

A. G. Shaper, D. G. Clayton, and J. N. Morris

There is a strong statistical association between cardiovascular mortality and the mineral content of drinking water; the softer the drinking water the higher the death rates. This inverse association between components of drinking water and cardiovascular death rates has been found in several countries since the initial report from Japan in 1957 which reported a close association between cerebrovascular death rates and the acidity of river drinking water. Table 1 indicates some of the countries in which this association has been reported. It is

Table 1. Some countries reporting an association between cardiovascular death rates and water components

Country	The water story Mortality group
Japan	Cerebrovascular
Sweden	Cerebrovascular (females). Degenerative HD
U.S.A.	All CVD; cerebrovascular, CHD, hypertensive HD
England/Wales	All CVD; cerebrovascular, CHD, "other" HD
Holland	C.H.D. (females)
Canada	C.H.D.
Finland	All CVD
Australia	C.H.D.; cerebrovascular disease
Ireland	All CVD

important to emphasise that the relationship is with cardiovascular disease *in general* not ischaemic heart disease in particular, and that different components of cardiovascular mortality are more clearly involved in some countries than in others. In Japan, cerebrovascular disease is the major association; in Sweden it is "myocardial degeneration" and in a review of studies in the United States, it is hypertensive heart disease which is most consistently correlated with water hardness. Clearly, some fundamental aspect of cardiovascular function is involved in the Water Story and the purpose of this brief communication is to draw attention to some of the possible factors concerned and to consider some of the problems and possibilities which the Water Story raise.

Some of the basic facts concerning the Water Story will be demonstrated using data from Great Britain, partly because the closest associations between death rates and water indices have been found in Great Britain and as a tribute to the late Margaret Crawford, whose work has provided such an impetus to international studies in this field.

Studies in Great Britain

In the 61 county boroughs of England and Wales with populations of 80,000 or over, the correlation coefficients between cardiovascular death rates and water hardness are negative and highly significant (Table 2). They are greatest with water calcium and with the carbonate fraction (reflecting temporary hardness); correlations with sodium are much lower and are negligible with magnesium.

Table 2. Associations between components of water hardness (1961) and death-rates (1958-64) men aged 45-64 in the 61 County Boroughs of England and Wales with a population of 80,000 or over in 1961

Water constituents p.p.m.	Correlation (r) with death-rates for:		
	Cardiovascular disease	Bronchitis	All "other" causes
Total solids	-0.61	-0.41	-0.23
Total hardness:	-0.65	-0.45	-0.26
Temporary hardness (carbonate)	-0.63	-0.48	-0.29
Permanent hardness (non-carbonate)	-0.51	-0.24	-0.10
Electrolytes (as ions):			
Calcium	-0.72	-0.55	-0.37
Magnesium	-0.02	+0.06	+0.15
Sodium	-0.24	-0.25	-0.11

The main subgroups of *cardiovascular disease* - cerebrovascular, ischaemic heart disease and "other" heart diseases - are all closely associated with water calcium, with correlation coefficients around -0.6 for male and females (Table 3). Correlations with other causes of death are also negative but are smaller. *Bronchitis* is also highly correlated with water hardness and calcium, but in Great Britain this association can be explained in terms of other factors, notably socio-economic conditions and industrialisation. *Infant mortality* is also negatively associated with water hardness and this is being investigated further.

Table 3. Associations between water calcium and local death rates at ages 45–64 (1958–64) in the 61 county boroughs of England and Wales with a population of 80,000 or over in 1961

Certified cause of death	Correlation (r) with water calcium p.p.m.	
	Males	Females
All cardiovascular disease	−0.72	−0.71
cerebrovascular	−0.62	−0.54
coronary	−0.59	−0.62
other heart	−0.60	−0.60

Table 4. Mean death-rates per 100,000 (1958–64) from cardiovascular disease at ages 45–64 years related to water calcium in the 61 county boroughs of England and Wales with total population of 80,000 or over in 1961

Water Calcium (p.p.m.)	Number of towns	Males	Females
< 10	8	751	355
10 - 39	24	721	330
40 - 69	9	636	306
70 - 99	13	633	281
100 +	7	546	248

Table 4 demonstrates the trend in cardiovascular death rates associated with the calcium content of the local drinking water in the 61 county boroughs in England and Wales. The male death rates are 37% higher in very soft towns compared with very hard towns. The proportional difference is even greater for females.

None of these findings, of course, is evidence of a direct causal relationship between drinking water and mortality; the correlation could be due to confounding factors. In a comprehensive search for such factors, over 100 indices of local social, economic, industrial and other environmental conditions were correlated with water hardness and calcium. There was no evidence that water hardness or calcium was merely reflecting other factors, and *rainfall* was the only variable closely associated with these water components. This is as expected; the high rainfall areas are mainly the soft-water areas and these areas have a high mortality from cardiovascular disease. However, a multiple regression study showed that, after allowing for other environmental and social factors, both water calcium and rainfall made significant separate contributions to the variation of cardiovascular death rates between the towns studied. The contribution made by rainfall remains perplexing; it could affect cardiovascular death rates through some component of water other than calcium or it could act independently.

In a situation like this, ideally it would be desirable to further explore the possibility of a direct causal relationship by experiments in which water hardness was changed in a community. This raises considerable problems; industrial and social as well as medical and technical. We have fortunately, in Great Britain, been able to take advantage of an 'experiment of opportunity' and death rates have been studied in the 83 county boroughs of England and Wales, in 11 of which the hardness of the water had changed, opportunely and for a variety of reasons, by 50 parts/10^6 or more, during the past 30 or so years (Table 5). A

Table 5. Proportional changes in mortality between 1948-54 and 1958-64 related to changes in water hardness in the large towns of England and Wales ages 45-64

	Water hardness Increased (5 towns)	Water hardness No change (72 towns)	Water hardness Decreased (6 towns)
	% change	% change	% change
Males Cardiovascular disease	+ 8.5	+ 11.2	+ 20.2
All other causes	- 10.8	- 13.0	- 12.4
Females Cardiovascular disease	- 14.9	- 11.8	- 9.0
All other causes	- 13.7	- 10.9	- 12.5

favourable effect on cardiovascular mortality was found where the drinking water had become harder compared with where it had become softer. Non-cardiovascular death rates were unaffected.

These findings suggest that there is a "water factor" affecting cardiovascular disease and we have to consider the possibility that there is a direct "cause-and-effect" association between the drinking water and cardiovascular disease; that there is some quality or component in the water affecting some major pathogenic processes.

Pathology. The association could be with any of one of the main processes in cardiovascular disease – hypertension, myocardial function, intravascular thrombosis or mural atheroma. In a comparison of the cardiac lesions in subjects dying in a soft water and a hard water town (Glasgow and London) there was no difference in the prevalence of extensive atheroma and severe stenosis in the coronary arteries between accident cases from the two areas, but significantly more ischaemic myocardial disease in the soft water areas. The findings suggested that a myocardial factor could be involved. Studies in Canada and the U.S.A. have indicated the higher death rates from ischaemic heart disease in soft water areas to be due to an excess of sudden deaths and recent work in Great Britain support this possibility. However, this is *not* the whole story; there remains a difference in CVD mortality in *non-sudden* deaths between hard and soft water towns.

Clinical. Because *all* subgroups of cardiovascular disease are involved in the Water Story, it is clear that whatever mechanism is involved must be common to ischaemic heart disease, cerebrovascular disease, hypertensive heart disease and those conditions labelled as "myocardial degeneration". Hypertension would seem to be the most likely common factor and in the search for differences in blood pressure levels and other risk factors for cardiovascular disease, we set up studies in 12 towns in England and Wales, 6 with very hard water and low CVD mortality rates, and 6 with very soft water and high CVD mortality rates. Clinical and biochemical measurements were made in 500 middle-aged sedentary workers resident in these towns.

There were significant differences found in heart rate, diastolic blood pressure and, to a lesser degree, blood cholesterol levels. With few exceptions, the results were surprisingly consistent for *heart-rate* and *casual diastolic pressure*; the cholesterol findings were less consistent. There was an interesting difference between the hard and soft water towns in the relation between age and blood pressure. There was little or no difference between the two groups at ages 40-50 years, but quite pronounced differences at ages 56-65 years. In the hard water groups mean diastolic pressure did not increase with age. It must be emphasised that this was an exploratory pilot study involving small numbers, in search of hypotheses, and that confirmation of these findings must be sought in larger and different studies. Meanwhile, we consider that the differences observed in mean blood pressure, heart rate and possibly blood cholesterol could account for a considerable proportion of the difference in cardiovascular mortality in the towns studied.

Discussion

There are two major suggestions arising from the evidence at present available; firstly, that hypertension is more prevalent in soft water areas; secondly, that a factor affecting myocardial function is involved. If we are to postulate a direct relationship between these two possible pathogenic aspects and the components of water, there are several mechanisms which have to be considered. The mineral content of water could be protective or injurious, soft waters could be carrying metal contaminants from pipes or soil, or other trace substances could be involved.

Calcium-Sodium-Magnesium Interrelationships

Calcium and magnesium are closely related – they compete for binding sites, they share absorption pathways and they could replace each other in some chemical relationship. Both are involved in enzymatic processes in heart muscle. Calcium in water could act by inhibiting the absorption of toxic elements or by providing an additional source of total calcium intake. There are suggestions from population studies in Japan, and from animal experiments, that a low calcium intake is associated with a greater prevalence of hypertension, particularly in females. High prevalence of hypertension has also been reported in populations living in areas with very high concentrations of sodium in the drinking water. Soft waters contain less calcium and more sodium than hard waters and artificial softening using base exchange methods can exaggerate this situation considerably. There is considerable epidemiological and experimental data linking the calcium-sodium-magnesium interrelationship to hypertension and this bulk electrolyte situation certainly deserves further examination in population studies and the laboratory. There are considerable difficulties in studying the electrolyte balance in free-living populations. Urinary excretion studies requiring frequent 24-hour collections constitute a major problem, and intake measurements are even more difficult. There is an overwhelming need for new methods in this field.

Lead

Plumbo-solvency from soft and acid waters has been a problem in Great Britain in the past and may still affect some soft water towns. We have found that the lead content of ribs was considerably higher in soft water areas as compared with hard warer areas in Great Britain and while it is unlikely that lead contamination could explain the "water story" it might be a contributory factor in some areas.

Cadmium

Cadmium dissolved from galvanized pipes might be a pathogenic factor and there is evidence from clinic-pathological and epidemiologic studies linking cadmium and hypertension. In a study of ribs from "sudden death" cases in Great Britain, significantly higher levels were present in ribs from the soft water areas.

Other trace elements are also being considered in the Water Story as some elements may have a protective effect by influencing lipid metabolism and arterial disease e.g. vanadium, manganese, chromium, lithium, while others such as lead, cadmium and cobalt are known to be harmful. Trace element studies comparing hard and soft water areas have not yet produced any consistent pattern of results and sampling and measurement techniques are far from standardised.

It is also possible that hard waters may be *protective* due to their mineral content. Calcium might inhibit the absorption of toxic substances and it has been shown that the absorption of lead, cadmium, zinc and chromium is inversely related to the concentration of calcium in the medium.

Conclusion. It is clear from these brief and speculative comments that there is no shortage of hypotheses to explain how the components of drinking water might affect cardiovascular function and disease. What is more important at the moment is to confirm the possibility that the Water Story involves the prevalence of hypertension and to further explore the myocardial aspects suggested by the differences in heart rate observed in the clinical study. It is also vital to take advantage of any experiments of opportunity provided by the softening or hardening of water supplies to a community. It may be premature to suggest the widespread hardening of water in those areas with soft water supplies, but it is probably not unreasonable to caution those who would soften a hard water supply.

THE METHODOLOGY OF INTERVENTION TRIALS

M. Steinbach

A multifactorial prevention trial, even of modest dimensions, is a complex enterprise of large scope. It involves ample resources, both human and material. Hence the design must be carefully analysed, in order not to waste these resources and to obtain maximum useful results. In the first table are given the main aims of the trial (Table 1). From the long list of items of its design I will only dwell

Table 1. General aims of a multifactorial intervention trial

---

1. Feasibility of such an enterprise on a large scale

2. The methodology

3. The psychological out-look:

   3.0. The responsiveness of the subject

   3.1. Attendance at periodical examination

   3.2. Adherence to recommendations

4. The medical out-look:

   4.1. Does intervention correct the risk factors?

   4.2. Does correction of risk factors reduce the specific morbidity and mortality?

---

on those of greater concern, that seem to me most suitable for discussion and most provocative. Once the decision is taken to direct such a trial against the degenerative cardiovascular diseases (atherosclerosis and hypertension) especially coronary heart disease, the first problem is the choice between a population at large, selected according to the home address, and an occupational one selected according to the place of work. After careful weighing the advantages and disadvantages we chose the population at large on account of its heterogeneity and hence its greater representativeness.

In regard to the size, the problems to be solved are the number and the manner
of randomization. For the determination of the number we can use the formula of
the Biometric Research Branch - Bethesda, published in the Final Report of the
National Diet-Heart Study, which, of course, is not the only one available. The
use of this formula implies previous knowledge of some experimental parameters:
d = the 5 year drop out rate, k = reduction of the 5 year event rate (p_e), f =
the length of time required to obtain maximum benefit of treatment, and to fix
a priori two statistical figures: α or type I or false positive error probability
that any rate difference between the experimental and control group could occur
by chance and β or type II or false negative error probability, i.e. the probability that the difference to be detected will not be missed, 1-β being the
power of the test. Assuming that d = 0.2, p_e = 0.05, k = 0.5 and f = 1 or 3, we
can derive the total sample sizes (the experimental and control groups together)
as shown in table 2.

Table 2. Total sample size for: p_e = .05; d = .20; k = .50

f	α = .01 β = .05	α = .01 β = .10	α = .05 β = .05	α = .05 β = .10
1	5,609	4,633	3,849	3,045
3	10,208	8,426	7,006	5,542

Our experimental group in Bucharest has 5.000 males aged 40-60, so that the total sample size will be 10.000. For randomization we prefer the two stage sampling with final exhaustive enumeration, the so-called "area sampling", because
of its simplicity and application to a middle size town with a homogenous population. One way is to randomize a small number of geographically limited units
and then to list within these units all the inhabitants we are interested in.
When the population is more heterogeneous, the best method is a stratified sampling.

The risk factors are the very core of any multifactorial intervention trial.
They should be accessible for detection and/or intervention. That is why we excluded, for instance, the behaviour pattern or the emotional stress (Table 3).

Table 3. Criteria: a) Evident or suspected influence
                   b) Accessible for detection and/or intervention

1. High blood cholesterol

2. High blood pressure

3. Smoking

4. Overweight

5. Diabetes

6. Minor nonspecific ECG abnormalities

7. Family history

The selection of risk criteria and cut-off points of the continuous variables
such as blood cholesterol, blood pressure, number of cigarettes per day, overweight - is a matter of arbitrary convention. This being the case, it would be

better in my opinion to be less strict in the choice of cut-off points and therefore enlarge the scope of intervention than to neglect some possible candidates
for heart disease. For blood cholesterol, for instance, we chose 220 mg/dl because the Framingham figures show two inflexion points: at 200 mg/dl (for the
30-49 age group) and at 240 mg/dl (for the 50-62 age group). In a recent paper
(1972) Fredrickson stated: "it may well be that a cholesterol concentration exceeding 220 at any age requres attention". Although 20 cigarettes a day is usually taken into account for segregating smokers at risk from other smokers or
nonsmokers, in the Western Collaborative Group Study 15 cigarettes daily were
shown to double the risk compared with non-smokers. For serum cholesterol, blood
pressure and overweight we differentiate 2 degrees of risk, more attention being
given to the highest. "Borderline hypertension" is defined as 140-150 mm Hg for
Systolic pressure and 90-94 mm Hg for diastolic pressure. The same principle
should be used for end points (Table 4) since separation of diagnostic criteria
can secure a greater flexibility for comparisons. A rigorous control group is a
prerequisite of any scientifically planned experience. But in the case of intervention trials we battle against two major difficulties: on is ethical — we cannot leave a man at high risk without treatment solely for the purpose of a good
control group; the second is practical — a group which has undergone an initial
screening for risks and diseases is no longer a genuine control group, psychologically uncontaminated. Detection at entry in only a small subsample is not of
great help. But I believe that most comparisons are possible using a control
group without an initial detection.

Table 4. End points

---

1. Myocardial infarction (fatal and nonfatal)

2. Cerebrovascular accident (fatal and nonfatal)

3. Sudden death

4. New coronary heart disease events

5. Other criteria for comparisons:

   — total mortality
   — total mortality minus neoplasms, accidents and
     respiratory diseases
   — mortality from cardiovascular diseases

Another controversial question is that of the doubleblind assessment. I am in
full agreement with the conclusions of the Final Report of the National Diet
Heart Study that in a mass field intervention trial a double-blind design "is a
formidable undertaking" and that a "mass field trial on a free-living population
can be undertaken with hope of success only with a non-double-blind design". In
a multifactorial trial the difficulties are still greater. The main reason is the
lack of motivation both in doctors and patients, as well as the difficulty of a
physician being unaware of a situation when the patient is aware of it.

The first method of intervention (Table 5) is to make the subject acquainted with
his situation. We use a green card for the subjects without risks, a yellow book
with the specification of risks at entry, some short advice for each risk correction and a record of the risk evolution and a red book for diseases (including
second degree risks).

Much time, money and man-power can be saved using a computer. The computer is an
efficient way of reducing the cost and of diverting the man-power towards strengthening the "intervention pressure", which is in turn a way of reducing cost,
by reducing k, the time necessary, for achievement of maximum treatment effect.
How the total expenses vary between enlarging the staff for this purpose and
reducing the k is a subject for a health operation research.

Table 5. Methods of intervention

---

1. Communication of periodic examinations results

2. Targeted health education ("written")

3. Consultation for additional explanations

4. Meetings and group discussions with subjects and
   their wives about risk factors (generally)

5. Meetings and group discussions with subjects and
   their wives about individual risk factors

6. Home visits

7. Medical advice for diet and drugs. Step-by-step
   approach

8. Personal discussions with the principal investigator

A. PRIMARY PREVENTIVE TRIAL IN GÖTEBORG, SWEDEN

G. Tibblin, L. Wilhelmsen, and L. Werkö

With a multiple logistic model it has been shown among randomly selected middle-aged men in Göteborg — the Men born in 1913 Study that it is possible to distinguish between a highest risk decile and a lowest risk decile; the formel running a risk of IHD (acute non-fatal myocardial infarction and acute fatal IHD) nearly 30 times higher than that of the latter (Wilhelmsen et al., 1973). Cholesterol, smoking and blood pressure are the necessary variables for this prediction.

If these three risk factors are casual, preventive measures offer great promise of reducing the high morbidity and mortality from IHD.

Purpose of Study

1. Is it possible to induce changes in the risk factors, cholesterol, smoking and blood pressure in a new sample of randomly selected population of middle-aged Swedish men?

2. Will these changes in these risk factors decrease the incidence of non-fatal and fatal myocardial infarction, stroke and the total death in the intervention group compared with a control group.

Method and the Study Population

The general design of the study is presented in Table 1. The subjects have been randomly divides into three groups, each comprising approximately 10.000 men. Group A is the intervention group, the two others (B and C) are the control groups. As the men are randomly allocated to the groups and the groups are large, it may be assumed that the initial risk profile is the same in all three groups. The examination began in 1970 with men born in 1915 and was completed during spring 1973 with those born in 1925. The effects on the risk factors are measured in the intervention and in a control group 4 years after they entered into the study.

Table 1. General design of the Primary Preventive Trial in Göteborg 1970 — Study group: All men born 1915-1922 and 1924-1925. N = 30,000

Groups	A N = 10 000	B N = 10 000	C N = 10 000

Investigation	Postal question-
	naire
	  Heredity
	  Heart symptoms
	  Physical activity
	    Occupation
	    Leisure-time
	  Smoking
	  Stress
	
	Examination
	  Height, weight,
	  blood pressure,
	  cholesterol
	  ECG
	
	Special question-
	naires and tests
	in sub-samples
		Postal question-
		naire
		  In random sub-
		  sample (to ensure
		  comparability)
		
		Examination
		  Same as in Group A
		  in sub-sample	

Treatment	Risk factors
	treated
	  High blood
	  pressure
	  High cholesterol
	  Smoking
	  (Physical inactivity)		

Rescreening after 4 years	Postal question- naire Check of results on risk factors	Postal question- naire Same as in Group A in sub-sample	
End points	Deaths, all causes Deaths, cause specific Non-fatal myocardial infarction Non-fatal stroke	in Groups A, B and C	

Participation Rate

The number and percentage of subjects in the intervention group who were sent the postal questionnaire, who answered it and who attended the screening examination are presented in Table 2.

Treatment

The treatment has been organized in special out-patient clinics. Table 3 shows the number of subjects in different risk groups. Patients who were already being treated for hypertension by other doctors constitute a certain problem. These patients were also invited to the diagnostic work-up and received information.

Treatment was only changed if it was considered necessary because of poor control of blood pressure.

Table 2. Number and percentage of subjects in the intervention group who were sent the postal questionnaire, who answered it, and who attended the screening examination. Men born 1915-1922 and 1924-1925

	N	%
Postal questionnaires sent	9.996	100
Postal questionnaires answered	8.393	84
Attended screening examination	7.600	76

Table 3. Allocation of subjects to treatment groups. Subjects are primarily allocated to the group with the lowest number. A smoker with hypertension will thus belong to group 1, etc N = 7.540

	N	%
1. Hypertension SBP ≥ 175 or DBP ≥ 115	980	13.0
2. Hypercholesterolemia ≥ 300 mg/100 ml[a]	694	9.2
3. Smoking ≥ 15 cigarettes per day	1.086	14.4
Total	2.760	36.6

[a]All subjects with cholesterol = 260-300 mg/100 ml are invited to attend a group information on diet.

Results concerning the adherence to the programme are acceptable — 91 per cent of the hypertensive subjects followed regular checkups one year after screening examination. From Table 4 it is clear that still 12 per cent had high blood pressure one year after the screening. All men with cholesterol values at screening (taken in the afternoon after at least 2 hours fasting) ≥ 300 mg/100 ml were re-investigated in the morning, and triglycerides and lipoprotein types were examined at the same time.

Diet information for groups of 7-10 men and their wives, or individually was given by a doctor and a dietician. Slides and booklets have been prepared for this purpose. If cholesterol value was high (≥ 300 mg/100 ml) in spite of dietary efforts over six months, clofibrate and/or nicotinic acid (according to lipoprotein type) was given.

The effect of the treatment is promising. In a studied group there is a significant drop in cholesterol from 311 to 272 mg/100 ml.

Table 4. Results of blood pressure control after 6 and 12 months in men born in 1915. Men with SBP ≥ 175 or DBP ≥ 115 allocated to treatment. N = 87

| | 6 months | | 12 months | |
	N	%	N	%
< 160/90	11	12	30	34
160/95 – 175/115	41	47	31	36
> 175/115	18	21	10	12
No therapy, BP acceptable	17	20	16	18
Total	87	100	87	100

All men who smoked ≥ 15 cigarettes were invited to a special antismoking clinic connected with the trial. The antismoking schedule started with an invitation to 40 smokers to an information meeting at which individual information on the results of the screening examinations was given. A short talk on the health consequences of smoking and the smoking mechanisms introduced a discussion. A series of slides and films about stopping smoking were used. The participants were then invited to group meetings (7-10 men) at one week intervals for further information about the antismoking programme recommended by us and for the delivery of chewing gum with nicotine, which is used as a substitute for smoking. The results with respect to stopping smoking is promising. 27% per cent were still non-smokers one year after the treatment started.

Evaluation of Effects

The end-points of the study are M.I. stroke and total death. In order to record deaths in the experimental and the control groups, all death certificates in the city of Göteborg are collected twice each month.

The overall autopsy rate for people below 65 years of age in the city is about 90 per cent. A myocardial infarction register has been in operation in Göteborg since 1968 and a stroke register since 1970. All clinically diagnosed cases of myocardial infarction and cerebro-vascular diseases are recorded from these registers. The staff of the registers do not know which group of the trial the patients belong to. The effect of the intervention can easily be measured as the difference in incidence of different end-points between the intervention group and the control groups. The incidence should be the same if the intervention was ineffective.

The trial is planned to continue for 10 years from the initial screening.

Summary

Swedish men aged 47-54 are usually interested in preventive measures. Three-fourth participate in a screening examination and most of the screened risk subjects take part in an attempt to change the risk factor in a favorable direction. It is also possible to reduce blood pressure and cholesterol and change the smoking habits among these men.

If these efforts are enough in order to change the morbidity and mortality we do not know yet.

THE HELSINKI MENTAL HOSPITAL STUDY
A PRIMARY PREVENTION TRIAL

Osmo Turpeinen

The Helsinki mental hospital study is a long-term dietary intervention trial conducted in two mental hospitals near Helsinki (Turpeinen et al., 1968, Miettinen et al., 1972).

In 1959 a cholesterol-lowering diet was introduced in one of the hospitals (hospital N), whereas the other hospital (hospital K) was kept on the normal hospital diet. Six years later the diets were reversed: hospital N was returned to the normal diet and hospital K was placed on the cholesterol-lowering diet. This dietary arrangement was followed for the second period of the study (1965-1971).

Table 1. Design of experiment

Time	Hospital N	Hospital K
First period	Experimental	Normal
1959-1965	diet	diet
Second period	Normal	Experimental
1965-1971	diet	diet

The experimental diet differed from the normal hospital diet in two important respects: ordinary milk was replaced by an emulsion of soybean oil in skim milk ("filled milk") and butter and ordinary margarine were replaced by a "soft" margarine with a high content of polyunsaturated fatty acids. The fatty acid compositions of these two diets were very different. The polyunsaturated/saturated fatty acid ratio (P/S ratio), which was 0.22-0.29 in the normal diet, was increased to 1.42-1.78 in the experimental one.

The subjects of the detailed study were men in the initial age range from 35-65 years. There were about 300 such subjects in each hospital. Subjects with patterns of coronary heart disease in their initial electrocardiogram were excluded in this part of the study.

The use of the experimental diet was associated with lowered serum cholesterol levels in both hospitals. The mean reductions as compared to the values on the normal hospital diet ranged from 12-18%.

Table 2. Mean serum cholesterol values

| Hospital | Mean serum-cholesterol (mmol/l) | | |
	1st period	2nd period	Difference
Males			
N	5.61	6.87	1.26
K	6.93	6.05	0.88
Females			
N	6.33	7.18	0.85
K	6.98	6.10	0.88

In the assessment of the incidence of coronary heart disease (CHD) the appearance of certain electrocardiographic signs (classified according to the Minnesota code) and the occurrence of coronary death were noted. These are end-points which can be observed with a fair degree of objectivity.

The incidence of CHD was found to be in both hospitals during the period of the experimental diet considerably lower than during that of the control diet. A comparison of the pooled diet periods with the pooled control periods revealed a clear-cut and statistically significant reduction of the CHD incidence associated with the use of the cholesterol-lowering diet.

In addition to the detailed investigation described above, also a larger mortality study was carried out. This comprised all patients admitted to the hospitals in the years 1959-1971, 10,612 patients in all.

In men, the use of the cholesterol-lowering diet was associated with considerably and significantly reduced mortality from CHD. Total mortality also was consistently lower on this diet, although the differences were too small for statistical significance.

Table 3. Age-adjusted death-rates per 1000 person-years

	C.H.D.	All diseases
Males		
Hospital N, period 1 (diet)	5.72	32.74
Hospital N, period 2 (control	12.97	36.64
Hospital K, period 1 (control)	15.18	35.27
Hospital K, period 2 (diet)	7.50	31.25
Pooled diet periods	6.61	32.00
Pooled control periods	14.08	35.96
Females		
Hospital N, period 1 (diet)	3.96	29.51
Hospital N, period 2 (control	7.74	30.00
Hospital K, period 1 (control	8.06	24.41
Hospital K, period 2 (diet)	6.46	28.59
Pooled diet periods	5.21	29.05
Pooled control periods	7.90	27.21

In women, the mortality from CHD also appeared to be lower during the diet period but the differences were small and not significant. In female total mortality no appreciable differences were found.

The mortality from malignant neoplasms showed no appreciable differences between the different dietary periods. Neither was there any indication that the use of the cholesterol-lowering diet would lead to an increased prevalence of gallstones.

THE CORONARY DRUG PROJECT — A SECONDARY PREVENTION TRIAL
THE CORONARY DRUG PROJECT RESEARCH GROUP*

R.J. Jones, Ch.R. Klimt, and J. Stamler

The Coronary Drug Project (CDP) has been in progress in the United States since 1966 as a collaborative study supported by the National Heart and Lung Institute (CDPRG**, 1973a). It involves 8,341 men age 30 to 64 years on entry in the study, participating in 53 clinical centers throughout the country.

This trial from its beginning has had three basic objectives: To evaluate long-term therapeutic efficacy of five pharmacologic regimens influencing serum lipids; to study the clinical course and prognosis of coronary artery disease; and to learn more about the effective conduct of large-scale multicenter trials of treatment for chronic disease. All patients before entry into the study had suffered one or more electrocardiographically documented myocardial infarcts (MI).

The main design characteristics of the CDP are:

1. Randomized allocation of patients to the five active treatment groups, and to the placebo control group.
2. Double blind design, i.e., the treatment unknown to the patients and the treating physician.
3. A detailed obligatory common protocol.
4. Every patient to be followed for a minimum of five years, and every patient to be followed until all have been observed for at least five years (to be accomplished by October, 1974).
5. As part of the common protocol, detailed provisions for quality control of data through use of a Central Laboratory, a single center for ECG reading using Minnesota Code criteria, a Coordinating Center, and a system of national committees.

The original treatment groups in the CDP were: Mixed conjugated equine estrogens in two dosage groups, 2.5 and 5.0 mg per day (ESG1 and ESG2); clofibrate, 1.8 mg per day (CPIB); dextrothyroxine, 6.0 mg per day (DT4); nicotinic acid, 3.0 mg per day (NICA); and lactose placebo (PLBO). All drugs were packaged in identical capsules and sealed; the common dosage was nine capsules per day, in a dosage of three t.i.d. For reasons of statistical power, men were randomly allocated to the five active treatment groups and placebo in a ratio of 1 to 1 to 1 to 1 to 1 to 2.5 — an average of 1,110 patients in each of the five active drug groups and 2,789 in the control group. Randomization was carried out separately for each of the 53 clinics and for two risk groups. Risk Group 1 was made up of patients who had suffered a single uncomplicated infarct; risk group 2, of patients who had had two or more infarcts, or only one infarct but with a complicated course (e.g., shock, secondary extension, pericarditis, congestive heart failure, thromboembolism, major arrhythmia).

The following conditions for inclusion in the study had to be fulfilled by a potential patient:

1. His age on entry had to be between 30 and 64 years.
2. There had to be a qualifying electrocardiogram documenting a past myocardial infarction, with survival for at least three months since most recent MI.
3. He had to be in New York Heart Association functional class I or II.

---

*Prepared for the Coronary Drug Project Research Group by Doctors Richard J. Jones, Christian R. Klimt and Jeremiah Stamler, and presented by Richard J. Jones, M.D.

**Abbreviation: CDPRG = Coronary Drug Project Research Group.

4. He must not have had heart surgery.
5. He must not have other major life-shortening disease, e.g., cancer.
6. He must not be on long-term anticoagulatns or on lipid-lowering drugs.
7. He must not be an insulin-dependent diabetic.
8. Also, he had to give his written consent after a thorough explanation of the design of the study and the potential side reactions of the drugs involved. The protocol also provided that study physicians were to use criteria for best modern medical care as the guiding basis for all treatment decisions concerning all patients.

The rate of recruitment was almost uniform over a three-year period between July, 1966 and October, 1969.

The following are among the many clinical events monitored at regular intervals: Death and cause of death, nonfatal cardiovascular complications (e.g., MI, acute coronary insufficiency, angina pectoris, congestive heart failure, ECG abnormalities, stroke thromboembolic disease), other illnesses; symptoms and signs of possible drug toxicity.

Clinical assessments have been performed at the following points in the study: three times in 4-week intervals before entry into the study and then every four months throughout the study. These include laboratory tests to determine blood lipid levels, to monitor toxicity and side reactions, and to check on adherence to medication. The annual examinations are more extensive than the two interim ones.

The statistical planning of the study yielded a sample size estimate of 8,379 patients (8,341 were actually recruited), based on the following assumptions: the probability that at the end of the trial and observed difference in total mortality between one of the active treatment groups and the control will be designated significant when in fact it is not was set at .01 (alpha); the probability that a true difference does exist but by chance is not observed was set at .05 (beta); and the minimal difference in mortality, as a percentage of placebo mortality, for which beta is equal to or less than .05 is .25. Since estimated 5-year mortiality for the placebo group was 30 per cent, this minimum reduction in mortality for a treatment group corresponded to a 5-year mortality rate of 22.5 per cent. The dropout and frank non-adherence rate after 5 years, estimated at no more than 30 per cent or 6 per cent per annum, was included in the sample size calculations. It was assumed that the methods of the study would assure essentially 100 per cent follow-up in terms of the primary mortality end point; in fact, vital status is unknown for only six of the 8,341 men after an average of five years of follow-up.

The many quantitative findings available for the CDP patients on entry are presented in detail in an already published report (CDPRG, 1973a). The following are a few key facts: On the average, the men were 52 years old; one per cent was under 35, 19 per cent between 60 and 64. Two-thirds were in risk group 1, i.e., had had only one uncomplicated infarction. The most recent MI occurred less than a year before entry for 31 per cent, and five or more years before entry for 20 per cent; mean time since last MI was 36 months, median time 23 months. Forty-seven per cent had a definite history of angina pectoris prior to admission. Over one-third were smoking cigarettes at entry.

As to the distribution of baseline serum cholesterol levels, 48 per cent were in the range equal to or greater than 250 mg/dl, 14 per cent, 300 or greater; the mean value was 251, the median 247; 50 per cent had serum triglycerides of 5.0 mEq/L or greater; 34 per cent of 6.0 or greater; the mean was 6.1, the median 5.0, with marked skewing to the right. As expected, these two lipid variables were significantly correlated ($r = 0.349$).

Detailed univariate and multivariate analyses of a host of baseline characteristics — demographic, medical historical, medical examination, ECG, X-ray, biochemical — verified that the randomization procedure had accomplished its purpose of establishing comparability among the six groups at entry.

Significant results are available as of this date in regard to the three major goals of the CDP. First, the clinical course and prognostic importance of various factors have been analyzed for patients in the placebo group with respect to four end points — mortality from all causes, mortality from coronary heart disease (CHD), sudden coronary death (defined as CHD death within 60 minutes of onset of symptoms), and incidence of major coronary events (nonfatal MI plus coronary death) (CDPRG, 1972a; 1972b, and unpublished date). There were 358 deaths (12.8%) among the 2,789 patients in the placebo group by the time this entire cohort had completed three years in the study, i.e., a mortality rate of 4.2 per cent per year. Of these 358 deaths, 336 (93.9%) were attributed to cardiovascular causes, 292 (81.6%) to coronary heart disease (CHD), of which 161 (45.0% of all deaths) were sudden deaths from CHD. There were 485 patients who suffered a major coronary event in the first three years of follow-up (17.4%, or an annual rate of 5.8%). Since 81.6 per cent of the deaths were due to coronary heart disease, factors related to this cause were generally related to mortality from all causes as well.

The method of stepwise linear regression was used to evaluate relationship of 40 baseline characteristics to three-year mortality (unpublished). This method first identifies the variable most highly correlated with mortality, and then successively selects additional variables on the same basis, after allowance for previously selected variables. The regression coefficients for the first five baseline variables selected by the stepwise computer program all showed t values (regression coefficients divided by their standard errors) greater than 4.00, indicating that each was strongly related to mortality even after taking account of the effects of the other four. These first five selected baseline variables were ST segment depression on the resting ECG recorded at the time of entry into the study, cardiomegaly diagnosed from the teleroentgenogram, New York Heart Association functional class II, ventricular conduction defects, and use of diuretics.

When an additional five variables were added, adjusted t values for the original five remained high (3.32 or greater), and the five additional variables had t values of 2.84 or greater. This second set of five variables were history of intermittent claudication, elevated serum cholesterol, frequent ventricular ectopic beats on the resting ECG, physical inactivity of leisure, and Q and/or QS abnormalities on ECG. When ten additional variables were included in the regression, the first ten continued to show high adjusted t values. Five of the second ten showed a significant positive relationship to mortality, with t values greater than 2.00. These were heart rate on resting ECG, number of previous MIs, systolic blood pressure, use of oral antidiabetic medication, and use of cigarettes at entry. The multiple correlation coefficient (R) for the five variable linear regression model was .27, for the ten variable .30, for the 20 variable .32. Little information was added when an additional 20 variables were included; none of these last 20 showed significant adjusted t values, no increase in R (the multiple correlation coefficient) was recorded due to addition of the last 20 variables.

The multiple logistic regression model was used to compute coefficients for the first ten factors selected by the linear regression model: ST segment depression, cardiomegaly, NYHA functional class II, ventricular conduction defects, use of diuretics, history of intermittent claudication, elevated serum cholesterol, frequent ventricular ectopic beats, physical inactivity during leisure hours, persistent Q and/or AS abnormalities. These coefficients were then used to calculate an individual score for risk of dying in three years for each of the 2,789 placebo patients, based on his baseline findings for these ten factors. (The logistic model, in contrast with the linear model, yields risk estimates between zero and one). The men were then classified into deciles of expected risk. There was a close fit between expected and observed mortality for each decile (Fig. 1) (unpublished). The men in the highest decile of expected risk accounted for 31 per cent of all observed deaths; the men in the two highest deciles for 50 per cent. The observed mortality rate for the highest decile of estimated risk was more than 12-times as high as that of the lowest. The average observed three-year mortality rate for the three lowest deciles of estimated risk was 5.2 per cent, or 1.7 per cent per year. This is a much lower rate than previously deemed possible for post-MI middle-aged men. This finding has extensive implications — e.g., in regard to insurability of good risk post-MI men, in regard to the limitations of coronary surgery as a means of improving life expectancy for such men.

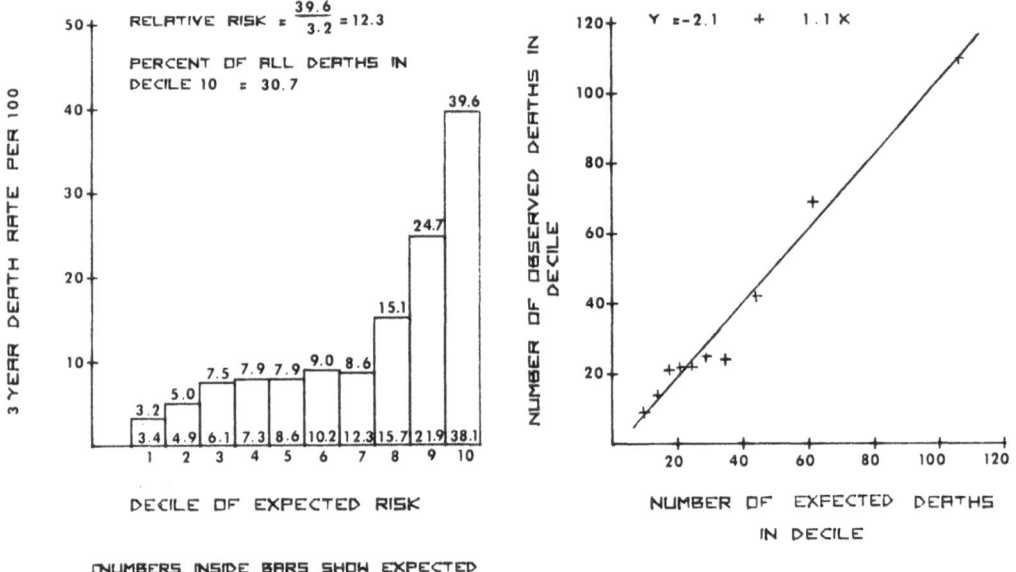

Figure 1. Expected and observed 3-year mortality for each decile of estimated risk, multiple logistic regression analysis with 10 variables — ST segment depression on resting ECG, cardiomegaly diagnosed from the teleroentgenogram, New York Heart Association functional class, ventricular conduction defects, use of diuretics, history of intermittent claudication, serum cholesterol, frequent ventricular ectopic beats on the resting ECG, physical inactivity of leisure, and Q and/or QS abnormalitites on ECG — 2,789 men, placebo group, Coronary Drug Project

In addition to this general analysis of the possible relationship of 40 baseline factors to three-year prognosis, detailed evaluation has confirmed that five elements of the post-MI recovery period resting ECG are independently related to risk — ST segment depression, Q and/or AS findings, ventricular conduction defects, ventricular premature beats, and heart rate (CDPRG, 1972a; 1972b). The findings with respect to ST segment depression, the first variable to be identified in the stepwise multiple linear regression analysis, are presented in Figure 2. The t value of 9.44 is the unadjusted t for the slope b from the univariate analysis; the t_a of 3.24 is after adjustment for 39 other factors, including other ECG variables. Fig. 2 also gives the data on Q-QS findings. Similar data for ventricular premature beats are presented in Figure 3. These data demonstrate unequivocally for the first time that ventricular dysrhythmia is prognostically important not only during the acute phase of an MI (e.g., in the coronary care unit), but also long-term, i.e., post recovery. Fig. 3 also gives the data on ventricular conduction defects, and Fig. 4 gives the findings on

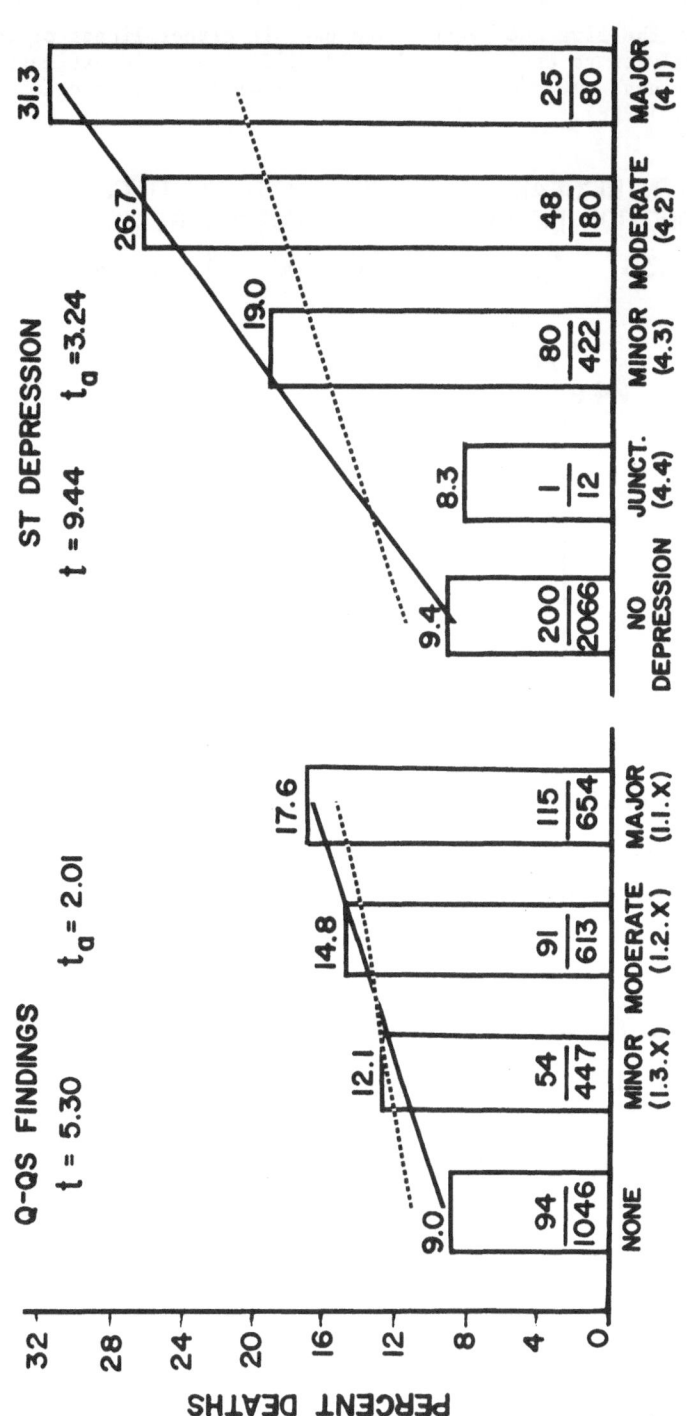

Figure 2. Analyses of relationship between Q-QS and ST depression findings in the baseline (entry) ECG and 3-year mortality from all causes in the 2,789 men of the placebo group. For information on the adjusted regression lines and their t values (t_a), see text

heart rate. When the five ECG factors are used in either linear or logistic multivariate analyses to estimate risk, wide differences in estimates across the deciles are obtained, and these correspond well with per cent deaths observed (Fig. 5) (CDPRG, 1972c).

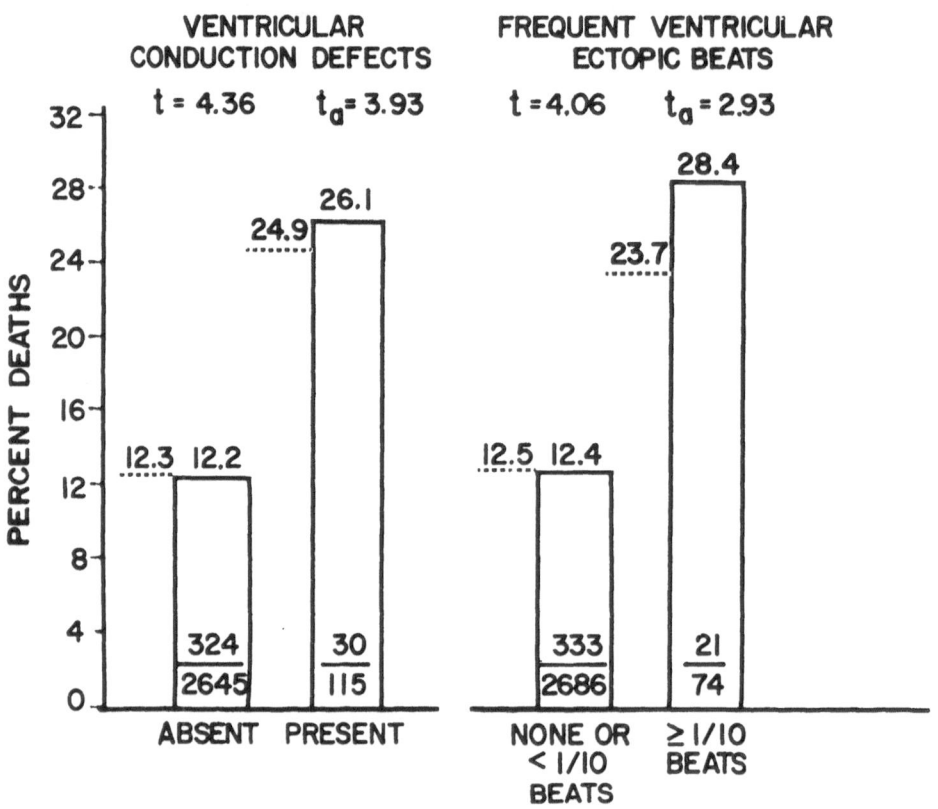

-------- ESTIMATED RATES ADJUSTED FOR 39 OTHER VARIABLES

Figure 3. Analyses of relationship between ventricular conduction defects and frequent ventricular ectopic beats in the baseline (entry) ECG and 3-year mortality from all causes in the 2,789 men of the placebo group. For information on the adjusted t (t_a), see text

Detailed analyses further demonstrate that in both univariate and multivariate analyses, serum cholesterol is significantly related to all four end points — mortality from all causes, mortality from sudden cardiac death, coronary mortality, and incidence of major recurrent coronary events (nonfata or fatal) (Fig. 6) (unpublished). This is also true at low, medium and high levels of serum triglycerides (Fig. 7). In contrast, baseline fasting serum triglycerides are not positively related to these and points. The highest mortality is in the group with high cholesterol and low triglycerides (Fig. 8). With statistical adjustment for the effect of other variables, triglycerides tend to have a *negative* relationship to mortality. This result is by no means inexplicable, since data are available indicating that hyperbetalipoproteinemia (with its pattern of hypercholesterolemia with little or no serum triglyceride elevation) may carry a greater risk of severe atherosclerosis and premature lethal CHD that hyperprebetalipoproteinemia (with its pattern of hypercholesterolemia with hypertriglyceridemia). This observation may in turn relate to the finding that betalipoprotein (low density lipoprotein) may more readily enter the arterial intima and be trapped there than prebetalipoprotein (very low density lipoprotein).

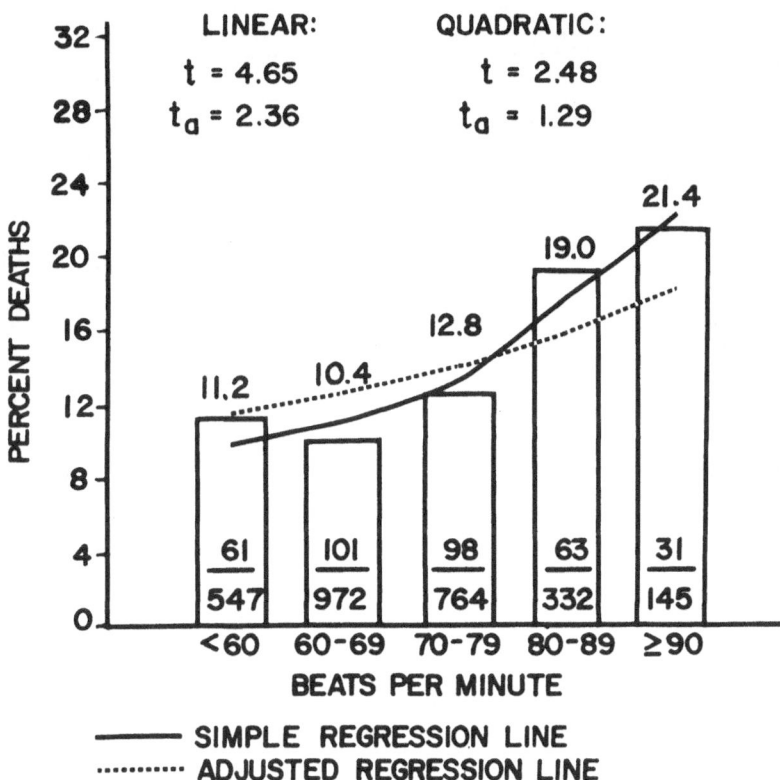

Figure 4. Analysis of resting heart rate findings in the baseline ECG and 3-year mortality from all causes in the 2,789 men of the placebo group. The regression lines are for the quadratic fit; the t values for this quadratic fit assess whether the regression equation with the quadratic term yields a significantly better fit than the linear regression equation

Finally, three major protocol changes have been made, all resulting from negative findings. The group given high dosage estrogen (5 mg per day) (ESG2) came to an early termination in May, 1970. There was a statistically non-significant excess in total mortality, CHD mortality, and sudden coronary death in the ESG2 group compared to the placebo group (Table 1) (CDPRG, 1970). Nonfatal infarctions were significantly more frequent than in the control group, as were nonfatal thromboembolic phenomena (e.g., thrombophlebitis and nonfatal pulmonary embolism), and this constellation of fatal and nonfatal findings led to cessation of this regimen. In addition, the cholesterol-lowering effect of this medication was modest, serum triglycerides rose significantly, and adherence was poor because of troublesome feminizing side effects.

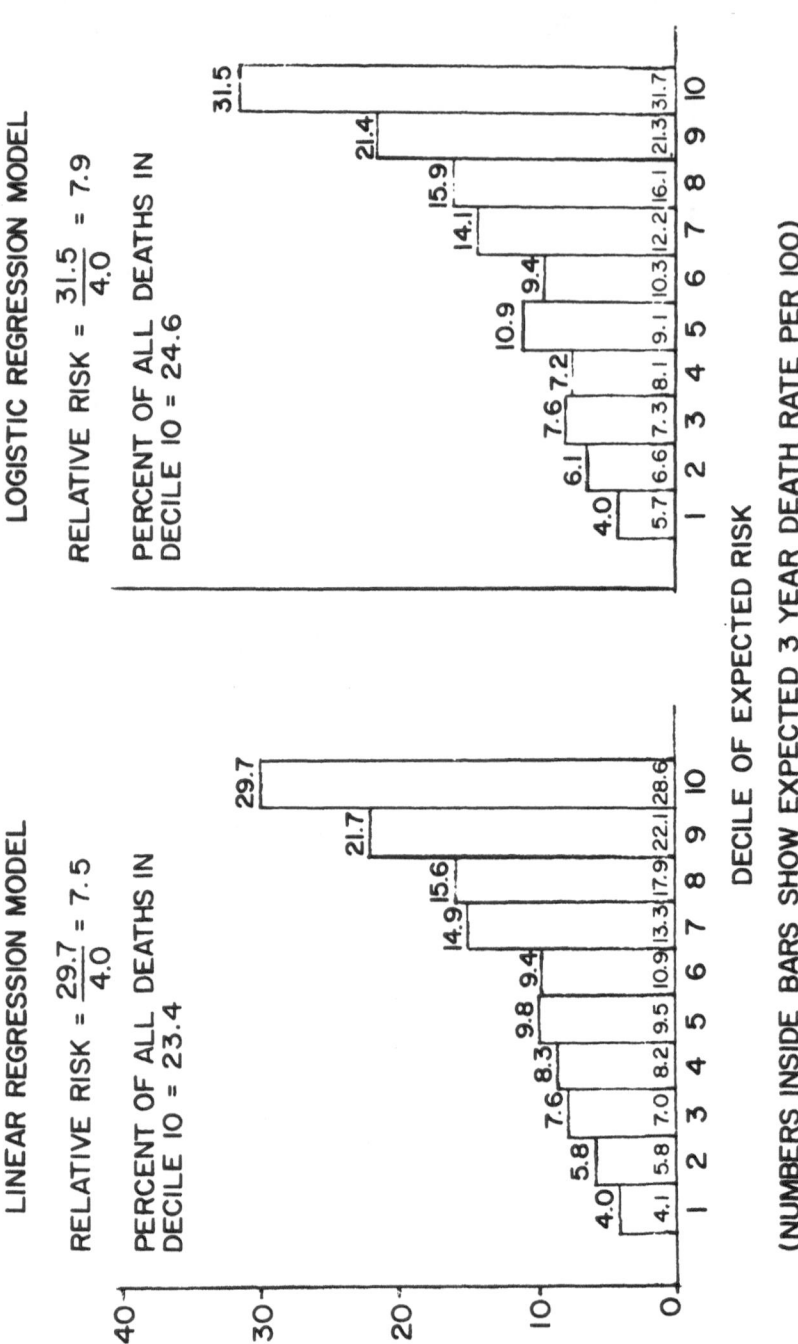

Figure 5. Expected and observed 3-year mortality for the placebo group; expected risk for each man was calculated based on the five foregoing ECG variables (see Figs. 2-4), using the multiple linear and multiple logistic regression models, and then ordering the men into deciles of expected risk

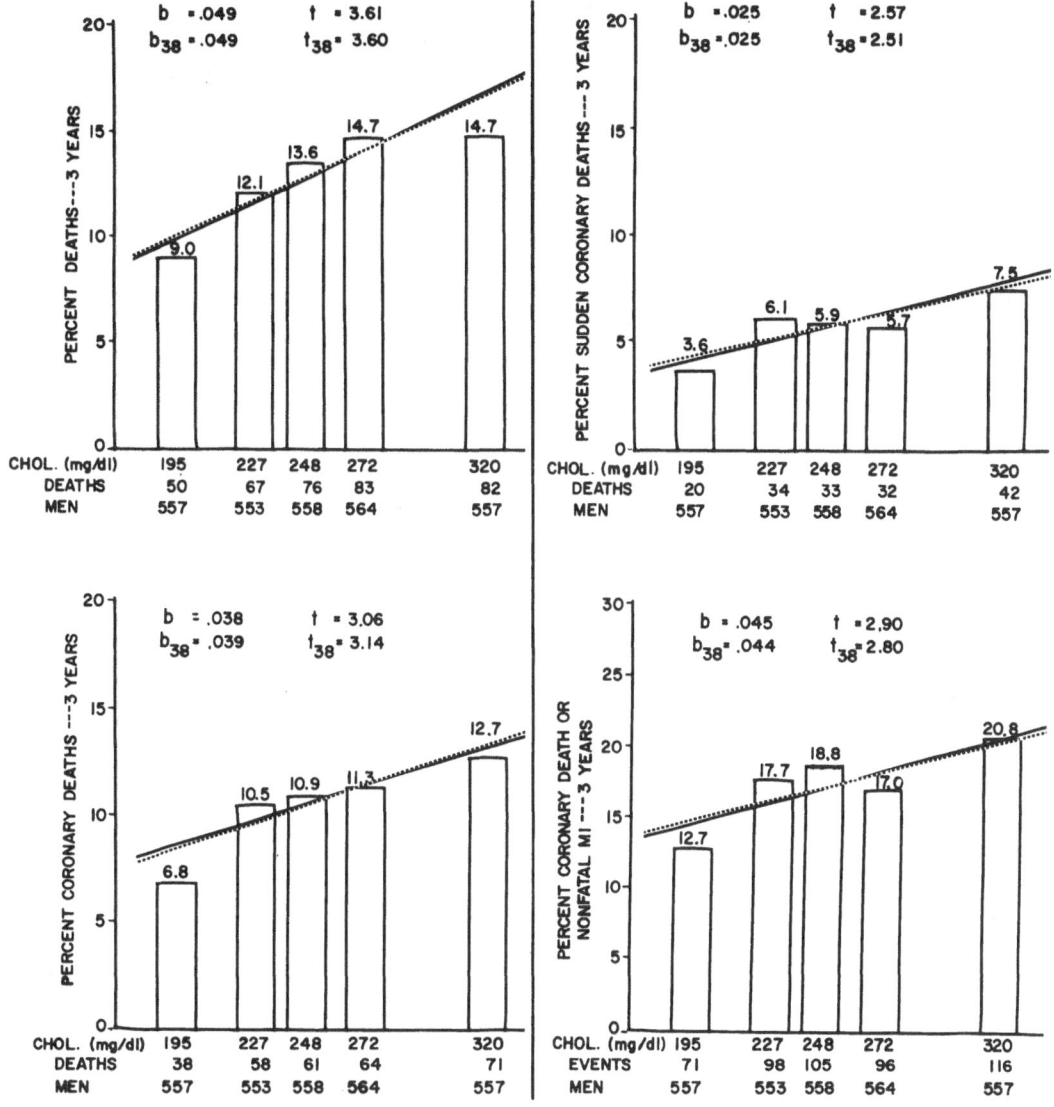

Figure 6. Analyses of relationship between baseline serum cholesterol level and 3-year rates for four stipulated endpoints for the 2,789 men of the placebo group. Cholesterol value for each man is the mean of his three baseline determinations at 4-week intervals. The two slopes in each graph are respectively the univariate and multivariate linear regression lines for the relationship between serum cholesterol and the stipulated endpoint; for the multivariate regression line, adjustment is made for the influence of 38 other variables on risk of mortality

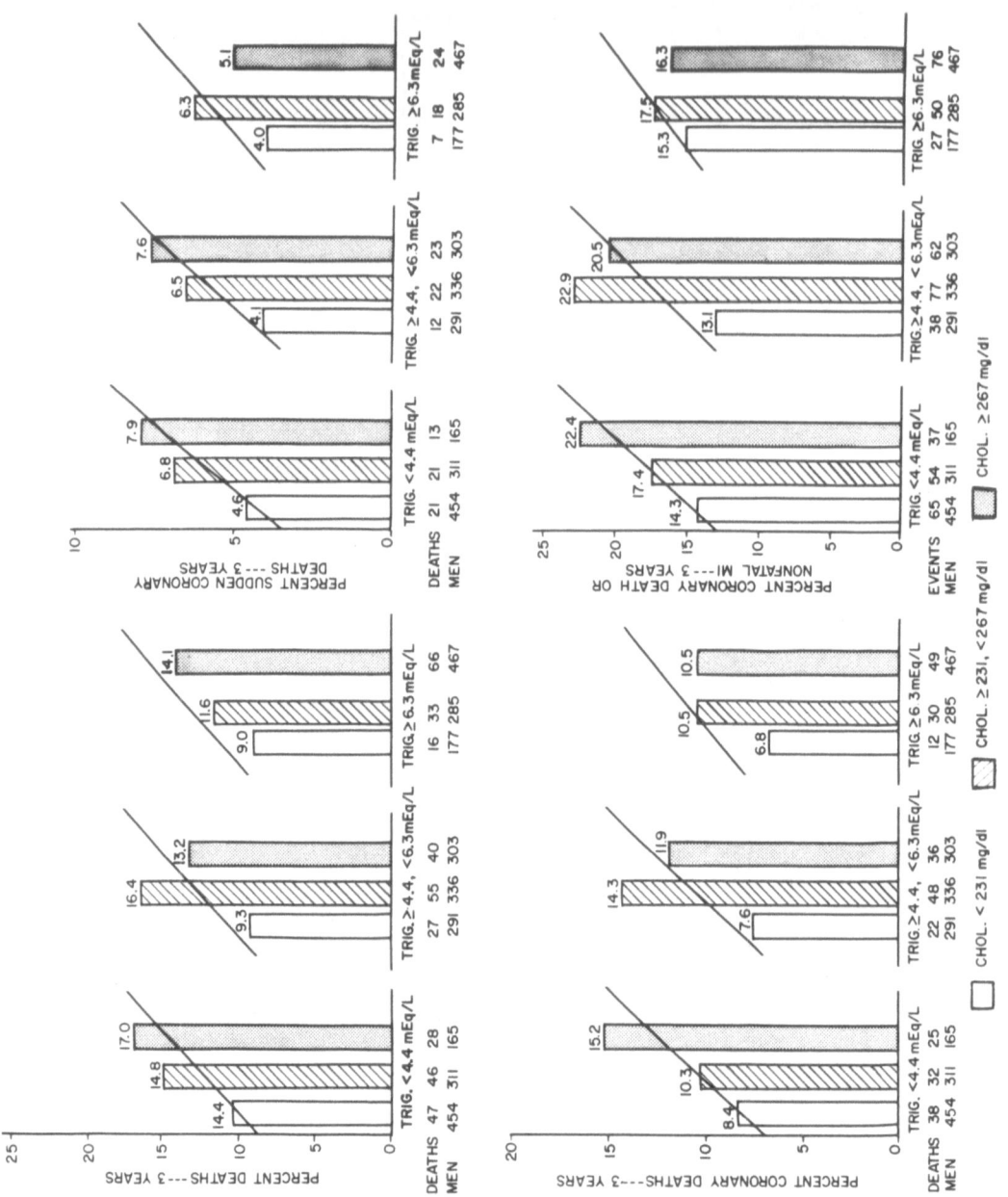

Figure 7. Analyses with serum fasting triglyceride levels controlled of relationship between baseline serum cholesterol level and 3-year rates for four stipulated endpoints for the 2,789 men of the placebo group. Cholesterol and triglyceride levels for each man are the means of his three baseline determinations at
4-week intervals. The slope lines are the linear regression lines of the relationship between serum cholesterol and the stipulated endpoints with serum
triglyceride levels simultaneously controlled

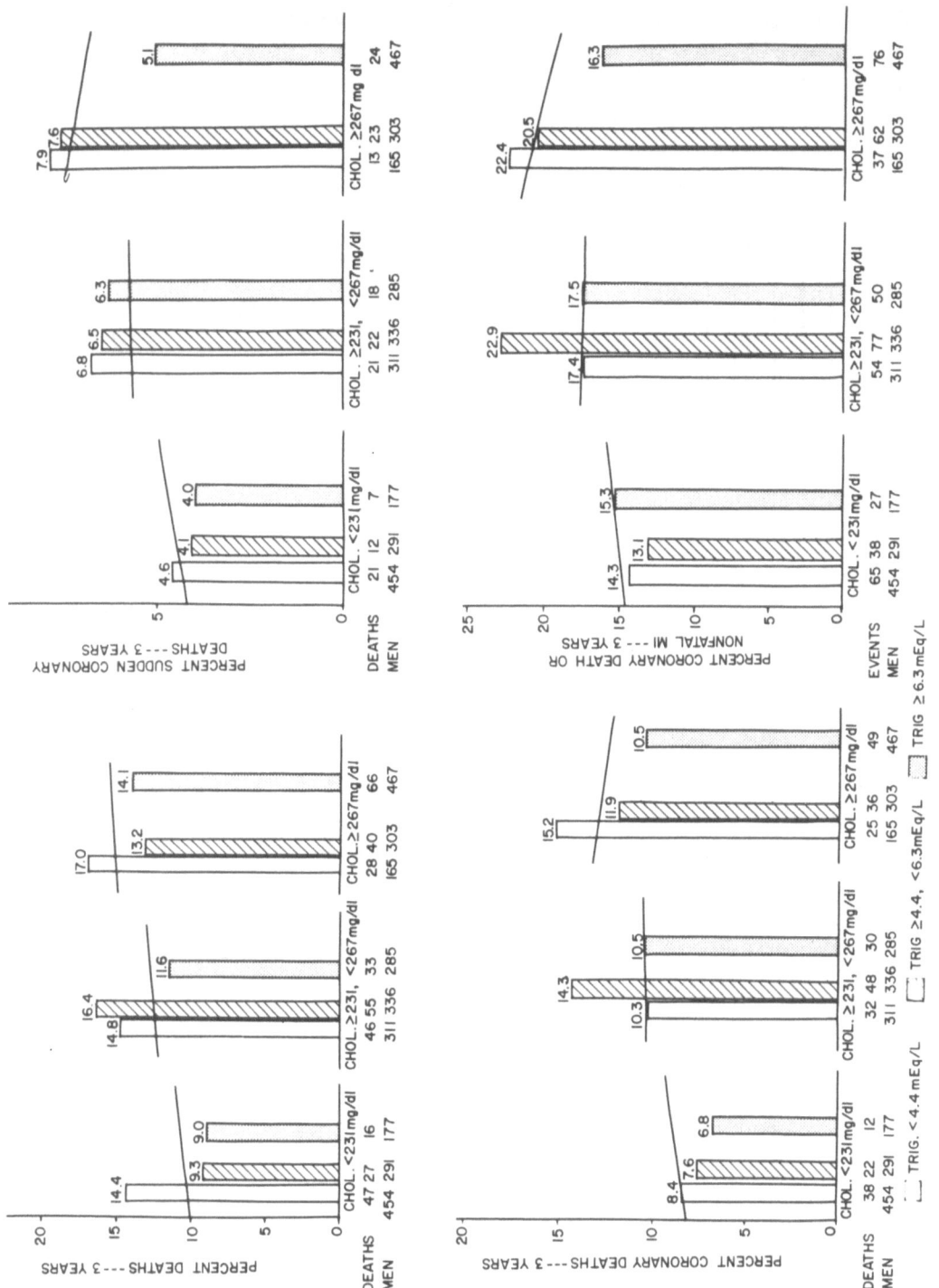

Figure 8. Analyses with serum cholesterol controlled of the relationship between baseline serum fasting triglyceride level and 3-year rates for four stipulated endpoints for the 2,789 men of the placebo group. Serum fasting triglyceride and cholesterol levels for each man are the means of his three baseline determinations at 4-week intervals. The slopes are the linear regression lines for the relationship between fasting serum triglycerides and the stipulated endpoints with serum cholesterol levels simultaneously controlled

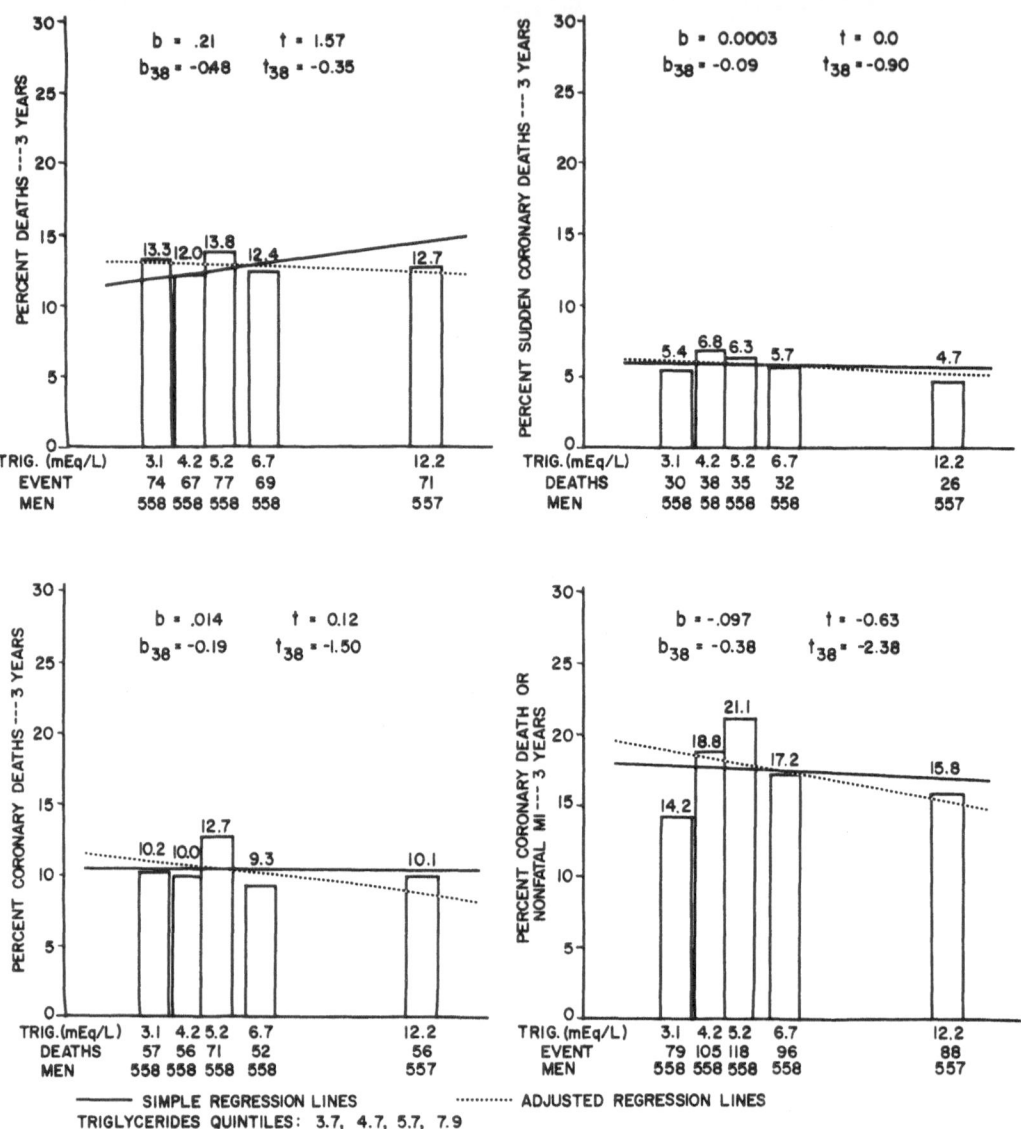

Figure 9. Analyses of relationship between baseline fasting serum triglyceride level and 3-year rates for four stipulated andpoints for the 2,789 men of the placebo group. Serum triglyceride value for each man is the mean of his three baseline determinations at 4-week intervals. The two slopes in each graph are respectively the univariate and multivariate linear regression lines for the relationship between fasting serum triglycerides and the stipulated endpoint; for the multivariate regression line, adjustment is made for the influence of 38 other variables on risk of mortality

Early in 1973, the lower dose estrogen regimen was also discontinued (CDPRG, 1973c). With an average follow-up of 56 months, the data indicated no evidence of a positive therapeutic effect in terms of the CDP's primary end point, mortality from all causes (Fig. 10 and Table 2) (CDPRG, 1973c), nor any likelihood of a positive effect by the end of the study. Moreover, based on small numbers of cases in both the ESG1 and placebo groups, there were suggestions of adverse trends with this estrogen regimen, in the form of excess incidence of venous thromboembolism and excess mortality from all cancers and particularly from lung

Table 1. Nonfatal and fatal events in 5.0 mg estrogen (ESG2) and placebo groups[a]

Event	ESG2 (total 1,119) No.	%	Placebo (total 2,788) No.	%	RBO[b]
Definite nonfatal MI[c]	63	6.2	82	3.2	0.015
MI incidence (definite nonfatal MI + coronary death)	123	11.0	209	7.5	0.13
Definite pulmonary embolism	17	1.5	10	0.4	0.045
Suspect and definite pulmonary embolism or thrombophlebitis	39	3.5	37	1.3	0.004
Coronary death	67	6.0	133	4.8	2.48
Sudden death	48	4.3	76	2.7	· 0.46
Total mortality	91	8.1	193	6.9	3.20

[a]All data in this and subsequent tables are as of Feb. 1. 1970, except for data in bottom row (second listing of "total mortality") in this table.

[b]RBO signifies relative betting odds (Bayesian approach [15]).

[c]MI signifies myocardial infarction. Denominators for nonfatal MI are 1,022 and 2,580 for ESG2 and placebo groups, respectively.

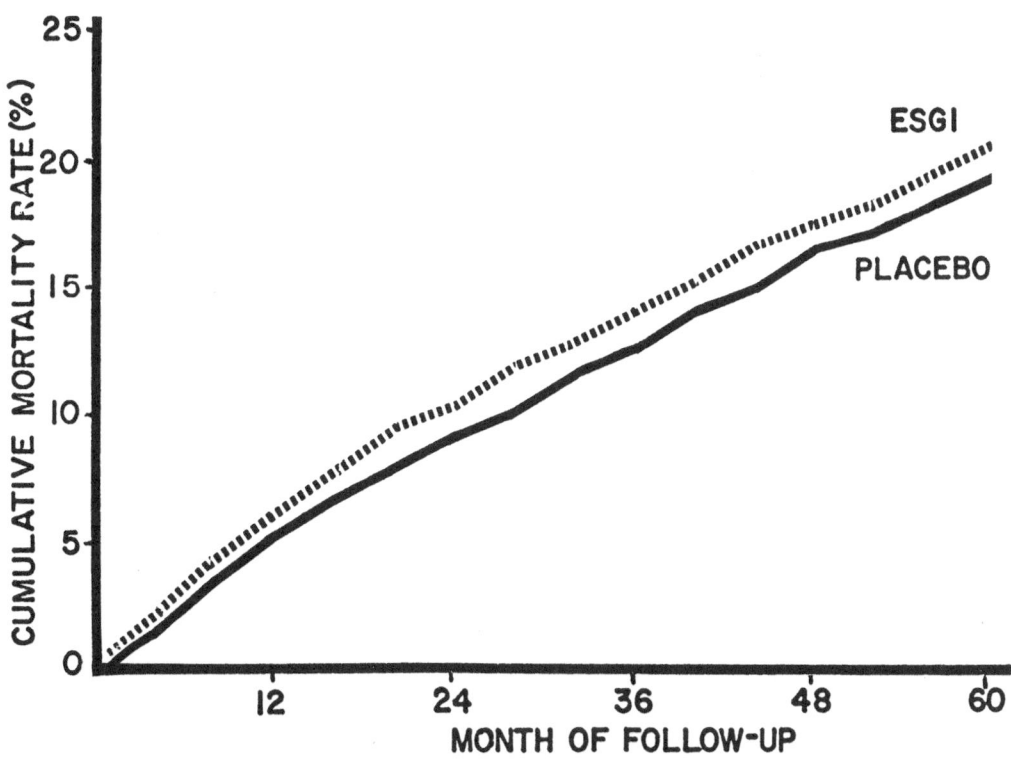

Figure 10. Life table cumulative rates for deaths from all causes for the placebo and lower dose (2.5 mg/day) estrogen group over 60 months of follow-up

cancers. As with the higher-dose estrogen group, cholesterol-lowering effect was slight and serum triglycerides tended to rise. Side effects were troublesome, leading a sizeable proportion of men to reduce or stop this medication.

Table 2. Nonfatal events and deaths by cause

Event	ESG1			Placebo					
	No.of men	No. with events	%	No.of men	No.with events	%	Z value	RBO (.25)	RBO (min.)
Death-all causes	1,101	219	19.9	2,789	525	18.8	0.76	5.82	1.00
Death-all cardio vascular (CV)[a]	1,101	190	17.3	2,789	481	17.2	0.01	7.61	1.00
Death-all non-cardiovascular	1,101	23	2.1	2,789	35	1.1	1.93	0.83	0.83
Death-cause unknown	1,101	6	0.5	2,789	9	0.3	1.01	1.09	1.00
Death-all CHD	1,101	162	14.7	2,789	410	14.7	0.01	6.29	1.00
Death-all sudden CV	1,101	82	7.4	2,789	246	8.8	-1.39	1.77	0.91
Death-all cancer	1,101	14	1.3	2,789	13	0.5	2.73	0.28	0.09
Death-lung cancer	1,101	6	0.5	2,789	4	0.1	2.23	0.72	0.38
Definite nonfatal myocardial infarction (MI)	1,059	121	11.4	2,693	306	11.4	0.05	2.46	0.92
Incidence (definite nonfatal MI or coronary death)	1,101	256	23.3	2,789	652	23.4	-0.08	4.86	1.00
Definite fatal or nonfatal pulmonary embolism	1,101	17	1.5	2,789	22	0.8	2.13	0.43	0.32
Definite or suspect fatal or nonfatal pulmonary embolism or thrombophlebitis	1,101	52	4.7	2,789	82	2.9	2.75	0.19	0.17

[a]Excludes sudden deaths attributed to noncardiovascular causes.

In December, 1971 treatment with d-thyroxine was stopped, despite sustained reduction in the intermediate end point — serum lipids (Fig. 11) (CDPRG, 1973c).
Total mortality was in excess over the control group, reaching almost statistically significant values (Fig. 12 and Table 3). Extensive analyses were done to
ascertain whether this excessive mortality tended to be concentrated in certain
subgroups. Large differences were found for the sizeable subgroups of patients
who either had had repeated infarcts or had survived one complicated infarct
(that is, risk group 2 patients), patients who had a definite history of angina
pectoris on entry in the study, and/or patients who on entry had a resting heart
rate of 70 or more per minute as determined from the baseline electrocardiogram.

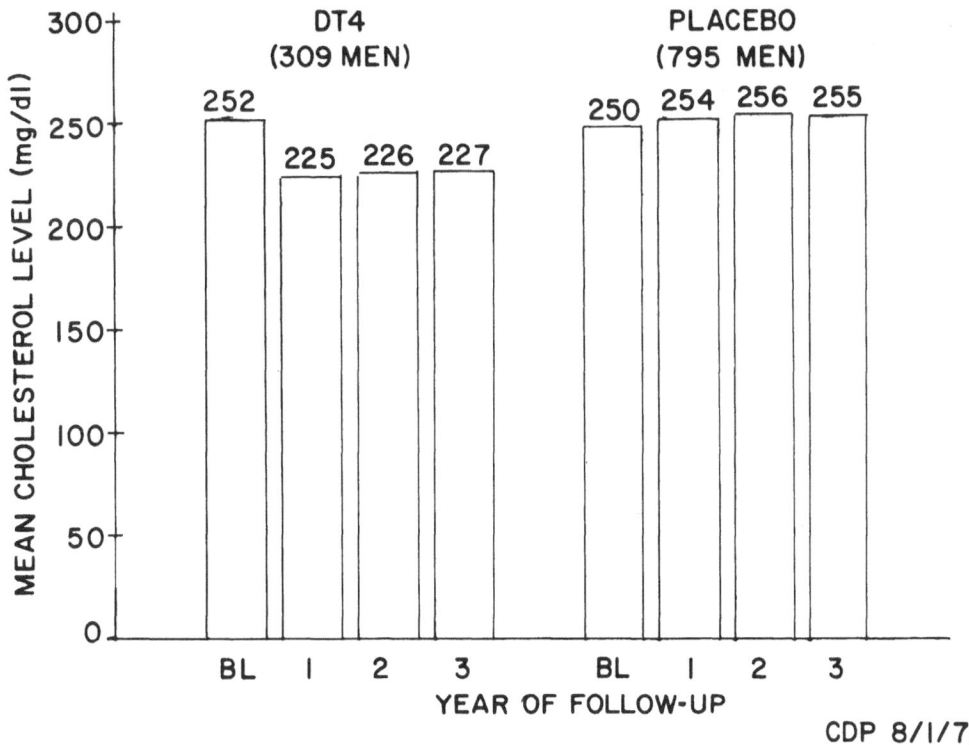

Figure 11. Mean levels of serum cholesterol at baseline and at annual intervals
for the dextrothyroxine and placebo groups respectively — cohort of patients
completing at least three years of follow-up

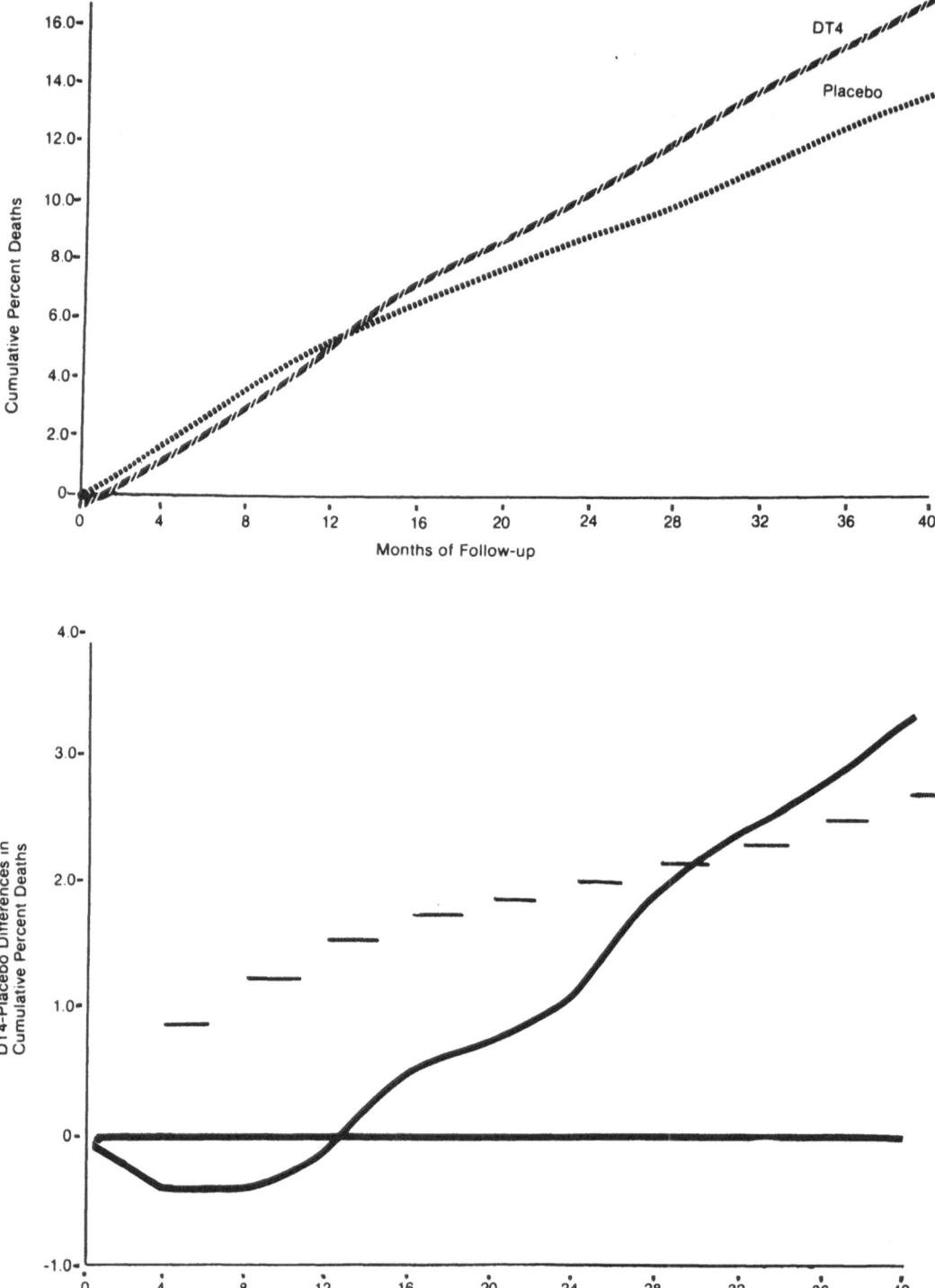

Figure 12. Life table cumulative rates for deaths from all causes for the dextrothyroxine and placebo groups over 40 months of follow-up (upper graph), and
the differences between the placebo and dextrothyroxine groups in these cumulative rates (lower graph). Broken lines in the lower graph denote two standard
error values at various time points

Table 3. Nonfatal events and deaths by cause, DT4 and placebo groups[a]

Event	DT4			Placebo			DT4 - Placebo S.E. of diff.	P.cent diff. DT4 - placebo Placebo
	No.of men	No.of events	Per-cent	No.of men	No.of events	Per-cent		
1. Death-all causes	1,083	160	14.8	2,715	339	12.5	1.88	+ 18.4
2. Death-all cardiovas-cular	1,083	146	13.5	2,715	317	11.7	1.54	+ 15.4
3. Death-non-cardiovas-cular	1,083	9	0.8	2,715	19	0.7	0.43	**
4. Death-cause unknown	1,083	5	0.5	2,715	3	0.1	2.13	**
5. Death-all CHD	1,083	119	11.0	2,715	274	10.1	0.82	+ 8.9
6. Death-sudden[b]	1,083	63	5.8	2,715	162	6.0	0.18	- 3.3
7. Definite nonfatal MI	1,053	89	8.5	2,618	202	7.7	0.75	+ 10.4
8. Major coron-ary events (Def. non-fatal MI + CHD death)	1,083	197	18.2	2,715	449	16.5	1.22	+ 10.3
9. All suspect or definite CV events (nonfatal or fatal)	1,083	736	68.0	2,715	1,758	64.8	1.88	+ 4.9

[a]Excludes 27 DT4 and 74 Placebo patients with frequent ectopic ventricular beats (FEVBs) at entry (1).

[b]Excludes sudden deaths attributed to non-cardiovascular causes.

**Per cent changes not calculated when per cent deceased is less than 1.0.

Among other things, this experience drives home the lesson that benefit; risk ratios for drugs for coronary disease cannot be predicted — in terms of decisive end points of morbidity and mortality over years — by their effects on any inter-mediate end point, e.g., serum lipids. Only that "late painful ordeal", the con-trolled mass field trial, can give a definitive answer, especially when — as with drugs — there is always bound to be some risk.

The key bodies of the Coronary Drug Project and their senior staff members are as follows:

---

*Deceased.

Ernest O. Theilen, M.D.; C. Basil Williams, M.D.; Stephen J. Herbert, M.D.; Fred
I. Gilbert, Jr., M.D.; Sidney A. Levine, M.D.; Louis B. Matthews, M.D.; Irving
Ershler, M.D.; Elmer E. Cooper, M.D.; Allan H. Barker, M.D.; Paul Samuel, M.D.

The Coronary Drug Project is proceeding as a Collaborative Study supported by
research grants and other funds from the National Heart and Lung Institute.

EVIDENCE FOR PREVENTION AND REGRESSION OF ATHEROSCLEROSIS IN MAN AND EXPERIMENTAL ANIMALS AT THE ARTERIAL LEVEL*

Robert W. Wissler and Dragaslava Vesselinovitch

In this presentation I intend to review very briefly the evidence that we have
found, both in the literature and in our own laboratory, that rather simple
measures can be effective both in *preventing the development* of atherosclerosis
and in *producing substantial regression* of atherosclerotic lesions, even when
they are rather far advanced.

Table 1. Selected studies showing anatomical evidence of prevention of
atherosclerosis in man and animals

Principal investigators and year	Species	Conditions of prevention	Evidence of prevention
Pick (1952)	Chicken	Estrogen and cholesterol	Prevents development of coronary atherosclerosis
Moskowitz (1956)	Rat	Estrogen and atherogenic diet	Lower blood cholesterol and smaller and less severe coronary artery lesions
Prichard (1966)	Pigeon	Estradiol valerate and cholesterol	Lower serum cholesterol level and less severe coronary atherosclerosis
Vesselinovitch (1967)	Rabbit	Hyperoxygenation and atherogenic diet	Lower serum cholesterol and less aortic disease as compared to rabbits on atherogenic diet
Wissler (1962)	Cebus Monkey	Diet low in cholesterol and high in unsaturated fats — corn oil	Lower blood lipids and fewer gross and microscopic lesions in aorta and coronary artery as compared to coconut oil and butter fat
Wissler (1965, 1971)	Rhesus Monkey	Prudent American diet	Very good correlation with serum cholesterol. Smaller and less severe lesions in the aorta and coronary arteries as compared to average American diet
McGill (1968)	Human	International study — correlation with calories and fat in diet	Less intimal surface involved with raised lesions in coronary artery and aorta. Very good correlation with serum cholesterol

*This study was supported in part by grants HE 2174, HE 6894, HE 12487 and HL
15062 from the National Heart and Lung Institute.

It is beyond the scope of this brief contribution to review comprehensively the abundant evidence that atherosclerosis at the lesion level can be prevented in experimental animals and man simply by keeping the serum cholesterol level low. Table 1 includes a few selected studies in 7 species including man that offer this kind of evidence. They are selected because the authors are very thoroughly acquainted with the work, either because they had the opportunity to monitor it while it was being done or because they participated in the studies directly. We think these studies offer abundant evidence that atherosclerosis can be prevented if the serum cholesterol level — especially that circulating as low density lipoprotein — remains low. This is true for susceptible species like the chicken, pigeon or rabbit, for resistant ones like the rat or Cebus monkey and for those intermediate in sensitivity such as the Rhesus monkey and man.

The case for regression of atherosclerotic lesions in man is much less well documented (Table 2). Thus far, positive reports of improved human atherosclerosis have been indirect or poorly controlled. Most of these reports have been based on studies of arteries in people who were subjected to severe dietary restrictions as a result of war or famine or who had chronic wasting diseases such as

Table 2. List of studies with evidence of regression of atherosclerotic lesions in man

Principal investigator (year)	Conditions of regression	Evidence of regression
Ashoff (1924)	Post world war I — semistarvation	Decrease in aortic atherosclerosis and re-absorption of lipids as compared to prewar autopsies
Wilens (1947)	Wasting disease 40-60 year old	Smaller and less severe lesions. Fewer lipid-containing phagocytes and in general less lipid in the intima. Lower coronary disease scores as compared to patients who died without loss of weight
Vartiainen (1946)	Post world war II — malnutrition	Less atherosclerosis in aorta, coronary and cerebral arteries. Decrease was greatest in 30-49 year age group, as compared to same age group at earlier period
Rivin (1954)	Carcinoma of the prostate and breast, estrogen treated	Diminution of coronary atherosclerosis was most prominent, as compared to patients not treated with estrogen
London (1961)	Metastatic carcinoma of the prostate treated with estrogen	Less severe lesions in aorta and significantly less coronary artery atherosclerosis as compared to patients not treated with estrogen
Buchwald (1967)	Ileal bypass operation	Lowering of atherosclerotic process as judged by lessening in anginal symptoms, xanthoma regression and apparent nonprogression of coronary and femoral atherosclerotic lesions as determined by angiography
McGill (1968)	Carcinoma — autopsy international study	Aortic atherosclerosis decreased as compared to many other control groups
Zelis (1970)	Hyperlipoproteinemias clofibrate treated	Improvement of peripheral circulation

Table 3. Regression studies showing reversal of *advanced* atherosclerotic lesions in experimental animals

Species & year	Principal investigator	Severity of lesions before regression	Regression conditions			Regression response
			Diet	Period (mos.)	Approx. serum chol. (mg/%)	
Rabbit ('28)	Anitschkow	Moderate	Low fat chow	24–36	–	Fibrous with less lipid
Rabbit ('67)	Wartman	Moderate	Chow & EDTA	1–1.5	205	Marked decrease in collagen
Rabbit ('68)	Vesselinovitch	Moderate	Chow + O_2 + cholestyramine	2	100	Marked improvement in all lesion components
Rabbit ('69)	Kjeldsen	Moderate	Chow + O_2	2.5	?	Moderate decrease in aortic lesions
Rabbit ('70, '71)	Vesselinovitch	Moderate	Chow + O_2 + estrogen	2.5	90	Marked improvement in all lesion components
Chicken ('49)	Horlick	Severe	Low fat starter mash	3.5	200	Moderate decrease in lipid in lesions
Pigeon (71,72)	Clarkson St. Clair	Severe	Cholesterol-free diet	2–8	348	Moderate decrease in lipid in lesions
Dog ('51)	Bevans	Severe	Low fat diet	2–4	200	Marked improvement in all lesion components
Dog ('68)	DePalma	Severe	Low fat diet & bile diversion	1.5–3	150	Marked decrease in aortic coronary & mesenteric lesions
Squirrel Monkeys ('67, '68)	Portman Maruffo	Moderate	Regular chow	3–5	–	Marked decrease in lipid in lesions
Rhesus ('70, '72)	Armstrong	Severe	Low cholesterol low fat or high corn oil	40	140	Marked decrease in lesion size and increase in lumen caliber
Rhesus ('73)	Vesselinovitch Jones	Severe	Low cholesterol low fat chow + W-1372	18	135	Marked decrease in all lesion components

cancer, with or without estrogen therapy. Nevertheless, the results shown in the 8 reports summarized in Table 2 all furnish either anatomical or functional evidence that atheromatous lesions in man may diminish under these conditions. Only the studies by Buchwald (1967) and those by Zelis et al. (1970) in patients subject to a high risk of progressive atherosclerosis show some tentative evidence of improvement of lesions as a result of a planned substantial therapeutic reduction of serum cholesterol levels.

Evidence is increasing that significant regression of atherosclerosis in experimental animals is possible. Some studies show reversal of even the most advanced atherosclerosis, characterized by complicated lesions containing a necrotic center, a fibrous cap, and many other features of the chronic fully developed lesion in man. Table 3 summarizes some of this data from 12 studies in 6 species. It is evident that in general the lesions were most reversible when the serum cholesterol could be lowered to levels under 150 mg% and under conditions that maintained these low levels for many months. Some of the most potent evidence comes from recent studies in Rhesus monkeys, because many of the lesions that existed at the beginning of therapy were advanced complex lesions containing a necrotic center, a thick fibrous cap and, in the case of the coronary arteries, moderate to servere narrowing of the lumens, But perhaps the most convincing part of the survey is that every species that has been studied under controlled conditions for regression potential has yielded some evidence that regression can be achieved under sustained therapeutic regimens.

The studies in the rabbit must be viewed in a special light. This species has been notably resistant to reversal of its rather singular type of atheromatous disease by simply removing cholesterol from the diet. Now a number of studies are showing that a low-fat, low-cholesterol diet combined with added therapeutic efforts such as an increase in ambient oxygen concentration, EDTA, cholestyramine, estrogen administration, or a combination of some of these factors, may yield a substantial and rather prompt reversal of the rabbit's stubborn form of atherosclerosis.

It appears that definitive studies of regression of atherosclerotic lesions are now feasible. Angiography and even more quantitative monitors of the atherosclerotic process (some of them non-invasive) which are now being developed are useful for studying the disease in man and animals. Swine and non-human primates provide excellent experimental models; severe atherosclerosis in these species resembles the disease in man very closely.

It is evident that much more work will be necessary in both man and animal models before we can confidently predict success or admit failure in the attempt to improve advanced atherosclerotic lesions in man. Nevertheless there is sufficient evidence at present to be optimistic that reversal can be achieved in the mammal if sustained cholesterol lowering to a level of 150 mg% or below can be achieved over a considerable period of time. It seems that this therapeutic goal will soon be reasonably attainable using the simple combination of a prudent diet and a bile salt sequestering agent.

LONG-TERM HYPOLIPIDEMIC TREATMENT IN THE PREVENTION OF RECURRENT CORONARY HEART DISEASE

Carlo Caruzzo

A long-term hypolipidemic therapy was tried on patients with Coronary Heart Disease (CHD) in order to evaluate its statistical influence on survival rates, the appearance of new myocardial infarctions during treatment, angina, and physical activity.

Material and Method

A total of 490 patients with non fatal myocardial infarct or angina pectoris was admitted to long-term study. 265 patients — 198 men (74.7%) and 67 women (25.3%) — were subjected to symptomatic therapy and correction of main coronary risk factors, including hyperlipidemia. For this purpose, subdivision into phenotypes in accordance with the Fredrickson-Levy-Lees classification (1967), was used. In the case of subjects observed before 1970, reliance was placed on determination of both serum cholesterol and triglycerides, conventional electrophoretic lipidogram, and blood sugar, with load curves where necessary. The control group formed by 225 patients — 147 men (65.3%) and 78 women (34.7%) — received the same treatment, except hypolipidemic therapy.

The mean age at entry into the study was 57.42 for the group receiving hypolipidemic treatment, and 59.19 years for the control group, with a standard deviation of observation of 9.87 and 9.09 respectively, and with a standard deviation of the mean of 0.61 for both groups, Blood pressure was normal in 129 subjects of the treated group (48.7%) and 96 subjects of the control group (42.7%); it was increased[1] in 136 subjects of the treated group (51.3%) and in 129 subjects of the control group (57.3%).

At the beginning of the study there was no significant difference in average values and in the percentage of pathological values of bloodsugar[2] in the treated group (101.5 mg/dl, with 43.4% pathological cases) and in the control group (102.1 mg/dl, with 38.8% pathological cases), of serum cholesterol[3] in the treated group (251.8 mg/dl, with 52.2% pathological cases) and in the control group (257.3 mg/dl, with 56.4% pathological cases), of serum triglycerides[4] in the treated group (187.0 mg/dl, with 49.2% pathological cases) and in the control group (176.2 mg/dl, with 45.5% pathological cases).

Both groups are then homogeneous, because of the opposite behavior with regard to the percentage of women and hypertension.

In confirmation of this, the theoretical survival curves, drawn homogeneously for both groups in relation to age and sex, obtained by comparison from ISTAT 1962 Mortality Tables on the same Piedmont and Aosta Valley healthy population, adjusted to initial composition and to changes in such composition, tend to be superimposed (Fig. 1). We must point out the fact that the percentage of patho-

---

[1] WHO definition: Systolic blood pressure ≥ 160 mmHg and/or diastolic blood pressure ≥ 95 mmHg.

[2] Enzymatic method. Maximal normal value 95 mg/dl.

[3] Watson method. Maximal normal value 240 mg/dl.

[4] Van Handel-Zilversmit method. Maximal normal value 150 mg/dl.

logical values of serum cholesterol and triglycerides is rather low (Blankenhorn et al., 1968; Heinle et al., 1969), approximately 50% in both groups, but many of the observed subjects, before the beginning of the study, had already followed hypolipidemic diets or therapies because of pathological values in their serum lipids.

There is a prevalence of myocardial infarctions in the group with hypolipidemic treatment (86 subjects equivalent to 32.4% against 54 subjects equivalent to 24% of the control group), but this is obviated by computing data both collectively and in the infarct subgroup. The maximum follow-up period was 19 years. The number of cases reported refers to the first year of treatment and decreases in subsequent years, because of mortality and differences in the period of observation. The average length of observation was 53.03 month with a standard deviation of 47.42 in the control group and 40.03 month with a standard deviation of 36.60 in the treated group, in which we observed a greater number of patients for a period shorter than one year.

Both groups of patients received the usual treatment for the main coronary risk factors (hypertension, diabetes, excessive or wrong diet, obesity, cigarette smoking, alcohol, physical inactivity), angina, and heart failure. In the hyperlipidemia-treated group, after phenotyping, the therapy shown in Table 1 (Parsons, 1965; Oliver et al., 1971; Krasno and Kidera, 1972; Boettiger et al., 1965; Caruzzo et al., 1963; Howard et al., 1971) was given. Treatment was continued for various periods in accordance with the seriousness of the case, strict adherence to medical prescriptions and the appearance of gastroenteric, hepatic, or other intolerance. The frequency of such intolerance, (Asdorph, 1971) expecially for nicotinic acid, justified a long-term lower dosage than that advised in the literature.

Table 1. Hypolipidemic treatment

Type of hyperlipidemia	Diet	Drug	Dose	Length of treatment
Hypercholesterolemia Type II (hyperbeta-lipoproteinemia)	low cholesterol low saturated fat high polyunsaturated fat	nicotinic acid	1.2gm/day	4-6 months/ year
Hypertriglyceridemia Type IV (hyperprebeta-lipoproteinemia)	low carbohydrates, specially low mono and di-saccharides no alcohol	clofi-brate	1.5gm/day	4-6 months/ year
Hypercholesterolemia and hypertriglyceridemia Type III (hyperbeta and prebeta-lipoproteinemia Type II b	low carbohydrates, specially low mono and di-saccharides no alcohol low cholesterol low saturated fat high polyunsaturated fat	clofi-brate and/or nic-otinic acid	1.5gm/day 1.2gm/day	4-6 months/ year
All patients, and in particular those with normal lipidemic pattern	moderately low cholesterol moderately low saturated fat moderately low mono and di-saccharides	phos-phatidyl choline	0.22-0.44 gm/day	during the periods of non treatment (4-6 months/year) long term (6-10 m./y.)
All patients, and in particular those with normal lipidemic pattern	moderately low cholesterol moderately low saturated fat moderately low mono and di-saccharides	heparin with small doses of nicotinamide	25mg/day	2-3 months/ year

Results

Survival. The overall survival curves for progressively diminishing groups of patients, were calculated in terms of compound probabilities derived from the probability of survival for each period. Fig. 1 shows the overall survival curves for both groups, compared with those of theoretical survival for groups of subjects homogeneous for age and sex with the previous groups, obtained by comparison from ISTAT 1962 mortality tables on the same healthy population. In different classes of observation (0-1, 1-2, etc.), on the analogy of mortality tables, we only considered complete years of follow-up.

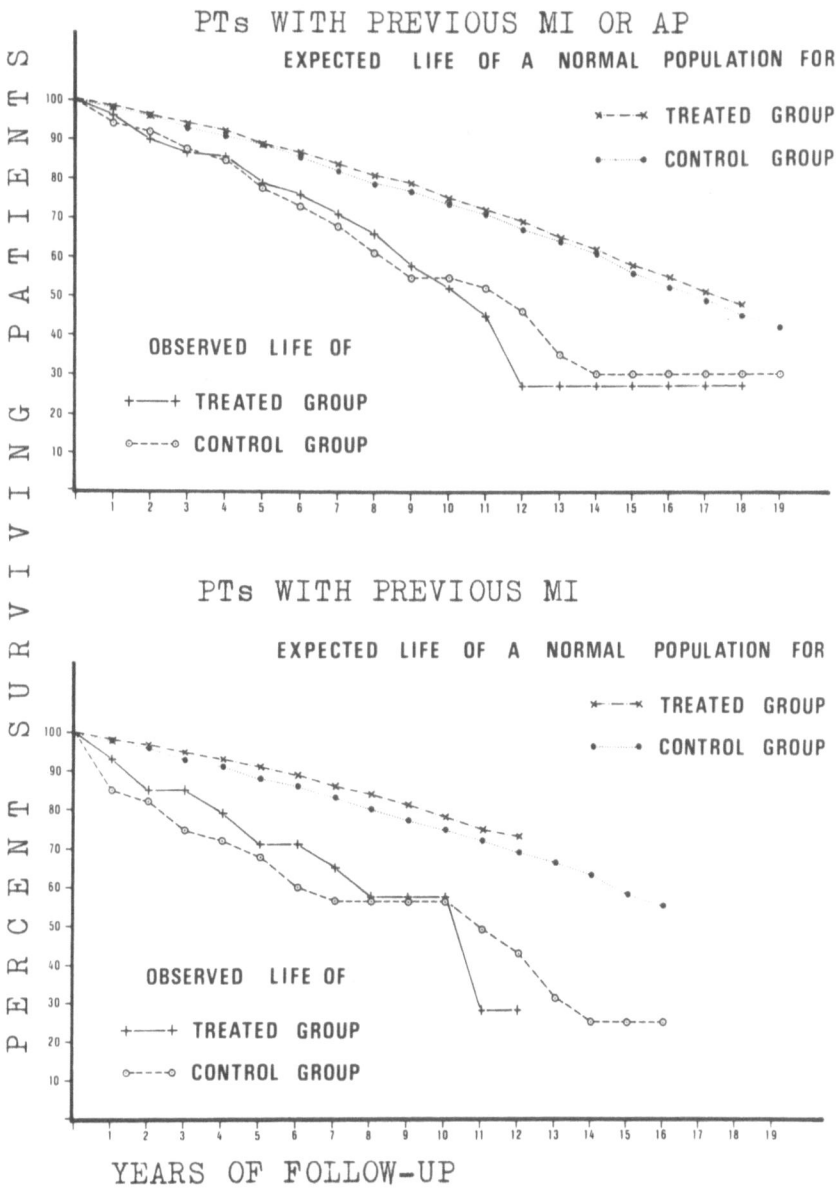

Figure 1. Percent survival rates in patients with previous non fatal Myocardial Infarction (MI) or Angina Pectoris (AP) (upper part of the figure), in patients with previous myocardial infarction and only (lower part of the figure), with or without hypolipidemic treatment, compared with the expected life of a normal population calculated according to the results of 1962 ISTAT Mortality Tables

The overall survival of the treated group does not show any significant differences from the control group. The mortality until the 10th year is about 45%; in our opinion it is difficult to lower this limit with any sort of medical and surgical treatment, (Master and Lasser, 1969; Zukel et al., 1969) which is why the natural mortality in the same healthy population in the equivalent period is about 25%.

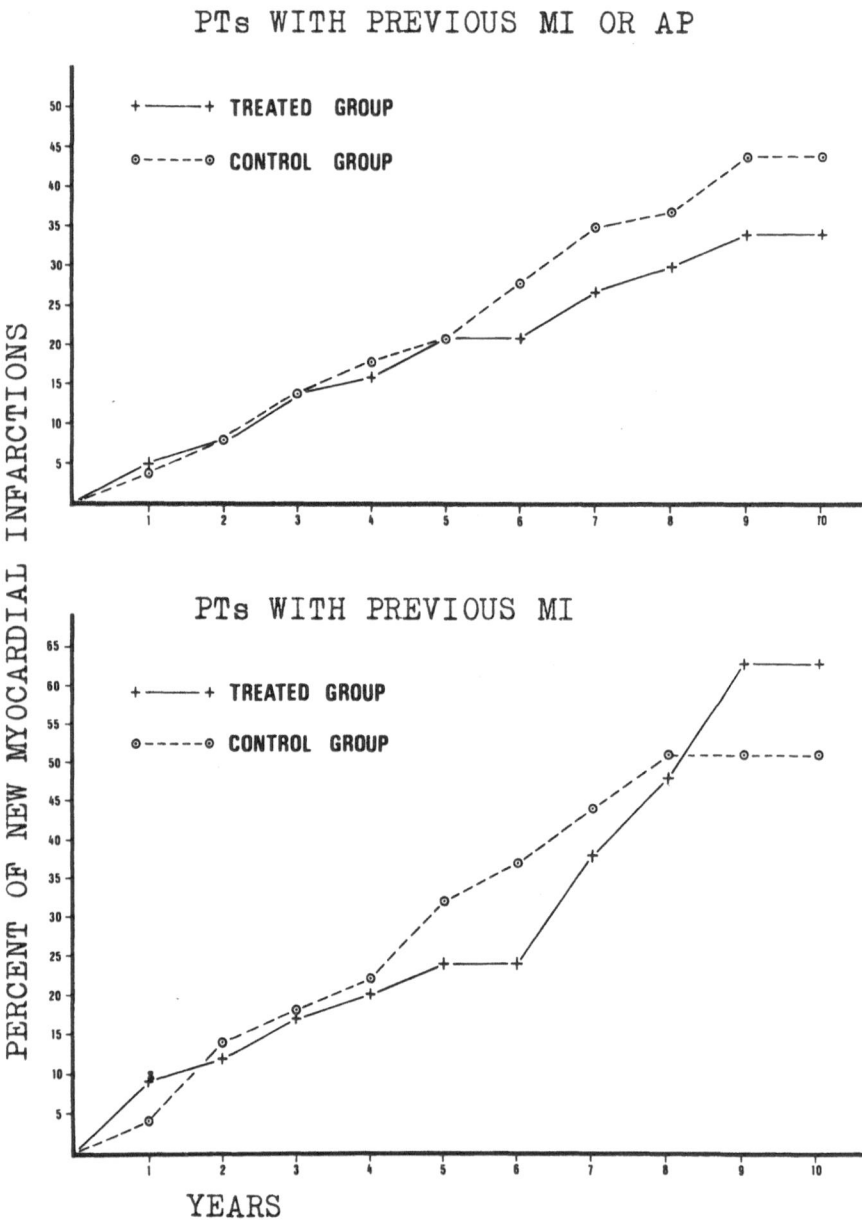

Figure 2. Percent of new fatal or nonfatal myocardial infarction during a ten-year-period of observation, in patients with previous Myocardial Infarction (MI) or Angina pectoris (AP) (upper part of the figure), and in patients with previous myocardial infarction (lower part of the figure), only with or without hypolipidemic treatment

Confinement of the analysis to nonfatal myocardial infarct cases resulted in finding a slightly better survival in the treated group up to the 10th year. After this time one can register an inversion of the phenomenon, but, at this point, the number of patients involved is insignificant.

Tests for significance, such as Student's t-test, were technically inapplicable to an analysis of such small differences in progressively smaller number of subjects. The test, in any case, wouldn't be significant.

It must be noted, lastly, that in Fig. 1 the theoretical percent curves of survival for both groups are very close, that is a substantial confirmation of the homogeneity for age and sex of both groups.

New Fatal or Nonfatal Myocardial Infarctions During the Period of Observation (Fig. 2). The curves are constructed in the way already described; compound probabilities are not applicable to an analysis of this kind. In the case of multiple episodes, only the first was included when compiling the diagrams.

The pattern for the percentage of new infarcts in the group with hypolipidemic treatment is much the same as that observed in the control group (Fig. 2). The same is true both for each of the two groups considered together and for patients with previous myocardial infarction only. Once again, for the same reasons exposed above, Student's t-test was inapplicable and, in any case, it would not be significant. It may, however, be noted that fewer infarctions were observed in the treated group after the 4th-5th year, a period of substantial homogeneity with the control group.

Table 2. Qualitative results: angina pectoris and physical activity before and after treatment of both groups

	General mean of hyperlipidemia untreated group x_1	General mean of hyperlipidemia treated group x_2	Difference between means $x_1 - x_2$	$\|t\|$ of difference of the means Ho: $x_1 - x_2 = 0$
Angina pectoris before treatment	2.618	2.879	− 0.261	3.172[a]
Angina pectoris after treatment	1.702	1.374	0.329	4.528[a]
Physical activity before treatment	2.529	2.642	− 0.113	1.700
Physical activity after treatment	1.982	1.491	0.492	6.840[a]
Angina pectoris before − Angina pectoris after	0.916	1.506	− 0.590	6.465[a]
Physical activity before − Physical activity after	0.547	1.151	− 0.604	7.991[a]

[a] The marked t are 1% significant.

Clinical Results. Our observation is now limited to only two elements: angina and physical activity. 4 classes were determined for angina[1] and 4 for physical activity[2]. Such an evaluation, essentially based on subjective criteria and in which placebo effect cannot be evaluated because of the lack of double-blind test, inapplicable to such a long-term study, is of course easily criticized.

In spite of these reservations, the analyses relative to the evaluation of angina and physical activity at the beginning of therapy and at the last observation, seem to be much more significant than the comparison between the survival percentage. Patients in the treated group, who at the start of the study presented a significantly higher degree of angina, had at the end of the study a significantly lower degree of angina than subjects in the control group. In much the same way, patients in the treated group began with a lower, though not statistically significant, degree of physical activity and they ended at a significant, higher degree. Table 2 shows the general means for angina or physical activity in both groups, before and after treatment, their difference and statistical significance t-test. The Table also shows individual differences relative to angina or physical activity, before and after treatment; the mean of these differences represents the average improvement of each group.

It will be seen that patients subjected to hypolipidemic treatment displayed a higher degree of improvement. Highly significant differences were observed for both angina and physical activity at the 1% level.

Conclusion

Long-term hypolipidemic treatment, as an addition to correction of the main coronary risk factors and symptomatic therapy, is devoid of significant influence on survival in coronary heart disease. The slight differences noted in subjects with previous nonfatal myocardial infarct were equally without significance. Appearance of first infarct in patients with angina or new infarction in subjects who suffered a previous one, occured with about the same frequency in both groups up to the fifth year, followed by a slight, nonsignificant increase in the untreated group between the fifth and the tenth year.

It may thus be deduced that hypolipidemic treatment was not sufficiently intensive or continuous, or, alternatively, that it is not a sufficient means of influencing either the evolution of advanced coronary atherosclerosis, or factors such as platelet aggregation, blood clotting, and fibrinolysis that were responsible for complications or death in our patients. In our view, further attempts at secondary preventive management should be directed towards such factors.

In spite of the necessary reservation for a possible placebo effect, subjective symptomatology of coronary heart disease, as represented by angina and physical activity, was much improved by hypolipidemic management, which resulted in considerable progress compared with the correction of all other risk factors and associated symptomatic therapy.

The activity of heparin at clarifying doses and of phosphatidylcholine, in our experience, seems to be very interesting, even if it is not truly objective. The eventual mechanism of these drugs in patients of this type is not yet known,

---

[1] I: no angina with ordinary physical activity; II: angina only with the more strenuous grades of ordinary activity; III: angina even with the milder forms of ordinary activity; IV: angina present even at rest.

[2] According to the criteria of N.Y.H.A. functional classification.

though hypotheses can be suggested (Caruzzo et al., 1963; Howard et al., 1971). Our experience is not sufficiently extensive to enable a judgment to be expressed with respect to the other drugs employed.

Summary

265 patients with CHD received, in addition to symptomatic therapy and the correction of main coronary risk factors, a long-term hypolipidemic treatment to see whether it had a significant effect on survival, the appearance of new myocardial infarctions during the follow-up period, angina, and physical activity. With regard to a group of patients who were subjected to the same treatment, except the hypolipidemic therapy, we can see that this former therapy: 1. Does not modify in a significant way the survival in treated subjects; 2. does not have a significant influence on the appearance of a myocardial infarct during the treatment; 3. produces, on the other hand, a clear improvement of angina and physical activity. The possible interpretations of such a behavior are discussed.

XVII

Dietary Management
of Hyperlipoproteinemias

WORKSHOP: Dietary Management of Hyperlipoproteinemias

Chairmen: R. Furman, USA
         G. Schlierf, West Germany

Participants: Y. Goto, Japan
             S. Grundy, USA
             G. Hartmann, Switzerland
             R. S. Lees, USA
             J. Lloyd, England
             M. Mancini, Italy
             G. Weber, Italy

Hyperlipidemias (hyperlipoproteinemias) have become one of the commonest metabolic syndromes. The incidence of hyperlipidemias in the general population, on
the basis of published data (Schlierf et al., 1972; Wood et al., 1972) and reports presented during this symposium, appears to range between 10 and 20%. Dietary factors, overnutrition in general and an increased consumption of specific
food-stuffs in particular, appear to be the most important factors responsible
for this dramatic increase in the manifestation rate of disorders which have been
almost unknown during the post-war years in many countries (Schettler, 1970) and
which are still rare in less affluent societies (Keys et al., 1970).

Calories

An interesting relationship between *calorie consumption and plasma lipid levels*
was pointed out by *G. Hartmann*. He put forward the hypothesis that the increase
of serum lipids with age in affluent societies is mainly due to a parallel increase in body-weight as shown in Fig. 1. In men the average increase of body-
weight between 20 and 40 years is about 12 kg and in the following 20 years only
about 2 kg. In women the inverse is true, although to a somewhat lower degree in
absolute amounts. Total serum lipids show a steep increase between the age of
20 and 40 in men, whereas the steep slope in women covers the age-range between
35 to 55, exactly paralleling the weight-curve.

Although the coincidence of these two pairs of curves must not have the significance of a cause and effect-relationship, the probability that the demonstrated
curves run parallel by chance is extremely small.

Furthermore, it can easily be shown, that calorie-dependent hyperlipidemias
(especially types III, IV and V) become manifest in men between the age of 20 and
40, that is during the greatest increase of excess body weight.

Dietary measures, therefore, are basic for management of the hyperlipidemias and
caloric restriction appears to be paramount. *M. Mancini, Italy* therefore reported on:

*Changes in plasma lipid concentration and in body weight in obese patients during
total fasting and low calorie intake.*

In his study, plasma concentrations of total cholesterol, triglycerides and FFA
were measured at regular intervals during a total fast lasting up to several
weeks in diabetic and non-diabetic obese subjects. Similar observations were made
during a 600 calorie diet prescribed for several months.

During the fasting regime the expected fall in plasma cholesterol and triglycerides, and the rise in plasma FFA were observed in the first 4 weeks but sub-

sequently, in spite of continued food deprivation, these concentrations tended to return towards the initial levels.

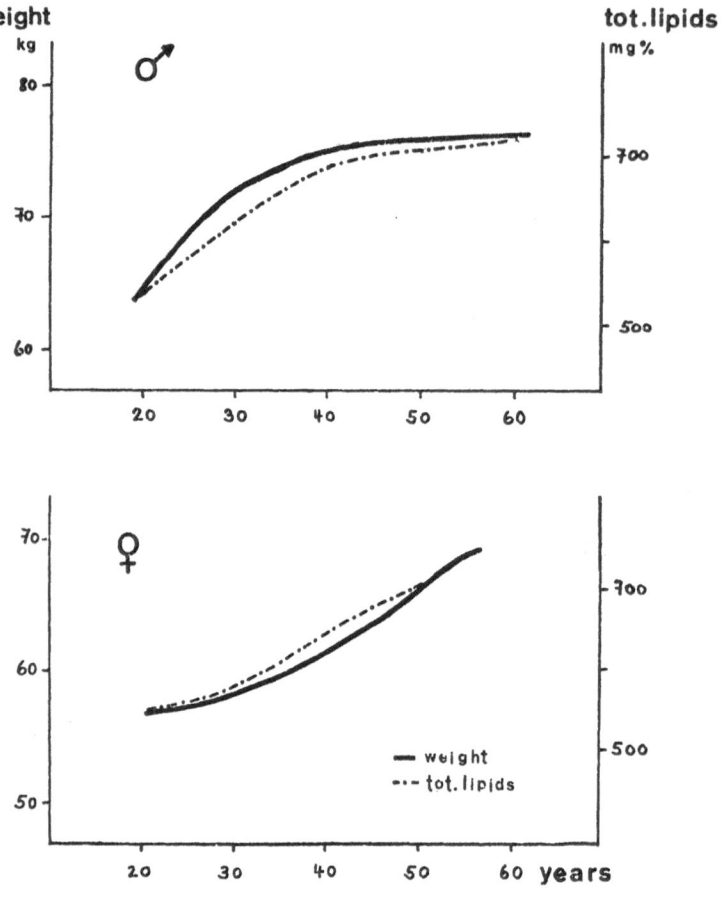

Figure 1. Body weight and total serum lipids in dependence of age in 1864 men and 363 women (Basle Study)

During the hypocaloric diet the hyperlipidemic obese patients showed significant decreases of both serum cholesterol and triglyceride concentrations.

The late rise in serum cholesterol concentration in prolonged fasting might have been due to a decreased fecal output of acidic and neutral steroids. The rise of triglycerides in the same circumstances might have been related to an increased FFA flux from adipose tissue or to a decreased plasma triglyceride removal by peripheral tissues.

Body weight was lost during total fasting at an almost constant rate averaging 267 g per day, except in the first week when there was a greater loss associated with sodium and water depletion. In the later weeks of the fast the daily body weight decrease was slightly lower than in the first eight weeks.

During the refeeding phase with a 600-900 kcal diet there was a net gain of weight in the first week which was coincident with sodium and water retention.

The mean body weight loss in the following 23 weeks of hypocaloric feeding was 65 g/day being slightly higher in the first 8 weeks of follow-up.

When the treatment consisted of a 600 kcal diet from the beginning again the weight loss was greater during the first week. Thereafter it tended to decrease from about 200 g per day in the second and third week to 42 g per day in the following weeks of treatment.

Decrease of body weight in obese patients reached -30% after one year of treatment by drastic calorie restriction; it was still -22% after two further years, during which clinical follow-up was interrupted.

When the treatment consisted of a 600-900 kcal diet from the beginning, body weight was 18% lower after 8 months, and was still 15% lower two years after the clinical follow-up was interrupted.

Dr. Mancini's findings demonstrate that drastic calorie restriction is well tolerated in gross obesity and long-term results are satisfactory.

Nearly 15 years of experience in the *dietary management of hyperlipidemia and coronary heart disease* have convinced *R.S. Lees, USA,* that both hyperlipidemia and atherosclerosis, at least in America, are due to the synergistic action of gluttony and sloth. Dr. Lees' approach to the dietary management of out-patients with hyperlipidemias and coronary heart diseases starts with a careful diet history.

The therapeutic diet is similar to the previous dietary preference but 700 calories below the individual demonstrated maintenance diet. The lipoprotein phenotypes of 141 consecutive patients referred to the out-patient clinic showed about 50% type II, about 40% type IV, and only a few percent type III and V patterns. In this variety of lipoprotein phenotypes the response to weight reduction was fairly uniform and satisfying, not only during the weight reduction period, but also after the patients were once again on diets which maintained body weights at lower levels. In a group of some 30 patients with various phenotypes and an average overweight of 15 - 20 pounds, this method of management resulted in achievement of a minimum of 10 - 15 pounds weight loss or in ideal body weight. There was a reduction in plasma lipids of all patients, the cholesterol lowering in type II being of the order of 20%, a dramatic lipid lowering occurring in type III and a 10% cholesterol and 50% triglyceride reduction in type IV. A subsequent study compared the effects of weight reduction with the use of clofibrate. In spite of decreased VLDL concentrations, total plasma cholesterol and triglycerides remained unchanged or even rose due to increases in LDL concentration in the "low LDL" subgroup. Caloric restriction was effective in both subgroups.

In summary, the obesity, which is so common in our population and which is the result of eating too much and burning too little, at least in the susceptible subjects is associated with hyperlipidemia and with atherosclerosis. The hyperlipidemia is markedly ameliorated by weight reduction in free living patients on ordinary solid diets. This amelioration compares favourably with that which can be obtained by at least one commonly used drug and is an important part and the first mode of therapy to be used in hyperlipidemia.

With regard to the *mechanism of the effect of weight reduction* on plasma lipid levels several possibilities have to be considered. One of these is reduction of the amount of adipose tissue and an increased adipocyte sensitivity to insulin, probably resulting in increased removal of VLDL. Conversely, as illustrated by the overfeeding experiments of Sims and co-workers, experimental obesity results in increase of adipocyte size, plasma triglycerides and insulin resistance. Another organ to be considered is the liver. It is known that in obesity there is a marked over-production of cholesterol (Miettinen, 1971) and also of triglycerides (Robertson et al., 1973). Furthermore, increased intake of calories in the obese state may overtax mechanisms for deposition of exogenous nutrients, thus contributing to hyperlipidemia. The latter factors rather than the reduction in adipose tissue mass would explain observations of rapid early lipid lowering as soon as negative calorie balance is established and before significant diminution of the adipose tissue mass has taken place.

Other Dietary Measures

While a weight reduction regimen is feasible and effective in four of five patients with hyperlipidemia, qualitative dietary changes have also to be considered, particularly in the familial type II patient. The polyunsaturated to saturated ratio, with weight reducing diets of little importance, achieves significance in dietary recommendations for segments of the population. In the experience of *A.G. Shaper*, England, a general recommendation to modify the fat intake resulted in a dietary change from a PS-ratio of 0.1 - 0.2 to 1.0. In his experience, cholesterol was reduced by 15%, triglyceride levels by 30%.

Reduction of dietary cholesterol is similarly effective irrespective of weight changes. Marked reduction of dietary cholesterol to a maximum of 200 - 300 mg/day is considered by Lees if plasma cholesterol levels do not respond satisfactorily to the initial hypocaloric regime.

Data on the deleterious effect of dietary cholesterol in rabbits were presented by *G. Weber*, Italy. He showed, that with the use of the scanning electron microscope changes can be demonstrated on the endothelial surface of rabbit vessels subjected to hypercholesterolemic diets for very short periods from 15 days to one month. The changes initiate near the origin of the collateral branches and are quite marked in this brief period. At the same time, the polysaccharide containing surface coat of the endothelial cells becomes markedly thickened. Interestingly in this rabbit model, a dissociation between vascular changes and hyperlipidemia can be demonstrated by glucocorticoid administration or injections of Tween 80.

The amount of carbohydrate, in Lees' experience, can be shown to affect plasma triglycerides in the experimental setting. Low carbohydrate diets, however, are poorly tolerated. Similar thinking applies to alcohol. There has been little effect by substitution of complex carbohydrate for simple carbohydrates, particularly due to a lack of acceptance of patients to reduce their sugar consumption.

Poly-Unsaturated Fatty Acids and Cholelithiasis

This topic was dealt with by *S. Grundy, USA*. In a recent report, Sturdevant et al., 1973 found that patients treated with diets containing unsaturated fats developed more cholesterol gallstones than did a control group which ingested mostly saturated fats. The mechanism for an increased likelihood of cholesterol gallstones on unsaturated fat diets was not apparent from this study. Grundy et al. have therefore attempted to determine whether unsaturated fats might alter the metabolism of cholesterol or bile acids so as to produce a lithogenic bile. The term "lithogenic bile" is defined as bile containing an excess of cholesterol relative to the solubilizing lipids — bile acids and phospholipids; in lithogenic bile, cholesterol exists in an unstable solution, and it is prone to precipitate to form gallstones.

Six patients were studied under metabolic ward conditions at the Veterans Administration Hospital, La Jolla, California. Each received a diet containing 40% of calories as lard for one month, and following this period, the patients were fed a diet containing 40% safflower oil for another month. During the last two weeks of each period, gallbladder bile was collected multiple times by duodenal intubation; bile was analyzed for lipid composition (cholesterol, bile acids and phospholipids). In 4 of 6 patients, gallbladder bile was unsaturated with cholesterol on lard, and it became more lithogenic on safflower oil — the lipid composition approached the limits of cholesterol solubility during the feeding of the oil. In another patient, bile was supersaturated with cholesterol throughout both study periods. Therefore, in some patients, at least, unsaturated fats seem to increase lithogenicity of gallbladder bile, and this effect may account for an increased prevalance of cholesterol stones on these fats.

In order to determine the mechanisms by which unsaturated fats lead to lithogenic bile, pool sizes of bile acids and hepatic secretion rates of biliary lipids were measured during constant infusion of liquid formula diets in the two periods. There was no decrease in bile acid pool sizes on unsaturated fats as compared to saturated fats and cholesterol secretion rates were not increased; these two alterations have been previously reported to contribute to the formation of lithogenic bile in patients with gallstones. The finding of lithogenic gallbladder bile on unsaturated fats occurring without alterations in bile acid pools or hepatic secretion of cholesterol suggests that an imbalance exists in secretion of these two lipids in the fasting state. Whether the liver secretes an excess of cholesterol during fasting or whether the bile acid pool is incompletely transferred into the gallbladder has not been determined.

Since the prevalence of gallstones has been on discussion, Dr. Turpeinen mentioned some observations his group has made in connection with the Finnish Mental Hospital study (Miettinen et al., 1972). Dr. Turpeinen found no difference between those patients who have been on the unsaturated diet and the control patients. The incidence of gallstones in the autopsy cases were just about the same and approximately 25% in both groups. It seems, that this is the percentage that the Californian investigators (Sturdevant et al.) have found in their experimental group and the striking figure is the rather low prevalence of gallstones in their control group. If one looks at the autopsy material that has been published from various parts of the world, the prevalence of gallstones in middle aged males runs usually about 25%.

Dietary Management of Type II Familial Hyperlipoproteinaemia in Children

June K. Lloyd, England confined her remarks to the dietary treatment of children who are heterozygous for familial hyperbetalipoproteinaemia (Type II) introducing a rather sobering experience into the workshop. In children perhaps even more than in adults, it is essential that any regime should be safe, acceptable to both child and parents, and maintain its effect in the long-term. To date, the only effect which can be measured in children is the hypocholesterolaemic effect, and even here there is no hard indication of the optimal serum cholesterol concentration one should aim for. Drash (1972) has suggested a value of 235 mg/100ml as the upper limit for "healthy children" in the United States. In familial hyperbetalipoproteinaemia it is probably overoptimistic to expect all children to achieve this low level. The really important long-term effect on the development of ischaemic heart disease will, of course, only come from prospective studies.

Of the 3 types of therapeutic measure available-diet, drugs, or a combination of the two, — it might be thought that diet would be the best for children, the dietary regime consisting (as for adults) of a reduction in the saturated fat intake with an increase in the intake of polyunsaturated fatty acids. Some concern has been expressed about the long-term safety of this regime and Dayton (1973) for instance would not recommend its use in general in children, although at present there would seem to be little good evidence that it is not safe.

When the other two criteria, acceptability and long-term efficacy are considered it has been Dr. Lloyd's experience that the regime is not acceptable to most of the children and as a consequence they do not adhere to it adequately, and the long-term results are poor in terms of maintaining satisfactory serum cholesterol concentrations. The children who have been treated come in the main from families in which parental motivation has been strong because of the early occurrence of ischaemic heart disease in one ore more members, and even in these families, in only 2 of about 25 children has diet remained the only form of treatment.

The reason for the non-acceptability of the diet is the necessity to restrict severely the intake of saturated fat (Segall et al., 1970). They have shown that the hypocholesterolaemic effect of the dietary regime has depended solely on the reduction in saturated fat intake, and that corn oil by itself has had no additional benefit. The data in the Table 1 shows the effect of two different regimes in respect of the amount of corn oil intake and demonstrates that the larger intake did not result in any greater hypocholesterolaemic effect. It is also clear from the mean values of serum cholesterol achieved on diet, and from the range of values, that many children were "inadequately" treated.

Table 1. Familial hyperbetalipoproteinaemia, effect of diet

Dietary Fat g/day, mean & range		Serum cholesterol mg/100 ml, mean & range		% Redn.
Sat. fat.	Corn oil	Pre-	On diet	
14	15	370	281	24
7 - 32	5 - 35	303 - 510	192 - 323	9 - 45
18	57	372	306	18
10 - 32	45 - 70	303 - 434	255 - 373	9 - 26

(From Segall, Lloyd, Fosbrooke & Wolff, 1970).

Lloyd has found this non-acceptability of the dietary regime to operate equally in pre-school children as in the older age groups and now no longer recommends diets except for those children in whom serum cholesterol concentrations are only slightly elevated (say to around 260-270 mg/100 ml) and in whom a modest reduction of around 10% may be adequate. She feels vindicated in her attitude by the relief with which children have accepted the somewhat unpalatable drug cholestyramine as a substitute for the dietary regime (West and Lloyd, 1973).

Observations on Hyperlipidemia and Diet in Japan

The difficulties in establishing "normal" lipid levels are illustrated by observations in Japan. The population mean now is 187 ± 44 mg/100 ml (mean ± SD). Treatment, according to Y. Goto starts with cholesterol levels greater than 230, and triglyceride levels greater than 150 mg%. These levels, as the Japanese diet and the rate of coronary heart disease, are rapidly changing: In 1955, the myocardial infarction mortality was 9.9 per 100,000, the fat intake averaged 18 g; in 1965, myocardial infarction mortality was up to 28.5 per 100,000 and the fat intake to 36 g, and in 1970 the myocardial infarction mortality increased to 37.9 per 100,000, the fat intake being 46.5 g. The milk consumption increased by a factor of 3.5 in 10 years, sugar and meat consumption by 1.5.

Difficulties in implementing dietary advice were also part of Dr. Goto's presentation. In his hyperlipidemia clinic, a diet similar for all types and modified from the American Heart Association diet has been used since 1969 at four different calorie levels and four levels of fat intakes (Table 2). The short- and long-term results in 24 out- and in 26 inpatients showed a reduction of both cholesterol and triglycerides, which was, however, significant only for cholesterol. Adherence is difficult since patients with hyperlipidemia usually do not have symptoms and usually cannot feel the success of dietary therapy. In addition, there is lack of knowledge in nutritional matters and difficulties of dietary practice. This could not be overcome by the introduction of a simple food exchange method, using symbols for calories, cholesterol and PS-ratio (Table 3).

Table 2. Effect of dietary treatment on serum lipids. Outpatients (N=24)

	Before	After	Lowest value
Cholesterol[a] (mg%)	258.3 $\pm$ 12.9[b]	238.5 $\pm$ 11.9	225.4 $\pm$ 11.9[b]
Triglyceride (mg%)	176.3 $\pm$ 55.6	159.6 $\pm$ 28.6	131.6 $\pm$ 23.4

	Inpatients (N=26)		
	Before	After	Lowest value
Cholesterol (mg%)	239.0 $\pm$ 12.4[b]	212.0 $\pm$ 10.8	205.7 $\pm$ 9.9[b]
Triglyceride (mg%)	265.0 $\pm$ 80.8	120.3 $\pm$ 13.6	118.8 $\pm$ 13.8

[a] Mean $\pm$ standard error. Lowest value: the lowest lipid concentration obtained.
[b] P .01.

Table 3. Effects of dietary treatment on serum lipids by using food exchange table. Outpatients (N=8)

	Before	After	Lowest value
Cholesterol[a] (mg%)	279.0 $\pm$ 17.8	275.3 $\pm$ 27.1	266.2 $\pm$ 25.9
Triglyceride (mg%)	178.4 $\pm$ 39.5	262.6 $\pm$ 54.2	230.1 $\pm$ 49.8

[a] Mean $\pm$ standard error.

Slight fall of cholesterol and considerable rise of triglycerides with food exchange method; rise of triglycerides due to the fact that patients chose carbohydrates for fats in order to reduce foods with unsaturated fat and cholesterol.

EFFECTS OF HYPOLIPIDEMIC REGIMES ON SERUM LIPOPROTEINS[*]

Lars A. Carlson, Anders G. Olsson, Lars Orö, Stephan Rössner, and
Göran Walldius

Introduction

There is a rapid development in the area of serum lipid lowering regimes. Diets,
drugs and other measures are used more and more frequently on more and more patients by more and more physicians. This increased use makes it mandatory that we
know in detail the effects and the side-effects of these various regimes, One important aspect on the effects of the so called serum lipid lowering regimes is the
effects on the *different* serum lipoprotein (LP) classes. Although it is well known
that the serum lipids are bound to proteins and thus exist as LP in blood and that
there are at least 3 major different LP classes we have surprisingly little knowledge about the effect of lipid lowering regimes on the concentration and composition of the LP classes. In fact it is not correct terminology to use expressions
such as "lipid lowering drugs", "cholesterol lowering drugs" or "triglyceride
lowering drugs". The correct terminology would be *LP lowering drugs* because it
is not the serum cholesterol that is reduced by e.g. nicotinic acid but the concentration of the whole β (and also pre- β) lipoprotein molecules in serum
(Carlson, 1969).

The three major LP classes, VLDL (very low density = pre- β), LDL (low density
= β) and HDL (high density = α), which are present in fasting serum all contain
the major serum lipid components cholesterol, triglycerides and phospholipids.
Since the concentration of the LP classes may vary independently of each other,
it is impossible by measurement of only total serum cholesterol and triglycerides
to estimate changes induced by drugs in the concentration of VLDL, LDL and HDL.
As a matter of fact one or two of the LP classes may have *increased* even if total
serum cholesterol decreases during treatment. Examples of this will be given
below.

There are four major indications for serum LP lowering regimes

1. Recurrent pancreatitis,
2. Xanthomas,
3. Primary prevention of IHD,
4. Secondary prevention of IHD.

Indications 1. and 2. are firmly established clinically. In recurrent pancreatitis
associated with hyperlipoproteinemia (HLP) of type V (Fredrickson et al., 1967;
Beaumont et al., 1970) LP lowering regims abolish the attacks and are life saving.
Likewise xanthomas present in patients having types II A, III, IV and V HLP
(Buxforf et al., 1974; Carlson, 1969) are reduced and may even disappear during
intensive LP lowering therapy. With regard to indications 3. and 4. it is not as
yet firmly established that treatment with LP lowering regimes prevents or delays

---

[*]Supported by grants from Svenska Margarinindustrins Förening för Näringsfysio-
logisk Forskning and from the Swedish Medical Research Council (19x-204).

Abbreviations: LP = lipoproteins, HLP = hyerlipoproteinemia, VLDL, LDL and HDL =
very low, low and high density LP, IHD = ischaemic heart disease, FFA = free
fatty acids, FIAT = fatty acid incorporation into adipose tissue.

ischaemic heart disease (IHD) and other atherosclerotic vascular diseases. However, studies with diets and drugs suggest that this is the case. From the quantitative point of view indications 1. and 2. comprise very small while 3. and 4. comprise very large groups.

LP Abnormalities in IHD

When LP lowering regimes are prescribed for primary or secondary prevention of IHD to patients with LP abnormalities it should be self-evident that the treatment should modify the LP spectrum into a "non-atherogenic" one. Although our present knowledge it quite insufficient concerning the specific role of the different LP classes for the development of IHD it seems reasonable that the goal should be to correct those LP abnormalities which are associated with IHD. In Table 1 we have summarized the differences between patients with IHD and normal subjects. Furthermore we have compared the LP levels in adult males and females considering the well known difference between the sexes with regard to IHD. VLDL is higher in IHD patients than in controls and also higher in males than in females. LDL is higher in IHD, but there is no significant sex difference. HDL, which sofar has not been paid much attention to in IHD, is lower in IHD and also consistently lower in males than in females.

From these differences between IHD and control subjects and between males and females treatment of HLP for primary or secondary prevention should induce the following changes in the serum concentration of the three major LP classes.

VLDL:	Decrease or if low unchanged,
LDL:	Decrease or if low unchanged,
HDL:	Increase or if high unchanged.

The facts in Table 1 suggest that changes in the opposite direction do not seem desirable.

Table 1. Summary of the characteristic differences in fasting serum lipoprotein levels between IHD patients and controls and between males and females

	IHD VS Controls	Males VS Females
VLDL	↑	↑
LDL	↑	=
HDL	↓	↓

Classification of HLP

Since there are different classes of LP it is not surprising that there should be different types of HLP depending on which class(es) of LP that is/are raised in concentration. Fredrickson, Lees and Levy introduced a system for classification of HLP into so called types based upon LP concentrations (Fredrickson et al., 1967). This has later been modified (Beaumont et al., 1970), which modification is now widely used. Chylomicrons, VLDL and LDL are the LP classes which are considered in this classification system. Concerning treatment of HLP one can ask if this system is a useful guideline to find the correct regime. In our opinion the typing system is useful in choosing therapy for the "extreme types", e.g.

in patients with type II A HLP with pronounced elevation of LDL or in type V
with massive chylomicronemia. In patients with moderate and borderline HLP the
usefulness of the typing system can be questioned as discussed below.

Earlier Studies on Drug Effects on LP

The explanation to the surprising fact that there are so few quantitative studies
on the effects of drugs on LP is that the techniques for LP analysis are still
rather cumbersome. There is, however, no escape from the fact that such analyses
have to be done on large patient materials over prolonged times with all forms
of treatment for HLP in order to evaluate the effects of a given regime in all
LP classes in the various types of HLP. One of the "classical" studies of drug
effects on LP in man is the one of Strisower et al where they studied the concentration of LDL and VLDL by analytical ultracentrifugation (Strisower et al.,
1970). Their results are summarized in Table 2. In Table 3 we have summarized
our own experience with the effects of nicotinic acid on serum LP over the last
ten years.

Table 2. Effect of clofibrate (1.5 g/day) on serum lipoproteins[a]

Group Nr.	Probable[b] Type	LDL	VLDL
1 N = 14	II A With tendon x.	NO	- 35 %
2 N = 21	II A No tendon x.	- 23 %	- 47 %
5 N = 5	II B	+ 32 % to - 30 %	- 57 %
3 N = 7	III	NO	- 71 %
4 N = 11	IV V	+ 59 %	- 64 %

[a]Analysed by analytical ultracentrifugation, data from Strisower et al. (1968).
[b]According to Fredrickson et al as modified by Beaumont et al. (1970).

Table 3. Effect of nicotinic acid[a] on serum lipoprotein levels

Type	LDL	VLDL	Chylo- microns
II A.	↓	↓	
II B	↓	↓	
III		↓↓	
IV	↑ or ↓	↓↓	
V	↑	↓↓	↓↓

[a]Effect is dose dependent, particularly on LDL (from Carlson et al. (1972a).

There is one aspect with these results which is important but has been neglected. That is the *increase* in LDL sometimes obtained with either clofibrate or nicotinic acid in type IV and type V HLP at the same time as VLDL is reduced (Table 2 and 3). Similar effects have also been observed by Wilson and Lees (1972) in a study on patients with HLP treated with both diet and clofibrate. As stated above an increase in LDL is an undesirable effect. The mechanism for these reciprocal changes in VLDL and LDL is not known. As described below it seems, however, possible to predict when LDL will increase during treatment in type IV and V HLP.

Examples of the Need for LP Analysis

The concentration of the different LP classes may vary independent of each other under physiologic conditions as well as during treatment. Determination of total serum cholesterol and triglycerides cannot define the effect of drugs on the serum LP spectrum. This will be examplified by the effects of two drugs; one — cholestyramine — a so called "cholesterol lowering" compound and one so called "triglyceride lowering" drug — oxandrolone.

Table 4 shows that cholestyramine reduced serum total cholesterol on the average by 24 per cent, while there was no significant effect on *total* serum triglyceride concentration. However, when we look at the effects on the LP a different picture emerges. The VLDL triglycerides and cholesterol had *increased* by 30%, while the LDL cholesterol and triglycerides had decreased by 33% and 20%. The lowering of LDL had thus masked the rise in VLDL when only *total* cholesterol and triglycerides were determined. When we then combined the cholestyramine treatment with clofibrate the increase in VLDL was turned into a decrease (-30%) and there is also a further reduction of LDL which was reduced over all by 39% with the combined treatment.

Table 4. Effect of cholestyramine (16 g/day of Questran®) on serum lipoproteins in hyperlipoproteinemia type II A (n = 13) and II B (n = 4)

	Cholesterol mg/100 ml Before	After	% Change	Triglycerides mmol/l Before	After	% Change
Serum	385	294	−24[a]	1.82	1.91	+ 5 ns
VLDL	23	30	+30[b]	0.77	1.01	+31[b]
LDL	286	193	−33[a]	0.74	0.59	−20[b]
HDL	53	53	0	0.22	0.23	+ 5 ns

ns = not significant.
[a] and [b] indicate that P is less than 0.001 and 0.01.

Results with the "triglyceride lowering" compound oxandrolone are given in Table 5. *Total* serum triglycerides were lowered by 30% while *total* cholesterol remained essentially unchanged. However, the LP analysis reveals that there were striking changes in all LP classes. The VLDL decreased considerably and so did HDL while LDL increased. This is a very instructive example of the necessity to perform LP analysis in the evaluation of a lipid lowering compound. The effects of oxandrolone on total serum triglycerides and cholesterol looked simple and attractive but the LP analysis revealed that the changes were quite complex. The exploration of the effects on the LP:s is thus not only of academic but also of considerable practical interest because as in the case of oxandrolone neither an increase in LDL nor a decrease of HDL seems to be a desirable therapeutic response.

Table 5. Effect of oxandrolone (7.5 mg/day) on serum lipoproteins in hyper-lipoproteinemia type II B (n = 4) and IV (n = 16)

	Cholesterol mmg/100 ml Before	After	% Change	Triglycerides mmol/1 Before	After	% Change
Serum	310	303	-2^{ns}	4.12	2.87	-30^{a}
VLDL	65	37	-43^{a}	2.97	1.93	-35^{a}
LDL	179	211	$+18^{b}$	0.66	0.78	$+18^{ns}$
HDL	43	28	-35^{a}	0.28	0.18	-36^{a}

ns = not significant.

[a] and [b] indicate that P is less than 0.001 and 0.01.

Interrelation Between VLDL and LDL

It is known that there sometimes exists reciprocal relation between the concentrations of VLDL and LDL. For example patients with type V HLP often have low levels of LDL which increase to normal when chylomicrons and VLDL levels are corrected. We have e.g. seen in a patient with extreme type V that LDL cholesterol increased from a very low level of 20 mg/100 ml to 130 mg/100 ml when VLDL triglycerides were reduced with nicotinic acid from 90 to 3 mmol/1 (Carlson et al., 1972a).

Furthermore also in type IV HLP treatment with clofibrate, nicotinic acid and diets may increase LDL when VLDL decreases which is a further example of this reciprocal relation. However, this behaviour is not a general rule as LDL and VLDL may also show parallel changes. Nicotinic acid has been shown to decrease both these LP:s and both increase with age. Since it is believed that VLDL is metabolized to LDL (Fig. 1), it would be expected that changes in the concentrations of VLDL and LDL would occur in parallel directions. The fact that the changes in concentration sometimes occur in a reciprocal way, sometimes in a parallel, indicates that the relation between VLDL and LDL is not as simple as in Fig. 1.

We have looked at the relation between LDL and VLDL in a group of subjects with HLP selected from a group of healthy persons because of a plasma cholesterol above 350 mg/100 ml or/and a plasma triglyceride above 3 mmol/1. This group thus represents the *entire* population of HLP in a population sample — moderate as well as excessive HLP:s — except type III HLP which were excluded. Fig. 2 reveals that there is a striking continuous reciprocal relation between LDL and VLDL, with increasing VLDL concentration LDL continuously decreases. It is indeed not appealing from the biological point of view to break this continuous relation. However, this is exactly what we are doing when we classify the HLP:s into types II A, II B and IV, because this classification implies that we use cut-off values for the "upper normal" limits of the concentrations of VLDL and LDL. In Figure 3 such cut-off limits have been applied to the LP of the persons in Fig. 2. A classification based upon "elevated" concentrations of LP seems questionable when one looks at Fig. 3, where it is apparent how this procedure breaks up the continuous relation between LDL and VLDL. Furthermore, the cut-off limits are certainly arbitrary and LP levels vary from day to day so that a person may "travel day by day from type to type of HLP", at least the moderate types of HLP.

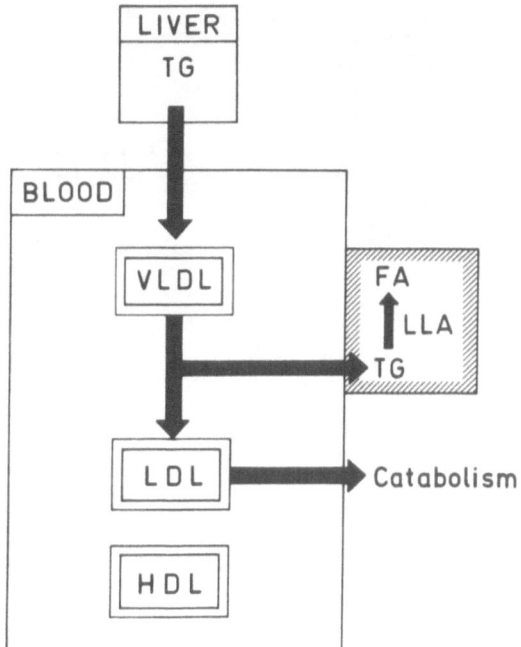

Figure 1. Metabolic relation
between VLDL and LDL ac-
cording to Levy et al. (1971)
(Major Metabolic Pathways of
Serum Lipoproteins)

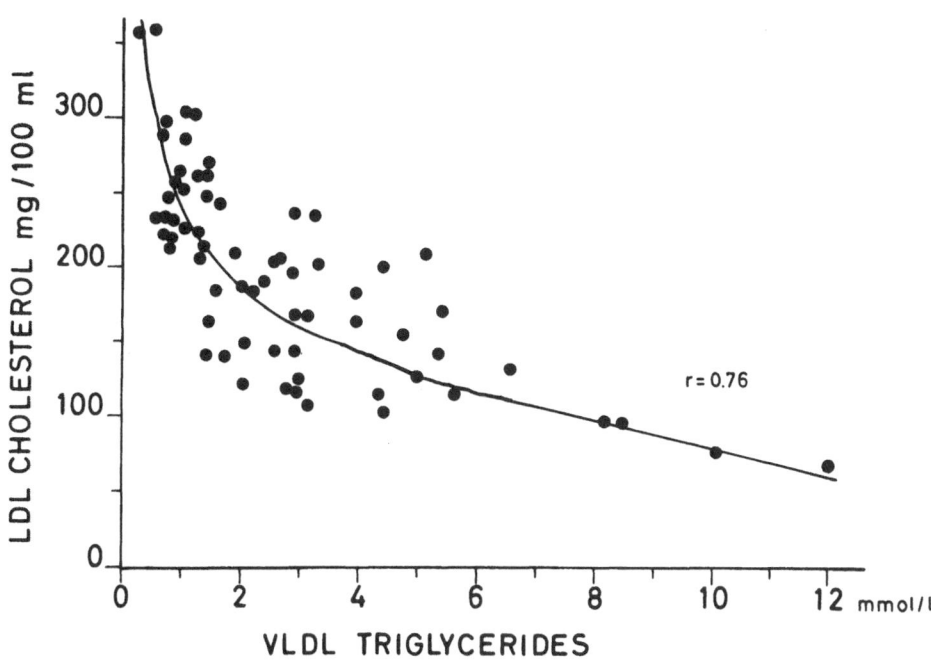

Figure 2. Relation between LDL-cholesterol and VLDL-triglycerides in a group of
healthy persons representing the *entire* population of HLP (except type III) in a
sample screened for serum concentrations of triglycerides and cholesterol. Note
the *continuous* reciprocal relation between LDL and VLDL

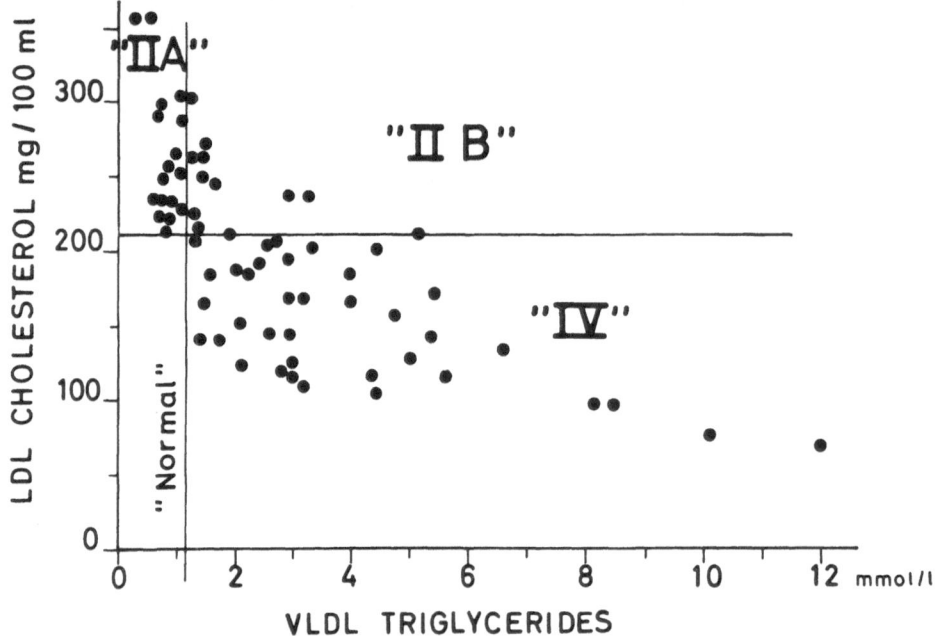

Figure 3. Cut-off values for the "upper normal" limit of VLDL-triglycerides (1.10 mmol/1) and of LDL-cholesterol (210 mg/100 ml) have been used for the population of HLP in Fig. 2 in order to classify the HLP into types IIA, II B and IV

Effects of Diet and Clofibrate on LP

The two LP lowering regimes which have least side effects and with which we have the longest experience are diet and clofibrate. The effects of these two regimes in the LP spectrum in the subjects in Figure 3 will be described. Simple dietary advice was given after LP analysis had been done. When LDL was high, a low saturated, high polyunsaturated diet low in cholesterol was prescribed. For subjects with high VLDL weight reduction and moderation with sugars were recommended. After two months of diet clofibrate was added for two months and LP analysis was performed. With this design we aimed at a practical and simple regime for lowering serum LP levels

The average results on the LP classes are shown in Tables 6, 7 and 8. The therapeutic response is rather uniform with regard to VLDL in which LP class both triglycerides and cholesterol are reduced by 50 - 76% in the three types of HLP. There were no major changes in the composition of VLDL concerning cholesterol and triglycerides. With regard to LDL the triglyceride response was also uniform with significant decreases of around 20% in the three types. The cholesterol response, however, varies. In type II A there was a reduction by 36%, in II B by 26%, but in type IV there was no significant effect. Thus the composition of LDL changes in different ways in the three types in a way which suggests that going from type II A to type IV the effects shift from primarily on S_f 0 - 12 to S_f 12 - 20. In HDL there was also a uniform and rather pronounced reduction of triglyceride concentration in all types, while the cholesterol content increased significantly in both II B and IV. There were thus changes not only in the levels of HDL but also in the composition of this LP which warrants further studies.

These average results of the treatment have thus shown different responses between the types with regard to the cholesterol content in LDL and HDL, while the triglycerides were fairly uniformly reduced in all LP classes in the three types of HLP. The *individual* response of the cholesterol content of VLDL and LDL is shown in Fig. 4. The cholesterol concentration in VLDL was reduced in all cases

in all types but one with type IV HLP. In type II A and II B HLP the LDL cholesterol decreased in all but one case. In type IV, however, the picture was quite
different. Some subjects had a pronounced increase, others showed a decrease and
some had no change in LDL cholesterol.

Table 6. Effect of diet and clofibrate (2 g/day of Atromidin®) on serum lipoproteins in hyperlipoproteinemia type II A (n = 16)

	Cholesterol mg/100 ml		% Change	Triglycerides mmol/1		% Change
	Before	After		Before	After	
Serum	376	256	− 32[a]	1.93	1.22	− 37[a]
VLDL	22	11	− 50[a]	0.78	0.39.	− 50[a]
LDL	265	169	− 36[a]	0.78	0.59	− 24[a]
HDL	66	63	− 5[ns]	0.29	0.17	− 41[a]

ns = not significant.
[a] P is less than 0.001.

Table 7. Effect of diet and clofibrate (2 g/day of Atromidin®) on serum lipoproteins in hyperlipoproteinemia type II B (n = 11)

	Cholesterol mg/100 ml		% Change	Triglycerides mmol/1		% Change
	Before	After		Before	After	
Serum	346	255	− 26[a]	3.27	1.52	− 54[a]
VLDL	45	14	− 69[a]	1.99	0.58	− 71[a]
LDL	254	187	− 26[a]	0.90	0.66	− 27[a]
HDL	47	54	+ 15[b]	0.25	0.20	− 20[c]

[a], [b] and [c] indicate that P is less than 0.001, 0.01 and 0.05.

Table 8. Effect of diet and clofibrate (2 g/day of Atromidin®) on serum lipoproteins in hyperlipoproteinemia type IV (n = 39)

	Cholesterol mg/100 ml		% Change	Triglycerides mmol/1		% Change
	Before	After		Before	After	
Serum	284	224	− 21[a]	5.22	1.84	− 65[a]
VLDL	73	22	− 69[a]	3.83	0.91	− 76[a]
LDL	151	138	− 8[ns]	0.77	0.62	− 19[a]
HDL	43	48	+ 12[a]	0.36	0.22	− 39[a]

ns = not significant.
[a] P is less than 0.001.

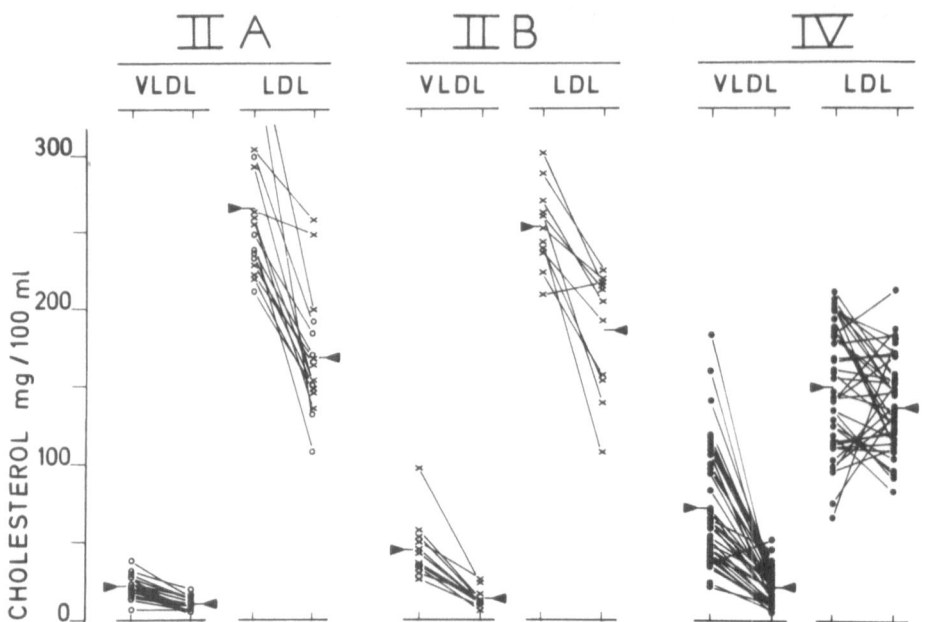

Figure 4. Individual response of VLDL, LDL and HDL cholesterol to diet and clofibrate in subjects with type II A, II B and IV HLP. The same subjects as in Fig. 2/3. Before treatment to left and after to right. Mean values are indicated

It is thus evident that in subjects with type II A and II B HLP treatment induced a parallel change in VLDL and LDL, both falling. In type IV there was sometimes a parallel change and sometimes a reciprocal change with decrease in VLDL but increase in LDL cholesterol. Since one of the characteristic differences between types II A and II B on one hand and type IV on the other is the concentration of LDL cholesterol with a mean value of 265, 254 and 151 mg/100 ml respectively, we looked at the changes induced in LDL (Δ LDL) by treatment in relation to the LDL concentration before treatment. Fig. 5 shows that there is a strong linear relation between these two parameters (r = 0.82).

The equation for the regression line is Δ LDL-cholesterol = -0.70 x LDL-cholesterol + 97.

This equation predicts that when pre-treatment LDL-cholesterol is below 138 mg/100 ml the Δ LDL-cholesterol will be positive, i.e. LDL-cholesterol will increase. When LDL-cholesterol is above this value the treatment will result in a negative Δ -value, i.e. a lowering of LDL-cholesterol.

These results are derived from this diet and clofibrate study. To see if it is a more general phenomenon that low LDL levels increase during treatment of HLP we studied nine patients with type V HLP in this regard, because this HLP, which is defined as fasting chylomicronemia and increased VLDL levels, almost always has low LDL levels. Fig. 6 shows the cholesterol content of the lipoproteins before and after treatment with either diet or nicotinic acid. In all nine patients the very high VLDL levels decreased and LDL, which was below the critical 138 mg/100 ml in all cases, increased. This response was independent of the kind of treatment. Furthermore, as shown in Fig. 7, the response of LDL appeared to fit the relation between Δ LDL and pre-treatment LDL just described (Fig. 5) for clofibrate diet. Thus this relation is not only valid for clofibrate but for treatments which in general lower VLDL. Since raising LDL is not a desirable effect, in seems necessary to measure LDL particularly in type IV before treatment. Combined treatment, e.g. with clofibrate and cholestyramine, may be the treatment of choice in type IV with LDL cholesterol below 140 mg/100 ml.

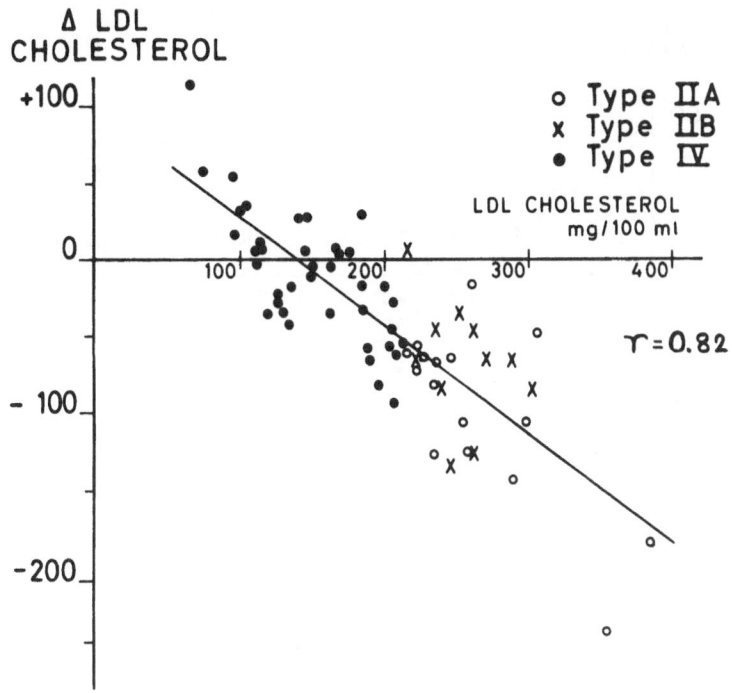

Figure 5. Relation between the changes in LDL (Δ LDL) concentration (mg/100 ml) induced by diet and clofibrate and the pre-treatment level of LDL. The linear relation existing for all three types of HLP predicts that when LDL-cholesterol is below 138 mg/100 ml there will be an increase in LDL

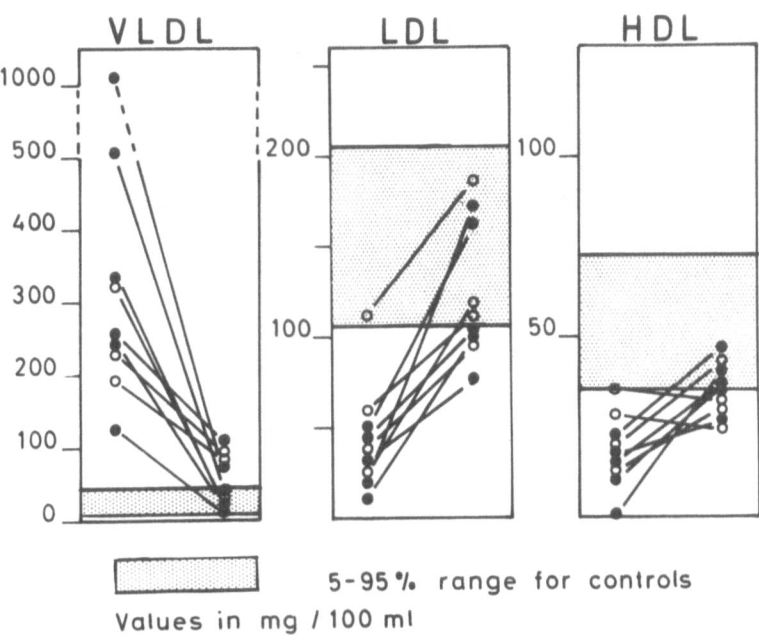

Figure 6. Effect of treatment with either diet (o-o) or nicotinic acid (•-•) (4.5 - 6 g/day) on the cholesterol concentration of VLDL, LDL and HDL in 9 patients with type V HLP. Before treatment to left and after to right. Observe the subnormal values for LDL and HDL before treatment

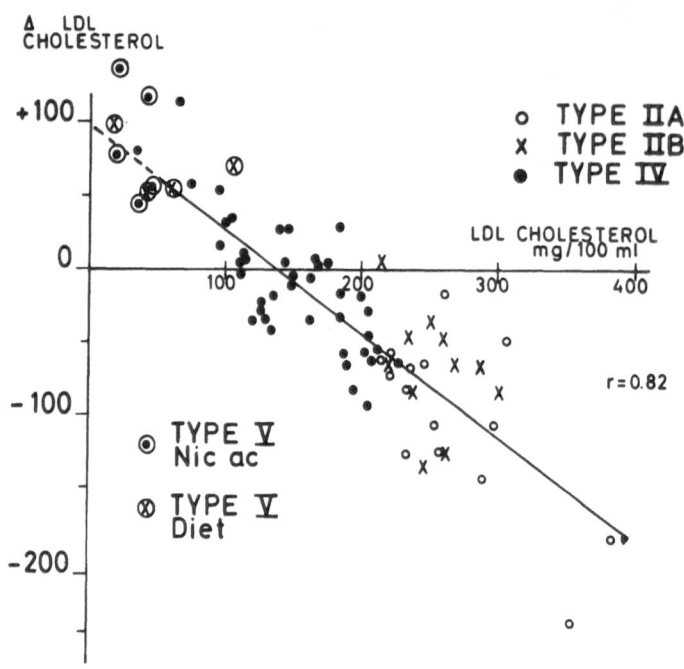

Figure 7. Relation between the changes in LDL (Δ LDL) induced in type V HLP
(Fig. 6) in relation to pre-treatment level of LDL. The regression line describes
the relation observed in Fig. 5 and the individual observations from that figure
are also included

Effect of Acute Changes of the Concentration of VLDL or LDL on the Interrelation

The reciprocal relation between VLDL and LDL (Fig. 2) can be explained if
LDL inhibits VLDL production or if VLDL stimulates LDL catabolism. Also when LDL
increases when VLDL is reduced may be explained if the high VLDL levels before
treatment had stimulated LDL catabolism, a stimulus which is reduced when VLDL
is reduced resulting in an increased LDL concentration. To study these possibilities we have in acute studies changed the concentration of either LDL or VLDL
to see if the change in concentration of one would affect the concentration of
the other according to the hypothesis above.

VLDL was raised by iv infusion of triglycerides as Intralipid®. Table 9 shows
that this as expected results in raised levels of VLDL. This is *followed* by a
decrease in LDL. This dynamic pattern fits with the hypothesis that the reciprocal relation between VLDL and LDL might be due to a stimulation of VLDL on LDL
catabolism.

On the other hand when LDL was reduced by a polyunsaturated diet no effect was
seen on VLDL (Fig. 8). When clofibrate was superimposed upon the diet VLDL decreased significantly within 24 hours and this was *followed* 24 hours later by a
increase in LDL cholesterol (Fig. 8). These results do not suggest that the concentration of LDL has any influence on VLDL but they are compatible with a stimulating effect of VLDL on LDL removal.

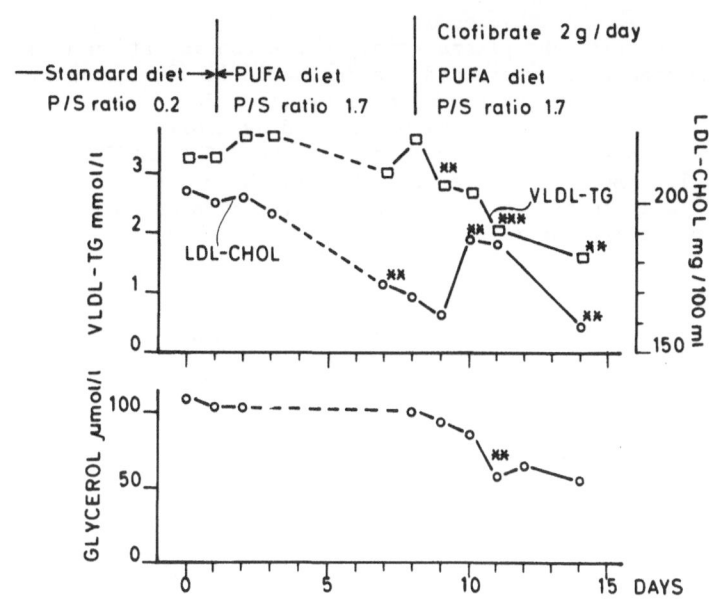

Figure 8. Average results from 5 patients with HLP treated on a metabolic ward with diets containing natural foods, body weights maintained constant. Fasting values for VLDL-triglycerides, LDL-cholesterol and free serum glycerol are given. *, ** indicate that the changes from preceding day were significant with P < 0.05 and 0.01

Table 9. Effect of IV infusion of Intralipid® on serum lipoproteins. Triglycerides (TG, mmol/l) and cholesterol (CHOL, mg/100 ml)

	VLDL		LDL_1		LDL_2		HDL	
	TG	CHOL	TG	CHOL	TG	CHOL	TG	CHOL
Fasting	2.4	37	0.09	10	0.33	112	0.22	41
Intralipid®								
1/2 hour	11.3	69	0.11	10	0.43	117	0.30	36
6 hours	9.3	101	0.15	14	0.55	94	0.36	36
24 hours	7.0	122	0.13	5	0.46	46	0.42	25

Adipose Tissue and HLP

Adipose tissue has two regulatory functions related to HLP. One is concerned with the *uptake* of triglycerides from blood and the other with *mobilization* of free fatty acids (FFA) into blood as depicted in Fig. 9. Defect removal, caused either by reduction in LLA or FIAT (see Figure 9) will raise VLDL concentrations. Since FFA are precursors to VLDL triglycerides in the liver, increased mobilization of FFA may cause increased levels of VLDL and subsequently of LDL. On the contrary a reduction of the flow of FFA may reduce VLDL and LDL. Nicotinic acid which lowers VLDL is known to reduce plasma FFA and to inhibit mobilization of FFA from adipose tissue by inhibiting lipolysis in adipose tissue. We have recently shown that clofibrate inhibits lipolysis in rat adipose tissue in vitro (Carlson et al., 1972b). Fig. 10 shows that when rats are fed clofibrate or tibric acid, the plasma triglyceride concentration is reduced. When adipose tissue from rats so treated was incubated in vitro, it can be seen that the fat mobilizing lipolysis was considerably reduced (Fig. 10). It is possible that part of the plasma VLDL lowering induced by clofibrate and other regimes is due to effects on adipose tissue causing reduced FFA mobilization, such as lowering of cyclic AMP. Compatible with this is the reduction of free glycerol in serum, which reflects fat mobilizing lipolysis in adipose tissue, early during clofibrate treatment (Fig. 8).

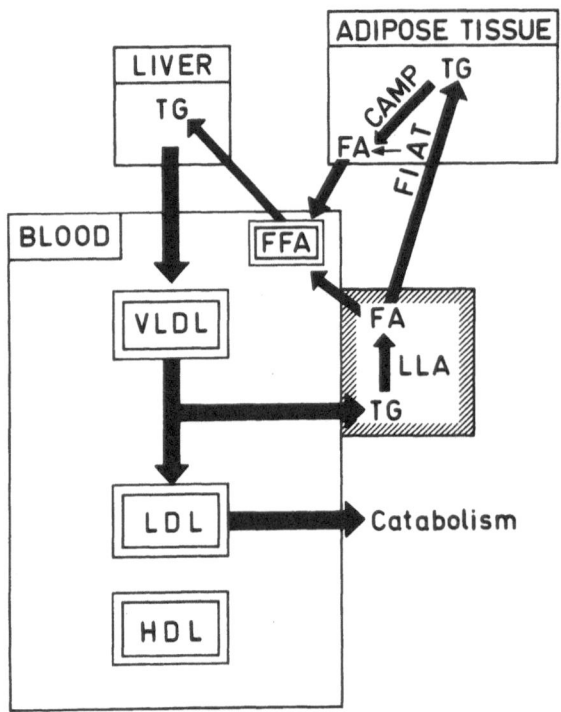

Figure 9. Schematic picture of the role of adipose tissue for the removal as well as for the secretion of VLDL (major metabolic pathways of serum lipoproteins)

Summary

1. The importance of evaluating effects of serum lipid lowering regimes not only on total serum cholesterol and triglycerides but also on the three major LP classes is stressed. Examples are given showing a) that even when total serum cholesterol is reduced some LP classes may have increased b) in spite of the fact that total cholesterol or total triglycerides may be unchanged one LP class may have increased and another decreased resulting in unchanged total levels.

2. A strong continuous, reciprocal relation between the concentrations of VLDL and LDL was found in a group of subjects representing a total population of HLP. The usefulness of classifying HLP by appliying cut-off points for "normal" LP levels was discussed against this continuous relation.

3. The effects of diet and clofibrate on LP levels in type II A, II B and IV and of diet or nicotinic acid in type V was described.

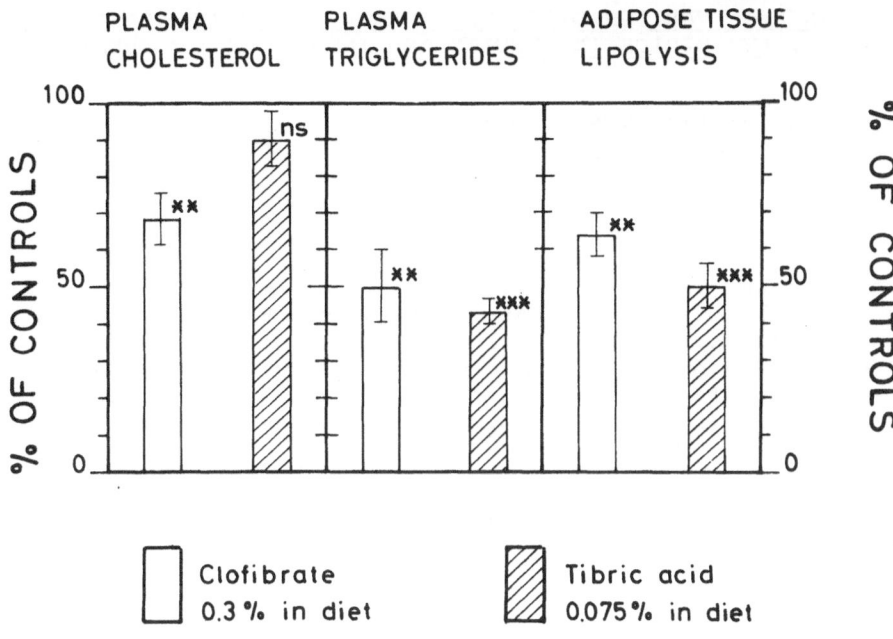

Figure 10. The effect of addition of clofibrate and tibric acid in the diet for
weeks to adult male rats on fasting serum lipids and on the lipolysis of adipose
tissue incubated in vitro

4. A linear relation was demonstrated between the changes in LDL-cholesterol
   induced by treatment and the pre-treatment LDL level. This relation predicts
   that when LDL is below 140 mg/100 ml there will be an *increase*, and when LDL
   is above this figure there will be a decrease in LDL cholesterol in response
   to diet, clofibrate and nicotinic acid.

5. Acute perturbations of LP levels by infusion of Intralipid®, by diet and by
   clofibrate suggested that the concentration of VLDL may influence the concentration of LDL and not the opposite.

6. The role of adipose tissue as a target organ for some lipid lowering regimes
   was discussed. Clofibrate was demonstrated to lower fat mobilizing lipolysis
   from adipose tissue in rats in vivo and reduces serum free glycerol in man.

INFLUENCE OF VARIOUS DIETS ON DIURNAL LEVELS OF PLASMA GLUCOSE, INSULIN, AND LIPIDS IN OBESITY AND INSULIN-INDEPENDENT DIABETICS

A.J. Houtsmuller, M.M.A. van den Broek-Boot, and
G.A.M. Peters

Until recently plasma cholesterol has been considered as one of the main causes of atherosclerosis. However, since improved methods became available for determination of other plasma lipids like triglycerides (TG) and free fatty acids (FFA) a connection between atherosclerosis and abnormal TG patterns was also observed. As atherosclerosis and myocardial infarction occur more frequently in diabetes a correlation with insulin secretion, hyperglycemia, and abnormal TG metabolism was to be expected. The purpose of this study was the investigation of the diurnal patterns of the parameters mentioned above during different feeding conditions in diabetics and nondiabetics.

Materials and Methods

Three groups of patients were studied, obese diabetics, lean diabetics (Malherbe et al., 1971), and insulin-independent obese controls (Mahler, 1971). All the patients were hospitalized and their body weight was maintained (± 0.5 kg). Each of them was submitted to three different isocaloric feeding periods of nine days each.

The composition of the diets was:

1. 50% saturated fat (butter), 30% starch
2. 50% unsaturated fat (2/3 linoleic acid), 30% starch
3. 50% starch, 30% mixed fats, proteins 20%

The diet sequence was chosen randomly. Blood was collected every tenth day and insulin, glucose, TG, and FFA were determined every two to four hours.

The patients received their diet in six equal portions, according to Schlierf et al. (1971).

Insulin was determined by a double antibody technique, glucose enzymatically, TG after Laurell, and FFA after Novak.

For statistical analysis Student's paired t-test was used (after analysis of variance). Statistical significance means $P < 0.05$.

Results

For each group of patients a plot was made for insulin, glucose, FFA, TG, and the 24 hours areas were determined.
These plots are summarized in Fig. 1 a-d, for each parameter per group.

Insulin. The highest plasma insulin areas were found in the obese diabetic group followed by the obese group, being lowest in the lean diabetic group.

Glucose. The plasma glucose areas were also highest in the obese diabetics, followed by the lean, being normal in the obese group.

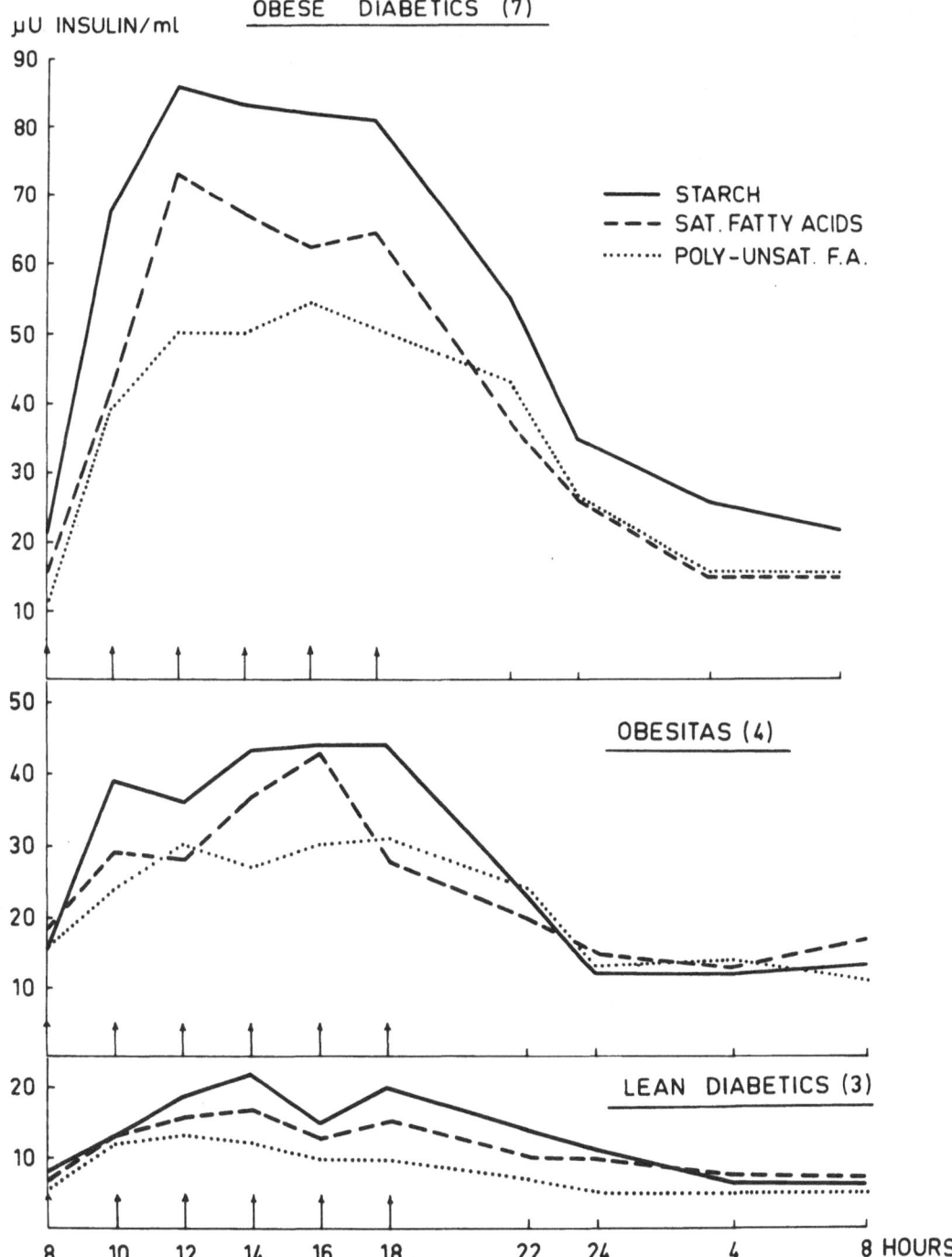

Figure 1. a) 24-hour-insulin area of obese diabetics, lean diabetics, and obese controls observed in 3 different isocaloric diet periods. For details see text

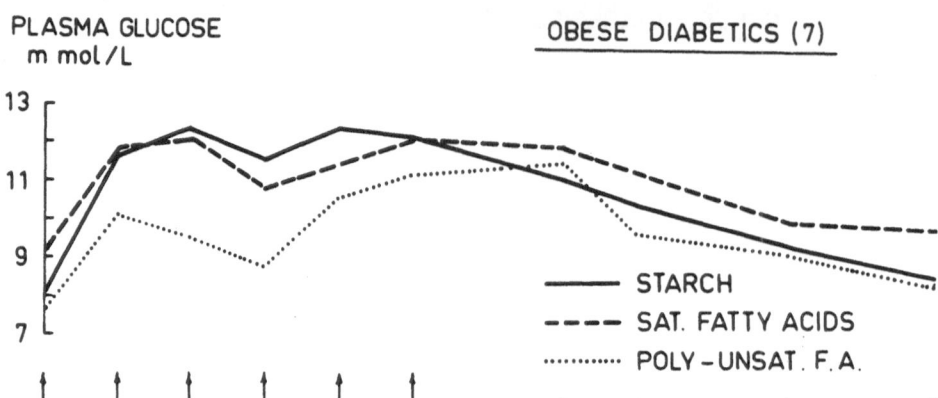

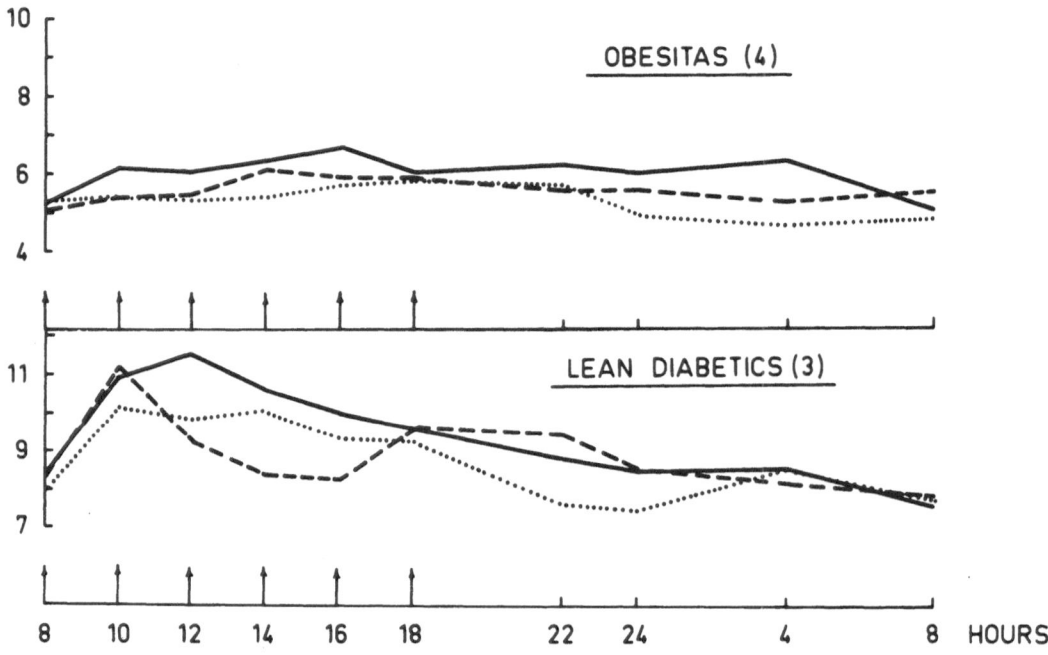

Figure 1. b) 24-hour-glucose area of obese diabetics, lean diabetics, and obese controls observed in 3 different isocaloric diet periods. For details see text

Triglycerides and FFA. TG were not determined in the lean group. As for the other groups, the plasma TG were much higher in the obese diabetic group. FFA fasting levels were higher in the obese group than in obese diabetics, being lowest in the lean diabetic group.
There was a different shape for the FFA plot in each group of patients. A sharp decrease in FFA level was observed in the first two to four hours, the decrease being largest in the obese group. After the last meal, FFA levels remained stable in both diabetic groups, however, in the obese group, a steady increase was observed during the night.

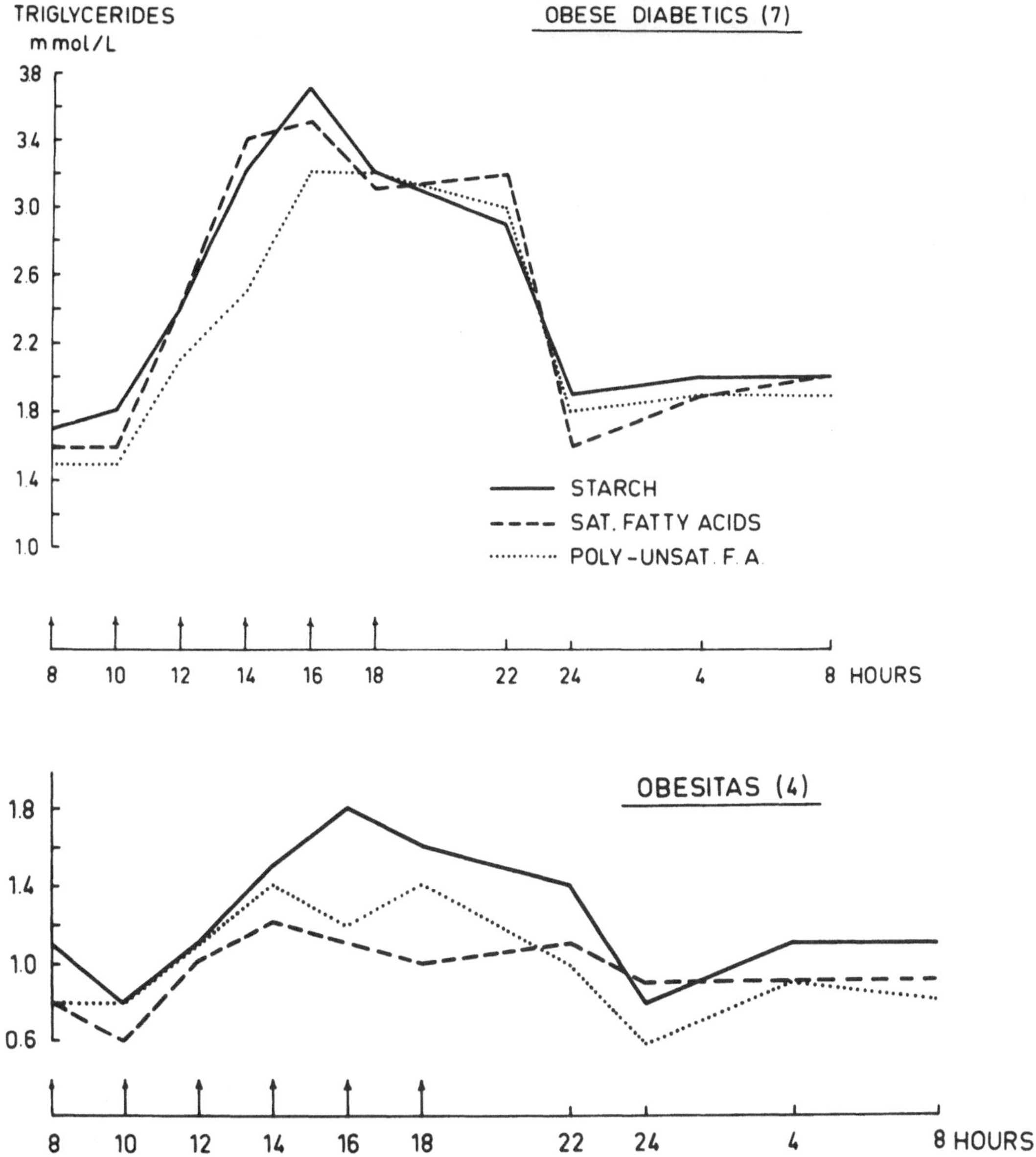

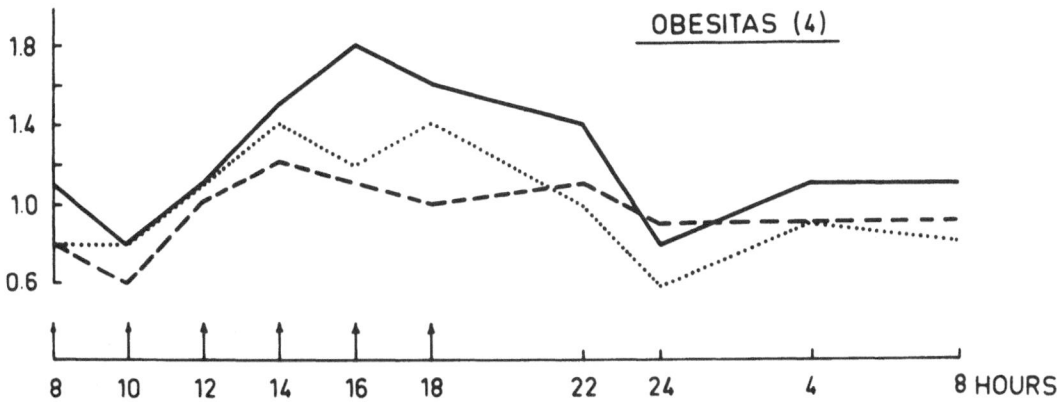

Figure 1. c) 24-hour-triglycerides area of obese diabetics and obese controls observed in 3 different isocaloric diet periods. For details see text

Influence of Diet

Insulin. In the diabetic groups, the 24-hour-insulin secretions (expressed as area) were higher in the starch diet compared with the linoleic acid diet ($P < 0.02$). The same differences are suggested in the obese group.

Glucose. The same observations were made for the glucose areas, being highest in the starch diet compared to the linoleic acid diet.

Triglycerides. A difference in the obese group was found only for the starch period, where TG were highest.
The FFA areas were all lowest in the starch period.

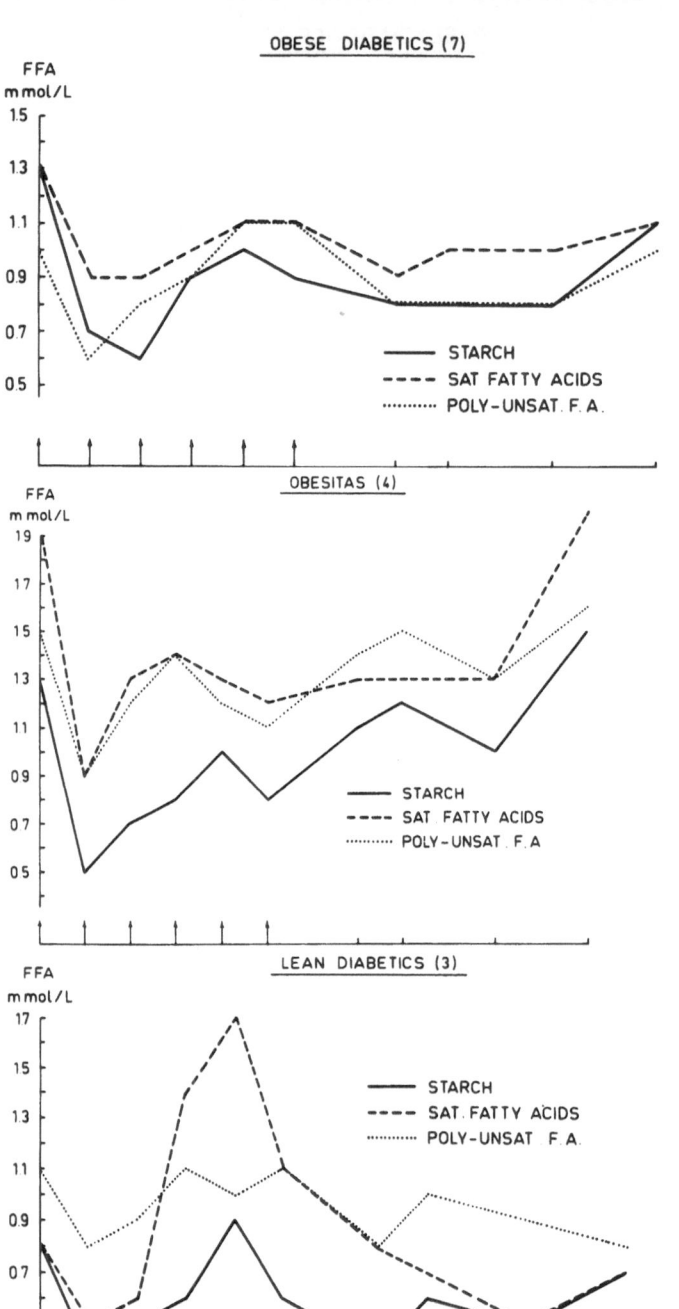

Figure 1. d) 24-hour-free fatty acids area of obese diabetics, lean diabetics, and obese controls observed in 3 different isocaloric diet periods. For details see text

Discussion

It is generally accepted that obese diabetics have lower insulin levels than comparable obese patients with regard to a 100 g glucose load.

This stimulant, however, is unphysiologic. We determined the 24-hour-insulin levels of obese and lean diabetics and obese patients, under the same circumstances. By comparing these data, we found much higher insulin levels in obese diabetic patients than in obesity. Observing glucose areas, this is to be expected because of the high glucose areas in obese diabetics.

However, for the same reason we expected the lean diabetics to have higher glucose areas than the obese diabetics on account of their low insulin levels. We found the opposite.

The most important data we consider to be the insulin secretion in different feeding periods. The lower insulin secretion in the linoleic acid period seems very promising in regard to the atherogenic action of insulin, found by Duff et al. (1954), Cruz et al. (1961), and Stout (1970) in animal experiments and the high insulin levels found in myocardial infarction (Malherbe et al., 1971).

Another remarkable effect was seen in the FFA data and plots. In obese and lean diabetics, a steady state is reached after the last meal, however, in the obese group, lipolysis is suggested during the night. The lower insulin levels in the obese group may play an important role in these phenomena.

In the obese diabetics, on the contrary, there might be a net TG uptake during the night, due to the still high insulin levels. TG decrease rapidly, while FFA remain at the same level. When we consider the findings of Mahler (1971) who discovered an insulin-sensitive triglyceride-splitting lipase in the aortic wall, regulating the accumulation of intracellular lipids, and recently confirmed by Gilbert and Galton (1973), the much lower insulin secretion in the linoleic acid period may explain the favourable results of the diet in atherosclerosis.

Summary

Controlled dietary studies were done on diabetic patients (obese and lean) and obesity, with diets of linoleic acid, starch, and saturated fatty acids. In starch diets, higher insulin secretions were observed compared to linoleic acid diets. This may explain the favourable results of linoleic acid diets in atherosclerosis, especially in diabetes.

POLYUNSATURATED RUMINANT FATS AND CHOLESTEROL METABOLISM IN MAN

Paul Nestel, Nathalie Havenstein, Trevor Scott, and Len Cook

We have previously described a lowering of the plasma cholesterol concentration in 5 or 6 subjects eating polyunsaturated ruminant fats (PRF) for 3 or 4 weeks (Nestel et al., 1973). Beef and dairy fats had been enriched with linoleic acid by feeding cattle supplemental crushed safflower seeds in which the oil droplets had been coated with formalin-treated casein. This prevents microbial hydrogenation of linoleic acid in the rumen; the fed linoleate is therefore absorbed unchanged, leading to linoleate levels of 20-30% in milk and meat fats. A diet in which all the fats were derived from these sources gave P/S ratios of 0.6 compared to 0.06 in an identical diet based on conventional ruminant fats (control diet). Since the 2 diets had similar amounts of cholesterol and contained fats of exclusively animal origin they were ideal for comparing the effects of polyunsaturated fatty acids on plasma lipid concentrations and on cholesterol metabolism. The first study had shown enhanced excretion of endogenous sterols during the third week of the PRF diet.

The second study was carried out in 8 healthy male students aged 15 - 24 yrs living on the metabolic ward. They ate the PRF diet for 6 weeks followed by the control diet for 6 weeks. Chromium oxide, 400 mg daily, served as marker of faecal flow. Plasma was collected 3 times weekly and faeces for the last 10 days of each period. During the last week of each diet, cholesterol absorption was measured once, by the oral administration of ^{14}C-β-sitosterol and ^3H-cholesterol.

The excretion of acidic and neutral steroids was quantified by gas chromatography and adjusted to a daily rate from the excretion of chromium oxide. Sterol degradation, assessed from the recovery of labeled betasitosterol, was minimal. The net sterol balance which, in the steady state, approximates cholesterol synthesis was calculated by subtracting the cholesterol intake from total sterol excretion. Cholesterol synthesis plus cholesterol absorption (derived from the relative recoveries of labeled sitosterol and cholesterol) equalled cholesterol turnover.

The plasma cholesterol levels fell when the PRF diet replaced the subjects' habitual diet (Fig. 1). During the last 10 days, the mean values were constant, (as were the body weights throughout), indicating a new steady state. When the control diet was introduced, the plasma cholesterol concentration rose at once. The PRF and control diets contained similar amounts of cholesterol and plant sterols, but differed in their P/S ratios: 0.70 versus 0.06. Thus the increment in the plasma cholesterol, which occurred to a significant degree in 6 of 8 subjects, could be attributed to the fall in P/S ratio. Changing to the control diet led to a significant mean increase of 9% in the group (p<0.001) (Table 1). The plasma triglyceride concentration also rose significantly by 15% when the PRF diet was replaced by the control diet (p<0.001). The change in the cholesterol level was close to the predicted difference estimated from the P/S ratios of the two diets (especially when only palmitate, myristate and linoleate were considered).

Despite the changes in plasma lipids, there were no overall differences in cholesterol metabolism (Fig. 2). Cholesterol absorption with the PRF and control diets were: (mean $\pm$ SD) 52 $\pm$ 4.0% and 54 $\pm$ 7.6% respectively (intakes 400 and 420 mg/day). Cholesterol synthesis for the PRF and control diets was 381 $\pm$ 160 and 366 $\pm$ 151 mg/day, giving values for cholesterol turnover of 584 $\pm$ 157 and 593 $\pm$ 154 mg/day respectively (for subjects weighing 67 kg on average). Bile acid excretion was 193 $\pm$ 85 and 208 $\pm$ 83 mg/day for PRF and control diets. None

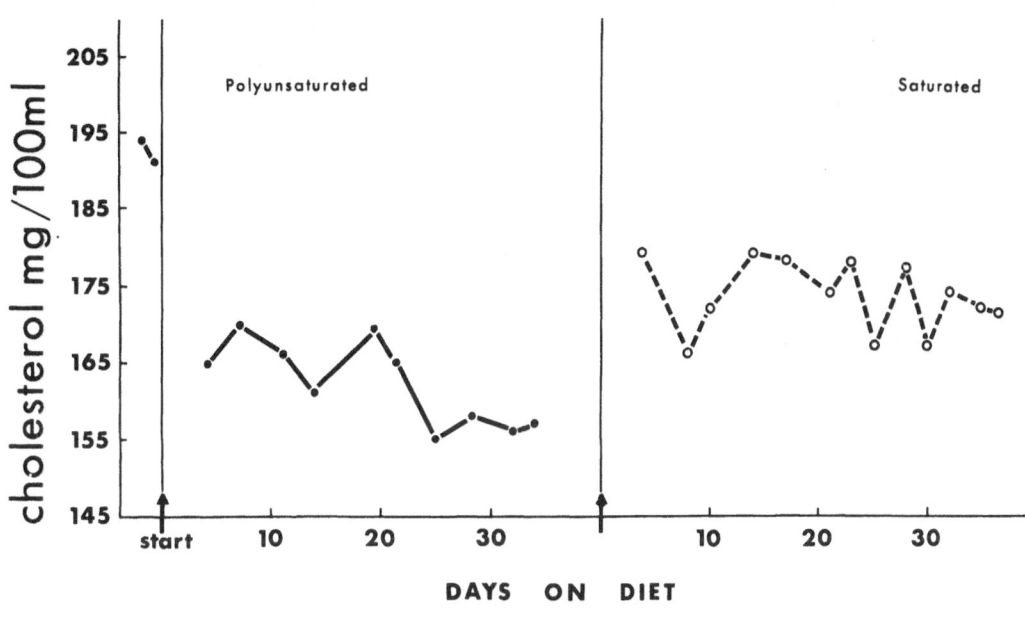

PLASMA CHOLESTEROL (mean 8 students)

Figure 1. Plasma cholesterol levels on the polyunsaturated ruminant and conventional ruminant diets

Table 1. Change in plasma lipids following substitution of saturated for polyunsaturated ruminant fats (PRF)

	Cholesterol		Triglyceride	
	mg/100 ml			
	PRF	Δ	PRF	Δ
	176	+14	116	+18
	182	+13	165	+35
	156	+ 6	70	+14
	172	+20	86	− 1
	187	+ 9	129	+29
	152	+24	114	+23
	108	+15	79	+15
	153	+ 3	92	+11
Mean (n=8)	160	+14 (9%)	106	+18 (17%)

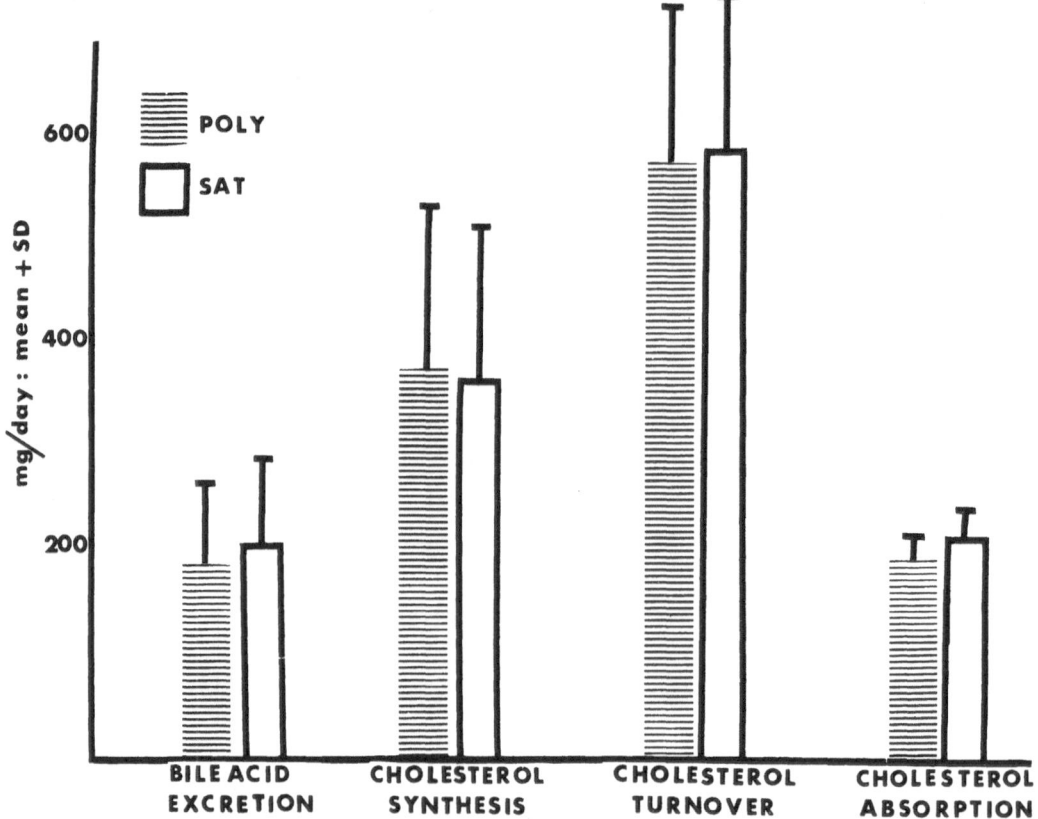

Figure 2. Cholesterol metabolism during the sixth week of each diet

of these differences, during the sixth week of each diet, were significant. This contrasts with the greater sterol excretion that we had observed previously during the third week of the PRF diet when the plasma cholesterol was still falling. It suggests a brief mobilization of cholesterol from the body which coincides with the reduction in the pool of plasma cholesterol. When this pool reaches a new equilibrium, total cholesterol turnover returns to its former rate.

XVIII

Drug Therapy of
Hyperlipoproteinemia

WORKSHOP: Absorbable Drugs

Chairmen: N. Zöllner, West Germany
          R. Paoletti, Italy

Participants: J. Davignon, Canada
             P. F. Spano, Italy
             N. Blaton, Belgium
             G. Crepaldi, Italy
             T. Shimamoto, Japan

Introduction (Prof. Zöllner)

Very few people have real good and real hard evidence with respect to long range clinical results. Experimental atherosclerosis is not part of what we have to discuss here. We hope to present facts and figures and that of course means that instead of discussing management of atherosclerosis we will have to discuss management of risk factors or of the expressions of risk factors.

We want to present a survey of the drugs available and how to evaluate them. Where we lack sufficient clinical experience in preventive trials with drugs we will discuss quantitatively assessible figures, but we want to stress long range effects because this is what really counts in management. If possible we want to indicate experiences in preventive or clinical medicine. In the patient, provided he is not taken out of his usual environment, fasting cholesterol values change little over short periods of time. During a recent study to be published we found the changes within a week to average 10.2 mg per 100 ml. The lower values were found during the second half of the week, possibly reflecting dietary habits during weekends and working days respectively (in two groups this difference was significant at the 99% and the 99.9% level!). However, there are individuals who exhibit serum cholesterol values remaining within the reproducability of the method which in our laboratory is $\pm$ 7.0 mg per 100 ml. Assuming that the possible changes of serum cholesterol during a week show a normal distribution, their standard deviation around the average of the week becomes 11.3 mg per 100 ml. From these data it may be concluded that under the conditions of a study in which before and during therapy blood samples are obtained at two different days of a week and analyzed in quadruplicate, changes must be 40 mg per 100 ml or more in order to be significant in an individual.

Smaller differences may become significant if groups of patients are tested. As an example, early work of *Knüchel* (1959) may be quoted, showing that in a selected group of patients a decrease of serum cholesterol from 262 $\pm$ 5.5 mg per 100 ml to 229 $\pm$ 6.2 mg per 100 ml may be significant at the two per cent level if the number of subjects is sufficient (n=30 in the study quoted).

The question must be asked if a small decrease of serum cholesterol, even if made statistically significant by a large number of trials, serves its therapeutic purpose. In xanthomatous diseases this is certainly not so. If normalization cannot be obtained, the decrease of serum cholesterol should amount to more than 100 mg per 100 ml in order to be called a therapeutic success of some sorts. This qualification however is more often met within groups of patients showing high initial values (Zöllner and Gudenzi, 1966). For this and similar reasons others prefer to express the therapeutic effect in per cent of the pretherapy levels. Similar objections are possible, since e.g. a 50 per cent decrease from 340 mg per 100 ml has another significance than from 900 mg per 100 ml. One might conclude that cholesterol levels before and during therapy should be recorded.

A number of other environmental factors is not as easily controlled as the dietary prescriptions. In order to exclude these it may become necessary to interrupt therapy by a placebo period. During the evaluation of a new drug such periods are certainly necessary.

REGRESSION OF XANTHOMAS AS A MEASURE OF THE EFFECTIVENESS OF TREATMENT IN PRIMARY HYPERLIPOPROTEINEMIAS

J. Davignon

Changes in size of skin xanthomas may serve as an index of the effectiveness of treatment in primary hyperlipoproteinemias. Some of these lesions may regress quite rapidly if the proper lipid-lowering regimen is applied; this is the case of the eruptive xanthomas found in types I and V as well as of most of the lesions found in type III hyperlipoproteinemia. Indeed in type III the pigmentation of the palmar creases, the pathognomonic discrete planar xanthomas distributed along the palmar creases, the punctate xanthomas at the fingertips or along the cubital edge of the palm as well as the tubero-eruptive xanthomas of the elbows may fluctuate spontaneously and are very sensitive to weight loss and other lipid lowering measures. In our experience these lesions may clear up completely in 6 to 12 months of treatment (Davignon, 1972). Xanthelasmas whether they are found in type III, IV, V or II are noted to regress more slowly. It has been reported that they may regress on a cholesterol lowering regimen in the absence of a significant change in plasma cholsterol which may start to go down as the xanthelasmas are disappearing (Palmer and Blacket, 1972). Tendon xanthomas are even more resistant to treatment and their regression is more difficult to assess. We have developed a standardized technique to measure the antero-posterior thickness of the Achilles tendon at the site where xanthomatous deposits are found, using a soft-tissue X-ray technique (Gattereau et al., 1973). This technique should prove useful to follow minute changes in tendon xanthomas. It is in patients homozygous for type II hyperbetalipoproteinemia however that the xanthomas are likely to regress the most slowly if at all with treatment. This has been true in 4 of the 5 homozygous patients we have been following over several years. Our experience with a 6 year old homozygous type II patient with angina pectoris would seem to indicate that a more rapid regression may be observed if strong cholesterol lowering measures are applied early in life. In this case an ileal bypass was performed at the age of 8 (probably one of the earliest ever carried out) and a marked regression was observed from the 2nd to the 8th month after surgery (Fig. 1). It is hoped that the changes observed at the level of xanthomas are also occurring in the arterial wall; improvement in the frequency and severity of anginal pain in this patient might be an indication that it does. Although scarce, there is some objective evidence in the literature that regression of atheromatous lesions may occur on a lipid lowering regimen both in type III (Zelis et at., 1970) and in type II (Ost and Stenson 1967; De Palma et al., 1970) hyperlipoproteinemia, so far however such findings have been reported only for peripheral arteries.

CLOFIBRATE AND DH-581 IN THE LONG TERM TREATMENT OF PRIMARY HYPERLIPOPROTEINEMIA

In the long term treatment of *primary* type II hyperlipoproteinemia one is confronted with the fact that diet has only a very limited effect on plasma cholesterol and that drugs have to be added to achieve any significant lowering of plasma lipids. Because of individual variations in response to drugs, it is often

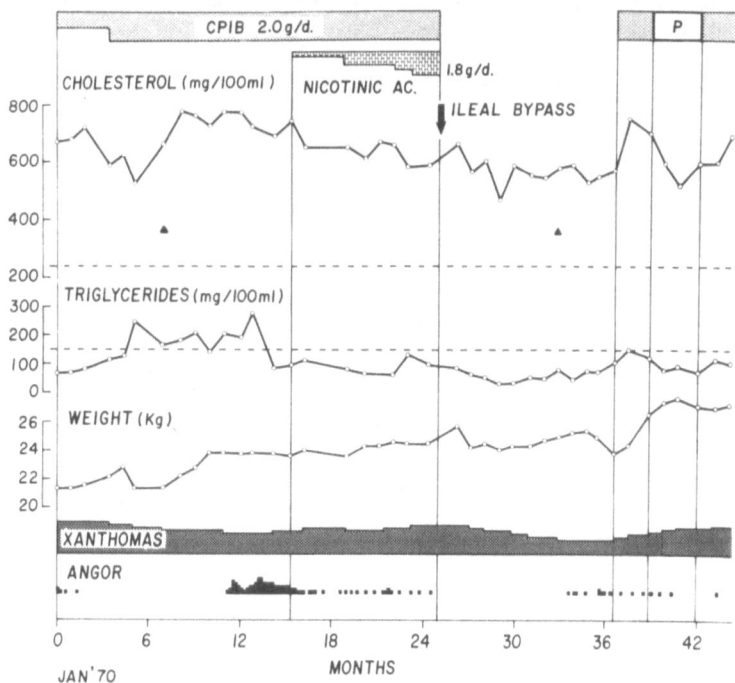

L.L. ♂ 6 YRS #1612 – TYPE II HOMOZYGOUS

Figure 1. This is the case of a 6 year old child with homozygous type II familial hyperbetalipoproteinemia, angina pectoris and intermittent claudication. A slight but temporary reduction of tuberous xanthomas was noticed during clofibrate (CPIB) and combined clofibrate and nicotinic acid therapy. Although plasma cholesterol was not markedly reduced after ileal bypass surgery a marked reduction of skin xanthomas was noticed as well as an improvement of the angina. After surgery addition of clofibrate caused a paradoxical increase in both plasma cholesterol and triglycerides on 2 occasions as well as an increase in size of the xanthomas. Note at the beginning of the study the escape to the cholesterol-lowering effect of clofibrate concomitant with a rise in triglycerides

necessary to proceed by trial and error until the most useful drug or combination of drugs is found for a given patient. Clofibrate (chlorophenoxyisobutyrate, CPIB) has not generally been proven very effective in primary type II hyperlipoproteinemia, however in our experience patients with a plasma triglyceride/cholesterol (TG/TC) ratio lower than 0.4 were more likely to be responsive to the cholesterol lowering effect of this drug than patients with a ratio equal to or above this value, whether they had tendon xanthomas or not (Davignon et al., 1971). Thus for instance a type IIa patient with a plasma cholesterol of 400 mg/ 100 ml and triglycerides of 60 mg/100 ml (TG/TC=0.15) is more likely to be responsive to the cholesterol-lowering effect of clofibrate and his plasma cholesterol may show a fall of up to 32%. This does not apply however, to the triglyceride-lowering effect of clofibrate which remains relatively good in type IIb. In this study, carried out over 3 years on 37 patients, great care was taken to eliminate type IV hyperlipoproteinemia by excluding patients with a TG/TC ratio greater than 0.8. Since then we have been using this ratio of 0.4 as a cut-off point to separate type IIa from type IIb patients. This relationship between cholesterol-lowering effect and TG/TC ratio was not observed in our 3 year study of DH-581 (probucol, Dow Chemical Co.) in 15 patients with primary type II hyperlipoproteinemia aged 27 to 51 years (mean: 39.8 ± 9.5, 8 females). The mean fall in plasma cholesterol was respectively 14.8% in 9 type IIa patients and 15.6% in type IIb patients. The individual falls in plasma cholesterol ranged from 3.7 to

Table 1. The effect of clofibrate on plasma cholesterol and triglycerides is compared with that of DH-581 in the same 10 patients with type II primary hyperlipoproteinemia. The cholesterol lowering effect of DH-581 is slightly greater than that of clofibrate. In contrast DH-581 does not share the triglyceride-lowering properties of clofibrate

	Clofibrate (2g/d)	DH-581 (1g/d)
Weeks on placebo	20.3 (9-44)[a]	14.1 (8-23)
Number of control samples	5.5 (3-9)	4.5 (3-7)
Weeks on drug	35.2 (16-16)	29.1 (21-38)
Number of samples on drug	7.4 (4-16)	8.3 (7-9)
Cholesterol: mean before and after	339→299	336→278
changes in mg/100 ml	-40 (-111+3)	-58 (-17-81)
changes in percentage	-11.8%	-17.3%
Number of patients with a p<0.005 fall	5	8
Triglycerides: mean before and after	132→95	112→121
changes in mg/100 ml	-37 (-87+4)	+ 9 (-29+115)
changes in percentage	-28.0%	+ 8.0%
Number of patients with a p<0.005 fall	3	0

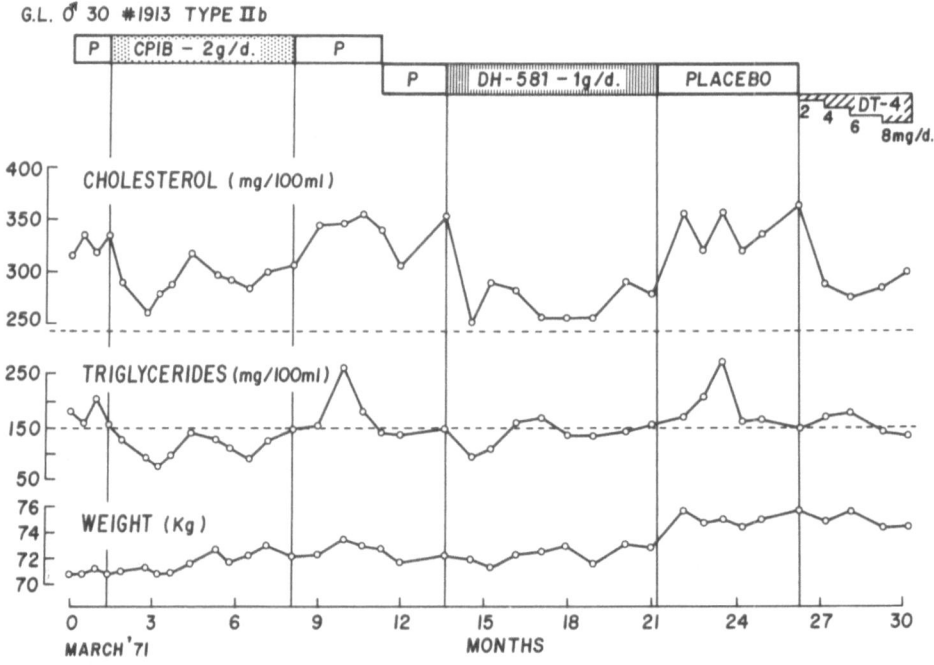

Figure 2. The lipid lowering effects of clofibrate (CPIB), DH-581 and dextrothyroxin (DT-4) are compared in a 30 year old type IIb patient. Note the more pronounced and sustained effect of DH-581 on plasma cholesterol, and the progressive development of resistance to the cholesterol-lowering effect of the other two drugs

25.5%. There was no significant effect on plasma triglycerides. In 10 of these patients we had the opportunity to compare the effect of DH-581 to that of clofibrate using the same single blind design. There were 6 type IIa patients and 4 type IIb. In this series the mean cholesterol fall was 11.5% on clofibrate and 17.5% on DH-581; for plasma triglycerides the changes were respectively -24.1 and +3.3% (Table 1). In one patient where clofibrate, DH-581 and dextro-thyroxin were sequentially assessed the fall in plasma cholesterol was respec-tively 12.6%, 20.0% and 10.4%, an escape being noted with both clofibrate and dextrothyroxin (Fig. 2). Thus DH-581 might prove to be as effective if not more effective than clofibrate in reducing plasma cholesterol in type II. Here again however the individual variation in response was important and it remains that in a given subject clofibrate might be at times more effective than DH-581.

DISPLACEMENT OF ALBUMIN BOUND TRYPTOPHAN BY CLOFIBRATE IN MAN

P.F. Spano, C.R. Sirtori, and R. Paoletti

Clofibrate (p-chlorophenoxyisobutyrate, CPIB) is highly bound to plasma proteins, has a relatively long half-life, 10-14 hours, in man (Thorp, 1963), and displaces oral anticoagulants from albumin binding sites (Solomon et al., 1967). We wanted to test whether CPIB could displace tryptophan from its plasma binding sites, thus increasing the availability of free tryptophan.

Tryptophan is the only circulating amino acid highly bound to serum proteins (McMenamy and Oncley, 1958); the tryptophan pool in brain is controlled by the free fraction of serum tryptophan (Gessa et al., 1972). There is ample evidence that the rate of synthesis of 5-hydroxytryptamine (5-HT) in brain is regulated principally by brain tryptophan, since the availability of this amino acid in the nervous tissues is considerably below the K_m of the first enzyme in 5-HT bio-synthesis, tryptophan hydroxylase (Eccleston et al., 1965). Treatments which cause increased synthesis of brain 5-HT all lead to significant increases in the concentration of brain tryptophan (Tagliamonte et al., 1971).

With previous experiments we have showed that in rats CPIB (200 mg.kg b.i.d. orally for 3 days) decreases total plasma tryptophan by about 70%, while increas-ing the free fraction by 50%; brain tryptophan and 5-hydroxyindole-acetic acid (5-HIAA) levels were also increased by 50% (Spano et al., unpublished). We report here the effects on plasma tryptophan levels of the clinically used dosage of CPIB on eight human volunteers, five of whom were hospitalised, and three leading a normal life.

Materials and Methods

Nine subjects volunteered for the study. Six were patients in hospital for non-acute medical reasons, and three were members of our research group. Five of the hospitalised patients had type IV and one a type V hyperlipoproteinemia (Fred-rickson et al., 1967), and one of the three out-patient volunteers had a type IV pattern.

The study lasted two weeks. During both weeks three blood samples were taken in the mornings of Monday, Wednesday and Friday under fasting conditions, and three samples at about 11.00 p.m. on the evenings of Sunday preceding the study and on Wednesday and Friday, in all patients. Seven subjects received CPIB during the first week, in two daily doses of 1 g, one in the morning and one before supper, beginning Monday morning and ending Friday afternoon; the following week they received identical placebos, according to the same schedule. One subject followed the opposite scheme, i.e., he received placebo the first week.

Blood was drawn in Vacutainer tubes containing EDTA (EDTA is known not to change total or bound tryptophan concentrations in plasma (McMenamy et al., 1961)), and free and bound tryptophan were determined in all samples, whereas cholesterol (Block et al., 1965), and triglycerides (McLellan, 1971) were assayed on the samples drawn on Monday and Friday mornings of both weeks.

Total tryptophan was determined on a plasma aliquot by a slight modification (Spano et al., unpublished) of the method of Denckla and Dewey (Denckla and Dewey, 1967). Free tryptophan was separated by centrifuging with a gas mixture (95% N_2 + 5% O_2) at 2,000 rpm for 204 at room temperature. The statistical significance of the differences was tested by two tailed t-test (Snedecor, 1956).

Results

Total tryptophan was merkedly decreased (between 50% and 70%) in all subjects during CPIB treatment and returned to normal at the beginning of the following week; the opposite pattern was followed by the only volunteer who received CPIB first (Fig. 1).

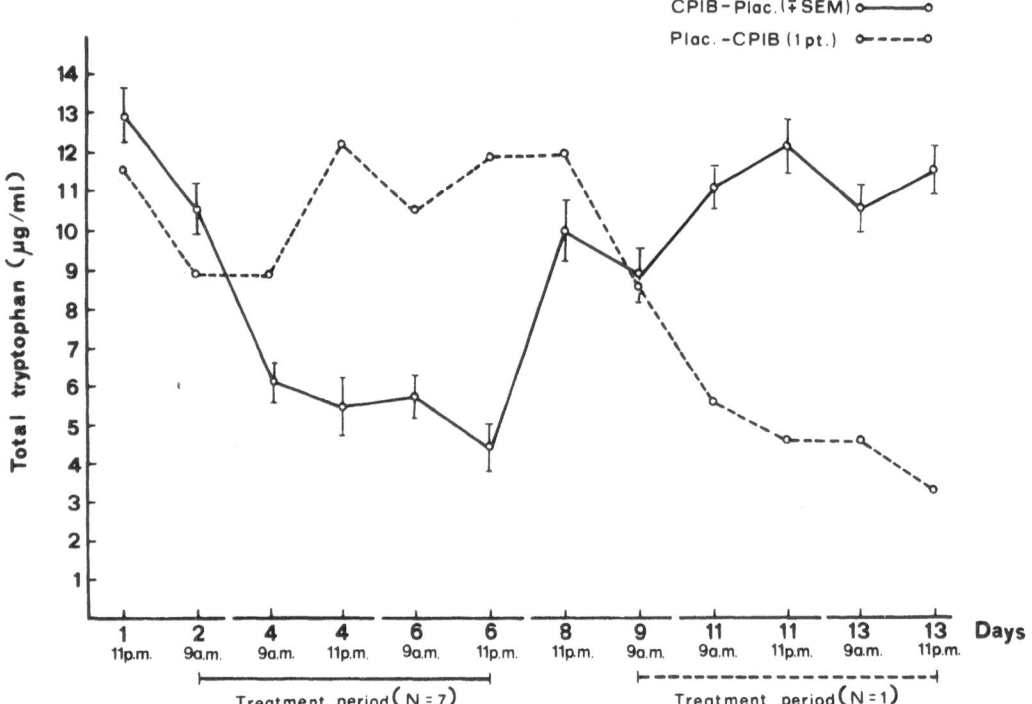

Figure 1. Total tryptophan levels during clofibrate and placebo treatments (o———o and o------o)

The percentage of free tryptophan was more than doubled in the samples taken in the mornings, and almost tripled in those taken in the evenings, during CPİB administration. These values returned to normal the week after the end of drug treatment (Fig. 2). Evening samples had always a higher level of free tryptophan, probably indicating that free tryptophan is regulated by a circadian rhythm (Fernström et al., 1971) also in humans, and that this is not altered by CPIB.

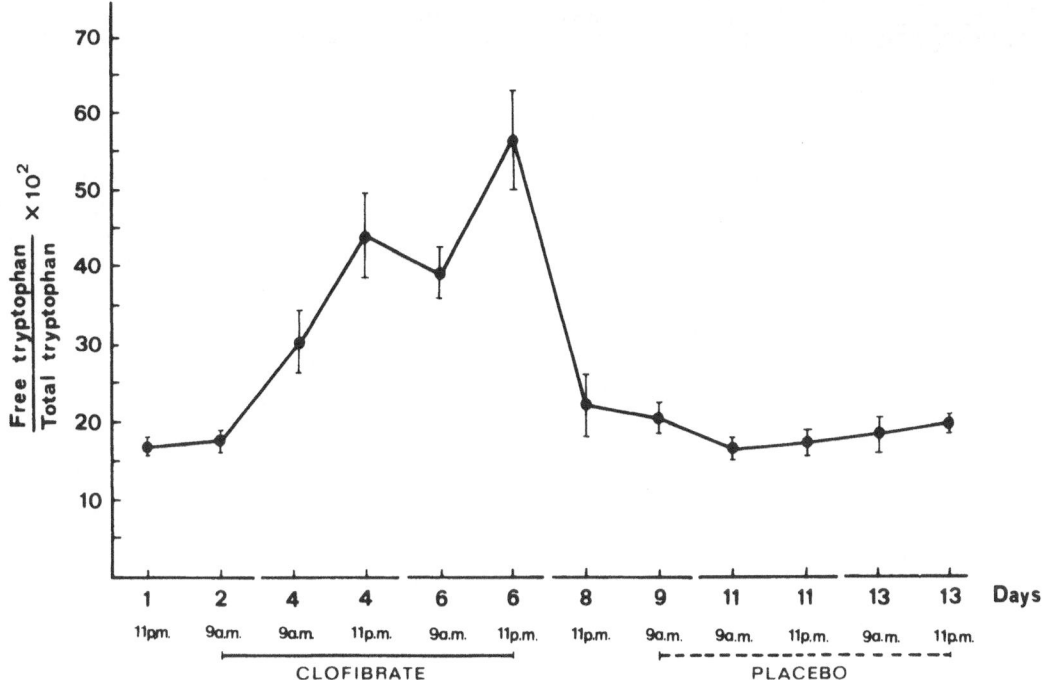

Figure 2. Percentage of free over total tryptophan during clofibrate and placebo treatments (all subjects pooled, x ——— x)

Plasma triglyceride levels were rapidly decreased by CPIB treatment, especially in the type V subjects. Cholesterol was only slightly decreased.

Discussion

Our data support the hypothesis that CPIB can decrease total plasma tryptophan in humans. This confirms our animal data and suggests also that in humans this treatment can stimulate brain 5-HT synthesis.

Free tryptophan levels were concomitantly significantly increased. Samples taken in the evenings had consistently higher concentrations of free tryptophan, indicating that CPIB does not alter the circadian rhythm of the free amino acid.

A lower concentration of tryptophan in the CSF and a lower free pool of serum tryptophan have recently been described in depressive patients (Aylward and Maddock, 1973; Coppen et al., 1972; 1973). Recent data has also shown that sodium salicylate can displace tryptophan from its plasma binding sites (Smith and Lakatos, 1971), as well as stimulate serotonin synthesis in rat brain (Tagliamonte, 1972). There is clinical evidence that salicylate, as well as other similar anti-rheumatic drugs, exert anti-depressive properties when evaluated with a psychiatric rating scale (Aylward and Maddock, 1973). Our data therefore, point out the possibility that CPIB may exert anti-depressant properties when administered alone or in combination with tryptophan, which is itself an anti-depressant.

Acknowledgements. The assistance and technical help of Drs. E. Agradi and E. Pappalettera, and Messrs. C.L. Galli, A. Ricci and L. Fassina are gratefully acknowledged.

MODES OF ACTION OF POLYUNSATURATED PHOSPHATIDYL CHOLINE AND RELATED COMPOUNDS ON LIPID METABOLISM AND ARTERIAL WALL

V. Blaton

Reduction of elevated plasma cholesterol, of oleic acid and of cholesterol oleate in the beta lipoproteins might logically be expected to prevent the development of atheromatous lesions or their progression. Essential phospholipids (poly unsaturated phosphatidyl choline, PU-PC) rich in linoleic and linolenic acid are known to have a blood lipid lowering effect and they reduce the accumulation of cholesterol esters in the intima.

There are different modes of action of phospholipid molecules on the arterial wall and on the plasma hyperlipoproteinaemia. According to Adams and Abdulla (1972) the phospholipid molecule plays an important role in the esterification of free cholesterol by the LCAT enzyme both in the arterial wall and in the plasma lipoproteins. He suggested that the donation of polyunsaturated fatty acids from phospholipids to cholesterol to form polyunsaturated cholesterol esters is more important in preventing atherosclerosis than the surface active dispersing properties. This hypothesis is supported by the data obtained from perfusing techniques according to Bowyer et al. (1967). Comparative studies on human subjects and on animals showed that the rate of hydrolysis is much higher for polyunsaturated than for saturated cholesterol esters.

In experimental atherosclerosis in rabbits Howard and Patelski (1972) observed a change of the aortic enzymes of hypercholesterolaemic rabbits treated with PU-PC. The activity of cholesterase was eight fold increased during the intravenous PU-PC therapy, while lipase and phospholipase were rather unaffected. The increase of cholesterase should lead to less arterial lipid deposition. The study of the intravenous treatment of patients with PU-PC was aimed to follow the influence on the plasma lipids, to control the preferential influence on the biochemical types of hyperlipoproteinaemia, and to compare the changes in individual lipoprotein classes after the intravenous injection of phosphatidylcholine.

Treatment of human hyperlipoproteinaemia with PU-PC lowers significantly plasma lipids, but acts selectively on the high cholesterol value. In type II and in type IV there was a signficant decrease of total cholesterol, but phospholipids decreased only significantly in type II. Triglycerides were not affected, (Blaton et al., (1972) and Peeters et al., (1973). Based on the integrated procedure for lipid and lipoprotein analysis (Blaton and Peeters, 1971) it could be demonstrated that alpha lipoproteins aswell as beta lipoproteins were decreased in concentration. Beta lipoproteins were more affected than alpha lipoproteins and were changed in their percentual lipid composition. Under influence of PU-PC plasma lipids were changed in their fatty acid composition. There was a decrease of the 18:1 / 18:2 ratio, especially in the cholesterolesters, which favours the metabolism of plasma cholesterol.

In view of the uncertainties of the effect of PU-PC on the hypertriglyceridemia, the effect of different PC-species on the lipoprotein lipase (LPL) in vitro was studied (Blaton and Peeters, 1973). The enzyme activation by PU-PC demonstrated the importance of chain length and double bonds of the fatty acid molecule.

The different modes of action demonstrated the anti-atherogenic effect of the PU-PC present as intact molecule and provide that some mechanisms may be operating in vivo.

TREATMENT OF HYPERLIPOPROTEINEMIA WITH METFORMIN

Crepaldi, Gaetano

A study has been performed in a group of 20 patients with endogenous hypertri-glyceridemia, 17 belonging to Fredrickson's type IV and three to type IIb. Eighteen males and two females. Mean age 45 years. Most of the patients were overweight with a mean weight of 118 $\pm$ 2 per cent of the ideal body weight. Glucose tolerance was reduced in 16 out of 20:1 showed fasting hyperglycemia and 7 chemical diabetes. No patient had insulin dependent diabetes. Before the period of treatment all patients were kept on balanced diet for at least two weeks in order to avoid body weight variations. The same diet was maintained throughout all the period of therapy.

Mean basal serum triglycerides were 464 $\pm$ 68 mg/100ml; mean serum cholesterol 271 $\pm$ 8 mg/100 ml. Mean fasting plasma glucose was 108 $\pm$ 9 mg/100 ml. After the controlled diet period of two weeks, all patients were treated with a standard dose of 2.55 g of metformin daily.

Serum cholesterol and triglycerides were controlled monthly together with fasting plasma glucose.

After the first month of treatment triglycerides decreased about 27% (313 versus 464 mg/100 ml). After a three month therapy serum triglycerides decreased to 256 mg/100 ml. with a diminution of about 37%. The difference to the basal values is statistically significant.

Behaviour of serum cholesterol follows that of triglycerides: 8% decrease after one month, 11% decrease after two and three months. Difference between basal and third month values is significant.

Fasting plasma glucose also diminished from 108 $\pm$ 9 to 93 $\pm$ 5 mg/100 ml.

During all the period of treatment no significant variation of body weight had been observed.

Side effects consisted mainly in gastrointestinal disturbances. Diarrhoea was present in about 10% of the patients.

These results are in accordance with those of Gustafson et al., (1971). The group of patients with hypertriglyceridemia (Type IV) treated by this author had mean basal triglycerides of 213 mg/100 ml, much lower in comparison to the values observed in our group of patients (464 $\pm$ 68 mg/100 ml).

TREATMENT OF ATHEROSCLEROTIC DISEASES WITH PYRIDINOLCARBAMATE

Takio Shimamoto

Pyridinolcarbamate has been designed to inhibit the influx of plasma substances including cholesterol bearing lipoproteins into the arterial wall by suppressing the contracting and swallowing activity of arterial endothelial cells as an endothelial-cell relaxant.

The contracting and swallowing activity of endothelial cells is elicited by administration of cholesterol, saturated fatty acids, angiotensin II, bradykinin, epinephrine, norepinephrine, serotonin, prostaglandin E1, and smoking in rhesus monkey and rabbit and it induces an acute infiltration of plasma substances such

as β-lipoprotein, fibrinogen and possibly pre-β-lipoprotein into the subenendo-
thelial space across the endothelial cells and a series of responses called "the
edematous arterial reaction".

Pyridinolcarbamate prevents the edematous arterial reaction and prevents the
atherosclerosis of cholesterol-fed rabbits. It has also a characteristic enhancing effect on glycolytic enzymes and TCA cycle enzymes of the intima and
media of the arterial wall of man and animals and markedly enhanced the repair
process of atheroma of rabbits.

Pyridinolcarbamate has been widely used in the treatment of atherosclerotic diseases in Argentine, Austria, Brazil, China, France, Hungary, Italy, Japan, Por-
tugal, Spain, Sweden, U.S.S.R. and many other countries, and many literatures,
not only from these countries, but also from Belgium, England, Germany and recently from U.S.A., are available, as summarized in Japanese Heart Journal 13:
537-562, 1972, Atherogenesis (edited by T. Shimamoto, F. Numano and G.M. Addison,
Excerpta Medica Amsterdam, 1973), and Cardiovascular Diseases (edited by Henry
I. Russek, University Park Press, Baltimore, 1974, p. 361-392).

BETA-PYRIDYLCARBINOL IN THE TREATMENT OF HYPERCHOLESTEROLEMIA

N. Zöllner

I don't want to got too deep into clinical aspects because that would be a retrospective judgement. However it may be stated that those who were successes
with respect to a sustained normalisation of serum cholesterol had a considerably better experience with respect to their coronary disease then those who
were nonresponders or non-takers of the drug.

From 1964 to 1966 78 patients with hypercholesterolemia were treated with β-pyridylcarbinol, the alcohol of nicotinic acid (Zöllner and Gudenzi, 1966). In 1969
49 of these patients were reexamined. Medical reports of 7 patients were known,
6 patients had died meanwhile, the fate of 15 patients is not known. 15 of these
49 patients had been taking β-pyridylcarbinol for 5 years. The serum-cholesterol
levels of these patients were significantly lower than those of the 34 patients
who had stopped the treatment with β-pyridylcarbinol. Of course one must keep
in mind that all facts mentioned come from a retrospective judgement. Still,
clinical signs of arteriosclerosis as angina pectoris or peripheral vascular
disease appeared to occur less often than in the control group. Following long
term application of β-pyridylcarbinol flushing of the face was only mentioned by
4 patients, 3 patients had complained about upper gastro-intestinal distress in
the beginning, which disappeared after antacid treatment. Liver function and
glucose tolerance were slightly impaired during the first months in a few patients; however when therapy was continued, these changes were no longer noted
(Zöllner et al., 1971).

EFFECT OF A NEW HYPOLIPIDEMIC, HYPOURICEMIC AGENT (HALOFENATE) IN HYPERLIPOPROTEINEMIC SUBJECTS

Stanley L. Altschuler and Donald Berkowitz

Hyperlipidemia and gouty arthritis are known risk factors in the development of coronary vascular disease (Hall, 1965), and the incidence of atherosclerosis is increased in hyperuricemic patients. It is well known that hyperuricemia is frequently associated with elevated lipids, particularly triglycerides and an agent with the ability to lower both of these serum levels would be valuable therapeutically.

Halofenate is known to have hypolipidemic effects (Berkowitz, 1972; Jepson et al., 1972; and Gilfillan, 1971) as well as hypouricemic actions (Jain,, 1970). The compound is a derivative of phenylacetic acid and is chemically very similar to clofibrate. Halofenate appears to be of low toxicity and is relatively well tolerated by patients. The most frequent side effects are gastrointestinal disorders and usually disappear without alteration of the dosage level. The most common symptoms are nausea or dyspepsia, but several of the patients have developed peptic ulcers.

This study was undertaken to evaluate the effects of halofenate on lipid and uric acid levels in patients with elevations of these parameters.

Methods

Fifty-seven patients, 33 male and 24 female, with type IV hyerlipidemia were selected for this study. The criteria for inclusion were pre-treatment cholesterol values greater than 275 mg and triglyceride levels greater than 175 mg. The age range was 24 to 65 years and the average age was 53 years. The initial part of the study was a double-blind comparison of the effect of halofenate versus probenecid. Treatment consisted of two tablets taken daily in the morning. Serum was collected after a 12 hour over-night fast and analyzed for cholesterol, triglyceride, and uric acid levels.

After the initial twelve week period the double-blind portion of the study was terminated and the results were tabulated. The patients treated with halofenate were continued on therapy, whereas the patients treated with probenecid were taken off therapy for eight weeks and were then adminstered halofenate. The results of the lipid and uric acid levels were tabulated in 12 week treatment periods. There were six treatment periods tabulated for the original halofenate group and four treatment periods completed for the probenecid to halofenate cross-over group.

Results

In Table 1 representing the first twelve week period, the serum triglycerides were decreased by 15% in 22 of 29 patients (76%) in the halofenate group. In the probenecid group the triglycerides were lowered by 15% in 5 of 28 patients (18%). This shows a highly significant response to halofenate in comparison with probenecid.

The serum cholesterol levels were reduced by 10% in only 3 of 29 patients (10%) taking halofenate and in 4 of 28 patients (14%) in the probenecid group. These results show that both drugs were ineffective in lowering cholesterol levels.

Table 1. A comparison of the effects of halofenate versus probenecid (number of patients with a significant response)

Treatment group	Number of patients	Triglyceride (15% reduction)	Cholesterol (10% reduction)	Uric acid (20% reduction)
Halofenate	29	22	3	23
Probenecid	28	5	4	25

For Triglyceride x^2 = 19.21, p < .001 (df = 1).
For Cholesterol x^2 = .19 (not significant).
For Uric acid x^2 = 1.11 (not significant).

The uric acid was lowered by 20% in 23 of 29 patients (79%) in the halofenate group and 25 of 28 patients (89%) in the probenecid treatment group. These results show that both drugs were effective in lowering uric acid levels and there is no significant difference in their effectiveness.

In Table 2 the mean values of the pre-treatment period and the first treatment period of halofenate (Group A), halofenate cross-over (Group B), and probenecid (Group C) are tabulated. It is apparent that the effect of halofenate on lowering triglyceride levels is significant in comparison to the effect of probenecid. Neither drug significantly altered the cholesterol levels, whereas both drugs were effective in lowering uric acid levels.

Table 2. Mean values for all clinical periods

	Pretreatment	Period 1	Period 2	Period 3	Period 4	Period 5	Period 6
Triglyceride							
Group A	370.9	258.4	321.7	253.7	283.8	245.0	209.8
Group B	328.2	181.4	147.4	146.9	142.0		
Group C	299.0	286.7					
Cholesterol							
Group A	341.8	351.3	338.4	331.8	306.4	336.8	325.7
Group B	336.8	301.5	296.5	296.7	279.5		
Group C	336.0	331.0					
Uric acid							
Group A	6.9	4.7	4.6	4.1	4.7	4.7	4.0
Group B	5.6	4.5	4.2	4.4	4.1		
Group C	6.8	4.6					

Group A = Halofenate.
Group B = Halofenate previously treated with probenecid.
Group C = Probenecid.

The mean values for pre-treatment and all clinical periods for the halofenate group and the halofenate cross-over group (Group B) are recorded in Table 2. Serum triglyceride was consistently lowered for both groups. Cholesterol was inconsistently lowered by halofenate. Uric acid was consistently lowered in both groups, more significantly in Group A than in Group B.

Table 3 demonstrates the effect of halofenate in each period for the three measured parameters. These results indicate the halofenate did not lose its potency over the 72 week duration of the study.

Table 3. Percent of patients showing acceptable decrease - by period

		Period 1	Period 2	Period 3
Cholesterol	Group A	10% (3/29)	25% (7/28)	21% (6/28)
(10% decrease)	Group B	48% (10/21)	41% (9/22)	45% (9/20)
Triglyceride	Group A	76% (22/29)	79% (22/28)	89% (25/28)
(15% decrease)	Group B	86% (18/21)	86% (18/21)	95% (19/20)
Uric acid	Group A	83% (24/29)	82% (23/28)	82% (23/28)
(20% decrease)	Group B	61% (13/21)	57% (12/21)	60% (12/20)

		Period 4	Period 5	Period 6
Cholesterol	Group A	60% (17/28)	29% (8/27)	48% (12/25)
(10% decrease)	Group B	80% (12/15)		
Triglyceride	Group A	79% (22/28)	80% (23/28)	92% (24/26)
(15% decrease)	Group B	85% (11/13)		
Uric acid	Group A	96% (27/28)	74% (20/27)	80% (21/26)
(20% decrease)	Group B	53% (8/15)		

Group A = Halofenate.
Group B = Halofenate previously treated with probenecid.

Discussion

On the basis of this study, halofenate appears to have a significant hypo-lipidemic action lowering triglyceride levels. Triglyceride was reduced significantly and consistently in 85% of the treatment periods for the patients taking halofenate. The compound improved cholesterol levels inconsistently.

An excellent hypouricemic response was confirmed in this investigation when the decrease in serum uric acid during halofenate treatment compared favorably with the response of patients treated with the known hypouricemic agent probenecid. The hypouricemic effect of halofenate on the cross-over group was dampened because the serum iric acid had not returned to the pre-treatment level registered prior to probenecid therapy. However, the mean values for the treatment periods were comparable to the mean values of the original halofenate group. The mode of action for this hypouricemic effect is thought to be uricosuric (Hutchinson, 1973).

A NEW ANTIATHEROSCLEROTIC AGENT, EG467. PRELIMINARY REPORT ON ITS EXPERIMENTAL AND CLINICAL TRIAL*

Takio Shimamoto, Toshiyuki Atsumi, Hiroshi Murase,
Tadahiro Sano, Fujie Numano, and Hiroh Yamazaki

EG467 is a nontoxic compound synthesized by the author with the cooperation of Prof. Ishikawa and his collaborators. The LD50 in rats and rabbits is over 5,000 mg/kg by oral administration and it is 3,500 mg/kg and over 2,500 mg/kg respectively by intraperitoneal administration. Long-term treatment of dogs and rats with 40 mg/kg and 200 mg/kg of EG467 for 10 months showed no recognizable toxicity, and the histological and electron microscopic analysis of all organs of these animals showed almost no change. No teratogenic nor carcinogenic effects have been observed during long-term treatment of rabbits with this compound. The solubility of this compound is relatively poor, but it is well absorbed by oral administration and an effect was easily obtained by oral administration.

The most important pharmacological effect of this compound is the inhibitory effect on the contraction of arterial endothelial cells (Shimamoto and Sunaga, 1972; Shimamoto and Numano, 1972; Shimamoto, 1972; Shimamoto and Sunaga, 1973; Shimamoto and Numano, 1973), which is induced by a single-dose treatment of rabbits or rhesus monkeys with epinephrine, norepinephrine, serotonin, bradykinin. angiotensin II, and cholesterol. The transendothelial transportation of plasma substances into the endothelial space is enhanced by the widened intercellular space induced by contraction of endothelial cells, and membrane flow and membrane vesiculation (Bennett, 1956) have been shown to be enhanced by contraction of endothelial cells (Shimamoto et al., 1972). These phenomena were inhibited by EG467. The acute infiltration of β-lipoprotein and IgG into the aortic wall of rabbits and rhesus monkeys, which is induced by contraction of the endothelial cells by various agents such as epinephrine, norepinephrine, angiotensin II, serotonin, and cholesterol, has been inhibited by pretreatment of test animals with 1 to 10 mg/kg of EG467 given orally.

However, no hypotensive effect was observed and no effect on smooth muscle of the gastrointestinal tract was noted, while contraction of bronchial smooth muscle and the spontaneous contracting and relaxing movement of rabbit uterus were slightly inhibited by EG467.

As shown in the Fig. 1, the primary and secondary aggregation of human platelets by ADP and epinephrine was shown to be inhibited by a relatively low concentration of EG467, which was added to the platelets suspended in platelet-rich plasma and incubated for 5 minutes at 37°C as shown in the table 1.

In one model (Kurai, 1965) of arterial type of experimental thrombosis in rabbits, pretreatment of animals by a single dose of 10 mg/kg of EG467, which is a therapeutic dose in man, exhibited a definite preventive effect against appearance of the experimental thrombosis. The weight of thrombi produced are statistically significantly less in animals pretreated with EG467 tahn in untreated animals as shown in the Fig. 2.

In rabbits, kept on 1% cholesterol pellets for 15 weeks, the concomitant and daily administration of EG467 in a dose of 1 and 10 mg/kg, which are therapeutic doses, exhibited a statistically significant and definite inhibitory effect on the appearance of fatty streaks in the aorta of rabbits and the p values were less than 0.01 and 0.01 respectively. As shown in the table, the larger dose: 10 mg/kg of EG467 exhibited a much more potent preventive effect than the lower dose: 1 mg/kg, and the difference between them was statistically significant as shown in the Fig. 3.

---

*Paper read on October 26, 1:45-2:00 p.m. (Chairman: S. Sailer).

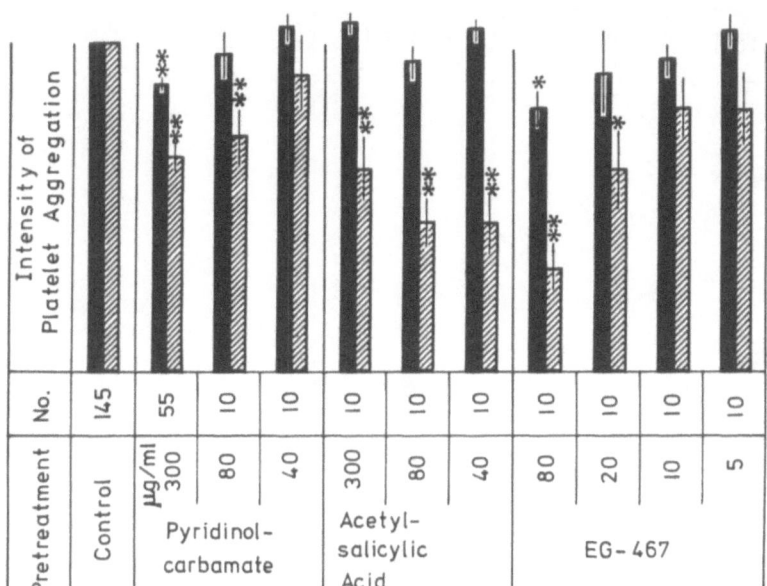

Figure 1. b) Effect of pretreatment on intensity of platelet aggregation induced by 1 µg/ml of epinephrine

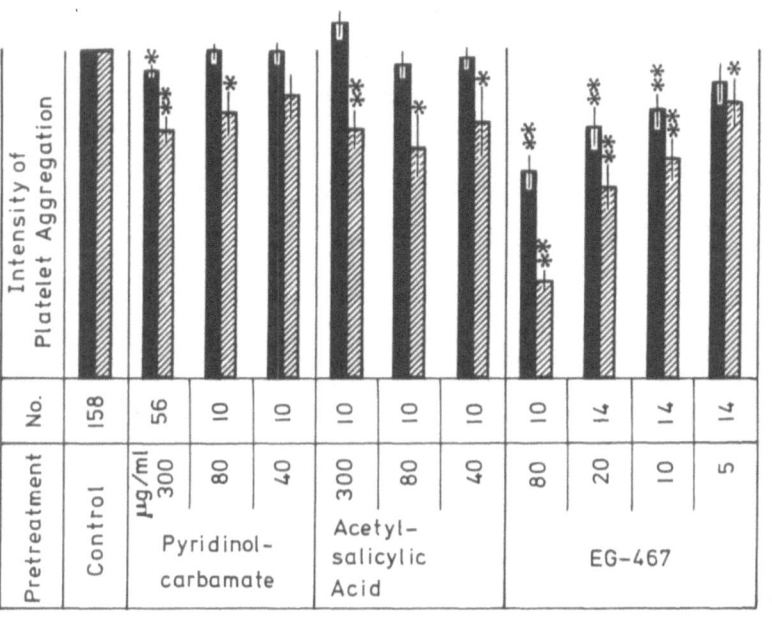

Figure 1. a) Effect of pretreatment on intensity of platelet aggregation induced by 3 x 10⁻⁶ M of ADP

■ Primary   ▨ Secondary

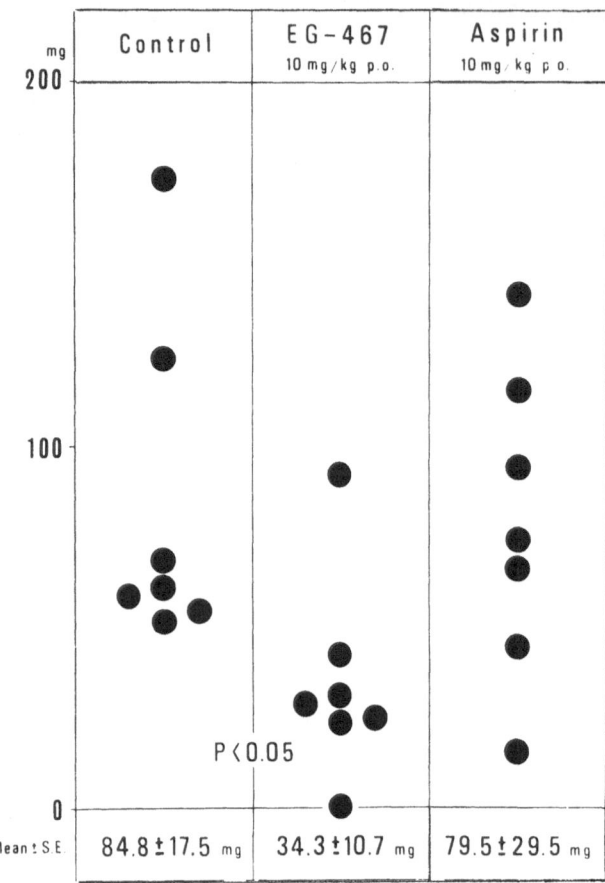

Figure 2. Weight of thrombus
in experimental model of
rabbit

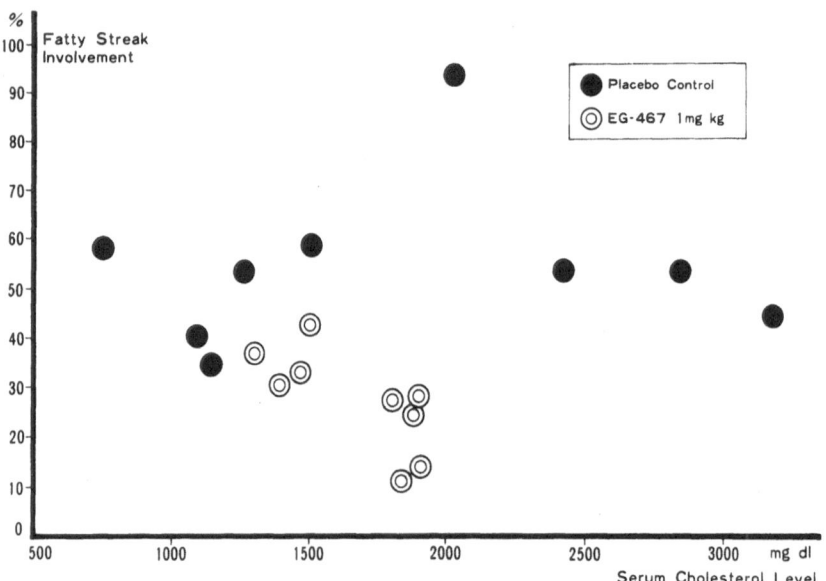

Figure 3. a) Preventive effect of EG-467 (1 mg/kg) against cholesterol induced
atherosclerosis

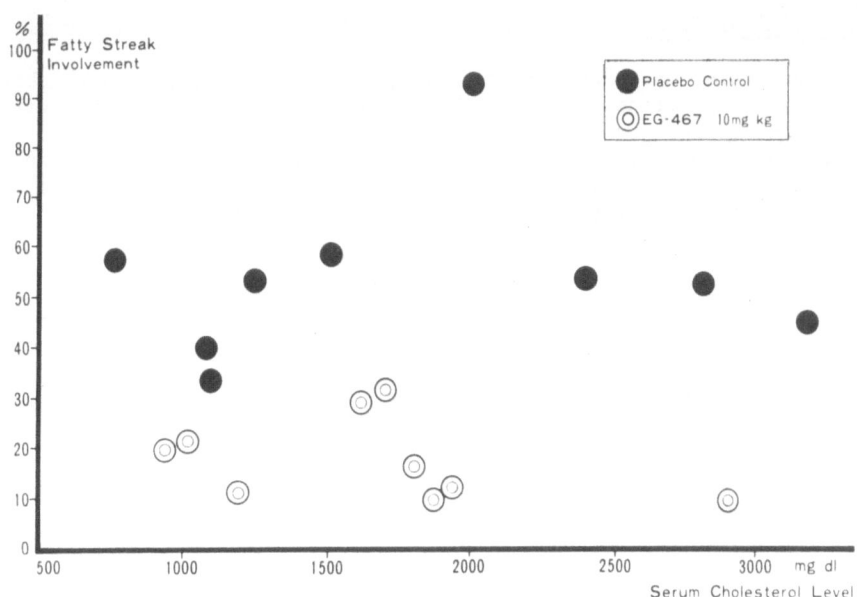

Figure 3. b) Preventive effect of EG-467 (10 mg/kg) against cholesterol induced atherosclerosis

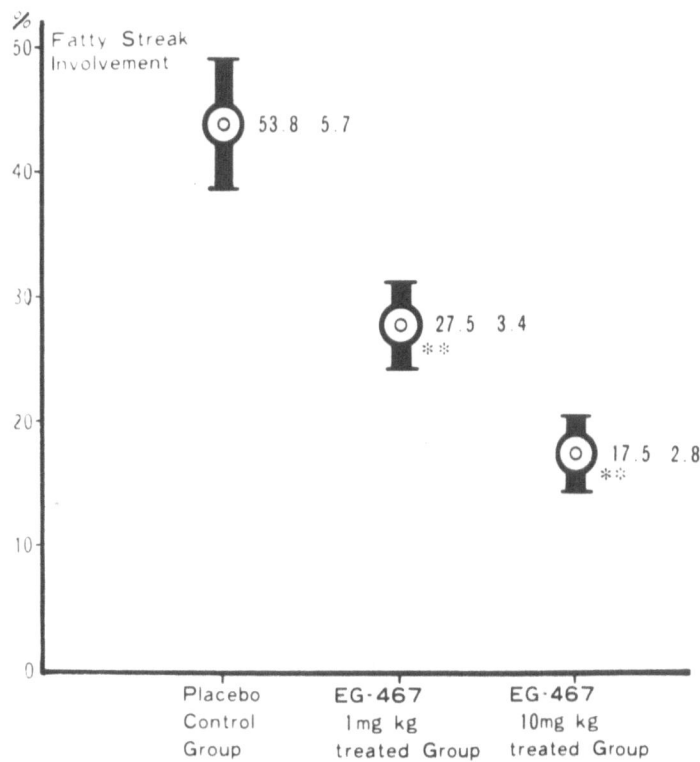

Figure 3. c) Fatty streak involvement (** = 0.01)

The Clinical Trial

The open study has been performed in patients suffering from cerebral atherosclerosis obliterans. The daily oral dose was 300 mg to 600 mg, divided into 3
individual doses and given after each meal.

Among the results in cerebral atherosclerosis, the slowly appearing improvement
of mental function, i.e. the degree of consciousness or the acuteness of attention, was quite impressive. The case history and the result of treatment in 2
representative cases are briefly reported below.

Case 1. J.K., 71-year-old, retired businessman (for 5 years). Three and half
years ago his behavior began to change and continued to change progressively. One
and half years ago he frequently could not recognize members of his family (wife
and daughter) and forgot their features and name, also his home, into which he
had moved 3 years before. These symptoms became worse since April of 1972. For
one year he was mumbling for a long time every day and showed no interest in
anything. His disorientation became marked and the trouble was that he very often
tried to go out with his suits wrapped in Furoshiki. He often asked or called
his dead father, mother, and sister, because he believed they were alive. No
motor, sensory, or reflex abnormality were noted.

On January 11, 1973, EG467 was started in daily dose of 300 mg. His daughter
recognized no change in the first three weeks. Thereafter his daughter found a
big difference, because he began to recognize his wife and daughter and did not
try to go out with his suits. However, the disorientation symptoms were still
marked. The time of murmuring became strikingly shorter. One month later, his
daughter found him watching the news broadcast on television for the first time
for almost 4 years. Cognitive impairment improved slightly.

Two month later, he no more mumbled or forgot his family members and did not call
his dead parents, but started quite correctly to answer questions such as about
his residence. The administration of EG467 was continued for 4 months and his
symptoms, disorientation and cognitive impairment, further improved without any
side effect.

Case 2. B.S. 69-year-old male. One year before, on April 10, he suffered from an
anginal attack. On June 6 he fell in the bathroom and thereafter he started to
be slightly inarticulate. In November 2, his wife died suddenly, and since then
he started to lose markedly interest and volition. On January 11, be suffered
from a chill, palpitation, and headache and on January 12 urinary and fecal incontinence set in.

On January 14 he was hospitalized. His answers and movements to questions were
markedly slow and almost without interest and volition to surroundings; however,
his consciousness was not much disturbed. No motor, sensory, or reflex abnormality were noted. However, disorientation and cognitive impairment were marked
and urinary and fecal incontinence was noted. January 26, 27, 28, 29 and 30, he
suffered from acute bronchopneumonia with fever of 38~39°C and because drowsy
for almost the whole day; he never tried to get out bed. The disorientation and
cognitive impairment became worse. Somtimes he had illusions and said "dog came
in" in the night.

On February 16, EG467 (daily dose 300 mg) was started. During one month almost
no change, but since March 15 his consciousness improved and his speech became
clear. Urinary and fecal incontinence started to decrease. On March 24 he was no
more incontinent and tried to walk for the first time. This he continued and he
desired to be active, for instance go to the lavatory. From March 28 he could
walk with a stick. Disorientation and cognitive impairment became markedly improved.

No side effect of EG467 was noted.

In patients suffering from angina of effort, the exercise ECG, besides the disappearance or marked diminution of anginal attacks or other symptoms, was recorded. In almost all 36 patients the anginal attack disappeared two to three weeks after the initiation of the treatment, and the exercise ECG markedly improved in 26 patients, while 10 cases remained unchanged. In 3 cases with the intermediate form of anginal attack, occurring mainly in the early morning or at midnight and accompanied by ST elevation, this disappeared on EG467, and during the past one year they are free from the symptom.

Of 10 patients suffering from intermittent claudication, 3 exhibited a remarkable prolongation of the claudication time two to three weeks after the initiation of the treatment, 4 exhibited a definite prolongation, and 3 remained unchanged, but no progression of the symptom was noted. In one patient suffering from cyanosis of all the toes of his left foot with severe pain, the administration of EG467 promptly reduced and abolished the pain, the cyanosis diminshed markedly and he steadily improved during one year of treatment.

EG467 was tolerated by all patients and 56 patients received it as long-term treatment for more than a year; no appreciable side effects have been observed in clinical and laboratory examinations at the University Hospitals.

Based on such evidence, double-blind trials have been planned and are going on in several institutions of Japan.

LONG-TERM CLOFIBRATE TREATMENT IN FAMILIAL HYPERLIPOPROTEINEMIAS

G. Crepaldi, D. Fedele, R. Fellin, and G. Briani

Clofibrate or ethyl-α-p-chlorophenoxyisobutyrate is a very effective lipid-lowering agent and is widely used in many types of hyperlipoproteinemia (Levy et al., 1969). It is more active in reducing triglycerides of VLDL than cholesterol of LDL. A reduction of platelet adhesiveness (Carson et al., 1963; Mustard, 1968) and a decrease of plasma fibrinogen (Cotton et al., ·1963) was reported. It also seems to increase fibrinolytic activity in plasma (Strivastava et al., 1963). Its value in the prevention of coronary atherosclerosis is currently being studied.

The exact mechanism of action whereby clofibrate lowers serum lipid concentration is not known.

The present study was carried out to evaluate the effectiveness of clofibrate in maintaining lower lipid levels for a prolonged period of time in patients with primitive hyperlipoproteinemias.

Material and Methods

Patients having undergone prolonged treatment included only those whose serum cholesterol or triglycerides were reduced to at least 15% or 25% respectively after a preliminary trial of three months and whose lipid values returned to normal levels after the drug was suspended.

The group of patients treated included 19 Type II patients, 14 patients with Type IV or V, 2 brothers and a sister with Type III.

Type II. This group had a mean age of 40 ± 3.7 and included 10 males and 9 females treated for a period of 24 to 36 months. The mean clofibrate dose was 2 g per day. The clinical features of these patients showed an elevated frequency of skin and tendinous xanthomas. Ischemic heart disease was present in 9 out of 19 patients.

Type IV and V. The fourteen patients of this group, 12 males and two females, were followed up for a period of 12 to 24 months. In this group of patients, mean age 47 ± 2.3 years, only two had eruptive xanthomas (Type V), three had abdominal pains, and overt diabetes was present in 5 out of 14. Ischemic heart disease was diagnosed in 7 out of 14.

Type III. Three patients with Type II, two brothers and a sister, were followed up for a period of 5 to 8 months. Two had tubero-eruptive xanthomas at the elbows and the knees.

Serum lipid analysis, agarose-gel electrophoresis, postheparin lipolytic activity, glucose tolerance test, and diet studies were performed in order to classify the patients. During treatment a hypocholesterolemic diet was given, adjusted to maintain a stable body weight.
Lipid analysis was performed every month and blood and liver function tests were done routinely.
After an initial one month control period, clofibrate was given in doses of 1.5-2 g per day, according to the weight of the patient. Only in childreen under 12 years the doses were 1 to 1.5 g/day.

Results

Type II patients with serum cholesterol basal values of 394 ± 23 mg/100 ml showed throughout the treatment period a decrease of -20.8+1.5% (P<0.05), with mean maximum decrease of -35.9+1.4%.

The percentage decrease of -20.8% corresponds to a diminution of serum cholesterol of -82 mg/100 ml; the decrease of serum cholesterol was 14% after one month, 17% after two months, 12% after 6 months, 24% after 12 months, 25% after 24 months, and 27% after 26 months.

Fig. 1 shows the mean percent decrease curve in three years of treatment.

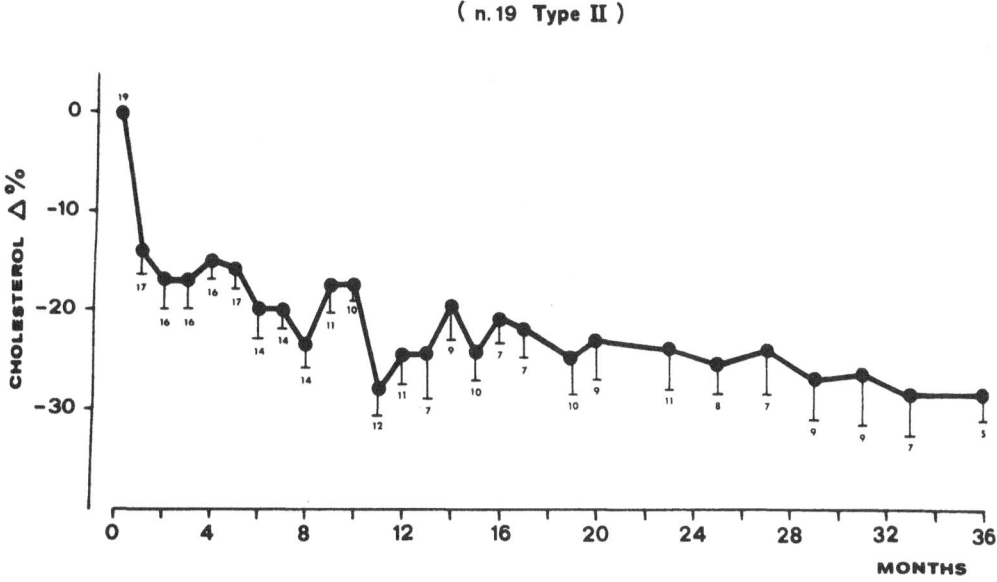

CLOFIBRATE

(n. 19 **Type II**)

Figure 1. Percent decrease of plasma cholesterol during 36 months of clofibrate treatment (Type II patients)

Type IV patients had a mean basal serum cholesterol value of 348 ± 23 mg/100 ml and serum triglycerides were 1203 ± 216 mg/100 ml. The mean percent decreases of serum cholesterol and triglycerides during the entire period of treatment were respectively -27.2+3.5% and -68.5+5.5%. All these decrements are highly significant and correspond to a decrease of 95 mg/100 ml cholesterol and a decrease of 824 mg/100 ml triglycerides.

Fig. 2 shows the two decrease curves of serum cholesterol and triglycerides respectively during the two years of the trial.

The patients with type III hyperlipoproteinemia belonged to the same family and the results reported refer to the treatment after eight months. Fig. 2 shows the mean percent decrease of serum cholesterol and triglycerides in these patients throughout the period of treatment. In these patients, with the same dosage of 2 g/day of clofibrate used in the other types of hyperlipemia, serum triglycerides and cholesterol normalized in a few weeks of treatment.

Tuberous and planar xanthomas decreased in size and sometimes disappeared in many of these patients.

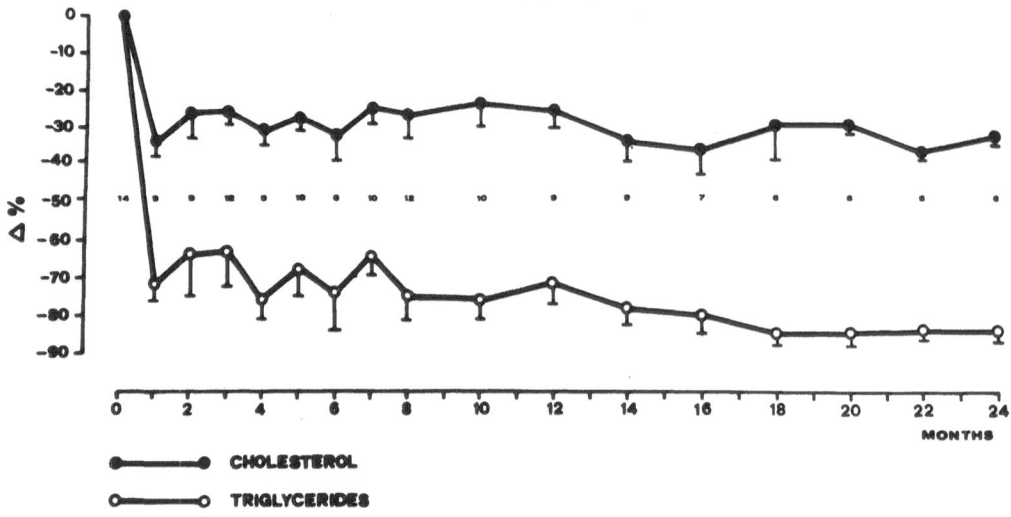

Figure 2. Percent decrease of cholesterol and triglycerides during 24 months of clofibrate treatment (Type IV – V patients)

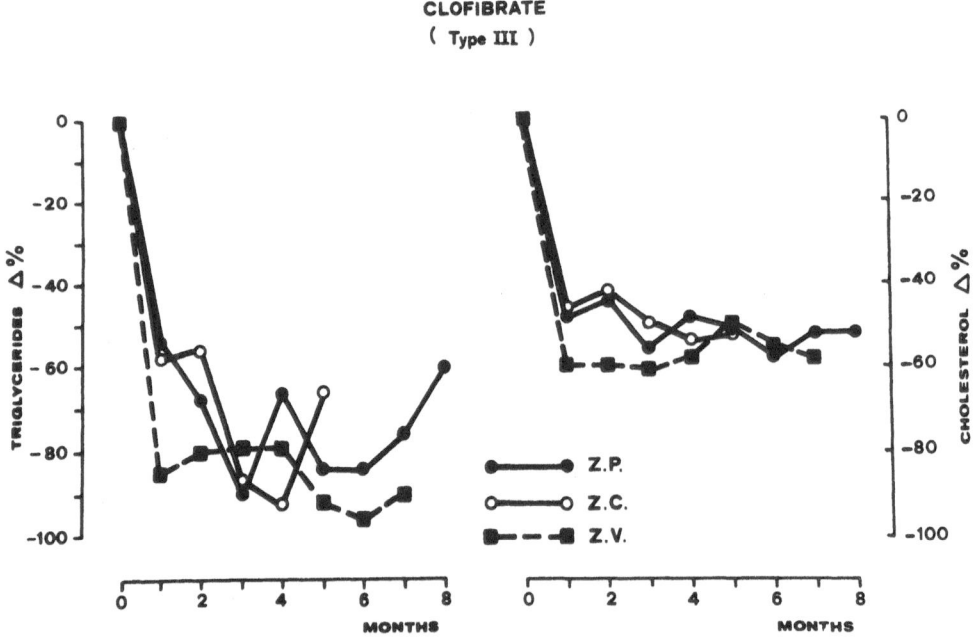

Figure 3. Percent decrease of cholesterol and triglycerides during 8 months of clofibrate treatment (Type III patients)

Side Effects

During all the period of treatment the drug was well tolerated and no toxic or allergic reactions occurred. In a few patients, gastrointestinal disturbances had been observed in the first weeks of treatment. Usually they disappeared without suspending the drug; only in two cases a transitory increase of serum transaminase was reported in the first two or three months of the trial.

One case, not included in the experimental group, deserves particular attention. After a few days of treatment this patient complained of violent pains in the legs; and there were increase of serum transaminase, proteinuria and myoglobinuria. These symptoms disappeared quickly on withdrawal of the drug. This case might be similar to those described by Langer and Levy (1968) as myositis.

Conclusions

The prolonged treatment with clofibrate of patients with different types of hyperlipoproteinemia confirmed that it is a very effective lipid-lowering agent and that absolute contraindications are unknown. The best results were obtained in the treatment of Type III in which the drug normalized serum lipid levels in a very short time, with depletion or disappearance of tuberous-eruptive xanthomas in a few months. These data confirm the data obtained by Levy et al., (1969) and Schlierf and Kahlke (1969) on the exceptional activity of the drug on broad beta disease.

The treatment of patients with Type IV is still very effective in maintaining a sustained lowering of serum triglyceride levels, confirming the previous data of Strisower and Strisower (1964) on endogenous hypertriglyceridemia and the more recent ones of Schlierf and Kahlke (1969) and Berkowitz (1971).

The mean percent decrease of serum cholesterol in patients with Type II is higher than that reported by other authors (Schettler et al., 1967; Levy et al., 1969). A significant diminution of serum cholesterol was reached after a few months therapy and it was constant throughout the whole period. Our results show that type II patients who respond to the preliminary three-month trial with clofibrate, usually can be continued on this therapy for many years. These data are in accordance with the findings of Berkowitz (1971).

Davignon (1971) found that the mean fall in serum cholesterol after one-year treatment was 20.1% in patients with Type IIa and 3.6% in patients with Type IIb.

The results of this study confirm the value of clofibrate as a lipid-lowering agent in the prolonged treatment of many types of hyperlipoproteinemia, including Type II.

: Management of Hyperlipoproteinemias with
Non-Absorbable Drugs

Chairmen: F.A. Gries, West Germany
                 T. Miettinen, Finland

Participants: G. Crepaldi, Italy
                 S.M. Grundy, USA
                 K.J. Hahn, West Germany
                 A.N. Howard, Great Britain
                 R.S. Lees, USA
                 J.K. Lloyd, Great Britain
                 T.M. Parkinson, USA

The workshop in the management of atherosclerosis was concerned with non-absorbable drugs. These agents act within the intestinal lumen interfering with cholesterol and bile acid absorption. The resulting enhanced elimination of cholesterol leads to reduction of plasma cholesterol, a phenomenon generally believed to inhibit or at least retard progression of atherosclerotic lesions in coronary and other arteries of patients with hypercholesterolaemia. The major ultimate aim of the therapy with non-absorbable hypocholesterolaemic drugs is to prevent clinical manifestations of atheromatosis such as sudden death and myocardial infarctions. No prospective controlled studies have been performed so far demonstrating that this goal can be achieved with hypocholesterolaemic drug therapy.

Since it was not the aim to cover the whole field of non-absorbable drugs, the workshop concentrated on cholesterol-lowering therapy in familial hypercholesterolemic (Type II) patients by the three bile acid sequestrant agents, cholestyramine, colestipol and Secholex, and drugs that inhibit cholesterol absorption such as sitosterol and neomycin, and the combination of non-absorbable with absorbable drugs.

BILE ACID SEQUESTRANTS

Mechanism of Action

As a basis for the understanding of the mode of action of non-absorbable agents, Grundy gave a short outline of the main pathways of cholesterol metabolism. Cholesterol synthesized primarily in the liver and intestine is equilibrated with the plasma and tissue cholesterol. The liver converts cholesterol into bile acids, which are secreted into the bile and largely reabsorbed in the distal third of the small intestine. They return through the portal circulation into the liver, where they exert a feed-back inhibition on the conversion of cholesterol into bile acids. In the gut mucosa bile acids inhibit cholesterol synthesis. Cholesterol can be excreted itself into the bile. One third to one half is re-absorbed. It returns via the enterolymphatic circulation to the liver, where it exerts a feed-back inhibition of its own formation from acetate. Interruption of intestinal reabsorption of bile acids has several consequences: 1. plasma cholesterol drainage into stools is markedly increased in the form of bile acids; 2. conversion of cholesterol to bile acids is enhanced; 3. plasma cholesterol is decreased; 4. the tissue cholesterol pool is diminished (e.g. xanthelasmata and xanthomata reduce in size); 5. cholesterol synthesis increases in the liver and intestine limiting the fall in plasma cholesterol. Inhibition of cholesterol

absorption has similar consequences except that the drainage of plasma cholesterol into stool is increased as cholesterol itself, bile acid synthesis being
unaffected. As a matter of fact plasma cholesterol concentrations can be significantly reduced in most hypercholesterolaemic patients by interruption of the
enterohepatic circulation of bile acids with bile acid-binding resins or surgical
ileal exclusion, as well as by inhibition of cholesterol absorption with neomycin
and plant sterols.

There is an overall relationship between bile acid excretion and plasma cholesterol-lowering. The association is, however, variable from patient to patient
apparently because the compensatory increase in hepatic and intestinal cholesterol synthesis may even prevent any decrease in plasma cholsterol; this appears
to be the case with some patients homozygous for familial type II hyperlipoproteinaemia. Nevertheless, in most hypercholesterolaemic patients the increase in
cholesterol synthesis is not sufficient to prevent a reduction in plasma cholesterol. There is also evidence that tissue pools of cholesterol can be decreased
by this treatment (Grundy).

Bile acid sequestering agents enhance cholesterol synthesis and turnover in experimental animals and human subjects. In contrast, although neomycin reduces
plasma and tissue cholesterol levels, it has inconsistent effects on cholesterol
turnover (Parkinson). An effect of bile acid sequestrants on cholsterol absorption as such can be shown in experimental animals (Parkinson, Howard) and may
also occur in man, depending on bile acid concentration in the intestine. However,
inhibition of cholesterol absorption is a minor effect of bile acid sequestrants
(Grundy).

Clinical Studies

Cholesterol Lowering Effect

The management of hypercholesterolaemic children offers a special problem and
was discussed by Dr. Lloyd. On a long-term basis any form of drug therapy can
only be justified in children with familial, hyper-β-lipoproteinaemia type II.
In the majority of these patients diet is inadequate for reduction of serum
cholesterol in the long-term. Untreated heterozygous individuals have a greatly
increased risk of death from ischaemic heart disease in early adult life, and
homozygous individuals develop coronary atheromatosis in childhood; they usually
die from myocardial infarction before reaching adult life. Any drug treatment
regimen in childhood, as indeed in adult life, should be effective, safe, and
acceptable to the patient and his relatives over the long-term. The recent availability of the bile acid sequestrant, cholestyramine, in more palatable form has
considerably enhanced its usefulness in paediatric practice. Cholestyramine given
in a mean dosage of 0.6 g/kg/day (range 0.3-1.1 g) with or without dietary modifications reduced serum cholesterol level by about 35%. The dose was correlated
positively with the faecal excretion of bile acids and percentage reduction of
serum cholesterol. Furthermore, cholestyramine given twice daily before breakfast and before the evening meal was as effective as an equal dose given in four
portions. The practical advantages of twice daily administration of cholestyramine are that the medicine need not be taken to school, and the drug can be
given under parental supervision.

In summary, to date these has not been any escape in the hypocholesterolaemic
effect of cholestyramine. The fact that dietary restriction of fat is not necessary has outweighed its relative unpalatibility. The finding that twice daily
administration is effective, makes its use even more acceptable for children.
Stein (Johannesburg) had similar good results in children below 15 years of
age, while the response of adoloscents was between 22 and 24% decrease, the difference most likely being due to better parental control of drugs and diet in
smaller than in older children.

From reports in the literature which were summarized by Grundy, in adults cholestyramine generally reduces plasma cholesterol from 15 to 30%, but greater reductions (30 - 50%) are frequently obtained in the hypercholesterolaemic groups.
Despite Lloyd's observation it is still uncertain whether there is a dose-re-
lationship above a dose of 10 g resin per day in adults (Grundy). With the ileal
by-pass operation, according to Buchwald, reported reductions are even greater.
Comparative studies have shown convincingly that the increase of faecal bile acid
excretion and the decrease of serum cholesterol is greater after ileal by-pass
than during cholestyramine (Miettinen). At the present time, ileal by-pass should
only be carried out in patients with primary hypercholesterolaemic type II, who
are resistant to drug therapy (Grundy, Stone, Chicago, Illinois). If it is planned, it should be performed early in life (Davignon, Montreal). Cholestyramine
response may be a good test of the effectiveness of ileal by-pass but resistance
to cholestyramine is no contraindication for the operation, since some homozygotes may respond better to ileal exclusion, and xanthomata may disappear in
these patients even when plasma cholsterol is not lowered markedly (Miettinen,
Crepaldi).

Experience gathered on 25 patients with type II hypercholesterolaemia (mean
plasma cholesterol 468 mg/100 ml), treated with the anion exchange resin colestipol, were reported by Crepaldi. The mean decrease of cholesterol during 12
months of treatment with 15 g per day was 53 mg/100 ml, three months' additional
treatment with 30 g per day resulting in a further decrease of 16 mg/100 ml; the
overall decrease was 15%. As can also be observed with cholestyramine, the decrease of serum cholesterol was associated with a significant increase in serum
triglycerides, a probable consequence of an accelerated production of VLDL by
the liver. Serum uric acid increased slightly by an unknown mechanism. The increase in triglycerides as well as data on a few individuals suggest the usefulness of combining colestipol with drugs inhibiting triglyceride production.

Parkinson reported a study evaluating the hypocholesterolemic activity and long-
term tolerance of 5 g of colestipol three times daily by 107 individual investigators following the same protocol. Subjects with the serum cholesterol level $\geq$
250 mg/100 ml (classified as type IIA or IIB) were randomly assigned to colestipol (1095 subjects) or placebo (1075 subjects); respective initial mean cholesterol values were 313 mg/100 ml and 308 mg/100 ml.

In the colestipol group, monthly mean cholsterol reductions ranged from 26 to
37 mg/100 ml and in the placebo group from 1 mg/100 ml to 14 mg/100 ml during
the treatment period of 24 months. A decrease of serum cholesterol of at least
15% was found in 40% of subjects in the colestipol group and in only 10 - 15% of
subjects in the placebo group, the difference being significant (p<0.005). Colestipol effects persisted during the entire 24 months. In contrast to observations
by Crepaldi, no consistent change was found in plasma triglycerides.

Ritland reported thet Secholex, 9 - 15 g per day for 18 months, lowered serum
cholesterol from 460 to 390 mg/100 ml (15% decrease). Side effects on renal or
hepatic function, and on the absorption of glucose, iron or vitamins were not
found. The glycine-taurine ratio in bile increased as it does in other situations,
where bile acid excretion is increased. Comparison of the effect of equal doses
of cholestyramine and Secholex on faecal steroid excretion revealed a higher bile
acid output with cholestyramine and a tendency to greater neutral sterol values
with Secholex; the total sterol excretion and cholesterol-lowering were almost
identical (Howard, Miettinen).

Treatment of Homozygous Type II

A rather unsolved problem is the treatment of homozygous patients with type II
hyperlipoproteinaemia since none of the known measures is satisfactory. Usually
combined therapy is tried. In a 16-year-old child, a combination of cholestyramine with diet, clofibrate, nicotinic acid or neomycin decreased cholesterol

from 1000 to 600 mg/100 ml and reduced xanthoma size, while in another child xanthoma developed despite a similar cholesterol-lowering regimes (Lloyd). Cholestyramine as well as ileal by-pass may occasionally cause a transient increase in plasma cholesterol in homozygous patients transiently (Grundy, Davignon), probably due to overcompensation of cholesterol synthesis after bile acid diversion. The increment in cholesterol may be reversed by addition of clofibrate or nicotinic acid (Davignon). It was never observed in heterozygotes, who apparently cannot compensate sufficiently for sterol losses in faeces, and therefore respond with a lowered plasma cholesterol (Grundy, Moutafis, Athens).

As Lees pointed out, one should be aware that homozygous patients do not respond uniformly to therapy. Some of them may respond to cholestyramine and diet quite well, while others do not (Stone). Lowering of cholesterol is not always identical with improvement of health, partly because a decrease of cholesterol by 40 - 50% leaves these patients still hypercholesterolaemic and does not necessarily prevent progression of coronary artery disease. But a lowering of cholesterol may, if not stop, at least retard the further worsening of atheromatous lesions. Too little is known about the dynamics of these lesions.

Combined Therapy

The conclusion of the fluent discussion was that because of compensatory increase in synthesis acceptable plasma cholesterol levels may not be obtained by diet and bile acid sequestrants alone. Therefore, the addition of drugs supposed to inhibit synthesis should be considered. Howard reported that, though in his studies on type II patients with moderately elevated cholesterol clofibrate alone had only little effect and Secholex lowered cholesterol by 19% only, a combination of Secholex (12 - 15 g/day) and clofibrate resulted in a decrease of more than 30%. The response was detected within 2 weeks and no rebound was observed, a finding confirmed by Scandinavian workers. The beneficial effect of the combination might be due to inhibition by clofibrate of resin-induced increase in synthesis of cholesterol. Since Secholex lowers LDL but has virtually no effect on VLDL, the combination of the resin with clofibrate is most useful in type IIB, where both LDL and VLDL are increased. Addition of nicotinic acid to cholestyramine treated patients also causes a further decrease in serum cholesterol (Miettinen).

Drug Interactions

Cholestyramine interferes with the absorption of drugs, as summarized by Hahn. As a matter of fact a reduction in the absorption of the anticoagulants warfarin and phenprocoumon have been well established when the two substances are administered simultaneously with cholestyramine or even if warfarin is taken three hours prior to the resin. The pharmacological effect on coagulation is reduced as well.

Absorption of chlorothiazide is not affected by the resin, while that of nicotinic acid and thyroxine is greatly impaired. Serum levels of digitoxin or digoxin are not affected if these cardiac glycosides are taken one and a half hours before administration of cholestyramine, however, digitoxin toxicity can be treated effectively by cholestyramine.

The resin may reduce absorption of iron salts and deficiency of vitamin K and folic acid has been observed in long-term therapy.

Side Effects of Therapy

The major side effects of bile acid sequestrants are functional in nature, and limited to the gastro-intestinal tract. The possible long-term side effects have not yet been thoroughly evaluated. Especially on large dosage a significant proportion of adult patients complain of various minor gastro-intestinal discomfort and constipation (Grundy, Parkinson). For instance in the multiclinical study reported by Parkinson, a 10.6% of the colestipol patients reported a functional gastro-intestinal complaint compared to 4.8% of the placebo patients. On the other hand, diarrhoea, the major complication of ileal exclusion, is mainly due to excessive quantities of bile acid in the colon and can be treated effectively with bile acid sequestrants. According to Lloyd abdominal discomfort and constipation have not been features in children. Slight malabsorption of fat has occurred but even on unrestricted diet the steatorrhoea (5.3 - 10.5 g/day) has been asymptomatic. Supplementary soluble vitamins have not been given, and so far there is no evidence of deficiency of vitamins A, D, E or K. Malabsorption of folic acid is evidenced by low serum and red cell folate concentrations. Though no child has become anaemic oral folic acid (5 mg/day) is now given to all children on long-term cholestyramine therapy. Growth rates of all the children in Lloyd's series have remained normal during the period studied. The theoretical possibility that long-term cholestyramine treatment may result in increased urinary oxalate excretion and hence renal calculi, requires further investigation.

In the study on colestipol (Parkinson) no significant abnormality was seen in hematology and blood chemistry data. The continuous diversion of bile acids might, however, enhance cholesterol gall stone formation. This possibility seems likely in view of the observation that patients subjected to ileal resection have a high prevalance of cholesterol stones. Thus far, there is no firm data to indicate that either ileal exclusion or bile acid sequestrants increase the incidence of gall stones. However, the bile becomes super-saturated with cholesterol in some patients treated with bile acid sequestrants, especially if these agents are combined with clofibrate. A greater rate of side effects may, however, be expected with combined therapy. When two or more drugs are used in combination transaminases, bilirubin, and the bromsulphthalein retention may be increased (Moutafis, Lees). Monitoring of liver function is necessary, especially with the combination of neomycin and clofibrate (Lees). However, no side effects except mild constipation in a few patients were observed with Secholex and clofibrate over several years (Howard).

The psychological implications of embarking upon life-long moderately unpleasant treatment in children as well as adults, who are symptom-free and outwardly healthy, has also to be considered (Lloyd). The anxiety in families with a strong family history of myocardial infarction tends to be considerable, particularly, when a parent has developed symptoms at an early age. In these cases, treatment may reduce the anxiety, even though one cannot, in our present state of knowledge, promise that the treatment will be effective in preventing or delaying the onset of heart disease.

Drugs that Inhibit Cholesterol Absorption

Lees stated that, though neomycin is an effective drug its usefulness in type II therapy has been poorly appreciated. It is given in doses of .5 - 2.0 g/day, which are well below those used for antibiotic purposes. At a dose of 1.5 g/day it decreases plasma cholesterol by 30 - 35% in adult patients with type II abnormality. When given with meals, few side effects are recorded; only three out of 42 patients had to stop the drug because of diarrhoea. Other complaints were metallic taste in the mouth or anorexia (6 out of 42 patients). Because the absorption of neomycin is low (1%) at the doses recommended for lipid lowering its plasma levels are below the toxic level and consequently no effects on hearing or renal function have been observed (Lees).

Sitosterols, a group of plant sterols found in plant oils, have been shown to lower serum cholesterol effectively by Grundy and coworkers. A preparation containing about 93% of β-sitosterol will be available in the near future. Except for occasional constipation there are no side effects of sitosterol. The average cholesterol-lowering in about 20 patients was 15%, the response varying from zero to 35%. In summary, both neomycin and sitosterols surely have a place in the treatment of type II hyperlipoproteinaemias (Lees).

Cardiovascular Benefit of Therapy

As mentioned before, no data on coronary artery disease in prospective studies with non-absorbable drugs are available. However, in general, therapy with bile acids sequestrants seems to be beneficial as may be derived from the first and preliminary results of the multiclinical study reported by Parkinson. At months 24 of the study 790 patients were still enrolled in the colestipol group and 768 patients in the placebo group. Of these 225 had completed at least 24 months of colestipol treatment and 210 placebo treatment. During this period there were 22 deaths of cardiovascular origin in the placebo group and only 10 deaths in the colestipol group. This difference is statistically significant at the 5% level by simple X^2-test. There was no significant difference in the distribution of patients by major disease diagnosis, such as atherosclerotic cardio-vascular disease, hypertension or diabetes mellitus between the two groups after randomization. Thus, although the study was not designed as a primary or secondary prevention trial, the data do suggest that colestipol may be protecting against cardiovascular death.

ENHANCEMENT OF CHOLESTEROL METABOLISM BY COLESTIPOL HYDROCHLORIDE IN EXPERIMENTAL ANIMALS

Thomas M. Parkinson, Thomas Honohan, John C. Schneider, Jr., Gary Elfring, and William A. Phillips

Colestipol hydrochloride (Colestid®, The Upjohn Company), a polyethylenepolyamine polymer with 1-chloro-2,3-epoxypropane, is a new bile acid sequestrant which lowers serum cholesterol levels in experimental animals (Parkinson et al., 1969; Marmo et al., 1970) and in man (Parkinson et al., 1969; Ryan and Jain, 1972; Glueck et al., 1972; Nye et al., 1972). Although type II, III and IV hyperlipoproteinemic subjects respond to the drug, it appears to be most effective in those with elevated serum cholesterol and normal or only slightly elevated triglycerides (type II). Triglyceride levels generally are not significantly affected by colestipol·HCl therapy.

Increased low density lipoprotein (LDL) levels in type II subjects appear to result from decreased LDL catabolism, rather than from increased synthesis or pool size (Langer et al., 1972). Also plasma cholesterol clearance was reported to be decreased in hypercholesterolemic subjects (Nestel et al., 1969) and fecal bile acid excretion was shown to be less in a family with hypercholesterolemia than in normal controls (Miettinen et al., 1967). Because of the efficacy of colestipol·HCl in type II hypercholesterolemia, animal studies were carried out to determine effects of the resin on various aspects of cholesterol metabolism, in particular those which are most important in regulating cholesterol turnover and bile acid excretion.

Two groups of male Upjohn:TUC(SD)spf rats weighing an average of 324 g, 15 rats per group, were fed semisynthetic diet containing 1% colestipol·HCl or diet alone. On day 15 of feeding each rat received intravenously 3.9 μCi [1,2-^{3}H]-cholesterol complexed with rat serum lipoproteins. Specific radioactivity of serum total cholesterol was measured by GLC and liquid scintillation spectrometry in blood samples obtained by sequential bleeding (Phillips et al., 1973) at 2 hours, 1, 3, 6, 10 and 14 days and at weekly intervals for a total of 7 weeks. Computer analysis of the turnover curves of serum cholesterol by a nonlinear estimation program indicated that the data could be fitted best to a 3-pool model (Goodman et al., 1973a). Enhancement of cholesterol turnover by colestipol·HCl is shown graphically in Fig. 1, which presents the semilogarithmic plots of mean serum specific activities vs. time for treated and control groups. Turnover parameters for each rat were calculated from computer analyses of individual turnover curves. In pool 1, the drug significantly increased cholesterol production rate (16.0 vs. 10.1 mg/day) and the excretion rate constant (0.79 vs. 0.53 day^{-1}) without significantly altering pool size or serum cholesterol concentrations. These results are compatible with an agent capable of interrupting the enterohepatic circulation of bile acids in the rat, which can compensate for increased bile acid loss by increasing cholesterol biosynthesis.

Effects of colestipol·HCl on cholesterol biosynthesis determined from mathematical analysis of the turnover data described above were confirmed by studies measuring the incorporation of [1-^{14}C]-acetate into cholesterol by homogenates of livers from rats fed 2% colestipol·HCl in the diet for 8 days. Pooled liver homogenates were incubated with [1-^{14}C]-acetate using standard procedure (Bucher and McGarrahan, 1956). Cholesterol digitonides were prepared from hexane extracts of homogenate hydrolyzed following incubation and were counted by liquid scintillation spectrometry. Colestipol·HCl feeding enhanced cholesterol synthesis approximately 2-fold compared to control animals (Table 1).

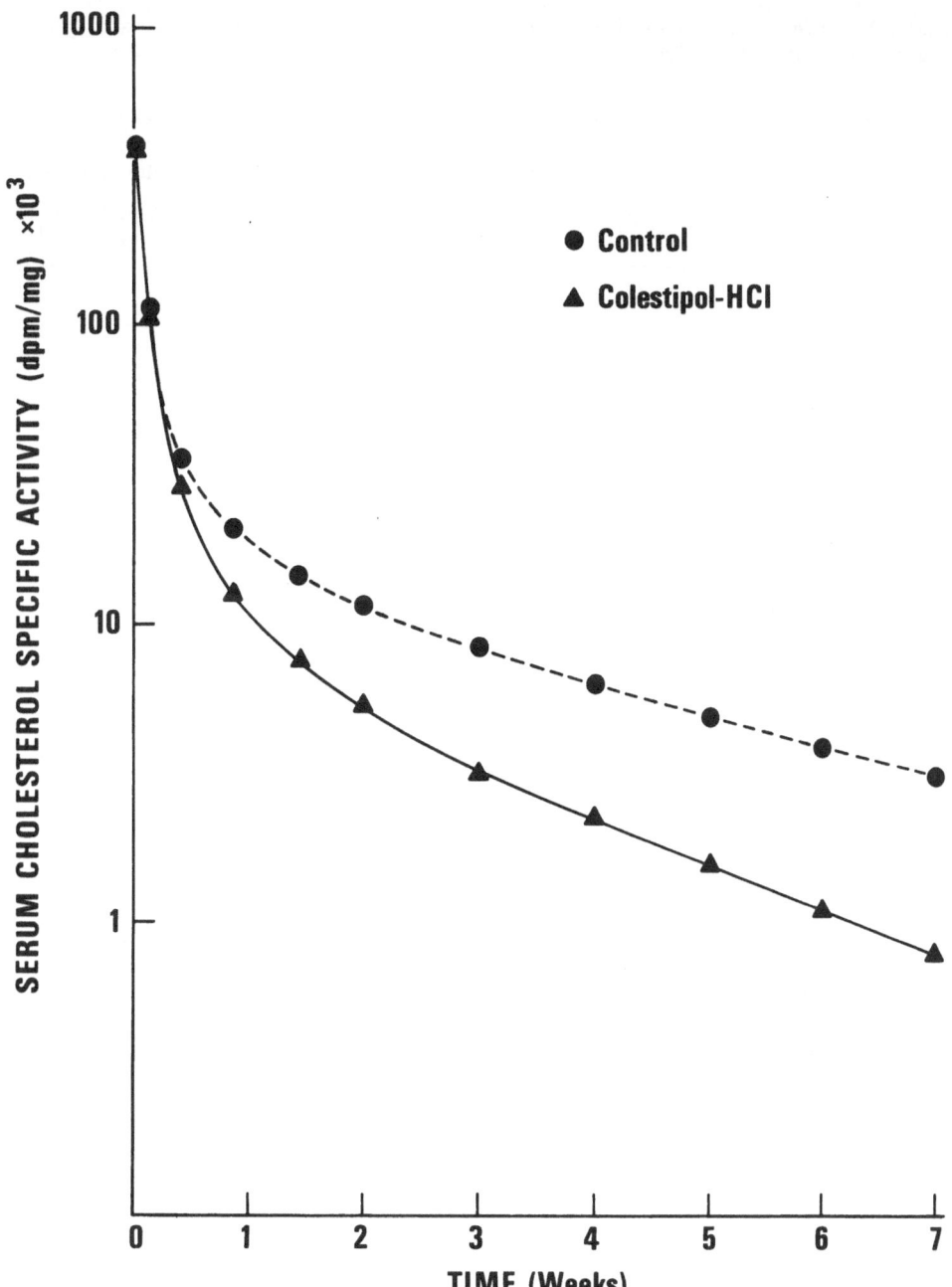

Figure 1

7α-Hydroxylation of cholesterol appears to be the first and rate-limiting step in bile acid synthesis (Danielsson et al., 1967). Since bile acids are the major products of cholesterol catabolism in man and the rat, cholesterol 7α-hydroxylase activity should be important in regulating cholesterol excretion. Effect of colestipol·HCl on 7α-hydroxylase activity of liver from rats fed 2% drug in the diet for 5 days was determined in general according to the methods of Berseus et al. (1969). The 20,000 X g supernatant fraction of liver homogenates was incubated with $[4-^{14}C]$-cholesterol. Extracts of homogenate were chromatographed on silica

Table 1. Effects of colestipol hydrochloride on hepatic cholesterol synthesis and cholesterol 7α-hydroxylase activity in rats

| Treatment | [1-^{14}C]-acetate incorporation into cholesterol | | [4-^{14}C]-cholesterol conversion to 7α-hydroxycholesterol | |
	dpm/mg protein/3 hr[a]	percent conversion[b]	nmoles/mg protein/hr[c]	percent conversion[d]
Diet	14,997	1.84	.008	0.51
Diet + 2% Colestipol·HCl	28,886	3.10	.014	1.03

[a]Means of duplicate samples.

[b]Dpm sterols/dpm acetate substrate X 100.

[c]Means of quadruplicate samples.

[d]Dpm 7α-hydroxycholesterol/dpm cholesterol substrate X 100.

Table 2. Effects of colestipol hydrochloride on fecal bile acid excretion in dogs

| Colestipol·HCl (mg/kg per day) | Total bile acids[a] | | | | | |
| | 69 days | | 6 months | | 12 months | |
	(µg/g feces)	(mg/96hrs)	(µg/g feces)	(mg/96hrs)	(µg/g feces)	(mg/96hrs)
Control	732	980	883	826	982	714
500	827	1008	1035	1073	2295[c]	2606[c]
1000	1447	2241[b]	1860[b]	2420[c]	2869[c]	3496[c]
2000	1480[b]	2380[b]	1960[c]	1862[c]	2881[c]	4161[c]
Standard Deviation(%)	36.7	37.1	29.8	21.8	15.0	45.4

[a]Sum of cholic, deoxycholic, lithocholic, 7-ketolithocholic and 7-ketodeoxycholic acids.

[b]Significantly different from control (p <0.05).

[c]Significantly different from control (p <0.01).

Reprinted from Parkinson et al., Atherosclerosis 17:167 (1973) by permission of Elsevier Scientific Publishing Co., Amsterdam.

gel thin layer plates and the spots corresponding to 7α-hydroxycholesterol were scraped off and counted by liquid scintillation spectrometry. 7α-hydroxylase activity expressed as either percent conversion of added cholesterol or n moles 7α-hydroxy-cholesterol formed per mg protein per hour, was increased approximately 2-fold by colestipol·HCl (Table 1).

Further evidence of enhanced bile acid production was obtained from dogs fed 500 - 2000 mg colestipol·HCl/kg daily in their food for 12 months. Four-day fecal collections were made beginning on day 69 and at 6 and 12 months. Samples were extracted and purified and fecal bile acids and neutral steroids were identified and quantitated by GLC (Parkinson et al., 1973). Total bile acid excretion was increased significantly in all treated dogs (Table 2). Deoxycholic acid was the major component, accounting for approximately 60% of the total in control dogs and increasing to about 75% under the influence of colestipol·HCl, with a proportional decrease in cholic acid. Total neutral steroids, consisting of cholesterol, desmosterol, campesterol, stigmasterol, β-sitosterol and mixtures of other isomeric plant sterols, were not increased significantly.

These data indicate that colestipol·HCl markedly increases bile acid fecal excretion and cholesterol turnover in experimental animals. Enhancement of fecal bile acid excretion by colestipol·HCl has been confirmed in man (Rubulis et al., 1972), and Goodman et al. (1973b) have found similar effects on cholesterol turnover rates in human subjects. Increase in cholesterol catabolism by colestipol·HCl, therefore, may in part explain the effectiveness of the drug in lowering serum cholesterol levels in type II hyperlipoproteinemia. Good patient acceptance and absence of serious side effects may make the drug eminently suitable for chronic therapy of this disorder, which is a major risk factor in the development of atherosclerotic vascular diasease.

XIX
Surgical Treatment of Arteriosclerosis

Chairmen: A. Senn, Switzerland
             M. Trede, West Germany

Participants: H. Denck, Austria
             B. Nachbur, Switzerland
             P. Waibel, Switzerland

The following brief reports by members of the panel on six aspects of the surgical treatment of arteriosclerosis will stress the indications for and the scope of operative therapy without going into technical details.

CHRONIC RENAL AND VISCERAL ARTERY STENOSIS: DIAGNOSIS AND INDICATION FOR VASCULAR RECONSTRUCTION

M. Trede

It is estimated that in 5% of all patients with diastolic hypertension the underlying aetiology is renovascular. The cause for renal artery stenosis is arteriosclerosis in 70% of cases.

The search for such a stenosis is relatively easy: rapid sequence urograms and isotope renograms serve as valuable screening tests in 80% of cases, whereas renal arteriography invariably confirms the anatomical lesion.

Far more problematical is the correlation of a stenosis with hypertension when one considers that 30% of cases with renal arterial stenosis are normotensive.

Split renal function studies, depending on a reduction of water and sodium excretion on the stenosed side, the Kaplan test depending on the hypertensive effect of angiotension infusion, and even the assay of renin in selectively catheterised renal veins — all show only imperfect correlation with changes in blood pressure after correction of renal artery stenosis.

The results of operation (from the literature and 121 own cases) help to define the indication for renovascular reconstruction. The ideal candidate should not be older than 40 years, the cause for stenosis should be fibromuscular hyperplasia rather than arteriosclerosis, the history of hypertension should not exceed 2 years and it should be resistant to medical therapy. Bearing these criteria in mind the blood pressure was normalised in 88% of cases with fibromuscular stenosis (as against 45% with arteriosclerosis) and in 77% of cases under the age of 40 (as against only 41% in those over 40 years of age).

Arteriosclerosis is the cause for chronic occlusions of the 3 main visceral arteries — coeliac, superior and inferior mesenteric — in 90% of cases. Excellent collateral connections between these vessels account for the fact that gradually developing stenoses in one or two of them often go unnoticed.

The indication for arteriographic study of the visceral arteries should be extended to include all cases of unsolved abdominal pain, recurrent peptic ulceration, chronic pancreatitis and possibly regional enteritis.

The indication for operation depends on the presence of abdominal symptoms (pain and malnutrition) coinciding with angiographic evidence of stenosis in 2 or more visceral arteries, in the absence of severe risk factors.

SURGICAL TREATMENT OF ACUTE ARTERIAL THROMBOSIS OF THE LIMBS

H. Denck

In the last 15 years 6682 patients with arterial occlusive disease have been
treated in the surgical department of the Lainzer Krankenhaus Vienna. 788 patients presented an acute arterial occlusion, in 88% due to arterial embolism,
in 12% due to arterial thrombosis in chronic occlusive vascular disease. Acute
occlusions in 63 patients with presenting arteriosclerotic lesions was explained
by a sudden drop of blood pressure, by a diminished cardiac output as for instance in myocardial insufficiency, changes of blood coagulation by oral contraceptives (4 times) etc. 11 times thrombosis occurred in an arteriosclerotic
aneurysm. A thrombectomy performed by Fogarthy catheter is frequently followed
by reocclusion. A more aggressive approach is therefore requested: thrombend-
arterectomy or a reconstructive procedure by by-pass technique. In patients in
bad general conditions an axillo-femoral or a femoro-femoral cross-over graft
performed in local anesthesia may be adequate to save a limb in unilateral iliac
thrombosis. Thrombosed arterial aneurysms must be excised or by-passed unless
recurrence is likely.

The differential diagnosis between embolism and thrombosis is very important.
While embolectomy can be performed easily with the Fogarty catheter by most surgeons, patients needing by-pass procedures or endarterectomy are best treated
by specialized vascular surgeons.

The amputation rate (29%) and the mortality (21%) in arterial thrombosis of the
limbs compared with the corresponding data of arterial embolism (6% and 4%)
illustrate the difficult problems in the surgical management of acute occlusions
in arteriosclerotic disease of the extremities.

Early operation of stenotic lesions may prevent acute ischemia and early des-
obliteration contributes to increase limb salvage rate and to lower morbidity
and mortality.

SURGICAL TREATMENT OF CEREBRO-VASCULAR INSUFFICIENCY

B. Nachbur

In cerebro-vascular disease the interest of the vascular surgeon is directed to
degenerative alterations of the accessible extra-cranial vessels from the aortic
arch to the base of the skull. Generally speaking — and with the exception of
Takayasu (pulseless) disease — obliterative lesions of the major branches of the
aortic arch rarely if ever give rise to irreversible localized cerebral damage.
The subclavian steal syndrome presenting as a temporary ischemic attack of the
hind brain is a case in point. This condition lends itself well to surgical correction (endarterectomy of the subclavian artery or by-pass procedure).

Internal carotid artery stenosis is of greater pathogenetic importance. It is
thought that 20 - 30% of strokes are essentially related to arteriosclerotic
disease of the internal carotid artery at the surgically accessible level of the
carotid bifurcation. Because in some cases the condition of the patient has been
worsened by surgery it has become necessary to classify as follows: 1. asymptomatic bruits, 2. transient ischemic attacks (TIA), 3. advancing stroke, 4. complete stroke. The indication for surgery in stage I is debatable and not generally accepted. Some authors favor endarterectomy in this stage as a protective
measure prior to major surgery elsewhere (i.e. open-heart or coronary surgery).
Carotid endarterectomy in expert hands is highly recommendable for stage II (TIA)

as the best method for prevention of frank stroke which is to be expected in 50%
of untreated patients within a 3-year-period. It seems that the improvement of
cerebral hemodynamics thus obtained is of less importance than the removal of a
potential source of microemboli. The latter probably consist of minute plateleft-
fibrin cholesterol complexes. In stage III it is technically possible and occasionally helpful to perform endarterectomy and extract distal thrombus within
the first 2 - 3 days but there is also the danger of ensuing hemorrhage into an
area of brain softening. This is the main reason why surgery is ungratifying in
stage IV.

CHRONIC ARTERIAL OCCLUSION OF THE LOWER EXTREMITIES

P. Waibel

The natural course of arterial disease in extremities is dependent on two factors,
the progressive circulatory disorder in the limb itself and circulatory disorders
in other parts of the body.

The circulatory disturbance in an extremity is generally divided in four stages
of intensity. These stages are important in surgical indications. Stage I means
stenosis or occlusion of arteries, but without symptoms. In stage II the patient
has intermittent claudication. In stage III skin blood flow is extremely reduced and ischemic rest pain is the main complaint of the patient, whereas in
stage IV necrosis or even gangrene are the sign of insufficient blood flow.

The scope of surgical treatment of vascular disease of the limbs is to improve
the fate of the patient's limb by reducing the amputation rate and, less important, to improve the walking ability. In stage III or IV the chance to lose
the involved limb is over 50% within one year. Results after surgery for vascular
disease of the limb show that death rate is not reduced, but fortunately also not
increased over that in nonoperative treatment. Mortality five years after aortoiliac reconstructions is 12%, after femoropopliteal reconstructions 12.6%. The
mortality is three times higher in stage III and IV after the same time. Most of
the fatalities are due to coronary heart disease or to cancer of the lung (1/3).

Results of reconstructive arterial surgery during the past ten years show that
it really improves not only walking ability, but in first order the fate of the
limb. Results are dependent of the site of reconstruction, the degree of initial
ischemia and hemodynamic factors. Patency rate is 73% after five and 31% after
ten years in aortoiliac reconstructions. It is even better after thrombendarterec-
tomy than after prosthetic bypass. Five years after femoropopliteal reconstructions 84% are still patent, 49% after ten years. Important is the amputation rate.
After aortoiliac reconstructions it is 3% within ten years. In the femoropopliteal area however it is 10% within five and 22% within ten years. If we consider
only reconstructions without prosthetic replacement not longer used in the femoropopliteal region, the figures are far below those after nonoperative treatment. This is not only true for degree III and IV but also for degree II ischemia.

The upper limb is affected by atherosclerosis in a smaller number of cases than
the lower limb, the natural compensation by collaterals is more effective,
therefore the number of reconstructive procedures for the arms is limited.
Indications for arterial surgery can be deduced by the results obtained: It is
dependent on the general condition of the patient, the site and extent of stenoses and occlusions, hemodynamic considerations and the degree of ischemia. All
these factors have to be evaluated and critically considered.

The indication is mandatory in stage III and IV, rest pain with or without necrosis or gangrene. It is relative in stage II, where we are aggressive in aortoiliac disease and less so in femoropopliteal occlusions. The better the general condition of the patient, the hemodynamic situation to be expected after reconstruction and the worse the circulatory disturbance in the extremity the more aggressive should surgical intervention be considered.

Summary

Surgeons are aware of the fact that at best they can treat only local manifestations of this generalised disease. Their therapy is purely symptomatic — arteriosclerosis itself cannot be influenced with the scalpel.
It is hoped that the excellent basic research work of the scientists gathered here in Berlin will make the prevention of arteriosclerosis possible thus reducing more and more the need for surgical interventions.

If nevertheless vascular surgery still does play an important role in the treatment of some sequelae of arteriosclerosis this has 5 reasons:

1. Modern techniques of vascular surgery, anaesthesiology not to mention the management of blood replacement and coagulation disorders, have reduced the risk of these procedures to an acceptable level — usually well below the risk inherent in an amputation or expectant treatment.
2. Most arterial lesions — particularly those involving the bigger, central vessels — are well localised and therefore amenable to local therapy.
3. The underlying disease itself progresses but slowly so that localised surgical reconstruction can improve the quality of the patient's life, even if it can hardly prolong his life-expectancy.
4. Whereas the aim of peripheral vascular surgery is the preservation of a functioning limb, life itself can be saved by vascular reconstruction of certain vital arteries: the carotid, coronary, renal or visceral vessels.
5. Finally the very progress that is being made in prophylaxis and medical treatment of arteriosclerosis encourages the surgeon in his endeavours to treat locally disabling manifestations of this disease.

Abstracts

1. EPIDEMIOLOGY

Lp(a) LIPOPROTEIN: QUANTITATIVE GENETIC ANALYSIS

John Albers and William Hazzard
Departments of Medicine and Biochemistry, University of Washington School of
Medicine, Seattle, WA/USA

Lp(a) lipoprotein [Lp(a)] has been suggested to be a qualitative autosomal dominant genetic marker in 30-45% of humans but this has been challenged in later
studies. In order to test this question a sensitive radial immunodiffusion assay
was developed with a lower limit of sensitivity of 1.5 mg%. Utilizing this technique, 78% (975 of 1251) of this Seattle population, which included 300 mother-
father-offspring triplets, had Lp(a) levels above 1.5 mg%. The distribution of
Lp(a) was skewed with a mean of 10 ± 13 mg% and a median of 6 mg%. Significant
correlations were found between mother-offspring (r=0.34), father-offspring (r=
0.40) and midparent-offspring (r=0.52), whereas no correlation was found between
parent-parent (r=0.04). Offspring's Lp(a) values more closely approximated midparent values rather than either parent. No significant correlation (p<.05) was
found between Lp(a) and either cholesterol, triglyceride or age. Thus, these data
suggest that Lp(a) exhibits continuous quantitative variation determined by multifactorial genetic mechanism.

HEREDITY, ENVIRONMENT AND BIOCHEMICAL CORONARY RISK FACTORS

Daniel Brunner, Shmuel Altman, Jacob Bearman
Donolo Institute of Physiological Hygiene, Tel Aviv University, Tel Aviv/Israel

The aim of this study was to investigate the interplay of hereditary and environmental influences on coronary risk factors such as serum cholesterol (CH), beta
cholesterol percentage (BCH), triglycerides (TGL) and uric acid (UA). In 5 Israeli
collective settlements all males and females 16-18 years old and their healthy
parents were examined. These settlements are a society without familial and household eating pattern, and therefore avoid confounding of genetical effects with
environmental nutritional influences. A total of 90 fathers, 90 mothers, 52 boys
and 38 girls were examined. Correlation coefficient, extreme quartile analysis
and analysis of variance of family data were determined for each possible pair of
family members with regard to CH, BCH, TGL, and UA.

The findings provided little or no support for a predominant genetical hypothesis
for the determination of CH, BCH, TGL. Only a relationship between fathers and
children presented a potential correlation. As to uric acid all three methods of
analysis provided a consistent pattern of distinct genetic influences. These
results do not predict what may emerge when children reach middle age.

ß-LIPOPROTEIN, TOTAL CHOLESTEROL AND TRIGLYCERIDES IN ICELANDIC MALES AGED 4-61 YEARS

David Davidson, Nikulas Sigfusson, Olafur Olafsson, Otto J. Björnsson, and
Þorstein Þorsteinsson
Heart Preventive Clinic, Reykjavik/Iceland

Since 1967 the Icelandic Heart Association has been conducting a prospective
health survey in the Reykjavik area. This paper reports the results of ß-lipoprotein (ß-LP), total cholesterol (CH) and triglyceride (TG) determinations in
2,203 males examined in the first stage (1967-'68) of this survey. The response

was 75%. ß-LP was measured with Hyland Beta-L-Test, total CH according to a modification of the method of Levine and Zak and TG according to the method of Kessler and Lederer, both the latter on Technicon Auto-Analyzer. The mean and s.d. for these three lipids were as follows:
ß-lipoproteins: 2.2±0.6 mm immunocrit
Cholesterol: 254±44 mg/100 ml
Triglycerides: 96±50 mg/100 ml

The CH and TG mean values increase with age up to approx. 50 years and then fall slightly. The ß-LP mean values are fairly independent of age. The age-specific correlation coefficents are low and decrease with age.

PROSPECTIVE STUDY OF CORD BLOOD CHOLESTEROL TO PREDICT LEVEL OF CHOLESTEROL AND TYPE II HYPERLIPOPROTEINEMIA IN ADOLESCENCE

Iqbal Krishan, Curtis G. Hames, Hermann A. Tyroler, Caroline Becker
Evans County Heart Research Project, Claxton, GA/USA

Cholesterol levels were determined for paired maternal and cord bloods from 571 consecutive live births occurring between January 1958 and July 1960 in a biracial community in rural Georgia. Mean cord blood cholesterol was 80.5 mg/100 ml, and was not associated with the level of maternal cholesterol for any of the four race-sex groups.

An historic prospective study was undertaken to determine the feasibility of using cord blood cholesterol to predict adolescent cholesterol level and Type II hyperlipoproteinemia. The population of 571 paired maternal and cord bloods was stratified into three groups according to the level of cord blood cholesterol: ≤68, 69-89, and ≥90 mg/100 ml. Recall of approximately equal numbers from these three groups was accomplished between September and November 1972. Fasting blood samples of adolescents were obtained for lipid determinations. Cord blood cholesterol levels did not predict adolescent cholesterol levels in any of the race-sex groups. Additionally, cord blood cholesterol levels did not predict the presence of Type II hyperlipoproteinemia in adolescence.

PREVALENCE OF TYPE II HYPERLIPOPROTEINEMIA IN BELGIAN POSTMEN

Willy Page, André van Melsen, Yvette van Melsen, Francine Vanderveiken, and Marcel Vastesaeger
Center of Preventive Cardiology for Belgian Postmen

Agarose gel electrophoresis and serum lipid determinations (total cholesterol, alpha cholesterol, triglycerides and phospholipids) were performed in 3,250 postmen, all volunteers, aged 20 to 65. An original method of assessment of Fredrickson's types in proposed, based on the estimation of the serum level of the lipoproteins, expressed in terms of their cholesterol content. According to this method the prevalence of type II is 18% (586 of 3,250) (14% type IIa, 4% type IIb). When taking age into account, there is a progressive rise of the prevalence of type IIa till the age of 50: 2% (3 of 154) at 20-24 and 23% (91 of 395) at 50-54, and a decrease during the sixth decade. The behaviour of type IIb seems to be rather different: slow progressive increase with maximal values at the age of 40-45 (6% - 39 of 668) and no marked decrease afterwards.

SERUM LIPIDS IN MEXICAN WORKERS

Eduardo Zorilla, Alfredo Hernández, Clementina Magos, L.G. Deysach, J.E. Dutt, and Pedro A. Serrano
Instituto Nacional de Cardiologia, Mexico City/Mexico

In a randomized age stratified sample of 500 active workers of a factory, the following were determined: blood pressure, blood glucose, resting electrocardiogram (ECG), serum total cholesterol and triglycerides and electrophoresis of lipoproteins. A subgroup of 311 males free of diabetes, obesity or ECG abnormalities was used to define "normal" lipid levels for four age groups: 20-29, 30-39, 40-49 and 50-59.

The 95th percentile cholesterol levels, in mg/100 ml, for such age groups were: 251, 298, 301, and 288. The corresponding triglyceride levels were: 226, 272, 365 and 217. Using arbitrary limits 9% of these men (28 of 311) had hypercholesterolemia (>275 mg/100 ml) and 22% (68 of 311) had hypertriglyceridemia (>200 mg/100 ml). Type II lipoprotein pattern was found in 8% of the entire sample (41 of 500); type IV in 20% (102 of 500); and types I, III, and V were absent.

The findings indicate similarity of normal lipid levels of Mexican males with those of other men who belong to so-called developed populations, and suggest a high prevalence of hyperlipoproteinemia among dwellers of Mexican cities.

PLASMA LIPID AND LIPOPROTEIN CONCENTRATIONS IN RURAL CALIFORNIAN COMMUNITIES

Peter Wood, Michael Stern, William Haskell, Nathan Maccoby, and John Farquhar
Departments of Medicine and Communication, Stanford University, Stanford, CA/USA

As part of an ongoing coronary disease risk modification study, a survey was conducted of 747 males and 932 females (18% Mexican-Americans) selected randomly from three towns, each of 15,000 population (Watsonville, Gilroy and Tracy). A probability sample of dwellings was identified, and all occupants aged 35-59 were asked to participate (78% response).

Fasting plasma total cholesterol for all males (mean$\pm$SD, 210$\pm$35 mg/100 ml) was not significantly different from all females (208$\pm$37 mg/100 ml), although women had somewhat lower values than men in the younger age groups, and higher values in the older age groups. A random sub-sample of men (n=147) and of women (n=97) indicated that lower density lipoprotein cholesterol was lower for females than for males (125$\pm$33 vs 139$\pm$31 mg/100 ml; p<0.005), while high density lipoprotein cholesterol was higher for women than for men (57$\pm$14 vs 43$\pm$10 mg/100 ml; p<0.001). Very low density lipoprotein cholesterol was lower in all females than in all males, as judged by lower mean fasting triglyceride levels (123$\pm$92 vs 146$\pm$108 mg/100 ml; p<0.001). Conclusion: similar mean cholesterol levels for men and women may conceal sizeable differences in levels of specific lipoproteins.

PRE-BETA$_1$-LIPOPROTEIN: RELATIONSHIP TO ANGIOGRAPHICALLY PROVEN CORONARY HEART DISEASE AND TO Lp(a) LIPOPROTEIN

Kåre Berg, Gösta Dahlén, Curt Erikson, Heikki Frich, Curt Furberg, and Mauri Wiljasalo
Institute of Medical Genetics, University of Oslo, Oslo/Norway

In a population study in the Boden area of Northern Sweden an association between coronary heart disease (CHD) and an extra pre-ß-lipoprotein (pre-ß$_1$-lipoprotein) band upon electrophoresis on cellulose acetate was found.

This association has been confirmed in a study of Finnish patients with angiographically proven CHD. Pre-ß₁-lipoprotein was present in the sera of 55% of 20
patients with CHD and in 23% of sera from 26 persons without demonstrable obstruction.

Certain properties of the pre-ß₁-lipoprotein suggested that it could be related
to the lipoprotein possessing the Lp(a) antigen (Lp(a) lipoprotein). Consequently,
this series of people was studied with respect to a possible association. A strong
positive association between occurrence of pre-ß₁-lipoprotein and Lp(a) lipoprotein was found ($0.0005 < P < 0.001$).

INCIDENCE OF POSTEXERCISE ISCHEMIC ST DEPRESSION AND CORRELATIONS WITH METABOLIC FACTORS IN A SCREENED POPULATION

Robert Cristol, Jean Cottet, and Jacqueline Lieper
Centre Recherche de l'Athérosclérose et C.I.E.M., Paris/France

Data from annual health examinations of 600 male, middle-aged, apparently healthy
subjects were recorded by the same examiner, and included age, weight index, dietary and smoking habits, arterial pressure, pre and postexertionnal E.C.G. and
fasting serum glucose, cholesterol, triglycerides and uric acid. After double
test of Master, 30 subjects (5%) exhibited ischemic ST depression (> 1 mm) and
51 other cases only suspect ST depression (0,5 to 1 mm). Significant differences
for both groups compared to age-matched control groups, appeared only for triglycerides. In comparing the whole ST depression group to the whole control
group, significant differences exist for cholesterol, triglycerides, glucose and
weight index, but not for uric acid.

PRE-BETA-1 LIPOPROTEIN IN ISCHEMIC HEART DISEASE

Gosta Dahlén, Curt Ericson, and Curt Furberg
Central Hospital, Boden/Sweden

In a population study performed in northern Sweden an extra pre-beta lipoprotein
fraction, designated the pre-beta-1 fraction, was found in about 20% among 1,600
middle-aged men. This fraction occured in men with normal as well as high serum
lipids. In two families further studied it appeared that the occurence of the
pre-beta-1 fraction is genetically determined. In a subsample of 286 men from
the oldest age-groups a significant correlation was found between the occurrence
of this fraction and the information from a postal questionnaire that the patient
suffered from pain or discomfort in his chest when walking uphill or hurrying.
An even stronger correlation was found when the occurrence of pre-beta-1 was correlated to the clinical diagnosis of typical or suspected angina pectoris. There
was no such correlation to the serum lipids. In a study of 20 patients with a
history of myocardial infarction about two thirds had the pre-beta-1 fraction.
Changes in lipoprotein fractions after a standard test meal indicates that the
pre-beta-1 fraction is metabolically active. There is no certain effect of
clofibrate on the occurrence of the fraction.

QUANTITATIVE AND QUALITATIVE SERUM LIPOPROTEIN IN ANALYSES IN HEALTHY MEN COMPARED WITH MALE MYOCARDIAL INFARCTIONS AND INTERMITTENT CLAUDICATION

Martin Eriksson and Lars A.Carlson
Geriatric Clinic, Uppsala/Sweden

57 myocardial infarctions (MI) and 57 intermittent claudication (PVD) were compared with 80 healthy men 30 - 70 years old randomly selected from the Uppsala
region with regard to their lipoprotein pattern.

The following main results were obtained. The mean concentration of both triglycerides and cholesterol was significantly elevated in VLDL and LDL in MI and
that of cholesterol in HDL significantly lowered in MI as well as PVD compared
to controls. The frequency (%) of types of hyperlipidemia was: Normal pattern
44/81, IIA 17/5, IIB 11/5, IV 25/9, III 4/0 (MI/controls).Normal pattern 70/81,
IIA 17/5 IIB 5/5, IV 5/9, III 1/0 (PVD/controls). The frequency (%) of sinking
pre-beta lipoprotein was 38/26 (MI/controls) and 41/26 (PVD/controls).

ON THE STUDY OF LIPID METABOLISM INDICES IN THE AGED

Nodar N. Kipshidze,and Ramaz B. Kurashvili
Institute of Therapy, Ministry of Health of the Georgian SSR, Tbilisi/UdSSR

50 inhabitants age 90 - 105 were studied to manifest lipid metabolism changes
with ageing. The control group consisted of 30 healthy persons as well as 50
patients with atherosclerotic cardiosclerosis, age 35 to 80. The results of the
investigations are as follows: free cholesterol level in the aged was 39 mg%,
in the healthy control group - 58 mg% and in the deseased control group - 69 mg%;
total cholesterol was - 193 mg%, 208 mg% and 338 mg% respectively in each of the
studied groups; and triglycerides were 116 mg% in the aged, 176 mg% and 341 mg%
in the control groups -healthy and diseased. With the most aged normal type of
hyperlipoproteinemia prevailed and with some of them V and I types (according to
Fredrickson). Thus the following points should be noted: the content of total
and free cholesterol, triglyceride levels were less than normal and considerably
lower than in young, mature and elderly persons with atherosclerotic cardiosclerosis. The data obtained show the absence of active atherosclerosis in aged.

PLASMA LIPOPROTEIN ABNORMALITIES IN NORMAL AND ATHEROSCLEROTIC SUBJECTS IN FOUR CITIES

Barry Lewis, Alan Chait, Celia Oakley, Dennis Krikler, Lars Carlson, M. Ericsson,
Jonas Boberg, Mario Mancini, Pasquale Oriente, E. Paggi, Horace Micheli, Bogdan
Malczewski, Arvid Weisswange, and Daniel Pometta
Royal Postgraduate Medical School, London/England

A multicentre study is in progress, 1. to assess frequency of hyperlipoproteinaemias in unselected patients with ischaemic heart disease (IHD) and peripheral
vascular disease (PVD); 2. to identify within and compare between apparently
healthy populations the frequency of hyperlipidaemias. Preparative ultracentrifugation is employed. In 220 men with IHD, raised very low density lipoprotein
(VLDL) cholesterol and triglyceride levels were commonest (e.g. in London and
Uppsala VLDL cholesterol 240 and 195%, VLDL triglyceride 225 and 185% of normal).
Raised VLDL occurred in 31, 25, and 20% of IHD patients in London, Uppsala and
Geneva respectively. Raised levels of low-density lipoprotein (LDL) or LDL and
VLDL were less common. Of 140 PVD patients, 30% in Uppsala, 54% in London had
hyperlipidaemia IV. Fat tolerance was impaired in IHD and PVD. Remarkably high
proportions of most communities had cholesterol levels > 300 mg/100 ml., triglyceride > 2.0 mM/L: in Uppsala (n = 80), Geneva (123), London (139) and Naples
(71). The proportions with higher cholesterol levels were 10, 6, 5, and 0%; those
with higher triglyceride levels were 25, 19, 18 and 15%.

HYPERLIPOPROTEINAEMIAS IN THE WEST OF SCOTLAND

Ross Lorimer, Thomas D.V. Lawrie, David Ballantyne, Victor Hawthorne, David
Greaves, Janet Jubb, and Henry G. Morgan
University Department of Medical Cardiology, Royal Infirmary, Glasgow/Scotland

A study was made of 4,474 apparently healthy males (ages 35-59) at work in the
West of Scotland. Investigations included fasting cholesterol, triglyceride,
electrophoresis and preparative ultracentrifugation. Lipoprotein typing was based
on the results. Subjects were divided into 'normal' and 'abnormal' on the basis
of blood pressure, ECG, cigarette smoking and obesity. The mean plasma cholesterol values in the total group varied only slightly with age whereas the highest
mean triglyceride value occurred in the 40-44 age group and then fell. Thirty-
eight point three per cent of the population had a cholesterol value above 240
mg% and 13.3% above 275 mg%. The overall prevalence of type II hyperlipoproteinaemia was 3.3% and of type IV was 12%. The prevalence of type II abnormality was
similar in the normal and abnormal subgroups but type IV was significantly less
prevalent in the normal (7.2%) than in the abnormal (14.1%). Seventeen per cent
of subjects who were obese, but otherwise normal, had a type IV abnormality. Thus
lipoprotein abnormalities occurred in 15% of an apparently healthy male population. These findings may be relevant to the high incidence of coronary heart
disease in the area.

HYPERLIPOPROTEINEMIA IN PATIENTS WITH MYOCARDIAL INFARCTION, ANGINA PECTORIS AND IN "NORMALS"

Uwe Stocksmeier
Working group for Long-Term Studies, Bernried-Höhenried/BRD

In 1,050 patients with hypercholesterinemia and/or hypertriglyceridemia we
analysed the Fredrickson classification by lipoprotein electrophoresis. In more
than 40% we found primary hyperlipoproteinemia. In the other, the most additional
disease has been diabetes mellitus; the other disease will be discussed. In the
"secondary-group" nearly 85% have had hypertriglyceridemia. In patients with
primary hyperlipemia more had type IV than II and III. Some cases with V will
be analysed. Difficulties of classification are shown.

THE PREVALENCE OF HYPERLIPOPROTEINAEMIAS IN A RANDOM SAMPLE OF MEN AND IN PATIENTS WITH ISCHAEMIC HEART DISEASE

Maurice C. Stone and Thomas B.S. Dick
Clinical Research Unit, Leigh Infirmary, Leigh, Lancashire/UK

Lipoprotein patterns were estimated by membrane filtration and nephelometry in a
random sample of men aged 30 - 69 years, and in an age matched group of male
patients with ischaemic heart disease (IHD). Abnormal lipoprotein patterns were
found in 19.4% of the random sample (55 of 283) and 40.4% of the IHD group (59 of
146).

The frequency distribution of the different types of hyperlipoproteinaemia was
similar in the two groups. In the random sample 17 of the 55 abnormal patterns
(31%) were type IIa, 7 (12.7%) were type IIb, 29 (52.7%) were type IV and 2
(3.7%) type V.

Severe hyperlipoproteinaemias (in which S_f 0-20 exceeded 700 mg/100 ml., or S_f
20-400 exceeded 500 mg/100 ml) were found in 3.2% of the random sample (9 of 283)
and 6.8% of the IHD group (10 of 146).

In the random sample, obese subjects (judged by skinfold thickness) had a significantly greater prevalence of hyperlipoproteinaemias (34%) than slim ones (9.0%). In the IHD subjects, however, the difference was smaller (48% v 29%) and not statistically significant. Slim IHD subjects had a three times greater prevalence of type IV than slim subjects in the random sample.

RELATION OF SERUM LIPOPROTEINS AND LIPIDS TO AORTIC ATHEROSCLEROSIS IN HYPERTENSIVE PATIENTS

Robert C. Tarazi and Lena A. Lewis
Cleveland Clinic Foundation, Cleveland, OH/USA

Serum lipids and lipoproteins were studied in 54 hypertensive patients of the Research Department; 21 males, 33 females, median age of 46 years (35 - 60 years). Twenty-eight of the 54 had atherosclerosis of the abdominal aorta as demonstrated by arteriography while 26 had no demonstrable lesions. There was no difference in the incidence of aortic atherosclerosis between hypertensives with essential hypertension and those with renal arterial disease. The incidence of abnormal serum lipoprotein patterns and elevated lipid levels was similar in hypertensives with (54.6% abnormal) or without (46%) aortic atherosclerosis. Serum lipid and lipoprotein abnormalities included those characteristic of types II-A, II-B and IV. No one type was characteristic of the hypertensives. In contrast, among normotensive subjects studied by coronary arteriography, lipid abnormalities were significantly more frequent in those with than without atherosclerosis (63% vs. 10%). Thus hypertension per se appeared a more dominant factor in aortic atherosclerosis than serum lipids and lipoproteins.

"RISK FACTORS" IN WEST-GERMAN PATIENTS WITH ANGIOGRAPHICALLY DOCUMENTED CORONARY HEART DISEASE

W. Kübler, D. Breithard, F.A. Gries, H. Klinger, Th. Koschinsky, F. Loogen, D. Schütz, and K.H. Vogelberg
1. Medizinische Klinik B, Düsseldorf/BRD

Among 541 patients who underwent coronary angiography "risk factors" were till now systematically analyzed in 71 subjects. The changes observed in the coronary arteries are graded into four groups of increasing severity. "Risk factors" are correlated with the grade of the severity of the coronary heart disease, the involvement of the number of coronary arteries and the changes on the peripheral circulation assessed by clinical routine methods. There is a significant relation between the graded severity of the coronary heart disease and arteriosclerosis of the peripheral arteries, the serum cholesterol, the number of "risk factors" present and type 0 and type II hyperlipoproteinemia. To date a significant relation between type IV hyperlipoproteinemia and the graded severity of the coronary heart disease could not be observed, furthermore, there is even no tendency of increasing blood pressure with more severe coronary lesions.

HYPERLIPOPROTEINAEMIA IN PATIENTS OF ACUTE MYOCARDIAL INFARCTION IN CHANDIGARH (INDIA)

M. Kumar, Avtar Singh, R.N. Chakravarti, and P.L. Wahi
Departments of Experimental Medicine and Internal Medicine, Post-graduate Institute of Medical Education and Research, Chandigarh/India

There are no reports available describing serum cholesterol, triglycerides, phospholipids and lipoprotein values of patients following acute myocardial infarction (AMI) in this part of the world where the dietary habits and socio-economic stress are different from that of the western world. This information may help to plan suitable diets after AMI and in retrospect to give dietetic counsel to the vulnerable group. Serial lipid (cholesterol, phospholipids and triglycerides) and lipoprotein (using cellulose acetate electrophoresis) profile was studied in patients of AMI for a period of at least 3 weeks to elucidate the changes in different lipid fractions with the clinical progress of the patients.

THE RELATIONSHIP OF RISK FACTORS TO ANGIOGRAPHIC APPEARANCES IN YOUNG PATIENTS WITH CARDIAC INFARCTION

Peter A. Valentine and Graeme J. Sloman
Royal Melbourne Hospital, Melbourne/Australia

Coronary angiography was performed and risk factors assessed in 45 patients who sustained cardiac infarction under 40 years of age. Coronary lesions were numerically scored according to severity of stenosis and also the longitudinal extent of disease.

There was a direct relationship between lipid concentration and angiographic score. This relationship held both for cholesterol and triglycerides, for all three coronary arteries whether considered separately or together and whether the occlusive process was assessed longitudinally or transversly.

Women and heavy smokers with normal blood lipids tended to have mild and discrete rather than diffuse involvement. Blood lipids were normal in all 6 patients with angiographically normal coronary arteries.

It would seem that there are at least two types of coronary lesions and that the type of lesion can be predicted from knowledge of risk factors present.

HYPERLIPOPROTEINAEMIA, PERIPHERAL VASCULAR DISEASE AND ECG ABNORMALITIES

David Ballantyne, Henry G. Morgan, and Thomas D.V. Lawrie
University Department of Medical Cardiology and University Department of Pathological Biochemistry, Royal Infirmary, Glasgow/Scotland

Three hundred and fifty three consecutive patients with peripheral vascular disease were investigated for hyperlipoproteinaemia. These were then correlated with electrocardiographic abnormalities. A hyperlipoproteinaemia was found in 32% of 266 males and in 47% of 87 females. In males, type IIa hyperlipoproteinaemia occurred in 7.5%, type IIb in 6.5% and type IV in 18% whereas in females type IIa hyperlipoproteinaemia was found in 29%, type IIb in 4.5% and type IV in 12.5%. One female had a type III. The prevalence of type IIa hyperlipoproteinaemia was significantly greater in females than males. No sex difference was found in the prevalence of types IIb or IV.

Twenty eight per cent had ECG evidence of myocardial ischaemia or infarction. The prevalence of type IIa and b hyperlipoproteinaemia was significantly greater in this group than in patients with a normal ECG. These findings suggest that in patients with peripheral vascular disease those with type IIa or b hyperlipoproteinaemia are more likely to have associated coronary heart disease.

LIPOPROTEIN PATTERNS IN PATIENTS WITH PERIPHERAL ARTERIAL DISEASE

Renato Fellin, Piergiorgio Settembrini, Giustina Briani, Silvio Marchetto, and
Gaetano Crepaldi
Clinica Medica Generale, Universita di Padua, Padua/Italia

A study of lipoprotein and lipid patterns was carried out in 58 male patients
with peripheral arterial disease (PAD) (mean age 51.4). Serum lipoproteins (LP)
were determined by micronephelometry. Serum cholesterol (TC) and triglycerides
(TG) were also evaluated. Comparison according to age classes were made with 68
normal males (mean age 48,9). Medium (M) particles (corresponding to Sf 20-400)
and TG were significantly higher in PAD patients than in controls (177±18 vs 111
±5 mg%; 183±16 vs 120±5 mg%, respectively). No significant differences were observed for small (S)particles (Sf 0-20), large (L) particles (Sf >400) and TC.
In PAD patients, 36% (21 of 58) LP patterns were considered abnormal as follows:
13 M (or type IV), two S (or type IIA); three SM (or type IIB), two ML and one
SML (or type V). Abnormal type M patterns, corresponding to Fredrickson's type IV,
appear to be the prevalent LP abnormality in patients with PAD.

RISK FACTORS AND ANGIOGRAPHICAL AMOUNT OF HUMAN ATHEROSCLEROSIS

Franco Pratesi, Alfrede Nuti, and Carlo Deidda
Institute of Angiology, Main Regional Hospital, Florence/Italy

200 patients suffering from atherosclerosis obliterans of the lower limbs were
divided into two groups on the basis of the amount of their atherosclerosis. This
amount was judged on the basis of angiographical examination, and not on the
basis of the clinical manifestations of the disease.

In the two groups the incidence of the following risk factors was studied:
1. blood pressure, 2. cholesterolemia, 3. beta/alpha in the lipoprotidemia,
4. tabagism, 5. diabetes.

The results indicate that the risk factors for the amount of atherosclerosis are
different from the risk factors for the gravity of the clinical manifestations in
atherosclerosis.

PRIMARY HYPERLIPOPROTEINEMIA AND OTHER "RISK FACTORS" IN PATIENTS WITH ARTERIAL OCCLUSIVE DISEASE OF THE LOWER LIMB

K.H. Vogelberg, H. Berger, F.A. Gries, Th. Koschinsky, W. Kübler, E. Schütz, and
Th. Stoltze
II. Medizinische Klinik und Poliklinik, Düsseldorf/BRD

In 72 patients with angiographically documented arteriosclerosis of the pelvic
and leg arteries the incidence of hyperlipoproteinemias and other "risk factors"
was examined. Extent and localization of the arteriosclerotic lesions were analyzed with respect to the occurence of the different "risk factors". Patients
with nicotin consumption as the only "risk factor" exhibited predominant arteriosclerotic lesions in the femoral arteries. With concomitant hyperlipoproteinemia
type II the pelvic arteries and with types II and IV the arteries of the lower
legs were in addition affected to a more severe degree. Type IV was more common
in patients over the age of 60 and often combined with obesity and abnormal glucose tolerance. In patients under the age of 60 years type II was predominant.
From these results a greater risk of arterial occlusive disease for patients with
type II compared with those of type IV can be suggested.

RELATIONSHIP OF PLASMA LIPIDS AND LIPOPROTEINS TO CEREBRAL ATHEROSCLEROSIS AND ECG FINDINGS

David Ballantyne, Kenneth W.G. Grossart, John P. Ballantyne, Alister Young, and Thomas D.V. Lawrie
University Department of Medical Cardiology, Royal Infirmary and Institute of Neurological Sciences, Glasgow/Scotland

The study was undertaken to investigate the interrelationship of plasma lipid and lipoprotein concentrations, coronary atheroma and cerebral atheroma in middle aged patients. Fasting plasma lipid and lipoprotein concentrations were measured and 12 lead ECG performed in 100 consecutive middle aged patients (57 males, 43 females - mean age 51) admitted for diagnostic carotid angiography. Forty patients had evidence of cerebral atheroma. Plasma lipid and lipoprotein concentrations in this group were similar to those found in the 60 subjects without cerebral atheroma. Twenty three of the 100 subjects had ECG changes indicative of myocardial ischaemia or infarction and mean plasma cholesterol and low density lipoprotein cholesterol concentrations were significantly higher in these patients compared to the value found in those with a normal ECG. These results indicate that there is no relationship between plasma lipid and lipoprotein concentrations and cerebral atheroma.

STUDIES ON SERUM LIPIDS IN ATHEROSCLEROTIC CEREBRO-VASCULAR DISEASE

Giustina Briani, Renato Fellin, Sebastiano Schiavon, and Gaetano Crepaldi
Clinica Medica Generale, Universita di Padua, Padua/Italia

Serum lipids and lipoprotein (LP), agarose gel electrophoretic patterns, were determined in 52 patients, aged over 60, with atherosclerotic cerebro-vascular disease (ACVD). As a comparison 83 controls of same age were considered. Group 60-69 ACVD patients showed a significant increase of serum triglycerides (TG) (in males 167 ± 20 vs 107 ± 7 mg%; in females 132 ± 14 vs 96 ± 8 mg%, respectively), and a significant decrease of serum cholesterol (TC) (in males 178 ± 9 vs 198 ± 5 mg%; in females 168 ± 10 vs 201 ± 5 mg%, respectively). Group >70 ACVD patients did not show any lipid abnormalities. Serum lipids increased in 35% (18 of 52) ACVD patients: in two TC increased, in 14 TG and in two TC and TG. LP electrophoresis showed a poor correlation between TG values and prebeta bands, that were often absent or slightly evident even with normal or elevated serum TG. These findings suggest some abnormalities of LP lipid contents in ACVD patients.

FREQUENCY OF MYOCARDIAL INFARCTION IN FAMILIES OF PATIENTS WITH HYPERTRIGLYCERIDEMIA

John Brunzell, Helmut Schrott, Joseph Goldstein, Arno Motulsky, and Edwin Bierman
Department of Medicine, University of Washington and VA Hospital, Seattle, WA/USA

Thre autosomal dominant forms of hyperlipidemia were identified by us in patients with myocardial infarction (MI). To compare the genetics of hypertriglyceridemia ($\uparrow$TG) in patients without MI to the earlier studies and to assess the frequency of MI in $\uparrow$TG, family studies were done on 56 patients referred for $\uparrow$TG. Three patients had non-familial $\uparrow$TG. Thirteen families were found to have pure Familial Hypertriglyceridemia (FHTG). Eleven had Familial Combined Hyperlipidemia (CHL), in which affected relatives had $\uparrow$TG and hypercholesterolemia together or elevations of cholesterol or TG alone.

Each genetic disorder appeared to segregate as a discrete autosomal dominant condition with full expression after 29 years of age. CHL was more common in the MI population, while FHIG was more common in the present series selected for $\uparrow$TG only.

MI was significantly more frequent in living hyperlipidemic relatives with CHL (7/26, 26.9%) than FHTG (2/40, 5.0%), or in normolipidemic relatives (2/84, 3.0%), or spouse controls (5/69, 5.8%). In 4/7 with CHL the MI occurred before the age of 40, as compared to two patients with FHTG (ages 50 and 60). These data substandiate the existence of Familial Combined Hyperlipidemia as a genetic entity and demonstrate its role as a risk factor for MI.

ISCHEMIC VASCULAR DISEASE IN FAMILIAL HYPERLIPOPROTEINEMIA WITH XANTHOMATOSIS. A STUDY OF 244 CASES

Bernard Jacotot, Philippe Sébastien, Violette Beaumont et Jean-Louis Beaumont
Unité de Recherches sur l'Athérosclérose de l'INSERM, Hôpital Henri-Mondor,
Créteil/France

A retrospective study on 244 cases of familial hyperlipoproteinemia with xanthomatosis was performed. The clinical features were related to coronary artery disease in most cases (58.8%) and to a lesser degree to arteriopathy of the lower limbs (18.8%) and cerebrovascular disease (15.2%). A total of 70% of patients had one or several arterial thrombosis.

In the present work, age of onset of the ischemic disease, sex ratio, topographic distribution and correlations of the different vascular diseases with other clinical and biological findings are investigated.

TYPE III HYPERLIPOPROTEINEMIA: A GENETIC STUDY WITH AN ACCOUNT OF THE RISKS OF CORONARY DEATH IN FIRST DEGREE RELATIVES

Hans Moser, Joan Slack, and Peter Borrie
M.R.C. Clinical Genetics Unit, London/England

From 25 index patients with type III hyperlipoproteinemia (HL), 20 families have been studied. Information has been obtained on all 98 first degree relatives (1st°Rels) of which 29 were dead. In 5 families one or more 1st°Rels had type III HL, including one parent. There was no consanguinity. The findings were not compatible with any simple Mendelian inheritance.

Investigation of fasting serum cholesterol and triglycerides, electrophoresis, lipid composition of VLDL and the distribution of lipoproteins on analytical ultracentrifugation showed no sign of bimodal segregation among 1st°Rels.

Life tables were used to examine the life experience of 1st°Rels. There was a small increase in risk of coronary death which was 1.8 times the expected risk in the general population. The increase was largely due to a 2.5 fold increase in coronary death among male relatives over 55 years. None of the increase was statistically significant. By comparison with the known high risk to 1st°Rels of patients with Familial type II HL there was a significantly lower coronary mortality rate in type III.

We conclude that the mode of inheritance of type III HL is polygenic with pronounced environmental influences and that the risk of coronary death among 1st°Rels is small.

SIGNS OF CORONARY AND PERIPHERAL ATHEROSCLEROSIS IN DIFFERENT TYPES OF ASYMPTOMATIC HYPERLIPOPROTEINAEMIA

Anders G. Olsson, Lars A. Carlson, Lars-Göran Ekelund, and Brita Eklund
King Gustaf V Research Institute, Stockholm/Sweden

In patients with hyperlipidaemia (IIL) but without symptoms of atherosclerosis the occurrence of signs of coronary insufficiency and obliterations of peripheral arteries was investigated. HL patients and controls (C) were selected from a health control. Serum was typed after separation in the preparative ultracentrifuge into VLDL, LDL and HDL and on paper electrophoresis. Exercise ECG and digital pulse plethysmography bilaterally on lower extremities were performed. The frequency of ischemic ST segment depressions differed between C (16%, 11 of 70) and type IIA (57%, 25 of 44), $p<0.001$, type IIB (72%, 18 of 25), $p<0.001$ and type IV (35%, 27 of 77), $p<0.01$. ST depressions occurred earliest in type IIB. Inclination time during digital plethysmography was prolonged in type IIA ($p<0.05$) and type IIB ($p<0.01$) above age 50 when compared to C.

In asymptomatic HL the occurrence of signs of coronary atherosclerosis is increased in type IIA, IIB and IV, type IIB being the most malignant one. Signs of peripheral atherosclerosis are seen in type IIA and IIB at ages above 50 years.

CORONARY AND PERIPHERAL ARTERY RESERVE IN DIFFERENT TYPES OF HYPERLIPOPROTEINEMIA

Jürgen Schneider, Achim Neitzert, Günther and Ortrun Mühlfellner, Peter Zöfel, Christian Eltze, Gerhard Fürst, and Hans Kaffarnik
Medizinische Poliklinik der Universität Marburg a.d. Lahn/BRD

In 194 outpatients with different types of hyperlipoproteinemia and in 181 normolipemic control patients occurrence of myocardial infarction (MI) was stated.

Coronary and peripheral artery reserve was studied in 100 hyper- and 61 normolipidemics out of these patients without manifestation of degenerative artery disease by ergometry and venous occlusion plethysmography.

The results obtained indicate that in groups with 56-58 years of mean age manifest MI is found predominantly in type IV patients and the surprising fact of high incidence of impaired reserve blood flow in type IIa.

CORONARY ARTERY DISEASE IN FAMILIAL TYPE II HYPERLIPOPROTEINEMIA: STUDY OF 116 KINDREDS

Neil Stone, Robert Levy, Donald Fredrickson, and Joel Verter
N.I.H., Bethesda, MD/USA

Conflicting data regarding Coronary Artery Disease (CAD) risk in type II, compel reassessment of risk in members of affected families, omitting propositi to avoid bias. The relatives over age 19 of 116 propositi with type II were chosen for analysis of CAD risk. In over 90% of the 754 living relatives, interview by one investigator and 12 lead electrocardiogram were obtained. In these, and in 295 deceased relatives, physician and hospital records were utilized as needed to determine CAD events. CAD was diagnosed in 29.6% of relatives with type II (II's) compared to 10.5% of normal relatives (N's)($p<.001$). The II's and N's did not differ significantly with regard to age distribution, sex, hypertension, smoking or diabetes. Angina pectoris by Rose questionnaire was noted in 21.9% of II's and 6.4% of N's. ($p<.001$.) Documented myocardial infarction (MI) occurred in 6% of II's versus 1% of N's. ($p=.002$) CAD death or MI occurred in 10.1% of II's contrasted with 1.8% of N's ($p<.001$). Life table analysis in males showed the cumulative probability (CP) of initial nonfatal CAD before age 40 to be 10.2% in II's and .5% in N's; before age 50 CP was 29% in II's compared with 4.4% in N's. CP of fatal and nonfatal CAD in males before age 40 was 16% in II's and .5% in N's. In this, the largest study of type II kindreds, thus far, CAD events occur more frequently and earlier in life in II's than in N's.

2. GENERAL ABSTRACTS

EXPERIMENTAL ATHEROGENESIS IN WISTAR RATS

Daniel Aubert, Jean-Claude Ferrand, Bernard Lacaze, Edouard Panak, Odile Pépin, and Marielle Podesta
Centre d'Etudes pour l'Industrie Pharmaceutique, Toulouse-Cedex/France

The aim of the study was to set up a pharmacological model for the induction of atheromatous lesions in rats.

Out of 1080 Wistar rats , 439 rats were used preliminarily to find out the best atherogenic regimen : oral Vitamin D_2, a relatively low cholesterol diet (0.5%), but no blockade of the thyroid function.

641 rats given this regimen showed:

- within the first week, a disruption of the elastic fibers and an increase in acid mucopolysaccharides in 70 - 90% of them according to the different batches;
- within one month the development of atheroma in the injured but regenerating wall;
- a marked increase in serum cholesterol (threefold) and a moderate one in triglycerides;
- on agar gel electrophoresis, a reversal of the pattern, with around 80% of ß and pre-ß lipoproteins.

After 6 weeks, cholesterol diet was discontinued, resulting in disappearance of lipidic deposits. Control animals (vitamin D_2 but no cholesterol) showed wall injury but no atheroma.

These atheromatous lesions, induced in an animal known as resistant, imitate most features of the early fatty streak of human atherosclerosis. The rapid onset of the lesions makes this model a suitable method for the screening of hypocholesterolemic agents.

A "PLASMA CHOLESTEROL INDEX" FOR THE MORE PRECISE PREDICTION OF ATHEROSCLEROTIC LESION FORMATION IN EXPERIMENTAL ANIMALS

David E. Bowyer, J. Stephen Cridland, Jeremy D. Pearson, Janice P. King, and Michael A. Reidy
Department of Pathology, University of Cambridge, Cambridge/England

Precise dietary production of atherosclerosis is complicated by genetically determined variability in induction of hypercholesterolaemia. This variation causes difficulties in predicting onset of lesions and assessing effects of treatments such as drugs.

We show that arterial lipid accumulation can be predicted more precisely by measuring a plasma cholesterol index, I b, from the area under the curve of plasma cholesterol concentration, C above a basal level, b, plotted against time, t:

$$I\ b = \int_{t1}^{t2} (C-b)dt \qquad g\ days/1.$$

At a critical value of I 100 (=200, in New Zealand White rabbits) there is a sharp increase in cholesterol esters and overt fatty streaks appear. If the arterial wall is damaged, lipid accumulation occurs before predicted by I. The method shows that accumulation of cholesterol esters occurs more rapidly than is usually supposed. It offers a technique for the study of factors which promote or diminish lesion formation without alteration of plasma cholesterol concentration.

STUDIES ON CHOLESTEROL ESTERASE ACTIVITY IN MONKEY AND RAT AORTA

P.I. Brecher, M. Kessler, and A.V. Chobanian
Boston University Medical Center, Boston, MA/USA

Cholesterol esterase activity has been examined in aortic tissue from rat and Rhesus monkey. Hydrolytic activity was observed in both microsomal and high speed supernatant fractions. The enzyme was cofactor independent, was not affected by the addition of bile salts, and was not readily reversible. The activity was not influenced by the addition of cholesterol but was inhibited by fatty acids. The mode of substrate introduction markedly influenced the degree of hydrolysis observed. Labeled cholesteryl esters introduced as acetone solutions were hydrolyzed to a relatively large extent while other forms of substrate introduction were less effective. Cholesteryl esters presented in the form of lipid droplets isolated from arterial lesions and from adrenal cells were not readily hydrolyzed by the aortic homogenates. Unsaturated fatty acid esters of cholesterol were hydrolyzed to a greater extent than the saturated esters in both high speed supernatant and microsomal fractions and in both normal and atherosclerotic aortas. No significant differences in cholesteryl ester hydrolysis were observed between normal or atherosclerotic monkey aorta.

EFFECT OF HYPERTENSION ON THE LIPID CONTENT AND METABOLISM OF DIFFERENT AREAS OF THE AORTIC INTIMA IN RABBITS

K.N. Bretherton, Allan J. Day, and S.L. Skinner
Department of Physiology, University of Melbourne, Parkville/Australia

Hypertension produced by cellophane perinephritis was studied for nine weeks in normal and cholesterol-fed (CF) rabbits. Increases in the cholesterol and lipid P content occurred in the arch, thoracic and abdominal segments of the aortas in both normal and CF rabbits. The concentration of cholesterol and of lipid P in the intima also increased in the CF rabbit, particularly in the thoracic segment (total cholesterol 227 and 35 μg/mg dry weight in hypertensive and normotensive respectively). Incubation in vitro of $(1-^{14}C)$ acetate and $(1-^{14}C)$-oleate with aortas from hypertensive and normotensive rabbits (CF and normal-fed) indicated increased incorporation of both these precursors into cholesterol ester with hypertension. The increased incorporation into cholesterol ester correlated with the intimal cholesterol concentration. Incubation in vitro of ^{32}P phosphate with aortas from normotensive and hypertensive rabbits indicated increased incorporation into lecithin with hypertension in the cholesterol-fed rabbit. No change in other phospholipid fractions was apparent.

ATHEROSCLEROTIC CHANGES IN CASES OF TRAUMATIC ACCIDENTAL DEATH

Daniel Brunner, Heinrich Karplus, and Izchak Metrani
Institute of Physiological Hygiene, Tel Aviv University, Tel Aviv/Israel

At the necropsis of 376 consecutive male cases of sudden traumatic accidental
death cross section at distances of 1 cm in each of the 3 main coronary branches
were performed, and the percentage decrease in luminal caliber calculated. Constriction of functional importance were indicated by score 5 for obstruction of
50-74%, score 6 for 75-89% and score 7 for more than 90% of the lumen or complete
occlusion. Scores of 7 in each of the 3 main vessels were found in 3 of 163 subjects aged 30-49, in 5 out of 81 aged 50-59, in 10 out of 64 aged 60-69, and in
10 out of 66 older than 70 years. The corresponding figures for subjects with
scores of 7 in two coronary arteries was 5, 8, 11 and 19. Close correlation between the severity of coronary narrowing and aorta arteriosclerosis and/or cerebral atherosclerosis as well as between heart weight and coronary atherosclerosis was found. Significant differences between subjects of European and non-
European origin were found. In subjects younger than 60 years there existed also
a correlation between ponderal index and narrowing of the right and the left
coronary artery, but not of the descending branch.

IN VIVO STUDY OF LYSIS OF THROMBO-EMBOLI IN INTRARENAL ARTERIES OF NORMAL AND LIPAEMIC MONKEYS

R.N. Chakravarti, S.P. Singh, M. Kumar, and K.C. Das
Departments of Experimental Medicine and Pathology, Post-graduate Institute of
Medical Education and Research, Chandigarh/India

Dynamics of lysis of standard dose of radioactive homologous fibrin clots introduced intraaortically in normal and high fat-cholesterol induced lipaemic monkeys
(Macaca mulatta) have been studied. Animals were laparotomised and injected near
the origin of left renal artery 3-4 million CPM of ^{125}I fibrin per animal. Monkeys were sacrificed up to 10 days postembolisation. Blood coagulation, euglobulin clot lysis time, ^{125}I counts in blood and kidneys were determined. Autoradiography and histopathology of kidneys were carried out to determine the thromboembolic index at various times. Half life of isotope both in kidney and blood of
the normal animals appeared to be less than that of the lipaemic monkeys. A good
correlation was found in radioactive counts, autoradiography and thrombo-embolic
index.

INCREASED FACTOR XIII ACTIVITY IN ENDOGENOUS HYPERTRIGLYCERIDEMIA

Mircea Cucuianu, Augustin Opincaru, Vasile Vasile, Titus Popescu
Medical Clinic I, Cluj/Roumania

When compared to values detected in 49 normal weight normolipemic subjects, factor XIII activity measured according to Heene was found to be increased in 102
hyperlipemic subjects with or without clinical atherosclerosis. This increase was
particularly obvious in hypertriglyceridemic patients (type II b and IV) while
factor XIII level was not significantly changed in pure hypercholesterolemia
(type II a). Hypertriglyceridemic patients also had higher levels of pseudo-
cholinesterase (PCE). Factor XIII activity was positively correlated with both
log. of serum triglyceride concentration (r = 490; p <0.01) and serum PCE (r =
742; p <0.01).
The hypothesis of an enhanced synthesis of proteins such as factor XIII and PCE
in the liver of subjects with endogenous hypertriglyceridemia is presented. Correction of hypertriglyceridemia by clofibrate therapy associated with low carbohydrate reduction diet was accompanied by a decrease of factor XIII activity but
had no effect on serum PCE levels.

SCANNING ELECTRON MICROSCOPY OF RABBIT AORTA STAINED WITH SILVER - A METHOD OF EVALUATING THE STRUCTURAL INTEGRITY OF THE ENDOTHELIUM

Peter F. Davies, Charles Twort, and David E. Bowyer
Department of Pathology, University of Cambridge, Cambridge/England

There is a need for a method of assessing the integrity of arterial endothelial cells. Treatment of rabbit aorta with silver salt solution stains what are believed to be intercellular junctions of endothelial cells. These silver lines have been viewed by scanning electron microscopy. Fixation at physiological pressure followed by dehydration on a frame to prevent contraction showed the endothelial cell layer as a flat sheet with the individual cells clearly outlined. There was little evidence of 'bridges' between cells when samples were carefully prepared. Disruption of cells during sample preparation or by various treatments led to the appearance of intercellular 'bridges' and loss of endothelial silver lines. These 'bridges' are considered to be artifacts of preparation resulting from contraction and partial folding of endothelial cells. The effects of deliberate disruption of endothelial cells by hypotonic solutions and by EDTA solutions are shown by this method.

LIPID COMPOSITION AND METABOLISM OF THROMBO-ATHEROSCLEROTIC LESIONS PRODUCED BY CONTINUED ENDOTHELIAL DAMAGE IN NORMAL RABBITS

Allan J. Day, Frank P. Bell, Sean Moore, and Robert Friedman
Department of Pathology, McMaster University, Hamilton, Ontario/Canada

Atherosclerotic lesions were produced by endothelial damage with polythene catheters inserted into the aorta in normal-fed rabbits. Two weeks after insertion, the mean concentrations of free and ester cholesterol in the lesions were 1,261 and 114 µg/mg of DNA respectively compared to 577 and 17 µg/mg of DNA in the adjacent normal intima. At four months free and ester cholesterol concentrations had risen in the lesion to 1,523 and 597 µg/mg of DNA respectively. Gas liquid chromatography indicated that the cholesterol esters in the lesion were higher in oleic acid and lower in linoleic acid than in the normal intima. Incorporation of $(1-^{14}C)$-oleic acid in the damaged aortas incubated in vitro showed that by two weeks two to three times as much oleic acid was incorporated into cholesterol ester in the lesion than in the normal intima. A similar increase was demonstrated at two months and four months. When ^{32}P-phosphate was used as precursor incorporation into lecithin was higher and into phosphatidyl inositol lower in the lesion than in the normal intima.

IN VITRO UPTAKE OF ^{125}I-LABELLED BETA-LIPOPROTEIN BY HEMODYNAMICALLY DIFFERENT AREAS OF RABBIT AORTA

Róbert Dénes, Sándor Virág. Antal Kóczé, and Mária Stützel
Semmelweis University of Medicine, Third Department of Medicine, Budapest/Hungary

Hemodynamic factors are supposed to influence the distribution of atheromatous lesions in the aortic wall. In our previous study we were able to correlate the in vitro incorporation of beta-lipoprotein with the species differences in susceptibility towards experimentally induced atherosclerosis. In our present investigations aortas of untreated rabbits were incubated in an in vitro system with ^{125}I-beta-lipoprotein. Following the incubation each aorta was cut into several pieces according to a previously established scheme. The radioactivity of each area was expressed as count/min/mg dry tissue. The results indicate a correlation between the hemodynamic pattern and the incorporation of labelled beta-lipoprotein.

DISTURBANCES IN PULMONARY GASEOUS EXCHANGE IN HYPERLIPOPROTEINEMIAS

Guiliano Enzi, Matteo Bevilacqua, and Gaetano Crepaldi
Clinica Medica Generale, Universita di Padua, Padua/Italia

Blood gas analysis at rest and after exercise, pulmonary diffusing capacity for
CO (DCO) and distribution of ventilation-perfusion ratio ($\dot{V}A/\dot{Q}$) were performed
in 19 hyperlipoproteinemic patients (Fredrickson's type I,II,IV). As controls 19
subjects, age paired, were considered. A significant reduction in arterial blood
O_2 tension (PaO_2) was observed in all types of hyperlipidemias. DCO resulted reduced in type IV. A significant negative correlation exists between plasma triglycerides and DCO values (r=0.5233). After exercise an increase of PaO_2 was observed up to normal values, which indicates a "venous admixture effect". Studies
with Xenon 133 excluded alterations in $\dot{V}A/\dot{Q}$ distribution. These disturbances in
pulmonary gaseous exchange (DCO reduction, PaO_2 reduction, venous admixture effect) can be explained by an alteration in the surfactant lipoprotein. The reduction in PaO_2 may be a co-factor in the pathogenesis of ischaemic heart disease
observed in hyperlipidemics.

HORMONE-STIMULATED LIPOLYSIS AND CYCLIC AMP SYNTHESIS: LACK OF A QUANTITATIVE RELATION

Guiliana Fassina, Paola Dorigo, and Rosa M. Gaion
Department of Pharmacology, University of Padua, Padua/Italy

A possible distinction between the sources providing energy to the successive
steps of hormone-sensitive lipolysis, was investigated in rat epididymal fat by
testing the influence of anoxia both on cyclic AMP (CAMP) synthesis and on
glycerol release stimulated by noradrenaline plus theophylline. In these experimental conditions a) the level of CAMP was increased to a concentration largely
sufficient for a maximum stimulation of lipolysis (ten to twenty times) while, in
contrast, the final lipolytic process was not stimulated. b) Glucose potentiated
the increasing effect of norepinephrine plus theophylline on CAMP level whereas
it was ineffective under aerobic conditions. c) Rotenone did not impair CAMP
accumulation. These data indicate that hormone-induced cyclic AMP synthesis may
be supported by anaerobic glycolysis, whilst the stimulation of lipolysis is dependent on oxidative phosphorylation. This possible dissociation of hormone effects on CAMP synthesis and on the lipolytic process suggests the importance of
a fine equilibrium between the metabolic sources of ATP for a suitable control
of lipid mobilization.

MICROANGIOPATHY IN HYPERLIPIDEMIAS

Elaine B. Feldman, Franklin Gluck, Anne C. Carter, Klaus F. Wellmann, and Bruno
W. Volk
Department of Medicine, SUNY Downstate Medical Center, Brooklyn, NY/USA

Microangiopathy may be the counterpart of atherosclerosis of large vessels. Increased incidence of atherosclerosis and glucose intolerance in hyperlipidemia,
and of all 3 factors in gout prompted measuring mean minimum basement membrane
width (MBMW) in lateral quadriceps needle biopsies (Williamson). Thirty-three
primary hyperlipoproteinemic patients (13 overt diabetes, 9 chemical diabetes,
11 normal 6h GTT), 19 gout patients (4 overt and 4 chemical diabetes, 11 normal
GTT, 50% hypertriglyceridemic), 12 overt and 3 chemical diabetes (lipids normal),
and 8 control subjects (lipids and GTT normal, no family history of diabetes)
were studied. Mean MBMW averaged 1118±67Å in 30 subjects with normal glucose
tolerance, and increased significantly (P<0.001) to 1557±105Å in overt diabetes
(29 patients). Both groups averaged 46 years of age. Linear regression of MBMW

with age occurred (14Å/yr, 0.01<P<0.001). Factorial analysis of variance indicated age (P=0.025), glucose intolerance (P=0.05) and gout (P=0.05) were significant influences, and that hyperlipidemia had no effect on MBMW. Uric acid levels did not correlate with MBMW (r=-011). Metabolic mechanisms for atherosclerosis may occur in gout and diabetes mellitus in addition to the factors in hyperlipidemia. Microangiopathy of hyperlipoproteinemias accompanies glucose intolerance indistinguishable from diabetes mellitus.

OXYGENATED STEROL ESTERS OF HUMAN ATHEROMA AND THEIR METABOLISM

John D. Gilbert, Andrew G. Smith, Charles J.W. Brooks, and W. Arthus Harland
Departments of Chemistry and Pathology, University of Glasgow, Glasgow/Scotland

Three structurally similar types of oxygenated sterol esters have been shown to occur regularly in diseased human aortas. These mainly comprise cholesterol esterified with hydroperoxy-, hydroxy- and keto-octadecadienoic acids. The structures of these compounds have been fully elucidated by combined gas chromatography-mass spectrometry. Their concentration increases with the severity of the disease. The presence of a glutathione peroxidase (EC.1.11.1.9), which can effect conversion of the hydroperoxides to hydroxy-esters, has been demonstrated in human and animal aortas. Its activity towards other lipid hydroperoxides has also been investigated.

Hydroxystearic acids, derived from the arterial cholesteryl hydroxy-esters, have been shown to be mixtures of optical isomers. It thus seems that the hydroperoxides are formed *via* a non-enzymic, possibly autoxidative process, and that in healthy tissue rapid enzymic reduction to hydroxy-esters keeps hydroperoxide concentrations at innocuous levels.

DEVELOPMENTAL AND SEX-LINKED MODIFICATIONS OF RAT'S AORTIC ENZYMES ACTIVITIES

Peter Hadjiisky, Jacqueline Renais, and Lucien Scebat
Cardiological Center, Boucicaut Hospital, Paris/France

35 enzyme activities (EA) linked with the glycolysis, pentose phosphate and glycogen pathways, TCA and esterolysis are histochemically studied and compared during the rat's ontogenesis. The changes observed suggest a progressive metabolic accentuation during the neonatal and prepubertal periods probably correlated with the increase of PO_2 and blood pressure after birth, with the growth and increased transparietal exchanges. The EA remain stable during the whole adult period. Their intensity is high (glycolysis-, esterolysis-diaphorases EA), moderate (aerobic oxidation-, and MPS-linked enzymes), or low (glycogen pathway-EA). The ageing is marked by a slight increase of the lysosomes-, glycolysis-, and lipogenesis-linked EA, and by a slight decrease of Krebs' cycle EA. The histoenzymatical differences between the sexes suggest some relations between sex and the histometabolic behavior of the aortic tissue.

GLYCOSOAMINOGLYCANS, COLLAGEN AND ELASTIN CONTENT IN AORTAS OF RABBITS FED ATHEROGENIC DIET AND AFTER ALLOXANE DIABETES

Janusz Hanzlik, Jeremiasz Tomaszewski, Jerzy Lopatynski, and Ireneusz Wolanski
Medical Department and Research Center, Medical School, Lublin/Poland

Influence of atherogenic diet and alloxan diabetes on composition of GAG fractions, collagen fractions and elastin content have been investigated. As result of these experiments we have found that atherogenic diet did not change GAG con-

tent. Alloxan diabetes itself and its combination with atherogenic diet caused
an increase of total GAG, especially of hyaluronic acid, heparan sulphate and
chondroitino-sulphates. Insoluble collagen content was diminished in intima and
media of aortas of animals fed atherogenic diet. Alloxan diabetes had no influence on collagen and elastin composition of aortic wall.

TOPOCHEMICAL STUDIES ON THE GLYCOSAMINOGLYCAN AND LIPID METABOLISM IN ARTERIAL TISSUE

M.H. Hodara, K.v. Figura, I. Filipovic, and E. Buddecke
University of Münster, Institute of Physiological Chemistry, Münster/BRD

Chemical and metabolic studies on multiple consecutive intima-media layers of
bovine and human aorta thoracica had the following results: The inner third of
the aorta contains 1.5 - 1.7 g glycosaminoglycans/100 g dry weight of tissue,
their concentration being reduced from intima to media to half of this value.
The distribution pattern of chondroitin sulfate (CS), dermatan sulfate (DS),
heparan sulfate (HS) and hyaluronate (HA) shifts within the individual layers,
characterized by a continuous decrease of the CS + DS/HS + HA-ratio from intima
to media. The maximum CS-DS-content present in the intimal layer (No. 1) of nonarteriosclerotic tissue changes to the subintimal layer (No. 2) in arteriosclerosis.

Analyses of lipids and their subfractions revealed significant differences between the tunica intima and the outer parts of the tunica media for bovine and
human aortae. Following ^{35}S-sulfate labelling by in vitro incubation of bovine
aorta the specific ^{35}S-radioactivity of all sulfated glycosaminoglycans show
striking reduction from intima to media. Likewise the incorporation of ^{14}C-
acetate into all lipid subfractions of the intima exceeds that of the media. The
higher incorporation of radioactivity into the intima glycosaminoglycans and
lipids is found to be the result of a more intensive metabolism of the intima
cells. In arteriosclerotic lesions (WHO I-II) an increased fatty acid synthesis
predominantly located in the intima is observed as compared with nonarteriosclerotic parts of the same aorta.

HUMAN ATHEROSCLEROTIC LESIONS FROM NORMO- AND HYPERLIPEMICS

Henry F. Hoff
Departments of Neurology and Pathology, Baylor College, Medicine, Houston,TX/USA

A histochemical and ultrastructural study was performed on atherosclerotic arteries from patients with known lipid profiles to determine if blood lipid
levels had any effect on localization of the apoprotein of low-density lipoproteins (apoLDL) and specific enzymes, or lesion type and structure. Arteries
(aorta, cerebral, coronary) were obtained from surgery or autopsy from six type
IV hyperlipoproteinemics and seven normolipemics. Histochemical techniques were
performed on cryostat sections to localize lipid, elastica, collagen, acid
mucopolysaccharides, DPN diaphorase, acid phosphatase, apoLDL. Adjacent tissue
was processed for electron microscopy. ApoLDL was mainly extracellular and
specific to plaque cores, areas positive for both acid mucopolysaccharides and
lipid, and on pseudoelastica fibers. Differences in overall lesion structure,
apoLDL and enzyme localization, and ultrastructural morphology were found to be
greater between individual lesions and arterial beds than between normo- and
hyperlipemics suggesting only minor effects of blood lipids on lesion structure.

CHANGES IN THE LEVEL OF PROSTAGLANDIN E$_2$ IN SKIN AND AORTA DURING EXPERIMENTAL ATHEROGENESIS IN THE RABBIT

S.L. Hsia, P.A. Berberian, and V.A. Ziboh
University of Miami School of Medicine, Miami, FL/USA

The involvement of prostaglandin E$_2$ (PGE$_2$) in atherogenesis was investigated. Control rabbits were fed rabbit chow while experimental animals an atherogenic diet of rabbit chow plus cholesterol (1% by weight) and cottonseed oil (2% by weight) for seven months. Specimens of aorta and skin were homogenized and incubated with ^{14}C-arachidonic acid. The ^{14}C-PGE$_2$ synthesized was identified by column and thin layer chromatography. The results indicated a threefold increase in PGE$_2$ synthesis by the intima-media preparations, and a twofold increase by skin preparations from the experimental animals. Determination of PGE$_2$ by gas-liquid chromatography showed that the skin of animals fed the atherogenic diet for five weeks contained 22 to 37 ng of PGE$_2$/mg protein, while skin from control animals contained 3 to 13 ng of PGE$_2$/mg protein. These results suggest the involvement of PGE$_2$ in atherogenesis and a parallelism in biochemical changes between skin and aorta.

AORTIC FIBROFATTY TYPE ATHEROSCLEROSIS FROM THROMBUS IN NORMOLIPIDEMIC RABBITS

Shao-nan Huang, Akinobu Sumiyoshi, Bernard I. Weigensberg, and Robert H. More
Department of Pathology, McGill University, Montreal/Canada

Polyethylene tubing induced massive, nonocclusive aortic thrombosis in normolipidemic rabbits. Evolution of the thrombi to typical fibrofatty atherosclerosis was observed as early as 4 weeks. The lesions persisted in animals maintained to 56 weeks. The complex cellular responses in injured aorta were characterized by an initial phase of cellular proliferation in intima that was followed by a phase of mixed cellular differentiation, then a phase of foam cell transformation and finally cellular necrobiosis. The electron microscopy elucidated the types of cellular infiltration and recognized the intimal smooth muscle cells in various phases of differentiation. The possible relationship of progenitor intimal smooth cells and the foam cells were supported. This model offers an opportunity to examine the morpho-kinetics of cell differentiation and modification, that may be correlated with the biochemical changes in atherogenesis in the normolipidemic state.

STUDIES ON THE MATERIAL TRANSPORT THROUGH THE VESSEL-WALL AND ON ITS EFFECTS ON THE DEVELOPMENT OF VASCULAR LESIONS

H. Jellinek, T. Kerényi, G. Elemér, and G. Horváth
Second Department of Pathology, Semmelweis Medical University, Budapest/Hungary

The permeability of the arterial wall was studied by the colloidal-iron method. Under different experimental conditions an increase of permeability was regularly observed. Experimental data were presented on the role of lymphatic drainage in material transport. In the same experiments the decrease in the intensity of ruthenium-red bindings by the external coat under pathological conditions was thought to be one of the possible explanations for the observed increase of permeability. The alkaline phosphatase network of the arteries was found enlarged in hypertension and narrow in hypoxia. Also this phenomenon was considered to have a role in the arterial wall's permeability. The initial disturbances in the nutrition of the arterial wall were followed by regeneration. The proliferative phenomena associated with the latter simulated the morphological appearance of arteriosclerosis.

THE EFFECTS OF CARBON MONOXIDE ON MYOCARDIUM ULTRASTRUCTURE CHANGES IN RABBITS AFTER A MODERATE, CHRONIC EXPOSURE

Knud Kjeldsen and Henrik Klem Thomsen
Department of Clinical Chemistry A Rigshospitalet, Copenhagen/Denmark

Rabbits were exposed to 180 ppm carbon monoxide for two weeks. Focal degenerative changes and necrozised areas were found in the myocytes of the left ventricle.

It is proposed that carbon monoxide in tobacco smoke is an important factor in the development of disperse myocardial fibrosis and may be responsible for the increased risk of myocardial infarction and sudden death seen in heavy smokers.

STUDIES OF SELECTIVE INTIMAL PERMEABILITY CHANGES IN CHOLESTEROL INDUCED ATHEROSCLEROSIS

Antal Kóczé, Sándor Virág, Róbert Dénes, and Mária Stützel
Semmelweis University of Medicine, Third Department of Medicine, Budapest/Hungary

Authors examined the permeability disturbances in early stages of cholesterol induced atherosclerosis by ^{125}I-beta-lipoprotein and ^{131}I-albumin. The adjoining adventitial surfaces of surviving rabbit aortic samples were stuck together by tissue adhesive. This way the selective intimal uptake of the aortic samples could be carried out. We found, that after a one week cholesterol supplemented diet the albumin uptake doubled, and that the beta-lipoprotein uptake did not change. After three to four weeks the inflow did not differ in the control and treated groups. In our opinion the permeability changes of the early phase are due to the endothel cell impairment. Later the media lesions become more expressed and exert an inhibitory effect on the higher albumin influx.

ENHANCED PLATELET AGGREGATION AS A RISK FACTOR IN ATHEROSCLEROSIS. STUDIES ON THE PROPERTIES OF A PLATELET AGGREGATING FACTOR

Hans J. Krzywanek and K. Breddin
Center of International Medicine, Department of Angiology, University, Frankfurt/BRD

Spontaneous aggregation of thrombocytes was studied using PAT I (morphological method) and recently PAT II (photometric registration). Platelet aggregation was greatly enhanced in 64% (166 of 262) of patients with a history of myocardial infarction, in 49% (133 of 273) of patients with peripheral arterial occlusions, and in 60% (282 of 472) of patients with diabetes of more than five years' duration, but only in 14.5% (79 of 545) of healthy individuals of all age groups.

Enhanced platelet aggregation is caused by a plasma factor, which has been identified as a high molecular weight protein, probably a fibrinogen derivative. It can be separated from patients' plasma by ethanol fractionation followed by gel chromatography. Its aggregating effect is not blocked by apyrase, indicating that it is independent of the action of ADP.

ADULT SWINE AS AN ANIMAL MODEL IN STUDIES ON ATHEROSCLEROSIS

Fred A. Kummerow, Takanobu Mizuguchi, Tadashi Arima, Shu-jen C. Yeh, and Byung H. Cho
Burnsides Research Laboratory, University of Illinois, Urbana, IL/USA

Four groups of 3 year old female swine were fed for 6 months a basal ration; the basal ration plus 20% corn oil; 20% of a margarine fat which contained 0% or one which contained 50% trans fatty acids. The basal diet of corn and soybean meal contained no cholesterol or saturated fat. The plasma, erythrocytes, heart, adipose, liver, adrenal and a portion of the aorta tissue of each individual animal was subjected to a total lipid analysis. The remaining portion of the aorta was stained with Sudan IV and the degree of atherosclerotic involved compared. The results indicated that fibrous plaques of varying degrees of severity were present in the aorta of all of the animals. The intima media layer of the aorta contained approximately the same amount of total lipid, cholesterol, cholesterol ester, triglycerides, free fatty acids and phospholipids. The average total plasma lipid and triglyceride levels in the heart tissue were highest in those fed the margarine fat which contained trans fatty acids. The adipose tissue of those fed corn oil contained significantly more linoleic acid (C18:2) although the plasma and the erythrocytes of all animals contained substantial amounts of C18:2.

EFFECT OF CYCLIC AMP AND RELATED DRUGS ON PLATELET BEHAVIOUR IN VIVO

P.M. Mannucci, C.A. Maggi, and G.C. Barbi
Haemophilia and Thrombosis Centre, Lipid and Metabolic Unit, University of Milano and Policlinico Hospital, Milano/Italy

The effect on platelet behaviour of purified cAMP and of its dibutyryl derivative has been studied in human volunteers on their intravenous injection. We have also studied whether known activators of adenylcyclase and inhibitors of phosphodiesterase such as theophylline, glucagon, vasopressin, isoprenaline and others, used alone or in combination, affect platelet behaviour *in vivo*. The platelet behaviour after these drugs has been correlated with the variations of the platelet level of cAMP. DB-cAMP (to a lesser extent, cAMP and isoprenaline) causes consistent inhibition of platelet aggregation induced by ADP, collagen and adrenaline. DB-cAMP also decreases platelet retention to glass beads and the release of PF_4 induced by the aggregating agents. The standardized bleeding time and the availability of PF_3 induced by kaolin were not affected. The other compounds were without effect at the dosage employed.

EARLY ARTERIAL LESIONS IN INFANCY AND CHILDHOOD

W.W. Meyer
Institute of Pathology, University of Mainz, Mainz/BRD

Gross calcifications of the internal elastic membrane in the common and internal iliac arteries have been found by a modified von Kossa technique in half of all newborn children that died in the first four weeks of life. After the age of one year the encrustations were present in all 40 cases studied. The calcium content of the lesions was confirmed by other histochemical methods. With a single umbilical artery not only calcifications but, moreover, gross atherosclerotic lesions have been demonstrated in the enlarged iliac arteries at the side of the single umbilical artery in children aged 13 months and four years. In the carotid siphon gross calcifications were present in all 30 children aged 1-16 years. The femoral artery is another common site of early calcific deposits in children. The calcifications represent the earliest gross arterial lesion indicating a very early injury which affects some predisposed arterial segments.

STRUCTURAL CORRELATES OF ENDOTHELIAL PERMEABILITY IN VARIOUS REGIONS OF RAT LARGE ARTERIES

Robert H. More, Istvan Hüttner, and Michel Boutet
Pathological Institute, McGill University, Montreal/Canada

Structural investigations of arterial endothelium of normotensive Sprague-Dawley rats using uranyl acetate treated and lanthanum permeated tissue preparations disclosed the presence of incomplete tight junctions. In addition, gap junctions in endothelium have been demonstrated for the first time. These observations have been made in four selected arterial regions (thoracic and abdominal aortas, and carotid and iliac arteries). Dissimilarities of incomplete tight junctions were, however, recognized which correlated with regional differences in permeability to the fine-structural protein tracer horseradish peroxidase.

STUDIES OF CORONARY ARTERIES IN DIFFERENT ETHNIC GROUPS AND CHILDREN OF DIFFERENT AGE GROUPS

Henry N. Neufeld and Zeev Vlodaver
Heart Institute, The Chaim Sheba Medical Center, Tel Hashomer and Tel Aviv University Medical School, Tel Aviv/Israel

Differences found in the incidence of coronary heart disease in different ethnic groups in Israel can be ascribed not only to different ways of life and diet but also to genetic factors. A study of comparative structural changes of coronary arteries of different ethnic groups in Israel was undertaken to investigate this latter hypothesis.

The following relevant factors have been shown to exist which could possibly explain the differences mentioned above:

1. Differences in histological development of coronary arteries among different ethnic groups.
2. Quantitative and qualitative differences in the histological development of coronary arteries between males and females without differences in two of the ethnic groups.
3. Differences in the structure of the coronary arteries in infants of some of the ethnic groups as compared with those of others.
These findings lend indirect support to the theory of an anatomical basis for the etiology of atherosclerosis.

LIPID METABOLISM IN AORTA OF RATS WITH STREPTOZOTOCIN-INDUCED DIABETES

H. Orimo, T. Sakurada, H. Okabe, A. Noma, and M. Murakami
Tokyo Metropolitan Geriatric Hospital, Tokyo/Japan

In an attempt to clarify the alteration in the aortic lipid synthesis in diabetes, rat aorta from streptozotocin-induced diabetes was incubated with ^{14}C-glucose and the incorporation of isotope in the lipid fractions was studied. After the incubation, lipid was extracted and the chloroform and methanol fractions were analysed for their composition and radioactivities.

In diabetic rats, in which streptozotocin (80 mg/kg) was given 4 days before sacrifice, the uptake of ^{14}C-glucose into both fractions was significantly decreased when compared with the controls.

However, these decreases were significantly inhibited when the rats were given simultaneous administration of Novolente insulin (15 μ/kg) and streptozotocin (80 mg/kg) for 4 days.

In rats in which streptozotocin (80 mg/kg) was repeatedly given for 1 month, the triglyceride content in the aorta was significantly decreased.

However, the uptake of ^{14}C-glucose into the aortic triglyceride was not significantly different from the controls.

These results suggest that the incorporation of ^{14}C-glucose into the aortic lipid was altered in diabetes and could be reversed by insulin.

STEROL-ESTER HYDROLASE ACTIVITY IN UNDISEASED AND ATHEROSCLEROTIC RABBIT AORTA

Jeremy D. Pearson and David E. Bowyer
Department of Pathology, University of Cambridge, Cambridge/England

Rates of hydrolysis of cholesteryl $(1-^{14}C)$ oleate and $(1-^{14}C)$ linoleate were determined in aortic homogenates from rabbits fed normal or atherogenic diets. Incubations with acetone-dispersed substrate were performed, lipids extracted and separated by thin layer chromatography. Concentrations of individual endogenous cholesteryl esters were found by chemical assay and gas liquid chromatography. The rates of hydrolysis of added, labelled, substrate (i.e. the turnover rate of each ester) did not vary with the degree of atherosclerosis (rate for cholesteryl oleate = 55±6 (22)*, rate for linoleate = 44±7 (23)). Recalculation of rates assuming complete equilibration of endogenous and exogenous ester indicated that the rate of hydrolysis of cholesteryl oleate rose significantly from <100 in undiseased tissue to >300 in diseased tissue, whereas the rate for linoleate was unchanged (55±9 (23)). This is because of the large increase in cholesteryl oleate (but not linoleate) concentration in diseased tissue. Thus, if endogenous cholesteryl ester in fatty streaks is accessible to the enzyme, an inadequate rate of sterol-ester hydrolysis cannot be the cause of cholesteryl ester accumulation.

---

*All rates are expressed as pmol/mg protein/h, and show Mean ± St.Error (no. Obs.).

THE FINE STRUCTURE OF REGENERATING AORTIC ENDOTHELIAL CELLS IN THE RAT

J.C.F. Poole
Sir William Dunn School of Pathology, Oxford/England

The structure of endothelial cells growing over organizing mural thrombi of the rat's aorta was examined in the electron microscope. The thrombi were induced by mechanical injury using a fine silk suture. Regenerating endothelial cells were found to contain filaments of two distinct types, appearing at different times and changing their spatial distribution as the cells matured. The smaller kind resembled smooth muscle myofilaments in size and spacing and in containing dense bodies. These were seen in the earliest regenerating endothelial cells examined, at first forming a continuous layer just deep to the cell surfaces but gradually separating into discrete bundles during the first six weeks after injury. The larger filaments had approximately twice the diameter of the smaller ones, were much more widely spaced and did not contain dense bodies. They were first seen five days after operation, at first widely distributed in the cytoplasm later becoming less numerous and grouped in small bundles.

INFLUENCE OF DIETARY FATS ON ATHEROSCLEROSIS, COAGULATION AND PLATELET PHOSPHOLIPIDS IN RABBIT

S. Renaud and P. Gautheron
INSERM, Unité 63, Lyon/France

Male rabbits were fed for six months, diets comprising cholesterol (0.1%) and either butter alone (10%) or butter (5%) plus cacao butter, coconut oil, olive oil, or corn oil (4.5%). These fats could be classified according to their atherogenicity as follows, in decreasing order: butter, olive oil, coconut oil, cacao butter and corn oil. The severity of the atherosclerotic lesions was significantly correlated with the plasma cholesterol (p<0.001). By contrast, the recalcification clotting time was shortest in cacao butter and butter and longest in rabbits fed olive oil and corn oil. Changes in coagulation, which resulted directly from the content of the dietary fats in stearic and linoleic acids, were correlated with the clotting activity (p<0.001) and the fatty acid composition (p<0.01) of the platelet fractions phosphatidyl serine + inositol, but not with the concentration of these fractions. Butter was the only fat able to induce severe alterations in coagulation, serum cholesterol and arterial wall morphology.

FUNCTIONAL CHARACTERIZATION OF ARTERIAL CELLS INVOLVED IN SPONTANEOUS ATHEROMA

Abel Lazzarini Robertson, Jr.
Division of Research, Cleveland Clinic Foundation, Cleveland, OH/USA

Identification of arterial cell types involved in the initial stages of human atheroma seems indispensible for a better understanding of its pathogenesis and eventual development of effective therapeutic measures.

Morphological criteria alone have proved to be of only relative value, even following the advent of electronmicroscopy-cytochemistry.

To avoid some of these shortcomings, newly developed organ culture techniques combined with use of arterial samples obtained during reconstructive vascular surgery have been applied to the isolation of human monoclonal diploid arterial cell populations for selective functional and ultrastructural studies.

In contrast to other species in which spontaneous atheroma is rare, cells isolated from the human arterial intima consist of at least two characteristic cell types with striking differences in their metabolic requirements and response to cytotoxic agents.

It is believed that these cytological differences may play important roles both in the development and progression of atherosclerosis in man.

VASCULAR STRUCTURE ELICITED BY PRUSSIAN BLUE PRECIPITATES OR BY PARTICULATE INJECTIONS

Simon Rodbard
Department of Cardiology, City of Hope Medical Center, Duarte, CA/USA

We have developed three techniques that provide information regarding vascular structure. 1. Tissues were perfused via an artery with saline containing ferrocyanate ion. Saline containing 1% ferric ion was then injected intraparenchymally (not intravascularly). Contact of ferric ion with ferrocyanide precipitates Prussian blue. Blue crystals were present throughout the extracellular spaces between the smooth muscle cells of adventitia and media, and it outlined the circumferential and radial arrangements of the vessel sheaths. 2. Liquid plastic containing pigment particulates was injected into the aortic wall taken at autopsy. Sections of these specimens showed that the pigment had been intruded into clefts between adjacent elastic lamina. 3. Liquid plastic was injected into the wall of the aorta. Tissue corrosion in KOH revealed that the liquid had spread between the elastic lamina of the wall, forming sheets. Casts of the adventitia showed numerous orifices which appeared to be the openings for vasa vasorum and related structures. These techniques offer new means for the study of the organization of the normal arterial wall at atheromata, at branchings, and other sites of local mechanical stresses.

PROTEIN PASSAGE THROUGH ENDOTHELIUM OF LARGE RAT ARTERIES DURING CATECHOLAMINE AND MECHANICALLY INDUCED HIGH AND LOW BLOOD PRESSURES

George Rona, Istvan Hüttner, and Robert H. More
Pathological Institute, McGill University, Montreal/Canada

High (140-220 mm Hg) and low (60-80 mm Hg) arterial blood pressures, monitored on a polygraph, were induced by infusion of catecholamines (norepinephrine and isoproterenol) as well as by mechanical means (aortic coarctation) in Sprague-Dawley rats. Fine-structural protein tracers (horseradish peroxidase and ferritin) were injected intravenously and localized later in the intima of selected arterial regions (thoracic and abdominal aortas, carotid and external iliac arteries) by electron microscopy. The results indicated that the passage of protein molecules through arterial endothelium is influenced by the level of the blood pressure. This effect, however, was modified by regional differences in permeability to protein tracers, being more evident in the thoracic aorta than in other selected regions, and tracer localization was not influenced by blood pressure levels in the iliac artery segment.

LESION FORMATION IN HYPERCHOLESTEREMIC PRIMATES FOLLOWING INTRAVASCULAR ENDOTHELIALIZATION

Russell Ross, Thomas Wight, and John Glomset

A series of primates (Macaca nemestrina) were fed a continuous high fat diet, resulting in a sustained hypercholesteremia (300 - 400 mg%). The animals were hypercholesteremic prior to injury and remained so for the duration of the experiment. Six weeks after becoming hypercholesteremic the endothelium of the right iliac artery and the abdominal aorta was removed with an intravascular (Fogarty) balloon catheter. Animals were sacrificed at six weeks, three months, six months, and nine months after deendothelialization. Both iliac arteries and the aorta were prepared for light and electron microscopy. Marked intimal thickening was seen in the right iliac and abdominal aorta in all animals by six weeks after injury. At all later intervals the right iliac vessel contained a proliferative lesion consisting of numerous lipid filled smooth muscle cells surrounded by connective tissue matrix. Small membrane bound globular appearing deposits were dispersed troughout the connective tissues. Numerous degenerating cells were present in the older lesions. Lipid was also seen in medial cells immediately subjacent to the internal elastic lamina. The uninjured left iliac arteries showed some lesion formation three month after starting the lipid diet. The lesions on the right side were more extensive than those on the left and were identical in appearance to the lipid filled fibrous plaque in man.

VASCULAR RETINAL ALTERATIONS OF HYPERLIPOPROTEINEMIA

Elisabeth Schäfer and Helmut Canzler
Augenklinik und Department für Innere Medizin der Medizinischen Hochschule,
Hannover/BRD

Alterations of retinal vascular system in 60 patients with hyperlipoproteinemia
(HLP) type II-IV (Fredrickson) are documented by colour and partial fluorescence
photophraphy.

We found, in a certain regularity, distinct tortuosity of the main retinal arteries, partly formed as corkscrews, partly as phenomenon of lash, omega-formed
branches, yellow-milky reflexes and often small dysphorical areas. These alterations we found specially connected with high beta-lipoproteins.
Contrary patients with high pressure showed a vascular course relativly straight,
constricted, sharp angled branches, very often atrophies of the pigment-epithelion
and in higher ages maculopathies. But real exsudates, composed of lipid material,
were only found in single cases. We noted one case of HLP without diabetes with
a large waxy plaque, which disappeared almost completely in a half a year.

We also found in 10 cases of young diabetes with HLP the same arterial tortuosity,
but no classical signs of diabetic retinopathy.

The alterations are interpreted as beginning angiopathy of retinal vases. We found
them already in a stadium of no other signs of arteriosclerosis. In case of young
diabetes with beginning changements of the arterial system the HLP probably may
be a factor of risk for the manifestation of diabetic retinopathy.

CHANGES IN PLATELET MORPHOLOGY INDUCED BY PLASMA FROM ISCHEMIC HEART DISEASE PATIENTS

Irwin J. Schatz and Irwin Gross
Department of Internal Medicine, University of Michigan Medical Center, An Arbor/
MI/USA

Platelets (PLT) change shape (from dendritic to spread) as they participate in
thrombosis. Ten patients with ischemic heart disease (IHDP), (6 acute infarction,
4 chronic), and 3 shock (noncardiogenic) patients (SP) had increased spread PLT
forms ($74\pm16.4\%$) compared to controls (P <.001), as seen on electron microscopy.
When PLT from 10 controls were exposed to IHDP plasma, spread forms increased
from $16.6\pm9.8\%$ to $54.0\pm16.4\%$ (P <.001), but there was no significant effect on
control PLT from SP plasma. Control PLT exposed to plasma from another control
group showed no change. When PLT from IHDP were incubated with normal plasma,
spread forms decreased ($80.3\pm15.3\%$ to $62.5\pm16.9\%$) (P <.025). In vivo, aspirin
(900 mg) caused marked suppression of spread PLT formation, and of plasma factor
activity in one patient with acute infarction.

We conclude a factor exists in the plasma of these IHDP, but not in SP, which
caused normal PLT to spread; contrariwise, normal plasma suppressed spread PLT
formation. Since the effect of plasma from acute IHDP, when compared to chronic
IHDP, was identical, this factor likely is not related to hormonal and/or therapeutic changes occurring during acute infarction.

ENDOTHELIAL CELL-CONTRACTION OF RABBIT AORTA INDUCED BY SINGLE-DOSE TREATMENT WITH CHOLESTEROL, EPINEPHRINE AND ANGIOTENSIN II

Takio Shimamoto and Fujio Numano
Institute for Cardiovascular Diseases, Tokyo Ika-Shika National University, Tokyo/ Japan

Single-dose treatment with cholesterol or epinephrine or angiotensin II was shown to induce the acute entry of ß-lipoprotein into the arterial wall of rabbit and rhesus monkey by immunofluorescent method by us. Among routes for the lipoprotein-entry, the intercellular one seemed most important for several reasons. Consequently we used 120 rabbits to count the number of contracted endothelial cells with nucleal pinch (Majno, 1969) after the above mentioned challenges. The vital fixation of endothelial cells of the aorta was performed under anesthesia with isotonic 2.5% glutaraldehyde (pH 7.4) infused through a catheter under a pressure of 110 mmHg. In aortic specimens from rabbits sacrificed 2 hours after cholesterol (1 g/kg p.o.) or 10 minutes after epinephrine (1 µg/kg i.v.) or angiotensin II (1 µg/kg i.v.) the contracted endothelial cells with pinch appeared in 6.2% ±1.1 (P <0.001), 4.1% ±1.2 (P <0.01) and 4.3% ±1.2 (P <0.01) of the cells counted respectively, while in specimens from animals receiving placebo or those challenged after Premarin (5 mg/kg i.v.) or pyridinolcarbamate (10 mg/kg p.o.) or EG 467 (1 mg/kg p.o.), there was no such cells. This evidence suggests the significance of endothelial cell contraction as a key mechanism in atherogenesis.

NON-HOMOGENEITY OF LIPID METABOLISM IN NORMAL AORTIC INTIMA-MEDIA

John B. Somer and Colin J. Schwartz
Department of Pathology, McMaster University, Hamilton/Canada

The experiments reported form part of a continuing study of areas of focal aortic Evans Blue uptake, previously shown to have an increased free cholesterol turnover. Young pigs were injected with dye and killed 2.5 hours later. Excised blue and white aortic segments were incubated in buffer with ^{14}C-1-acetate at 37°C. Tissues were washed and homogenized in chloroform:methanol (2:1). Lipids were separated by thin-layer chromatography, eluted and counted. Incorporation of acetate in total lipid was significantly greater in blue than in white areas (p <0.025). This increase was apparent in each lipid fraction. Additionally, the percentage of label incorporated in phospholipid was significantly greater in blue areas, a difference resulting from an increased proportion of label incorporated in phosphatidyl choline. Saponification studies indicated that most of the ^{14}C-1-acetate was incorporated into fatty acid. These findings suggest that there is a greater synthesis of fatty acids in blue than in white areas of the normal young pig aorta.

FIBRINOLYSIS AND PLATELET AGGREGATION IN ATHEROSCLEROSIS AND THROMBOANGIITIS OBLITERANS

Niculae Stancioiu and Maria-Lorena Scrobohaci
Center of Assistance to Cardiac Patients (ASCAR), Bucharest/Roumania

Euglobulin clot lysis time (ECLT), platelet aggregation (PA) by ADP and Norepinephrine (NE), cholesterol, ß-lipoproteins, total lipids, fibrinogen were carried out from the venous and arterial (when concomitant sampling was possible) or only venous blood of 25 peripheral (atherosclerosis obliterans -AO), 15. coronary atherosclerosis (CA), 15 with AO and CA, 20 thromboangiitis obliterans (TO) and 18 healthy subjects (HS). In other 18 AO and 14 TO patients fibrinolysis inhibitors (FI) were measured. Arterio-venous differences were statistically significant for ECLT both in AO and TO and PA by ADP in AO and not significant for the remaining groups and determinations. ECLT, FI and PA were much increased in patients groups, compared to HS. Significant differences were found between TO and AO concerning ECLT and PA by NE much higher in the first and FI and PA by ADP in the second disease. No cause-to-effect relationship between hyperlipemia and fibrinolysis and PA was found.

VARIATIONS OF BRAIN ENZYMATIC ACTIVITIES IN EXPERIMENTAL ATHEROSCLEROSIS

Gino Toffano, Pietro Gonzato, and Ferrante Aporti
Research Laboratories - FIDIA, Abano Terme/Italy

Rabbits under atherogenic diet for 40 days have an increase of the aortic cholesterol over 90%. These rabbits show appreciable changes of membrane-bound and of cytoplasmic enzymes. In the case of the membrane-bound enzymes such as the Mg^{++} dependent and the Na^+, K^+-stimulated ATPase, there is an increase of activity of about 50% in the case of cytoplasmic enzymes such as the pyridoxal phosphate-dependent glutamate and the dopa decarboxylase, there is a decrease of activity of about 20%. These changes may be related to the phospholipid and fatty acid content of membranes. The prevention of brain injury by treatment with brain cortex phospholipids is under investigation.

MECHANICS OF RABBIT AORTA WITH EXPERIMENTALLY INDUCED ATHEROSCLEROTIC LESIONS

Andrus Viidik
Institute of Anatomy, University of Aarhus/Denmark
Sören Björkerud and Göran Bondjers
Department of Histology, University of Göteborg/Sweden

Atherosclerotic lesions were induced by superficial mechanical injury in aortas of rabbits in order to provide information on mechanical factors in atherogenesis and relate them to gross structural composition. 12 weeks after injury the sizes of aortic ring specimens and their stress-strain behavior were recorded and the morphology of the lesions defined. The size was dependent of the type of lesion present as was the rupture site. The weakest point was always the lesion, some types of them being weaker than others. This pattern was influenced by cholesterol feeding, to which some of the animals were subjected during third and fourth week after injury, and resulted in areas devoid of endothelium, which were particularly sensitive to strain and ruptured more easily. The aortic rings with healing lesions, especially those from cholesterol-fed animals, were mechanically heterogenous, while intact ones were homogenous. The mechanical inferiority of the lesions may be an important factor preventing repair, possibly by dilatation of mechanically weak segments.

STUDIES ON EXPERIMENTAL ATHEROSCLEROSIS BY IMMUNOFLUORESCENCE

Kenneth W. Walton
Department of Experimental Pathology, University of Birmingham, Birmingham/England

It has been established by the use of immunofluorescence that the principal vehicle transporting lipid into human atherosclerotic lesions is serum low-density lipoprotein (LDL). The purpose of the present study was to see whether a similar technique could be applied to the arterial lesions of lipid-fed rabbits. Frozen sections from the arteries of rabbits fed a diet containing 1% cholesterol, or 20% beeflard without added cholesterol, were examined after treatment with fluorescein-labelled sheep anti-rabbit LDL and after staining with Oil red O. Arterial lesions developed more quickly and extensively on the cholesterol-diet than in beef-fat fed animals and contained more lipid-filled cells. In both groups there was close correspondence between extracellular lipid reactive with Oil red O and rabbit LDL as delineated by immunofluorescence. Some fat-filled cells reacted brightly, some weakly and some failed to react. These findings are closely similar to those reported in human lesions and are compatible with an insudative mechanism of atherogenesis in the lipid-fed rabbit.

ULTRASTRUCTURAL OBSERVATIONS IN RABBIT AORTIC ENDOTHELIAL SURFACE IN EARLY CHOLESTEROL EXPERIMENTAL ATHEROGENESIS AND DURING A COMBINED TREATMENT WITH TWEEN 80 AND CHOLESTEROL

Giargio Weber, Piera Fabbrini, and Loretta Resi
Pathological Anatomy Institute, University of Siena, Siena/Italy

Endothelial aortic surface of guinea-pigs, rabbits and rats is covered with a Concanavalin-A reactive glycidic coat (Bernhard and Avrameas' method). This coat, in early experimental cholesterol atherogenesis in rabbit, shows after 15 days of treatment a remarkable increase in its thickness, while later on it diminishes or disappears. Where the endothelial surface has lost its reactivity, a deposit of plasmatic material, admixed with circulating cells, takes place. An increase in the aortic Concanavalin-A reactive coat thickness may be found in ultrathin sections examined in TEM, after one month of a combined treatment with cholesterol and Tween 80 (inducing in rabbits a heavy cholesterol storage in parenchymal organs, the arterial wall involvement being negligible).

STATISTICAL MODEL OF PROGRESS AND DISTRIBUTION PATTERN OF ATHEROSCLEROSIS

W.-W. Höpker, E. Nüssel, F.-J. Hehl, G. Köhler, and K. Kayser
Institute of Pathology and Institute of Industrial and Social Medicine of the University of Heidelberg, Heidelberg/BRD

A statistical model of progress and distribution pattern of atherosclerosis is presented, in which anamnestic, clinical and morphological influence factors were included and were concluded with the help of factor analysis. The vessels of 90 autopsied men were measured. The computation of these data could verify the following hypotheses:

1. Atherosclerosis is a disease which acts in different vessel regions with different power and quality.
2. With the help of defined measure of the vessels we got relations between the singular vessel regions and the different risk factors.
3. We could also relate different histological criteria in different modus and different combinations with the risk criteria.
4. Furthermore we studied what kind of influence factors in combination with the individuality of anatomy and pulse are combined with what kind of risk criteria. We found different constellations between the localisation and the hypertension, diabetes and smoking too. With the help of this model the complex development of atherosclerosis in different vessel regions under the influence of different risk factors can be described.

THE AFFECTION OF AORTA AND METABOLIC CHANGES IN CHOLESTEROL AND GLUCOSE ADMINISTRATION

Noosrat Khamidovich Abdullajev and Bachodyr Guljamov
The Institute of Regional Medicine, Laboratory of Pathological Physiology,
Tashkent/USSR

The aim of the investigation is the comparison of the character and the degree of metabolic changes in carbohydrates and lipids administration. Cholesterol and glucose were given to rats and rabbits per os during 4-6 months both separately and in combination. The changes of aortic intima and lipids metabolism indices (summary lipids, cholesterol and its fractions, free fatty acids, -lipoproteins, ketone bodies content in blood and lipolytic activity of aortic wall) were more manifested after cholesterol administration, then after administration of cholesterol and glucose and they were feebly marked when only glucose was given. We can suppose that in atherosclerosis development of the main pathogenetic role belongs to the changes of carbohydrates and lipids metabolism.

A DIRECT EFFECT OF INSULIN ON PLASMA TRIGLYCERIDE RELEASE BY THE LIVER

Gérald Alcindor and Recaredo Infante
Liver Research Unit (INSERM U-9), Paris/France

It is established that insulin can influence the hepatic triglyceride (TG) production through a decreased influx of NEFA. The possibility of a direct effect of the hormone on the TG synthesis or/and release by the liver was investigated.

The kinetics of plasma TG secretion were studied in fasted rats after saline or insulin injection together with Triton WR 1339 (blocking TG output from plasma) and ^{3}H-palmitic acid in order to label the liver and plasma triglycerides.

The results show: a) Insulin decreases the TG secretion by the liver; b) the kinetics of TG secretion under insulin do not follow the kinetics of NEFA level variations; c) in the period of maximal hormonal effect the liver releases a minimum amount of TG with a very high specific radioactivity compared to the controls; d) in vivo injected insulin partly inhibits the hydrolysis of reserve TG by intracellular lipase (pH 4.5) as studied by incubation of liver homogenates in vitro.

Inhibition of TG secretion by the liver after insulin administration seems to be the consequence of a decrease in the intracellular fatty acid pool size due to: 1) inhibition of intracellular lipolysis of reserve TG and 2) decreased influx of plasma NEFA.

EFFECT OF HALOFENATE ON SERUM LIPIDS AND URIC ACID

W. Aronow, J. Vangrow, W. Nelson, J. Pagano, and N. Papageorge's
University of California, Irvine, CA/USA

The effect of halofenate on serum lipids and uric acid was evaluated in 48 patients with hypertriglyceridemia. One month after dietary control and a two month control period, 25 patients received placebo and 23 patients received halofenate for 48 weeks in a double-blind study. Four of 17 ASHD patients (24%) on placebo and one of 18 ASHD patients (6%) on halofenate died of myocardial infarction (P >0.05). Halofenate lowered the mean serum triglyceride level 49% from the control period in comparison with placebo (P <0.01) but did not affect the mean serum cholesterol level. Halofenate decreased the mean serum uric acid level 35% from the control period in comparison with placebo (P <0.01). Forty-one patients, including 28 with ASHD, remained in this study for another 48 weeks. All received halofenate. One of 28 ASHD patients (4%) died of myocardial infarction. Halofenate decreased the mean serum triglyceride level in 27 of 41 patients (66%) ≥15% compared to the control period (if previously on halofenate) or compared to the control plus placebo period (if previously on placebo). Halofenate decreased the mean serum uric acid level in 35 of 41 patients (85%) ≥20% compared to the control period (if previously on halofenate) or compared to the control plus placebo period (if previously on placebo). Halofenate is especially of value in treating patients with hypertriglyceridemia and hyperuricemia.

7-BETA-(^{3}H)-7-ALPHA-OH CHOLESTERYLOLEATE: A PRECURSOR IN BILE ACID BIOSYNTHESIS

Gerd Assmann, Howard Sloan, and Donald S. Fredrickson
NIH, Bethesda, MD/USA

Analyses of post-mortem samples of liver, spleen and adrenal of patients with Wolman's disease revealed accumulation of 7 α -OH cholesterylesters. In addition, 7ß-OH-, 7 Keto-, 5-6 α epoxy- and 5-6 ß epoxy cholesterolesters were isolated and identified by gas chromatography, mass- and NMR spectroscopy. To establish a physiological role of cholesterylesters in bile acid biosynthesis, 7ß-(^{3}H)-7 α -OH cholesteryloleate and (4-^{14}C) cholesteryloleate were synthesized and administered i.v. (^{3}H/^{14}C ratio: 1.4/1) into a bile fistula dog. Over half of the radioactivity was recovered in bile acids within 24 h. The ^{3}H/^{14}C ratio in chenodesoxycholic and cholic acids were 5/1 and 2.9/1, respectively. In addition, 7 α -OH cholesterylester-hydrolase activity was found in the cytosol of rat liver cells. Wolman's disease is known to be associated with esterase deficiency and malabsorption is one of its chief clinical features. The present findings suggest that 7 α -OH cholesterylester may normally be an important precursor of bile acids. Furthermore, we suggest that synthesis of bile acids is likely severely impaired in Wolman's disease, an hypothesis which has not yet been tested. Several of the 5, 6 or 7 oxygenated sterols may be auto-oxidation products, though we failed to detect them in tissues of controls or patients with Tangier disease or cholesteryl ester storage disease.

AGGLUTINATION OF LIPID PARTICLES IN AUTOIMMUNE HYPERLIPIDEMIA (AIH)

Jean-Louis Beaumont and Liliane Lorenzelli
Unité de Recherches sur l'Athérosclérose de l'INSERM, Hôpital Henri-Mondor, Créteil/France

In AIH, the release of the lipids carried by serum lipoproteins is restrained by the antibody reactivity of immunoglobulins (Ig) which inhibit lipolysis either by reacting with the enzymes (for ex. heparin lipase) or the substrate (lipoproteins).

In the latter type, agglutination of lipid particles may be visible to the naked eye or by microscope in milky serum stored for 24 hours at + 4oC.

This phenomenon reminds of agglutination of red cells in autoimmune anemias. Its immunological mechanism can be demonstrated by in vitro reproduction with synthetic or natural lipidic particles and the Ig extracted from spontaneous agglutinates.

An in vitro, activated lipidic emulsion agglutination test (ALEA) was developed with natural and synthetic emulsions coated with different antigens. The test may be used with an antiglobulin reagent in order to detect non agglutinating antibodies.

Spontaneous agglutination and ALEA test are useful for the detection and study
of AIH.

VARIATIONS IN CARBOHYDRATE COMPOSITION OF HUMAN SERUM LOW DENSITY LIPOGLYCO-PROTEINS

Pieter van der Bijl
Gaubius Institute, Health Research Organisation TNO, Leiden/The Netherlands

The carbohydrate composition of human serum low density lipoglycoproteins (LDL),
has been investigated. LDL fractions were isolated, by ultracentrifugation, from
sera of 12 apparently healthy adults in the age group 23 to 42 and from pool serum
obtained from several hundred normal adults between the ages 16 and 90. Delipidation of the fractions, followed by methanolysis, re-N-acetylation, silylation
and gas-liquid chromatography, gave the amounts of different monosaccharide residues present in each apoLDL fraction. Total carbohydrate content and relative
amounts of monosaccharide residues present in the LDL fractions of five males
and five females, corresponded well with the values obtained from the poolserum
fraction. Significant differences were observed between the results obtained for
the fractions described above, especially in glucose and N-acetylglucosamine content, and the analysis figures for two apoLDL fractions isolated from the serum
of one male and one female. Structural differences, as a result of variations in
the carbohydrate composition, between LDL isolated from the sera of apparently
healthy adults, are therefore possibly present.

TURBIDIMETRIC ESTIMATION OF TRIGLYCERIDE-RICH LIPOPROTEINS AFTER PRECIPITATION BY SODIUM LAURYL SULFATE

Meier Burstein and Harold R. Scholnick
Centre National de Transfusion Sanguine, Paris/France

With appropriate concentration of sodium lauryl sulfate VLDL and chylomicrons
are precipitated from normal and abnormal human sera and float on centrifugation.
This precipitation occurs at 35°C and requires the presence of a non dialyzable
thermolabile serum factor. Only triglyceride-rich lipoproteins are precipitated
while LDL, HDL and LP-X form with SLS soluble complexes.

Based on this selective precipitation, a turbidimetric procedure for estimation
of VLDL plus chylomicrons was developed.

The SLS turbidity values are normal in type II patients and high in type III and
IV. The highest values were obtained in grossly lipemic sera (post prandial, type
V). In clear sera the value increases with the level of serum triglycerides and
with the amount of VLDL estimated either by agarose electrophoresis (pre beta) or
by a specific anti VLDL serum. There is no correlation with the level of cholesterol or phospholipids.

STRUCTURAL ALTERATIONS OF VERY LOW DENSITY LIPOPROTEINS OF RABBITS DURING CHOLESTEROL FEEDING

Germán Camejo, Virgilio Bosch, and Amado López
Centro de Biofísica y Bioquímica, Instituto Venezolano de Investigaciones
Científicas (IVIC), Caracas/Venezuela

The lipoproteins with density less than 1.019 g/ml (VLDL) of rabbits made hypercholesterolemic by cholesterol feeding were fractionated by gel filtration. The

amount of each fraction obtained, VLDL-1 and VLDL-2, was found to be related to
the degree of hypercholesterolemia. Differences were found in the percentage
composition, size, and flotation rate of VLDL-1, and VLDL-2. However, the apolipoproteins of the two fractions were similar. Control rabbits were injected
with VLDL-1 and VLDL-2 with ^{14}C-cholesterol. The rate of disappearance from plasma of VLDL-1, the larger particles, was faster than that of VLDL-2. After 30
minutes, cholesterol injected associated with VLDL-1 was found in VLDL-2, on the
other hand VLDL-2 cholesterol was not transferred to VLDL-1 in vivo. Hexane could
easily extract cholesterol associated with VLDL-1 (the large particles) but not
that of VLDL-2. Treatment of VLDL-2 with pronase renders its cholesterol hexane-
extractable, suggesting that the different protein content of VLDL-1 and VLDL-2
is the basis for their difference in stability. It is postulated that a possible
relationship between structure, stability, and metabolic fate of this abnormal
lipoproteins exists.

VERY LOW DENSITY LIPOPROTEINS FROM CHOLESTEROL FED ANIMALS AND THEIR RELATIONSHIP TO EXPERIMENTAL ATHEROSCLEROSIS

Charles E. Day and Bradford Barker
Diabetes and Atherosclerosis Research, The Upjohn Company, Kalamazoo, MI/USA

Little information exists on serum lipoproteins of cholesterol fed animals. We
examined the serum lipoproteins from male cholesterol fed New Zealand white rabbits, White Carneau pigeons, Japanese quail and cholesterol cholic acid fed rats.
Most of the increase in cholesterol from fasted serum was attributable to very
low density lipoproteins (VLDL), d<1.006 g/ml. VLDL consisted of 60% cholesterol
(free + esterified) with an esterified to free molar ratio near 3. VLDL protein,
triglyceride, and phospholipid were relatively constant for the four species at
10%, 8%, and 21%, respectively. Material precipitating with polyanions such as
heparin was increased several-fold over control levels as measured turbidi-
metrically. Cholesterol fed rabbit VLDL + LDL was labeled with ^{125}I and incubated with freshly excised aortic tissue, collagen and elastin. Significant
binding of lipoprotein was found in all cases. Mucopolysaccharides readily precipitated these lipoproteins. These results suggest that VLDL from cholesterol
fed animals are a primary component of atherogenesis because they carry a heavy
load of cholesterol esters in a physical state which readily reacts physico-
chemically with arterial tissue and its structural components.

SOME ASPECTS OF THE RETINO-CEREBRAL HAEMODYNAMICS IN ATHEROSCLEROSIS

Marieta Dumitrache, Mircea P. Popescu, and Afrodita Craiu
Clinica de Oftalmologie, Spitalul Coltea, Bucuresti/Roumania

In atherosclerosis some changes of the cerebral haemodynamics are in direct correlation with the changes of the retinal blood vessels, elements which are able
to be studied by some objective research methods.

The measuring of the *ophthalmic* arterial pressure and of the retino-humeral index
are criteria for the retino-cerebral atherosclerosis evolution appreciation.

In this paper we present some aspects of spontaneous and post-therapeutic evolution of the retino-cerebral vascular equilibrium in atherosclerosis based on the
correlation between the general chemical context, biochemical aspect, ophthalmo-
scopic aspect of the FO and ophthalmodynamometry, by observing 60 patients with
different degrees of atherosclerosis from the Coltea Clinic Bucharest.

THE FATE OF ISOLATED APOLIPOPROTEINS IN THE RAT

Shlomo Eisenberg and Daniel Rachmilewitz
Department of Medicine "B", Lipid Research Laboratory, Hebrew University-
Hadassah Medical School, Jerusalem/Israel

Studies on the metabolism of rat plasma lipoproteins have shown that the fate of
the various apoproteins is heterogenous. To determine whether the metabolism of
isolated apolipoproteins is similar to that of the same proteins in lipoproteins,
we have prepared five ^{125}I-labeled apolipoprotein groups of VLDL and HDL origin.
Apolipoproteins were separated by gel filtration on Sephadex G-150. Following injection of labeled apoproteins to rats, 90-95% of the radioactivity was associated with lipoproteins (d<1.21). The distribution of ^{125}I-apoproteins between
VLDL and HDL, 5 min after the injection, differed considerably and the ratio
ranged from 0.02 (for the A proteins) to 0.30 (for the C proteins). The T 1/2 of
three different HDL apoprotein fractions in circulation was 5-10, 10.5 and 11 hrs.
The distribution of isolated apoproteins among lipoproteins and their T 1/2 in
circulation closely resembled that of the same apoproteins after injection of
intact lipoproteins. It is concluded that isolated apoproteins are incorporated,
at least in part, into preformed lipoproteins and share the metabolic fate of the
native lipoprotein-protein.

INSULIN SECRETION IN HUMAN ENDOGENOUS AND EXPERIMENTAL HYPERTRIGLYCERIDEMIA

Domenico Fedele, Antonio Tiengo, Michele Muggeo, and Gaetano Crepaldi
Clinica Medica Generale, Universita di Padua, Padua/Italia

Interpretation of hyperinsulinism observed in endogenous hypertriglyceridemia is
still controversial. In 13 hyperlipemics (mean triglycerides 1554±253 mg%),
the insulin (IRI) response to arginine infusion is significantly higher (47 vs
31 µU/ml at 30 minutes; 23 vs 15 µU/ml at 60 minutes), than that obtained in the
same patients after triglyceride (TG) reduction by clofibrate treatment (mean TG
384±51 mg%). A positive correlation was found between basal TG and the IRI peak
after arginine. In 11 controls IRI levels during experimental hyperlipemia (Intralipid infusion) did not significantly vary. Also IRI response to arginine during
Intralipid (mean TG 907 mg%) was higher, but not significantly, than that obtained
during saline infusion. The IRI response reduction following TG decrease in hyperlipemics does not appear related to an improvement of glucose utilization or body
weight variations.

SPECIES DIFFERENCES IN AFFINITY OF VERY LOW DENSITY LIPOPROTEIN PEPTIDE FOR RADIO-ACTIVE IODINE; METABOLISM OF HUMAN AND RAT VLDL

Noel Fidge and Paul Nestel
Department of Clinical Science, Australian National University, Canberra/
Australia

Labeling characteristics of rat, pig and human VLDL were found to differ markedly
with radioactive iodine using 3 techniques, 1. iodine monochloride method, 2.
chloramine-T method and 3. enzymatic radioiodination with lactoperoxidase. All
techniques produced good labeling of human VLDL with 80-95% of the radioactivity
bound to protein, in contrast to 30-60% with rat and pig VLDL. Increasing the
atoms of iodine per molecule of protein (I/R ratio) using ICl (technique 1) led
to higher percent protein labeling especially with rat VLDL (at I/P of 12-16,
65-70% was protein-bound but at I/P 1-3, only 33-50%).

When human and rat VLDL with I/P ranging from 0.5-15 were injected into rats,
catabolic rates were similar at I/P ranging from 0.5-6 but degradation rates

increased with higher I/P ratios. Exchange of the small C proteins between VLDL
and HDL proceeded at similar rates in vivo in rats for both human and rat VLDL
with I/P 0.5-6. Similar results were observed for a transfer of apo-B protein
from VLDL to LDL with both preparations.

HOW FATS IN FOOD MAY ALTER CHOLESTEROL METABOLISM

R. Fraser and R.W. Wissler
Department of Pathology, University of Sydney, Sidney/Australia

Ratios of free cholesterol (FC) to cholesterol esters (CE) in thoracic duct
lymph (TDL) from rabbits fed varying amounts of cholesterol (C) and triglycerides
(TG) were estimated to study the influence of dietary TG on C metabolism. TDL was
collected from 15 groups of 4-7 animals 6 hours after feeding 50 μc cholesterol-
1,2 ^{3}H in 50 g chow, containing by weight 0,0.8 or 2% C and 0.15 or 30% various
TG. The radioactivity in FC:CE was compared after separation by thin-layer chromatography. At constant levels of dietary C, FC:CE increased as dietary TG increased. Of fats studied, coconut oil caused the greatest increase. At constant
levels of a TG, TC:CE decreased as dietary C and total C in TDL increased. Differences in FC:CE between groups were highly significant, e.g. 0.16±0.01 (SEM)
from animals fed 2% C and 0% TG and 4.39±0.70 from 0% C and 30% TG. The surface
of chylomicrons carries diffusable FC while their core contains CE to be metabolized by the liver, perhaps inhibiting synthesis of C.

INSULIN, CARBOHYDRATE AND LIPID INTERRELATIONSHIPS IN ISCHEMIC HEART (HD) AND THROMBOTIC CEREBROVASCULAR DISEASE (ITCVD)

Menard M. Gertler, Hillar E. Leetma, Russell Koutrouby, and Robert G. Guthrie
New York University Medical Center, New York, N.Y./USA

Carbohydrate and lipid metabolism were evaluated during oral glucose tolerance
tests (GTT) in 65 IHD and 61 ITCVD males and in healthy age-matched controls
(± 3 years). Abnormal GTT, usually accompanied by type IV hyperlipoproteinemia,
was higher in IHD (37%) and ITCVD (70%) than in controls (19% and 34% respectively). Immunoreactive insulin (IRI) response in IHD with abnormal GTT and ITCVD
showed elevated and delayed peaks at two hours. Free fatty acid response in IHD
and ITCVD had a significantly lower rebound at three hours. All subjects with
abnormal GTT had significantly higher and lagging lactate levels at two and three
hours. Abnormal GTT was neither related to relative weight nor to elapsed time
from onset of IHD or ITCVD. Canonical correlations revealed that IRI is the common denominator in both carbohydrate and lipid abnormalities in IHD and ITCVD.
Discriminant function analyses were developed to identify and separate IHD and
ITCVD prone individuals.

STUDIES ON THE PHOSPHOLIPID GROUPS ON THE SURFACE OF LOW DENSITY LIPOPROTEINS

Santibrata Ghosh, Mukul K. Basu, and John S. Schweppe
Department of Biochemistry, Northwestern University, Medical School, Chicago, IL/
USA

The nature and distribution of ionic groups on the surface of low density lipoprotein, important in its interaction with the constituents of arterial wall,
were studied by electrophoretic methods combined with phospholipase D digestion
of LDL and binding of a fluorescent probe with LDL. Electrophoresis at pH 6.8
showed that low concentrations of $CaCl_2$ (∼20 mM) may reverse the charge of LDL
isolated from normolipemic individuals (LDL-N) suggesting the existence of phos-

pholipid (PL) groups exposed to the aqueous environment. LDL isolated from type II
hyperlipidemics (LDL-II), required a lower concentration of $CaCl_2$ for charge
reversal. In absence of ether, phospholipase D liberated, in one hour, 40% of the
total available choline from LDL-N, and about 60% from a pooled sample of LDL-II.
As expected, the net charge of LDL was rendered more negative by the digestion.
Fluorescence of ANS (1-anilino-8-naphthalene sulphonate) in LDL solution was enhanced markedly in the presence of Ca^{++}, again reflecting the role of the PL
groups on the surface of LDL. In 1.4 mM $CaCl_2$ the number of binding sites for ANS
was 198, compared to a total of about 550 PL groups per mole of LDL (m.w. $2.2 \cdot 10^6$).
LDL-II showed a slightly higher fluorescence than LDL-N.

METABOLISM OF PLASMA VERY LOW DENSITY LIPOPROTEIN (VLDL) BY ISOLATED ADIPOCYTES

Richard C. Gross
Department of Medicine, University of California-San Diego, La Jolla, CA/USA

Impaired removal of triglyceride (TG) from plasma VLDL may be important in the
genesis of hyperlipoproteinemia. To study regulation of this process, isolated
rat epididymal adipocytes from fed animals were incubated with human VLDL labeled with glyceryl trioleate-1-^{14}C. After 15 min incubation, fat cells contained
5-8% of medium radioactivity per 10^6 cells. Radioactivity appeared in all cell
lipid classes, with >80% in TG between 2 and 15 min. Radioactivity in medium TG
decreases by 30-50% in 15 min. Free fatty acid radioactivity rose as high as 25%
of total medium radioactivity during the first 5 min, but fell thereafter. The
role of lipoprotein lipase (LPL) was assessed using diethyl-p-nitrophenylphos-
phate, diisopropylfluorophosphate and apolipoprotein Ala. These inhibitors of
lipase activity depressed hydrolysis of medium TG to a greater degree (30-80%)
than they depressed incorporation of radioactivity into cells (25-60%). Though
hydrolysis of medium TG was inversely proportional to concentration of apolipoprotein Ala, cell uptake radioactivity was inhibited by 25% regardless of Ala
concentration. These studies demonstrate that rat adipocytes avidly hydrolyze
human VLDL TG and incorporate their fatty acids. Fatty acid incorporation is partly controlled by rate of TG hydrolysis, but may depend on other factors as well.

DEFICIENCY OF LIPOPROTEIN A (LP-A), THE MAJOR LIPOPROTEIN FAMILY OF HUMAN PLASMA HIGH DENSITY LIPOPROTEINS

A. Gustafson, W.J. McConathy, and P. Alaupovic
Department of Medicine I, University of Göteborg, Göteborg/Sweden and
Lipoprotein Laboratory Oklahoma Medical Research Foundation, Oklahoma City,OK/USA

Plasma lipids of a 47 year-old female patient with diffuse plane xanthoma were
characterized by normal cholesterol, slightly reduced phospholipid and variable,
but elevated triglyceride. Whereas the total protein contents of LVDL and LDL
were within the normal limits, that of HDL accounted for only 1% (1.8 of 200) of
normal values. The VLDL and LDL consisted of lipoprotein B (LP-B) and lipoprotein
C (LP-C) present both in the form of association complexes and as separate entites.
The HDL consisted only of separable LP-B and LP-C; the major LP-A family and/or
its A-I and A-II polypeptides were absent. In addition to skin lesions, the patient exhibited splenomegaly, hepatomegaly and coronary insufficiency. The tonsils
had a normal appearance. Despite the absence of LP-A, the LCAT activity was still
one-half of its normal value; the CE/FC ratio and the fatty acid composition of
cholesterol esters were normal. The unique biochemical and clinical features of
this disorder of lipid transport seem to warrant its designation as LP-A deficiency.

SUBFRACTIONATION OF HIGH DENSITY LIPOPROTEINS IN RELATION TO CHOLESTEROL ESTER-IFICATION IN VITRO

A. Gustafson and S.O.Olofsson
Departments of Medicine and Medical Biochemistry, University of Göteborg, Göteborg/Sweden

The function of the enzyme lecithin-cholesterol-acyl-transferase (LCAT) is to esterify cholesterol in plasma, preferentially in high density lipoproteins (HDL), utilizing the beta fatty acid of lecithin.

A procedure is described for the isolation of LCAT substrate with the enzyme. The incubation of the substrate-enzyme complex caused a release of new lipoprotein subfractions in proportions to the cholesterol esterification.

From human plasma, added with a SH-blocking agent, HDL fractions were isolated and purified by sequential preparative ultracentrifugation, gel filtration on Sepharose 4 B and column chromatography on hydroxyl apatite. The incubation of the HDL fraction gave cholesterol esterification, a reduced lecithin/sphingomyelin ratio and the production of lipoprotein subfraction. One subfraction contained lysolecithin and the thin precipitin line antigenic determinant of lipoprotein A and another subfraction newly formed cholesteryl ester and apo-lipoprotein A and C peptides.

It is suggested that the thin immuno-precipitin line peptide of lipoprotein A is the carrier of the LCAT substrate.

CHARACTERIZATION OF THE RAT C-APOLIPOPROTEINS

Peter N. Herbert, Herbert G. Windmueller, and Richard S. Shulman
NIH, Bethesda, MD/USA

The C-apolipoproteins from rat plasma HDL have been isolated and characterized. The delipidated apolipoproteins were fractionated by gel and ion-exchange chromatography and characterized by polyacrylamide gel electrophoresis, and amino acid, sialic acid and terminal group analyses. The rat C-I apoprotein, like its human equivalent, was rich in lysine (16%) and contained no tyrosine. It also lacked valine, had COOH-terminal alanine and NH$_2$-terminal aspartic acid. C-II in the rat, like its human counterpart, had COOH-terminal glutamic acid and NH$_2$-terminal threonine. The rat C-III apoprotein, like its human homologue, was found in two polymorphic forms differing in sialic acid content (0 and 3 moles of sialic acid/mole of protein, respectively). The rat C-III apoprotein contained no histidine, and had COOH-terminal proline and NH$_2$-terminal aspartic acid. Rat HDL also contained a protein of C-apoprotein size (6,000 - 10,000 M.W.) that had no apparent human equivalent. This protein was very rich in glutamic acid (21%), had no histidine, and had COOH-terminal alanine and a blocked NH$_2$-terminus.

The striking interspecies homology of the rat and human C-apolipoproteins suggests a much greater functional specificity than has been defined to date, and indicates the opportunities resident in studies of the comparative biochemistry and evolution of the plasma apolipoproteins.

ACUTE SERUM LIPOPROTEIN CHANGES INDUCED BY A HIGH CARBOHYDRATE DIET

Richard J. Jones
Department of Medicine Pritzker School of Medicine, University of Chicago,
Chicago, IL/USA

Sixteen patients with hyperlipemic fasting serum have been studied in a research
unit where they were given a eucaloric formula diet for 7 days containing 20-26%
of calories as protein and 60-70% as saccharide. Daily fasting serum samples were
subjected to sequential centrifugation for isolation of 4 lipoprotein fractions
(HDL, LDL, VLDL and S_f >400) and measurement therein of cholesterol (C), phospholipid (PL) triglyceride (TG) and protein (PR).

Nine patients showed greater levels of the serum TG than 400 mg% after 2 to 4
days of formula diet. With this carbohydrate induction of hyperlipoproteinemia
dramatic quantitative and qualitative changes could be demonstrated in each lipoprotein fraction. VLDL and S_f >400 C increased at least two-fold while HDL and
LDL C decreased 53-70%. Increasing levels of TG were seen in each lipoprotein
fraction, although the greatest increases (2-3%) were seen in VLDL and S_f >400.
Although C/TG showed some decrease in VLDL, a much more striking C/TG decrease
was seen in LDL. Reductions of C/PL and C/PR were also seen consistently in LDL.
Thus, with this carbohydrate induction of hypertriglyceridemia, there is a reduction in amount of TG rich, C poor LDL as well as increased amounts of TG rich,
C poor, PR poor VLDL.

TREATMENT OF HYPERURICEMIA AND HYPERLIPIDEMIA WITH MK 185 A DERIVATIVE OF CLOFIBRATE

Ch. Keller, G. Wolfram, and N. Zöllner
Medical Polyclinic University of Munich, Munich/BRD

Patients with a mixed type of hyperlipidemia frequently suffer also from hyperuricemia. Both diseases are known to induce cardiovascular and kidney diseases
and should therefore be treated early in their course and as long as the patient
is alive. So far the two metabolic changes could only be treated with different
drugs. In a double blind study with 23 patients we compared the new derivative of
clofibrate, halofenate MK 185, with a known uricosuric agent probenecid. Both
drugs were given in one daily dose of 1.0 mg by month after 6 weeks of placebo
treatment; 11 patients took MK 185, and 12 patients probenecid for 24 weeks. The
study ended with a 3 month - cross over period. The uric acid levels were lowered
sufficiently in both groups from an average pretreatment level of 7.4 mg per 100
ml with a mean of 0.4 to 5.2 mg per 100 ml with a mean of 0.3. The plasma levels
remainded low when the MK-group changed to probenecid but increased when the
probenecid-group took placebo again. Triglycerides were also lowered by MK 185
from 450 mg per 100 ml with a mean of 80 to 300 mg per 100 ml with a mean of 90,
but this finding was not quite as consistent as in uric acid levels. Cholesterol
was influenced by neither drug. The new drug was well tolerated by all patients
treated.

INVESTIGATION OF THE LIPOPROTEINS AND APOLIPOPROTEINS FROM PATIENTS WITH A-BETA-LIPOPROTEINEMIA DURING FASTING AND FOLLOWING THE INTRAVENOUS INFUSION OF TRI-GLYCERIDES

Gerhard Kostner, Hans Bohlmann, and Anton Holasek
Institute of Medical Biochemistry, University of Graz, Graz/Austria

The serum from patients with abetalipoproteinemia was examined in order to evaluate how the absence of LpB would affect the distribution of lipoprotein families

in various density classes. Serum lipoproteins were isolated at density 1.063 and 1.063-1.21. After total delipidization, different polypeptides were separated and characterized by immunochemistry, electrophoresis and amino acid analysis. All apoproteins were present in HDL fractions with the exception of one apoC peptide. The relative distribution was similar to normals. In density fraction 1.063 only apoAI peptide could be demonstrated. Following a high triglyceride load, a shift of some polypeptide from HDL to fractions of lower density was observed. The total amount of individual polypeptides remained unchanged. It was therefore concluded that an intravenous administration of triglycerides does not promote the de novo biosynthesis of apoA and apoC polypeptides in these patients.

ISOLATION AND CHARACTERIZATION OF DIFFERENT LIPOPROTEIN FAMILIES OF HUMAN SERUM HIGH DENSITY LIPOPROTEINS

Gerhard Kostner and Pierre Alaupovic
Institute of Medical Biochemistry, University of Graz, Graz/Austria

According to the "family concept" lipoprotein density classes of human serum represent a mixture of different lipoprotein entities characterized by individual protein moieties. After total delipidization, at least eight nonidentical polypeptides can be demonstrated in high density lipoproteins (HDL). In order to evaluate in which manner these polypeptides participate in the assembly of different molecules in HDL, we separated several families from HDL by column chromatography precipitation and immunoadsorption. The major family in HDL_2 and HDL_3 was found to be LpA with apoAI and apoAII as constitutive polypeptides. The ratio apoA:apoAII was different for LpA in HDL_2 and in HDL_3. From HDL_2 a lipoprotein was isolated containing only apoAI peptides. In addition 1PB and LpC were isolated from the HDL fraction and were identified employing standard chemical and physical-chemical methods. It was concluded that HDL is a mixture of three different lipoprotein families LpA, LpB and LpC and that LpA exists in several subgroups.

DENSITY DISTRIBUTION OF PLASMA LIPOPROTEINS IN RHESUS MONKEYS: DIFFERENTIAL EFFECT OF AN ATHEROGENIC DIET IN MALES AND FEMALES

Norman L. Lasser and Joseph F. Allebaugh
Department of Medicine, College of Medicine and Dentology of N.J., N.J. Medical School, Newark, NJ/USA

Rhesus monkeys were fed an atherogenic diet containing 1.2% cholesterol (chol.) and 22% fat. The density distribution of plasma lipoproteins (LP) was examined by measuring the cumulative appearance of LP chol. in supernatant fractions following ultracentrifugation at densities progressively increased by small increments. Plasma lipid values at the beginning of the experiment (control) and at one month were, respectively: chol. 144 and 595 mg/dl and triglyceride 42 and 49 mg/dl. In control plasma 5 mg/dl chol. was found in d <1.006 (VLDL), 10 in d 1.006-1.030 (IDL), 30 in d 1.030-1.060 (LDL), and 76 in d 1.060-1.21 (HDL). At one month in males 32 mg/dl chol. was found in VLDL, 306 in IDL, 70 in LDL, and 77 in HDL. Corresponding values in females were 30, 288, 167, and 69 mg/dl. The same fractions were analyzed with regard to lipid apoprotein and immunological composition, and these results confirmed in monkeys on the diet for 13 months. It is concluded that feeding an atherogenic diet results in an increase in LDL of a lower than normal density in rhesus monkeys, with a greater effect in males.

QUANTITATION OF APOLIPOPROTEINS IN VLDL AND LDL SUBFRACTIONS OF NORMAL AND HYPERLIPOPROTEINEMIC (TYPE II-A) SUBJECTS

D.M. Lee
Oklahoma Medical Research Foundation, Oklahoma City, OK/USA

The purpose of this study was to quantify the soluble (S) (ApoA and ApoC) and the insoluble (I) (ApoB) apolipoproteins of VLDL, LDL_1 (1.006-1.019 g/ml), LDL_2 (1.019-1.053 g/ml) and LDL_3 (1.053-1.063 g/ml) from normal and hyperlipoprotein-emic (Type II-A) subjects. Apolipoproteins separated by a delipidization proce-dure were quantified gravimetrically. ApoC was the predominant S protein in VLDL and LDL_1, whereas ApoA was present only in trace amounts; in LDL_2 and LDL_3, ApoA amounted to 14-40% of the S protein content. The average percent composition of S and I apolipoproteins in normal VLDL was 45 and 55%, in LDL_1 38 and 62%, in LDL_2 6 and 94%, and in LDL_3 20 and 80%, respectively. In type II patients, the only deviation from these compositional patterns was noticed in LDL_1 (27 and 73%, respectively). The most significant difference between normal and type II patients was the protein concentrations of LDL_1 and LDL_2. The average ApoB concentrations of LDL_1 and LDL_2 from type II patients (10 and 120 mg%) were twice as high as those from normal subjects (5 and 67 mg%). Similarly, the concentration of S apo-lipoproteins in LDL_2 from type II patients was 10 mg%, while that from normals was 4-5 mg%.

LIPOPROTEIN LIPASE ACTIVITY IN HUMAN ADIPOSE TISSUE

H. Lithell, J. Boberg, H. Hedstrand, P.-H. Iverius, and A.-M. Östlund
Departments of Geriatrics and Medical Chemistry, Uppsala University, Uppsala/
Sweden

Adipose tissue lipoprotein lipase (LDL) activity is a factor of importance for serum triglyceride (TG) removal and probably of importance for development of hyperlipoproteinaemia. An emulsion of soybean-oil containing glycerol-tri-^{14}C-1-oleate with phospholipid as emulsifier has been tested as substrate for LPL from percutaneously taken human adipose tissue biopsies. The optima for pH and ionic strength are the same for LPL from several sources tested. An inhibitory effect is present with whole serum or delipidated VLDL apo-C as emulsion activa-tors. However, no such inhibition occurs with D_2 (r-glu). In an incubation vol-ume of 1.2 ml LPL activity increased linearly with wet weight up to 25 mg. Glycine 2M-NaOH buffer (pH 8.6) is superior to other tested buffers for stability of en-zyme activity at 37°C.
Adipose tissue from 36 men 59 years of age was incubated in triplicate. The LPL activity in normal men (serum TG 2.46 mmol/1) was between 12 and 36 mU/g and in men with hypertriglyceridaemia the range was 5-23 mU/g. A significant negative correlation (r = -0.87) was found between LPL activities in adipose tissue and serum TG concentrations in hypertriglyceridaemic men but not in men with normal serum TG concentrations.

CHOLESTEROL TOLERANCE TEST AS AN INDICATOR OF DIETARY IMPLICATION IN PLASMA CHOLESTEROL LEVELS

Haruo Nakamura, Ichiro Takeuchi, Yoshiharu Ehata, Hiroshi Shigematsu, Yoichi
Umetada, Yasuteru Tonomo, Tsutomu Hara, and Noboru Irie
Department of Medicine, Keio University, Tokyo/Japan

Dietary cholesterol is known to affect the plasma lipids with considerable vari-ations depending upon subjects.
The present study was carried out to establish a practical and clinical procedure to evaluate the varying response of plasma cholesterol to its dietary intake.

Plasma cholesterol was measured in certain intervals after 3 g of cholesterol ingestion with or without radio-iodinated cholesterol. Increment of plasma cholesterol
was generally highest in 8 to 24 hours samples. The magnitude of response of
plasma cholesterol to the ingestion appeared to be proportional to the extent of
dietary effect of exogenous cholesterol on the plasma concentration.

DIFFERENTIAL EFFECTS OF GLUCOSE AND ETHANOL ON ADIPOSE TISSUE LIPOPROTEIN LIPASE ACTIVITY IN MAN

Peter Nilsson-Ehle
Department of Physiological Chemistry, University of Lund, Lund/Sweden

A moderate dose (30 g/m^2) of glucose to young healthy volunteers induced a rapid,
significant increase of adipose tissue lipoprotein lipase activity to 180% of
initial fasting values after 2 h. A significant decrease in plasma triglyceride
levels occurred. After a moderate ethanol load (60 g), adipose tissue lipoprotein lipase decreased continuously to 43% of initial values after 6 h, which was
significantly lower than in controls fed water. Concomitantly, plasma triglycerides increased to 167% of initial levels.
Adipose tissue lipoprotein lipase is considered a major factor regulating triglyceride uptake from plasma. The results thus indicate that defective lipoprotein
removal may cooperate with the increased lipoprotein secretion from the liver
in the development of hyperlipemia after a single dose of ethanol. After glucose
intake on the other hand, the increased uptake in adipose tissue, probably in
combination with decreased lipoprotein secretion from the liver, results in a
net decrease in plasma triglyceride levels.

FIBRINOGEN AND FIBRINOLYSIS BEHAVIOUR IN HYPERLIPEMIC SUBJECTS AND IN PATIENTS WITH CORONARY HEART DISEASE

Dal Palù[1], W. Donadon[1], and E. Tonolli[2]
[1]Clinica Medica, [2]Istituto di Biochimica ad Ematologia, Policlinico Borgo Roma,
Verona/Italia

Fibrinogen (F) and euglobulin lysis time (ELT) was determined in three groups of
subjects: a) healthy normolipemic subjects n.152; b) hyperlipemic subjects without ischaemic heart disease (IHD) n.89; c) hyperlipemic and normolipemic patients
with IHD n.79. These groups were compared according to three age classes (20-34;
35-49; 50-64). In group a) mean F levels significantly increase with age; on the
contrary mean ELT values do not significantly change. In groups b) and c), compared with group a),. mean F levels and ELT were significantly higher only in the
first two age classes but not in the third class. Mean F levels and ELT were not
significantly different between group b) and c) in all age classes. More over no
significant differences were found between hyperlipemic and normolipemic patients
of group c). It is concluded that: 1) hyperlipemic and IHD patients exhibit, compared with controls, a similar increase of F levels and ELT; 2) this increase in
IHD subjects is independent of the coexistence of hyperlipemia.

ISOLATION OF FIVE LIPOPROTEIN DENSITY CLASSES BY ZONAL ULTRACENTRIFUGATION

Josef Patsch, Sigurd Sailer, Friedrich Sandhofer, Gerhard Kostner, and Herbert
Braunsteiner
Medical Department, University of Innsbruck, Innsbruck/Austria

In order to separate uncontaminated and intact lipoproteins (LP) quantitatively
within 26 hours, a modification of the rate zonal ultracentrifugation technique

was developed (Beckman model L2-65B, Ti-14 rotor). This method consists of two steps:

1. A non-linear density gradient of NaBr in the range of 1.0-1.4 with four grades (1.00, 1.17, 1.30, 1.40) was constructed (Beckman gradient pump model 141). Heparin plasma was adjusted to a density d=1.40, introduced into the rotor at its periphery, and centrifuged at 41,000 rpm, 15°C for 24 hours. By means of this technique, HDL_2 and HDL_3 were isolated quantitatively from LP d < 1.063 and proved to be uncontaminated by albumin (double immunodiffusion).

2. A linear density gradient (NaBr 1.0-1.3) was formed. The LP fraction (d < 1.063) was adjusted to a density of 1.30, introduced into the rotor's periphery, and centrifuged at 42,500 rpm, 15 C for 140 minutes. A quantitative isolation of VLDL plus chylomicrons, LDL, and other LP classes, such as "intermediate LP" (type III), was achieved.

COMPARATIVE STUDY OF HIGH DENSITY PLASMA LIPOPROTEINS AND APOPROTEINS IN CHIMPANZEE AND MAN

Hubert Peeters, Raphael Vercaemst, and Victor Blaton
Simon Stevin Instituut, Brugge/Belgium

Because diet induced hyperbetalipoproteinemia in chimpanzees simulates human type II hyperlipoproteinemia, the validity of the chimpanzee as an experimental model for comparative investigation of lipoprotein turnover and metabolism requires the analysis of the properties of chimpanzee plasma lipoproteins and their compositional apoproteins. The report describes isolation, characterization and delipidation of HDL_2 and HDL_3 and a fingerprint of their polar and apolar lipids. Apo-polypeptides are obtained by electrofocusing in 8 M urea and on Sephadex G-200. N-terminal and C-terminal amino acid residues and the aminoacid composition of apoproteins and of their subunits and polypeptides are analyzed on a Beckman 120 AAA. Molecular weights are determined on SDS-polyacrylamide. Two main polypeptides, R-Glutamine I and R-Glutamine II and their polymorphic forms are identified, minor peptides with C-terminal residues as R-serine, R-alanine, R-valine, were detected. Relationships between the apoproteins of HDL_2 and HDL_3 in human and non human primates confirm the validity of the chimpanzee as a model.

THE METABOLISM OF CHOLESTERYL ESTER-RICH REMNANT PARTICLES IN NORMAL-FED AND CHOLESTEROL-FED RABBITS

Trevor G. Redgrave
Department of Physiology, University of Melbourne, Parkville/Australia

Rabbits but not rats rapidly become hypercholesterolaemic when fed cholesterol. The hypercholesterolaemic response of rabbits was investigated by examining the metabolism of remnant particles which are important in transport of exogenous cholesterol to the liver. In normal-fed (NF) rabbits cholesteryl ester-rich remnant particles were formed from thoracic duct lymph lipoproteins and metabolised in the usual way. In cholesterol-fed (CF) rabbits the recovery of injected cholesteryl ester label was significantly less than in NF rabbits. The recovery of total cholesterol label was not significantly reduced however and the reason for low recovery of esterified cholesterol in CF rabbits was rapid hydrolysis of remnant particle cholesteryl ester, apparently occurring in the liver. In CF rats there was no enhancement of hydrolysis of remnant particle cholesteryl ester. These findings suggest that the activity of hepatic cholesteryl ester hydrolase might account for different responses of rats and rabbits to dietary cholesterol. Direct measurements of hepatic enzyme activities support the finding of increased hydrolytic activity in CF rabbits.

LIPOPROTEINS IN HUMAN PERIPHERAL LYMPH

Drago Reichl and Josef J. Pflug
Medical Research Council Lipid Metabolism Unit, Hammersmith Hospital, London/
England

The composition of lipoproteins from human peripheral lymph was analyzed in order
to improve our understanding of their transfer across the vascular wall. Peripheral lymph was obtained by cannulating a lymphatic trunk on the dorsum of the
foot. Lymph was subjected to sequential preparative ultracentrifugation under
conditions used for the separation of plasma VLDL, LDL and HDL. Free and esterified cholesterol and triglycerides were determined in these fractions of lymph
and the results compared with those obtained by analysis of the plasma lipoproteins obtained from each subject. There were no detectable lipids in the fraction
of lymph corresponding to plasma VLDL. The composition of lipids in the fractions
floating at densities of plasma LDL and plasma HDL differed from the corrrespond-
ing values in plasma lipoproteins. These results preclude a significant transfer
of intact plasma lipoproteins from the blood to peripheral lymph.

THE INTRAVENOUS FAT TOLERANCE TEST (IVFTT): A DIAGNOSTIC TOOL

Stephan Rössner
Department of Internal Medicine and Nutrition Unit, Karolinska Hospital, Stock-
holm/Sweden

An i.v. fat tolerance test simple enough to be used in clinical routine has been
developed using a soybean oil emulsion. *Method:* The fat emulsion is given as a
single dose injection (0.1 g fat/kg body weight). Light scattering of plasma is
then analyzed nephelometrically. The elimination is of the first order and the
IVFTT is expressed as %/min. *Results*: IVFT is negatively correlated to the plasma
TG concentration. The IVFT is significantly correlated to endogenous plasma TG
turnover. In hyperlipidaemias wide variations of IVFT at the same plasma TG concentrations were found suggesting varying fractional turnover rates. The plasma
TG lowering effect of drugs (clofibrate analogues, oxandrolone and nicotinic acid)
has been accompanied by an improved IVFT suggesting increased peripheral elimination of plasma TG. Oral contraceptives increase plasma TG concentration without
affecting IVFT, suggesting that an increased plasma TG secretion causes the
plasma TG rise. *Conclusion*: IVFTT can be of use in experimental metabolic studies,
during treatment with drugs affecting plasma TG concentrations and a complement
in the classification of hyperlipoproteinaemia.

CHARACTERISTICS OF A NEW LIPOPROTEIN PHENOTYPE-COMBINED HYPERLIPOPROTEINEMIA

Herbert G. Rose, Paul Kranz, Murray Weinstock, Joseph Juliano, and Jacob I. Haft
VA Hospital, Bronx, NY/USA

Combined elevation of plasma low-density lipoproteins (LDL) and very-low density
lipoproteins (VLDL) can be a genetic manifestation (CHL). The mode of inheritance
is unsettled, particularly of the LDL elevation, but we favor polygenic determination. To further test the genetic postulate, and also to define the relationship of CHL to the Type IV disorder, we have studied two groups of subjects with
VLDL elevation.

17 Type IV subjects have been matched with 19 CHL subjects with regard to weight,
age, sex, and relative body weight. VLDL cholesterol is higher in Type IV (80.6
$\pm$ 7.0 mg% vs. 58.9 $\pm$ 5.2 p <0.01) while LDL cholesterol is higher in CHL (215 $\pm$
5.3 mg% vs. 129 $\pm$ 5.4 p <0.001). LDL apoprotein levels, determined by radioimmunoassay, also appear higher. Distribution of LDL levels appears bimodal, although

skewness in the Type IV subjects suggests overlap. Despite elimination of acquired causes and matching of LDL-related variables, some subjects (CHL group) maintain higher LDL. This supports genetic determination. CHL subjects manifest a higher incidence of abnormal glucose tolerance test responses, but have a similar high frequency of hyperuricemia and obesity.

EFFECTS OF 3-HYDROXY-3-METHYLGLUTARIC ACID ON CHOLESTEROL METABOLISM IN VITRO AND IN VIVO

Marianne Rouge, Hans Lengsfeld, and Fred Gey
F. Hoffmann-La Roche & Co., Ltd., Basel/Switzerland

Confirming Hamprecht et al. (1971) 3-hydroxy-3-methylglutaric acid (HMGA) reduces the incorporation of ^{14}C-acetate into cholesterol in rat liver homogenate: HMGA at 2×10^{-4} M results in about 50% inhibition. Under the present conditions HMGA inhibits rat liver microsomal 3-hydroxy-3-methylglutaryl-coenzyme A reductase (HMG-CoA reductase) non-competitively. Structurally related di- or tricarboxylic acids are ineffective. In intact rats repeated oral or i.p. application of HMGA changes significantly neither the incorporation of injected ^{14}C-acetate or ^{3}H$_2$O into liver cholesterol nor HMG-CoA reductase activity. Oral or i.p. application of HMGA for two weeks (1-3mmoles/kg before the diurnal active phase of the animals or twice daily) to rats, mice, golden hamsters or guinea pigs does not lower plasma cholesterol. Therefore, in vivo HMGA may fail to reach inhibiting levels at the site of cholesterol synthesis.

In conclusion, more efficient analogues of HMG-CoA are needed for inhibition of cholesterol synthesis in vivo at its key step.

ISOLATION AND CHARACTERIZATION OF THE "INTERMEDIATE" (TYPE III) LIPOPROTEIN

Sigurd Sailer, Josef Patsch, Friedrich Sandhofer, and Herbert Braunsteiner
Medical Department, University of Innsbruck, Innsbruck/Austria

Diagnostic problems of type III hyperlipoproteinemia cause contradictory reports concerning incidence of this disease as well as chemical and immunological properties of the lipoprotein (LP) typical for type III. In seven patients suspected for type III by means of agarose gel electrophoresis, a quantitative isolation of VLDL, "intermediate" LP, and LDL was achieved by zonal ultracentrifugation (linear density gradient NaBr 1.00-1.30, 42 500 rpm, 140 minutes, 10 C). The "intermediate" LP was found between VLDL and LDL. Its plasma concentration was 80-387 mg/100 ml; its ratio to LDL was 0.25-3.0; it contained (range) 32-43% cholesterol, 13-28% triglycerides, 21-26% phospholipids, and 19-24% protein. Apo-LP-B and Apo-LP-B, but not Apo-LP-A were detectable (double immunodiffusion). The "intermediate" LP migrated slightly faster than LDL (in agarose gel electrophoresis) and floated completely only at a density of d=1.035 (angle head rotor, 130 000 g, 18 hours). This method allows an exact diagnosis of the type III hyperlipoproteinemia and a quantitative preparation of the "intermediate" LP.

LOCALISATION OF PORCINE LIPOPROTEINS IN THROMBI AND IN AORTA

P.John Scott, G. Dennis Calvert, and D. Norman Sharpe
Department of Medicine, University of Auckland, School of Medicine, Auckland/ New Zealand

These studies tested the hypothesis that physical characteristics in part determine localisation of lipoproteins (LPs) in thrombi and artery walls. Zonal centrifugation separated two LPs species closely related in density but of differing physical characteristics. Apoprotein was radio-iodinated with 125-I. 125-I-LP was injected into pigs, or introduced into pig blood used to form thrombi in Chandler's tubes.

Localisation of 125-I-LP was determined by direct counting, histochemistry and autoradiography. Both LPs were associated with the red cell mass of thrombi in vivo and in vitro, rather than platelet aggregates. Lipid from these LPs is unlikely to accumulate in arterial intima from incorporation of purely platelet thrombi. Distribution differences of the two LPs in pig aorta correlated with differences in aorta structure and mucopolysaccharide content. Physical differences between LPs, rather than size, may account for differences in distribution of LP within artery wall.

APOLIPOPROTEIN AND LIPOPROTEIN HETEROGENEITY

Bernard Shore, Antone Salel, Virgie Shore, Robert Zelis, and Dean Mason
Biomedical Division, University of California, Livermore, CA/USA

Genetic, metabolic, dietary and other factors van affect composition of the major lipoprotein (LP) classes as well as their concentration in plasma. In sera in which the major very low density lipoprotein (VLDL, d <1.006) species are of ß-mobility in agarose electrophoresis and are enriched in cholesteryl esters, the VLDL and LDL_2 (d 1.006-1.019) are enriched in an arginine-rich apoLP. In type III VLDL (elevated) and LDL_2 (elevated) and in hypothyroid VLDL (not elevated) and LDL_2 (elevated), there is an enrichment in this apoLP. In rabbits fed excess cholesterol, the VLDL (elevated) are of ß-mobility and are greatly enriched in the arginine-rich proteins(s) and cholesteryl esters and very low in triglycerides. The VLDL and LDL_2 of types II, IV and normal, but not III, persons on low cholesterol diets often have no excess arginine-rich apoLP. The VLDL and LDL_2 (both elevated) of type IV sera giving a double pre-ß band contain little of this apoLP and relatively more apoVLDLser than usual. The arginine-rich apoLP may be one of several associated primarily with cholesterol transport and metabolism; other apoLPs may be involved primarily in metabolism of triglycerides or other lipids. Variations in LP composition as well as concentration may reflect the homeostasis of these metabolic pathways.

CHOLESTEROL METABOLISM IN HYPERLIPOPROTEINEMIAS IN MAN

Harbhajan S. Sodhi and Bhalchandra J. Kudchodkar
Department of Medicine, University of Sastatchewan, Saskatoon/Canada

An analysis of published and our own unpublished data indicated that there was no significant difference in the absorption of dietary cholesterol between normal subjects and patients with different hyperlipoproteinemias. Absorbed cholesterol caused inhibition of endogenous synthesis in normal subjects as well as in patients with types IIa, IIb, IV, and V hyperlipoproteinemia. The absorbed cholesterol appeared to replace rather precisely the decrease in endogenous synthesis. Furthermore, the catabolism of absorbed and synthesized cholesterol was identical. This is in accord with our hypothesis that dietary cholesterol removed by the liver enters the same pool as the cholesterol synthesized in the liver. Cholesterol synthesis in type IIa was subnormal and in types IIb, IV, and V it was greater than normal. Correspondingly, the fecal excretion of total steroids was also less in type IIa and freater than normal in types IIv, IV, and V. The ratio of neutral to acidic fecal steroids, however, was identical in all except type V. These observations support our hypothesis that catabolism of endogenous cholesterol in man is greater in conditions associated with hyper-pre-ß-lipoproteinemia than in conditions where the pre-ß-lipoprotein is low or normal.

ISOELECTRIC FRACTIONATION OF PLASMA HIGH DENSITY LIPOPROTEINS

Harbhajan S. Sodhi, Govindaswamy S. Sundaram, and Samuel L. MacKenzie
Department of Medicine, University of Saskatchewan, Saskatoon/Canada

Preparative isoelectric focusing of several samples of high density lipoproteins (HDL_2) gave identical resolution profiles. Approximately 10 protein peaks with reproducible isoelectric points were observed. When fractions containing only the 2 middle peaks were pooled, concentrated, and rerun, they appeared in the same location and with the same isoelectric points. When all fractions were pooled and tested by analytical ultracentrifugation and agarose electrophoresis, the material was indistinguishable from the original HDL_2. The pooled fractions from each major peak indicated differences in the proteins (by acrylamide gel electrophoresis) and in their protein to cholesterol and protein to phospholipid ratios. The pooled peaks also differed in their ultraviolet and infrared spectra. They reacted with HDL antisera.

These results suggest that the architecture of HDL_2 depends, at least in part, on critical ionic bonds, which are destroyed under conditions prevailing in isoelectric focusing. The data also indicate that HDL_2 includes protein components differing in electric properties as well as in cholesterol and phospholipid binding.

CHOLESTERYL ESTER METABOLISM IN LIVER AND BLOOD PLASMA OF VARIOUS ANIMAL SPECIES

Kjell Torgeir Stokke
Institute of Clinical Biochemistry, University of Oslo, Rikshospitalet, Oslo/
Norway

Enzymes taking part in formation and breakdown of cholesteryl esters (CE) may correlate with the tendency to develop hypercholesterolemia and atherosclerosis. In eight different animal species the activities of the following enzymes were determined: 1. the plasma lecithin:cholesterol acyltransferase (LCAT); 2. the liver microsomal acyl-CoA:cholesterol acyltransferase; and 3. the liver lysosomal acid cholesterol esterase. The latter enzyme may take part in hydrolysis and elimination of lipoprotein CE.

The activities of these enzymes differed considerably in the various animal species. The highest LCAT activity was observed in monkey and man, whereas calf displayed rather low activity. In human liver no acyl-CoA:cholesterol acyltransferase activity could be demonstrated, and in liver from guinea pig very low activity was observed. This constrasts to the high activity found in rat liver. The highest cholesterol esterase activity was observed in rabbit and calf liver, whereas hydrolytic activity in rat, guinea pig, dog and swine was rather low.

ENDOGENOUS TRIGLYCERIDE TRANSPORT IN HYPERTRIGLYCERIDEMIA – THE EFFECT OF PHENFORMIN

R.W. Stout, D. Porte Jr., J.D. Brunzell, and E.L. Bierman
Department of Medicine, University of Washington, Seattle, WA/USA

The effect and mechanism of action of phenformin was studied in 9 subjects with endogenous hypertriglyceridemia. On a fat-free high carbohydrate formula diet, administration of phenformin, 50 mg b.d. for 2 weeks, resulted in a fall in both triglyceride (mean % change -14.3%, $p < 0.01$) and cholesterol (-12.6%, $p < 0.01$), very low density lipoproteins being reduced by the drug. Insulin, which enhances triglyceride synthesis, was also reduced by phenformin (-23.3%, $p < 0.001$) as were the triglyceride precursors, free fatty acids (FFA) and glucose. The fall in

FFA levels (-16%, p <0.01) was accompanied by a reduction in FFA turnover (-26.5%, p <0.001). Endogenous triglyceride removal rate (a measure of triglyceride production) measured during a prolonged heparin infusion, decreased in 8 subjects (13.4%, p <0.05), although the kinetics of TG removal were unchanged. Thus phenformin lowers triglyceride levels by reducing endogenous triglyceride production; this effect may be due to the reduction in insulin, glucose and free fatty acids.

EPIDEMIOLOGICAL STUDY ON HYPERLIPIDEMIA AMONG JAPANESE

Motoo Tsushima, Eiichiro Asano, Yoshiya Hata, Yasuhiko Homma, Yoichi Umetada, Noriaki Nakaya, and Yuichiro Goto
Department of Medicine, School of Medicine, Keio University, Tokyo/Japan

Atherosclerotic vascular diseases are known to frequently develop in certain types of hyperlipidemias. An epidemiological study on hyperlipidemias has been conducted in two farm villages and a fishing village in Japan since 1969. An anabolic steroid has been employed as lipid lowering agent to assess whether it would decrease the morbidity. Regarding the prevalence and the mortality of atherosclerotic diseases, neither cerebral thrombosis nor myocardial infarction have been recognized in anabolic steroid group. Cerebral bleeding appeared to have close association with hypercholesterolemia, high blood pressure and obesity, and cerebral thrombosis had close relationship to hypercholesterolemia and high blood pressure.

CHOLESTEROL AND TRIGLYCERIDE COMPOSITION OF VERY LOW AND LOW DENSITY LIPOPROTEINS IN HYPERLIPOPROTEINEMIAS

B. Vessby, L.A. Carlson, and H. Hedstrand
Department of Geriatrics, University of Uppsala, Uppsala/Sweden

The lipoprotein pattern in serum was studied in healthy 50 year old men to define normal limits for the ratios between cholesterol (CH) and triglycerides (TG) in very low density lipoproteins (VLDL) and low density lipoproteins (LDL) and TG content in LDL. From the same sample men with hyperlipoproteinemias (HL) were also studied. The analysis was performed by consecutive spins in an ultracentrifuge at d. 1.006 and 1.063 to isolate VLDL and LDL followed by CH and TG determinations. Whole serum, top and bottom fractions at d. 1.006 were also analysed on agarose gel electrophoresis. All HL types had high LDL TG. Type III had the highest ratio CH/TG in VLDL, the lowest in LDL and the highest LDL TG. Type IV also had significantly lower ratio in LDL than normals. Patients who in addition to the normal pre-ß band had a slow moving band in the top fraction on electrophoresis also showed high CH/TG ratio in VLDL, a low ratio in LDL and increased LDL TG when compared to patients with the same type of HL but without "slow pre-ß" occurring in about 20% of this population may a lipoprotein of "intermediary type" related to the "floating ß" in type III HL.

STUDY OF AN INTRAVENOUS FAT TOLERANCE TEST WITH INTRALIPID IN HUMAN SUBJECTS

Kazunari Wada, Rhyuhei Sakaguchi, Koichi Murakami, and Junichi Mise
Department of Medicine, Yamaguchi University School of Medicine, Ube/Japan

An intravenous fat tolerance test with Intralipid was performed on 130 human subjects. The exogenous triglyceride removal rate, K_2 value, was determined by micronephelometry. The relation of K_2 value to post-heparin lipolytic activity (PHLA) and TG were studied with reference to the following factors determined simultaneously in the same individuals: cholesterol, plasma albumin, blood sugar, age, body weight, height, obesity (% increment of body weight) and L/O ratio (% increment of linoleic to oleic acid ratio calculated at 30 minutes after the Intralipid injection) of plasma NEFA.

The calculated partial correlation coefficients and "t" values indicated that there were partial correlation between K_2 and fasting triglyceride ($r = -0.6277$, $p < 0.05$) and between K_2 and age ($r = -0.4983$, $p < 0.10$). The results obtained by multiple regression analysis was that K_2 value was changed by such factors as TG and age.

From the above mentioned factors, two principle components were determined by "principle component analysis". The factors which had relatively high coefficients in the first component were K_2, obesity, TG, cholesterol and body weight, and the factors in the second component were PHLA, albumin and age. These statistical findings suggest that each of the two principle components has its own distinctive pathophysiological properties and K_2 value gives better and also different clinical information from that obtained by the measurement of PHLA.

EFFECT OF HEPARIN ON THE KINETICS OF GUINEA PIG AND HUMAN POSTHEPARIN LIPASE ACTIVITY

Thomas F. Whayne, Jr.
Oklahoma Medical Research Foundation, Oklahoma City, OH/USA

Lipoprotein lipase (LPL) is essential for metabolism of circulating triglycerides (TG). Allosteric control of postheparin (PH) lipase TG substrate activation by heparin was suggested previously. The purpose of this study was to explore further the control mechanism and investigate its role in man. Rat HDL was added to guinea pig (GP) PH serum assays containing constant TG, and the effect of heparin evaluated. Increase in GP PH serum lipase activity produced by HDL resembled a Michaelis-Menten hyperbola. Heparin addition, 0.8 unit/ml, changed this to an S-shaped curve. As heparin was increased, the S-shaped curve shifted to the right with decreased V_{max}. Next, human VLDL was added to human PH serum assays with and without in vitro heparin. VLDL increased human PH serum lipase activity as a Michaelis-Menten hyperbola. Heparin addition, 3.2 unit/ml, changed this to an S-shaped curve. As heparin was increased, the S-shaped curve shifted to the right with decreased V_{max}. All S-shaped curves with GP and human PH serum gave straight lines when plotted by the Hill equation linear form. Thus, heparin altered kinetics of lipase activity and increased Hill equation K. These data provide more evidence for an allosteric effect of heparin on PH serum lipase activity and suggest such control in man through this mechanism. Control of LPL in human lipid transport is undergoing further study using purified enzyme.

A GENERATIONAL STUDY OF LIPIDS AS A POSSIBLE PREDICTOR OF CLINICAL ATHEROSCLEROSIS

Asher Woldow, J. Cohen, and L. Parry
Philadelphia Geriatric Center, Philadelphia, PA/USA

Predictability of abnormal lipids in a multi-generational study beginning with an aged population (average 82 years) is being investigated. This study is being done at the Philadelphia Geriatric Center where problems in completing such a study are less than in an average community. There are over 700 residents living under reasonably similar environment including dietary habits. Complete family histories and physicals are obtained and laboratory findings, including lipid typings and glucose profiles are being accumulated. Here we find it easier to bring in the family members who visit their parents frequently. So far we have over 600 people generated by 95 residents, including 4 generations, in the initial preliminary study. Initial studies suggest there is a predictability of lipid factors in the first and second generations (average ages 82 and 58 respectively) and between second and third generations (average ages 58 and 34 respectively). The results are more predictable when spouses are included. The correlation is somewhat less between generations one and three suggesting probable environmental factors. The findings are more consistent with cholesterol as compared to triglycerides. By increasing the number if family members included, the weighting of unequal family numbers may be eliminated.

THE VALUE OF CASUAL PLASMA LIPID DETERMINATIONS IN POPULATION SCREENING

Peter Wood, Woodrow Myers, Herbert Klein, and Morris Bunow
Department of Medicine, Stanford University, Stanford, CA/USA

To study the potential mass screening use of casual plasma lipid values (no attempt to prescribe fasting), 157 male and 286 female cannery workers (aged 25-79) were examined. An 8 a.m. fasting blood sample was drawn, after which a normal breakfast was eaten followed by the usual morning's work. A "casual" blood sample was then drawn at midday. Each participant's plasma samples were analyzed together in pairs for total cholesterol (TC) and triglycerides (TG) by Auto-Analyzer I.

Male TG levels (mean±SD, mg/100 ml) surpassed female levels in both fasting (147±105 vs 121±85) and casual (237±177 vs 169±124) states. Arbitrary "upper limits of normal" were set for fasting and casual TG levels, respectively: male, 174/249 mg/100 ml; female, 149/199 mg/100 ml. The casual data then indicated the following percentages of true negatives, true positives, false negatives and false positives, respectively: males, 68, 21, 3 and 8%; females, 72, 16, 5 and 7%. Fasting and casual TC levels were very similar ($r = 0.97$, for each sex).

Conclusions: a) male casual TG values exceeded those for females of similar age; b) casual TG values provided a useful guide to fasting levels in mass screening; c) casual and fasting TC levels were virtually identical.

INHIBITION BY DIMETHYLBIGUANIDE OF THE INCORPORATION OF 4-^{14}C CHOLESTEROL IN THE AORTA OF THE RABBIT

René Agid, Georges Marquié and Max Lafontan
Institut de Physiologie, Université P. Sabatier, Toulouse/France

Since we showed that dimethylbiguanide (DMB) attenuated to a large extent the lipidic perturbations caused by cholesterol in rabbits, the influence of DMB (120 mg/kg/day) upon incorporation of cholesterol ^{14}C (10 μc) in the aorta and other tissues was studied. Administration of DMB reduced the incorporation of ingested cholesterol ^{14}C after 24 hours by 50 to 70% in plasma, liver, bone marrow and aorta, compared with normal animals. But since intestinal absorption of cholesterol was also diminished in the same proportion, cholesterol ^{14}C was injected in the blood in another set of experiments. On this occasion DMB brought about the same reduction of the specific activity of cholesterol ^{14}C in the aorta, but not in other tissues. These results fit our previous finding that DMB attenuates lipidic infiltration of the tissues and experimental atherosclerosis in the rabbit.

A.C. Arntzenius, H.A. van Geuns, T.L. Mellema, J. Meijer, D.P. Sluyter, and
K. Styblo
The Royal T.B. Association and Heart Foundation, The Hague/Netherlands

The purpose of this study is to investigate the usefulness of chest clinics in
combating coronary heart disease. Medical and paramedical personnel received 4
months training in standardized screening and intervention procedures. Use is
made of questionnaires on the family history and symptoms; a 12-lead resting ECG
is read clinically as well as coded by Minnesota Code. Blood pressure,cholesterol,
glucose intolerance, height and weight, urine and chest X-ray films are examined
and results are grouped in scores. In subjects with elevated risk factors intervention on smoking, eating and exercise habits is carried out by district nurses
on home visits; the risk factors are reexamined every 3 months. Results of first
examination show that of 4,000 subjects, aged 20-50 years, one-third had low,
one-third borderline elevated and one-third had elevated risk factors. Results
of intervention on 1,200 subjects with elevated risk factors reexamined at 3 and
6 months will be presented. Authors feel that preliminary results are encouraging.

NICOTINIC ACID PLUS BETA-BLOCKERS IN TREATMENT OF HYPERLIPOPROTEINAEMIAS

Pietro Avogaro, Carlo Capri, Cazzolato Guiseppe
Ospedale Regionale Generale, Venezia/Italia

Association between N.A and beta-B has proved synergic in animals to inhibit
FFA release and epinephrine-induced hypertriglyceridaemia. 11 patients type II A
and 6 type IV underwent a treatment for four periods of one month each (1 with
placebo; 1 with N.A (750 mg/day); 1 with beta-B (60 mg/day); 1 with N.A (250
mg/day) plus beta-B (20 mg/day). Patients weight has not significatively varied
($\pm$ 2 Kg.). Cholesterol has proved significatively reduced in type II by beta-B
plus N.A (-8.7%) and by N.A (-11.8%) and in type IV only by N.A (-5.5%). In the
type IV triglycerides have been reduced by beta-B plus N.A (-33.2%). These data
support the hypothesis of a major effect of the two drugs in reducing hyper-
glyceridaemia. This goal is achieved without any unpleasant side-effect due to
the very low doses employed.

EFFECT OF COLESTID ON SERUM LIPIDS OF PATIENTS WITH TYPE IV HYPERLIPOPROTEINEMIAS

Gaetano Bazzano and Gail Bazzano
Department of Medicine, St. Louis University and City Hospital Unit II, St. Louis,
MO/USA

Colestid, a synthetic organic bile sequestrant polymer, has been recently shown
to be effective in the reduction of plasma cholesterol and ß-lipoprotein cholesterol in familial Type II hyperlipoproteinemia (JAMA 222:676, 1972). We report
now the serum cholesterol, triglycerides and body weight in 47 patients with Type
IV hyperlipoproteinemia. Twenty-five of these patients were given Colestid (15
gm/day), while the remaining were given Avicel (8.1 gm/day) as a placebo. Laboratory data were collected monthly during the first year and every two months
thereafter. The serum cholesterol levels appeared to decrease 22% at the end of
one year and a further 10% at the end of the second year. These changes are significant at a confidence level of 95% with a p <.01, both at the end of the first
and second year. A lower, statistically not significant decrease in serum cholesterol was also observed in the placebo group. Triglycerides and body weight

showed a decreasing trend not present in the placebo group. It appears therefore that Colestid may be a useful agent in the treatment of Type IV hyperlipoproteinemias.

PROTECTIVE EFFECTS OF PENTAERYTHRITOLTETRANICOTINATE AGAINST EXPERIMENTAL ATHEROSCLEROSIS IN HYPERLIPEMIC RABBITS

Ralph Brattsand
AB Bofors Novel-Pharma, Mölndal/Sweden

The correlation between serum cholesterol (chol.) and degree of aortic fat infiltration was studied in rabbits fed chol. at different levels. A correlation existed in the serum chol. region 300-1000 mg/100 ml but not above the latter level. Hyperlipemia was induced by dietary administration of chol. in a normal diet, or of coconut oil resp. butter in a semisynthetic diet. These diets gave different degrees of hyperchol.-emia, hyper-TG-emia and aortic changes. Addition of pentaerythritoltetranicotinate (niceritrol, INN) 0.5% in the diet reduced serum as well as aortic chol. levels. The protection in aorta was also tested with exclusion of the serum lipid reduction. This was achieved by giving the niceritrol-treated animals extra dietary fat so that the same serum LD- and VLD-lipoprotein levels were attained. Even then niceritrol gave 35% (P <0.01) lower levels of free and esterified chol. in aorta. The investigations indicate that the niceritrol-induced inhibition in aorta is caused by a reduction of serum LD- and VLD-lipoproteins as well as by other factors.

REDUCTION OF HYPERLIPIDEMIA IN HUMANS WITH DH-581 (PROBUCOL)

Frank L. Canosa, Adolfo M. Aparicio, and Edwin Boyle, Jr.
Miami Heart Institute, Research Division, Miami Beach, FL/USA

To determine the effectiveness of probucol in reducing serum cholesterol and triglycerides, 116 hyperlipidemic patients were given 500 mg of the drug orally b.i.d. Twenty-seven of these patients have completed two years and eighty-one have completed one year of treatment. Examinations were done at monthly intervals for two months and every two months thereafter. No dietary changes were requested of the patients. No toxicity or changes in body weight were observed. Marked xanthelasma and xanthoma reductions were noted in some subjects. Evaluation was made by comparison of pre-treatment control values of cholesterol and of triglycerides with treatment values up to twenty-four months. For the total group of 116 patients, a reduction in serum cholesterol from 301 to 262 mg% (P <.0001) was observed after one month, and the cholesterol did not vary significantly from the reduced levels in subsequent months, being relatively more effective in phenotype II than in IV. Triglyceride response was erratic and inconsistent.

It is concluded that probucol is effective in reducing cholesterol in hyperlipidemic humans with no significant side effects.

LONG TERM TREATMENT OF PRIMARY HYPERLIPOPROTEINAEMIA WITH D,L-ALPHA-METHYL-THYROXINE-ETHYLESTER (CG 635)

Helmut Canzler, F. Arnold Gries, Hans-Dieter Miß, Theodor Koschinsky, and Karl Jahnke
Department Innere Medizin der Medizinischen Hochschule Hannover, 2. Medizinische Klinik der Universität Düsseldorf, Städtische Krankenanstalten Wuppertal, Düsseldorf/BRD

Recent studies on D, L-alpha-methylthyroxine-ethylester (CG 635) showed lowering effects on serum cholesterol and triglyceride levels. For a therapeutical trial received 52 out-patients with primary hyperlipoproteinaemia (HLP) 40 - 60 mg of CG 635 interrupted by placebo periods. The intake was controlled by measurement of plasma iodine levels. 12 out of 31 patients with HLP type II a and II b, according to Fredrickson, showed lowering cholesterol effects of 20 - 40%, four 10 - 20% and 15 none. In eight out of 19 patients with HLP type IV and V a sufficient decrease of cholesterol and triglycerides in serum was observed. In three patients cholesterol levels only were lowered, while in eight patients no effect of the substance was seen. In two patients with HLP type III the therapy failed. 20 out of 27 cases successfully treated were observed for 6 - 18 months. An optimal decrease by serum lipids seems to be reached 8 - 12 weeks after initiation of therapy and kept constant in most of the cases all over the observation time. In several patients the serum lipids increased again moderately or returned to the original level during long term therapy. Rebound effects after discontinuation were not observed. Relevant side effects were not noticed. The best therapeutic effects were seen in excessive primary HLP type II a.

TEN YEARS' EXPERIENCE WITH CHOLESTYRAMINE IN THE TREATMENT OF HYPERLIPIDEMIAS

H. Richard Casdorph
Lipid Research Foundation, Long Beach, CA/USA

During the past ten years we have treated over 200 hyperlipidemic patients by the long-term administration of cholestyramine (Questran). This represents over 2,500 patient-months of therapy. Serum cholesterols were reduced an average of 20% (from 337 to 257 mg%)(range 7-57%). Cholesterols were performed by automated method. Statistical significance at the P .01 level. Serum triglycerides have not been significantly altered by this drug. One hundred type II patients obtained an average reduction of serum cholesterol of -20% (from 337 to 257 mg%) (range 7-57%). A new method of administering the resin in a single daily dose unrelated to meals indicates that this simplified method is approximately equally as efficacious in reducing the serum cholesterol. There has been no evidence of malabsorption of vitamins A, D or E. There has been some reduction in the prothrombin times. No bleeding phenomena. Side effects consist of constipation, epigastric distress and acute pancreatitis.

A PALATABLE BILE ACID SEQUESTRANT REDUCES CHOLESTEROL

Elmer E. Cooper
Santa Rose Medical Center, San Antonio, TX/USA

Colestipol is an insoluble, nonabsorbable, copolymer with a bile acid binding capacity. It prevents reabsorption of cholates from intestinal tract into the enterohepatic circulation causing a net loss of bile acids, and therefore of cholesterol, from the body. In 141 hyperlipidemic subjects studied for 104 weeks, five g three times daily lowered serum cholesterol levels by an average of 40 mg per 100 ml. A comparable group of 69 hyperlipidemics on placebo showed on average no change in serum cholesterol. Serum triglycerides were not significantly altered. The high molecular resin is not absorbed from the gastrointestinal tract producing a slight increase in fecal volume. Blood chemistries, serum enzymes, prothrombin times, hematology, urinalysis, and body weights were not changed. There was no fat-soluble vitamin interference or ophthalmological effects. Colestipol is a tasteless and odorless copolymer and has a high acceptability of therapy. Side effects were limited to occasional bloating, gas, and constipation. While types II, III, and IV hyperlipidemics responded effectively, type II was most often promptly and consistently markedly reduced. Colestipol is a safe, effective, palatable hypolipidemic agent.

INCREASED RATE OF OXYGEN TRANSPORT FROM BLOOD TO TISSUES AFTER HEPARIN IN ATHEROSCLEROTIC PATIENTS

Hyman Engelberg
Beverly Hills, CA/USA

Using an ear oximeter and maximum breathholding, the effect of heparin upon the rate of transfer of oxygen from the blood to the tissues was determined in 41 atherosclerotic patients. It was increased after heparin in 23 individuals, unchanged in 12, and decreased in 6. In the entire group of patients there was an increase of 14% in the average rate of oxygen transfer. In general heparin increased the rate of oxygen transfer in those subjects whose control values were below average. These results indicate that in some atherosclerotic individuals there is interference, which is removed by heparin, with the transfer of oxygen from the blood to the tissues.

PRIMARY SCREENING FOR ANTIHYPERLIPIDEMIC AGENTS

Hiroshi Enomoto and Rainer Zschocke
Nippon Shinyaku Co., Ltd., Kyoto/Japan and Klinge & Co., Munich/BRD

To develop a rapid and efficient primary screening system for hypolipemic activity, the following test models were applied and their efficacy evaluated: in vitro and in vivo lipid mobilization, Triton - and fructose - induced hyperlipidemia (T- and F-test respectively), and the normolipemic rat (N-test). Male Sprague Dawley and Wistar rats, 180-220 g b.w., were compared in the N-test and found to respond similarly to lipid lowering agents. Compounds were given in isotonic agar either i.p. (T-test) or p.o. (in vivo lipolysis, F- and N-test). Optimal conditions for the N-test were a three-day treatment, blood collection on the fourth day four to six hours after the last dose, and food withdrawal during the same time period. In the F-test conditions were similar except for the inclusion of 10% fructose in the drinking fluid during the last 48 hours and a 16 hours fast prior to bleeding. For all compounds tested the triglyceride (TG)-lowering effect in the F-test was significantly correlated with the TG - and cholesterol (TC)-decreasing activity observed in the N-test ($2\alpha < 0.01$, N = 86). The TC-lowering effect in the T-test was significantly correlated to lipid lowering activity in the N-test ($2\alpha < 0.05$, N = 207). This correlation did not persist, however, when values of below 20% inhibition in the T-test were excluded, indicating a high incidence of false positive results with the T-test. Antilipolytic activities in vitro and in vivo were not correlated to either of the other tests. It is concluded that the F- and N-test are best suited for the rapid screening of prospective hypolipemic compounds. The value of the T-test is doubtful, while in vivo and in vitro lipid mobilization are regarded unsuitable for this purpose.

CHOLESTEROL SYNTHESIS IN MINI PIGS. INFLUENCE OF DIET AND HYPOLIPIDEMIC DRUGS

Wolfram Kaiser, Klaus Stocker, and Dieter Brechenmacher
Medizinische Poliklinik der Universität, München/BRD

The most commonly used animal in studies for cholesterol synthesis is the rat. The lipid metabolism of the mini pig seems to be more similar to that of the human species. By determining the 7-dehydrocholesterol concentration in the serum after blocking 7-dehydrocholesterol reductase with AY 9944 the in vivo choles- terol synthesis in mini pigs was measured during physiologic, different dietary and hypolipidemic drug managements. High cholesterol intake or fasting is based on a feedback mechanism of cholesterol synthesis. Pectin, algin or tomatine in- creases synthesis. a-chloro-phenoxy-isobutyrate leads to significant decreases whereas nicotinic acid or ß-pyridylcarbinol shows no changes in cholesterol syn- thesis. These results are discussed in relation to published views on regulation of cholesterol metabolism in rats and humans.

EFFECTS OF DIETS, IODOCASEIN, AND CLOFIBRATE ON HUMAN LIPOPROTEIN METABOLISM

Noboru Kimura, Seiki Nanbu, Hiroo Goda, and Hironori Toshima
Internal Medicine, Kurume University School of Medicine, Japan

Plasma lipoproteins (LP) have been studied in hyperlipidemic subjects who under- went hypolipidemic diet, iodocasein, or clofibrate treatment. Plasma lipids and individual LP-lipids and protein were measured at the beginning and the end of treatment periods. To investigate a synthesis of LP, we have measured an atom % of ^{15}N in each LP fractions at 6 hours after administration of ^{15}N-glycine. After these therapies the per cent change in both LDL-cholesterol (Chol) and tri- glyceride (TG) generally paralleled those in plasma. The rise in LDL-^{15}N con- centration without change in LDL protein was found after the diet therapy but there was no change in this after clofibrate treatment. Oppositely change in this was found after iodocasein therapy following the diet therapy. TG and Chol in VLDL absolutely decreased without in proportion to change in those in plasma, 30% ± 6 and 51% ± 12, respectively. Both VLDL-C/P, C/^{15}N and TG/P, TG/^{15}N ratio were decreased after each treatment. The change of LDL synthesis caused by dietary change or drug treatment reflects changes in plasma lipids. The absolute reduction of VLDL lipids without change of protein and VLDL synthesis may be an important factor in the change of LDL.

ON CLINICO-EXPERIMENTAL PHARMACOTHERAPY OF ISCHEMIC CARDIOPATHIES

S.G. Kobaladze
Chair of Internal Medicine, Medical Institute, Tbilisi/USSR

The object of the work - experimental and clinical evaluation of efficiency of intensain and sustac. As criteria served: in experiment - a morphological study of cardiac muscle after an experimental infarction of myocardium, in clinic - polycardiographic, radiokymographic and biochemical investigation (acid-base balance, electrolytic balance, gaseous blood contents, coagulating and anti- coagulating blood systems). Under the action of above-mentioned preparations in experiment processes of compensatory order are observed - formation of vascular network, massive preservation of muscular fibres, increased retrograde flow of blood and lymph, formation of closing arteries. In patients with ischemic heart disease under the action of intensain and sustac is observed regulation of acid- base balance and electrolytic balance, as well as of gaseous blood contents with parallel positive changes in cardiodynamics.

TREATMENT OF PRIMARY HYPERLIPOPROTEINAEMIA TYPE II COMPARING DL-α-METHYLTHYROXINE-
ETHYLESTER, D-THYROXINE AND A COMBINATION OF D-THYROXINE + TRIIODTHYRONONE

T. Koschinsky, F.A. Gries, K.H. Vogelberg, H. Miss, K. Jahnke, H. Canzler, F.A.
Horster, J. Herrmann, W. Wildmeister, and H.L. Krüskemper
2. Medizinische Klinik, University of Düsseldorf, Düsseldorf/BRD

38 patients with primary hyperlipoproteinaemia type II (31 type IIa, 7 type IIb)
were treated as follows: 8 weeks placebo, 12 weeks 40 mg DL-methylthyroxine-
ethylester (CG 635)/day, 8 weeks placebo, 20 weeks 2-4-6 mg D-thyroxine + 0.5-1-
1.5 mg triiodthyronine (EMD 26-916)/day, 8 weeks placebo, 20 weeks 4-6-8 mg D-
thyroxine (DYNO)/day, 8 weeks placebo.

In patients with type IIa serum cholesterol was lowered by CG 635 (56 mg/100 ml
or 21%), in relation to dose by EMD 26-916 (170 mg/100 ml or 34%) and in relation
to dose by DYNO (65 mg/100 ml or 16%). In patients with type IIb cholesterol was
lowered to a lesser degree. The effect on triglycerides was irregular and minute
in both types.

The ^{127}I Pb was raised by CG 635 to 50-70 µg/100 ml, by EMD 26-916 and by DYNO in
relation to dose to 10 - 30 µg/100 ml. The ^{127}I Pb normalized during each placebo
period.
Total-thyroxine (T) and the effective thyroid ratio were measured also.
EMD 26-916 lowered cholesterol most effectively.

CLINICAL DIAGNOSIS OF EARLY ATHEROSCLEROSIS OF THE LOWER EXTREMITIES

Jiří Linhart, Rudolf Dejdar, Jiří Spáčil, and Anna Hlavová
Institute for Clinical and Experimental Medicine, Prague/Czechoslovakia

Since the importance of diagnostic methods has not been clarified, noninvasive
techniques were compared with angiography. Arterial murmurs indicated atherosclerosis with a high specificity but limited sensitivity. Abnormal segmental
pulse wave velocity and/or crest time were highly specific and sensitive. Maximal
calf blood flow after ischemic exercise was lower in patients with atheromatous
plaques than in control subjects. Angiography was capable of demonstrating initial
atheromatosis even in small arteries of the leg and foot provided there was adequate anaesthesia with a normal blood pressure and satisfactory skin temperature.
It is concluded that the noninvasive methods are of considerable value for screening, whereas angiography remains the method of choice in the selected subjects.

RELATIONSHIPS BETWEEN ADRENAL STEROIDS AND LIPID METABOLISM AFTER EXERCISE

A. Lopez-S., Charles Wingo, and John Hebert
Louisiana State University Medical School, New Orleans, LA/USA

In previous experiments in animals it was shown that voluntary exercise produces
a significant increase in adrenal size; in humans, an increase was observed in the
urinary excretion of dehydroepiandrosterone and its metabolites androsterone and
etiocholanolone. We have now studied the effect of exercise on adrenal steroid
metabolism and found in rats after 10 weeks of exercise a small change in the
activity of adrenal Δ^5-3 β -hydroxy-steroid-dehydrogenase (from 116 to 140 µg
androstenedione formed/30 minute/mg protein) and a significant increase in the
activity of hepatic Δ^4-5 α (β)-steroid reductase (from 13 to 15 µg androstenedione
metabolized/hr/mg protein). At the same time there was a disappearance of hepatic
glucose-6-phosphate dehydrogenase isoenzymes known to be inhibited "in vivo" and
"in vitro" by dehydroepiandrosterone. In humans we have found a negative correlation between etiocholanolone and serum cholesterol (r = -0.32) and etiocholanolone and β plus pre-β-lipoprotein cholesterol (r =-0.37). These studies suggest

that adrenal steroids may regulate the effect of exercise on lipid metabolism through their effect on the activity of hepatic glucose-6-phosphate-dehydro-genase.

THE EFFECT OF 3-5 CYCLIC ADENOSINE-MONOPHOSPHATE UPON EXPERIMENTAL AORTIC SCLEROSIS IN RABBITS INDUCED BY EPINEPHRINE WITH THYROXIN

George F. Mikulicich, Tom Y. Oester, Fred Buddingh, and Peter Jepson
Loyola University School of Medicine and Hines Veteran Administration Hospital, Chicago,IL/USA

Epinephrine inj., i.v. (50 mcg/kg) and thyroxine (0.2 mg/kg), given daily results in animals, surviving 10 days or more, in severe sclerotic changes of the thoracic and often abdominal aorta as demonstrated in voluminous publications of the last 3 decades. We studied the effect of high i.v. doses of 3-5 cyclic AMP (10 - 20 mg/kg) with and without diphosphoesterase inhibitors such as theophylline and papaverine given daily prior to epinephrine thyroxin inj. It did not inhibit the development of sclerosis, but prolonged substantially the time of survival and inhibited the early development of congestive heart failure as seen in animals without 3-5 cyclic AMP. There was no difference between 3-5 cyclic and 3-5 di-butyryl AMP in same doses. Both have also not inhibited the invariable loss of weight due to thyrotoxic state. In prior studies we could inhibit the epinephrine-thyroxin aortic sclerosis with alpha blocage by phentolamine, which inhibits intracell., 3-5 cyclic AMP release.

EFFECTS OF DEXTROTHYROXINE ON HYPERLIPIDEMIA AND EXPERIMENTAL ATHEROSCLEROSIS IN BEAGLE DOGS

Rajiva Nandan, Jerry D. Fisher, Paul J. Garvin, Charles E. Ganote, and Robert B. Jennings
Baxter Laboratories, Inc., Morton Grove, IL/USA

Beagle dogs, 24 $\pm$ 6 months old fed a thiouracil-free semisynthetic diet containing hydrogenated coconut oil and cholesterol (SS diet) for 12 months developed marked hyperlipidemia and severe atherosclerosis. The effects of dextrothyroxine ($D-T_4$) therapy on these changes were studied.

Dogs in Group I (four male, three female) were fed SS diet alone. Dogs in Group II (four male, five female) and III (three male, four female) were given SS diet plus single daily oral doses of $D-T_4$ in tablet form (one-tenth and five-tenths mg/kg body weight, respectively). Three untreated control dogs (Group IV, one male, two female)were fed Purina dog meal for 12 months. Group I developed marked elevation of serum cholesterol, triglyceride, phospholipid, and ß-lipoprotein and severe atherosclerosis in large and small arteries. Intimal fatty lesions were always present in the abdominal aorta and many of its branches. Large and small coronary arteries showed similar lesions. The degree of surface involvement appeared to be directly related to circulating lipid levels. $D-T_4$ produced a significant dose related lowering of serum lipids and markedly decreased the severity of aortic and coronary artery lesions. Dogs in Group IV developed neither hyperlipidemia nor atherosclerosis.

COMPARATIVE HISTOENZYMATIC AND MICROCHEMICAL STUDIES ON THE ANTIATHEROSCLEROTIC
EFFECT OF PYRIDINOLCARBAMATE AND ESTROGEN ON PHOSPHOFRUCTOKINASE AND MALATE
DEHYDROGENASE IN THE ARTERIAL WALL (IN VIVO AND IN VITRO)

Fujio Numano, Kinya Moriya, Masahiko Kobayashi, Shoko Yamazawa, Tomoe Kuroiwa,
Takeo Takahashi, Atsushi Sagara, and Takio Shimamoto
Tokyo Ika-Shika National University, Tokyo/Japan

Pyridinolcarbamate (PDC) and estrogen (EST), both of which exhibit a preventive
effect against plasma infiltration into arterial wall induced by chemical or
mechanical stresses exhibit a preventive effect against atherosclerosis. However,
histoenzymatic studies on glycolytic and TCA cycle enzymes in aortic wall revealed a different inclination, that is, increased activities with PDC and decreased activities with EST under cholesterol feeding. Microbiochemical analysis
of PFK and MDH in aortic wall exhibited a statistically significant decreased
activity in both intima and media compared with normal diet ones. PDC treated
animals exhibited almost the same activities as that of normal diet ones. On the
other hand, EST exhibited statistically decreased activity in media of aortic
wall. In vitro experiments revealed the same inclination of both substances in
these enzyme activities. These studies suggest the different mechanisms of both
substances to exert the common vascular permeability inhibiting effect and anti-
atherosclerotic effect.

EFFECT OF PENTAERYTHRITOLTETRANICOTINATE (PERYCIT®) ON PLASMA LIPIDS AND LIPO-
PROTEINS AND A COMPARISON WITH NICOTINIC ACID

Lars Orö, Anders Olsson, and Stephan Rössner
Department of Internal Medicine, Karolinska Hospital, Stockholm/Sweden

One group of 32 ambulant patients with various atherosclerotic diseases was
treated with Perycit® (P) 3 g daily for 3 months and 4.5 g daily for another 3
months. Plasma cholesterol and triglycerides (TG) decreased significantly and the
higher dose was more effective. The plasma TG fall was not associated with an
increase in the i.v. fat tolerance. Lipoprotein analyses showed that the cholesterol conc. decreased in the VLD and LD fractions. In the HD fraction there was
an increase. The plasma TG fall was mainly due to changes in the VLD lipoproteins.
The response to the treatment was qualitatively the same in type IIA and IIB as
in type IV (Fredrickson types). P. was compared with nicotinic acid (N.A.) in
another group of 44 patients previously treated with N.A. for 10-90 months. The
cholesterol lowering effect of P. was significantly better than that of N.A.
Uric acid concentration was also followed in all patients and was not affected
by P. but was increased by N.A. treatment.

TWO-YEAR STUDY OF A NEW CHOLESTEROL-REDUCING AGENT (PROBUCOL) IN HYPERLIPIDEMIC
HUMANS

William B. Parsons Jr.
Jackson Clinic and Foundation, Madison, WI/USA

Probucol [4,4-(isopropylidenedithio)bis (2,6-di-t-butylphenol] was studied in 50
hyperlipoproteinemic individuals (32 type II, 12 type IIB, 5 type IV, 1 type V).
After 3 baseline lipid tests, each received 500 mg (2 tablets) twice a day for
2 years, with serum cholesterol (C) and triglyceride (T) measurements every 4
weeks. Mean C values (partial resumé) were:

					Months of Probucol Administration			
Type	No.	0	1	2	4	8	12	18	20
II	32	298	240	240	237	235	241	248	246
II B	12	305	259	246	260	237	257	244	233
IV	5	265	225	216	228	215	232	241	248
V	1	409	340	384	209	266	232	298	243

Mean C and T levels before and during 24 months of probucol therapy were:

		Before		During Probucol Therapy			
Type	No.	C	T	C		T	
II	32	298	110	242	(−19%)	101	(− 8%)
II B	12	305	214	249	(−18%)	199	(− 7%)
IV	5	265	427	227	(−14%)	426	(−−−−)
V	1	409	1227	307	(−25%)	852	(−30%)

Probucol caused neither side effects nor toxic effects on hematologic, renal, or hepatic function. It reduces serum cholesterol, probably by interference with biosynthesis of cholesterol between the acetate and mevalonate steps, with little effect on triglycerides.

EFFECT OF POLYUNSATURATED PHOSPHATIDYL CHOLINE ON REGRESSION OF ATHEROSCLEROSIS IN BABOONS

Jerzy Patelski and Alan N. Howard
Medical Academy, Poznan and Department of Investigative Medicine, University of Cambridge, Cambridge/England

Previous work has shown that intravenous polyunsaturated phosphatidyl choline (PUPC) from soya would reduce the incidence and severity of aortic atherosclerosis experimentally induced in baboons. In the current work, the possible effect of PUPC on the regressions of lesions was examined. Aortic atherosclerosis was induced by feeding 1% cholesterol and injecting bovine serum albumin on 5 occasions 16 days apart. After six months, a control diet was given and the baboons injected with either saline (10 ml) or PUPC (10 g in 10 ml) thrice weekly for four months. PUPC had no effect on regression as measured by aortic staining or cholesterol content. Aortic lipolytic enzymes showed wide individual variation but the trend was for a decrease in glycerol ester hydrolase and increase in cholesterol ester hydrolase activity. In addition, acyl Co A: cholesterol acyl transferase was inhibited. It is concluded that the mechanism of action of PUPC is to inhibit the formation of aortic cholesterol esters.

METABOLIC EFFECTS OF XANTHINOL NIACINATE

E.J. Pinter and C.J. Pattee
Subdepartment of Endocrinology and Metabolism, Reddy Memorial Hospital, Montreal/ Canada

This study attempts to describe some metabolic actions of xanthinol niacinate (XN) and compare these with the effects of nicotinic acid (NA). 22 volunteers were involved, seven with hyperlipidemia were given XN orally (1350 mg/day), and five normals were studied with single iv injection of 1500 mg XN. Total fat, triglyceride, cholesterol and corticosteroids were determined and kinetic studies of plasma free fatty acids (FFA) done using the method of successive measured injections of ^{3}H-palmitic acid. Kinetic studies were also made in ten subjects given 500 mg iv NA. In hyperlipidemia six out of seven showed a hypolipidemic effect. Kinetic studies demonstrated a biphasic response of FFA consisting of an initial drop in FFA pool and production (3623 $\pm$ 450 → 2211 $\pm$ 510 μEq and 928 $\pm$ 60 → 652 $\pm$ 84 μEq/min) followed by a marked prolonged increase (2211 $\pm$ 510 → 12839 $\pm$ 1250 μEq and 652 $\pm$ 84 → 2533 $\pm$ 214 μEq/min). Plasma corticoids rose progressively. Identical changes were found after NA. Conclusions: While XN and NA lead to amelioration of hyperlipidemia they exert profound and potentially hazardous metabolic action: a biphasic change of FFA with marked prolonged net increment predominating. FFA stimulation connected with the use of XN and NA should be considered with caution when treating patients with peripheral vascular and coronary heart disease.

PDX CHLORIDE THERAPY IN HYPERBETALIPOPROTEINAEMIA

Ståle Ritland, Åke Lanner, Olav Fausa, Jan P. Blomhoff, and Egil Gjone
Medical Department A, Rikshospitalet, Oslo/Norway

Intestinal absorption and jejunal bile acid concentration were studied before and during treatment with an anion exchange resin, PDX chloride. Four females and 5 males (mean age 26 years) with familial hyperlipoproteinaemia type II A were treated with 9 g daily for 3 months and 15 g daily for 9 months. The mean serum cholesterol decreased from 461 to 392 mg/100 ml (15%), the mean serum triglycerides increased from 73 to 105 mg/100 ml (44%), whereas phospholipids were unchanged. During treatment only small changes within normal limits occurred in serum electrolytes, albumin, gammaglobulin, some of the clotting factors, liver and renal function tests, absorption of iron, glucose, vitamin B_{12}, folic acid, gastric acid output and in the fecal excretion of fat and nitrogen. The jejunal bile acid concentration after meal and the glycine/taurine ratio increased significantly. The mechanism of this changed ratio has not been investigated.

No side effect of the drug was demonstrated.

CLINICAL EXPERIENCES WITH α-METHYLTHYROXINE ETHYLESTER, A NEW LIPID-LOWERING AGENT

Wolfgang Schwartzkopff, Helke Hoffmann, Jaak Nijssen, and Vollrad Etzel
Westend Clinic, Free University, Berlin/BRD

Lipid-lowering and cardiogenic effects of α-methylthyroxine ethylester (CG 635) were clinically tested on cardiac patients in two double-blind cross-over studies. In the first study 120 patients were given a placebo or 40 mg CG 635/day in five phases of five weeks' duration each. Cardiac complaints, morning and evening pulse rate, nitroglycerin consumption, serum triglycerides, blood sugar, liver function and other parameters were determined. Median serum cholesterol decreased by 60 mg/100 ml in 14 (73%) of the 19 patients whose median serum cholesterol was more than 300 mg/100 ml and by 50 mg/100 ml in 18 (56%) of the 32 patients whose median serum cholesterol was 251-300 mg/100 ml. The remaining patients had median serum cholesterol less than 250 mg/100 ml (41 pat.) or were not to evaluate. CG 635 had no statistically significant effect on pulse rate and did not alter liver function. Possible substance related transitory increase in cardiac complaints were noted in one subject. Analogous results were obtained in a second study on 180 patients treated with CG 635 for three months.

THE EFFECT OF THE ADMINISTRATION OF POLYUNSATURATED PHOSPHOLIPID ON PLASMA LIPIDS IN MAN

J. Skořepa, M. Fučik, P. Mareš, and H. Todorovičová
Fourth Department of Medicine, Faculty of Medicine, Charles University,
Prague/Czechoslovakia

Atherosclerotic patients were administered polyunsaturated phosphatidyl choline; its effect on the level of cholesterol and its esters in plasma was followed. Administered perorally, it made the level of plasmatic cholesteryl linoleate rise in 11 patients out of 12 (P <0.01). The level of total cholesterol was seen to drop (P <0.01). The drop was at the expense of the unesterified proportion. It is probable that free cholesterol diminishes as a result of increased esterification with linoleic acid. Polyunsaturated phospholipid takes part in the transacylation. The administration of polyunsaturated phosphatidyl choline seems to have an effect on the metabolism of lipids similar to that of a diet containing unsaturated vegetable oils but without their adverse qualities, i.e. the need for high doses and high caloric intake. A considerable part of linoleic acid combined in a triglyceride is apparently lost through ß-oxidation and is thus unable to function as an essential fatty acid.

EFFECT OF CHLOROPHENOXYISOBUTYRATE ON PYRUVATE AND LIPOPROTEIN METABOLISM IN TYPE IV HYPERLIPIDEMIC SUBJECTS

H.B. Stähelin, J. Th. Locher, and R. Maier
Department of Internal Medicine, Kantonsspital University of Basel, Basel/
Switzerland

Six male patients with type IV hyperlipidemia who had previously been receiving treatment with the Al-salt of chlorophenoxyisobutyric acid (alufibrate) or placebo were injected with $[1-^{14}C]-$ or $[2-^{14}C]$-pyruvate (1-P, 2-P). The exhalation of total CO_2 and $^{14}CO_2$ was monitored to estimate indirectly acetyl-CoA formed from 1-P and the oxidation of 2-P through the TCA-cycle. Incorporation of 2-P into VLDL, LDL and HDL lipids was measured subsequent to separation by ultracentrifugation. Considerably more $^{14}CO_2$ was exhaled after 1-P than after 2-P. (14% vs. 5.8%). As compared with placebo, alufibrate did not affect total CO_2 exhalation, only slightly diminished the oxidation of 1-P and increased the oxidation of 2-P by 25%. Thus, alufibrate appears to diminish the availability of acetyl-CoA for fatty-acid synthesis. Drug treatment reduced the serum concentration of VLDL by 53% (911 to 431 mg/100 ml serum, p <0.01) by decreasing VLDL-lipid turnover by 25% (p <0.05) and by increasing the net removal rate by 30% (p <0.01). No effect on LDL and HDL lipids was detected. Total serum cholesterol was reduced by 15% (316 to 274 mg%) and serum triglycerides by 44% (723 to 402 mg%).

INTESTINAL ALTERATION OF STEROLS IN PATIENTS: IMPLICATIONS FOR BALANCE STUDIES

M.T. Ravi Subbiah, Mary C. Naylor, and Bruce A. Kottke
Mayo Clinic and Mayo Foundation, Rochester, MN/USA

To compare the simultaneous conversion of cholesterol and specific plant sterols into their 5ß-reduction products and to evaluate the relationship between recovery and bacterial degradation of ß-sitosterol, 10 hyperlipoproteinemic patients on solid diets underwent sterol balance studies using a mixture of plant sterols (1 g/day) and chromium sesquioxide (1.5 g/day) as fecal flow markers. Sterols were measured by combined TLC and GLC.
Salient features noted included: (1) A 20% difference between the recoveries of campesterol and ß-sitosterol, even when corrected with Cr_2O_3 as a fecal flow

marker (campesterol, $67.7\pm18.7\%$; ß-sitosterol, $88.6\pm23.6\%$); this observation and confirmatory studies in the pigeon and chicken suggest that sterol absorption decreases in the order $C_{27}>C_{28}>C_{29}$. (2) The ratios of fecal cholesterol and of the plant sterols to their bacterial degradation products were not the same in any of the patients; in vitro studies of fecal homogenates showed similar conversion of [^{14}C]ß-sitosterol and [^{3}H]cholesterol to 5ß-stanols. (3) ß-Sitosterol recovery was not related to bacterial conversion of sterols; this was also confirmed by in vitro studies of fecal homogenates using [^{14}C]cholesterol. We conclude that these observations should be taken into consideration in the interpretation of sterol balance studies.

ON THE FACTORS AFFECTING EARLY RESULTS OF DIETARY MANAGEMENT IN HYPERLIPO-PROTEINEMIA

Jiři Válek, Dušan Grafnetter, and Zdenka Slabochová
Institute of Clinical and Experimental Medicine, Prague/Czechoslovakia

The paper deals with studies on the effect of a diet (polyunsaturated-saturated fatty acids ratio - P/S 1.6) on blood lipids in hyperlipoproteinemia during a three week follow up period (a total of 28 patients). In a group of eight subjects where a delayed immunoreactive insulin (IRI) rise after a 100 g glucose was found, beta cholesterol increased for 3.4% from the mean level of 188.0 mg% as compared to the drop of -14.3% from the mean 199.7 mg% in remaining subjects. Triglycerides dropped to -9.7% from the mean 244.0 mg%. With reference to another group (six from 17) treated with a diet of a P/S ratio 0.2 it is suggested that impaired insulin activity might contribute either to the decreased efficiency of the lipid lowering diet or to endogenous increases of lipemia occurring at the food composition intake common in our country.

DESTRUCTION OF PLATELETS BY FATTY ACIDS AND ITS PREVENTION BY PHOSPHATIDYLCHOLINE

Ellen Weber, Eberhard Morgenstern, Erhard Walter, Theo Pfleiderer, and Klaus-Jürgen Hahn
Abteilung für Klinische Pharmakologie, Medizinische Universitätsklinik, Heidelberg/BRD

The enzymatically measured ATP content of pig platelets was chosen to demonstrate the cell damaging effect of fatty acids (FA) and to study its prevention by phosphatidylcholine (PCh). Saturated FA with 4 to 16 carbon atoms led to a decrease in platelet ATP which is directly correlated to the concentrations used and related in a more complex manner to the length of the carbon chain. Saturated FA with 18 carbon atoms and more did not change the ATP level whereas testing five different unsaturated FA with 16 and 18 carbon atoms showed a pronounced decrease. PCh prevented the destructive action of saturated FA excepting 4C and 6C provided both substances were added to the cell suspensions after emulsifying them simultaneously. Preincubation of the platelets with PCh or EDTA did not diminish the action of FA. The preventive effect of PCh is attributed to its marked surface properties. A hydrophilic coat is formed around the emulgated lipid particles thus reducing their affinity to the lipophilic platelet outer membrane.

LIPID-LOWERING EFFECT OF HEMOPERFUSION WITH AMBERLITE XAD- 2 RESIN

Achim Weizel and Hikmat Y. Rizk
Medizinische Universitätsklinik Heidelberg, Heidelberg/BRD

Resin hemoperfusion has been used in barbiturate intoxication. In vivo studies in one patient and in dogs showed a 25-40% reduction of total cholesterol (TC) and triglyceride (TG) levels after therapy. In vivo studies confirmed this effect with a 5-20% reduction of TC, the TG reduction was 15-30%. In vitro studies with isolated lipoproteins showed a reduction of TG in all fractions (VLDL: 35-70%, LDL 20-40%, HDL 30-60%). The TC reduction was 10-30% in VLDL, 20-50% in LDL, and 8-20% in HDL. There was no change in the protein concentration.

Amberlite resin seems to be a potent lipid-lowering agent which interferes with TG and cholesterol metabolism.

MULTIVARIATE ANALYSIS OF RISK FACTORS AND PRIMARY PREVENTION OF CORONARY HEART DISEASE IN MIDDLE-AGED SWEDISH MEN

Lars Wilhelmsen, Hans Wedel, and Gösta Tibblin
Medical Department I, Sahlgren's Hospital, Göteborg/Sweden

For the prospective study of risk factors for CHD 973 men all aged 50 were recruited from a general Swedish urban population. Of the 855 participants, 834 were CHD free on entry, and have been observed for 9 years and 4 months. All except 2 out of 55 deaths were autopsied. Twenty-five nonfatal and 19 fatal cases of CHD occurred.

By a multiple logistic model 9 probable risk factors were analysed. Serum cholesterol, smoking, systolic blood pressure, dyspnea and conviction for drunkenness were significantly related to CHD but not serum triglycerides, hematocrit or geographical mobility (place of birth). Physical inactivity during work showed a slight tendency to relationship.

The most important risk factors (high cholesterol, high blood pressure and smoking) are treated in a primary preventive trial comprising 10,000 intervention subjects and 20,000 control subjects randomly selected from the total male population aged 47-55. The screening examination is completed. The possibilities to intervene on the risk factors are discussed.

THE USE OF TUBERCULOSIS DISPENSARIES FOR THE DETECTION OF AND INTERVENTION IN SUBJECTS WITH ELEVATED RISK FACTORS FOR CORONARY HEART DISEASE. A FEASIBILITY STUDY

A.C. Arntzenius, G.J.M. Boerma, H.A. van Geuns, T.L. Mellema, D.P. Sluyter, and K. Styblo
The Royal T.B. Association and Heart Foundation, The Hague/The Netherlands

The purpose of this study is to investigate the usefulness of chest clinics in combating coronary heart disease. Medical and paramedical personnel, trained in standardized techniques to measure and register risk factors make use of a questionnaire, ECG, blood pressure, cholesterol, glucose tolerance test, weight, height, urine tests and chest X-ray films.

In subjects with elevated risk factors intervention on smoking, eating and exercise habits is carried out by district nurses on home visits; the risk factors being re-examined every three months.

Results of first examination show that of 4,000 subjects, aged 20-50 years, one-third had low, one-third had borderline elevated and one-third had elevated risk factors.

Results of intervention on 1,200 subjects with elevated risk factors at three and six months retesting will be presented.
Authors feel that preliminary results are encouraging.

INCORPORATION OF ^{14}C-L-LEUCINE INTO LIVER PROTEINS AND LIPOPROTEINS OF CARBON TETRACHLORIDE TREATED RATS

Carlos Arreaza, Virgilio Bosch
Instituto de Medicina Experimental, Universidad Central, Caracas/Venezuela

Inhibition of lipoprotein synthesis by CCl_4 has been proposed as a mechanism of fatty liver production in the rat. To study this problem CCl_4 was given per os to fasting rats. Three and 24 hours after, liver slices were incubated for two hours in Krebs-Ringer buffer containing ^{14}C-1-leucine. The slices were then homogenized and suspended in solutions of appropriate densities to obtain very low density (VLDL), low density (LDL), high density (HDL) lipoproteins and proteins with density >1.210 g/ml. This was performed by preparative ultracentrifugation using a source of carrier lipoproteins hyperlipemic rat plasma. The fractions were precipitated, avoiding contaminating radioactivity from free leucine, tRNA and lipids. Samples were counted by a liquid scintillation method. Treated rats showed more than a fourfold activity of controls in VLDL, LDL and proteins with density >1.210 g/ml. No difference was found in HDL. No lipoprotein synthesis inhibition by CCl_4 was found in this study.

GLASS ADHESIVENESS AND NUMBER OF PLATELETS IN PATIENTS WITH CORONARY HEART DISEASE

Emilia Babei, Elena Ungureanu, and Emilia Cristea
Institute of Public Health and Medical Researches, Jassy/Roumania

Glass adhesiveness (modified Rovatti method) and the number of platelets (technique of Poppa, Enache, Nicoară) were studied in 523 subjects, out of which 55 normal subjects, 57 afflicted by inflammatory and endocrine disturbances or by gastro-duodenal ulcers and 411 subjects suffering from coronary heart disease. Adhesiveness in the patients was evidently modified in relation to the normal values. Yet it was less modified in painless or hypertensive coronary disease and highly modified in painful coronary diseases. It was also found that in angina pectoris and in the intermediate syndrome increased pathologic values were dominant, while in myocardial infarction increased and decreased pathologic values were equal. The number of platelets does not present any significant statistical aspects.

THE CHEMISTRY AND SERUM STEROL LOWERING PROPERTIES OF 1- {2- [4'-(TRIFLUOROMETHYL)-4-BIPHENYLYLOXY]ETHYL} SECONDARY AMINES

F.L. Bach
Medical Research, Cyanamid International
B.D. Johnson and E. Cohen
Metabolic Disease Therapy Section, Lederle Laboratories, Division of American Cyanamid Co., Pearl River, NY/USA

A structure-activity relationship correlates the pK_A values and the molecular volumes of the terminal amino groups with high activity in this new series of

4,4'-biphenyl derivatives. The cyclohexyamino residue in the most active non-steroidal hypocholesterolemic agent synthesized in this study, N-{2-[4'-(tri-fluoromethyl)-4-biphenylyloxy]ethyl}cyclohexylamine monohydrochloride (CL 77,724), has a pK_A value of 8.2 and a molecular volume lying in the region of 109 cubic Ångstroms. Compound CL 77,724 lowers serum sterol levels significantly compared to controls when administered orally at 0.00003% (0.18 mg drug/600 g feed) of the diet in rats. Although this biphenyl derivative has hormonal-like activity, its usefulness in the treatment of human atherosclerosis remains questionable, since one of its modes of action is interference with the *in vivo* conversion of 7-de-hydrocholesterol to cholesterol in animals.

HISTOLOGICAL CHANGES IN THE AORTA AND BIOCHEMICAL ALTERATIONS IN NORMOTENSIVE AND HYPERTENSIVE RATS AFTER LIGATION OF THE THORACIC DUCT

Günter Bartsch, Norbert Müller, and Hartmut Cremer
A. Nattermann & Cie. GmbH, Cologne and Department of Pathology, University of Bonn, Bonn/BRD

Renal hypertension was produced by a constricting clip around the left renal artery. Subsequently the thoracic duct was ligatured just before its entry into the left angulus venosus. Observations were made up to 109 days after ligation. Ligature of the thoracic duct in normo- and hypertensive rats induced morphological changes of the aortic wall. At first, histological alterations impressed as edematous thickening of the adventitia. Next, the edema penetrated into media and intima, and in addition, vacuolated smooth muscle cells were demonstrable. The gradual disappearance of the edema was accompanied by a slight adventitial fibrosis. Renal hypertension induced a moderate elevation of serum lipids. Ligation of the thoracic duct modified the lipid content of the liver and promoted a severe hyperlipemia in hyper- and normotensive animals.

LEFT VENTRICULAR HYPERTROPHY AND HYPERTENSIVE HEART DISEASE IN EVANS COUNTY, GEORGIA

Robert Beaglehole, H.A. Tyroler, John Cassel, Al Bartel, Curtis Hames, and Siegfried Heyden
School of Public Health, UNC, Chapel Hill, NC/USA

The prevalence and incidence of electrocardiographical left ventricular hypertrophy (LVH/ECG) and of hypertensive heart disease (HHD) is reported for the biracial population of Evans Co., Georgia, as a follow-up to previous attempts to explain the differing prevalence and incidence of ischaemic heart disease (IHD) in blacks (B) and whites (W). Minnesota Code 3:1 is the criterion for LVH and its association with hypertension indicates HHD.

The prevalence of LVH/ECG is strongly associated with levels of systolic and diastolic blood pressure (BP), and controlling for BP there is a weaker association with age. At each level of BP, age, and Quetelet Index, LVH/ECG is significantly higher in blacks than in whites, and in males (M) than in females (F). The prevalence of HHD increases with age and is also higher in blacks and in males. The incidence of HHD for the following groups is: WM, 2.4% (21 of 878), WF, 1.3% (12 of 928), BM, 6.7% (28 of 419), BF, 5.3% (28 of 526); blacks are more prone than whites to develop LVH with the development of hypertension.

This study indicates that hypertension has a different atherogenic risk factor meaning for blacks and whites; it predicts HHD in blacks and IHD in whites.

ANTIATHEROGENIC ACTION OF THERAPEUTICAL PHYSICAL PROCEDURES

Laszlo Birek, Zoltan Rakosfalvy, Eva Kotay-Lakatos
Physiotherapeutic and Rehabilitation Clinic, Tîrgu-Mures/Roumania

While searching for new mechanisms in physiotherapy, the authors followed in hundred subjects the variation of those parameters, which when significantly disturbed, play a determining role in the human atherogenesis. After general massage, Charcot' showers, brush-baths, dry frictions we noticed a significant increase of the heparinemia and blood-LPL-activity, whence global coagulability, platelet-adhesiveness and aggregability clearly indicated a decreasing tendency, as compared with pre-procedural levels. A procedure applied for three weeks led to the normalisation of pathological cholesterol levels. The main mechanism underlying this process, as verified by our animal experiments, seems to be the release of heparin, resulting from the degranulation of skin mast-cells, due to the thermo-mechanical energy of the procedure used. The authors termed this phenomenon as "endoheparinisation" and consider that their observations substantiate its use in the prevention and therapy of the atherosclerotic disease.

SCREENING AND EARLY DIAGNOSIS OF ATHEROSCLEROSIS

F.H. Bonjer, J. Baart, G.J.H. Dresen, C.A.M. Hendriks, A.E. Leuftink, and E. van Westreenen
Department of Cardiology, University of Leiden, Leiden/The Netherlands

If a substantial reduction in coronary mortality is to be achieved, coronary candidates will have to be detected and provided with advice and guidance. Cooperation of 12 occupational health services in the Netherlands made it possible to develop a screening procedure for the early detection of risk factors for ischaemic heart disease. A questionnaire and measurements of height, weight and blood pressure, a 12-lead ECG and spirometry are handled by nurses and technicians. Blood is collected from fasting subjects for the determination of glucose, serum cholesterol and total lipids. All screening data are processed with the aid of a central computer and integrated into a coronary risk profile. Advices are given in order to reduce risk factors.

Up to date screening data of about 6,500 male subjects (40-65 yrs) have been analysed. Results: mean systolic blood pressure rises concurrently with age like in the Framingham study, but mean values are 7-9 mm Hg higher. Serum cholesterol values differ considerably between Western (low) and Eastern (high) part of the Netherlands. Mean values exceed those of Framingham by 30 mg%. Systolic bloodpressure correlates positively with overweight, serum lipids and LVH (in those over 45 yrs).

MOFETTE THERAPY AND CO_2 WATERBATHS FOR THE TREATMENT OF ATHEROSCLEROSIS OBLITERANS

Zoltán Brassai, Endre Horváth, László Ferencz, and Géza Benedek
Clinic of Internal Medicine II, Tîrgu-Mureş/Roumania

In Covasna, Roumania, postvolcanic CO_2 gas emanations are used in the form of mofette therapy (twice daily) and CO_2 waterbaths (once daily) for the treatment of atherosclerosis obliterans. The authors have studied in seventy male patients with atherosclerosis obliterans (all without gangrene) the haemodynamic modifications of extremities (measured walking distance, skin temperature, radioactivity measurements after injection of ^{131}I) and the elimination of urinary catecholamines during treatment. The results indicated that the arterial blood supply to the feet was definitely enhanced after CO_2 therapy for all patients, thus promoting the formation of collateral circulation. The elimination of urinary catecholamines was significantly diminished (p<0.01).

GUIDELINES FOR FOOD CHOICES FOR FAT MODIFIED DIETS. A USEFUL TOOL FOR NUTRITIONISTS

Helen B. Brown and Marilyn Farrand
Cleveland Clinic Foundation, Cleveland, Ohio, and National Heart and Lung Institute, Bethesda, MD/USA

Fat-modified diets applied to large populations require loose structure and adaptability to world-wide cultures and life styles. Often recommendations for choosing foods are rigid without consideration for individual preferences and needs. Guidelines are presented to provide a rationale for food selection. The diet prescription is converted from percent calories of major nutrients to grams. Common foods are divided into five groups according to their nutrient composition with emphasis on their fat and cholesterol content. Basic foods are chosen from the five groups to fit into the diet prescription insuring nutritional balance as well as lipid lowering effect. By this means the diet may be individualized by the occasional use of foods ordinarily not advised. Some may be used in addition to basic foods, others may be substituted for them. A mathematical method for checking food choices with the diet prescription is provided.

SYPHGMORECORDINGS AS A NONINVASIVE ASSESSMENT OF ARTERIAL COMPLIANCE: RESULTS IN NORMAL WEST AFRICANS

Raymond Carlisle, I.E. Samson, and Angela R. Cooke
Department of Medicine, University College Hospital, Ibadan/Nigeria

Atherosclerosis is recognised to have an exceptionally low prevalence in West Africans. Arterial wall assessment suitable for wide-spread application will of necessity be noninvasive. Syphgmorecordings were taken for a representative sample of 19 West African subjects free of circulatory disease, at rest in a supine position. Serum cholesterol was determined in each case. The rate of brachial arterial pressure rise, dP/dt init., was found to be: mean 1,635 torr/sec, SE 145 (for the initial 2/3 of the upstroke as calculated by linear regression). Values already determined for Swedish subjects give: mean 749 torr/sec, SE 74.5.

It is concluded that peripheral factors are most important in determining dP/dt during early ejection, since the difference between the two groups studied indicates increased compliance for the West African compared with the Swedish subjects.

EFFECT OF PROBUCOL IN LOWERING SERUM CHOLESTEROL

Donald McCaughan
Department of Cardiology, Veterans Administration Hospital, West Roxbury, and Harvard Medical School

The purpose of this study was to determine the cholesterol lowering effect of Probucol compared with a matched group of placebo patients. Ninety patients were started on drug and thirty on placebo and followed for one year. Cholesterol values were determined at two monthly intervals and compared with three pretreatment values. The mean change in serum cholesterol for patients on drug was - 16.2% viz - 10.4% on the placebo group from pretreatment values. Side effects were minor. It is concluded that probucol is an effective and safe cholesterol lowering agent.

EFFECT OF THE PROTRACTED ADMINISTRATION TO RABBITS OF ASPIRIN IN ASSOCIATION WITH CHOLESTEROL

Gheorghe Chera, Sofia Dolinescu, Gabriela Volcinschi, Iuliu Nitulescu, Stefan Hărăgus, Mircea Cucuianu, and Ion Zagreanu
Institute of Public Health and Medical Research, Jassy, and First Medical Clinic, Cluj/Roumania

Aspirin, which is known as exerting an antiadhesive action on the blood platelets and, according to some authors a diminution of cholesterolemia, was administrated per os to rabbits as pure substance in daily doses of 60 mg/kg during 6 months or as its Na salt in daily doses of 300 mg/kg during 3 months and associated in both cases with a daily dose of 0.300 g/kg cholesterol. Aspirin did not influence the level of blood cholesterol and has not modified the evolution of the atherogenic process induced by the cholesterol administered alone. It has intensified the liver steatosis and has favored the appearance of centrolobular necroses, hastening the process of fibrosis. The neutralisation of aspirin as a sodic salt did diminish its ulcerogenic action on gastric mucosa.

A NEW CONCEPT: A DYNAMIC ROLE OF DIETARY FAT ON SERUM LIPIDS AND ATHEROSCLEROSIS

Wu Chun-Chung and Huang Te-Hsiu
Department of Medicine, Taiwan University Hospital, Taipei/Taiwan

To investigate the effects of lard, a series of experiments were carried out.

1. A group of rabbits were fed first on lanolin diet and after the cholesterol levels reached 800 mg/dl, it was substituted with lard diet for 8 weeks. 2. A lard diet feeding group of rabbits was fed for 15 months. 3. One lot of rabbits was fed on lard mixed with lanolin diet for four months. 4. 12 persons were kept on low cholesterol diet added with 100 gm of lard daily for six days. A marked decrease of serum cholesterol levels was seen in the first experiment, insignificant change of lipid levels in the second, a marked increase of lipid levels in the third, and insignificant change of lipid levels in the fourth. It failed to induce marked atherosclerotic change throughout the experiments. These variable results may suggest the potential dynamic effects of lard, either decrease, balance or increase, in the serum lipid levels according to the fecal free fatty acid excretion and cholesterol content in the diet.

SHEAR FORCES AND THE LOCALIZATION OF AORTIC ATHEROSCLEROTIC LESIONS IN RABBITS

J.F. Cornhill and Margot R. Roach
Department of Biophysics, University of Western Ontario, London, Ontario/Canada

The predilection for atherosclerotic lesions to occur at branches has led to the development of two haemodynamic theories of atherogenesis. One postulates that lesions occur in low shear regions proximal to, whereas the other postulates that lesions occur in high shear regions distal to a branch. To test these theories, atherosclerosis was induced in five rabbits by feeding them 90 egg yolks over a period of 60 days in addition to rabbit pellets ad lib. The aortic periorificial lesions were visualized by gross Sudan III staining and their size and position were mapped on polar coordinates. Sudanophilic lesions were found surrounding 86% of the aortic ostia. In the descending aorta, 1% of the lesions occurred in low shear areas proximal to, whereas 99% occurred in the high shear areas distal to a branch. Therefore, under the above experimental conditions, the atherosclerotic lesions occurred in areas of high shear.
Supported by the Ontario Heart Foundation.

DIFFUSIBLE FRACTION OF SERUM CHOLESTEROL

Stephen I. Csögör
Medical Research Center, Tîrgu Mures/Roumania

If human serum is mixed with paraffin oil, some of the lipids diffuse into oil.
It therefore seems that serum lipids have two fractions, one strongly bound by
lipoprotein structures, and the other loosely bound and diffusible in an oil
phase. I designated the loosely bound fraction "diffusible". Small molecules,
because of their association with plasma proteins, lose their initial diffusion
properties. The distribution of protein-bound lipids is limited according to the
distribution of their carriers. To obtain data concerning the amount of plasma
cholesterol supplied to tissues the diffusible fraction must be determined. Our
data demonstrate an increase in the diffusible fraction of serum cholesterol in
atherogenic conditions. Healthy females show lower values than males. Highest
levels of diffusible cholesterol were observed in maturity-onset diabetes, broad-
beta disease, and type IV hyperlipoproteinemia. Diffusible cholesterol is a good
indicator of antiatherogenic therapy.

INCREASED FACTOR XIII ACTIVITY IN ENDOGENOUS HYPERTRIGLYCERIDEMIA

Mircea Cucuianu, Augustin Opincaru, Vasile Vasile, and Titus Popescu
Medical Clinic I, Cluj/Roumania

Since factor XIII is known to delay fibrinolysis in vitro, its activity was investigated according to the method of Heene in 102 hyperlipemic patients in
comparison to 49 normolipemic normal weight subjects. Factor XIII activity was
found to be significantly increased in hyperlipemic patients with or without
clinical atherosclerosis. When the type of hyperlipoproteinemia was taken into
consideration it was found that factor XIII level was only slightly changed
(1222 ± 120 u) in pure hypercholesterolemia (type II-a) as compared to aged
matched controls (1147 ± 150 u). Fibrin stabilizing activity was obviously increased in endogenous hypertriglyceridemia (1510 ± 170 u). Correction of hypertriglyceridemia by clofibrate therapy associated to a low carbohydrate reduction diet was accompanied by a decrease of factor XIII level. The hypothesis
about an enhanced synthesis of factor XIII in the liver of hypertriglyceridemic
patients is presented.

ONTOGENETICALLY DETERMINED FEATURES OF THE NORMAL ARTERIAL WALL AND LOCALIZATION OF THE ATHEROSCLEROTIC PLAQUE

Fritz Dalith
Pathoradiological Research Institute, Tel-Aviv University Medical School,
Tel-Hashomer/Israel

The prevailing theory regarding the localization of the atherosclerotic plaque is
that locally increased haemodynamical stress acts upon a previously intact arterial wall. Some workers have already attributed the primary role to pre-existing
focal medial thinning. Additional support for the concept of a prime defect of
the vascular wall has emerged from studies at this Institute. Focal alterations
of the arterial wall texture at six particular sites of the aortic arch and the
brachiocephalic arteries have been demonstrated in young individuals. Microscopically these lesions show: a) circumscribed thinning of the tunica media.
b) structural and histochemical changes in cells, fibres and ground substance,
and c) focal thickening of the tunica adventitia. These changes, already present
at birth, appear to be located where embryological vascular structures have been
disconnected from persistent branchial artery derivatives. It is suggested that

they represent ontogenetically determined alteration in the texture of the normal arterial wall. The location of these developmental defects, as seen in the young subjects, corresponds to the preferential sites of atherosclerotic plaques in the elderly.

THE AGING OF THE ARTERIAL WALL. HISTOLOGIC AND ENZYMATIC EXPERIMENTAL STUDY

Modeste Dallocchio, Jacky Larrue, Michel Rabaud, Gabriel Razaka, René Crockett, and Henri Bricaud
Unité de Recherches de Cardiologie U8-INSERM- Hôpital du Tondu, Bordeaux/France

The thoracic aorta of 250 rabbits aged from 1 to 24 months was studied for its histologic and enzymatic evolution. The morphologic, enzymatic and histometabolic data enable one to establish a chronology in the severity of the lesions. A high elevation of the deshydrogenase activities is related to the cellular proliferation located in the internal third of the aortic media. *The center* of the fibrous chondroid or calcified lesions is characterized by decreasing ATPase and deshydrogenase activities, whereas *the periphery* of these lesions by increasing deshydrogenase activities. An intense alkaline phosphatase activity is noted at the periphery of the lesions early in the chondroid stage. Confrontation of enzymatic data and of spontaneous histologic modifications noted in animals of different ages enables one to analyse the metabolic alterations reflecting the aging of the arterial wall. In general, histologic and metabolic alterations correlate with the principal disorders of the arterial wall noted during the various types of experimental atherosclerosis.

JAPANESE QUAIL IN ATHEROSCLEROSIS RESEARCH

Charles E. Day and Walter W. Stafford
Diabetes and Atherosclerosis Research, The Upjohn Company, Kalamazoo, MI/USA

Japanese quail (*Coturnix coturnix japonica*) were investigated as a potential new animal model for atherosclerosis research. After 10 days on a diet containing 2% cholesterol, serum cholesterol levels rose from an initial 254 mg/dl to 667 mg/dl. This increase was due mostly to a cholesterol-rich very low density lipoprotein. A group of 77 birds (35 females, 42 males) were fed the cholesterol diet for 15 weeks after which their thoracic aortas were examined for grossly visible atherosclerotic lesions. Total incidence of visible lesions was 44% (34 of 77). The incidence in males and females was 48% (20 of 42) and 40% (14 of 35), respectively. Severity of lesions was extremely variable but greater in males; 7 males manifested lesions so severe that the lumen was almost occluded. Histologically, atherosclerotic aortas exhibited intimal thickening with cellular proliferation and lipid deposition. In another experiment with 96 male birds aortic cholesterol levels were measured by GLC at monthly intervals after cholesterol feeding began. The first visible lesions and statistically significant increase in cholesterol (free and esterified) were both seen at 3 months. No lesions have been seen in the arteries of 60 control birds. The coturnix quail is a promising new animal model for basic atherosclerosis research.

CLASSIFICATION OF PRIMARY HYPERLIPIDEMIAS USING DIETETIC SEQUENCE STUDIES

Gérard Debry, Pierre Drouin, Denis Guisard, and Luc Méjean
Départment de Nutrition, Université I de Nancy et Groupe de Recherches de Nutrition et de Diététique, INSERM U 59, Nancy/France

The authors present their method for the classification of hyperlipidemias using 6 isocaloric, isoprotidic dietetic sequences each lasting 3 weeks: 1. balanced with alcohol, 2. balanced without alcohol, 3. hyperglucidic, hypolipidic without alcohol, 4. hyperlipidic, hypoglucidic without alcohol, 5. balanced with alcohol, 6. balanced without alcohol. 70 hyperlipidemic non diabetics, having a constant weight during all the sequences could be divided into 34 pure hypercholesterol-emias, 10 MIXED hypertriglyceridemias, 19 hypertriglyceridemias sensitive to alcohol, and 7 hypertriglyceridemias sensitive to carbohydrates. Under these conditions with a normal caloric diet the nutritional sensitivity is negligible for the hypercholesterolemias, slight for the mixed hyperlipemias, and elevated for the hypertriglyceridemias sensitive to alcohol or to carbohydrates. The posologic and therapeutic usefulness of this method is evident.

THE EFFECT OF HUMAN GROWTH HORMONE (STH) ON FATTY ACID METABOLISM IN HUMANS

Herwig Ditschuneit, Ulrich Klör, Dorothea Rakow, Jens-D. Faulhaber, and Hans Ditschuneit
Department of Metabolism and Nutrition, University Ulm, Ulm/BRD

In recent experiments in vitro with fat tissue of rats and humans we could de-monstrate that STH of high purity has no lipolytic effect. Also, the sensitivity of the tissue against lipolytic substances were not stimulated by these STH-preparations. To investigate this STH in vivo comparative studies were performed with infusions of STH and heparin in human beings. During the infusions the fol-lowing substances in blood were measured: FFA, ß-hydroxybutyric acid, glucose and insulin. From the results we can conclude that STH primarily stimulates the FFA-oxidation with secondary increase of ketone body formation. These results are of great interest because STH play an important role in pathogenesis of athero-sclerosis as we have recently shown.

ON THE RELATED EVOLUTION OF SOME EXPERIMENTAL ATHEROSCLEROSIS LESIONS

Sofia Dolinescu and Acad. Iulius Nitulescu
Institute of Public Health and Medical Research, Jassy/Roumania

The atherosclerosis was produced in rats through the associated administration during 10 days of epinephrine with cholesterol or with vitamin D. In the first instance the prevalent trouble was a lipidic accumulation, in the second calcium deposits. In both cases the first alterations appeared in the media with sub-sequent endothelial extension. Myocardic infarctions were frequently met. The development of the lesions was followed by biochemical and histoenzymatic de-terminations made after 48 hours from the cessation of the administration and also after a lapse of time of 1-2 years. It is concluded that the lesions continue a protracted, extensive evolution long after the disparition of their induction and after the normalisation of the serum biochemical alterations.

TREATMENT OF PERIPHERAL ISCHEMIC DISEASES BY THE IMPROVEMENT OF THE FLOW PROPERTIES OF BLOOD

Albrecht H. Ehrly
Department of Internal Medicine, Division Angiology, University of Frankfurt, Frankfurt/BRD

The conventional non-surgical therapy of peripheral vascular diseases by several drugs (vasodilators) has not been very successful in the past. The improvement of the flow properties of blood including a decrease in blood viscosity ba a snake venom preparation (Arwin) seems to be a helpful new therapeutical concept. 24 hours after starting Arwin therapy the viscosity of blood and plasma, measured by different rheological methods, was decreased. Simultaneously, red cell aggregation and plasma fibrinogen concentration were reduced. A decrease in blood viscosity is followed by an increase in peripheral blood flow as could be shown by vein plethysmography. The improvement in the flow properties of blood, which could be maintained for some weeks by daily intravenous injections can be correlated to a clear improvement in the clinical status of the patients suffering from peripheral ischemia.

INCREASED CAPILLARY PERFUSION OF BLOOD THROUGH A 8 MICRON TEST SYSTEM BY PHOSPHOLIPIDS

Albrecht M. Ehrly and Rainer Blendin
Department of Internal Medicine, Division of Angiology, University of Frankfurt, Frankfurt/BRD

The mode of action of the so-called 'essential' phospholipids in the treatment of peripheral arteriosclerosis is still discussed. Suggesting that the capillary perfusion of the vessel wall may play a role in the pathogenesis of arteriosclerosis and basing on the connection between capillary perfusion and ischemia in vascular diseases, we studied the influence of 'essential' phospholipids on the microrheology of blood. In healthy volunteers, a single dose of 750 mg was given intravenously. Blood was collected from the antecubital vein before and 15, 30 and 45 minutes after administration. Blood was measured in a 8 micron filter apparatus. After the injection of phospholipids the number of filtrated erythrocytes was increased about 25% as compared to the controls. This indicates an improved filtrability of blood. The mechanism of this effect is unknown.

DIELECTRIC STUDIES ON BETA-LIPOPROTEINS

C.G. Essex, E.H. Grant, G.L. Mills, R.J. Sheppard, Joan Slack, and G.P. South
Queen Elizabeth College, Middlesex Hospital Medical School and M.R.C. Clinical Genetic Unit, London/England

Differences in structure of low density lipoproteins have been investigated by the combined use of analytical ultracentrifugation and dielectric measurements in five controls and four heterozygotes and two homozygotes with familial hyperbetalipoproteinaemia.

Measurements of dielectric constant have been made on lipoproteins in aqueous solutions in a coaxial line at frequencies between 300 and 1200 MHz, a radio frequency bridge below 10 MHz and with a Time Domain Reflectometer.

In the controls the specific decrement at 800 MHz was 0.107-0.111, in the heterozygotes 0.112-0.120 and in the homozygotes 0.122 and 0.124 ml/mg.
The results indicate that no difference in molecular shape can account for the differences in specific decrement but the findings are consistent with an increased quantity of bound water associated with the ß-lipoprotein molecules in the abnormal samples.

HYPOLIPIDEMIC THERAPY AND GLUCOSE TOLERANCE

Elaine B. Feldman, Franklin Gluck, and Anne C. Carter
Department of Medicine, SUNY Downstate Medical Center, Brooklyn, NY/USA

Possible improvement in glucose tolerance with hypolipidemic drug therapy was investigated in 20 hypertriglyceridemic patients in a double-blind study of halofenate vs clofibrate. Semi-annual 6h oral glucose tolerance tests for 1-2 yrs. measured plasma glucose, insulin, growth hormone, FFA and glycerol, fasting cholesterol, triglycerides and lipoprotein Type. Mean control values were: triglycerides 451 mg/100 ml; fasting, 1h and 2h glucose 95, 185 and 164 mg/100 ml; peak insulin 95 µU/ml. Lipoprotein Types were: IIb, 2; III, 2; IV, 12; V, 2; VI, 2. Eleven patients were chemical diabetics (5 obese); 9 patients were normal (4 obese); 13 patients were atherosclerotic (7 chemical diabetics). With therapy, triglycerides declined 30%. At 48 wks, 79% of patients had normal glucose tolerance with mean 1h and 2h glucose decreased 14 and 17 mg/100 ml below control values. At 96 wks, 83% of patients had normal glucose tolerance, 1h and 2h glucose were 10 and 28 mg/100 ml below control values. Peak insulin decreased 12 µU/ml. Basal FFA declined with therapy. Body weight changes were insignificant. Halofenate effects on glucose, insulin and FFA exceeded clofibrate. Association of improved glucose tolerance with effective lipid lowering may provide additional rationale and mechanisms for hypolipidemic drug therapy, and decrease additional risk factors in atherosclerosis.

STRUCTURE-ACTIVITY RELATIONSHIPS IN THE HYPOLIPIDEMIC PHENYLACETALS OF THE GLYOXYLIC ACID

János Fischer, József Borsy, Tamás Fodor, József Rákóczi, and Andrea Maderspach
EGYT Pharmacochemical Works and Pharmaceutical Research Institute, Budapest/ Hungary

About 100 new glyoxylic acid phenylacetals (I) have been synthesized to find new hypolipidemic agents. The first part of the compounds was open-chain derivatives. Their activity was found to be in correlation with their aromatic character. Among the various ring variations the 4-chloro substitution was the most advantageous. Among the derivatives containing carboxylic groups the following molecules had favourable activity: N-isopropyl-bis (4-chlorophenoxy)-acetamide and bis (4-chlorophenoxy)-acetyl-urea. The second part of the compounds syntesized were heterocyclic derivatives of I. Both groups of the compounds displayed a significant blood lipid lowering effect in rats at dose levels of 3-30 mg/kg respectively.

OPTIMUM ENZYME DIAGNOSIS OF MYOCARDIAL INFARCTION

Robert S. Galen and S. Raymond Gambino
Columbia-Presbyterian Medical Center, New York, NY/USA

While the prevention of atherosclerosis is clearly the way to attack the problem of myocardial infarction, we are nonetheless faced with an ever increasing number of hospital admissions with the diagnosis of "rule out M.I.". Serial measurement of serum enzymes and isoenzymes have become well established as aids in the diagnosis of myocardial infarction. The optimum combination and sequence of available assays has not been clearly defined. We have made serial kinetic measurements for 10 days of ALT, AST, HBD, LD and its isoenzymes in 50 patients with documented myocardial infarction. We have also measured these enzymes in 50 patients undergoing general or open heart surgery where postoperative rises in enzymes interfere with the accurate laboratory evaluation of possible myocardial infarction. Our results are integrated into a model designed to measure the predictive value of these enzyme tests.

LARGE SCALE STUDY OF AN IMPROVED SCREENING TEST FOR ATHEROGENIC HYPERLIPIDEMIAS

J.L.De Gennes, G. Turpin, and J. Truffert
Endocrinologic Clinic, C.H.U. Pitié-Salpêtrière, Paris/France

For improving detection and identification of ambiguous systematic comparison of conventional lipid parameters Total Cholesterol (TC) by Babson technic; Triglycerides (TG) by Van Handel and Zilversmit technic; electrophoretic pattern by paper electrophoresis of Lees and Hatch) was performed at the 8th and 12th hour of an overnight fasting. Simply the dinner, taken at home, was postponed between 11, 30 and 12h PM and standardized (1200C : 48% of glucids, 36% of lipids and 17% of protids). While no significative changes of these parameters was registered in 88 control subjects of both sexes (age range 20 to 65 mean 39), and in 72 certified type II (21 with tendinous xanthomas). Marked and significative changes in TG concentration and TG rich lipoproteins was registered in 62 cases of type III and type II + IV, and 4 cases of massive type IV. The major interest of the test was to discover abnormalities of TG at the 8th hour in 41 cases looking like pure type II at the 12th hour; and combined abnormalities of TG and CT in 22 subjects looking falsely normal at the 12th hour despite obvious signs of accelerated atheromatosis.

A NEW ANTIGENIC COMPOUND IN HUMAN AORTIC TISSUE ? : ANTIGEN Ao

Jean Gras, Janine P. Bringuier, and Philippe Courpron
University Claude Bernard, Lyon/France

The presence of a particular antigenic compound in aortic tissue is a new argument for immunological theories on atherosclerosis. The soluble proteins of human aorta were extracted in saline solution, and rabbit immunsera were prepared. The gel immunodiffusion technic 'shows, with crude immunsera, the presence of proteins with identical antigenic character to human serum proteins. Moreover, fibrinogen, C-reactive protein and an unknown component are detected. After immunabsorption of immunsera against serum, liver and human fibrinogen, all precipitation lines disappear except one. This unknown fraction is not detected in spleen, kidney, myocardium and striated muscle. It seems that this fraction would be probably proper to human aortic wall, but verifications concerning the presence of this antigen in other arterial tissues are now carried out.

NO INFLUENCE OF CHOLESTYRAMINE ON THE ABSORPTION OF ß-METHYL-DIGOXIN IN MEN

Klaus-Jürgen Hahn and Katharina Reindell
Medizinische Universitätsklinik, Heidelberg/BRD

The exchange resin cholestyramine, which reduces elevated serum cholesterol levels, interferes with the gastrointestinal absorption of several drugs among others also with digitoxin. Since many patients with coronary complications of hyperlipoproteinemia type II require digitalisation, knowledge on interaction with other cardiac glycosides is necessary. The effect of cholestyramine on the absorption of ß-methyl-digoxin was studied in six male hospitalized patients in a controlled single blind study using a randomized cross over repetition design. Blood levels of the tritium labelled compound following the sole or combined intake with cholestyramine were determined in intervals for 48 hours. There were no significant differences in the course of the blood levels. A comparison of the areas under the curves yields a 5.8% reduction of drug absorption by the resin, which is not statistically significant.

RADIOCIRCULOGRAPHIC DIAGNOSIS OF INTERMITTENT VERTEBROBASILARY INSUFFICIENCY

Stefan Hărăguş, Ioan Muresan, George Uza, Tiberius Holan, and Marcel Micluţia
Medical Clinic I, Cluj/Roumania

The value of radiocirculography with ^{51}Cr injected into the cubital vein for the diagnosis of intermittent vertebrobasilary insufficiency (IVI) has been assessed in 64 atherosclerotic patients and in ten healthy control subjects. Two dilution curves have been obtained by means of two detectors (occipital and precordial). On the basis of the Stewart Hamilton principle the cardiac output was calculated and the ratio between areas of the two curves was used for the assessment of the relative cerebral blood flow (RCBF). In control subjects the mean RCBF was 882.4 ml/min. This was not significantly modified in Biemond position (maximal rotation and flexion of the head). In patients with IVI mean RCBF was normal or decreased in anteroposterior position, decreasing with more than 20% (mean decrease 296 ml/min.) in Biemond position. The obtained data were in agreement with clinical and angiographic findings. The method was easy to perform. It is useful for the precocious etiopathogenic diagnosis of IVI.

THE EFFECT OF CLOFIBRATE ON THYROXINE METABOLISM

W. Arthur Harland and J. Stewart Orr
Department of Pathology, Western Infirmary, and Department of Clinical Physics and Bioengineering, Glasgow/Scotland

Experiments were performed to study the effect of clofibrate on thyroxine metabolism in rats. Clofibrate (0.2% diet) was fed for 3 weeks and then thyroxine secretion rates and tissue concentrations of thyroxine were estimated using a new radiothyroxine method. Clofibrate caused a small reduction in serum Protein Bound Iodine concentration and a rise in thyroxine concentration in the liver. Substantially increased hepatic flux of thyroxine was associated with increased biliary thyroxine clearance. Thyroxine flux in other tissues was slightly reduced. The significance of these results will be discussed.

LONG-TERM EFFECT OF ALUFIBRATE (ALUMINIUM-[BIS-ALPHA-PARACHLOROPHENOXY-ISOBUTYRATE]) IN VARIOUS TYPES OF HYPERLIPIDEMIAS

Georges Hartmann and Johannes Stähelin
Medizinische Universitätsklinik, Inselspital, Bern/Schweiz

The effect of alufibrate has been investigated in 67 primary hyperlipidemias (45 men and 22 women). The study included 16 types II-A, 25 II-B, 2 III, 18 IV, and 6 V. The daily doses of alufibrate were 1.5-2.0 g. Evaluation was made by comparison of results from the 4th week of treatment on with pretreatment values. The drug-effect in the group of responders (mean treatment 390 days) was (%±SD):

Type	Chol	TG	Non-Responders
II-A	-16.2± 7.6	--	7/9
II-B	-13.3± 5.5	-34.2±15.9	8/17
III	-39.9	-51.6	0/2
IV	-15.1±12.2	-51.9±13.2	4/14
V	-27.6± 15.0	-67.1±12.6	1/5

The effect of alufibrate seems to be of the magnitude as that of clofibrate. The number of responders is relatively high in type II-A and II-B.

EFFECT OF ESSENTIAL PHOSPHOLIPIDS ON ELEVATED BLOOD LIPID LEVELS

Gert Hevelke, Eva Grott, Roman Zappe, and Konrad Machalke
Siekertal Hospital, Bad Oeynhausen/BRD

52 subjects with elevated blood lipid levels were treated with 500 mg essential phospholipids three times daily for six weeks. Total lipids, cholesterol (free and esterified cholesterol) and triglycerides were estimated and lipid electrophoresis carried out.

The following criteria were used to assess possible side effects: SGOT, SGPT, Gamma-GT, ESR, urine analysis, blood sugar, blood pressure and pulse rate.

After six weeks of treatment a significant fall of systolic and diastolic blood pressure, of triglycerides, cholesterol and of raised lipid electrophoresis levels was registered.

Side effects were not observed.

FAMILIAL LECITHIN: CHOLESTEROL ACYL-TRANSFERASE (LCAT) DEFICIENCY, LIGHT AND ULTRASTRUCTURAL STUDIES

Torstein Hovig and Egil Gjone
Electron Microscopic Laboratory, Institute of Pathology and Medicine, Department A, Rikshospitalet, Oslo/Norway

Ultrastructural studies of negatively stained plasma from a patient with LCAT-deficiency revealed presence of membranes in a fingerprint pattern and stacks of discs. Biopsies from kidneys revealed presence of membranes and membrane-surrounded particles in the glomerular capillaries; within the lumina, in the basement membrane and in the mesangial regions. The capillary endothelium was damaged and partly detached, but no thrombi was observed. Membrane structures were observed in the liver, especially in the perivascular regions where fibrosis was noted. In the spleen numerous so-called "sea-blue" histiocytes were noted, and ultrastructurally they contained granules composed of concentrically arranged membranes. Arteries and veins revealed presence of membranes in the subendothelial regions. It is concluded that pathological lipoproteins may leak out through the vessel wall and cause vessel and tissue damage. LCAT-deficiency may represent a model of vascular damage caused by abnormal lipoprotein particles, leading to atheromatous changes.

SERUM LIPOPROTEINS IN PATIENTS TREATED WITH HYPOLIPAEMIC DRUGS DETERMINED BY NEPHELOMETRY

Alan N. Howard and Rupert J. Courtenay Evans
Department of Investigative Medicine, University of Cambridge, and Addenbrooke's Hospital, Cambridge/England

Nephelometry has been suggested as a quantitative method for the assay of serum triglycerides. Together with a serum cholesterol determination, it can be used to calculate the concentration of low density (LD), very low density (VLD) lipoproteins and chylomicrons, the values of which correlate well with analytical ultracentrifugal analysis. The aim was to investigate the use of this procedure in patients treated with certain hypolipaemic drugs. Using the Thorp-Stone nephelometer the serum of patients treated with poly-(2-(diethylamino)ethyl) polyglycerylene dextran hydrochloride (PDX chloride) showed chiefly a marked decrease in LD. Those treated with clofibrate showed a reduction in both LD and VLD where the latter was elevated. A combination of both drugs gave a greater decrease in LD than each independently, and a decrease in VLD when elevated. It is concluded that the combination therapy is valuable in Type IIa and IIb hyperlipoprotein-aemia.

THE INDUCTION OF SPONTANEOUS MYOCARDIAL NECROSIS AND FIBROSIS IN FAT-FED RABBITS

Huang Te-Hsiu and We Chun-Chung
Department of Medicine, Taiwan University Hospital, Taipei/Taiwan

To induce spontaneous myocardial necrosis and fibrosis, a series of fat diets was given to rabbits. 1. Two groups of rabbits were kept on 1% cholesterol diet for four months at different temperatures, 16°C and 32°C respectively. 2. Three groups of rabbits were fed on cholesterol diet added with 10 ml of different fats, safflower oil, lard and butter respectively for four months. 3. Three groups of rabbits were fed on lanolin diet added with the same amount of different fats, ricebran oil, lard and lanolin for four months. 4. Another group of rabbits was fed with lard 10 ml daily for 15 months. Increased frequency of myocardial necrosis was seen in the first experiment of the group kept at 16°C and less in the group at 32°C. No necrosis was seen in the second experiment whereas increased frequency of fibrosis was seen, and these changes were less marked in the third, and neither myocardial change nor coronary atherosclerosis was seen in the fourth. These data suggest myocardial necrosis can be easily induced by sole cholesterol feeding at low temperature. However adding fat will retard the process, it increased the frequency of fibrosis, and even without direct influence on the myocardial damage by sole lard feeding.

LIPID FRACTIONS OF LOW DENSITY LIPOPROTEINS IN CARDIOVASCULAR DISEASES

Peter Ilinov and Serafim Popnikolov
Chair of Cardiology, Centre of Cardiovascular Diseases, Medical Academy, Sofia/
Bulgaria

To characterize the physico-chemical status of serum lipids in cardiovascular patients, lipid fractions of low density lipoproteins (LDLP) have been estimated by the following method: fallout of LDLP with 0.5 M $CaCl_2$ and dextran sulfate; extraction with chloroform-methanol mixture; separation of lipids by thin-layer chromatography; estimation (in %) of separate lipid fractions through bichromate reagent. The 140 patients studied – 24 with recent MI and arterial hypertension (AH), 41 with chronic ischaemic heart disease (CIHD), 43 with AH, 15 with hyperlipoproteinaemias and 20 healthy controls were then separated into three main groups according to triglycerides (group I<18%, group II with 18-28%, group III >28%), with three subgroups in each one according to the cholesterol/phospholipid ratio (a<1, 2; b with 1, 2-1, 4; c>1, 4). The group distribution of patients (e.g. predominantly with recent MI in group Ia; with CIHD in group IIIa) suggests a possible diagnostic and prognostic value of this test.

LIPIDS IN A LONG-TERM TRIAL WITH A BIPHASIC OESTRADIOL VALERIANATE-NORGESTREL PREPARATION IN POST-MENOPAUSAL WOMEN

K. Irsigler, H. Lageder, W. Schneider, and K. Matt
The 1st Medical Clinic (Head: Prof.Dr.E.Deutsch) and the 1st Gynecological
Clinic of Vienna (Head: Prof.Dr.E.Gitsch), Vienna/Austria

In 20 postmenopausal women (10 after hysterectomy + ovarectomy) hormonal treatment was given to compensate loss or reduction of ovarial function.

A biphasic substitution with 11 days of estrogen (2 mg oestradiol-valerianate) and 10 days of estrogen + 0.5 mg DL-norgestrel was given with a free interval of 7 days for each cycle. After 1 cycle with placebo 7 cycles with medication were followed by 1 cycle placebo again with regular controls.

Several haematologic and metabolic parameters were evaluated. There was no rise in serum-cholesterol or triglycerides nor any change of the lipoprotein pattern after longterm treatment.

	control	5th cycle (11th days)	(21st days)
Triglycerides	107 ± 44	104 ± 44	91 ± 35
Cholesterol	251 ± 53	249 ± 57	238 ± 59

EFFECT OF ALLIUM SATIVUM L. ON SERUM CHOLESTEROL OF HEALTHY INDIVIDUALS

Medard Kerekes, Delia Nicoară, and Stephen Csögör
Medical Research Center, Tîrgu-Mures/Roumania

The action of Allium sativum L. (garlic) on serum cholesterol was investigated, in clinically healthy persons, during two different seasons. In the first experiment, carried out in April, seven persons consumed daily 3 g of garlic, during the evening meal, while four were controls. After one month, the mean of total serum cholesterol decreased with 29.2 mg% in the experimental group, while in the controls a decrease of 6.1 mg% occurred, the difference being significant. The second experiment was carried out in December, in the conditions described, comprising 14 treated persons and 11 controls. The mean of total serum cholesterol decreased with 10.9 mg% in the experimental group, an increase of 1.7 mg% occurring in the controls (non-significant difference). Garlic seems to have a lowering effect on serum cholesterol in healthy individuals.

METABOLIC AND MORPHOLOGIC ASPECTS OF HYPERTRIGLYCERIDEMIA IN LIVER DISEASE

Ulrich Klör, Dieter Paulini, Ulrich Staudacher, Hans H. Ditschuneit, and Hans Ditschuneit
Zentrum für Innere Medizin, Universität Ulm, Ulm/BRD

In severe liver cell damage a triglyceride (TG) rich lipoprotein (LP) fraction has been observed which has the characteristics of a LDL. Measurements of lipoprotein lipase (LPL) by a modification of the method of Fredrickson and electron microscopy of the LDL of liver patients were undertaken to elucidate the mechanism of hypertriglyceridemia. In 30 patients with liver cell damage the LPL was reduced to less than half the normal values. Electron microscopy of the LDL fraction prepared by ultracentrifugation revealed polycyclic, chylomicron-like particles (CLP) up to 5000 A in diameter closely surrounded by normal LDL. The same CLP were found together with normal chylomicra in the VLDL plus chylomicra fraction of these patients.
Our results indicate that a diminished degradation of TG rich particles caused by a low LPL may be responsible in part for the elevated TG values. The accumulation of the TG rich CLP may contribute to the hypertriglyceridemia, too.
Some evidence suggests that CLP are partially metabolised chylomicra or "remnants" which cannot be taken up, as is normally the case, by the damaged liver.

MULTIFACTORIAL PREVENTION OF ISCHAEMIC HEART DISEASE. A FEASIBILITY STUDY

Marcel Kornitzer and Robert Streulens
Department Cardiologie, Hôpotal St. Pierre, Bruxelles/Belgique

Risk scores based on age, systolic blood pressure, blood cholesterol and smoking habits were assigned to 199 male employees, aged between 40 and 60. The subjects were divided at random into two groups. The "prevention group" received advice about obesity, blood cholesterol, systolic hypertension and cigarette smoking. These subjects were re-examined after 4, 8 and 12 months, whereas subjects in the control group after twelve months only. No medication was prescribed by our team. Advice concerned diet and habits. As regards relative weight a reduction of 6% or more was observed in 20% of the prevention group and in 7% of the control group (P<0.01). For subjects with an initial cholesterol level of 250 mg% or more, there was a fall of 11% or more in 34.4% of the subjects in the prevention group, against only 20.7% of the subjects in the control group (0.1<P<0.05). Systolic blood pressure dropped by 6% or more in 35% of the subjects in the prevention group, compared to 21% in the control group (P<0.05). As regards cigarette smoking, 26% of the subjects in the prevention group who had smoked more than 5 cig. a day, changed this habit. The corresponding figure was 13% in the control group (0.1<P<0.05). There were few dropouts: 88% attendance at the annual check-up. It is possible to modify various risk factors simultaneously in a population of male employees by giving prevention advice every four months.

GLYCOSPHINGOLIPIDS OF LIPOPROTEIN CLASSES IN HYPERLIPIDEMIA

Terrence T. Kuske
Department of Medicine, Medical College of Georgia, Augusta, GA/USA

Data obtained on plasma of 12 healthy, 16 hyperlipoproteinemic and three Gaucher subjects demonstrate that glycosphingolipids (GSL) are present in very low density lipoproteins (VLDL), and levels are increased in hyperlipoproteinemia. GSL were isolated chromatographically from ultracentrifugally separated VLDL and infranatant fractions, and quantitated by acid hydrolysis and anthrone determinations.

Increased quantities of glucosyl ceramide (GL-1), lactosyl ceramide (GL-2), trihexosyl ceramide (GL-3) and globoside (GL-4) were found in the increased VLDL of ten hyperlipoproteinemic patients, and in the infranate in three patients with elevated low density lipoproteins. GL-1 levels in five hyperlipoproteinemics were comparable to the two to threefold increase observed with Gaucher's disease. Trihexosyl ceramide levels in one patient approximated the threefold increase reported for Fabry's disease. GSL levels declined in proportion to the lipoprotein levels in five patients evaluated after treatment.

GL-1, GL-2 and GL-3 content of VLDL in normal and hyperlipoproteinemic patients was proportional to the total lipid, and correlated at highly significant (P= <.001) levels. Content of all GSL were significantly correlated with infranatant total lipid. These data suggest the GSL are structural components of lipoproteins.

ARTERIOSCLEROSIS IN PYRIDOXINE DEFICIENT SPONTANEOUS HYPERTENSIVE RATS (SHR)

Fumio Kuzuya and Noboru Yoshimine
Third Department of Internal Medicine, Nagoya University School of Medicine, Showa-Ku, Nagoya/Japan

In 6th and 7th International Congress of Gerontology in Copenhagen and Vienna, authors reported arteriosclerosis in various organs in pyridoxine deficient monkeys. In this papers, authors investigated the arteriosclerosis in spontaneous hypertensive rats (SHR) kept on pyridoxine deficient diet for 6 months. The arteriosclerotic fibrous plaque and thrombosis were found in pyridoxine deficient SHR but not in SGR kept on normal diet. On the other hand, hypertensive thickness or proliferative changes of elastic fibre of aortic and arterial wall were prominent in spontaneous hypertensive rats kept on normal diet or pyridoxine deficient diet but not in other strain rats.

STUDIES ON THE STRUCTURE OF HUMAN PLASMA HIGH DENSITY LIPOPROTEIN

Peter Laggner, Karl Mueller, and Gerhard Kostner
Institut für Röntgenfeinstrukturforschung am Forschungszentrum, and Institut für Medizinische Biochemie der Universität Graz, Graz/Austria

The LpA fraction of human plasma high density lipoprotein HDL_3 of mol.wt.200,000 which is homogeneous with respect to its protein constituents was studied in solution by X-ray small angle scattering. Scattering curves were obtained from different solvent electron densities by using different concentrations of sucrose. The analysis based on Fourier transformation and theoretical model curve fitting resulted in a spherical particle of 96 Å diameter. The electron density distribution shows an outer high electron density shell of 11 Å thickness which reflects the surface location of the polypeptides and the phospholipid polar head groups. The low electron density core of 37 Å radius indicates an extended conformation of the cholesterol esters thus forming a spherical micellar structure together with the hydrocarbon chains of the phospholipids.

CHARACTERIZATION OF ASSOCIATED AND FREE FORMS OF LP-B IN LOW DENSITY LIPOPROTEINS OF NORMAL HUMAN PLASMA

D.M. Lee and P. Alaupovic
Oklahoma Medical Research Foundation, Oklahoma City, OK/USA

Structure of LDL was studied by physical-chemical and immunological methods. Whereas the LDL_1 (d 1.006-1.019 g/ml) subfractions gave completely or partially fused precipitin lines, the LDL_2 (d 1.019-1.063 g/ml) exhibited separate lines with antibodies to LP-B and LP-C. The molecular weight of LDL_1 was 4.7×10^6 daltons and those of LDL_2 subfractions $2.9-3.0 \times 10^6$ daltons. The ApoC accounted for 38% of the protein content of LDL_1, but only 7% of that of LDL_2. Antiserum to LP-C caused a complete coprecipitation of LP-B and LP-C in LDL_1, but not in LDL_2. A preparation of LDL_1 was isolated ultracentrifugally from the immuno-precipitate of whole serum with anti-LP-B; this lipoprotein consisted of LP-B and LP-C and had a molecular weight of 4.4×10^6 daltons. These results indicate a fundamental difference between the LDL_1 and LDL_2 subfractions. In the former, lipoprotein families exist in the form of association products, whereas in the latter they occur as separate entities. The higher molecular weight of LDL_1 is due to the association of LP-B and LP-C in a structural entity containing more triglyceride than the separate LP-B and LP-C families of LDL_2.

CALORIGENIC ACTIVITY OF D-THYROXINE AND D-TRIIODOTHYRONINE IN COMBINATION

Götz Leopold, Zdenek Simane, and Herbert Nowak
Medical Research (E. Merck), Darmstadt/BRD

In initial clinical trials D-thyroxine (DT 4) and D-3, 5, 3'-triiodothyronine (DT 3) in combination (4:1) lower effectively serum cholesterol levels in type II hyperlipoproteinemia without cardiac side effects which are observed using either

DT 3 or DT 4 alone. As cardiac side effects correlate with the calorigenic activity (CA) of thyreomimetic drugs it was tried to reproduce the clinical observations in an animal model. A mouse anoxia method was used and evaluated by analysis of variance.

The relations in CA obtained: LT 3 250-fold > DT 3; LT 4 100-fold > DT 4; DT 3 5-fold > DT 4.

The combination DT 4/DT 3 (4:1) as compared in doses of equivalence to DT 3 or DT 4 alone exerted only one third of the CA of the single components. – An indication for a lesser CA of the combination can also be observed comparing the body weight gains in rats (normo- and hyperlipemic or propylthio-uracil-loaded) treated with DT 3, DT 4 or DT 4/DT 3 (4:1) over two weeks.

RESPIRATORY AND GLYCOLYTIC DISORDERS OF THE MYOCARDIUM OF RATS RECEIVING A DIET SUPPLEMENTED WITH VITAMIN D-2 OR WITH EGG YOLK OR THESE SUPPLEMENTS ASSOCIATED

G. Leporda, Constantsa Haller, and S. Freund
Institute of Public Health and Medical Research, Jassy/Roumania

Wistar rats receiving a diet supplemented with vitamin D-2 (600.000) I.U./kg for 6 or 12 days) or egg yolk (2 g daily for 4 months), or these two supplements together presented besides morphological changes of atherosclerosis type disorders of the respiratory and glycolitic metabolism of the myocardium: decoupling tion of P/O and increased production of lactate. The above diets have favoured an increase of the acidity of the inner medium of the myocardium cells and the growth of the concentration of pyridinnucleotides which contributes to the synthesis of fatty acids and lipid substances which played an important role in the pathogenesis of atherosclerosis.

COMPARATIVE STUDY WITH BIS/4-CHLOROPHENOXY/-ACETYL-UREA AND CLOFIBRATE ON HYPER-LIPEMIAS INDUCED BY IMPAIRED CARBOHYDRATE METABOLISM

Andrea Maderspach, József Borsy, and János Fischer
Research Institute for Pharmaceutical Chemistry, Budapest/Hungary

Hyperlipemia was induced in normal rats by fructose or alloxan administration. Fructose, via a direct effect on liver triglyceride formation results in an elevated serum lipid concentration. The investigated compounds decreased the elevated triglyceride level but bis/4-chlorophenoxy/-acetyl-urea was approximately ten times as potent as clofibrate. Alloxan diabetes is known to be associated with high serum lipid levels. Bis/4-chlorophenoxy/-acetyl-urea resulted in a dose dependent lipid lowering effect and decreased the abnormal blood glucose concentration while clofibrate had no influence on alloxan hyperlipemia.

SCANNING ELECTRON-MICROSCOPIC AND ULTRAHISTOCHEMICAL STUDIES ON ANGIOPATHY-MODELS OF THE MINIATURE-PIG

Markwart Marshall, Hans Hess, and Marita Mallasch
Medizinische Poliklinik, Universität München/BRD

Experimental animals were Hanford miniature pigs whose arteries were gained in narcotic state in their original tension. Besides scanning electronmicroscopy of the endothelium, the biogenous amines in the inner layers of the vessels were analysed by argentaffin and chromaffin reactions through X-ray microanalysis. It could be demonstrated that the epinephrine content amounts to no more than ten per cent of the norepinephrine content and that the norepinephrine content is lower in the thoracic aorta than in the coronary, carotid and femoral artery and in the abdominal aorta. Ice and epinephrine provocation were used as angiopathy models in femoral and carotid arteries. Every provocation leads to adhesions of platelets. Acetylsalicylic acid inhibits these adhesions.

CHOLESTEROL AND TRIGLYCERIDES AFTER LONG-TERM INFUSION OF FRUCTOSE, SORBITOL AND XYLITOL

Fritz Matzkies, Gerhard Berg, Dietrich Bergner, and Hanne Bickel
Department of Medicine, University of Erlangen-Nuremberg/BRD

After oral administration of different carbohydrates the observation was made that fructose causes a marked rise in triglycerides compared with other sugars (Zakin, 1967). We examined whether following paranteral application of carbohydrates the concentration of serum lipoproteins was also altered. 36 healthy fasting male subjects received continous infusions of 10 per cent electrolyte-free solutions of fructose (n=12), sorbitol (n=12) and xylitol (n=12) lasting six hours. Triglycerides (Kreutz and Eggstein) and cholesterol (Liebermann and Burchard) were determined before and at the end of the experiment. Statistical evaluation revealed that following the infusion of fructose, sorbitol and xylitol no significant changes in triglycerides were observed. Cholesterol concentration, too, was not altered by xylitol and fructose but was significantly lowered ($p < 0.001$) by sorbitol.

BLOOD INSULIN AND GLUCOSE REGULATION DURING PRIMARY HYPERLIPIDEMIAS

Luc Méjean, Pierre Drouin, Denis Guisard, Jean-Paul Pointel, and Gérard Debry
Département de Nutrition Université I de Nancy et Groupe de Recherches de Nutrition et de Diététique, Inserm U 59, Nancy/France

The glucose tolerance test and the intravenous tolbutamide test with radioimmunologic assay of the blood insuline were administered to a group of 96 hyperlipidemic non diabetics who had been classed by electrophoresis analysis and by dietetic sequences: 42 hypercholesterolemias (12 obese, 30 non obese) 21 mixed hyperlipidemias (8 obese, 12 non obese), 27 hypertriglyceridemias sensitive to alcohol (7 obese, 20 non obese), 6 hypertriglyceridemias sensitive to carbohydrates (4 obese, 2 non obese). The occurence of latent diabetes was elevated, in the following order of importance: hypercholesterolemias, mixed hypertriglyceridemias sensitive to carbohydrate or to alcohol. Hyperinsulinemia was frequent, and was found in the obese and the non obese. The reduction of hyperlipidemia by appropriate diet normalized the hyperglycemia and the hyperinsulinemia and provided an additional proof of the glucose-fatty acid interactions.

EARLY GROSS CALCIFICATIONS AND EARLY LIPID DEPOSITS IN RELATION TO THE PREFORMED ARTERIAL STRUCTURES

W.W. Meyer
Institute of Pathology, University of Mainz, Mainz/BRD

A combined gross staining of early calcific and lipid deposits has been used for demonstration of their initial localisation in larger arterial segments and for the evaluation of their histotopographic interrelations. In the large muscular arteries and in the iliac arteries the patterns of early calcifications largely depend on the differentiation of the subendothelial elastic structures and the system of gaps which develop in the internal elastic membrane during the growth.

In the carotid siphon the calcifications initially appear in the thick subendothelial networks. In contrast, the early lipid deposits become first visible in the intimal cushions at the concave parts of the curves. Even in the straight segments of the carotid arteries the peculiar patterns of the lipid infiltration depend on definite structural differences of the individual arterial sectors. The remodeling of the arterial wall which results from calcification also influences the localisation of the subsequent lipid deposits.

EFFECT OF CLOFIBRATE AND NAFENOPIN ON THE RESPONSE TO THE INTRAVENOUS FAT TOLERANCE TEST AFTER SHORT AND LONG TERM TREATMENT

Horace Micheli, Arved Weisswange, Bogdan Malzcewski, and Daniel Pometta
Unité de Diabétologie, Département de Médicine, Hôpital cantonal, Genève/Suisse

A single injection of a fat emulsion was performed in 37 hyperlipemic and 29 normolipemic subjects and the fractional elimination rate (K2) determined. Under treatment with clofibrate or nafenopin, the test was repeated either within 24 hr. or one month later. Administration of 2 g clofibrate for 24 hr had no significant effect on K2 (n=8), whereas 1.5 g/day for one month increased K2 by 30% (p <0.05; N310). During that time fasting serum triglycerides (TG) decreased by 28% (p < 0.01). In contrast to clofibrate, nafenopin (300 mg/day) increased significantly the fractional removal rate by 28% (p <0.001; n=32) within 24 hr and by 44% (p < 0.001; n=16) after one month of treatment. Fasting TG decreased by 22% (p <0.001) amd 40% (p <0.001) respectively. The increased elimination rate of a fat emulsion may partly explain the hypolipemic action of both drugs. Individual results show differences that stress the heterogeneity of hyperlipemias of the same type.

MODIFICATION OF THE BIOCHEMICAL STRUCTURE OF MYOCARD AND AORTIC WALL IN ATHEROSCLEROSES

Ioana Mogos-Tănase and Maria Popescu

Qualitative modifications of the thiolic groups were recorded at the voltage level by polarography with automatic recording from the hydrosoluble proteins isolated from myocard and aorta in 50 cases (47 to 72 years old) with atherosclerosis. The tissue was removed immediately after death. After the tryptic hydrolysis of the proteins from myocard and aorta, valine, alanine, and leucine from the myocard and methionine, and lysine from the aorta could not be chromatographically separated. In 40 of the cases choline and linoleic acids have not been identified in the glycero-phosphatide fraction of the aorta. The results were compared and statistically assessed with those obtained in an equal number of controls 40 years old who died by violent death. The importance of the knowledge of the tissular and plasmic constituents biochemical structure for the prognosis of atherosclerosis is discussed.

MODIFICATIONS IN THE STRUCTURE OF PLASMA LIPIDS IN ATHEROSCLEROSIS

Ioana Mogos-Tănase, Maria Popescu, and Gh. Mogos
"D. Danielopolu" Institute of Normal and Pathologic Physiology, Bucharest/Roumania

In a number of 100 patients with atherosclerosis ranging from 40 to 75 years total lipids, non-esterified fatty free acids, cholesterol, triglycerides, phospholipids, lecithine, sphingomyelin and plasmic ß-lipoproteins were followed up by chromatographic and chemical methods. The results were compared with those obtained in similar method conditions in an equal number of control patients of the same age and sex. In 60 cases the phospholipids and lecithin content were found under the normal values. In 40 cases choline, sphingosine, oleic and linoleic acids were not chromatographically isolated in the plasmic fraction from phospholipids, lecithin and sphingomyelin.

The physiological and pathological significance of the plasmic lipids in athero-sclerosis is discussed.

COMPARISON OF EFFECTS OF MUCOPOLYSACCHARIDES UPON SPONTANEOUS AND INDUCED ATHERO-SCLEROSIS IN MONKEYS, RATS, RABBITS, AND HUMAN PATIENTS WITH CORONARY ARTERIO-SCLEROTIC HEART DISEASE

Lester M. Morrison, Benjamin H. Ershoff, Gurwant S. Bajwa, O. Arne Schjeide, Roslyn B. Alfin-Slater, and Norbert L. Enrick
Institute for Arteriosclerosis Research, Loma Linda University School of Medicine, Los Angeles, CA/USA

A ten year comparative study is presented on the effects of various acid muco-polysaccharides including heparin, chondroitin-4 and 6-sulfates, chondroitin poly-sulfates and heparinoids upon the spontaneous and the diet-induced atherosclerosis of squirrel monkeys, the diet-induced coronary atherosclerosis of rats and rabbits.

These results, pathological changes and therapeutic results are compared to those observed in human patients with demonstrable coronary arteriosclerotic heart dis-ease treated successfully by mucopolysaccharides since 1942.

The acid mucopolysaccharide chondroitin-4-sulfate shows approximately the same statistically significant ratio of reduction to one-sixth that of controls in mortality and morbidity rates for atherosclerotic monkeys and rats as demonstrated for human coronary arteriosclerotic heart disease.

ATHEROSCLEROTIC SIGNS OF THE LATERAL TONGUE-VESSELS

Casile Mülfay
Department of Ear Nose and Throat, Medical and Pharmaceutical Institute, Tîrgu-Mureş/Roumania

The evolution of atherosclerosis of the lateral tongue-vessels was investigeted, discussing its clinical and diagnostic importance. As a consequence of fine and abundant vessel-supply, the latero-inferior surface of the tongue is uniformly pink, in youth. Usually, during the fourth decade, punctiform nodules appear, which histopathologically correspond to dilated vessels, and thrombi, respective-ly. With ageing, an increasing number of blood-vessels obliterate and disappear. In aged, decreased blood-supply leads to pallor and advancing atrophy of the region. The examination of the lateral tongue-vessels supplies valuable informa-tion regarding the vascular system. Distribution, extent, and degree of throm-botic ischemia have a decisive importance in the evaluation of vitality and biol-ogical age.

ASSESSMENT OF THE ACTIVATION OF FACTOR VII, A MEANS TO ESTIMATE INTIMAL PATENCY

A.D. Muller, R. Gonggrijp, and H.C. Hemker
Laboratory for Cardiovascular Research, University Hospital, Leiden/The Nether-lands

Blood coagulation factor VII is the one that triggers thrombin formation via the extrinsic pathway. Thrombinformation is essential for the genesis of a platelet thrombus. A thrombus forms at the site of an intimal lesion, it forms at those places where factor VII activator is present. The activation of factor VII therefore may be a crucial event in the origin of a thrombus, and constitute.the link between the events in the intima, the soluble coagulation factors and the platelet reaction. We established that factor VII_a is a serine esterase, and that factor VII is its proenzyme. We found a means of assessing both the total potential yield of factor VII_a (i.e. the content of the proenzyme) and the concentration of factor VII_a present in the sample. The degree of activation of factor VII in the circulating plasma therefore can be estimated. The activation ratio rises with age and is correlated with intimal patency. The most common cause for its rise is atherosclerotic damage of the intima. A high degree of activation is also found as a complication of malignant disease.

MITOCHONDRIAL ENZYMATIC AND MORPHOLOGICAL CHANGES DURING ATHEROSCLEROSIS

Marvin Murray and Danny Helton
University of Louisville, Louisville, KY/USA

Mitochondrial enzymatic and morphologic changes occurring in the human abdominal aorta were studied as a function of the degree of atherosclerosis as defined by the World Health Organization. The following organelles were isolated by differential centrifugation: mitochondria, mitochondria containing lipid droplets and lipid vesicles. Mitochondria and mitochondria containing lipid droplets were isolated from normal and fatty streak. As the degree of atherosclerosis increased so did the number of mitochondria containing lipid droplets and lipid vesicles. Morphologically, the sequence suggested formation of lipid vesicles from normal mitochondria. This hypothesis was reenforced by observation of mitochondrial marker enzymes in high specific activity and total activity in altered mitochondria and the lipid vesicle fraction. Lipid accumulation and concurrent necrosis by these mitochondria may be one focal point leading to the development of the atherosclerotic plaque.

VINCAMIN EFFECTS ON CEREBRO-VASCULAR DISEASES

G. Nappi, G.M. Kauchtschischvili, and G. Bono
Clinica Neuropatologica, Università di Pavia, Pavia/Italia

Vincamin, an alkaloid from the plant Vinca minor L., has been administrated and compared with Placebo in patients with chronical cerebro-vascular insufficiency, all having clinical and instrumental (cerebralplethysmography and ophthalmo-dynamography) data of haemodynamic disorders regarding single hemisphere.- Vincamin was administrated i.v. (15 mg), i.M. (15 + 15 mg x 10 days), orally (20 mg x 3 x 10 days).- The significant decrease of bihemispheric and/or biophthalmic differences observed after i.v. administration appears larger and more evident after a 20 days administration. Waves getting symmetrical were observed a clinical disorders reducing. Authors conclude Vincamin action consists in vasoregulation and in metabolic effects: regional cerebral blood flow increase and in O_2 utilization.

CLINICAL EXPERIENCE WITH DH 581, A NEW CHOLESTEROL LOWERING COMPOUND

David T. Nash
Syracuse, NY/USA

DH 581, a new cholesterol lowering drug, was studied in thirty adults for over one year in a double blind study. There were seventeen females and thirteen males.

Seven were studied initially with placebo for three months. The mean of three fasting cholesterol and triglyceride determinations prior to therapy was used as the baseline. Monthly determinations of lipids, physical examinations and screening test for hematological, renal, and hepatic toxicity were performed. Lipoprotein phenotyping by paper electrophoreses, electrocardiograms, and opthalmological examinations were performed prior to and after three months of therapy. All patients on therapy received 500 mg of DH 581 twice a day. There was an approximately 15% drop in cholesterol for the entire group studied on DH 581. Twenty-two of the patients experienced a cholesterol drop of 12% or more and are considered responders. Their average response was 19%. Eight non-responders averaged a 3% drop in cholesterol.

MUCOPOLYSACCHARIDES IN THE PROPHYLAXIS OF ATHEROSCLEROSIS, AS RELATED TO HYPER-DYSLIPIDEMIA AND FIBRINOLYSIS

Pietro de Nicola and Francesco Nicrosini
Institute of Gerontology and Geriatrics, University of Pavia, Pavia/Italy

In rabbits given 1.5 g/day cholesterol and an extractive mucopolysaccharidic complex (EMC) for 60 to 90 days a significant reduction of total lipids, triglycerides and total steroids in blood, liver and aorta, and of enzymes in blood has been observed. The reduced oxygen consumption under these conditions was normalized. Similar results were obtained also in experimental poisoning with CS_2 and CCl_4. In humans the hyperlipidemia due to 1 g/kg of butter and 400 ml of milk was considerably reduced and an activation of fibrinolysis took place after 2, 4 and 6 hours if the EMC was administered. In 289 aged atherosclerotic patients given EMC for 15 to 40 days a significant reduction of lipidic fractions was observed. An increase of fibrinolytic activity and a reduction of total and lipoprotein activity was observed after giving ^{131}I triolein+EMC.

THE POSSIBLE ROLES OF BIOELECTRIC PHENOMENA IN ATHEROGENESIS

Roland D. Paegle
Department of Pathology, New York University School of Medicine, New York, NY/USA

Special attention is given in this review of the studies on bioelectric phenomena to the possibility that piezoelectric potentials may be of sufficient magnitude in certain morphologic configuration to produce microthrombi on the intimal surfaces of arteries and arterioles or to cause electrophoretic mobility or electrical field flow fractionation of proteins, lipoproteins and mucopolysaccharides and thus to contribute to the formation of the various deposits seen in the arteriosclerotic plaques. Collagen deposition at the cathode and stabilization by salt has been noted in-vitro.

The piezolectric effect in biological tissues is ascribed to the stress-induced polarization of uniaxilly oriented collagen, elastin and DNA. It is different from potentials and from the streaming potentials. Due to continuous pulsation, the arterial wall components are exposed to repeated mechanical stress more than any other collagen rich tissue of the human body. Hence, the effects could be expected to 1. be more marked in the cardiovascular system and 2. increase with age. The large scale surveys of aging humans have documented that atherosclerosis, including fibrosis and diffuse fibrous thickening of the human aorta, are age related.

DISSIMILARITIES BETWEEN FATTY STREAK AND LARGE CALCIUM DEPOSIT MORPHOLOGY AND DISTRIBUTION IN HUMAN AORTAS

Roland D. Paegle
Department of Pathology, New York University School of Medicine, New York, NY/USA

The locations of the fatty streaks were determined in 152 aortas and compared to the distribution of the macroscopic calcium salt deposits in arteriosclerotic plaques. Direct visualization of the light yellow fatty streaks in the unfixed, flattened and air dried specimens and use of roentgenograms (Siemens X-ray tube at 5ma, 12KV and no filter) avoided the possibility of dissolving any of the lipids, proteins or minerals during fixation. The lesions which were graded on a 0-4+scale included: a) fatty streaks, b) grumous, ulcerating atheromas, c) mural thrombi and clots. The per cent of ostia with fatty streaks and/or calcific deposits were also calculated.
The zonal distribution of the fatty streaks in the posterior walls of the thoracic segments not only differed markedly from the random distribution of the calcium deposits, but occurred in much younger individuals. The band of fatty streaks in the posterior portion of the thoracic aorta constituted the main group of early lipid deposits which regressed with age without evoking complicated plaques. The larger calcium deposits in the thoracic as well as abdominal aortas usually were irregular in shape and differed markedly from the fine streaks and delicate network of the early lipid deposits seen in young individuals.

EFFECT OF ETHANOL ON THE SYNTHESIS AND SECRETION OF LIPOPROTEINS

Joachim Papenberg, Ekbert Ast, Ursula Garbe, and Monika Daumann
Medizinische Universitätsklinik Heidelberg, Heidelberg/BRD

In humans ethanol causes type IV hyperlipoproteinemia with hyper-pre-ß-lipoproteinemia and hypertriglyceridemia. As compared to controls patients with Zieve syndrome and with primary type IIb and type IV hyperlipoproteinemia ethanol causes a markedly higher elevation of pre-ß-lipoproteins with hypertriglyceridemia. These observations in humans are compared with experiments on lipoprotein synthesis and secretion of the isolated perfused fed rat liver. Here it could be demonstrated that ethanol inhibits pre-ß-lipoprotein synthesis and secretion as it was also reported for albumin and transferin synthesis. This discrepancy of the ethanol effects on pre-ß-lipoprotein secretion in humans and in the in vitro system of the isolated rat liver is discussed.

CHARACTERIZATION OF NORMAL HUMAN LIPOPROTEINS, ISOLATED BY RATE ZONAL ULTRACENTRIFUGATION

Josef Patsch, Gerhard Kostner, and Sigurd Sailer
Medical Department, University of Innsbruck, Innsbruck/Austria

Differing data with regard to the composition of plasma lipoproteins (LP) can be explained at least partly by not quite complete separation of the LP density classes by ultracentrifugation in the angle head rotor. By means of rate zonal ultracentrifugation, LP of normal fasting humans of both sexes were separated ($n=29$, $\bar{x} \pm$ S.D.).

LP	Conc. mg/100 ml	Chemical composition, % w/w			
		Chol	TG	PL	Protein
VLDL	66 ± 35	14 ± 3	53 ± 7	20 ± 3	12 ± 4
LDL	244 ± 51	41 ± 3	8 ± 2	26 ± 3	26 ± 3
HDL$_2$	95 ± 32	23 ± 3	7 ± 3	29 ± 4	40 ± 5
HDL$_3$	245 ± 37	16 ± 2	4 ± 2	27 ± 3	53 ± 5

After delipidation, Apo-LP were identified by polyacrylamide gel electrophoresis and by quantitative immunochemical methods. Each LP fraction was albumin free (Ouchterlony). In particular, in all fractions of the density range of LDL besides Apo-B always Apo-A and Apo-C were detectable. The ratio A-I/I-II was much higher in HDL_2 (10:1) than in HDL_3 (4:1). A-III was present in HDL_3, but in no instance in HDL_2.

CHARACTERIZATION AND QUANTITATION OF THE ABNORMAL LIPOPROTEIN OCCURRING IN CHOLESTASIS

Walter Petek, Gerhard Kostner, and Anton Holasek
Institute of Medical Biochemistry, University of Graz, Graz/Austria

The abnormal serum lipoprotein (Lp-X) appearing in patients with cholestasis was investigated. Lp-X was isolated by a combined procedure employing preparative ultracentrifugation, column chromatography; and immunoadsorption. The resulting Lp-X preparation reacted only with antibodies to Lp-C and Lp-X. The apoproteins of Lp-X reacted with antibodies to Lp-A, Lp-C, and albumin. The apoproteins obtained from these patients reacted with antiserum against either IgA or IgG or both. When the individual apoproteins, immunoglobulins, and albumin of the Lp-X was quantitated by radial immunodiffusion and densitometric scanning of poly-acrylamide gels, it was shown that more than 50% of the protein was present as apoCI. The content of albumin varied from 5 to 15%. The remaining proteins were shown to consist of other apoC and apoA peptides as well as immunoglobulins. Lp-B or apoB could not be demonstrated in Lp-X.

PROPERTIES OF ABNORMAL SERUM LIPOPROTEINS IN CHOLESTASIS

J. Picard, D. Veissière, and F. Bertrand
Laboratoire de Biochimie, Faculté de Médecine Saint-Antoine, Paris/France

Abnormal lipoproteins were detected in serum from patients with cholestasis by immunoelectrophoretic procedure using a specific immunoserum. They were isolated by gel filtration on a Biogel column. These abnormal lipoproteins contained about 60% of phospholipids and 2% of proteins. Several antigenic determinants appeared after delipidation. One protein component was identified as the serum albumin which represents less than 15% of protein moiety. Two antigenic determinants were found in the non-albumin apolipoprotein and identified as apolipopeptides A and C. The fatty acid composition of phospholipids was also different in the cholestasis abnormal lipoproteins and in the normal serum lipoproteins. In experimental cholestasis abnormal lipoproteins were also observed. They have the same properties as in human cholestasis.
In hepatitis with cholestasis abnormal serum lipoproteins were also detected. The composition of abnormal serum lipoproteins in hepatitis with cholestasis was not found in the same proportion. These results suggest the abnormal lipoproteins plurality.

QUANTITATIVE ASPECTS OF PLASMA FREE FATTY ACID CHANGES FOLLOWING IV HEPARIN

E.J. Pinter, and C.J. Pattee
Subdepartment of Endocrinology and Metabolism, Reddy Memorial Hospital, Montreal/Canada

Heparin induces elevation of plasma free fatty acids (FFA); this was implicated in the production of arrhythmias and intracellular deposition of fat. Five volunteers were given 50 USP units/kg of heparin iv. FFA production, utilization and pool sizes were determined with the method of successive measured injections of albumin bound ^{3}H palmitic acid, twice before and at two, 20 and 30 minutes following the iv heparin up to 60 minutes. Preheparin kinetic data were: FFA production: 835 ± 70 µEq/min; FFA utilization: 830 ± 94 µEq/min; pool size: 3089 ± 256 uEq. At three minutes post heparin FFA production and pool reached a peak: 1623 ± 150 µEq/min and 6024 ± 540 µEq respectively; utilization rates also increased: 1369 ± 124 µEq/min (due to mass action effect). By the twentieth minute following heparin FFA pool was still 5460 ± 490 µEq.. Utilization rates however exceeded production at this time. It is concluded that iv heparin is followed by a rapid and short lived addition of FFA to the circulating pool amounting to 2935 µEq net gain at peak, based on a 788 µEq/min addition to the prevailing FFA production rate. FFA increments are considerable and are comparable to those seen with potent adipokinetic hormones. These changes are non physiological with regard to energy needs and may be harmful; they are of short duration, however.

L-DOPA AND FAT MOBILIZATION

E.J. Pinter, and G. Tolis
Subdepartment of Endocrinology and Metabolism, Reddy Memorial Hospital, Montreal/ Canada

15 volunteers of both sexes (eight lean and seven grossly obese) were given a single 500 mg oral dose of L-DOPA and blood specimens were obtained at -30 minutes, 0, 1, 1.2, 1.4, 2, 2.5, 3, 3.4, 4, 5 and 6 hours after administration for determinations of plasma free fatty acids (FFA) by the Trout method, growth hormone (GH) by radioimmunoassay, cortisol (C) and glucose. Results and conclusions: There was a marked increase of FFA reaching a peak at 3.4 hours (480±90 → 970±150 µEq/L) with high levels persisting at 6 hours. Four out of seven grossly obese showed no increase of FFA. GH reaches a peak at two hours (1.5±1 ng/ml →12.2±4.5 ng/ml). There was no increase of GH in four of seven obese, the same subjects who had exhibited no FFA rise. C levels showed undisturbed diurnal decline. Blood glucose remained stable. L-DOPA is a potent adipokinetic agent; the mechanism of action is most likely dependent on GH rise, as shown by the FFA vs GH changes in the obese. Consequences of stimulated adipokinesis (thrombogeneicity, hyperlipidemia, impaired carbohydrate tolerance) may be considered in chronic use of L-DOPA.

PLETHYSMOGRAM PATTERNS IN OBLITERANT ATHEROSCLEROSIS OF THE LOWER LIMBS

Pavel Pites, Alexandra Iancu, and George Uza
Institute of Public Health and Medical Research, Cluj/Roumania

The possibility of a distal detection of the arterial obstructions of the lower limbs by means of vasculogram pattern analyses was studied. The investigations were based on the study of the digital plethysmogram in 200 patients with atherosclerotic chronic obliterant arteriopathy in different evolutive stages. The correlation of the obtained data with other laboratory data permitted to delineate certain plethysmogram patterns occurring in arteriopathic patients, different from those obtained in controls: a rounded, flattened, "saw teeth" aspect with only slight oscillations. The data of our investigations furnish important aid in the diagnostic and therapeutical survey of chronic obliterant arteriopathy, as an improved digital plethysmogram pattern always reflects an improved clinical state.

PARIETAL ELASTASE: ROLE OF INHIBITORS WHEN ASSESSING ITS ACTIVITY

Michel Rabaud, Jacky Larrue, René Crockett, Modeste Dallocchio, and Henri Bricaud
Unité de Recherches de Cardiologie U8-I.N.S.E.R.M., Hôpital du Tondu, Bordeaux/
France

The role of elastase in the arterial wall biology was studied in rabbits using
isotopic and immunologic technics. The existence of a parietal elastase is probable; nevertheless it is difficult to demonstrate its specific activity because
of existing tissular inhibitor, homologous to serum glycoproteins. The injection
of elastase in large dose to rabbits induces, during the following minutes, a
breaking down of the serum inhibitor which comes back to subnormal values two
hours after. On the other hand repeated injection of small doses of elastase
induces a significant augmentation of the inhibitor correlated with rising titers
of circulating antibodies against the injected elastase. The administration of
cholesterol, simultaneously or not, while using the same doses of elastase, inter-
fers significantly with the inhibitor. These alterations of the inhibiting activities facilate the catabolic properties of the enzyme.

Our results stress some new aspects of elastase in its role in arterial wall
pathology.

DIETARY MANAGEMENT OF HYPERLIPOPROTEINEMIA TYPE I

Anna D. Rakow, Ulrich Klör, Doris Leupold, and Hans Ditschuneit
Zentrum für Innere Medizin und Kinderheilkunde, Universität Ulm, Ulm/BRD

A two years follow-up of two brothers age three and six years with type I under
different diets showed that a reduction of triglyceride (TG) values below 1000mg%
could not be achieved under outpatient conditions. Under a diet with normal fat
content the lipoprotein pattern showed a predominance of chylomicra (TG 3000-
8000 mg%). A low-fat-high-carbohydrate (CHO) diet caused a drop of TG to between
1000 and 1500 mg% and a significant decrease of chylomicra, but there was a dramatic increase of VLDL. A relatively good proportion of chylomicra and VLDL was
obtained with a diet consisting of 27% fat, 27% CHO and 36% protein. One third of
the fat was given as medium chain (MCT) and two thirds as long chain (LCT) triglyceride. Since the analysis of the fatty acid pattern in plasma and adipose
tissue had shown that the proportion of linoleic acid was only about half normal,
5 g of saturated fat were replaced by safflower oil. The administration of a protein rich bread allowed a suitable diet in spite of the high protein content.

A long time follow-up will show whether it is more reasonable 1. to lower the
chylomicra by reducing the LCT intake or 2. to lower the VLDL level by restriction of dietary CHO.

STUDIES ON THE PRECIPITATION OF LIPOPROTEIN BY HEPARIN

Agaram Subba Rao
Postgraduate and Research Institute, Bowring and Lady Curzon Hospitals, Bangalore/
India

Heparin can precipitate serum lipoprotein fraction in presence of calcium ions,
in vitro. To find out whether endogenous heparin from Mast cells, present in the
walls of blood vessels and capillaries, can act similarly in vivo, conditions for
such precipitation have been studied. Extent of precipitation was followed by
optical density of the resultant solution. Heparin could precipitate the lipoprotein at 60 IU per 100 ml. The amount of precipitate was not proportional to
calcium concentration and the curve of optical density versus calcium concentra-

tion was of S-Type. The precipitation started at 6.3 mEq/l and considerable precipitation occurred at 9 to 10 mEq/l. Calcium requirement to get a given optical density was reduced in general, in the test serum of high lipoprotein content. It was also reduced by 1 mgEq/l when pH was reduced by 0.2 units. The results indicate the possibility of endogenous heparin being implicated in the precipitation of plasma lipoprotein, - in which form cholesterol and phospholipids are transported, - and therefore in atheromatous plaque formation.

SERUM LIPOPROTEIN AND LIPOPROTEIN-CHOLESTEROL RATIO AS ATHEROGENIC INDEX

Chitradurga Ramachandra Rao and Agaram Subba Rao
Post-Graduate and Research Institute, Bowring and Lady Curzon Hospitals,
Bangalore/India

A low density serum lipoprotein fraction has been estimated using heparin as precipitant in presence of calcium cholride (0.025 M), in 49 normals and 46 subjects suffering from I.H.D. The lipoprotein fraction is found to be significantly increased in subjects with I.H.D. compared to the normals (P <0.05). Similar increase is found in the ratio of this lipoprotein fraction to total cholesterol, and the increase is highly significant (P <0.01). However cholesterol to phospholipid in the subjects with I.H.D. is not significant (P >0.05). These studies indicate that the levels of lipoprotein fractions as estimated by precipitation with heparin and the ratio of this lipoprotein fraction to total cholesterol can be used as useful atherogenic indices.

MANIFESTATIONS OF VASCULAR CHANGES IN DIABETES MELLITUS

W. Redisch, E.N. Terry, L.R. Rouen, and R. Camerini-Davalos
New York Medical College, New York, NY/USA

The high incidence of occlusive arterial disease in diabetics has been established. The purpose of this study was to relate microangiopathy to the prevalence of atherosclerosis. 825 active patients of a metropolitan diabetes clinic were screened and evaluated for manifestations of micro- and macroangiopathy; plethysmography, capillary microscopy and angiography were used selectively; skin and muscle biopsies were obtained at different stages of diabetes. Incidence of occlusive arterial disease was 41.2%. Microangiopathy was present in 60.3%, only 44.9% of whom has macro-angiopathy as well. In vivo- and biopsy microscopy showed features specific for diabetic microangiopathy. This microangiopathy may be a major factor in the high incidence of atherosclerosis in diabetes.

EFFECTS OF BASIC ALUMINUM CLOFIBRATE ON IIa AND IIb HYPERLIPOPROTEINEMIA

Suzanne Ripoll, Willy Page, Francine Vanderveiken, Marcel Vastesaeger, and Marc Ricoeur
Centre d'Etudes pour l'Industrie Pharmaceutique, Toulouse/France

Thirty-two hyperlipidemic patients (typed as IIa and IIb) have been treated with aluminum clofibrate, in order to evaluate the long-term effect of clofibrate (51 weeks) and to detect possible drawbacks of a four weeks discontinuation of therapy.

Sixteen biological tests, especially lipids, hemostasis and serum enzymes were performed eight times during the trial.

Results confirm the efficiency of clofibrate on lipid fractions and, in addition, show:

- a slight decrease in blood sugar,
- a marked and significant decrease in fibrinogen,
- no effect on platelet count and normotest,
- no effect on serum enzymes,
- a decrease in pre-beta and beta-cholesterol as expected, but an absolute increase in alpha cholesterol. A possible mode of action of clofibrate is discussed in the light of these findings: clofibrate would favour the catabolism of pre-beta and beta-lipoproteins into alpha-lipoproteins,
- a rebound of every biological parameter occurred on discontinuation of treatment. This shows that long-term and uninterrupted therapy is imperative.

BIDIMENSIONAL IMMUNOELECTROPHORESIS OF HUMAN SERUM LOW AND VERY LOW DENSITY LIPOPROTEINS PARTIALLY DELIPIDATED

S. Salmon. G. Lastra, I. Beucler, M. Ayrault-Jarrier, and J. Polonovski
Laboratoire de Biochimie, C.H.U. Saint-Antoine, Paris/France

This method has the advantage to dissociate and to reveal the lipoprotein's different proteinic chains.

First electrophoresis is performed in 1% agarose in veronal buffer. A second one is then carried perpendicularly in agarose containing antiserum, in the same buffer.

By this method very low density lipoproteins (VLDL) Sf 20-400 partially delipidated with ether, show several precipitin curves using anti VLDL antisera. This same fraction gives immunological specific curves of low density lipoproteins (LDL) with anti LDL antisera, and of high density lipoproteins (HDL) with anti HDL antisera. The other curves are specific of the VLDL. Precipitin curves obtained with LDL Sf 0-12, partially delipidated with ether against anti LDL antisera are not all revealed when we use anti VLDL sera.

This method gives specific means to follow different lipoprotein proteinic chains during their dissociation or their degradation.

PROPHYLAXIS OF THROMBOSIS BY INHIBITORS OF PLATELET AGGREGATION (EXPERIMENTAL AND CLINICAL FINDINGS)

Inge Scharrer and Klaus Breddin
Department of Angiology, Center of Internal Medicine, University of Frankfurt, Frankfurt/BRD

The mechanism by which aggregation inhibitors act is not yet clearly understood. Our own investigations of the effect of acetylsalicylic acid make it likely that its long lasting effect is caused by the acetylation of plasma proteins of large molecular weight with long half life. Acetylsalicylic acid, sulfipyrazone and some pyrimidopyrimidine compounds and combinations of these drugs with each other or with anticoagulants have been tested in clinical trials. Our own trials and the studies published so far have made likely an antithrombotic effect in the arterial and to a lesser degree in the venous system.

RELATIONSHIP BETWEEN SERUM LIPOPROTEINS AND LIVER ENDOPLASMIC RETICULUM (E.R.)

Ole Arne Schjeide
Department of Biology, Northern Illinois University, De Kalb, IL/USA

Comparison was made of the composition of total lipids and fatty acids (F.A.s) of serum lipoproteins in the chicken during growth and maturation of the liver E.R. as it takes place during embryogenesis and in the adult bird in response to estrogen treatment. Activity of acyl: Co A ligase (EC 6.2.1.3.) for saturated F.A.s was relatively high during initial phase of E.R. proliferation whereas F.A. activation of the liver E.R. with respect to unsaturated F.A.s increased as its growth rate slowed. Correlated with this enzymatic pattern was an increase in the ratio of unsaturated F.A.s to saturated F.A.s in the total serum lipid. An increase in serum triglyceride associated with VLDL was also noted upon completion of stimulation of E.R. in the adult bird. Synthesis and secretion of individual VLDL complexes, as measured by uptake of lysine - ^{14}C, occurred within 10 minutes. Since its apparent rate of synthesis was very similar to that of other serum proteins, the magnitude of synthesis appears to be related to numbers of synthetic sites on the E.R.

APOLIPOPROTEINS IN THE GENETICALLY OBESE HYPERLIPOPROTEINEMIC ZUCKER FATTY RAT

Gustav Schonfeld
Cynthia Felski, Lipid Research Center, Washington University, St. Louis, MI/USA

Hyperlipoproteinemia (HL) in the fatty rat (Fa) may serve as a model of some human HL. To understand pathophysiology, we measured the levels and characterized the compositions of lipoproteins (Lp) of Fa. Lp isolated from male rats by ultracentrifugation (VLDL d<1.006, LDL 1.006-1.063, HDL 1.063-1.21), were analyzed for triglycerides (TG), cholesterol (chol), phospholipids (PL) and protein. Apolipoproteins (ApoLp) were quantified by polyacrylamide elctrophoresis and gel filtration. Body weights of Fa were 160% of controls (C). Total TG were 1111 & 105, chol 189 & 78, PL 388 & 160 (n=12, p<0.01). VLDL, LDL and HDL (TG+chol+PL+ protein) of Fa and C were 623 & 87, 105 & 62 and 468 & 241 mg/dl, respectively (n=4, p<0.02). VLDL of Fa had more TG (78 vs 60%), less protein (6 vs 16%), and 3 times normal amounts of fast migrating no.5 and 6 peptides (Koga et al) than C. No.5 and 6 peptides in LDL and HDL were 140 & 170% of C. Slow bands 2 and 3 were decreased in all Lp of Fa.

Conclusions: a) In Fa all Lp are elevated, especially the VLDL, which are enriched in TG. b) Lp of Fa contain more no.5 and less no.3 peptides than C. c) Whether the altered compositions reflect abnormal synthesis or catabolism is under study.

THROMBOSIS AND ATHEROSCLEROSIS: EVOLUTION OF LIPID PROFILES DURING ORGANIZATION OF PULMONARY THROMBOEMBOLI

Colin J. Schwartz, Jan H. Craig, and Frank P. Bell
Department of Pathology, McMaster University, Hamilton/Canada

The ultra-structure and lipid composition of organizing artificial autologous pulmonary thrombo-emboli were studied in the pig. No net lipid accumulation was observed, although thrombi had, at 4 weeks, transformed into fibrofatty plaques in which smooth muscle cells were prominent. Unesterified cholesterol and phospholipids together accounted for more than 85% of the total lipid; esterified cholesterol, triglycerides and free fatty acids each comprised less than 5% of total lipid at all time periods. During organization, esterified cholesterol content showed a slight increase. Sphingomyelin and lecithin, the predominant phospholipids, showed no increase during organization. Aortic plaques, however, contained greater amounts of esterified cholesterol and sphingomyelin; additionally, the fatty acid profiles of esterified cholsterol, sphingomyelin, and lecithin from aortic lesions and organizing thrombi differed. This study has shown that the lipid profile of organizing thrombi does not evolve towards that characteristic of the atheromatous plaque, and suggests that plaque lipids are largely derived from a source other than thrombi.

HYPERLIPIDEMIA AND LIPID RETENTION IN RABBIT FEMORAL HEAD

Theodore Nicholas Siller
Donner Building McGill University, Montreal/Canada

The role of hyperlipidemis in alcoholic osteonecrosis is not yet clear. Groups of 20% alcohol, 1% cholesterol, and a diet with both, were compared with controls. Serum triglyceride, free fatty acid, and cholesterol levels at start and at sacrifice up to 3 months, were done. A gravimetric method for total bone fat was used. Cholesterol gave high levels of all fractions but low bone fat. Alcohol showed high triglyceride and the highest bone fat. Together, high serum values, similar to cholesterol alone, were seen but with more bone fat. Cholesterol induces hyperlipidemia, but alcohol reflects mainly triglyceride elevation. This latter Type IV hyperlipidemia gives increased deposition and retention of fat in bone. Gross fat embolism, often cited in alcoholic osteonecrosis, need not be evoked for increased lipid retention in bone.

ATHEROMATOUS EMBOLI-INDUCED NECROSIS IN RABBIT FEMORAL HEADS

Theodore Nicholas Siller
Donner Building, McGill University, Montreal/Canada

Simulation of human embolization of atheromatous debris from the abdominal aorta was done to determine if this is a cause of a vascular necrosis. Human material or plain cholesterol crystals were infused into the femoral artery by peristaltic pump with the opposite hip as a control. Radioactive cholesterol was used in some cases to tag debris and undecalcified autoradiographic bone sections produced. Labelled material persisted up to 6 months. Various degrees of bone death occurred and by 10 months massive necrosis was seen with a mosaic pattern, without collapse or cystic changes. The mechanism may be due to low grade sclerosis by cholesterol or esters but not by vascular occlusion.

POTENTIATING OF LIPID LOWERING ACTIVITY OF CLOFIBRATE BY COMBINING WITH VERY LOW DOSES OF 3-PYRIDIL-CARBINOL IN RATS

Zdenek Simane and Herbert Nowak
Medical Research (E. Merck), Darmstadt/BRD

Some combinations of lipid lowering agents act synergistical so that a satisfactory therapeutic response can be obtained with lower doses, thus eliminating the undesirable side effects. To find out the optimal dosage and relation between the components of such a combination, the present study on the effects of clofibrate and 3-pyridylcarbinol (PC) in normo- and hyperlipemic rats was done. In general, the combination of both drugs appears to be more effective in decreasing the serum levels of cholesterol, triglycerides and phospholipids than the single components. The hypolipemic activity of clofibrate can be enhanced by such low doses of PC which alone are not able to decrease cholesterol or triglycerides. The optimal relation of clofibrate to PC found was 20:1. With increasing the dosis of the PC component no further improvement of the lipid lowering activity of the mixture was reached.

FIBRINOLYTIC ACTIVITY OF THE ARTERIAL WALL AND ATHEROSCLEROTIC DISEASE, HISTO-CHEMICAL AND HEMATIC DISTRICTUAL INVESTIGATIONS

Marcello Tesi and Luciano Caramelli
Department of Angiology, Main Regional Hospital of S.Maria Nuova, Florence/Italy

The present investigation concerns the evaluation of the fibrinolytic activity of the arterial wall during atherosclerotic disease. It was carried out in atherosclerotic patients with obliterations at different levels of the arterial route, and in control subjects of the same age.

1. Histochemical investigations. Different sections of arterial wall (aorta, iliac, femoral popliteal and tibial arteries) were studied. The tissue plasminogen activator was evaluated by the method of Todd, that consents to observe the distribution of this enzyme in the different tunica of the arterial wall.

2. Hematic investigations. In the lower limb district, the acetylcholine fibrinolytic test was carried out by the method of Tesi and Caramelli, that consents to evaluate the fibrinolytic potentials of the different districts examined.

The test for the lower limb district is carried out as follows:
a) The basal fibrinolytic activity is determined. That is, we determine the arterial and venous femoral lysis.
b) The districtual lysis is activated. 30 mg of acetylcholine are then injected into the femoral artery.
c) The fibrinolytic activity is evaluated in dynamic conditions. Then we determine the arterial and venous femoral lysis, 5 minutes following the stimulation (intra-arterial injection of acetylcholine).

The results achieved in basal conditions, did not prove differences between the two groups examined. The results achieved in dynamic conditions revealed in the control subjects a higher fibrinolytic activity than that presented by the atherosclerotic patients.

ASSESSMENT OF AGING - A NEW RISK FACTOR FOR MYOCARDIAL INFARCTION

Gösta Tibblin
Medical Department I, Sahlgren's Hospital, Göteborg/Sweden

Purpose of the study is to show that assessment of aging is of value in the study of the development of CHD. Data are from 1. 40 male myocardial infarction patients aged 48-50 and 50 controls from population samples of the same age and sex. 2. a cross-sectional study of 1100 men aged 50 and 60 years. The myocardial infarction patients differ significantly in reaction time, vibration sense, skin wrinkles, memory, hearing, accommodation and sinus arrhythmia. In this age-homogenous group the MI-patients are biological older compared to controls. In the cross-sectional study subjects of the same age with hypercholesterolemia, hypertriglyceridemia, hypertension and smoking also were more biological to the development of MI and can mirror a mechanism which can be responsible both for the development of the disease and the risk factors. Support for this hypothesis is the findings that in the prospective population study of 973 men born in 1913, the risk factors cholesterol, blood pressure, triglycerides not only were related to death in CVD but also to non-cardiovascular deaths.

CLINICAL RESEARCH ON THE ANTI-SCLEROTIC AND ANTI-THROMBOTIC ACTION OF GLUCURONIL-GLUCOSAMIN-GLICANE

Rinaldo Turpini
Institute of Clinical Medicine, University of Pavia, Pavia/Italy

A clinical research has been carried out on the anti-sclerotic and anti-throm-botic action of an extractive heparinoid having a high clarifying and anti-dis-lipidic power, namely Glucuronil-glucosamin-glicane sulphate. Its action on blood vessels and on hematochemical characters has been studied by means of an analysis of four groups of parameters. The patients, of an age between 55 and 80, were kept under control for 10 days and then treated with 18 mg/day of active substance for 50 days. All the parameters used have been determined at the beginning of the ob-servation period, after 10 days and after 50 days. The results show a clear im-provement, achieved through: a) a reduction of aphasia phenomena, motor-nerves troubles, weakness, dizziness; b) reduction of cholesterol, triglycerid and beta-lipoproteins in the serum; c) activation of the plasminogen and reduction of the platelet's aggregation; d) reduction of the sludge endovascular phenomenon and increase of the number of open capillary vessels. The reduction of vascular insufficiency is statistically significant.

TRANSPORT OF CHOLESTEROL AND TRIGLYCERIDE IN LYMPH CHYLOMICRONS AND VLDL

George Vahouny, M.Blenderman, and C.R. Treadwell
George Washington Medical Center, Washington/USA

The relative roles of chylomicrons and VLDL in lymphatic transport of absorbed cholesterol esters and triglycerides was studied in rats of both sexes. Lymph was collected in two hour periods from normal and puromycin-treated rats which re-ceived an intraduodenal infusion of oleic acid-1-^{14}C and cholesterol-7α-^{3}H fol-lowed two hours later with leucine-1-^{14}C. Following lipoprotein separation and extraction, the patterns of lipid and protein labelling were determined. The fol-lowing results were obtained:

1. About 10% of the ^{14}C-triglyceride in lymph was in VLDL, and while the chylo-micron labelling decreased with time, that in VLDL remained constant. In con-trast, cholesterol in chylomicrons and VLDL increased with time, with about 10% of the absorbed cholesterol in the VLDL.

2. The role of VLDL transport of cholesterol was of greater significance in fe-male rats.

3. 60% of leucine incorporation into lipoprotein was in the VLDL fraction in the first 2 hours. The protein labelling in VLDL, chylomicrons and LDL diminished at later times, while that in HDL and residual protein increased.

4. Puromycin inhibition of lipid transport was only on lymph VLDL of female rats, while its effect on protein synthesis was evident in all protein fractions.

MITOCHONDRIAL DNA EXTRACTED FROM THE ATHEROSCLEROTIC RABBIT AORTIC WALL

Dimitri Vekhoff, Michel Claire, and Bernard Jacotot
Unité de Recherches sur l'Athérosclérose de l'INSERM, Hôpital Henri-Mondor, Créteil/France

In any type of tissue, the mitochondria may show changes in their structure and enzymatic properties in response to alterations in physiological conditions.

The mitochondria have been shown to be the cellular site where most of the fatty acids synthesis take place in rabbit aorta.

In fact, the question regarding atherosclerosis is to know how lipogenesis is regulated within vascular tissues.

The contents of nucleic acids in aortic mitochondria and the structural aspects of DNA's isolated by the modified method of Borst are comparatively investigated.

According to the obtained data, we may conclude that enzymatic regulation probably cannot be accomplished without the participation of the mitochondrial gene.

EVOLUTIONS OF ATHEROGENICITY IN MEN AND WOMEN WITH AGE AND COMPARISON WITH HYPERLIPAEMIA

G. Verdonk
Department of Internal Medicine, State University of Ghent, Ghent/Belgium

In connection with the known difference in men and women with respect to atherosclerotic complications, a systematic study is made concerning the evolution of atherogenicity as a function of age.

It is concluded from this study that:

- in cases of atherosclerosis, complicated with diabetes or obesity, a more pronounced unfavourable evolution with age in women as in men, is stated.
- in cases of infarction, the atherogenicity in men and women seems to be independent of the age in which the infarction occurs. The atherogenicity in female patients seems more injurious in all age-groups.
- patients with hyperlipaemia, presenting atherosclerotic lesions can be classified, in general, as type II and III. In type II we state, besides a generally increased atherogenicity in comparison with pure or complicated atherosclerosis that the main deviation occurs at the level of cholesterol, while the triglycerides turn out less unfavourable. In type III the deviation occurs principly at the level of the pre-beta lipids and the total cholesterol and to a lesser extent at the level of the triglycerides.

EFFECTS OF LIPOSTABIL THERAPY ON PLASMA CHOLESTEROL, LIPIDS, AND FIBRINOGEN AND ON PLATELETS ADHESIVENESS

Roman Vlaicu, Ioan Crîsnic, and Caius Zamora
First Medical Clinic, Cluj/Roumania

A modification of the plasma cholesterol, lipids, and fibrinogen and of the platelets adhesiveness in atherosclerotic patients has been noticed already. 21 atherosclerotic patients were treated with Lipostabil for a period of 75 days. Before and after the treatment the above mentioned parameters were measured.
A significant decrease of the plasma lipids ($p < 0.01$) and of the platelets adhesiveness ($p < 0.02$), a decrease of the cholesterol level ($p < 0.05$), and a non significant modification of the plasma fibrinogen ($p < 0.2$). It was concluded that Lipostabil may influence some atherogenetic factors.

17-BETA-ESTRADIOL AND TESTOSTERONE SERUM LEVELS IN PATIENTS WITH MYOCARDIAL INFARCTION AND PERIPHERAL ARTERIAL DISEASE

Hermann Wagner, Karsten Böckel, Norbert Wenning, and Werner H. Hauss
Medical Clinic and Policlinic, Westf. Wilhelms University, Münster, Münster/BRD

The effect of estrogens and androgens on the lipid and vessel wall metabolism in case of atherosclerosis has often been reported. On the other hand little is known on the secretion of androgens and estrogens in patients with atherosclerotic disease. Therefore 17-beta-estradiol and testosterone serum levels before and after stimulation with human chorionic gonadotropin (HGG) were measured in same aged, healthy patients (n=29), and in patients with myocardial infarction (n=22) as well as with peripheral arterial disease (n=39). The hormones were determined by radioimmunological methods. The investigations have shown that the serum levels of testosterone of the healthy control group in comparison with those of patients with myocardial infarction and peripheral arterial disease were significantly lower, whereas the serum levels of 17-beta-estradiol were significantly higher in the atherosclerotic group. The results will be discussed.

XANTINOL NICOTINATE THERAPY IN EXPERIMENTAL PULMONARY FIBRIN EMBOLISM

P.L.Wahi, K.D. Boruah, and R.N. Chakravarti

Departments of Internal Medicine and Experimental Medicine, Post-graduate Institute of Medical Education and Research, Chandigarh/India

The therapeutic effect of xantinol nicotinate (XN) has been evaluated in rabbits subjected to pulmonary fibrin embolism since this drug has been claimed to be a powerful fibrinolytic agent. Two groups of 18 rabbits each were administered intravenously a standard dose of autologous fibrin clots. While animals in the control group received isotonic saline, those in the experimental group received (XN) intravenously (100 mg/Kg) immediately after fibrin administration and thereafter daily. Animals were sacrificed ater 2 hrs, 6 hrs and 7 days following embolisation. Histopathological studies on lungs were carried out using various stains including special fibrin stains. Pulmonary embolic index was determined. (XN) improved the general condition of the animals, reduced mortality and significantly lowered the pulmonary embolic index at each time interval studied.

EARLY PROLIFERATION OF MEDIA MUSCLE CELLS OF THE AORTA AFTER ATHEROGENIC DIETS OF DIFFERENT COMPOSITION

Kurt Wegener, Konrad Heilmann, Walter Hofmann, and Wilhelm-Wolfgang Höpker
Institute of Pathology, University of Heidelberg, Heidelberg/BRD

Do different atherogenic diets influence the proliferation of media muscle cells? 4 groups (A, B, C, D) of 26 rats each were fed an atherogenic diet of different composition for 13 days. A: Cholesterol + BAPN (beta-amino-proprio-nitril); B: Cholesterol; C: BAPN; D: normal food. 2 animals of every group were sacrificed every day 1 hour after injection of 100 μCi H-3-thymidine. Paraffine-sections and autoradiogramms. A: Proliferation begins 7-8 days after feeding and shows an constant ascent to the 13th day. B: The same as in group A. C: Proliferation begins at the 8th day after feeding but at a lower rate as in A and B. The ascent is much lower. D: No proliferation. In all groups histologically remarkable changes of the vessel wall are absent.

Media muscle cells take part in early reactions of the vessel wall after atherogenic diet. Cellular changes begin earlier than histological changes of the vessel wall. Cholesterol is an important factor in starting cell proliferation.

PROTEIN BINDING AND MOVEMENT OF STEROIDS: SIGNIFICANCE OF ALBUMIN

Ulrich Westphal
Department of Biochemistry, University of Louisville School of Medicine, Louisville, KY/USA

It is suggested that the steroid-binding serum proteins have an important function
in facilitating permeation of the steroid hormones from the site of synthesis
through the capillary walls into the blood stream. The process is comparable to
a dialysis through a semipermeable membrane. The rate of dialysis of cortisterone
through such membrane was found to increase substantially when serum albumin or
other steroid-binding proteins were added to the outside buffer solution.

A second function of serum albumin is seen in accelerating the dissociation of
high-affinity complexes of steroids with proteins such as corticosteroid-binding
globulin (CBG). Human serum has approximately 1000 times more albumin than CBG
molecules. About half of the dissociation energy is saved, and the dissociation
rate increased, if albumin interacts with CBG, and albumin instead of the buffer
accepts the steroid. As evidence, the presence of serum albumin has been found
to greatly accelerate the dissociation of steroids from CBG.

GLUCOSE TOLERANCE, INSULIN RESPONSE AND LIPID ABNORMALITIES IN THE AGED INDIVIDUAL

Asher Woldow, Bernard Shapiro, Jacob J. Cohen, and George Kollmann
Philadelphia Geriatric Center and Department of Nuclear Medicine, Albert Einstein
Medical Center, Philadelphia, PA/USA

The significance of glucose tolerance and insulin response to blood lipid levels
in the aged population and eventual relationship to coronary artery disease is
yet to be defined. In a group of 97 elderly patients (average age 82) the relationship of the above parameters was studied. Two hour glucose tolerance curves
were drawn and the insulin response on each blood sample was determined. The
curves of each were plotted on graph paper and the area under the curves was
determined as the glucose to insulin (G/I) ratio. These results were compared to
cholesterol and triglycerid levels as well as lipid typing. There was a poor linear correlation of glucose tolerance to lipid abnormalities when compared alone.
Insulin response did show a relative correlation to lipid abnormalities particularly with triglyceride levels. However, we noted that when the glucose-insulin
or G/I ratio was considered and compared to lipid levels the best correlation
was found. High G/I ratios showed only 20% lipid elevations and with low G/I
ratios there was a 55% correlation with lipid abnormalities. The results suggest
the significance of abnormal metabolism in the aged population.

CELL DAMAGE CAUSED BY XANTHINE OXIDASE TREATED BY FOLIC ACID

Kurt A. Oster
Park City Hospital, Bridgeport, CT/USA

A mechanism for the initiation of myocardial cell damage has been established by
the demonstration of plasmalogen depletion in the cell membrane through ectopic
xanthine oxidase. Xanthine oxidase has been found in pathological heart tissue
but not in the normal myocardium. The damage to the cell would be one of disturbance of the normal equilibrium of the phospholipid composition of the cell
membrane by enhancing the sphingomyelin content of the membrane and diminishing
the plasmalogen component. This change in the cell membrane will influence the
active transport of ions, creating problems of arrhythmia by a disarray of sodium
and potassium. A new therpeutic approach for the prevention of the proliferation
of the continuing cell damage created by ectopic xanthine oxidase was found in
the xanthine oxidase-inhibiting properties of large doses of folic acid, which
has been used for this purpose for the first time. Forty patients with severe

atherosclerotic changes have been treated successfully with folic acid doses, between 40-80 mg, for the last three years. Folic acid had no toxic effect in large doses and may become, one day, the "penicillin equivalent" for the treatment of amenable atherosclerotic clinical manifestations.

SYNTHESIS OF LOW DENSITY (LDL) AND VERY LOW DENSITY LIPOPROTEINS (VLDL) AND APOLIPOPROTEINS BY HUMAN ARTERIES

William Hollander and John Paddock
B.U. Medical Center, Boston, MA/USA

The capacity of human arteries to synthesize LDL, VLDL and their apolipoproteins was studied by incubating arterial tissue removed at surgery or autopsy with ^{3}H-leucine or ^{3}H-leucine and ^{14}C-acetate. Following incubation for 4 hours, the lipoproteins were extracted from the intima with saline and separated by differential density ultracentrifugation. Arterial LDL and VLDL were identified chemically, immunochemically and by gel filtration and analytical ultracentrifugation. Following delipidation and solubilization of arterial LDL and VLDL in sodium dodecyl sulfate the apoproteins were isolated by gel filtration, acrylamide electrophoresis and identified by amino acid composition, sedimentation coefficient and immunochemical reactivity to antisera to apoLDL, apoHDL and apoVLDL including alanine apoVLDL (D-3). Radiochemical analyses of the isolated arterial lipoproteins revealed incorporation of ^{3}H-leucine and ^{14}C-acetate into both the protein and lipid moieties of LDL and VLDL. The incorporation of ^{3}H-leucine into the apoproteins of LDL and VLDL was demonstrated by the precipitation of ^{3}H-apoproteins by specific antisera and by the isolation of ^{3}H-leucine from the ^{3}H-apoproteins by split stream amino acid analysis. Conclusion: Arterial synthesis of LDL and VLDL may contribute to the deposition of these lipoproteins in diseased arteries.

REGULATION OF CHOLESTEROL SYNTHESIS. INHIBITION OF RAT HEPATIC 3-HYDROXY-3-METHYLGLUTARYL-COENZYME A REDUCTASE BY A BILE BETA-LIPOPROTEIN

Victor W. Rodwell and Donald J. McNamara
Department of Biochemistry, Purdue University, West Lafayette, IN/USA

A component of bovine bile which inhibits the acitivity of 3-hydroxy-3-methyl-glutaryl-CoA (HMG-CoA) reductase [EC 1.1.1.34], the key regulated enzyme of hepatic cholesterogenesis, has been isolated and its properties studied.

At least 2 bile components decreases conversion of acetate to mevalonate, and hence to cholesterol. Physiological levels of bile acids inhibit cholesterogenesis from acetate or from mevalonate, but don't inhibit rat liver HMG-CoA reductase or HMG-CoA synthase [EC 4.1.3.5]. HMG-CoA reductase is, however, inhibited by crude bile. The active principle, isolated from bovine bile in an essentially homogeneous state as judged by gel electrophoresis, is a high M.W. lipoprotein (p = 1.024). While its lipid composition parallels that of a serum β-lipoprotein, it appears not bo be present in bovine serum. Inactivation of HMG-CoA reductase by the purified β-lipoprotein, a function of time, of lipoprotein concentration and of microsomal protein concentration, is decreased several fold by HMG-CoA plus NADP, but not by either substrate alone. Possible roles for this lipoprotein in regulation of HMG-CoA reductase and of hepatic cholesterogenesis will be discussed.

EFFECTS OF DIETARY PROTEIN ON PLASMA CHOLESTEROL LEVELS IN RABBITS FED CHOLESTEROL-FREE SEMISYNTHETIC DIETS

Robert M.G. Hamilton and Kenneth K. Carroll
Department of Biochemistry, University of Western Ontario, London/Canada

When rabbits are transferred from a natural diet to a cholesterol-free, low fat, semisynthetic diet their plasma cholesterol levels increase from ~70 to ~200 mg/100 ml. The present studies are part of an investigation of different non-lipid components of the diet to determine the cause of this elevation. Semisynthetic diets containing isonitrogenous amounts of protein from various source were fed to groups of 5-6 male New Zealand white rabbits for 28 days. Diets containing skim milk powder, casein or lactalbumin gave average plasma cholesterols of 200 mg/100 ml or higher. With defatted fish protein, beef protein and pork protein, the plasma cholesterols averaged 190, 160 and 110 mg/100 ml respectively. When vegetable proteins such as wheat gluten, peanut protein or soybean protein were used, the levels were similar to or lower than those observed with the natural diet. Addition of 15% by weight of either butter or corn oil to the soybean diet made little difference to the plasma cholesterol level. These results indicate that the source of dietary protein is an important factor in determining the level of plasma cholesterol in this experimental model.

LIPOPROTEIN UPTAKE BY RAT AORTIC SMOOTH MUSCLE CELLS IN TISSUE CULTURE

Edwin L. Bierman, Olga Stein and Yechezkiel Stein
Department of Medicine B, Lipid Research Laboratory Hadassah University Hospital;
Department of Experimental Medicine and Cancer Research Hebrew University-Hadassah Medical School, Jerusalem/Israel

Lipoprotein (LP) metabolism was studied in pure cultures of smooth muscle cells (SMC), grown from intimal-medial segments of young adult rat aorta and compared to that in aortic fibroblasts (F) grown from adventitia. These two aortic cell types were clearly distinguishable by growth characteristics and morphology. Ultracentrifugally prepared rat plasma very low density lipoproteins (VLDL) and high denstiy lipoproteins (HDL), labeled with I^{125} in their protein moiety, were taken up linearly during 48 hours by both cell types in stationary growth phase. Incorporation was proportional to LP concentration in the medium (20-120 µg LP protein/10^6 cells) and ranged from 0.1% (VLDL by SMC) to 0.5% (HDL by F). Despite multiple washings, a large fraction of LP radioactivity associated with cells was surface bound and trypsin releasable. VLDL and HDL activity was localized intracellularly in SMC by electron microscopic radioautography. In pulse-chase studies with SMC exposed to HDL, non-protein, non-iodine radioactivity was found in the medium. These results suggest that aortic SMC can incorporate and catabolicze lipoproteins.

THE ARTERIAL SMOOTH MUSCLE CELL: INSULIN STIMULATION OF CELL PROLIFERATION

R.W. Stout, E.L. Bierman, and R. Ross
Departments of Medicine and Pathology, University of Washington, Seattle, WA/USA

Proliferation of smooth muscle cells is a charaoteristic feature of the early lesions of atherosclerosis. As plasma insulin levels are frequently elevated in patients with atherosclerosis, the effect of insulin on cell proliferation was studied, using smooth muscle cells cultured from thoracic aortae of one-year-old monkeys (Macaca nemistrina). Insulin, added to the culture medium in concentrations of 10, 100, 1000 and 10,000 µU/ml, resulted in successively greater stimulation of growth which was highly significant by analysis of variance (p <0.001). There was a significant linear relationship between the logarithm of the insulin dose and the proliferative response. Serum from which insulin had been removed stimulated growth less well (p <0.05) than whole serum at the same concentration. The effect of insulin (100 µU/ml) was partially inhibited by dibutyryl cyclic AMP at a concentration of 10^{-5}M, and completely by 5 x 10^{-5}M, suggesting that cyclic AMP may have a role in this insulin action. Thus insulin in physiological concentrations can stimulate proliferation of arterial smooth muscle cells in culture.

STRUCTURE OF NASCENT HIGH DENSITY LIPOPROTEIN (HDL)

Robert L. Hamilton, Mary C. Williams, Richard J. Havel, and Christopher J. Fielding
Cardiovascular Research Institute and Department of Anatomy, University of California, San Francisco, CA/USA

To determine the molecular structure and mechanism of formation of plasma HDL, we compared nascent HDL from two sources. HDL from rat liver Golgi apparatus have α-elctrophoretic mobility and appear as bilayer or vesicular structures by electron microscopy (EM). Plasma HDL are ~115 Å spheres by EM. HDL from perfused rat liver are similar to plasma HDL by EM and polypeptide composition but have ~40% less cholesteryl ester (CE). Inhibition (~85%) of lecithin-cholesterol acyl transferase (LCAT) in perfusate leads to nascent HDL composed mainly of polar lipids and proteins with ~85% less CE than plasma HDL. In negative stains, these nascent HDL are 46 Å by 190 Å discs which form rouleaux similar to the major HDL of LCAT-deficient patients. In thin section, HDL discs show trilaminate staining like cell membranes and lecithin bilayers. We propose that liver secretes nascent HDL as bilayer discs, the edge of which is sealed by polypeptides. LCAT converts the Beta-acyl moiety of surface lecithin and cholesterol to non-polar CE which penetrates the central hydrocarbon region of the disc. A droplet of CE forms as LCAT continues to act thereby separating the original bilayer structure of the disc to form an oily core enclosed by a phospholipid-cholesterol-protein monolayer.

STUDIES OF THE ACTIVE SITE OF AN APOLIPOPROTEIN

R.S. Shulman, L.A. Witters, and P.N. Herbert
NIH, Bethesda, MD/USA

The primary structures of three of the human apolipoproteins have been determined and the studies described were designed to identify the segment of the proteins most active in lipid binding. Using apolipoprotein C-III as a model, the susceptibility of the apoprotein to tryptic digestion after recombination with phospholipid was evaluated. The COOH-terminal half (residues 41-79) that normally yields three tryptic peptides was found resistant to tryptic cleavage when C-III was combined with phospholipid; and this peptide was isolated intact from the tryptic digest. As judged by ultracentrifugal and circular dichroic criteria, this peptide was demonstrated to recombine with phospholipid in a manner analogous to intact C-III. The three tryptic peptides normally obtained from residues 41-79 did not demonstrate this property. Moreover, this peptide (41-79) was prepared by an independent method. Taking advantage of the original residue at position 40, the lysine residues of C-III were reversibly blocked with citraconic anhydride and the molecule was enzymatically cleaved into two halves by tryptic digestion. After deacylation at acid pH, the two halves of the protein were isolated. The results described above were confirmed with peptide 41-79 so obtained.

IMPROVED EXTRACTION AND PURIFICATION OF LIPOPROTEIN LIPASE BY AFFINITY CHROMATOGRAPHY FROM PIG ADIPOSE TISSUE

Andre Bensadoun, Christian Ehnholm, Daniel Steinberg, and W. Virgil Brown
Department of Medicine, School of Medicine, University of California, San Diego,
La Jolla, CA/USA

Lipoprotein lipase was purified from acetone powders of pig adipose tissues.
Acetone powders were extracted with 1.5 M NaCl, 0.005 M Na veronal pH 7.4 buffer
which was six times more effective as a means of elution of lipoprotein lipase
than the commonly employed 0.025 M NH4OH-NH4Cl pH 8.6 buffer. Most of the purification was accomplished by affinity chromatography on Sepharose 4B columns containing covalently bound heparin. At this step, the preparation was purified
3,000- to 4,000-fold. This purified enzyme binds reversibly to columns containing
concanavalin A covalently bound to Sepharose. Lipolytic activity was eluted from
concanavalin A-Sepharose column with linear gradients of NaCl and methyl Alpha-
D-glycopyranoside. Isoelectric focusing yielded a single major peak of activity
with a pI of 4.0. The crude enzyme showed a 20-fold stimulation by serum whereas
that purified by isoelectric focusing exhibited a complete dependence on the
presence of serum activator in the medium. Of the three very low density lipoproteins studied, only apoLp-glu could substitute for serum as an activator. In
the presence of serum in the assay system, apoLp-ser was as potent an inhibitor
of lipoprotein lipase as apoLp-ala.

POLYUNSATURATED FATTY ACIDS AND ISCHAEMIC HEART DISEASE IN VENEZUELA

Virgilio Bosch, Carlos Arreaza, Cecilia Santana, and Gonzalo Peters
Universidad Central Caracas/Venezuela

It has been shown that patients with ischaemic heart disease (IHD) have lower
plasma linoleate concentration than normals. This subject is of interest in Vene-
zuela where sesame oil is extensively used as foodstuff. Fifty one IHD patients
without infarction from the University Hospital and 46 normal adults were studied.
Plasma lipids were extracted with chloroform/methanol (2:1 v/v) and resolved into
cholesterylesters (CE),triacylglycerides (TG) and phospholipids (PL) by thin
layer chromatography. Methylesters were analyzed by gas-liquid chromatography.
In IHD patients linoleic and oleic acids amounted to 45 and 24 per cent composition of fatty acids in CE as compared to 51 and 21 respectively in controls.
Linoleic acid also was decreased in PL of female patients but not in males. In
our study even patients with IHD had higher percentage of linoleate in CE than
values reported for normal persons on other countries. Differences presented are
highly statistically significant.

IN VIVO AND IN VITRO BINDING OF HYPOLIPIDEMIC DRUGS TO SERUM LIPOPROTEINS

Jean-Louis Beaumont, Christiane Dachet, Violette Beaumont and Jean-Claude Buxtorf
Unité de Recherches sur l'Athérosclérose de l'I.N.S.E.R.M. Hôspital Henri-Mondor,
Créteil/France

The previously reported binding of clofibrate and several related drugs (SU
13.437, GP 45.699, MK 185) to serum lipoproteins was studied in vivo after absorption of a therapeutic dose and in citro during dialysis experiments using C_{14}
labeled and non labeled drugs.

In vivo, although their major part is bound to albumin, an average 5% of the
drugs is bound to the low density lipoproteins, specially of the 1.019-1.063
class. The molar ratio of drug to protein is about 1 for albumin and reaches 25
or more for lipoproteins.

In vitro, alpha- and beta-lipoproteins bind the drugs. When they are used in very low concentrations, the binding is reversible and the interaction meets an equilibrium. With high concentrations, irreversible changes in the beta-lipoprotein appear when the molar ratio of drug to protein exceeds 100. The damaged beta-lipoproteins release part of their phospholipids and all their free cholesterol.

It is thought that this hitherto unknown interaction may alter the physiological function of lipoproteins and throw some new light on the mode of action of the hypolipidemic drugs.

REFERENCES

ABDULLA, Y. H., ADAMS, C. W. M.: Sulphydryl dependence of arterial lecithin: cholesterol transacylase. Atherosclerosis 12, 319 (1970).

ABDULLA, Y. H., ORTON, C. C., ADAMS, C. W. M.: Cholesterol esterification by transacylation in human and experimental atheromatous lesions. J. Atheroscler. Res. 8, 967 (1968).

ABRAHAMSEN, A. F.: Survival of ^{51}Cr-labelled human platelets. Oslo: Universitets-forlaget (1969).

ACHESON, J., DANTA, G., HUTCHINSON, E. C.: Controlled trial of dipyridamole in cerebral vascular disease. Brit. Med. J. 1, 614 - 615 (1969).

ADAMS, C. W. M.: Vascular histochemistry in relation to the chemical and structural pathology of cardiovascular disease. London: Lloyd-Luke 1967.

ADAMS, C. W. M.: Tissue changes and lipid entry in developing atheroma. In: Ciba Foundation Symposium on Mechanisms in the Development of Early Atheroma, London, 1972. Atherogenesis: Initiating factors, p. 5 - 37. (Ciba Foundation Symposium 12). Amsterdam: Associated Scientific Publishers, 1973.

ADAMS, C. W. M., ABDULLA, Y. H.: Polyunsaturated phospholipids and experimental atherosclerosis. In: Phospholipide p. 44 (SCHETTLER, G., Ed.) Stuttgart: Thieme 1972

ADAMS, C. W. M., BAYLISS, O. B., ABDULLA, Y. H., MAHLER, F. R., ROOT, M. A.: Lipase, esterase and triglyceride in the aging human aorta. A quantitative histochemical and biochemical study. J. Atheroscler. Res. 9, 87 - 102 (1969).

ADAMS, C. W. M., BAYLISS, O. B., IBRAHIM, M. Z. M.: A hypothesis to explain the accumulation of cholesterol in atherosclerosis. Lancet 1962 1, 890.

ADAMS, C. W. M., MORGAN, R. S., BAYLISS, O. B.: No regression of atheroma over one year in rabbits previously fed a cholesterol enriched diet. Atherosclerosis 18, 429 (1973).

ADAMS, G. H., SCHUMAKER, V. N.: Polydispersity of human low-density lipoproteins. Ann. N. Y. Acad. Sci. 164, 130 (1969).

ADAMS, G. H., SCHUMAKER, V. N.: Equilibrium banding of low-density lipoproteins III. Studies on normal individuals and the effects of diet and heparin-induced lipase. Biochim. Biophys. Acta 210, 462 (1970).

ADAMS, W. C., GAMAN, E. M., FEIGENBAUM, A. S.: Breed differences in the response of rabbits to atherogenic diets. Atherosclerosis 16, 405 - 411 (1972).

ADLERSBERG, D.: Hypercholesterolemia with predisposition to atherosclerosis: An inborn error of lipid metabolism. Am. J. Med. 11, 600 (1951).

ADLERSBERG, D., PARETS, A. D., BOAS, E. P.: Genetics of atherosclerosis. J. Amer. med Ass. 141, 246 (1949).

ADLERSBERG, D., SCHAEFER, L. E.: The interplay of heredity and environment in the regulation of circulating lipids and in atherogenesis. Am J. Med. 26, 1 (1959).

ADMIRAND, W. H., SMALL, D. M.: The physicochemical basis of cholesterol gallstone formation in man. J. Clin. Invest. 47, 1043 (1968).

AGID, R., MARQUIE, G.: Effets préventifs du NN-diméthylbiguanide sur le développement de l'athérosclérose induite par le cholestérol chez le lapin. C. R. Acad. Sc. Paris 261, 793 (1965).

AHRENS, E. H., Jr., HIRSCH, J., OETTE, K., FARQUHAR, J. W., STEIN, Y.: Carbohydrate-induced lipemia. Trans. Assoc. Am. Physicians 74, 134 (1961).

AKANUMA, Y., KUZUYA, T., HAYASHI, M., IDE, T., KUZUYA, N.: Positive correlation of serum lecithin: cholesterol acyl-transferase activity with relative body weight. Europ. J. Clin. Invest. 3, 136 (1973).

ALADJEM, F., LIEBERMAN, M., GOFMAN, J. W.: Immunochemical studies on human plasma lipoproteins. J. Exp. Med. 105, 49 (1957).

ALAUPOVIC, P.: Recent advances in metabolism of plasma lipoproteins: chemical aspects. Progr. Biochem. Pharmacol. 4, 91 (1968).

ALAUPOVIC, P.: Apolipoproteins and lipoproteins, Atherosclerosis 13, 141 - 146 (1971).

ALAUPOVIC, P.: Conceptual development of the classification systems of plasma lipoproteins. In: Protides of the biological fluids 19, 9 (PEETERS, H., Ed.) Oxford: Pergamon Press 1971.

ALAUPOVIC, P., KOSTNER, G., LEE, D. M., McCONATHY, W. J., MAGNANI, H. N.: Peptide composition of human plasma apolipoproteins A, B and C. Exposés Ann. Biochem. Med. 31, 145 (1972).

ALAUPOVIC, P., LEE, D. M., McCONATHY, W. J.: Studies on the composition and structure of plasma lipoproteins. Distribution of lipoprotein families in major density classes of normal human plasma lipoproteins. Biochim. Biophys. Acta 260, 689 (1972).

ALAUPOVIC, P., SANBAR, S. S., FURMAN, R. H., SULLIVAN, M. L., WALRAVEN, S. L.: Studies of the composition and structure of serum lipoproteins. Isolation and characterization of very high density lipoproteins of human serum. Biochemistry 5, 4044 (1966).

ALBERS, J., CHEN, C. H., ALADJEM, F.: Human serum lipoproteins. Evidence for three classes of lipoproteins in S_f 0-2. Biochemistry 11, 57 (1972).

ALBERS, J. J., HAZZARD, W. R.: Immunochemical quantification of the human plasma Lp(a) lipoprotein., Lipids (in press).

ALBRINK, M. J.: Triglycerides, lipoproteins, and coronary artery disease. Arch. int. Med. 109, 345 (1962).

ALBRINK, M. J., MAN, E. B.: Serum triglycerides in coronary artery diasease. Arch. intern. Med. 103, 4 (1959).

ALBRINK, W. S., ALBRINK, M. J.: The hyperlipidemia of lymphoma-bearing hamsters. Yale J. of biol. medicine 43, 288 (1971).

ALCINDOR, L. G., INFANTE, R., SOLER-ARGILAGA, C., RAISONNIER, A., POLONOVSKI, J., CAROLI, J.: Induction of the hepatic synthesis of β-lipoproteins by high concentrations of fatty acids. Effect of actinomycin D. Biochim. Biophys. Acta 210, 483 (1970).

AMENTA, J. S., WATERS, L. L.: The precipitation of serum lipoproteins by mucopolysaccharides extracted from aortic tissue. Yale J. Biol. Med. 33, 112 (1960).

ANDERSON, T. W.: Mortality from ischemic heart disease: Changes in middle-aged men since 1900. J. Amer. med. Ass. 224, 336 (1973).

ANDERSON, T. W., LE RICHE, W. H., McKAY, J. S.: Sudden death and ischaemic heart disease. Correlation with hardness of local water supply. New Engl. J. Med. 280, 805 - 807 (1969).

ANGEL, A., FARKAS, J.: Structural compartments in adipose cells. In: Adipose tissue: Regulation and metabolic function, p. 152 - 161. London: Academic Press 1970.

ANITSCHKOW, N. N.: Über die Veränderungen der Kaninchenaorta bei experimenteller Cholesterinsteatose. Beitr. path. Anat. 56, 379 (1913).

ANITSCHKOW, N. N.: Über die Rückbildungsvorgänge bei der experimentellen Atherosklerose. Verhandl. deutsch. path. Gesellsch. 23, 473 (1928).

ANITSCHKOW, N. N.: A history of experimentation on arterial atherosclerosis in animals. In: Arteriosclerosis: A Survey of the Problem, p. 271 (COWDRY, E. V., Ed.). MacMillan, New York: 1933.

ANTONOVSKY, A.: Social and cultural factors in coronary heart disease: An Israel-North American sibling study. Isr. J. med. sci. 7, 1578 (1971).

ARDLIE, N. G., GLEW, G., SCHWARTZ, C. J.: Influence of catecholamines on nucleotide-induced platelet aggregation. Nature 212, 415 - 417 (1966).

ARDLIE, N. G., SCHWARTZ, C. J.: A comparison of the organisation and fate of autologous pulmonary emboli and of artificial plasma thrombi in the anterior chamber of the eye, in normocholesterolaemic rabbits. J. Path. Bact. 95, 1 -18 (1968).

ARFORS, K.-E., HINT, H. C., DHALL, D. P., MATHESON, N. A.: Counter-action of platelet activity at sites of laser-induced endothelial trauma. Brit. Med. J. 4, 430 - 431 (1968).

ARMSTRONG, M. L., CONNOR, W. E., WARNER, E. D.: Xanthomatosis in rhesus monkeys fed a hypercholesterolemic diet. Arch. Pathol. 84, 227 - 237 (1967).

ARMSTRONG, M. L., MEGAN, B. M.: Lipid depletion in atheromatous coronary arteries in rhesus monkeys after regression diets. Circ. Res. 30, 675 (1972).

ARMSTRONG, M. L., MEGAN, M. B.: Arterial fibrous proteins in cynomolgus monkeys after atherogenic and regression regimens. Circulation 48, Suppl. 4, 41 (1973).

ARMSTRONG, M. L., WARNER, E. D.: Morphology and distribution of diet-induced atherosclerosis in rhesus monkeys. Arch. Pathol. 92, 395 - 401 (1971).

ARMSTRONG, M. L., WARNER, E. D., CONNOR, W. E.: Regression of coronary atheromato-
sis in rhesus monkeys. Circ. Res. 27, 59 - 67 (1970).
ARONOW, W. S., DENDINGER, J., ROKAW, S. N.: Heart rate, carbon monoxide level af-
ter smoking high-, low- and non-nicotine cigarettes. A study in male patients
with angina pectoris. Ann. Int. Med. 74, 697 (1971).
ARTERIOSCLEROSIS: A report by the National Heart and Lung Institute Task Force on
Arteriosclerosis. DHEW Publication No. (NIH) 72 - 137. Vol. 1 (June 1971).
ARTHUR, J. B.: Five year study by a group of physicians of the Newcastle upon
Tyne Region: Trial of clofibrate in the treatment of ischaemic heart disease.
Brit. Med. J. 4, 767 - 775 (1971).
ASCHOFF, L.: Lectures in Pathology. New York: Hoeber 1924.
ASHFORD, T. P., FREIMAN, D. G.: Platelet aggregation at sites of minimal endo-
thelial injury. Amer. J. Path. 53, 599 - 607 (1968).
ASSMANN, G., BREWER, H. B., Jr.: Lipid-protein interactions in high-density lipo-
proteins. Proc. Natl. Acad. Sci., USA 71, 989 - 993 (1974).
ASSMANN, G., BREWER, H. B., Jr.: A molecular model of High Density lipoproteins.
Proc. Natl. Acad. Sci. USA 71, 1534 (1974).
ASSMANN, G., HIGHET, R. J., SOKOLOSKI, E. A., BREWER, H. B., Jr.: Nuclear/magnetic
resonance spectroscopy of native and recombined lipoproteins. Proc. Natl. Acad.
Sci. USA (in press).
ASSMANN, G., KRAUSS, R. M., FREDRICKSON, D. S., LEVY, R. I.: Characterization,
subcellular localization, and partial purification of a heparin-released⸴tri-
glyceride lipase from rat liver. J. Biol. Chem. 248, 1992 (1972).
ASSMANN, G. KRAUSS, R. M., FREDRICKSON, D. S., LEVY, R. I.: Positional specificity
of triglyceride lipases in post-heparin plasma. J. Biol. Chem. 248, 7184 -
7190 (1973).
ASSMANN, G., SOKOLOSKI, E. A., BREWER, H. B., Jr.: ^{31}P Nuclear magnetic resonance
spectroscopy of native and recombined lipoproteins. Proc. Nat. Acad. Sci. USA
71, 549 (1974).
ASTRAND, I.: Prognostic value of exercise electrocardiogram in older men. Scand.
J. Clin. Lab. Invest. 23, 271 - 276 (1969).
ASTRUP, P.: Some physiological and pathological effects of moderate carbon monoxide exposure. British med. J. 4, 447 (1972).
ASTRUP, P., KJELDSEN, K., WANSTRUP, J.: Enhancing influence of carbon monoxide on
the development of atheromatosis in cholesterol-fed rabbits. J. Atheroscler.
res. 7, 343 - 354 (1967).
ASTRUP, P., KJELDSEN, K., WANSTRUP, J.: Effects of carbon monoxide exposure on the
arterial wall. Ann. N. Y. Acad. Sci. 174, 294 (1970).
ATSUMI, I., ISOKANE, N., HONDA, Y., MITSUDA, M., SHIMAMOTO, T.: Studies on atherosclerosis obliterans, tibialis anterior blood flow measured by 133 Xe clearance method and its clinical evaluation, Jap. Circ. J. 35, 1220 (1971).
AURELL, CRAMER, K., RYBO, G.: Serum lipids and lipoproteins during long-term administration of an oral contraceptive. Lancet 1966 I, 291.
AVOY, D. R., SWYRYD, E. A., GOULD, R. G.: Effects of CPIB with and without androsterone on cholesterol biosynthesis in rat liver. J. Lipid Res. 6, 369 (1965).
AYLWARD, M., MADDOCK, J.: Plasma-tryptophan levels in Depression. Lancet 1973 I,
936.
AYRAULT-JARRIER, M., LEVY, G., POLONOVSKI, J.: Etude des -lipoprotéins sériques
humaines par immunoélectrophorèse. Bull. Soc. Chim. Biol. 45, 703 (1963).
AYRES, S. M., GIANNELLI, S., Jr., MULLER, H.: Carboxyhemoglobin and access to
oxygen. Arch. Environ. Health 26, 8 (1973).
BAGLIO, C. M., FARBER, E.: Reversal by adenine of the ethionine-induced lipid
accumulation in the endoplasmic reticulum of the rat liver: a preliminary report. J. Cell Biol. 27, 591 - 601 (1965).
BAILEY, J. M.: Regulation of cell cholesterol content. In: Atherogenesis: Initiating factors. (CIBA Foundation Symposium, Vol. 12, new series), p. 63 - 92
(1973).
BAILEY, J. M., BUTLER, J.: Anti-inflammatory drugs in experimental atherosclerosis.
Part 1. Relative potencies for inhibiting plaque formation. Atherosclerosis
17, 515 - 522 (1973).
BALIS, J. U., HAUST, M. D., MORE, R. H.: Electron microscopic studies in human
atherosclerosis. Cellular elements in⸴aortic fatty streaks. Exp. Mol. Path.
3, 511 - 525 (1964).

941

BARKER, W. C., DAYHOFF, M. O.: Detecting distant relationships: Computer methods and results. In: Atlas of protein sequence and structure (DAYHOFF, M. O., Ed.) Vol. 5, p. 101 - 107. Silver Spring, Maryland: The National Biomedical Research Foundation 1972.

BARNARD, P. J.: Pulmonary arteriosclerosis and cor pulmonale due to recurrent thromboembolism. Circulation 10, 343 - 361 (1954).

BAROLDI, G.: Acute coronary occlusion as a cause of myocardial infarct and sudden coronary heart death. Amer. J. Cardiol. 16, 859 - 880 (1965).

BAROLDI, G.: Significance of arterial obstructive lesions in early diagnosis of coronary heart disease. Adv. Cardiol. 8, 49 - 66 (1973).

BAROLDI, G., MANION, W. C.: Microcirculatory disturbances and human myocardial infarction. Amer. Heart J. 74, 173 (1967).

BAR-ON, H., KOOK, A. I., STEIN, O., STEIN, Y.: Assembly and secretion of very low density lipoproteins by rat liver following inhibition of protein synthesis with cycloheximide. Biochim. Biophys. Acta 306, 106 (1973).

BAR-ON, H., ROHEIM, P. S., STEIN, O., STEIN, Y.: Contribution of floating fat triglyceride and of lecithin towards formation of secretory triglyceride in perfused rat liver. Biochim. Biophys. Acta 248, 1 (1971).

BAR-ON, H., STEIN, O., STEIN, Y.: Multiple effects of cycloheximide on the metabolism of triglycerides in the liver of male and female rats. Biochim. Biophys. Acta 270, 444 - 452 (1972).

BARTER, P. J., CARROLL, K. F., NESTEL, P. J.: Diurnal fluctuations in triglyceride, free fatty acids, and insulin during sucrose consumption and insulin infusion in man. J. Clin. Invest. 50, 583 (1971).

BARTER, P. J., NESTEL, P. J.: Plasma free fatty acid transport during prolonged glucose consumption and its relationship to plasma triglyceride fatty acids in man. J. Lipid Res. 13, 483 (1972).

BARTER, P. J., NESTEL, P. J.: Precursors of plasma triglyceride fatty acids in obesity. Metabolism 22, 779 (1973).

BARTER, P. J., NESTEL, P. J., CARROLL, K. F.: Precursors of plasma triglyceride fatty acid in humans. Effects of glucose consumption, clofibrate administration and alcoholic fatty liver. Metabolism 21, 117 (1972).

BASSO, L. V., HAVEL, R. J.: Hepatic metabolism of free fatty acids in normal and diabetic dogs. J. Clin. Invest. 49, 537 (1970).

BAUM, D., GUTHRIE, R. BRUNZELL, J. D., VOGEL, W. C., BIERMAN, E. L.: Triglyceride abnormality in infantile hypothyroidism. Amer. J. Dis. Child. 125, 612 - 613 (1973).

BAUMGARTNER, H. R.: The role of blood flow in platelet adhesion, fibrin deposition, and formation of mural thrombi. Microvascular Res. 5, 167 - 179 (1973).

BAUMGARTNER, H. R.: The subendothelial surface and thrombosis. Proc. IV. Internat. Congress on Thrombosis and Haemostasis, Vienna, Austria. p. 42 (1973).

BAUMGARTNER, H. R., STUDER, R.: Gezielte Überdehnung der Aorta abdominalis am normo- und hypercholesterinaemischen Kaninchen. Pathol. Microbiol. 26, 129 (1963).

BEAUMONT, J. L.: L'hyperlipidémie par auto-anticorps anti-beta-lipoprotéines: Une nouvelle entité pathologique. C. R. Acad. Sc. Paris, Série D. 261, 4563 (1965).

BEAUMONT, J.L.: Une gamma-A globuline de myélome douée d'une activité spécifique anti-lipoprotéines. L'auto-anticorps anti-Pg. C. R. Acad. Sc. Paris, Série D. 263, 2046 (1966)

BEAUMONT, J. L.: Gamma-globulines et hyperlipidemies l'hyperlipidemie par auto-anticorps. Ann. Biol. Clin. 27, 10 and 611 (1969).

BEAUMONT, J. L.: Un deuxième type d'auto-anticorps anti-lipoprotéines de myélome: l'IgG anti-Lp Al. Sa. C. R. Acad. Sc. Paris, Série D. 269, 107 (1969).

BEAUMONT, J. L.: Autoimmune hyperlipidemia. An atherogenic metabolic disease of immune origin. Rev. Frse Etudes Clin. & Biol. 15, 1037 (1970).

BEAUMONT, J. L.: Le phénomène d'agglutination des particules lipidiques dans les hyperlipidémies par auto-anticorps. Le test d'agglutination des émulsions lipidiques activées (AELA). C. R. Acad. Sc. Paris, Série D. 272, 2404 (1971).

BEAUMONT, J. L., BAUDET, M. F.: Présence d'un phospholipide dans le site Pg que révèle l'IgA myélomateuse anti-lipoprotéines (anti-Pg). C. R. Acad. Sc. Paris, Série D. 266, 969 (1968).

BEAUMONT, J. L., BAUDET, M. F., DELPLANQUE, B., PERON, F.: L'hémagglutination passive au chlorure de chrome. Son emploi sans diluant macromoléculair. Pathologie et biologie. 17, 429 (1969).

BEAUMONT, V., BEAUMONT, J. L.: L'hyperlipidémie expérimentale par immunisation chez le lapin. Pathologie et Biologie. 16, 869 (1968).

BEAUMONT, V., BEAUMONT, J. L.: Hyperlipidemia and tumors: the hyperlipidemia of lymphoma-bearing hamsters. Forthcoming in: Biomedicine.

BEAUMONT, J. L., BEAUMONT, V., ANTONUCCI, M.: Présence d'un auto-anticorps anti-beta-lipoprotéines dans le sérum d'un lapin ayant une hyperlipidemie par immunisation (l'hyperlipidémie par auto-anticorps expérimentale). C. R. Acad. Sc. Paris, Série D, 268, 1830 (1969).

BEAUMONT, J. L., BEAUMONT, V., JACOTOT, B.: Un nouveau cas d'hyperlipidémie par auto-anticorps. Son traitement par la D-pénicillamine. Bull. Soc. Med. Hopitaux de Paris 118, 709 (1967).

BEAUMONT, J. L., BEAUMONT, V., LEMORT, N., ANTONUCCI, M.: Les auto-anticorps de myélome. Etude comparée de deux types: l'IgA anti-Lp P. G. et l'IgG anti-Lp A. S. Annales de Biologie Clinique 28, 387 (1970).

BEAUMONT, J. L., CARLSON, L. A., COOPER, G. R., FEJFAR, Z., FREDRICKSON, D. S., STRASSER, T.: Classification of hyperlipidaemias and hyperlipoproteinaemias Bull. Wld. Hlth Org. Bull. Org. mond. Santé 43, 891 - 915 (1970).

BEAUMONT, J. L., DELPLANQUE, B.: Méthode de purification d'anticorps de lapin anti-beta-lipoproteines humaines à partir de précipités spécifiques. Immunochemistry 6, 489 (1969).

BEAUMONT, J. L., JACTOT, B., BEAUMONT, V.: L'hyperlipidémie par auto-anticorps. Une cause d'athérosclérose. La Presse Medicale 75, 2315 (1967).

BEAUMONT, J. L., JACTOT, B., BEAUMONT, V.: L'hyperlipidémie par auto-anticorps. Son pouvoir athérogène. In: Le Rôle de la Parei Artérielle dans l'Athérogénèse Vol. 1, p. 507 - 524. Paris: Colloque CNRS (1968).

BEAUMONT, J. L., JACTOT, B., VILAIN, C., BEAUMONT, V.: Présence d'un auto-anti-corps anti-beta-lipoprotéines dans un sérum de myélome. C. R. Acad. Sc. Paris, Série D. 260, 5960 (1965).

BEAUMONT, J. L., LEMORT, N.: Une immunoglobuline anti-héparine dans un sérum hyperlipidémique (Une nouvelle variété d'hyperlipidémie par auto-anticorps). C. R. Acad. Sc. Paris, Série D. 271, 2452 (1970).

BEAUMONT, J. L., LEMORT, N.: Les immunoglobulines anti-héparine. Un facteur de thromboses, d'hyperlipidémies et d'athérosclérose. Forthcoming in: Pathologie et Biologie.

BEAUMONT, J. L., LORENZELLI, L.: L'auto-anticorps antilipoprotéines (anti-Pg) du gamma-A myélome avec hyperlipidémie. Méthode d'isolement et de purification à partir des compléxes circulants. Annales de Biologie Clinique 25, 655 (1967).

BEAUMONT, J. L., LORENZELLI, L.: Le phénomène d'agglutination des particules lipidiques. Son intérêt en séro-immunologie. Pathologie et Biologie 20, 357 (1972).

BEAUMONT, J. L., LORENZELLI, L., DELPLANQUE, B.: Emploi d'un détergent pour la purification d'anticorps anti-lipoprotéines. Immunochemistry 7, 131 (1970).

BECKER, C. G.: Tropomyosin of smooth muscle (Manuscript in preparation).

BECKER, C. G., MURPHY, G. E.: Demonstration of contractile protein in endothelium and cells of the heart valves, endocardium, intima, arteriosclerotic plaques and Aschoff bodies of rheumatic heart disease. Am.J. Path. 55, 1 (1969).

BECKER, C. G., NACHMAN, R. L.: Contractile proteins of endothelial cells, platelets and smooth muscle, Am. J. Path. 71, 1 (1973).

BECKMAN, L., OLIVECRONA, T.: Serum-cholesterol and ABO and Lewis bloodgroups. Lancet 1970 I, 1000.

BEHRMAN, H. R., McDONALD, G. J., GREEP, R. O.: Regulation of ovarian cholesterol esters: evidence for the enzymatic sites of prostaglandin-induced loss of corpus luteum function. Lipids 6, 791 (1971).

BELL, F. P., ADAMSON, I. L., SCHWARTZ, C. J.: Aortic endothelial permeability to albumin: Focal and regional patterns of uptake and transmural distribution of ^{131}I-albumin in the young pig. Exp. Molec. Path. In press (1974a).

BELL, F. P., GALLUS, A. S., SCHWARTZ, C. J.: Focal and regional patterns of uptake and the transmural distribution of ^{131}I-fibrinogen in the pig aorta in vivo. Exp. Molec. Path. In press (1974 b).

BELL, F. P., SOMER, J. B., CRAIG, I. H., SCHWARTZ, C. J.: Patterns of aortic
Evans Blue uptake *in vivo* and *in vitro*. Atherosclerosis 16, 369 - 375
(1972).

BENDITT, E. P., BENDITT, J. M.: Evidence for a monoclonal origin of human atherosclerotic plaques. Proc. Natl. Acad. Sci. USA, 70, 1753 - 1756 (1973).

BENNETT, H. S.: The concepts of membrane flow and membrane vesiculation as mechanisms for active transport and ion pumping. J. Biophysic. and Biochem.
Cytol. 2, 99 (1956).

BENNETT, L. L., KREISS, R. E., LI, C. H., EVANS, H. M.: Production of ketosis
by the growth and adrenocorticotropic hormones. Amer. J. Physiol. 152, 210
(1948).

BENSADOUN, A., EHNHOLM, C., STEINBERG, D., BROWN, W. V.: Improved extraction
and purification of lipoprotein lipase by affinity chromatography from pig
adipose tissue. This volume p. 937.

BENSADOUN, A., EHNHOLM, C., STEINBERG, D., BROWN, W. V.: Purification and
characterization of lipoprotein lipase from pig adipose tissue. J. Biol.
Chem. (in press) 1973.

BERENSON, G. S., RADHAKRISHNAMURTHY, B., DALFERES, E. R., Jr., SRINIVASAN, S.
R.: Carbohydrate macromolecules and atherosclerosis. Human Path. 2, 57
(1971).

BERENSON, G. S., RADHAKRISHNAMURTHY, B., FISHKIN, A. F., DESSAUER, H., ARQUEM-
BOURG, P.: Individuality of glycoproteins in human aorta, J. Atheroscler.
Res. 6, 214 - 223 (1966).

BERG, K.: A new serum type system in man - the Lp system. Acta path. microbiol.
scand. 59, 369 - 382 (1963).

BERG, K.: Further studies on the Lp system. Vox sang. 11, 419 - 426 (1966).

BERG, K.: The Lp system. Series Haematol. 1, 111 (1968).

BERGMAN, E. N., HAVEL, R. J., WOLFE, B. M., BOHMER, T.: Quantitative studies
of the metabolism of chylomicron triglycerides and cholesterol by liver
and extrahepatic tissues of sheep and dogs. J. Clin. Invest. 50, 1831
(1971).

BERGSTROM, S., CARLSON, L. A., WEEKS, J. R.: The prostaglandins: A family of
biologically active lipids. Pharmacol. Rev. 20, 1 (1968).

BERKOWITZ, D.: Long-term treatment of hyperlipidemic patients with clofibrate.
J. Amer. Med. Ass. 218, 1002 - 1005 (1971).

BERKOWITZ, D.: Clinical experiences with halofenate, a new hypolipidemic and
hypouricemic agent. Circulation 46 (suppl. II), 256 (1972).

BERMAN, H. J.: Anticoagulant-induced alterations in haemostasis, platelet
thrombosis, and vascular fragility in the peripheral vessels of the hamster
cheek pouch. In: Anticoagulants and Fibrinolysins, p. 95 - 107 (McMILLAN,
R. L., MUSTARD, J. F., Eds.). MacMillan Co. of Canada Ltd. 1961.

BERNOULLI, D.: Hydrodynamica, sive, de viribus et motivibus fluidorum commen-
tarii. J. R. Dulsecker (1738).

BERSEUS, O., DANIELSSON, H., EINARSSON, K.: Enzymatic transformations of the
steroid nucleus in bile acid synthesis. In: Methods in Enzymology, XV,
p. 551 (CLAYTON, R. B., Ed.). New York: Academic Press 1969.

BESTERMAN, E. M. M., GILLETT, M. P. T.: Inhibition of platelet aggregation by
lysolecithin. Atherosclerosis 14, 323 - 330 (1971).

BEVANS, M., DAVIDSON, J. D., KENDALLS, F. F.: Regression of lesions in canine
arteriosclerosis. Arch. Pathol. 51, 288 (1951).

BIER, D. M., HAVEL, R. J.: Activation of lipoprotein lipase by lipoprotein
fractions of human serum. J. Lipid Res. 11, 565 (1970).

BIERMAN, E. L.: Insulin and hypertriglyceridemia. Israel J. Med. Sciences 8,
303 - 308 (1972).

BIHARI-VARGA, M.: Thermoanalytical assay of glycosaminoglycans. Acta Biochim.
et Biophys. 6, 271 (1971).

BIHARI-VARGA, M., SIMON, J., GERÖ, S.: Identification of glycosaminoglycan
lipoprotein complexes in atherosclerotic aorta intima by thermoanalytical
methods. Acta Biochim. Biophys. Acad. Sci. Hung. 3, 365 - 377 (1968).

BILHEIMER, D. W., EISENBERG, S., LEVY, R. I.: Abnormal metabolism of very low
density lipoproteins in type III hyperlipoproteinemia. Circulation 44,
Suppl. II, 56 (1971).

BILHEIMER, D. W., EISENBERG, S., LEVY, R. I.: The metabolism of very low density lipoprotein proteins I. Preliminary in vitro and in vivo observations. Biochim. Biophys. Acta 260, 212 - 221 (1972).

BIÖRCK, G., BOSTRÖM, H., WIDSTRÖM, A.: On relationship between water hardness and death rate in cardiovascular diseases. Acta med. scand. 178, 239 - 252 (1965).

BIRNSTINGL, M. A., BRINSON, K., CHAKRABARTI, B. K.: The effect of short-term exposure to carbon monoxide on platelet stickiness. Brit. J. Surg. 58, 837 - 839 (1971).

BJÖRKERUD, S.: Reaction of the aortic wall of the rabbit after superficial longitudinal, mechanical trauma. Virchows Arch. Abt. A Path. Anat. 347, 197 - 210 (1969 a).

BJÖRKERUD, S.: Atherosclerosis initiated by mechanical trauma in normolipidemic rabbits. J. Atheroscler. Res. 9, 209 - 213 (1969 b).

BJÖRKERUD, S.: Preparative, staining, and microscopic techniques for the study of whole artery segments. Atherosclerosis 15, 147 - 152 (1972).

BJÖRKERUD, S.: Potential of regulation of arterial smooth muscle function by endothelium - a review. Proc. Workshop Conference "The Smooth Muscle of the Arterial Wall", Heidelberg, West-Germany, Oct. 29 - 31, 1973. Plenum Press. 1974 (in press).

BJÖRKERUD, S., BONDJERS, G.: Arterial repair and atherosclerosis after mechanical injury. Part 1: Permeability and light microscopic characteristics of endothelium in non-atherosclerotic and atherosclerosis lesions. Atherosclerosis 13, 355 - 363 (1971).

BJÖRKERUD, S., BONDJERS, G.: Arterial repair and atherosclerosis after mechanical injury. Part 2: Tissue response after induction of a total local necrosis (deep longitudinal injury). Atherosclerosis 14, 259 - 276 (1971).

BJÖRKERUD, S., BONDJERS, G.: Endothelial integrity and viability in the aorta of the normal rabbit and rat as evaluated with dye exclusion tests and interference contrast microscopy. Atherosclerosis 15, 285 - 300 (1972).

BJÖRKERUD, S., BONDJERS, G.: Arterial repair and atherosclerosis after mechanical injury. Part 5: Tissue response after induction of a large superficial transverse injury. Atherosclerosis 18, 235 - 255 (1973 a).

BJÖRKERUD, S., BONDJERS, G.: Uptake, accumulation, and removal of cholesterol in the normal and atherosclerotic arterial wall. Nutr. Metabol. 15, 27 - 36 (1973 b).

BLACKBURN, H., TAYLOR, H., KEYS, A.: Prognostic significance of the post-exercise electrocardiogram. Amer. J. Cardiol. 25, 85 (1970).

BLACKET, R. B., LEELARTHAEPIN, B., PALMER, A. J., WOODHILL, J. M.: Coronary heart disease in young men: A study of seventy patients with a critical review of etiological factors. Aust. New Zeal. J. Med. 3, 39 (1973).

BLAKELY, J. A., GENT, M.: Platelets, drugs and longvity in a geriatric population. In: Platelets, Drugs and Thrombosis, (HIRSCH, J., CADE, J. F., GALLUS, A. S., SCHÖNBAUM, E., Eds.), New York: S. Karger (1974) (in press).

BLANKENHORN, D. H., CHIN, H. P., LAU, F. Y. K.: Ischemic heart disease in young adults. Metabolic and angiographic diagnosis and the prevalence of type IV hyperlipoproteinemia. Ann. Int. Med. 69, 21 (1968).

BLATON, V., HOWARD, A. N., GRESHAM, G. A., VANDAMME, D., PEETERS, H.: Lipid changes in the plasma lipoproteins of baboons given an atherogenic diet. Part I. Changes in the lipids of total plasma and of alpha and beta lipoproteins. Atherosclerosis 11, 497 (1970).

BLATON, V., PEETERS, H.: Integrated approach to plasma lipid and lipoprotein analysis. In: Blood Lipids and Lipoproteins, Chap. 6, p. 304 (NELSON, G., Ed.). New York: Wiley 1971.

BLATON, V., PEETERS, H.: Integrated approach to plasma lipid and lipoprotein analysis. In: Blood Lipids and Lipoproteins, Chapter 6, p. 369. (NELSON, G., Ed.). New York: J. Wiley and Sons 1971.

BLATON, V., PEETERS, H.: Effect of unsaturated phosphatidylcholine on the lipoprotein lipase activity in vitro. This volume p. 565.

BLATON, V., VANDAMME, D., PEETERS, H.: Chimpanzee and Baboon as Biochemical Models for Human Atherosclerosis. In: Goldsmith and Moor-Jankowski. Medical Primatology. Part III, p. 306 - 312. Basel: Karger 1972.

BLATON, V., VANDAMME, D., PEETERS, H.: The effect of essential phospholipids on plasma lipid and fatty acids in hyperlipidemia. Verhandl. deutschen Gesellschaft. Innere Med., Wiesbaden 78, 1242 (1972).

BLATON, V., VERCAEMST, R., VANDECASTEELE, N., CASTER, H., PEETERS, H.: Isolation and partial characterization of chimpanzee plasma high density lipoproteins and their apolipoproteins. Biochemistry. 1974 (in press).

BLATT, J. M., EISENBERG, S., STEIN, O., STEIN, Y.: Phospholipases in arterial tissue. V. Comparison of the activity of phosphatide acyl-hydrolase and sphingomyelin choline phosphohydrolase in aortae of male, female and ovariectomized rats. Biochim. Biophys. Acta 231, 327 (1971).

BLOCK, W. D., JARRETT, K. J., LEVINE, J. B.: Use of a single color reagent to improve the automated determination of serum cholesterol. In: Automation in Analytical Chemistry. p. 345, New York: Mediad, (SKEGGS, L. T., Jr. Ed.)(1965).

BLOOR, C. M.: Hereditary aspects of coronary atherosclerosis. In: Atherosclerosis and coronary heart disease: The Twenty-forth Hahnemann Symposium, p. 1. (LIKOFF, W., SEGAL, B. L., INSULL, W., Jr., and MOYER, J. H., Eds.). New York: Grune and Stratton 1972.

BLUMENTHAL, S.: Prevention of atherosclerosis, Amer. J. Card. 31, 591 (1973).

BOBERG, J., CARLSON, L. A.: Determination of heparin-induced lipoprotein lipase activity in human plasma. Clin. Chim. Acta 10, 420 (1964).

BOBERG, J., CARLSON, L. A., FREYSCHUSS, U., LASSERS, B. W., WAHLQUIST, M. L.: Splanchnic secretion rates of plasma triglycerids and total ans splanchnic turnover of plasma free fatty acids in men with normo- and hypertriglyceridemia. Europ. J. Clin. Invest. 2, 454 (1972).

BÖTTCHER, C. F. J.: Lipids of the human arterial wall. In: Drugs affecting Lipid Metabolism, p.54 (GARATTINI, S. and PAOLETTI, R., Eds.) Amsterdam: Elsevier 1961.

BÖTTCHER, C. J. F., VAN GENT, C. M.: Changes in the composition of phospholipids and of phospholipid fatty acids associated with atherosclerosis in the human aortic wall. J. Atheroscler. Res. 1, 36 (1961).

BOETTIGER, L. E., CARLSON, L. A., ENGSTADT, L., OROE, L.: The effects of long-term heparin treatment in ischaemic heart disease. J. Atheroscler. Res. 5, 253 (1965).

BOLTON, C. H., HAMPTON, J. R., MITCHELL, J. R. A.: Nature of the transferable factor which causes abnormal platelet behaviour in vascular disease. Lancet 1967 II, 1101 - 1105.

BOLZANO, K., SANDHOFER, F, BRAUNSTEINER, H.: The effects of oral administration of sucrose on the turnover rate of plasma free fatty acids and on the esterification rate of plasma free fatty acids to plasma triglycerides. Horm. Metab. Res. 4, 439 (1973).

BONDJERS, G., BJÖRKERUD, S.: Fluorometric determination of cholesterol and cholesteryl ester in tissue on the manogram level. Anal. Biochem. 42, 363 (1971).

BONDJERS, G., BJÖRKERUD, S.: Arterial repair and atherosclerosis after mechanica injury. Part 4: Uptake and composition of cholesteryl ester in morphologically defined regions of atherosclerotic lesions. Atherosclerosis 15, 273 (1972).

BONDJERS, G., BJÖRKERUD, S.: Cholesterol accumulation and content in regions with defined endothelial integrity in the normal rabbit aorta. Atherosclerosis 17, 71 - 83 (1973 a).

BONDJERS, G., BJÖRKERUD, S.: Arterial repair and atherosclerosis after mechanical injury. Part 3: Cholesterol accumulation and removal in morphologically defined regions of aortic atherosclerotic lesions in the rabbit. Atherosclerosis 17, 85 - 94 (1973 b).

BONNER, M. J., MILLER, B. F., KOTHARI, H. V.: Lysosomal enzymes in aortas of species susceptible and resistant to atherosclerosis. Proc. Soc. Exp. Biol. Med. 139, 1359 (1972).

BORENZSTAYN, J., ROBINSON, D. S.: The effect of fasting on the utilisation of chylomicron triglyceride fatty acids in relation to clearing factor lipase (lipoprotein lipase) released by heparin in the perfused rat heart. J. Lipid Res. 11, 111 (1970).

BORN, G. V. R.: Quantitative investigations into the aggregation of blood platelets. J. Physiol. 162, 67^P (1962).

BORN, G. V. R., HONOUR, A. J., MITCHELL, J. R. A.: Inhibition by adenosine and by 2-chloroadenosine of the formation and embolization of platelet thrombi. Nature 202, 761 (1964).

BOSTRÖM, H., WESTER, P. O.: Trace elements in drinking water and death rate in cardiovascular disease. Acta med. scand. 181, 465 - 473 (1967).

BOTTI, R. E., RATNOFF, O. D.: The clot-promoting effect of soaps of long chain saturated fatty acids. J. Clin. Invest. 42, 1569 - 1577 (1963).

BOUCH, D. C., MONTGOMERY, G. L.: Cardiac lesions in fatal cases of recent myocardial ischaemia from a coronary care unit. Brit. Heart J. 32, 795 - 803 (1970).

BOUVIER, C. A., ROSNER, P., BERTHOUD, S., RITSCHARD, J., SCHERRER, J. R., HAUSSER, E.: Anomalie du comportement plaquettaire lors d'infarctus du myocarde. Cardiologie 50, 232 (1967).

BOWYER, D. E., HOWARD, A. N., GRESHAM, G. A.: Lipid synthesis in perfused normal and atherosclerotic rabbit aorta Biochem. J. 103, 54 (1967).

BRADFORD, R. H., FURMAN, R. H.: Plasma Post-Heparin Lipolytic Activity in Hyperchycomicronemia (Fat-Induced Lipemia). Biochim. Biophys. Acta 164, 172 (1968).

BRADFORD-HILL,A.: Principles of Medical Statistics,p.22,London:Lancet Ltd. 1961.

BRADY, R. O.: The genetic mismanagement of complex lipid metabolism. Bull. N. Y. Acad. Med. 47, 173 (1971).

BRANWOOD, A. W., MONTGOMERY, G. L.: Observations on the morbid anatomy of coronary artery disease. Scott. Med. J. 1, 367 - 375 (1956).

BRAUN-FALCO, O., KELLER, CH., ZÖLLNER, N.: Xanthoma formation and other tissue reactions to hyperlipidemias. Proceedings of the International Symposium on Xanthoma Formation and Other Tissue Reactions to Hyperlipidemias, (Basel, München, Paris, London, New York, Sydney: Karger 1972).

BRECHER, P., BRAGA-ILLA, F., CHOBANIAN, A. V.: The metabolism of cholesterol esters in rat adrenal cell suspensions. Endocrinology 93, 163 - 172 (1973).

BRECHER, P., KESSLER, M., CLIFFORD, C., CHOBANIAN, A. V.: Cholesterol ester hydrolysis in aortic tissue. Biochim. Biophys. Acta 316, 386 (1973).

BRECHER, P. I., TERCYAK, A., CHOBANIAN, A. V.: Increased cholesterol esterification by different enzyme systems in atherosclerotic aortic tissue. Circulation 7 & 8, IV-78 (1973).

BREDDIN, K.: Über die gesteigerte Thrombocytenagglutination bei Gefäßkranken. Schweiz. Med. Wschr. 95, 655 (1965).

BREDDIN, K.: Die Thrombozytenfunktion bei hämorrhagischen Diathesen, Thrombosen und Gefäßkrankheiten. Thrombos. Diathes. haemorrh. (Stuttg.) Supp. 27 (1968).

BREDDIN, K., SCHARRER, I.: Klinische Ergebnisse der Behandlung mit Acetylsalicylsäure bei Gefäßkranken. Folia angiologica 21, 187 (1973).

BREWER, H. B., Jr., LUX, S. E., RONAN, R., JOHN, K. M.: Amino acid sequence of human apoLP-Gln-II (apoA-II), an apolipoprotein isolated from the high-density lipoprotein complex. Proc. Nat. Acad. Sci. USA 69, 1304 (1972 a).

BRINDLEY, D. N., HUBSCHER, G.: The intracellular distribution of the enzymes catalysing the biosynthesis of glycerides in the intestinal mucosa. Biochim. Biophys. Acta 106, 495 (1965).

BROCHS, H.: Experimentelle undersogelsen over lipoidaflezringen i coronarteriene hos kaniner. Thesis, Copenhagen: 1945.

BROWN, D. F.: Blood lipids and atherogenesis. Amer. J. Med. 46, 691 (1969).

BROWN, D. F., DAUDISS, K.: Hyperlipoproteinemia. Prevalence in a free-living population in Albany, New York. Circulation 47, 558 (1973).

BROWN, D. F., KINCH, S. H., DOYLE, J. T.: Fasting and postprandial serum triglyceride levels in health and in ischemic heart disease. J. Atheroscler. Res. 6, 232 (1966).

BROWN, M. S., DANA, S. E., GOLDSTEIN, J. L.: Regulation of 3-hydroxy-3-methylglutaryl coenzyme A reductase activity in human fibroblasts by lipoproteins, Proc. Nat. Acad. Sci. USA 70, 2162 - 2166 (1973).

BROWN, M. S., DANA, S. E., GOLDSTEIN, J. L.: Regulation of 3-hydroxy-3-methylglutaryl coenzyme A reductase activity in cultured human fibroblasts: Comparison of cells from a normal subject and from a patient with homozygous familial hypercholesterolemia. J. Biol. Chem. 249, 789 - 796 (1974).

BROWN, M. S., GOLDSTEIN, J. L.: Familial hypercholesterolemia: Biochemical, genetic and pathophysiological considerations. Adv. Intern. Med. In press.

BROWN, W. V., BAGINSKY, M. L.: Inhibition of lipoprotein lipase by an apoprotein of human very low density lipoprotein. Biochem. Biophys. Res. Commun. 46, 375 (1972).

BROWN, W. V., LEVY, R. I., FREDRICKSON, D. S.: Studies of the proteins in human plasma very low density lipoproteins. J. Biol. Chem. 244, 5687 (1969).

BROWN, W. V., LEVY, R. I., FREDRICKSON, D. S.: Further characterization of apo-lipoproteins from the human plasma very low density lipoproteins. J. Biol. Chem. 245, 6588 (1970).

BRUNZELL, D., PORTE, D., BIERMAN, E. L.: Evidence for a common saturable removal system for dietary and endogenous triglyceride in man. J. Clin. Invest. 50, 15 a (1971).

BRUSCHKE, A. V. G., PROUDFIT, W. L., SONES, F. M.: Progress study of 590 consecutive nonsurgical cases of coronary disease followed 5 - 4 years. Circulation 47, 1147 - 1163 (1973).

BUCHER, N. L. R., McGARRAHAN, K.: The biosynthesis of cholesterol from acetate-1-^{14}C by cellular fractions of rat liver. J. Biol. Chem. 222, 1 (1956).

BUCHWALD, H.: The development of the sub-total ileal bypass operation as a therapeutic approach to hypercholesterolemia and atherosclerosis: A review. Diseases Chest 51, 459 (1967).

BUCK, R. C.: Uptake of radioactive sulphate by arteries of normal and cholesterol-fed rabbits. J. Histochem. Cytochem. 3, 435 (1955).

BUCK, R. C.: Intimal thickening after ligature of arteries. Circ. Res. 9, 418 - 426 (1961).

BUCK, R. C., ROSSITER, R. J.: Lipids of normal and atherosclerotic aortas. A chemical study. Arch. Path. 51, 224 (1951).

BUCKELL, M.: The effect of citrate on euglobulin methods of estimating fibrinolytic activity. J. Clin. Path. II, 403 (1958).

BUCKLEY, J. T., DELAHUNTY, T. J., RUBINSTEIN, D.: The relationship of protein synthesis to the secretion of the lipid moisty of low density lipoprotein by the liver. Canad. J. Biochem. 46, 341 - 349 (1968).

BUDDECKE, E.: Untersuchungen zur Chemie der Arteriewand. V: Darstellung und chemische Zusammensetzung von Mucopolysacchariden der Aorta des Menschen. Z. Physiol. Chem. 318, 33 (1960).

BULLOCK, B. C.: Comparison of coronary artery atherosclerosis in Macaca arctoides (Stumptail Macaque) and Cercopithecus aethiops (African green monkey). Fed. Proc. 32, 315 (1973).

BULLOCK, B. C., LEHNER, N. D. M., CLARKSON, T. B., FELDNER, M. A.: Response of three species of nonhuman primates to an atherogenic diet. Circulation 46, Supp. II, 251 (1972).

BUNGENBERG DE JONG, J. J., MARSH, J. B.: Biosynthesis of plasma lipoproteins by rat liver ribosomes. J. Biol. Chem. 243, 192 (1968).

BURCH, G. E., TSUI, C. Y., HARB, J. M.: Pathologic changes of aorta and coronary arteries of mice infected with coxsackie B$_4$ virus. Proc. Soc. exp. biol. med. 137, 657 (1971).

BURKE, J. S., URIUHARA, T., MACMORINE, D. R. L., MOVAT, H. Z.: A permeability factor released from phagocytosing PMN-leukocytes and its inhibition by protease inhibitors. Life Sciences 3, 1505 - 1512 (1964).

BURNET, M.: The clonal selection theory of antibody production. Vol. 1. New York: Oxford University Press 1959.

BURSTEIN, M., SCHOLNICK, H. R., MORFIN, R.: Rapid method for the isolation of lipoproteins from human serum by precipitation with polyanions. J. Lipid Res. 11, 583 (1970).

BURTON, A. C.: Relation of structure to function of the tissues of blood vessels. Physiol. Rev. 34, 619 (1954).

BUTCHER, R. W., BAIRD, C. E., SUTHERLAND, E. W., Jr.: Effects of lipolytic and antilipolytic substances on adenosine 3', 5'-monophosphate levels in isolated fat cells. J. Biol. Chem. 243, 1705 (1968).

BUTCHER, R. W., HO, R. J., MENG, H. C., SUTHERLAND, E. W.: Adenosine 3', 5'-monophosphate in biological materials. J. Biol. Chem. 240, 4515 (1965).

BUXTORK, J. C., BEAUMONT, V., JACOTOT, B., BEAUMONT, J.-L.: Regression de xanthomes et medicaments hypolipidemiants. Atherosclerosis 19, 1 (1974).

CADE, J. F., HYNES, D. M., REGOECZI, E., HIRSH, J.: Effective thrombolysis by streptokinase in low dosage. Circulation 46, Suppl. II, 54 (1972).

CAHN, R. D., KAPLAN, N. O., LEVINE, L., ZWILLING, E.: Nature and development of lactic dehydrogenase. Science 136, 962 (1962).

CALAY, R., JONNIAUX, G., KOCHELEFF, P., SOBET, L., BASTENIE, P. A.: Dextrothyroxine therapy for the disordered lipid metabolism of preclinical hypothyroidism. Lancet 1971 I, 205 - 206.

CALIMBAS, T. D.: Requirement for a carrier protein in sterol conversions by a protozoan. Federation Proc. 31, 430 (1972).

CALIMBAS, T. D.: Characteristics of a protozoan enzyme system catalyzing conversion of cholesterol to Δ5,7,22-cholestatrienol. Federation Proc. 32, 519 (1973).

CAMERINI-DAVALOS, R. A., EHRENREICH, T., PATEL, D., OPPERMANN, W.: Nephropathy in spontaneously diabetic mice and its possible prevention by pyridinolcarbamate (PDC). In: Atherogenesis II, p. 223 (SHIMAMOTO, T., NUMANO, F., ADDISON, G. M., Eds.). Excerpta Medica, 1973.

CAMERINI-DAVALOS, R. A., OPPERMAN, W., MITTI, R., EHRENREICH, T.: Studies of vascular and other lesions in KK mice. Diabetologia 6, 324 (1970).

CAMPBELL, D. J., DAY, A. J., SKINNER, S. L., TUME, R. K.: The effect of hypertension on the accumulation of lipids and the uptake of (^{3}H)cholesterol by the aorta of normal-fed and cholesteriol-fed rabbits. Atherosclerosis 18, 301 - 319 (1973).

CAMPBELL, D. J., SKINNER, S. L., DAY, A. J.: Cellophane perinephritis hypertension and its reversal in rabbits: Effect on plasma renin, renin substrate and renal mass. Circ. Res. 33, 105 - 115 (1973).

CAMPBELL, D. J., SKINNER, S. L., DAY, A. J.: Suppression of plasma renin by atherogenic levels of serum cholesterol in rabbits. Clinical Science and Molecular Medicine 45, 565 - 569 (1973 a).

CAPLAN, B. A., SCHWARTZ, C. J.: Increased endothelial cell turnover in areas of in vivo Evans blue uptake in the pig aorta. Atherosclerosis 17, 401 - 417 (1973).

CARLSON, L. A.: Studies on the incorporation of injected palmitic acid-1-^{14}C into liver and plasma lipids in man. Acta Soc. Med. Upsalien. 56, 3 (1960 c).

CARLSON, L. A.: Serum lipids in men with myocardial infarction. Acta med. scand. 167, 399 (1960 b).

CARLSON, L. A.: The effect of nicotinic acid treatment on the chemical composition of plasma lipoprotein classes in man. Drugs Affecting Lipid Metabolism. Advances in Experimental Medicine and Biology 4, 327 - 338 (1969).

CARLSON, L., BOTTIGER, L. E.: Ischemic heart disease in relation to fasting values of plasma triglycerides and cholesterol. Stockholm prospective study. Lancet 1972 I, 865.

CARLSON, L. A., ERIKSSON, I., WALLDIUS, G.: A case of massive hypertriglyceridemia and impaired fatty acid incorporation into adipose tissue glycerides (FIAT) both corrected by nicotinic acid. Acta Med. Scand. 194, 363 (1973).

CARLSON, L. A., FRÖBERG, S., ORÖ, L.: A case of massive hypertriglyceridemia corrected by nicotinic acid or nicotinamide therapy. Ather. 16, 359-368 (1972).

CARLSON, J. P., McCOY, K. E., DEMPSEY, M. E.: Squalene and sterol carrier protein: Model for lipoprotein structure and function; role in control of cholesterol synthesis. Circulation 48, IV - 70 (1973).

CARLSON, L. A., OLSSON, A. G.: Hyperlipidemia and its management. In: Modern Trends in Cardiology (OLIVER, M. F., Ed.), 1973.

CARLSON, L. A., RÖSSNER, S.: A methodological study of an intravenous fat tolerance test with Intralipid ^{R} emulsion. Scand., J. Clin. Invest. 29, 271 (1972).

CARLSON, L. A., WALLDIUS, G., BUTCHER, R. W.: Effect of chlorophenoxyisobutyric acid (CPIB) on fat-mobilizing lipolysis and cyclic AMP levels in rat epididymal fat. Atherosclerosis 16, 349 - 357 (1972).

CARO, C. G.: Transport of material between blood and wall in arteries. Ciba Foundation Symposium 12 (New Series). Atherogenesis: Initiating Factors, p. 127 Amsterdam: Assoc. Scientific Publishers 1973.

CARO, C. G.: Transport of ^{14}C-4 cholesterol between intra-luminal serum and artery wall in isolated dog common carotid artery. Journal of Physiology 233, 37^P (1973).

CARO, C. G., FITZ-GERALD, J. M., SCHROTER, R. C.: Atheroma and arterial wall shear: Observation, correlation and proposal of a shear dependent mass transfer mechanism for atherogenesis. Proc. Roy. Soc. Lond. B. 177, 109 (1971).

CARREL, A.: La technique operatoire des anastamoses vasculaires, et la transplantation des visceres. Lyon Medical. 98, 859 (1902).

CARREL, A.: The surgery of blood vessels. Bull. Johns Hopkins Hosp. 18, 18 (1907).

CARREL, A., LINDBERGH, C. A.: The culture of organs. Harper and Row (Hoeber) 1938.

CARROLL, K. K.: Diet, cholesterol metabolism, and atherosclerosis. J. Amer. Oil Chemists' Soc. 44, 607 - 614 (1967).

CARROLL, K. K.: Plasma cholesterol levels and liver cholesterol biosynthesis in rabbits fed commercial or semi-synthetic diets with and without added fats or oils. Atherosclerosis 13, 67 - 76 (1971).

CARSON, P., McDONALD, L., PICKARD, S., PILKINGTON, T., DAVIES, B., LOVE, F.: Effect of Atromid on platelet stickiness. J. Atheroscler. Res. 3, 623 (1963).

CARTER, C. O.: Genetics of common disorders. Brit. med. Bull. 25, 52 (1969).

CARTER, S. A.: Indirect systolic pressures and pulse waves in arterial occlusive disease of the lower extremities. Circulation 37, 624 (1968).

CARTER, S. A.: Clinical measurement of systolic pressures in limbs with arterial occlusive disease. J. A. M. A. 207, 1869 (1969).

CARTER, S. A.: Investigation and treatment of arterial occlusive disease of the extremities. Clin. Med. 79, 12 - 24, 15 - 22 (May, June) (1972 a).

CARTER, S. A.: Response of ankle systolic pressure to leg exercise in mild or questionable arterial disease. New Engl. J. Med. 287, 578 (1972 b).

CARUZZO, C., TARTARA, D., PAGANO, P. G., PELLEGRINI, A., COSTANZO, F., GRANDE, A.: Was bedeutet der Anstieg des Serum-Cholesterinspiegels unter der Behandlung mit hochungesättigten Fettsäuren? Med. Welt 10, 526 (1963).

CASDORPH, H. R.: Treatment of the hyperlipidemic states, p. 416. Springfield: Charles C. Thomas 1971.

Catecholamine column test kit instructions. Bio-Rad Laboratories, Richmond, Calif.

CAVALLERO, C., TUROLLA, E., RICEVUTI, G.: Cell proliferation in the atherosclerotic plaques of cholesterol fed rabbits. Part 1: Colchicine and (^{3}H)thymidine studies. Atherosclerosis 13, 9 - 20 (1971).

CAZENAVE, J.-P., PACKHAM, M. A., GUCCIONE, M. A., MUSTARD, J. F.: Inhibition of platelet adherence to a collagen-coated surface by non-steroidal anti-inflammatory drugs, pyrimido-pyrimidine and tricyclic compounds, and xylocaine. J. Lab. Clin. Med. 83, 797 (1974).

CAZENAVE, J.-P., PACKHAM, M. A., MUSTARD, J. F.: Quantitation of platelet adherence to damaged surface of rabbit aorta. Circulation 48, Suppl. IV-56 (1973).

CEMBRANO, J., LILLO, M., VAL, J., MARDONES, J.: Influence of Sex Difference and Hormones on Elastin and Collagen in the Aorta of Chickens. Circulation Res. VIII, 527 (1960).

CHANDLER, A. B.: In vitro thrombotic coagulation of the blood. A method for producing a thrombus. Lab. Invest. 7, 110 - 114 (1958).

CHANDLER, A. B.: Thrombosis and the development of atherosclerotic lesions. In: Atherosclerosis p. 88 - 93 (Jones,R.J.,Ed.). New York: Springer-Verlag 1970.

CHAPMAN, M. J., MILLS, G. L., TAYLAUR, C. E.: Effect of a lipid-rich diet on the properties and composition of lipoprotein particles from the Golgi apparatus of guinea pig liver. Biochem. J. 131, 177 (1973).

CHEEK, D. B.: Overgrowth of Lean and Adipose Tissues in Adolescent Obesity. Ped. Res. 4, 268 (1970).

CHEEK, D. B., HILL, D. E.: Muscle and Liver Cell Growth: Role of Hormones and Nutritional Factors, Fed. Proc. 29, 1503 (1970).

CHEN, R. M.: Effects of hyperlipemic rabbit serum and its lipoproteins on proliferation and lipid metabolism of rabbit aortic medial cell in vitro. Dissertation for degree of Doctor of Philosophy, University of Chicago 1973.

CHEN, R., DZOGA, K.: Sequential lipid accumulation in rabbit aortic medial cells incubated in hyperlipemic serum. Fed. Proc. 32, 856 (1973).

CHEN, R., DZOGA, K., BORENSZTAJN, J., WISSLER, R. W.: Effect of hyperlipemic lipoproteins on the lipid accumulation of rabbit aortic medial cells in vitro. Circulation 46, II - 253 (1972).

CHEN, R. M., GETZ, G. S., FISHER-DZOGA, K., WISSLER, R. W.: Effect of hyperlipemic serum on lipid biosynthesis and efflux of rabbit aortic medial cells in vitro. Circulation 48, IV - 152 (1973).

CHEN, R. M., GETZ, G. S., FISHER-DZOGA, K., WISSLER, R. W.: Effects of hyperlipemic serum on proliferation and detachment rate of rabbit aortic medial
cells. Submitted for presentation at 1974 Federation Meetings.

CHERNICK, S., SRERE, P. A., CHAIKOFF, I. L.: The metabolism of arterial tissue.
II. Lipide syntheses: The formation in vitro of fatty acids and phospholipides by rat artery with ^{14}C and ^{32}P as indicators. J. Biol. Chem. 179, 113
(1949).

CHESNEY, C. M., HARPER, E., COLMAN, R. W.: Human platelet collagenase. J. Clin.
Invest. 53; 1647 - 1654 (1974).

CHESTERTON, C. J.: Distribution of cholesterol precursors and other lipids among
rat liver intracellular structures. J. Biol. Chem. 243, 1147 - 1151 (1968).

CHIANG, B., PERLMAN, L. V., FULTON, M., OSTRANDER, L. D., Jr., EPSTEIN, H.: Predisposing factors in sudden cardiac death in Tecumseh, Michigan. A prospective study. Circulation 41, 31 - 37 (1970).

CHIN, H. P., BLANKENHORN, D. H.: Separation and quantitative analysis of serum
lipoproteins by means of electrophoresis on cellulose acetate. Clin. Chem.
Acta 20, 305 (1968).

CHMELAR, M., CHMELAROVA, M.: Lipolytic effect of insulin and other hormones in
vitro in aortic tissue of experimental animals. Experientia 24, 1118 (1968).

CHOBANIAN, A. V.: Effects of sex hormones on phospholipid, RNA and protein synthesis in the arterial intima. J. Atheroscler. Res. 8, 763 (1968).

CHOBANIAN, A. V., GERRITSEN, G. C.: Glucose metabolism in diabetic hamster aorta.
Circulation 44, II - 13 (1971 a).

CHOBANIAN, A. V., GERRITSEN, G. C.: Cholesterol metabolism in the diabetic hamster. J. Clin. Invest. 50, 19 a (1971 b).

CHOBANIAN, A. V., MANZUR, F.: Metabolism of lipid in the human fatty streak lesion. J. Lipid Res. 13, 201 - 206 (1972).

CHOI, J. H., HAUST, M. D., WYLLIE, J. C., MORE, R. H.: The presence of albumin
in human normal intima and atherosclerotic lesions demonstrated by fluorescent antibody techniques. Lab. Invest. 15, 1125 - 1126 (1966).

CHUNG, J., SCANU, A. M., REMAN, F.: Effect of phospholipids on lipoprotein lipase
activation in vitro. Biochim. Biophys. Acta 296, 116 (1973).

CLAESSON, M. H.: Dye exclusion as a method of differentiating between living and
dead lymphoid cells. In vivo and in vitro studies. Acta Morphol. Neerl. -
Scand. 9, 1 - 11 (1971).

CLAIRE, M., JACOTOT, B., BEAUMONT, J. L.: Characterization of lipid classes associated with elastin isolated from normal and pathological human aorta. In:
Protides of Biological Fluids 22 (PEETERS, H., Ed.). London: Pergamon Press,
1974 (in preparation).

CLARKSON, B.: Animal Models of Atherosclerosis. In: Advances in Veterinary Science and Comparative Science. Vol. 16, p. 151 - 173 (BRANDLY, C. A. and CORNE-
LIUS, C. E., Eds.). New York: Academic Press 1972.

CLARKSON, T. B., KING, J. S., LOFLAND, H. B., FELDNER, M. A.: Changes in pathologic characteristics and composition of plaques during regression. Circulation
44, II - 48 (1971).

CLARKSON, T. B., LOFLAND, H. B.: Effects of cholesterol-fat diets on pigeons susceptible and resistant to atherosclerosis. Circ. Res. 9, 106 - 109 (1961).

CLARKSON, T. B., LOFLAND, H. B., BULLOCK, B. C.: Effect of type of dietary fat on
sterol distribution and metabolism in squirrel monkeys. Circulation 39, III-5
(1969).

CLARKSON, T. B., LOFLAND, H. B., BULLOCK, W. C., GOODMAN, H. O.: Genetic control
of plasma cholesterol. Arch. Path. 92, 37 - 45 (1971).

CLARKSON, T. B., MIDDLETON, C. C.: Naturally occurring atherosclerosis in birds.
Ann. N. Y. Acad. Sci. 127, 685 - 693 (1965).

CLARKSON, T. B., PRICHARD, R. W., NETSKY, M. G., LOFLAND, H. B.: Atherosclerosis
in pigeons. Its spontaneous occurrence and resemblance to human atherosclerosis. Arch. Pathol. 68, 143 (1959).

COBURN, R. F.: The carbon monoxide.body stores. Ann. N. Y. Acad. Sci. 174, 11
(1970).

COCHRANE, C. G.: Studies on the localization of circulating antigen-antibody complexes and other macromolecules in vessels. I: Structural studies. J. of exper. medicine 118, 503 (1963).

COCHRANE, C. G.: Mechanisms involved in the deposition of immune complexes in tissues. J. of exper. medicine 134, 75 (1971).

COHEN, L., BLAISDELL, R. K., DJORDJEVICH, J., ORMISTE, V., DOBRILOVIC, L.: Familial xanthomatosis and hyperlipidemia and myelomatosis. American J. of medicine 40, 299 (1966).

COLLINS, G. H.: Glial cell changes in the brainstem of thiamine-deficient rats. Amer. J. Pathol. 50, 791 - 814 (1967).

CONNOR, W. E.: The acceleration of thrombus formation by certain fatty acids. J. Clin. Invest. 41, 1199 - 1205 (1962).

CONNOR, W. E., HOAK, J. C., WARNER, E. D.: Massive thrombosis produced by fatty acid infusion. J. Clin. Invest. 42, 860 - 866 (1963).

CONNOR, W. E., WITIAK, D. T., STONE, D. B., ARMSTRONG, M. O.: Cholesterol balance and fecal neutral steroid and bile acid excretion in normal men fed dietary fats of different fatty acid composition. J. Clin. Invest. 48, 1363 (1969).

CONSTANTINIDES, P.: Experimental Atherosclerosis, p. 43. Amsterdam: Elsevier edit. 1965.

CONSTANTINIDES, P.: Experimental Atherosclerosis, p. 66. Amsterdam: Elsevier edit. 1965.

CONSTANTINIDES, P., ROBINSON, M.: Ultrastructural injury of arterial endothelium. III: Effects of enzymes and surfactants. Arch. Path. 88, 113 - 117 (1969).

COOKE, P. H., SMITH, S. C.: Smooth muscle cells: The source of foam cells in atherosclerotic White Carneau pigeons. Exp. Mol. Pathol. 8, 171 (1968).

COOMBS, R. R. A., FRANKS, D., GURNER, P. W., POLLEY, M. J., RICHARDS, C. G.: Studies on mixed agglutination with special reference to the A antigen and the physical properties of the operative antibodies. Immunology 8, 182 (1965).

COPPEN, A., BROOKSBANK, B. W. L., PEET, M.: Tryptophan concentration in the cerebrospinal fluid of depressive patients. Lancet 1972 I, 1393.

COPPEN, A., ECCLESTON, E.G., PEET, M.: Total and free tryptophan concentration in the plasma of depressive patients. Lancet 1973 II, 60 - 63.

COPPEN, A., PRANGE, A. J., WHYBROW , P., NOGUERA, R.: The comparative antidepressant value of L-tryptophan and imipramine with and without attempted potentiation by liothyronine. Arch. Gen. Psychiatr. 26, 234 - 241 (1972).

CORNFIELD, J.: Discriminant functions. Rev. Intern. Statist. Inst. 35, 2 (1967).

CORNFIELD, J., MITCHELL, S.: Selected risk factors in coronary disease. Arch. Environ. Health 19, 382 (1969).

CORNWELL, D. G., GEER, J. C., PANGANAMALA, R. V.: Development of atheroma and the lipid composition of the deposit. In: Encycl. Pharmacol. Ther., Sect. 24. Pharmacology of lipid transport and atherosclerotic process (MASORO, E. J., Ed.). Oxford: Pergamon Press 1973 (In press).

CORONARY DRUG PROJECT RESEARCH GROUP: The coronary Drug Project: Initial findings leading to modifications of its research protocol. J.A.M.A. 214, 1303 (1970).

CORONARY DRUG PROJECT RESEARCH GROUP: The prognostic importance of the electrocardio gram after myocardial infarction. Experience in the Coronary Drug Project. Ann. Intern. Med. 77, 677 (1972).

CORONARY DRUG PROJECT RESEARCH GROUP: The Coronary Drug Project: Findings leading to further modifications of its protocol with respect to dextrothyroxine. J. A. M. A. 220, 996 (1972).

CORONARY DRUG PROJECT RESEARCH GROUP: The Coronary Drug Project: Design, methods and baseline results. Circulation 47, Suppl. 1 (1973).

CORONARY DRUG PROJECT RESEARCH GROUP: Prognostic importance of premature beats following myocardial infarction. Experience in the Coronary Drug Project. J. A. M. A. 223, 1116 (1973).

CORONARY DRUG PROJECT RESEARCH GROUP: The natural history of myocardial infarction in the coronary drug project: Prognostic importance of serum lipid levels. (in press).

CORONARY DRUG PROJECT RESEARCH GROUP: The Coronary Drug Project: Findings leading to discontinuation of the 2.5 mg/d estrogen group. J.A.M.A. 226, 652 (1973).

CORONARY DRUG PROJECT RESEARCH GROUP: Factors influencing long-term prognosis
after recovery from myocardial infarction - Three-year findings of the Coronary Drug Project. J. Chron. Dis (In press).

COTTON, R. C., BLOOR, K., ARCHIBALD, G.: The effect of pyridinol carbamate treatment on the platelet response to ADP in patients with peripheral atherosclerosis, Brit. J. Surg. 59, 313 (1972).

COTTON, R. C., WADE, E. G., SPILLER, G. W.: The effect of Atromid on plasma fibrinogen and heparin resistance. J. Atheroscler. Res. 3, 648 (1963).

COWAN, W. K.: Genetics of duodenal and gastric ulcer. Clin. Gastroenterol. 2, 539
(1973).

COX, G. E., TAYLOR, C. B., COX, L. G., COUNTS, M. A.: Atherosclerosis in rhesus
monkeys. II: Hypercholesterolemia induced by dietary fat and cholesterol.
Arch. Path. 66, 32 (1958).

CRAIG, I. H., BELL, F. P., GOLDSMITH, C. H., SCHWARTZ, C. J.: Thrombosis and
atherosclerosis; the organization of pulmonary thromboemboli in the pig. Macroscopic observations, protein, DNA, and major lipids. Atherosclerosis 18,
277 - 300 (1973).

CRAWFORD, D. W., BECKENBACH, E. S., BLANKENHORN, D. H., SELZER, R. H., BROOKS,
S. H.: Grading of coronary atherosclerosis: Comparison of a modified IAP
visual grading method and a new quantitative angiographic technique. Atherosclerosis (In press).

CRAWFORD, M. D.: Hardness of drinking-water and cardiovascular disease. Proc.
Nutr. Soc. 31, 347 - 353 (1972).

CRAWFORD, M. D., GARDNER, M. J., MORRIS, J. N.: Mortality and hardness of local
water-supplies. Lancet 1968 I, 827 - 831.

CRAWFORD, M. D., GARDNER, M. J., MORRIS, J. N.: Changes in water hardness and
local death-rates. Lancet 1971 II, 327 - 329.

CRAWFORD, M. D., GARDNER, M. J., MORRIS, J. N.: Cardiovascular disease and the
mineral content of drinking water. Brit. med. Bull. 27, 21 - 24 (1971).

CRAWFORD, M. D., GARDNER, M. J., MORRIS, J. N.: Water hardness, rainfall and cardiovascular mortality. Lancet 1972 I, 1396 - 1397.

CRAWFORD, T., CRAWFORD, M.D.: Prevalence and pathological changes of ischaemic
heart disease in a hard-water and in a soft-water area. Lancet 1967 I, 229 -
232.

CROCKET, R., DALLOCHIO, M., RAZAKA, G., Bricaud, H., BROUSTET, P.: Etude biolog-
ique du sérum chez le lapin, au cours de l'immunisation par antigène aortique.
Revue de L'atherosclerose 10, 44 (1968).

CRUNKHORN, P., WILLIS, A. L.: Cutaneous reactions to intradermal prostaglandins.
Brit. J. Pharmacol. 41, 49 - 56 (1971).

CRUZ, A. B., AMATUSIO, D. S., GRANDE, F., HAY, L. J.: Effect of intra-arterial
insulin on tissue cholesterol and fatty acids in alloxan diabetic dogs. Circ.
Res. 9, 39 (1961).

CUCUIANU, M. P., NISHIZAWA, E. E., MUSTARD, J. F.: Effect of pyrimido-pyrimidine
compounds on platelet function. J. Lab. Clin. Med. 77, 958 - 974 (1971).

CUDKOWICZ, L., ARMSTRONG, J. B.: The blood supply of malignant pulmonary neoplasms. Thorax 8, 152 - 156 (1953).

CURRAN, R. C., CRANE, W. A. J.: Mucopolysaccharides in the atheromatous aorta.
J. Path. Bact. 84, 405 (1962).

DAHLEN, G., ERICSON, C., FURBERG, C., LUNDKVIST, L., SVÄRDSUDD, K.: Studies on an
extra pre-beta lipoprotein fraction. Acta med. scand. suppl. 531 (1972).

DAHME, E., KALICH, J., KAISER, E., FREYTAG VON LORINGSHOVEN, K., STAVROU, D.:
Studie zur Arteriosklerosegenese beim Hanford-Miniaturschwein unter normalen
und experimentellen Bedingungen. Atherosclerosis 14, 153 - 168 (1971).

DALFERES, E. R., Jr., RUIZ, H., KUMAR, V., RADHAKRISHNAMURTHY, B., BERENSON, G.
S.: Acid mucopolysaccharides of fatty streaks in young human male aortas,
Atherosclerosis 13, 121 - 131 (1971).

DALY, M. M.: Effect of hypertension on lipid composition of rat aortic intima-
media. Circ. Res. 31, 410 (1972).

DANES, S.: Cell culture and genetic disease. Hosp. Practice 4, 88 (1969).

DANIELLI, J. F., DAVSON, H.: A contribution to the theory of thin films. J. Cell.
Comp. Physiol. 5:4, 495 (1935).

DANIELSSON, H., EINARSSON, K., JOHANSSON, G.: Effect of biliary drainage on individual reactions in the conversion of cholesterol to taurocholic acid. Europ.
J. Biochem. 2, 44 (1967).

DANOWSKI, T. S., KHURANA, R. C., GONZALES, A. R., FISHER, E. R.: Capillary basement membrane thickness and the pseudodiabetes of myopathy. Amer. J. Med. 51,
757 - 766 (1971).

DAOUD, A.S., FRITZ, K. E., JARMOLYCH, J.: Increased DNA synthesis in aortic explants from swine fed high cholesterol diet. Exp. Mol. Pathol. 13, 377 (1970).

DAOUD, A. S., FRITZ, K. E., JARMOLYCH, J., AUGUSTYN, J. M.: Use of aortic medial
explants in the study of atherosclerosis. Exp. Mol. Pathol. 18, 177 (1973).

DAOUD, A. S., FRITZ, K. E., SINGH, J., AUGUSTYN, J. M., JARMOLYCH, J.: Production
of mucopolysaccharides, collagen and elastic tissue by aortic medial explants.
Proc. Int. Wksp. Arterial Mesenchyme and Arteriosclerosis (In press).

DARMADY, J. H., FOSBROOKE, A. S., LLOYD, J. K.: Prospective study of serum cholesterol levels during first year of life. Brit. Med. J. 2, 685 - 688 (1972).

DAVIDOFF, F., TISHLER, S., ROSOFF, C.: Marked hyperlipidemia and pancreatitis
associated with oral contraceptive therapy. New Engl. J. Med. 289, 552
(1973).

DAVIES, B. J.: Disc electrophoresis. Ann. N. Y. Acad. Sci. 121, 404 (1964).

DAVIGNON, J.: Treatment of primary hyperlipoproteinemias with drugs. Modern Med.
Canada 27, 605 - 615 (August 1972).

DAVIGNON, J., AUBRY, F., NOEL, C., LAPIERRE, Y., LAFORTUNE, M.: Heterogeneity of
familial hyperlipoproteinemia type II on the basis of fasting plasma trigly-
ceride/cholesterol ratio and plasma cholesterol response to ethyl p-chlorophenoxyisobutyrate. Rev. Can. Biol. 30, 307 - 318 (1971).

DAY, A. J., BELL, F. P., MOORE, S., FRIEDMAN, R.: Lipid composition and metabolism of thrombo-atherosclerotic lesions produced by continued endothelial
damage in normal rabbits. Circ. Res. (submitted for publication in 1973).

DAY, A. J., GOULD-HURST, P. R. S.: Cholesterol esterase activity of normal and
atherosclerotic rabbit aorta. Biochim. Biophys. Acta 116, 169 (1966).

DAY, A. J., TUME, R. K.: Incorporation of (^{14}C) oleic acid into lipid by foam
cells and by other fractions separated from rabbit atherosclerotic lesions.
Atherosclerosis 11, 291 (1970).

DAY, A. J., WAHLQVIST, M. L.: The uptake and metabolism of ^{14}C-labeled oleic acid
by atherosclerotic lesions in rabbit aorta. A biochemical and radioautographic study. Circ. Res. 23, 779 (1968).

DAY, A. J., WAHLQVIST, M. L.: Localization by autoradiography of phospholipid
synthesis in rabbit atherosclerotic aorta. Exp. Molec. Pathol. 11, 263 (1969).

DAY, A. J., WAHLQVIST, M. L., CAMPBELL, D. J.: Differential uptake of cholesterol
and of different cholesterol esters by atherosclerotic intima in vivo and in
vitro. Atherosclerosis 11, 301 - 320 (1970).

DAYTON, S.: Dietary prevention of heart disease. Lipid Metabolism and Atherosclerosis. Proceedings of Symposium of Netherland Society for Cardiology (COTTON,
D., Ed.). Excerpta Medica (1973).

DAYTON, S., HASHIMOTO, S.: Origin of fatty acids in lipids of experimental rabbit
atheroma. J. Atheroscler. Res. 8, 555 (1968).

DAYTON, S., HASHIMOTO, S.: Recent advances in molecular pathology: a review. Cholesterol flux and metabolism in arterial tissue and in atheromata. Exp. Mol.
Pathol. 13, 253 - 268 (1970).

DAYTON, S., HASHIMOTO, S.: Origin of cholesteryl oleate and other esterified
lipids of rabbit atheroma. Atherosclerosis 12, 371 (1970).

DEAMER, D. W., KRUGER, F. A., CORNWALL, D. G.: Total liver protein and amino acid
incorporation into liver protein in orotic acid-induced fatty liver. Biochim.
Biophys. Acta 97, 147 - 149 (1965).

DE GENNES, J. L. et al.: Thrombose de la carotide interne après un seul cycle de
contraceptifs oraux au troisieme mois du post partum chez une femme de 27 ans
présentant une hyperlipidémie familiale. Soc. Med. Hôpitaux Paris 118, 899
(1967).

DE HAAS, J. H.: Primary Prevention of Coronary Heart Disease. Heart 4, 3 (1973).

DEJEDAR, R., ROUBKAVA, H., CACHOVAN, M., et al.: Comparison of postmortem angiograms with macroscopic and microscopic findings in the femoral and popliteal
arteries. Arch. für Kreislaufforschung 54, 309 (1967).

DE LALLA, O. F., GOFMAN, J. W.: Ultracentrifugal analysis of serum lipoproteins. In: Methods of Biochemical Analysis, Vol. 1, p. 459 (GLICK, D., Ed.). New York: Interscience 1954.

DE MEIS, L., MAROJA, R.: Release of an esterase from liver upon heparin injection. Quart. J. Exp. Physiol. 52, 174 - 183 (1967).

DEMPSEY, M. E.: Cholesterol biosynthesis in liver tissue. In: Chemistry of brain development, 31 - 39. New York: Plenum 1971.

DEMPSEY, M. E.: Cholesterol Biosynthesis in vitro. In: Pharmacology of hypolipidemic agents. Berlin: Springer-Verlag 1974 a (In press).

DEMPSEY, M. E.: Regulation of steroid biosynthesis. Ann. Rev. Biochemistry 1974 b (In press).

DEMPSEY, M. E.: Sterol carrier protein. In: Sub-unit enzymes: Biochemistry and function. New York: Dekker 1974 c (In press).

DEMPSEY, M. E., RITTER, M, C., LUX, S. E.: Functions of a specific plasma apolipoprotein in cholesterol biosynthesis. Fed. Proc. 31, 430 (1972).

DENCKLA, W. D., DEWEY, H. K.: The determination of tryptophan in plasma, liver, urine. J. Lab. Clin. Med. 69, 160 - 169 (1967).

DE PALMA, R. G., HUBAY, C. A., INSULL, W., Jr., ROBINSON, A. V., HARTMAN, A. H.: Progression and regression of experimental atherosclerosis. Surg. Gynec. Obstet. 131, 633 - 647 (1970).

DE PALMA, R. G., HUBAY, C. A., VOGT, C. J., INSULL, W., HARTMAN, P. H., ROBINSON, A. V.: Regression and prevention of experimental atherosclerosis: Effects of diet and bile diversion in the dog. Surg. Forum 19, 308 (1968).

DEUPREE, R. H., FIELDS, R. I., McMAHAN, C. A., STRONG, J. P.: Atherosclerotic lesions and coronary heart disease: Key relationships in necropsied cases. Lab. Invest. 28, 252 - 262 (1973).

DEUTSCHER, S., OSTRANDER, L. D., EPSTEIN, F. H.: Familial factors in premature coronary heart disease - A preliminary report from the Tecumseh Community Health Study. Amer. J. Epidem. 91, 233 (1970).

DE WULF, H., HERS, H. G.: The role of glucose, glucagon and glucocorticoids in the regulation of liver glycogen synthesis. Eur. J. Biochem. 6, 558 (1968).

DIDISHEIM, P., OWEN, C. A., Jr.: Effect of dipyridamole (Persantin) and its derivatives on thrombosis and platelet function. Thromb. Diath. Haemorrh. Suppl. 42, 267 - 275 (1970).

DIETERICH, R.A., VAN PELT, R. W., GALSTER, W. A.: Diet-induced cholesteremia and atherosclerosis in wild rodents. Atherosclerosis 17, 345 - 352 (1973).

DIETSCHY, J. M., WILSON, J. D.: Regulation of cholesterol metabolism. New Engl.J. Med. 282, 1128 (1970).

DIXON, F. J., SCHULTZ, R. T., MILGROM, F.: Cardiac lesions in rabbits injected with autologous gamma-globulins. Lab. Invest. 14, 2056 (1965).

DOCK, W.: The predilection of atherosclerosis for the coronary arteries. JAMA 131, 875 - 878 (1946).

DOLE, V. P.: A relation between non esterified fatty acids in plasma and the metabolism of glucose. J. Clin. Investig. 35, 150 (1956).

DOLL, R., HILL, A. B.: Mortality in relation to smoking: Ten years observations of British doctors. Brit. Med. J. 1, 1399 (1964).

DOYLE, J. T., DAWBER, T. R., KANNEL, W. B., HESLIN, A., SANDRA, KAHN, H. A.: Cigarette smoking and coronary heart disease. Combined experience of the Albany and Framingham studies. New Engl. J. Med. 266, 796 (1962).

DOYLE, J. T., DAWBER, T. R., KANNEL, W. B., KINCH, S. H., KAHN, H. A.: The relationship of cigarette smoking to coronary heart disease; the second report of the combined experience of the Albany, N. Y., and Framingham, Mass., studies. Am. Med. Ass. J. 190, 886 - 890 (1964).

DRASH, A.: Atherosclerosis, cholesterol and the paediatrician. J. Pediat. 80, 693 (1973).

DRILL, V. A.: Oral contraceptives and thromboembolic disease I. prospective and retrospective studies. Amer. Med. Assoc. J. 219, 583 - 592 (1972).

DUFF, G. L., BRECHIN, D. J. H., FINKELSTEIN, W. E.: The effect of alloxan diabetes on experimental cholesterol atherosclerosis in the rabbit. IV: The effect of insulin therapy on the inhibition of atherosclerosis in the alloxan-diabetic rabbit. J. Exper. Med. 100, 371 (1954).

DUFF, L., McMILLAN, G. C.: Effect of alloxan diabetes on experimental cholesterol atherosclerosis in the rabbit. J. exp. Med. 89, 611 - 630 (1949).

DUGAN, F. A., RADHAKRISHNAMURTHY, B., BERENSON, G. S.: Enzymograms of glyco-protein preparations from connective tissue. Enzymologia 33, 215 - 223 (1967).

DUGDALE, M., MASI, A. T.: Hormonal contraception and thromboembolic disease: effects of the oral contraceptives on hemostatic mechanisms. A review of the literature. J. Chronic Diseases 23, 775 - 790 (1971).

DUGUID, J. B.: Thrombosis as a factor in the pathogenesis of coronary atherosclerosis. J. Path. Bact. 58, 207 - 212 (1946).

DUGUID, J. B.: Thrombosis as a factor in the pathogenesis of aortic atherosclerosis. J. Path. Bact. 60, 57 - 61 (1948).

DULIN, W. E., WYSE, B. H.: Diabetes in the kk mouse. Diabetologia 6, 317 (1970).

DUNCAN, L. E., BUCK, K., LYNCH, A.: The effect of pressure and stretching on the passage of labelled albumin into canine aortic wall. J. Atheroscler. Res. 5, 69 - 79 (1965).

DUNCAN, L. E., CORNFIELD, J., BUCK, K., LYNCH, A.: The effect of blood pressure on the passage of labelled plasma albumin into canine aortic wall. J. Clin. Invest. 41, 1537 - 1545 (1962).

DUPONT, J., DUPONT, J. C., FROMENT, A., MILON, H., VINCENT, M.: Selection of three strains of rats with spontaneously different levels of blood pressure. Biomedicine 1, 36 - 41 (1973).

DURY, A.: Lipid distribution and metabolism in two areas of aorta of normal and cholesterol-fed rabbits. Proc. Soc. Exp. Biol. Med. 94, 70 (1957).

DYERBERG, J., HJORNE, N.: Quantitative plasma lipoprotein estimation by agarose gel electrophoresis. Clin. Chim. Acta. 28, 203 (1970).

DZOGA, K., JONES, R., VESSELINOVITCH, D., WISSLER, R. W.: Use of enzyme labeled antibodies to identify smooth muscle cells in tissue culture. Fed. Proc. 29, 444 (1970).

DZOGA, K., VESSELINOVITCH, D., FRASER, R., WISSLER, R. W.: The effect of lipoproteins on the growth of aortic smooth muscle cells in vitro. Am. J. Path. 62, 32 a (1971).

EATON, R. P., BERMAN, M., STEINBERG, D.: Kinetic studies of plasma free fatty acid and triglyceride metabolism in man. J. Clin. Invest. 48, 1560 (1969).

ECCLESTON, D., ASHCROFT, G. W., CRAWFORD, T. B. B.: 5-Hydroxyindole metabolism in the rat brain. A study of intermediate metabolism using the technique of tryptophan loading. J. Neurochem. 12, 493 - 503 (1965).

EDELSTEIN, C., LIM, C. T., SCANU, A. M.: The serum high density lipoproteins of Macacus rhesus. II. Isolation, purification, and characterization of their two major polypeptides. J. Biol. Chem. 248, 7653 (1973).

EDHOLM, O. G., HOWARTH, S., SHARPEY-SCHAFER, E. P.: Resting blood flow and blood pressure in limbs with arterial obstruction. Clin. Sci. 10, 361 (1951).

EDWARDS, P. A.: Effect of adrenalectomy and hypophysectomy on the circadian rhythm of β-hydroxy-β-methylglutaryl coenzyme A reductase activity in rat liver. J. Biol. Chem. 248, 2912 - 2917 (1973).

EGELRUD, T.: Reversible binding of lipoprotein lipase from hen adipose tissue to insolubilized heparin. Biochim. Biophys. Acta 296, 124 (1973).

EGELRUD, T., OLIVECRONA, T.: The purification of a lipoprotein lipase from bovine skim milk. J. Biol. Chem. 247, 6212 (1972).

EGELRUD, T., OLIVECRONA, T.: Purified bovine milk (lipoprotein) lipase: activity against lipid substrates in the absence of exogenous serum factors. Biochim. Biophys. Acta 306, 115 (1973).

EGGEN, D. A., SOLBERG, L. A.: Variation of atherosclerosis with age. Lab. Invest. 18, 571 - 579 (1968).

EGGEN, D. A., STRONG, J. P., NEWMAN, W. P., III: Experimental atherosclerosis in primates: A comparison of selected species. Ann. N. Y. Acad. Sci. 162, 110-119 (1969).

EHNHOLM, C., BENSADOUN, A., BROWN, W. V.: Separation and partial purification of two types of triglyceride lipase from swine post-heparin plasma. J. Clin. Invest. 52, 26 a (1973).

EHNHOLM, C., GAROFF, H., RENKONEN, O., SIMONS, K.: Protein and carbohydrate composition of Lp(a) lipoprotein from human plasma. Biochemistry 11, 3229 (1972).

EHNHOLM, C., GAROFF, H., SIMONS, K., ARO, H.: Purification and quantitation of the human plasma lipoprotein carrying the Lp(a) antigen. Biochim. Biophys. Acta 236, 431 (1971).

EHNHOLM, C., SHAW, W., GRETEN, H., BROWN, W. V.: Purification from human plasma of a heparin-released lipase with activity against triglyceride and phospholipids. J. Biol. Chem. (Submitted for publication 1973).

EINARSSON, K., HELLSTRÖM, K.: The formation of bile acids in patients with three types of hyperlipoproteinaemia. Europ. J. Clin. Invest. 2, 225 (1972).

EINARSSON, K., HELLSTRÖM, K., KALLNER, M.: The effect of clofibrate on the elimination of cholesterol as bile acids in patients with hyperlipoproteinaemia type II and IV. Europ. J. Clin. Invest. 3, 345 (1973).

EISENBERG, S., BILHEIMER, D. W., LEVY, R. I.: The metabolism of very low density lipoprotein proteins. II. Studies on the transer of apoproteins between plasma lipoproteins. Biochim. Biophys. Acta 280, 94 (1972).

EISENBERG, S., BILHEIMER, D.W., LEVY, R. I., LINDGREN, F. T.: On the metabolic conversion of human plasma very low density lipoproteins to low density lipoproteins. Biochim. Biophys. Acta 326, 361 (1973).

EISENBERG, S., BILHEIMER, D. W., LINDGREN, F., LEVY, R. I.: On the apoprotein composition of human plasma very low density lipoprotein subfractions. Biochim. Biophys. Acta 260, 329 (1972).

EISENBERG, S., STEIN, O., STEIN, Y.: Phospholipases in arterial tissue. VI. The role of growth and age in the development of phosphatidylacyl-hydrolase activity in aortic tissue. Biochim. Biophys. Acta 231, 505 (1971).

EISENBERG, S., STEIN, Y., STEIN, O.: Phospholipases in arterial tissue. II. Phosphatide acyl-hydrolase and lysophosphatide acyl-hydrolase activity in human and rat arteries. Biochim. Biophys. Acta 164, 205 (1968).

EISENBERG, S., STEIN, Y., STEIN, O.: Phospholipases in arterial tissue. III. Phosphatidyl acyl-hydrolase, lysophosphatide acyl-hydrolase and sphingomyelin choline phosphohydrolase in rat and rabbit aorta in different age groups. Biochim. Biophys. Acta 176, 557 (1969 a).

EISENBERG, S., STEIN, Y., STEIN, O.: Phospholipases in arterial tissue. IV. The role of phosphatidyl acyl-hydrolase, lysophosphatide acyl hydrolase, and sphingomyelin choline phosphohydrolase in the regulation of phospholipid composition in the normal human aorta with age. J. Clin. Invest. 48, 2320 (1969 b).

ELIASSON, R., BYGDEMAN, S.: Effect of dipyridamole and two pyrimido-pyrimidine derivatives on the kinetics of human platelet aggregation and on platelet adhesiveness. Scand. J. Clin. Lab. Invest. 24, 145 - 151 (1969).

ELKELES, R. S., HAMPTON, J. R., MITCHELL, J. R. A.: Effect of oestrogens on human platelet behaviour. Lancet 1968 2, 315 - 318.

ELMFELDT, D., WILHELMSEN, L.: A study of representative post-myocardial infarction patients aged 27 - 55. In: Preventive Cardiology p. 129 (eds. TIBBLIN, G., KEYS, A., and WERKÖ, L.). New York: J. Wiley and Sons 1972).

EMMONS, P. R., HARRISON, M. J. G., HONOUR, A. J., MITCHELL, J. R. A.: Effect of dipyridamole on human platelet behaviour. Lancet 1965 a II, 603 - 606.

EMMONS, P. R., HARRISON, M. J. G., HONOUR, A. J., MITCHELL, J. R. A.: Effect of a pyrimidopyrimidine derivative on thrombus formation in the rabbit. Nature 208, 255 (1965 b).

EPSTEIN, F. H.: Hyperglycemia: A risk factor in coronary heart disease. Circulation 36, 609 (1967).

EPSTEIN, F. H.: Epidemiologic aspects of atherosclerosis. Atherosclerosis 14, 1 (1971).

EPSTEIN, F. H.: Glucose intolerance and cardiovascular disease. Triangle 12, 3 (1973).

ERHARDT, L. R., LUNDMAN, T., MELLSTEDT, H.: Incorporation of ^{125}I-labelled fibrinogen into coronary arterial thrombi in acute myocardial infarction in man. Lancet 1973 II, 387 - 390.

ERIKSSON, M., CARLSON, L. A.: Quantitative and qualitative serum lipoprotein analyses in healthy men compared with male myocardial infarctions and intermittent claudication. This volume p. 838.

ESTERLY, J. A.: Observations on the possible relationship of hypertension, increased arterial permeability to blood cells, and atherogenesis. New Physician 14, 145 - 151 (1965).

EVANS, G.: Effect of platelet-suppressive agents on the incidence of amaurosis fugax and transient cerebral ischemia. In: Cerebral Vascular Diseases, Eighth

Conference, p. 297 - 300 (McDOWELL, F. H., and BRENNAR, R. W., Eds.). New York: Grune and Stratton 1973.

EVANS, G., PACKHAM, M. A., NISHIZAWA, E. E., MUSTARD, J. F., MURPHY, E. A.: The effect of acetylsalicylic acid on platelet function. J. Exp. Med. 128, 877 - 894 (1968).

EVANS, R. L., PELLEY, J. W., QUENEMOEN, L.: Some simple geometric and mechanical characteristics of mammalian blood vessels. Amer. J. Physiol. 199, 1150 - 1152 (1960).

FAERGEMAN, O., DAMGAARD-PEDERSEN, F.: Increase of post-heparin lipase activity by oxandrolone in familial hyperchlomicronemia Scand. J. Clin. Lab. Invest. 31, 27 - 31 (1973).

FAHEY, J. L., LAWRENCE, M. E.: Quantitative determination of 6.6 S γ-globulins, β2A-globulins and γ1-macroglobulins in human serum. J. Immunol. 91, 597 (1963).

FAIRBANKS, G., STECK, T. L., WALLACH, D. F. H.: Electrophoretic analysis of the major polypeptides of the human erythrocyte membrane. Biochemistry 10, 2606 (1971).

FAJANS, S. S.: What is diabetes? Med. Clin. N. Amer. 55, 793 (1971).

FAJANS, S. S.: Current unsolved problems in diabetes management. Diabetes 21 (Suppl. 2), 678 (1972).

FALCONER, D. S.: The inheritance of liability to certain diseases estimated from the incidence among relatives. Ann. Hum. Genet., Lond.,29, 51 (1965).

FALOONA, G. R., STEWART, B. N., FRIED, M.: The effects of actinomycin D on the biosynthesis of plasma lipoproteins. Biochemistry 7, 720 (1968).

FARBER, E.: Ethionine fatty liver. Advances Lipid Res. 5, 119 - 183 (1967).

FARQUHAR, J. W., GROSS, R. C., WAGNER, R. M., REAVEN, G. M.: Validation of an incompletely coupled two-compartment nonrecycling catenary model for turnover of liver and plasma triglyceride in man. J. Lipid Res. 6, 119 (1965).

FEDERMAN, J. L., GERRITSEN, G. C.: The retinal vasculature of the Chinese hamster: A preliminary study. Diabetologia 6, 186 (1970).

FEINLEIB, M.: Genetic epidemiology of coronary heart disease. Paper presented at the 24th Annual Meeting, American Society of Human Genetics, Philadelphia 1972.

FELDMAN, S. A., HO, K. J., LEWIS, L. A., MIKKELSON, B., TAYLOR, C. B.: Lipid and cholesterol metabolism in Alaskan Arctic Eskimos. Arch. Path. 94, 42 (1972).

FELT, V., BENES, P.: The incorporation of (4-^{14}C) cholesterol into different cholesterol esters of rat aorta in vitro. Biochim. Biophys. Acta 176, 435 (1969).

FERNSTRÖM, J. D., LAZIN, E., WURTMAN, R.: Daily variations in the concentrations of individual amino acids in rat plasma. Life Sci. 10, 813 - 819 (1971).

FIELDING, C. J.: Purification of lipoprotein lipase from rat post-heparin plasma. Biochim. Biophys. Acta 178, 499 (1969).

FIELDING, C. J.: Human lipoprotein lipase I, Purification and substrate specifity. Biophys. Acta 206, 109 (1970).

FIELDING, C. J.: Further characterization of lipoprotein lipase and hepatic post-heparin lipase from rat plasma. Biochim. Biophys. Acta 280, 569 (1972).

FIELDING, C. J.: Kinetics of lipoprotein lipase activity: effects of the substrate apoprotein on reaction velocity. Biochim. Biophys. Acta 316, 66 (1973).

FIELDING, J., FIELDING, P. E.: Purification and substrate specificity of lecithin cholesterol acyl transferase from human plasma. FEBS letters 15, 355 (1971).

FILIPOVIC, I., BUDDECKE, E.: Increased fatty acid synthesis of arterial tissue in hypoxia. Eur. J. Biochem. 20, 587 (1971).

FILIPOVIC, I., KRESSE, H., BUDDECKE, E.: ATP-controlled fatty acid synthesis in cultured arterial fibroblasts. Eur. J. Biochem. 36, 541 (1973).

FISCHER, G. M.: In vivo effects of estradiol on collagen and elastin in rabbit aorta. Endo. 91, 1227 (1972).

FISCHER, G. M., LLAURADO, J. G.: Collagen and elastin content in canine arteries selected from functionally different vascular beds. Circulation Res. 19, 394 (1966).

FISCHER-DZOGA, K., CHEN, R., WISSLER, R. W.: Effects of serum lipoproteins on the morphology, growth and metabolism of arterial smooth muscle cells. Proceedings of the Workshop on Arterial Mesenchyme and Arteriosclerosis, New Orleans, 1973 (In press).

FISCHER-DZOGA, K., JONES, R. M., VESSELINOVITCH, D., WISSLER, R. W.: Increased mitotic activity in primary cultures of aortic medial smooth muscle cells after exposure ro hyperlipemic serum. This volume p. 193.

FISCHER-DZOGA, K., JONES, R. M., VESSELINOVITCH, D., WISSLER, R. W.: Ultrastructural and immunohistochemical studies of primary cultures of aortic medial cells. Exp. Molec. Path. 18, 162 (1973 a).

FISHER, C. M.: Observations of the fundus oculi in transient monocular blindness. Neurology 9, 333 - 347 (Mineapolis 1969).

FISHER, E. R., FISHER, B.: Effect of induced atherosclerosis on fresh and lyophilised aortic homografts in rabbits. Surgery 40, 530 (1956).

FISHER, W. R.: The characterization and occurence of an Sf 20 serum lipoprotein. J. Biol. Chem. 245, 877 (1970).

FLATZ, G.: Serum-cholesterol, ABO blood-groups and haemoglobin type. Genetic influences on the serum-cholesterol level. Humangenetik 10, 318 (1970).

FLORENTIN, R. A., NAM, S. C.: Dietary-induced atherosclerosis in miniature swine. I. Gross and light microscopy observations: Time of development and morphologic characteristics of lesions. Exp. and Mol. Path. 8, 263 (1968).

FLORENTIN, R. A., NAM, S. C., LEE, K. T., LEE, K. J., THOMAS, W. A.: Increased mitotic activity in aortas of swine after three days of cholesterol feeding. Arch. Pathol. 88, 463 - 469 (1969).

FOLCH, J.: A simple method for the isolation and purification of total lipids from animal tissue. J. Biol. Chem. 226, 497 (1957).

FOLCH, J., ASCOLI, I., LEES, M., HEATH, J. A., LEBARON, F. N.: Preparation of lipid extracts from brain tissue. J. Biol. Chem. 191, 833 (1951).

FOLCH, J., LEES, M., SLOANE-STANLEY, G. H.: A simple method for the isolation and purification of total lipids from animal tissues. J. Biol. Chem. 226, 497 - 509 (1957).

FOMONS, S., BARTELS, D. J.: Concentration of cholesterol in serum of infants in relation to diet. Amer. J. Dis. Child. 99, 27 (1960).

FORTE, T. M., NICHOLS, A. V.: Application of electron microscopy to the study of plasma lipoprotein structure. Adv. Lipid Res. 10, 1 (1972).

FORTE, G. M., NICHOLS, A. V., GLAESER, R. M.: Electron microscopy of human serum lipoproteins using negative staining. Chem. Phys. Lipids 2, 396 (1968).

FORTE, T. M., NORUM, K. R., GLOMSET, J. A., NICHOLS, A. V.: Plasma lipoproteins in familial lecithin: cholesterol acyltransferase deficiency: structure of low and high density lipoproteins as revealed by electron microscopy. J. Clin. Invest. 50, 1141 (1971).

FOWLER, P. B. S., SWALE, J., ANDREWS, H.: Hypercholesterolemia in borderline hypothyroidism stage of premyxoedema. Lancet 1970 II, 488 - 491.

FRANCIS, T., Jr., EPSTEIN, F. H.: Survey methods in general populations. Milbank Mem. Fund. Quart. 43, 333 (1965).

FRANZBLAU, C., FARIS, B., KAGAN, H. M., SCHMID, K.: Interaction of glycoprotein with collagen. Circulation 48, IV - 79 (1973).

FREDRICKSON, D. S.: A physician's guide to hyperlipoproteinemia. Modern Concepts Cardiovascular Dis. 16, 31 (1972).

FREDRICKSON, D. S.: Plasma lipoproteins and apoproteins. Harvey Lecture, February 15, 1973.

FREDRICKSON, D. S., GOTTO, A. M., LEVY, R. I.: Familial lipoprotein deficiency. In: Metabolic basis of inherited disease, 3rd edition, p. 493 (STANBURY, J. B., WYNGAARDEN, J. B., and FREDRICKSON, D. S., Eds.). New York: Mc Graw-Hill Book Co. 1972).

FREDRICKSON, D. S., LEVY, R. I.: Familial hyperlipoproteinemia. In: The Metabolic Basis of Inherited Disease, 3rd ed., p. 545 (STANBURY, J. B., WYNGAARDEN, J. B., and FREDRICKSON, D. S., Eds.). New York: Mc Graw-Hill 1972.

FREDRICKSON, D. S., LEVY, R. I., LEES, R. S.: Fat transport in lipoproteins: an integrated approach to mechanisms and disorders. New Engl. J. of Med. 276, 34, 94, 148, 215, 273 (1967).

FREDRICKSON, D. S., Levy, R. I., LINDGREN, F. T.: A comparison of heritable ab-
    normal lipoprotein patterns as defined by two different techniques. J. Clin.
    Invest. 47, 2446 - 2457 (1968).
FREDRICKSON, D. S., LUX, S. E., HERBERT, P. N.: The apolipoproteins. Adv. Exptl.
    Med. Biol. 26, 25 (1972).
FREDRICKSON, D. S., ONO, K., DAVIS, L. L.: Lipolytic activity of post-heparin
    plasma in hyperglyceridemia. J. Lipid Res. 4, 24 (1963).
FREEMAN, C. P., WEST, D.: Complete separation of lipid classes on a single thin-
    layer plate. J. Lipid Res. 7, 324 (1966).
FREIS, E. D.: Effect of antihypertensive treatment on morbidity (Part 2). Milbank
    Mem. Fund. Quart. 47, 153 (1969).
FRENCH, J. E.: Thrombosis as a factor in atherosclerosis. Angiology 17, 590 - 592
    (1966).
FRENCH, J. E., JENNINGS, M. A., FLOREY, H. W.: Morphological studies on athero-
    sclerosis in swine. Ann. N. Y. Acad. Sci. 127, 780 - 799 (1965).
FRIEDBERG, CH. K.: Erkrankungen des Herzens, p. 1224. Stuttgart: Georg Thieme
    Verlag 1959.
FRIEDEWALD, W. T., LEVY, R. I., FREDRICKSON, D. S.: Estimation of the concentra-
    tion of low density lipoprotein cholesterol without the use of the prepara-
    tive ultracentrifuge. Clinical Chemistry 18, 499 (1972).
FRIEDMAN, M.: Pathogenesis of coronary artery disease. New York: Mc Graw-Hill 1969.
FRIEDMAN, M., BYERS, S. O.: Experimental thrombo-atherosclerosis. J. Clin. Invest.
    40, 1139 - 1152 (1961).
FRIEDMAN, M., BYERS, S. O., ST. GEORGE, S.: Origin of lipid in experimental throm-
    boatherosclerosis. J. Clin. Invest. 41, 828 - 841 (1962).
FRIEDMAN, M., BYERS, S. O.: Endothelial permeability in atherosclerosis. Arch.
    Pathol. 76, 99 - 105 (1963).
FRITZ, K. E., JARMOLYCH, J., DAOUD, A. S., PETERS, T., Jr.: Factors influencing
    DNA synthesis and degradation present in swine serum and aortic tissue. Exp.
    Mol. Pathol. 16, 54 (1972).
FROLICH, E. D., TARAZI, R. C., DUSTAN, H. P.: Re-examination of the hemodynamics
    of hypertension, Amer. J. Med. Sci. 257, 9 - 23 (1969).
FRY, D. L.: Acute vascular endothelial changes associated with increased blood
    velocity gradients. Circ. Res. 22, 165 - 197 (1968).
FRY, D. L.: Certain chemorheologic considerations regarding the blood vascular
    interface with particular reference to coronary artery disease. Circulation
    Suppl. IV 39/40, 38 - 57 (1969).
FRY, D. L.: Responses of the arterial wall to certain physical factors. In Ciba
    Foundation Symposium on Mechanisms in the Development of Early Atheroma.
    Atherogenesis: Initiating factors, pp. 93 - 125. (Ciba Foundation Symposium
    12). Amsterdam: Associated Scientific Publishers 1973.
FUERTES - DE LA HABA, A., CURET, J. O., PELEGRINA, I., BANGDIWALA, I.: Thrombo-
    phlebitis among oral and nonoral contraceptive users. Obstet. Gynecol. 38,
    259 - 263 (1971).
FUHRMANN, W.: Arteriosclerose; Erkrankungen der Koronargefäße. In: Humangenetik:
    Ein kurzes Handbuch in fünf Bänden. Vol. III/2, p. 508 (BECKER, P. E., Ed.).
    Stuttgart: Thieme 1972.
FUJINAMI, T., OKADO, K., SENDA, K., SUGIMURA, M., KISHIKAWA, M.: Experimental
    atherosclerosis with ascorbic acid deficiency. Jap. Circ. J. 35, 1559 - 1565
    (1971).
FUKUI, K.: Clinical results of pyridinolcarbamate treatment of hemiplegics in
    Kakeyu Hospital. In: Atherogenesis. Excerpta Medica, p. 239 (1969).
FULLER, G. C., LANGNER, R. O.: Elevation of aortic proline hydroxylase: a bio-
    chemical defect in experimental arteriosclerosis. Science 165, 987 - 990
    (1970).
FULTON, G. P., AKERS, R. P., LUTZ, B. R.: White thrombo-embolism and vascular
    fragility in hamster cheek pouch after anticoagulants. Blood 8: 140 - 152
    (1953).
GAEBLER, O. H.: Further studies of anterior pituitary extracts. J. Biol. Chem.
    100, 46 (1930).
GALTON, D. J.: Regulation of supply of glycerol phosphate for lipogenesis in hu-
    man adipose tissue. Clin. Science 36, 505 (1969).

GALTON, D. J., BRAY, G. A.: Studies on lipolysis in human adipose cells. J. Clin. Invest. 46, 621 (1967).

GALTON, D. J., WILSON, J. P. D., KISSEBAH, A. H.: The effect of adult diabetes on glucose utilisation and esterification of palmitate by human adipose tissue. Europ. J. Clin. Invest. 1, 399 (1971).

GANESAN, D., BRADFORD, R. H., ALAUPOVIC, P., Mc CONATHY, W. J.: Differential activation of lipoprotein lipase from human post-heparin plasma, milk and adipose tissue by polypeptides from human apolipoprotein C. Fed. Eur. Biochem. Soc. Letters 15, 205 (1971).

GANESAN, D., BRADFORD, R. H., ALAUPOVIC, P., Mc CONATHY, W. J.: Activation of lipoprotein lipase from human postheparin plasma by specific polypeptides of human serum apolipoproteins. Fed. Proc. 30, 208 (1971).

GANGULY, M., CARNIGHAN, R. H., WESTPHAL, U.: Steroid-Protein Interactions. XIV. Interaction between Human α_1-Acid glycoprotein and Progesterone. Biochemistry 6, 2803 - 2814 (1967).

GARBASCH, C., CHRISTENSEN, B. C.: Scanning electron microscopy of aortic endothelial cell boundaries after staining with silver nitrate. Angiologica 7, 365 (1970).

GARDAIS, A., PICARD, J., HERMELIN, B.: Glycosaminoglycans distribution in aortic wall from five species. Comp. Biochem. Physiol. 44 B, 507 - 515 (1973).

GAST, C. F.: Influence of aspirin on hemostasis. Rheum. Dis. 23, 500 (1964).

GATTEREAU, A., DAVIGNON, J., LANGELIER, M., LEVESQUE, H. P.: An improved radiological method for the evaluation of Achilles tendon xanthomatosis. Canad. M. A. J. 108, 39 - 43 (1973).

GAYNOR, E.: Hormonally altered thrombogenicity in rabbit iliac arteries. Proc. 16th Annual Meeting American Society of Hematology, p. 39 (1973).

GEDDA, L., POGGI, D.: Sulla regolazione genetica del colesterolo ematica (Uno studio su 50 coppie gemellari MZ e 50 coppie DZ). Acta genet. med. (Roma) 9, 135 (1960).

GEER, J. C., CATSULIS, C., Mc GILL, H. C., Jr., STRONG, J. P.: Fine structure of the baboon aortic fatty streak. Am. J. Pathol. 52, 265 - 286 (1968).

GEER, J. C., HAUST, M. D.: Smooth muscle cells in atherosclerosis. Monogr. on Atheroscler., Vol. 2. Basel: Karger 1972.

GEER, J. C., Mc GILL, H. C., ROBERTSON, W. B., STRONG, J. P.: Histologic characteristics of coronary artery fatty streaks. Lab. Invest. 18, 565 - 570 (1968).

GEER, J. C., McGILL, H. C., STRONG, J. P.: The fine structure of human atherosclerotic lesions. Amer. J. Path. 38, 263 - 287 (1968).

GEER, J. C., PANGANAMALA, R. V., NEWMAN, H. A. I., CORNWELL, D. G.: Arterial wall metabolism. In: The pathogenesis of atherosclerosis, p. 200 - 213 (WISSLER, R. W., and GEER, J. C., Eds.). Baltimore: Williams and Wilkins 1972.

GEERTINGER, P., SORENSEN, H.: Complement and Arteriosclerosis. Atherosclerosis 18, 65 - 71 (1973).

GENT, A. E., BROOK, C. G. D., FOLEY, T. H., MILLER, T. N.: Dipyridamole: a controlled trial of its effect in acute myocardial infarction. Brit. Med. J. 4, 366 - 368 (1968).

GENTON, E., WEILY, H. S., STEELE, P. P.: Platelets, drugs and heart disease. Can. Med. Assoc. J. 108, 463 (1973).

GERMUTH, F. G., SENTERFIT, L. B., POLLACK, A. D.: Immune complex disease. I. Experimental acute and chronic glomerulonephritis. Johns' Hopkin Med. Journal 120, 225 (1967).

GERÖ, S.: Allergy and autoimmune factors. In: Atherosclerosis, p. 655 (SCHETTLER, F. G., and BOYD, G. S., Eds.). Amsterdam: Elsevier 1969.

GERÖ, S.: Demonstration of autoantibodies in cardiovascular diseases by vascular and other antigens. 6th European Congress of Cardiology. In: Revista Espanola de Cardiologia, Madrid, 1972.

GERÖ, S., GERGELY, J., DEVENYI, T., JAKAB, L., SZEKELY, J., VIRAG, S.: Role of mucoid substances of the aorta in the deposition of lipids. Nature (Lond.), 187, 152 (1960).

GERÖ, S., GERGELY, J., JAKAB, L., SZEKELY, J., VIRAG, S.: Comparative immunoelectrophoretic studies on homogenates of aorta, pulmonary arteries and inferior vena cava of atherosclerotic individuals. J. Atheroscler. Res. 1, 88 - 91 (1961).

GERÖ, S., VIRAG, S., BIHARI-VARGA, M., SZEKELY, J., FEHER, J.: Role of mucopoly-saccharides in the deposition and metabolism of lipids. Prog. biochem. Pharmacol. 2, 290 (1967).

GERRITSEN, G. C., DULIN, W. E.: Characterization of diabetes on the Chinese hamster. Diabetologia 3, 74 (1967).

GERTLER, M. M., LEETMA, H. E., SALUSTE, E., ROSENBERGER, J. L., GUTHRIE, R. G.: Ischemic heart disease: Insulin, carbohydrate and lipid interrelationships, Circulation 46, 103 (1972).

GERTLER, M. M., WHITE, P. D.: Coronary heart disease in young adults. Cambridge, Mass.: Havard University Press 1954.

GERTLER, M., WHITE, P. D., CADY, L. D., WHITER, H. H.: Coronary heart disease. A prospective study. Amer. J. med. Sci. 248, 377 (1964).

GESSA, G. L., BIGGIO, G., TAGLIAMONTE, A.: Brains serotonin turnover; dependence on free tryptophan concentration in plasma. Fed. Proc. 31, 599 (1972).

GEYER, G.: Ultrahistochemie. Stuttgart: Fischer 1969.

GIBOFSKY, A., JAFFE, E. A., FOTINO, M., BECKER, C. G.: Identification and comparison of histocompatibility antigens on fresh and cultured human vascular endothelium and lymphocates. (Manuscript in preparation).

GILBERT, C. H., GALTON, D. J.: The presence of a hormone-sensitive cyclase system in the rat aorta and its relation to lipolysis. Atheroscler. 18, 257 (1973).

GILBERT, J. B., MUSTARD, J. F.: Some effects of atromid on platelet economy and blood coagulation in man. J. Atherosclerosis Res. 3, 623 - 633 (1963).

GILFILLAN, J. L., HUNT, V. M., HUFF, J. W.: Hypolipemic properties of 2-Aceto-amidoethyl (p-chlorophenyl) (M-trifluoromethylphenoxy) acetate in the rat. Proc. Soc. Exp. Biol. Med. 136, 1274 - 1276 (1971).

GIORDANO, A. R., SPRARAGEN, S. C., HAMEL, H.: A model for the rapid production of atheromatous lesions in rabbits. Lab. Invest. 22, 94 - 99 (1970).

GIRARD, A., ROHEIM, P. S., EDER, H. A.: Lipoprotein synthesis and fatty acid mobilization in rats after partial hepatectomy. Biochim. Biophys. Acta 248, 105 (1971).

GLAGOV, S.: Hemodynamic risk factors: mechanical stress, mural architecture, medial nutrition, and the vulnerability of arteries to atherosclerosis. In: The pathogenesis of atherosclerosis, p. 164 - 199 (WISSLER, R. A., and GEER, J. C., Eds.). Baltimore: Williams and Wilkins 1972.

GLAGOV, S., ROWLEY, D. A., KOHUT, R. J.: Atherosclerosis of human aortas and its coronary and renal arteries. Arch. Path. 72, 558 (1961).

GLASER, G., MAGER, J.: Biochemical studies on the mechanism of action of liver poisons. II. Induction of fatty livers. Biochim. Biophys. Acta 261, 500 (1972).

GLAUMAN, H., DALLNER, G.: Lipid composition and turnover of rough and smooth microsomal membranes in rat liver. J. Lipid Res. 9, 720 - 729 (1968).

GLOMSET, J. A.: The plasma lecithin : cholesterol acyltransferase reaction. J. Lipid Res. 9, 155 - 167 (1968).

GLOMSET, J. A.: Plasma lecithin : cholesterol acyltransferase. In: Blood lipids and lipoproteins: Quantitation, composition, and metabolism. p. 745 (NELSON, G. J., Ed.). New York: Wiley-Interscience 1972.

GLOMSET, J. A., NICHOLS, A. V., NORUM, K. R., KING, W., FORTE, T.: Plasma lipoproteins in familial lecithin : cholesterol acyltransferase deficiency. J. Clin. Invest. 52, 1078 (1973).

GLOMSET, J. A., NORUM, K. R.: The metabolic rate of lecithin: cholesterol acyltransferase: Perspectives from pathology. Advances in Lipid Res. 11, 1 (1973).

GLOMSET, J. A., NORUM, K. R., NICHOLS, A. V., KING, W. C., MITCHELL, C. D., APPLEGATE, K. R., GJONE, E., GONG, E. M.: Plasma lipoproteins in familial lecithin : cholesterol acyltransferase deficiency. Effects of dietary manipulation. (To be submitted).

GLUECK, C. J.: Effects of oxandrolone on plasma triglycerides and postheparin lipolytic activity in patients with types III, IV and V familial hyperlipoproteinemia. Metabolism 20, 691 (1971).

GLUECK, C. J., BROWN, W. V., LEVY, R. I., GRETEN, H., FREDERICKSON, D. S.: Amelioration of hypertriglyceridemia by pregestational drugs in familial type V hyperlipoproteinemia. Lancet 1969 I, 1290.

GLUECK, C. J., HECKMAN, F., SCHOENFELD, M., STEINER, P., PEARCE, W.: Neonatal familial type II hyperlipoproteinemia: Cord blood cholesterol in 1800 births. Metabolism 20, 597 (1971).

GLUECK, C. J., LEVY, R. I., FREDRICKSON, D. S.: Norethindrone acetate, postheparin lipolytic activity, and plasma triglycerides in familial types I, III, IV, and V hyperlipoproteinemia - studies in 26 patients and five normal persons. Ann. Int. Med. 75, 345 - 352 (1971).

GLUECK, C. J., LEVY, R. I., GLUECK, H. I., GRALNICK, H. R., GRETEN, H., FREDRICKSON, D. S.: Acquired type I hyperlipoproteinemia with systemic lupus erythematosus, dysglobulinemia and heparin resistance. Am. J. Med. 47, 318 (1969).

GLUECK, C. I., Mc KENZIE, M. R., GLUECK, C. J.: Crystalline IgG protein in multiple myeloma: identification effects on coagulation and on lipoprotein metabolism. J. of Lab. and Clin. Medicine 79, 731 (1972).

GLUECK, C. J., SCHEEL, D., FORD, S., STEINER, P. M.: Colestipol and cholestyramine resin: comparative effects in familial type II hyperlipoproteinemia. J. Amer. med. Ass. 222, 676 (1972).

GLUECK, C. J., TSANG, R., FALLAT, R., BUNCHER, C. R., EVANS, G., STEINER, P.: Familial hypertriglyceridemia: Studies in 130 children and 45 siblings of 36 index cases. Metabolism 22, 1287 (1973).

GODFREY, R. C., STENHOUSE, N. S., CULLEW, K. J., BLACKMAN, V.: Cholesterol and the child: Studies of the cholesterol levels of Bussleton school children and their parents. Austr. pediatr. J. 8, 72 (1972).

GOFMAN, J. W., DE LALLA, O., GLAZIER, F., FREEMAN, N. K., LINDGREN, F. T., NICHOLS, A. V., STRISOWER, E. H., TAMPLIN, A. R.: Serum lipoprotein transport system in health, metabolic disorders, atherosclerosis and coronary artery disease. Plasma 2, 413 - 486 (1954).

GOFMAN, J. W., RUBIN, L., Mc GINLEY, J. P., JONES, H. B.: Hyperlipoproteinemia. Am. J. Med. 17, 514 (1954).

GOFMAN, J. W., YOUNG, W.: The filtration concept of atherosclerosis and serum lipids in the diagnosis of atherosclerosis. In: Atherosclerosis and its origin, p. 197 - 229 (SANDLER, M., and BOURNE, G. H., Eds.). New York: Academic Press 1963.

GOLDSMITH, H. L.: The flow of model particles and blood cells and its relation to thrombogenesis. In: Progress in hemostasis and thrombosis, Vol. 1, p. 97 - 139 (SPAET, T. H., Ed.). New York: Grune and Stratton 1972.

GOLDSMITH, J. R.: Carbon monoxide and coronary heart disease. Ann. Intern. Med. 71, 199 (1969).

GOLDSTEIN, J. L., ALBERS, J. J., HAZZARD, W. R., SCHROTT, H. G., BIERMAN, E. L., MOTULSKY, A. G.: Genetic and medical significance of neonatal hyperlipidemia. J. Clin. Invest. 52, 35 a (1973 c).

GOLDSTEIN, J. L., BROWN, M. S.: Familial hypercholesterolemia: Identification of a defect in the regulation of 3-hydroxy-3-methylglutaryl coenzyme. A reductase activity associated with overproduction of cholesterol. Proc. Nat. Acad. Sci. 70, 2804 (1973).

GOLDSTEIN, J. L., HARROD, M. J. E., BROWN, M. S.: Homozygous familial hypercholesterolemia: Specificity of the biochemical defect in cultured cells and feasibility of prenatal detection. Amer. J. Hum. Genet. (In press).

GOLDSTEIN, J. L., HAZZARD, W. R., SCHROTT, H. G., BIERMAN, E. L., MOTULSKY, A. G.: Hyperlipidemia in coronary heart disease. I. Lipid levels in 500 survivors of myocardial infarction. J. Clin. Invest. 52, 1533 (1973 a).

GOLDSTEIN, J. L., MOTULSKY, A. G.: Genetics and endocrinology. In: Textbook of endocrinology, 5th ed. (WILLIAMS, R. H., Ed.). Philadelphia: W. B. Saunders 1974 (In press).

GOLDSTEIN, J. L., SCHROTT, H. G., HAZZARD, W. R., BIERMAN, E. L., MOTULSKY, A. G.: Hyperlipidemia in coronary heart disease. II. Genetic analysis of lipid levels of 176 families and delineation of a new inherited disorder, combined hyperlipidemia. J. Clin. Invest. 52, 1544 - 1568 (1973).

GOMORI, G.: The distribution of phosphatase in normal organs and tissue. J. Cell. Comp. Physiol. 17, 71 - 74 (1941).

GOODMAN, DeW, S.: Cholesterol ester metabolism. Physiol. Rev. 45, 747 (1965).

GOODMAN, DeW, S., NOBLE, R. P.: Turnover of plasma cholesterol in man. J. Clin. Invest. 47, 231 (1968).

GOODMAN, DeW, S., NOBLE, R. P., DELL, R. B.: Three-pool model of the long-term turnover of plasma cholesterol in man. J. Lipid Res. 14, 178 (1973).

GOODMAN, DeW, S., NOBLE, R. P., DELL, R. B.: The effects of colestipol resin and of colestipol plus clofibrate, on the turnover of plasma cholesterol in man. J. Clin. Invest. 52, 2646 (1973).

GORE, I., FUJINAMI, T., SHIRAHAMA, T.: Endothelial changes produced by ascorbic deficiency in guinea pigs. Arch. Path. 80, 371 (1965).

GORE, I., TANAKA, Y., FUJINAMI, T., GOODMAN, M. L.: Aortic acid mucopolysacchari- des and collagen in scorbutic guinea pigs. J. Nutr. 87, 311 (1965).

GOTTESMAN, I. I., SHIELDS, J.: Genetic theorizing and schizophrenia. Brit. J. Psychiat. 122, 15 (1973).

GOTTO, A. M., Jr.: Recent studies on the structure of human serum low-and-high- density lipoproteins. Proc. Natl. Acad. Sci. 64, 1119 (1969).

GOTTO, A. M., BROWN, W. V., LEVY, R. I., BIRNBAUMER, M. E., FREDRICKSON, D. S.: Evidence for the identity of the major apoprotein in low density and very low density lipoproteins in normal subjects and patients with familial hyper- lipoproteinemia. J. Clin. Invest. 51, 1486 (1972).

GOTTO, A. M., LEVY, R. I., FREDRICKSON, D. S.: Preparation and properties of an apoprotein derivative of human serum β-lipoprotein. Lipids 3, 463 (1968 a).

GOTTO, A. M., LEVY, R. I., JOHN, K., FREDRICKSON, D. S.: On the protein defect in abetalipoproteinemia. New Engl. J. Med. 284, 813 - 818 (1971).

GOTTO, A. M., LEVY, R. I., ROSENTHAL, A. S., BIRNBAUMER, M. E., FREDRICKSON, D. S.: The structure and properties of human beta-lipoprotein and beta-apopro- tein. Biochem. Biophys. Res. Commun. 31, 699 (1968 b).

GRABOWSKI, G. A., DEMPSEY, M. E., HANSON, R. F.: Role of the squalene and sterol carrier protein (SCP) in bile acid synthesis. Fed. Proc. 32, 520 (1973).

GRAFNETTER, D., SHIMAMOTO, T., NUMANO, F.: Blood and tissue lipids during the treatment of rats with high-fat diet, calciferol and pyridinol-carbamate. In: Atherogenesis II, Excerpta Medica, 1973, p. 122 (SHIMAMOTO, T., NUMANO, F., and ADDISON, Eds.).

GRAHAM, R. C., GRIFFIN, R.: Arthus synovitis with horseradish peroxidase as anti- gen: sequential participation of platelets and leucocytes. Brit. J. Exp. Path. 53, 578 - 585 (1972).

GRANT, E. H., SHEPPARD, R. J., MILLS, G. L., SLACK, J.: A dielectric investiga- tion of the water of hydration of low density lipoproteins in familial hyper- beta-lipoproteinaemia. Lancet 1972 I, 1159.

GREENE, M. L.: Clinical features of patients with the "partial" deficiency of the X-linked uricaciduria enzyme. Arch. intern. Med. 130, 193 (1972).

GREENHALGH, R. M., ROSENGARTEN, D. S., MERVART, I., LEWIS, B., CALNAN, J. S., MARTIN, P.: Serum lipids and lipoproteins in peripheral vascular disease. Lancet 1971 II, 947.

GREIG, H. B. W.: Inhibition of fibrinolysis by alimentry lipaemia Lancet 1956 II, 16.

GRESHAM, G. A., HOWARD, A. N.: Aortic rupture in the turkey. J. Atherosclerosis Res. 1, 75 (1961).

GRESHAM, G. A., HOWARD, A. N.: Vascular lesions in primates. Ann. N. Y. Acad. Sci. 127, 694 - 701 (1965).

GRETEN, H.: Post-heparin plasma phospholipases in normals and patients with hyperlipoproteinemia. Klin. Wschr. 50, 39 - 41 (1972).

GRETEN, H.: Enzymatic degradation of plasma lipoproteins. In: Exposés Annuels de Biochimie Médicale, p. 161 - 181 (POLONOVSKI, J., Ed.). Paris: Masson et Cie 1972.

GRETEN, H., LEVY, R. I., FALES, H., FREDERICKSON, D. S.: Hydrolysis of diglyceri- de and glyceryl monoester diethers with "lipoprotein lipase". Biochim. Bio- phys. Acta 210, 39 (1970).

GRETEN, H., LEVY, R. I., FREDRICKSON, D. S.: Evidence for separate monoglyceride hydrolase and triglyceride lipase in post-heparin human plasma. J. Lipid Res. 10, 326 - 330 (1969).

GRETEN, H., SNIDERMAN, A. D., CHANDLER, J. G., STEINBERG, D., BROWN, W. V.: Evi- dence for the hepatic origin of a canine post-heparin plasma triglyceride lipase. FEBS Letters 42, 157 (1974).

GRETEN, H., WALTER, B.: Purification of rat adipose tissue lipoprotein lipase. FEBS Letters 35, 36 (1973).

GRETEN, H., WALTER, B., BROWN, W. B.: Purification of a human postheparin plasma triglyceride lipase. FEBS Letter 27, 306 (1972).

GRIMBY, G., BJURE, J., AURELL, M., EKSTRÖM-JODAL, B., TIBBLIN, G., WILHELMSEN, L.: Work capacity and physiologic responses to work. Men Born in 1913. Amer. J. Cardiol. 30, 37 - 42 (1972).

GROSS, L., EPSTEIN, E. Z., KUGEL, M. A.: Histology of the coronary arteries and their branches in the human heart. Amer. J. Pathol. 10, 253- 274 (1934).

GROSS, R. C.: Lipoprotein triglyceride metabolism in cultured human fibroblasts. Clin. Res. 20, 191 (1972).

GRUNDY, S. M., AHRENS, E. H., Jr.: Measurement of cholesterol turnover, synthesis, and absorption in man, carried out by isotope kinetic and sterol balance methods. J. Lipid Res. 10, 91 (1969).

GRUNDY, S. M., AHRENS, E. H., Jr., DAVIGNON, J.: The interaction of cholesterol absorption and cholesterol synthesis in man. J. Lipid Res. 10, 304 (1969).

GRUNDY, S. M., AHRENS, E. H., Jr., SALEN, G.: Interruption of the enterohepatic circulation of bile acids in man: comparative effects of cholestyramine and ileal exclusion on cholesterol metabolism. J. Lab. Clin. Med. 78, 94 (1971).

GUNN, G. C., DOBSON, H. L., GRAY, H.: Studies of pulse wave velocity in potential diabetic subjects, Diabetes 14, 489 (1965).

GUNNING, A. J., PICKERING, G. W., ROBB-SMITH, A. H. T., RUSSELL, R. R.: Mural thrombosis of the internal carotid artery and subsequent embolism. Quart. J. Med. 33, 155 - 195 (1964).

GUPTA, P. P., TANDON, H. D., RAMALINGASWAMI, V.: Experimental atherosclerosis in rabbits with special reference to reversal. J. Path. 101, 309 - 317 (1970).

GURPIDE, E., MANN, J., SANDBERG, E.: Determination of kinetic parameters in a two-pool system by administration of one or more tracers. Biochemistry 3, 1250 (1964).

GUSTAFSON, A., ALAUPOVIC, P., FURMAN, R. H.: Studies of the composition and structure of serum lipoproteins: physical-chemical characterization of phospholipid-protein residues obtained from very-low-density human serum lipoproteins. Biochim. Biophys. Acta 84, 767 (1964).

GUSTAFSON, A., ALAUPOVIC, P., FURMAN, R. H.: Studies of the composition and structure of serum lipoproteins. Separation and characterization of phospholipid - protein residues obtained by partial delipidization of very low density lipoproteins of human serum. Biochemistry 5, 632 (1966).

GUSTAFSON, A., BJÖRNTORP, P., FAHLEN, M.: Metformin administration in hyperlipidemic states. Acta Med. Scand. 190, 491 (1971).

GUTSTEIN, W. H., FARRELL, G. A., ARMELLINI, C.: Blood flow disturbance and endothelial cell injury in preatherosclerotic swine. Lab. Invest. 29, 134 - 149 (1973).

GUTSTEIN, W. H., PARL, F.: Ultrastructural changes of coronary artery endothelium associated with biliary obstruction in the rat. Am. J. Pathol. 71, 49 - 60 (1973).

GUTSTEIN, W. H., SCHNECK, D. J., APPLETON, H.: Mechanism of plasma lipid increases following brain stimulation. Metabolism 18, 300 - 310 (1969).

GUZMAN, M. A., Mc MAHAN, C. A., Mc GILL, H. C., et al.: Selected methodologie aspects of the international atherosclerosis project. Lab. Invest. 18, 479 (1968).

HADJIISKY, P., SCEBAT, L., RENAIS, J., CACHERA, J. P., BUBOST, C., LENEGRE, J.: Altérations morphologiques des vaisseaux coronaires de deux homotransplants cardiaques de longue durée chez l'homme. Rev. Europ. Etudes Clin. and Biol. 16, 596 (1971).

HAEREM, J. W.: Sudden coronary death; the occurrence of platelet aggregates in the epicardial arteries of man. Atherosclerosis 14, 417 - 432 (1971).

HAEREM, J. W.: Platelet aggregates in intramyocardial vessels of patients dying suddenly and unexpectedly of coronary artery disease. Atherosclerosis 15, 199 - 213 (1972).

HAFT, J. I., FANI, K.: Intravascular platelet aggregation in the heart induced by stress. Circulation 47, 353 - 358 (1973).

HAFT, J. I., KRANZ, P. D., ALBERT, F. J., FANI, K.: Intravascular platelet aggregation in the heart induced by norepinephrine. Microscopic studies. Circulation 46, 698 - 708 (1972).

HALE, A. J., HALL, T., CURRAN, R. C.: Electron-microprobe analysis of calcium, phosphorus and sulphur in human arteries. J. Path. 93, 1 (1967).

HALL, A. P.: Correlation among hyperuricemia, hypercholesterolemia, coronary didease and hypertension. Arth. Rheumat. 8, 846 – 852 (1965).

HAMILTON, R. L., Jr.: In: Post-heparin plasma lipase from the hepatic circulation Ann Arbor, Mich.: University Microfilms 1964.

HAMILTON, R. L., HAVEL, R. J., KANE, J. P., BLAUROCK, A. E., SATA, T.: Cholestasis: lamellar structure of the abnormal human serum lipoprotein. Science 172, 475 (1971).

HAMMOND, E. C., GARFINKEL, L., SEIDMAN, H.: Longevity of parents and grandparents in relation to coronary heart disease and associated variables. Circulation 43, 31 (1971).

HAMMOND, M. G., FISHER, W. R.: The characterization of a discrete series of low density lipoproteins in the disease, hyper-pre-beta-lipoproteinemia. J. Biol. Chem. 246, 5454 (1971).

HAMPTON, J. R., MITCHELL, J. R. A.: Effect of aggregating agents on the electrophoretic mobility of human platelets. Brit. Med. J. 1, 1074 – 1077 (1966).

HAND, R. A., CHANDLER, A. B.: Atherosclerotic metamorphosis of autologous pulmonary thromboemboli in the rabbit. Amer. J. Path. 40, 469 – 486 (1962).

HANSEN, A. P.: Abnormal serum growth hormone response to exercise in juvenile diabetics. J. Clin. Invest. 49, 1467 (1970).

HARA, I., KUZUYA, F.: Lipoprotein lipase. Protein, Nucleic acid and Enzyme Suppl. 8, 79 (1967).

HARARY, I., FARLEY, B.: In vitro studies on single beating heart cells. I. Growth and organization. Exp. Cell Res. 29, 451 (1967).

HARARY, I., GERSCHENSON, L. E., HAGGERTY, D. F., Jr., DESMOND, W., MEAD, J. F.: Fatty acid metabolism and function in cultured heart and HeLa cells. In: Lipid metabolism in tissue culture cells. Wistar Inst. Symp. Monogr. 6, p. 17 (ROTHBLAT, G. H., and KRITCHEVSKY, D., Eds.).   : Wistar Inst. Press 1967.

HARDIN, N. J., MINICK, C. R., MURPHY, G. E.: Experimental induction of atheroarteriosclerosis by the synergy of allergic injury to arteries and lipid rich diet. III. The role of earlier acquired fibromuscular intimal thickening in the pathogenesis of later developing atherosclerosis. Amer. J. Pathol. 73, 301 (1973).

HARKER, L. A., SLICHTER, S. J.: Studies of platelet and fibrinogen kinetics in patients with prostetic heart valves. New Engl. J. Med. 283, 1302–1305 (1970).

HARKER, L. A., SLICHTER, S. J.: Platelet and fibrinogen consumption in man. New Engl. J. Med. 287, 999 – 1005 (1972).

HARKER, L. A., SLICHTER, S. J.: Arterial thromboembolism quantitation and prevention. Proc. IVth Internat. Congress on Thrombosis and Haemostasis, Vienna, Austria. p. 170 (1973).

HARLAN, W. R., GRAHAM, J. B., ESTES, H.: Familial hypercholesterolemia: A genetic and metabolic study. Medicine 45, 77 (1966).

HARLAN, W. T., Jr., WINESETT, P. S., WASSERMAN, A. T.: Tissue lipoprotein lipase in normal individuals and in individuals with exogenous hypertriglyceridemia and the relationship of this enzyme to assimilation of fat. J. Clin. Invest. 46, 239 – 247 (1967).

HARLAND, W. A., HOLBURN, A. M.: Coronary thrombosis and myocardial infarction. Lancet 1966 II, 1158 – 1160.

HARPEL, P. C.: Studies on the interaction between collagen and a plasma kallikreinlike activity. Evidence for a surface-active enzyme system. J. Clin. Invest. 51, 1813 – 1822 (1972).

HARRISON, C. V.: Experimental pulmonary arteriosclerosis. J. Path. Bact. 60, 289 – 293 (1948).

HARRISON, M. J. G., MARSHALL, J., MEADOWS, J. C., RUSSELL, R. W. R.: Effect of aspirin in amaurosis fugax. Lancet 1971 II, 743 – 744.

HARVALD, B., HAUGE, M.: Coronary occlusion in twins. Acta genet. med. (Roma) 19, 248 (1970).

HARVIE, N. R., SCHULTZ, J. S.: Studies of the Lp-lipoprotein as a quantitative genetic trait. Proc. Nat. Acad. Sci. 66, 99 (1970).

HASHIMOTO, S., DAYTON, S.: Transfer of cholesterol and cholesteryl esters into wall of the rat aorta in vitro. J. Atheroscler. Res. 6, 580 (1966).

HASHIMOTO, S., DAYTON, S., ALFIN-SLATER, R. B.: Esterification of cholesterol by homogenates of atherosclerotic and normal aortas. Life Sci. 12 (II), 1 (1973).

HASHIMOTO, H., TILLMANNS, H., SARMA, J. S. M., MAO, J., HOLDEN, E., BING, R. J.: Lipid metabolism in perfused human nonatherosclerotic coronary arteries and saphenous veins. Atherosclerosis 19, 35 (1974).

HASLAM, R. J.: Role of adenosine diphosphate in the aggregation of human blood platelets by thrombin and by fatty acids. Nature 202, 765 (1964).

HASS, G. M.: Elastic tissue. Arch. Pathol. 27, 334 (1939).

HASS, G. M.: Observations on vascular structure in relation to human and experimental atherosclerosis. In: Symposium on atherosclerosis, p. 24 - 32. Publication 338, National Academy of Sciences - National Research Council, Washington, D. C. 1955.

HATCH, F. T., LEES, R. S.: Practical methods for plasma lipoprotein analysis. Advan. Lipid Res. 6, 1 (1968).

HATCH, F. T., LINDGREN, F. T., ADAMSON, G. L., JENSEN, L. C., WONG, A. W., LEVY, R. I.: Quantitative agarose gel electrophoresis of plasma lipoproteins: A simple technique and two methods of standardization. J. Lab. Clin. Med. 81, 946 - 960 (1973).

HAUSS, W. H., GERLACH, U., JUNGE-HÜLSING, G., THEMANN, H., WIRTH, W.: Studies of the monospecific mesenchymal reaction and the transit zone in myocardial lesions and atherosclerosis. Ann. N. Y. Acad. Sci. 156, 207 (1969).

HAUST, M. D.: Electron microscopic and immuno-histochemical studies of fatty streaks in human aorta. In: Proceedings of International Symposium on Recent Advances in Atherosclerosis. In: Progr. Biochem. Pharmacol. Vol. 4, p. 429 - 437 (MIRAS, S. J., HOWARD, A. N., and PAOLETTI, R., Eds.). Basel, New York: Karger 1968.

HAUST, M. D.: The morphogenesis and fate of potential and early atherosclerotic lesions in man. Human Pathol. 2, 1 - 29 (1971).

HAUST, M. D.: Arteriosclerosis. I.: Concepts of Disease. Textbook of Pathology, chap. 17 (BRUNSON, J. G., and GALL, E. A., Eds.). New York: MacMillan Co. 1971.

HAUST, M. D., CHOI, J. H., WYLLIE, J. C., MORE, R. H.: Demonstration of albumin in human atherosclerotic lesions by the fluorescent antibody technique. Circ. 32, Suppl. II, 17 (1965).

HAUST, M. D., MORE, R. H.: The thrombotic basis of arteriosclerosis. The Heart Bulletin 9, 90 - 92 (1960).

HAUST, M. D., MORE, R. H.: Significance of the smooth muscle cell in atherogenesis. In: Evolution of the atherosclerotic plaque, p. 51 - 63 (JONES, R. J., Ed.). Chicago, London: The University of Chicago Press 1963.

HAUST, M. D., MORE, R. H.: Development of modern theories on the pathogenesis of atherosclerosis. In: The pathogenesis of atherosclerosis, p. 1 - 19 (WISSLER, R. W., and GEER, J. C., Eds.). Baltimore: The Williams and Wilkins Co. 1972.

HAUST, M. D., MORE, R. H., BENCOSME, S. A., BALIS, J. U.: Electron microscopic studies in human atherosclerosis. Extracellular elements in aortic dots and streaks. Exp. Mol. Pathol. 6, 300 - 313 (1967).

HAUST, M. D., WYLLIE, J. C., MORE, R. H.: Atherogenesis and plasma constituents I. Demonstration of fibrin in white plaques by the fluorescent antibody technique. Am. J. Path. 44, 255 - 267 (1964).

HAVEL, R. J.: Conversion of plasma free fatty acids into triglycerides of plasma lipoprotein fractions in man. Metabolism 10, 1031 (1961).

HAVEL, R. J.: Typing of hyperlipoproteinemias. Atherosclerosis 11, 3 (1970).

HAVEL, R. J., EDER, H. A., BRAGDON, J. H.: The distribution and chemical composition of ultracentrifugally separated lipoproteins in human serum. J. Clin. Invest. 34, 1345 - 1353 (1955).

HAVEL, R. J., FELTS, J. M., VAN DUYNE, C. M.: Formation and fate of endogenous triglycerides in blood plasma of rabbits. J. Lipid Res. 3, 297 - 308 (1962).

HAVEL, R. J., FIELDING, C. I., OLIVECRONA, T., SHORE, V. G., FIELDING, P. E., EGELRUD, T.: Cofactor activity of the protein components of human very low density lipoproteins in the hydrolysis of triglycerides by lipoprotein lipase from different sources. Biochemistry 12, 1828 (1973).

HAVEL, R. J., GORDON, R. S., Jr.: Idiopathic hyperlipemia: Metabolic studies in an affected family. J. Clin. Invest. 39, 1777 (1960).

HAVEL, R. J., KANE, J. P.: Primary dysbetalipoproteinemia: predominance of a specific apoprotein species in triglyceride-rich lipoproteins. Proc. Nat. Acad. Sci. USA 70, 2015 (1973).

HAVEL, R. J., KANE, J. P., BALASSE, E. O., SEGEL, N., BASSO, L. V.: Splanchnic metabolism of free fatty acids and production of very low density lipoproteins in normotriglyceridemic and hypertriglyceridemic humans. J. Clin. Invest. 49, 2017 (1970).

HAVEL, R. J., KANE, J. P., KASHYAP, M. L.: Interchange of apolipoproteins between chylomicrons and high density lipoproteins during alimentary cipemia in man. J. Clin. Invest. 52, 32 (1973).

HAVEL, R. J., NAIMARK, A., BORCHGREVINK, F.: Turnover rate and oxidation of free fatty acids of blood plasma in man during exercise: studies during continuous infusion of palmitate-1-^{14}C. J. Clin. Invest. 42, 1054 (1963).

HAVEL, R. J., SHORE, V. G., SHORE, B., BIER, D. M.: Role of specific glycopeptides of human serum lipoproteins in the activation of lipoprotein lipase. Circ. Res. 27, 595 (1970).

HAWKINS, R. I.: Smoking, platelets and thrombosis. Nature 236, 450 – 452 (1972).

HAY, R. V., POTTENGER, C. A., REINGOLD, A. L., GETZ, G. S., WISSLER, R. W.: Degradation of ^{125}I-labelled serum low density lipoprotein in normal and estrogen-treated male rats. Biochem. Biophys. Res. Commun. 44, 1471 (1971).

HAYASE, K., MILLER, B. F.: Lipase activity in the human aorta. J. Lipid Res. 11, 209 (1970).

HAYASHI, M., NAKAJIMA, Y., FISHMAN, W. H.: The cytochemic demonstration of β-glucuronidase emplying naphthol AS-BI glucoronide and hexazonium pararosanilin J. Histochem. and Cytochem. 12, 293 (1964).

HAZZARD, W. R., BIERMAN, E. I.: Aggravation of broad –B disease (type II hyperlipoproteinemia) by hypothyroidism. Arch. Intern. Med. 130, 822 – 828 (1972).

HAZZARD, W. R., BRUNZELL, J. D., NOTTER, D. T., SPIGER, M. J., BIERMAN, E. L.: Estrogens and triglyceride transport: increased endogenous production as the mechanism for the hypertriglyceridemia of oral contraceptive therapy. In: Progress in Endocrinology. Proceedings, IV Int. Cong. of Endocrinology 1972.

HAZZARD, W. R., GOLDSTEIN, J. L., SCHROTT, H. G., MOTULSKY, A. G., BIERMAN, E. L.: Hyperlipidemia in coronary heart disease. III. Evaluation of lipoprotein phenotypes of 156 genetically defined survivors of myocardial infarction. J. Clin. Invest. 52, 1569 (1973).

HAZZARD, W. R., PORTE, D., Jr., BIERMAN, E.: Abnormal lipid composition of very low density lipoproteins in diagnosis of broad-beta disease. Metabolism 21, 1009 (1972).

HEARD, B.E.: An experimental study of thickening of the pulmonary arteries of rabbits produced by the organisation of fibrin. J.Path.Bact.64,13-19 (1952).

HEIKINHEIMO, R., JÄRVINEN, K.: Acetylsalicylic acid and arteriosclerotic-thromboembolic diseases in the aged. J. Amer. Geriatrics Soc. 19, 403 – 405 (1971).

HEINLE, R. A., LEVY, R. I., FREDRICKSON, D. S., CORLIN, R.: Lipid and carbohydrates abnormalities in patients with angiographically documented coronary artery disease. Am. J. Cardiol. 24, 178 (1969).

HELIN, P., LORENZEN, I., GARBARSCH, C., MATTHIESSEN, M. E.: Arteriosclerosis in rabbit aorta induced by noradrenaline. The importance of the duration of the noradrenaline action. Atherosclerosis 12, 125 – 132 (1970).

HELIN, P., LORENZEN, I., GARBARSCH, C., MATTHIESSEN, M. E.: Arteriosclerosis in rabbit aorta induced by mechanical dilation. Biochemical and morphological studies. Atherosclerosis 13, 319 – 331 (1971).

HEMKER, H. C., KAHN, M. J. P.: Reaction sequence of blood coagulation. Nature 215, 1201 (1967).

HEPTINSTALL, R. H.: The effects of high blood cholesterol on the pulmonary arterial changes produced in rabbits by the injection of blood clot. Brit. J. Exp. Path. 38, 438 (1957).

HERBERT, P. N., SHULMAN, R. S., LEVY, R. I., FREDRICKSON, D. S.: Fractionation of the C-apoproteins from human plasma very low density lipoproteins. Artifactual polymorphism from carbamylation in urea-containing solutions. J.Biol. Chem. 248, 4941 (1973).

HEREMANS, J.: In: Les globulines sériques du système gamma. Leur nature et leur pathologie, p. 227. Bruxelles: Arscia S. A. 1960.

HERMELIN, B., PICARD, J., LEVY, P., GARDAIS, A.: Turnover of sulfated glycosaminoglycans in rat aortic wall. 1973 (In press).

HERRMANN, R. G.: Effect of platelet aggregation inhibitors on bleeding time. Can. Med. Assoc. J. 108, 454 - 455 (1973).

HESS, H.: Neue Überlegungen zur Physiopathologie obliterierender Angiopathien. Fortschr. Med. 88, 833 - 838 and 923 - 928 (1970).

HESS, H., FROST, H.: Argumente für eine einheitliche Pathogenese ätiologisch unterschiedlicher arterieller Verschlußprozesse. Verh. Dtsch. Ges. f. Kreislaufforschung, p. 333. Darmstadt: Dietrich Steinkopff-Verlag 1969.

HESS, H., MALLASCH, M., MARSHALL, M., KLINGELE, H.: Ultrahistochemische Untersuchungen mit Röntgenmikroanalyse: Nachweis biogener Amine in menschlichen Thrombocyten. Klin. Wschr. 50, 776 (1972).

HESS, R., SCARPELLI, D. G., PEARSE, A. G. E.: The cytochemical localisation of oxydative enzymes J. Biophys. Biochem. Cytol. 4, 753 - 761 (1958).

HESS, R., STÄUBLI, W.: The development of aortic lipidosis in the rat. A correlative histochemical and electron microscopic study. Amer. J. Path. 43, 301 - 335 (1963).

HILDEN, M., AMRIS, C. J., STARUP, J.: The haemostatic mechanism in oral contraception. Acta Obstet. Gynecol. Scand. 46, 562 - 571 (1967).

HIRSH, J., BUCHANAN, M., GLYNN, M. F., MUSTARD, J. F.: Effect of streptokinase on hemostasis. Blood 32, 726 - 737 (1968).

HO, K. J., TAYLOR, C. B.: Comparative studies on tissue cholesterol. Arch. Path. 86, 585 (1968).

HOAK, J. C., CONNOR, W. E., WARNER, E. D.: Thrombogenic effects of albumin-bound fatty acids. Arch. Pathol. 81, 136 - 139 (1966).

HOEPFNER, E.: Über Gefäßnähte, Gefäßtransplantation und Reimplantation von amputierten Extremitäten. Arch. f. Klin. Chir. 70, 417 (1903).

HOFF, H.F.: Human intracranial atherosclerosis. Amer.J.Pathol.69,421-438 (1972).

HOKANSON, D. E., MOZERSKY, D. J., SUMNER, D. S., STRANDNESS, D. E., Jr.: Ultrasonic arteriography. A new approach to arterial visualization. Biomed. Eng. 6, 420 (1971).

HOKIN, L. E., HOKIN, M. R.: Effects of acetylcholine on the turnover of phosphoryl units in individual phospholipids of pancreas slices and brain cortex slices. Biochim. Biophys. Acta 18, 102 (1955).

HOLLANDER, W., PADDOCK, J.: Synthesis of low density (LDL) and very low density lipoproteins (VLDL) and apolipoproteins by human arteries. Circulation 48, IV - 16 (1973).

HOLMAN, E.: Abnormal arteriovenous communications. Springfield, Ill.: Charles C. Thomas 1968.

HOLMAN, R. L., Mc GILL, H. C., STRONG, J. P., GEER, J. C.: The natural history of atherosclerosis. The early aortic lesions as seen in New Orleans in the middle of the 20th century. Am. J. Pathol. 34, 209 - 235 (1959).

HOLMSEN, H., DAY, H. J., STORMORKEN, H.: The blood platelet release reaction. Scand. J. Haematol. Suppl. 8, 1 - 26 (1969).

HONOUR, A. J., ROSS-RUSSELL, R. W.: Experimental platelet embolism. Brit. J. Exp. Path. 43, 350 - 362 (1962).

HOOD, B.: Antihypertensive treatment and myocardial infarction. In: Preventive Cardiology, p. 83 (TIBBLIN, G., KEYS, A., and WERKÖ, L., Eds.). London: Halstead Bass 1972.

HOOD, B., JANSSON, G., HEDSTRAND, H., ABERG, H.: Hypertension and vascular damage in the coronary and other vascular areas. In: Early phases of coronary heart disease: Possibility of prediction. Skandia International Symposium, (WALDENSTRÖM, J., LARSSON, T., and LJUNGSTEDT, N., Eds.). Stockholm: Nordiska Bokhandelns 1973.

HORCH, U., KADATZ, R., KOPITAR, Z., RITSCHARD, J., WEISENBERGER, H.: Pharmacology of dipyridamole and its derivatives. Thromb. Diath. Haemorrh. Suppl. 42, 253 - 266 (1970).

HORLICK, L.: Platelet adhesiveness in normal persons and subjects with atherosclerosis. Effect of high fat meals and anticoagulants on the adhesive index. Amer. J. Cardiol. 8, 459 - 470 (1961).

HORLICK, L., KATZ, L. N.: Retrogression of atherosclerotic lesions on cessation of cholesterol feeding in the chicken. J. Lab. Clin. Med. 34, 1427 (1949).

HORNSTRA, G.: Dietary fats and arterial thrombosis. In: Dietary fats and thrombosis (RENAUD, S., and NORDÖY, A., Eds.). Haemostasis 2, p. 21 - 52. Basel: S. Karger 1973/74.

HORNSTRA, G., CHAIT, A., KARVONEN, M. J., LEWIS, B., TURPEINEN, O., VERGROESEN, A. J.: Influence of dietary fat on platelet function in men. Lancet 1973 I, 1155 - 1157.

HORNSTRA, G., VENDELMANS-STARRENBURG, A.: Induction of experimental arterial occlusive thrombi in rats. Atherosclerosis 17, 369 - 382 (1973).

HOUGIE, C.: Thromboembolism and oral contraceptives. Amer. Heart J. 85, 538 - 545 (1973).

HOVIG, T.: Release of a platelet-aggregating substance (adenosine diphosphate) from rabbit blood platelets induced by saline "extract" of tendons. Thromb. Diath. Haemorrh. 9, 264 - 278 (1963).

HOWARD, A. N.: Recent advances in nutrition and atherosclerosis. In: Atherosclerosis: Proceedings of the Second International Symposium, p. 408 - 413 (JONES, R. J., Ed.). 1969.

HOWARD, A. H., BLATON, V., VANDAMME, D., VAN LANDSCHOOT, N., PEETERS, H.: Lipid changes in the plasma lipoproteins of baboons given an atherogenic diet. Part 3. A Comparison between lipid changes in the plasma of the baboon and chimpanzee given atherogenic diets and those in human plasma lipoproteins of Type II hyperlipoproteinaemia. Atherosclerosis 16, 257 - 272 (1972).

HOWARD, A. N., GRESHAM, G. A.: Dietary Aspects of Atherosclerosis and Thrombosis. Int. J. for vit. Res. 38, 546 - 559 (1968).

HOWARD, A. N., GRESHAM, G. A., JONES, D., JENNINGS, I. W.: The prevention of rabbit atherosclerosis by soyabean meal. J. Atherosclerosis Res. 5, 330 - 337 (1965).

HOWARD, A. N., PATELSKI, J.: Effect of intravenous polyunsaturated phosphatidylcholine in experimental atherosclerosis. Verhandl. deutschen Gesellsch. Innere Med. (Wiesbaden) 78, 1245 (1972).

HOWARD, A. N., PATELSKI, J., BOWYER, D. E., GRESHAM, G. A.: Atherosclerosis induced in hypercholesterolaemic baboons by immunological injury; and the effects of intravenous polyunsaturated phosphatidyl choline. Atherosclerosis 14, 17 (1971).

HOWARD, C. F., Jr.: De novo synthesis and elongation of fatty acids by subcellular fractions of monkey aorta J. Lipid Res. 9, 254 - 261 (1968).

HOWARD, C. F., PORTMAN, O. W.: Hydrolysis of cholesteryl linoleate by a high speed supernatant preparation of rat and monkey aorta. Biochim. Biophys. Acta 125, 623 (1966).

HOWES, E. L., Jr., Mc KAY, D. G., MARGARETTEN, W.: The participation of the platelet in the vascular response to endotoxemia in the rabbit eye. Amer. J. Path. 70, 25 - 44 (1973).

HÜTTNER, I., BOUTET, M., MORE, R. H.: Studies on protein passage through arterial endothelium. II. Regional differences in permeability to fine structural protein tracers in arterial endothelium of normotensive rat. Lab. Invest. 28, 678 - 685 (1973).

HÜTTNER, I., MORE, R. H., RONA, G.: Fine structural evidence of specific mechanism for increased endothelial permeability in experimental hypertension. Amer. J. Path. 61, 395 - 405 (1970).

HUGHES, A. F. W.: Studies on the area vasculosa of the embryo chick; the influence of the circulation on the diameter of the vessels. J. Anat. 72, 1 - 17 (1937).

HUGHES, A., TONKS, R. S.: Intravascular platelet clumping in rabbits. J. Path. Bact. 84, 379 - 390 (1962).

HUGUES, J.: Accolement des plaquettes aux structures conjonctives périvasculaires. Thromb. Diath. Haemorrh. 8, 241 - 255 (1962).

HUNTER, R.: Standardization of the Chloramine-T method of protein iodination. Proc. Soc. Exp. Biol. Med. 133, 989 (1970).

HURST, J. W., LOGUE, R. B.: The heart, arteries and veins, p. 1072. New York, London: Mc Graw-Hill 1966.

HUTCHINSON, J. C., WILKINSON, W. H.: The uricosuric action of halofenate (MK-185) in patients with hyperuricemia or uncomplicated primary gout and hyperlipidemia. Atherosclerosis 18, 353 - 362 (1973).

HUTTUNEN, J. K., AQUINO, A. A., STEINBERG, D.: A purified triglyceride lipase, lipoprotein in nature, from rat adipose tissue. Biochim. Biophys. Acta 224, 295 (1970).

HUTTUNEN, J. K., STEINBERG, D.: Activation and phosphorylation of purified adipose tissue hormone-sensitive lipase by cyclic AMP-dependent protein kinase. Biochim. Biophys. Acta 239, 411 (1971).

HUTTUNEN, J. K., STEINBERG, D., MAYER, S. E.: ATP-dependent and cyclic AMP-dependent activation of rat adipose tissue lipase by protein kinase of rat adipose tissue lipase by protein kinase from rabbit skeletal muscle. Proc. Nat. Acad. Sci. (USA) 67, 290 (1970).

HUTTUNEN, J. K., STEINBERG, D., MAYER, S. E.: Protein Kinase activation and phosphorylation of a purified hormone-sensitive lipase. Biochem. Biophys. Res. Commun. 41, 1350 (1970).

HYUN, J., STEINBERG, M., TREADWELL, C. R., VAHOUNY, C. V.: Cholesterol esterase: a polymeric enzyme. Biochem. Biophys. Res. Commun. 44, 819 (1971).

IGANTOWSKI, A.: Über die Wirkung des tierischen Eiweißes auf die Aorta und die parenchymatösen Organe der Kaninchen. Virchows Arch.f.path.Anat.u.Physiol. (1909).

ILEBEKK, A., MJÖS, O. D.: Effect of nicotine on severity of acute myocardial ischemic injury in dogs. Scand. J. Clin. Lab. Invest. (In press).

IMAI, H., LEE, K. T., PASTORI, S., PANLILIO, E., FLORENTIN, R., THOMAS, W. A.: Atherosclerosis in rabbits. J. Exp. Mol. Path. 47, 273 (1966).

IMAI, Y., MATSUMURA, H.: Genetic studies on induced and spontaneous hypercholesterolemia in rats. Atherosclerosis 18, 59 - 64 (1973).

INFANTE, R., ALCINDOR, G., RAISONNIER, A., PETIT, D., POLONOVSKI, J., CAROLI, J.: Biosynthèse des lipoprotéines plasmatiques par le foie en régéneration. Biochim. Biophys. Acta 187, 335 - 344 (1969).

INGERMAN, C., SMITH, J. B., KOCSIS, J. J., SILVER, M. J.: Arachidonic acid induces platelet aggregation and platelet prostaglandin formation. Fed. Proc. 32, 219 abs. (1973).

INMAN, W. H. W., VESSEY, M. P.: Investigation of deaths from pulmonary, coronary, and cerebral thrombosis and embolism in women of child-bearing age. Brit. Med. J. 2, 193 - 199 (1968).

INMAN, W. H. W., VESSEY, M. P., WESTERHOLM, B., ENGELUND, A.: Thromboembolic disease and the steroidal content of oral contraceptives. A report to the committee on safety of drugs. Brit. Med. J. 2, 203 - 209 (1970).

INSULL, W., Jr.: Lipids in arteriosclerotic arterial tissues of man in Atherosclerosis and Coronary Heart Disease, p. 20 (LIKOFF, W., SEGAL, B.L., INSULL, W., Jr., and MOYER, J. H., Eds.). New York: Grune and Stratton 1972.

INSULL, W., Jr., HATA, Y., MEAKIN, J. D., MARCHANT, L.: Morphology of lipid rich organelles in tissues of man and rat. Scanning electron microscopy/1971, Part I. Proceedings of the Fourth Annual Scanning Electron Microscope Symposium, p. 337 - 344. Chicago: Illinois Institute of Technology Research Institute 1971.

IREY, N. S., NORRIS, H. J.: Intimal vascular lesions associated with female reproductive steroids. Arch. Pathol. 96, 227 - 234 (1973).

JACKSON, I. M., Mc KIDDIE, M. T., BUCHANAN, K. D.: Influence of blood-lipid levels and effect of prolonged fasting on carbohydrate metabolism in obesity. Lancet 1971 II, 450.

JACKSON, R. L., GOTTO, A. M., Jr., LUX, S. E., JOHN, K. M., FLEISCHER, S.: Human plasma high density lipoprotein. Interaction of the cyanogen bromide fragments from apolipoprotein glutamine II (A-II) with phosphatidylcholine. J. Biol. Chem. 248, 8449 (1973 a).

JACKSON, R. L., MORRISETT, J. D., POWNALL, H. J., GOTTO, A. M., Jr.: Human high density lipoprotein, apolipoprotein glutamine II. The immunochemical and lipid-binding properties of apolipoprotein glutamine II derivatives. J. Biol. Chem. 248, 5218 (1973 b).

JACKSON, R. L., TAUNTON, O. D., GALLAGHER, J. G., HOFF, H. F., GOTTO, A. M., Jr.: A comparison of the physical, chemical and immunochemical properties of low density lipoproteins from pig and man. J. Biol. Chem. 1973 (In press).

JACOBI, E., HAGEMANN, G., POLIWODA, H.: Eine In-Vitro-Methode zur Bestimmung der Thrombozytenadhäsivität. Thrombos. Diathes. haemorrh. (Stuttg.) 26, 192 (1971).

JACOBI, E., HAGEMANN, G., POLIWODA, H.: Some investigations into Clinical Pathophysiology of Platelet Adhesiveness. In: Erythrocytes, Thrombocytes, Leukocytes (GERLACH, E., MOSER, K., DEUTSCH, E., WILMANNS, W., Eds.). Stuttgart: G. Thieme 1973.

JACOTOT, B., BEAUMONT, J. L., MONNIER, G., SZIGETI, M., ROBERT, B., ROBERT, L.: Role of elastic tissue in cholesterol deposition in the arterial wall. Nutrition and Metabolism. Proc. Internat. Symp. on xanthomata formation and other tissue reactions to hyperlipidemias 15, 46 (1973).

JACOTOT, B., MONNIER, G., BEAUMONT, J. L.: In vivo incorporation of dietary ^{14}C-cholesterol in rat serum lipoproteins and transfers in connective tissue. Clin. Chim. Acta 33, 95 (1971).

JAFFE, E. A., HOYER, L. W., NACHMAN, R. L.: Synthesis of anti hemophilic factor antigen by cultured human endothelial cells. J. Clin. Invest. 52, 2757 (1973).

JAFFE, E. A., NACHMAN, R. L., BECKER, C. G., MINICK, C. R.: Culture of human endothelial cells derived from umbilical veins. J. Clin. Invest. 52, 2745 (1973).

JAIN, A., RYAN, J. R., HAGUE, D., Mc MAHON, F. G.: The effect of MK-185 on some aspects of uric acid metabolism. Clin. Pharmacol. Therap. 11, 551 - 557 (1970).

JANADO, M., MARTIN, W. G.: Molecular heterogeneity of a pig serum low-density lipoprotein. Can. J. Biochem. 46, 875 (1968).

JANADO, M., MARTIN, W. G., COOK, W. H.: Separations and properties of pig serum lipoproteins. Can. J. Biochem. 44, 1201 (1966).

JANSEN, H., HÜLSMANN, W. C.: Long-chain acyl-CoA hydrolase activity in serum: Identity with clearing factor lipase. Biochim. Biophys. Acta 296, 241 - 248 (1973).

JANUSKEVICHIUS, Z., BLOOZHAS, J.: Clinical trial of pyridinolcarbamate. In: Atherogenesis II, Excerpta Medica, 1973, p. 311.

JARETT, L., STEINER, A. L., SMITH, R. M., KIPNIS, D. M.: The involvement of cyclic AMP in the hormonal regulation of protein synthesis in rat adipocytes. Endocrinology 90, 1277 (1972).

JARMOLYCH, J., DAOUD, A. S., LANDAU, J., FRITZ, K. E., Mc ELVENE, E.: Aortic medial explants. Cell proliferation and production of mucopolysaccharides, collagen and elastic tissue. Exp. Mol. Pathol. 9, 171 (1968).

JENKINS, C. S. P., PACKHAM, M. A., GUCCIONE, M. A., MUSTARD, J. F.: Modification of platelet adherence to protein-coated surfaces. J. Lab. Clin. Med. 81, 280-290 (1973).

JENNINGS, R. B.: Early phase of myocardial ischemic injury and infarction. Amer. J. Cardiol. 24, 753 (1969).

JENSEN, J., BLANKENHORN, D. H., CHIN, H. P., STURGEON, P., WARE, A. G.: Serum lipids and serum uric acid in human twins. J. Lipid Res. 6, 193 (1965).

JENSEN, J., BLANKENHORN, D. H., KORNERUP, V.: Coronary disease in familial hypercholesterolemia. Circulation 36, 77 (1967).

JEPSON, E. M., SMALL, E., GRAYSON, M. F., BANCE, G., BILLIMORIA, J. D.: A comparative study of a new drug MK-185 with clofibrate in the treatment of hyperlipidaemias. Atherosclerosis 16, 9 - 14 (1972).

JERSILD, R. A., Jr.: A time sequence study of fat absorption in the rat jejunum. Am. J. Anat. 118, 135 - 162 (1966).

JESSE, M. J., HENNEKENS, C. H., FERRER, P. L., BLUMENTHAL, S.: Blood pressure in Newborns, Neonates and Infants. (In preparation).

JESSE, M. J., HENNEKENS, C. J., FERRER, P. L., BLUMENTHAL, S.: Serum Lipids in Families of Men with Premature Infarction: A Case Control Study. (In preparation).

JESSE, M. J., HENNEKENS, C. H., FERRER, P. L., BLUMENTHAL, S.: Risk Factors in Progeny of Men with Premature Myocardial Infarction: A Discriminant Function Analysis. (In preparation).

JEZKOVA, Z., POKORNY, J.: The appearance of a wide variety of antibodies in atherosclerosis. Angiologica 4, 359 (1967).

JIMENEZ, S. A., PROCKOP, D. J.: Specific inhibition of collagen synthesis in rat granulomas by the incorporation of the proline analogue cis-4-hydroxyproline into intracellular collagen. J. Clin. Invest. 50, 49 A (1970).

JØRGENSEN, L.: The role of platelet embolism from crumbling thrombi and of platelet aggregates arising in flowing blood. In: Thrombosis, p. 506 – 533. (SHERRY, S., BRINKHOUS, K. M., GENTON, E., and STENGLE, J. M., Eds.). Washington: Nat. Acad. Sciences 1969.

JØRGENSEN, L.: Mechanisms of thrombosis. Pathobiology Annual (1971).

JØRGENSEN, L., HAEREM, J. W., CHANDLER, A. B., BORCHGREVINK, C. F.: The pathology of acute coronary death. Acta Anaesth. Scand. (Suppl.) 29, 193 – 199 (1968).

JØRGENSEN, L., HOVIG, T., ROWSELL, H. C., MUSTARD, J. F.: Adenosine diphosphate-induced platelet aggregation and vascular injury in swine and rabbits. Amer. J. Path. 61, 161 – 170 (1970).

JØRGENSEN, L., PACKHAM, M. A., ROWSELL, H. C., MUSTARD, J. F.: Deposition of formed elements of blood on the intima and signs of intimal injury in the aorta of rabbit, pig, and man. Lab. Invest. 27, 341 – 350 (1972).

JØRGENSEN, L., ROWSELL, H. C., HOVIG, T., GLYNN, M. F., MUSTARD, J. F.: Adenosine diphosphate-induced platelet aggregation and myocardial infarction in swine. Lab. Invest. 17, 616 – 644 (1967).

JØRGENSEN, L., ROWSELL, H. C., HOVIG, T., MUSTARD, J. F.: Resolution and organization of platelet-rich mural thrombi in carotid arteries of swine. Amer. J. Path. 51, 681 – 719 (1967).

JOHNSON, B. C., EPSTEIN, F. H., KJELSBERG, M. O.: Distributions and familial studies of blood pressure and serum cholesterol levels in a total community – Tecumseh, Michigan. J. Chron. Dis. 18, 147 (1965).

JOHNSON, L. D., MOSKOWITZ, M. S.: Inhibition of cholesterol esterase hydrolytic activity in hog aorta. Circulation 38, Suppl. VI., 11 (1968).

JOHNSON, R. C., SHAH, S. N.: Evidence for two soluble noncatalytic proteins in hepatic microsomal cholesterol synthesis. Biochem. Biophys. Res. Commun. 48, 105 – 111 (1973).

JOIST, J. H., LLOYD, J. V., MUSTARD, J. F.: Availability of platelet factor 3 activity in suspensions of washed platelets. Proceedings IIIrd Congress. The International Society on Thrombosis and Haemostasis. Washington, D. C., p. 210 (1972).

JONES, A. L., OCKNER, R. K.: An electron microscopic study of endogenous very low density lipoprotein production in the intestine of rat and man. J. Lipid Res. 12, 580 – 589 (1971).

JONES, A. L., RUDERMAN, N. B., HERRERA, M. G.: Electron microscopic and biochemical study of lipoprotein synthesis in the isolated perfused rat liver. J. Lipid Res. 8, 429 – 446 (1967).

JONES, R. J.: Atherosclerosis: Proceedings of the Second International Symposium. New York: Springer-Verlag 1970.

KADAR, A., ROBERT, B., ROBERT, L.: Etude biochimique et électromicroscopique des microfibrilles du tissu conjonctif. Pathol. Biol. 21, 80 – 88 (1973).

KAGAN, A., RHOADS, G. C., ZEEGAN, P. D., NICHAMAN, M. Z.: Coronary heart disease among men of Japanese ancestry in Hawaii: The Honolulu Heart Study. Isr. J. med. Sci. 7, 1573 (1971).

KAHN, E. B., EDWARDS, C. N.: Smoking and youth: Contributions to the study of smoking behaviour in high school students. Journal of School Health 40, 561 – 562 (1970).

KAJIMA, M., POLLARD, M.: Arterial lesions in gnotobiotic mice congenitally infected with LCM virus. Nature 224, 188 (1969).

KAKITA, C., JOHNSON, P. J., PICK, R., KATZ, L. N.: Relationship between plasma cholesterol level and coronary atherosclerosis in cholesterol-oil fed cockerels. Atherosclerosis 15, 17 – 29 (1972).

KALANT, N., TEITELBAUM, J. I., COOPERBERG, A. A.: Dietary atherogenesis in alloxan diabetes. J. Lab. Clin. Med. 63, 147 (1964).

KAN, K. W., RITTER, M. C., UNGAR, F., DEMPSEY, M. E.: The role of a carrier protein in cholesterol and steroid hormone synthesis by adrenal enzymes. Biochem. Biophys. Res. Commun. 48, 423 – 429 (1972).

KAN, K. W., UNGAR, F.: Characterization of an adrenal activator for cholesterol side chain cleavage. J. Biol. Chem. 248, 2868 (1973).

KANE, J. P.: A rapid electrophoretic technique for identification of subunit species of apoproteins in serum lipoproteins. Anal. Biochem. 53, 350 (1973).

KANEKO, Y.: Plasma renin activity and prognosis of essential hypertension, Jap. Circ. J. 36, 995 (1972).

KANNEL, W. B., CASTELLI, W. P., GORDON, T., Mc NAMARA, P. M.: Serum cholesterol, lipoproteins, and the risk of coronary heart disease. Ann. intern. Med. 74, 1 (1971).

KANNEL, W. B., CASTELLI, W. P., Mc NAMARA, P. M., SORLIE, P.: Some factors affecting morbidity and mortality in hypertension, Milbank Memorial Fund Quarterly 47, Part 2, 116 (1969).

KANNEL, W. B., DAWBER, T. R.: Atherosclerosis as a pediatric problem. J. Ped. 80, 544 (1972).

KANNEL, W. B., SKINNER, J. J., Jr., SCHWARTZ, M. S., SHURTLEFF, D.: Intermittent claudication. Incidence in the Framingham Study. Circ. 41, 875 (1970).

KAO, V. C. Y., WISSLER, R. W.: A study of the immunohistochemical localization of serum lipoproteins and other plasma proteins in human atherosclerotic lesions. Expl. Molec. Path. 4, 465 (1965).

KAO, V. C. Y., WISSLER, R. W., DZOGA, K.: The influence of hyperlipemic serum on the growth of medial smooth muscle cells of rhesus monkey aorta in vitro. Circulation 38, VI - 12 (1968).

KAPLAN, A., JACQUES, S., GANT, M.: Effect of long-lasting epinephrine on serum lipid levels. Am. J. Physiol. 191, 8 - 12 (1957).

KAPLAN, A. P., SCHREIBER, A. D., AUSTEN, K. F.: Isolation and reaction mechanisms of human plasma plasminogen activator and its precursor. Fed. Proc. 31, 624 abs. (1972).

KARAM, J. H., GRODSKY, G. M., PAVLATOS, F. C., FORSHAM, P. H.: Critical factors in excessive serum-insulin response to glucose. Obesity in maturity-onset diabetes and growth hormone in acromegaly. Lancet 1965 I, 286.

KASS, E. H., ZINNER, S. H.: How early can the tendency towards hypertension be detected? Milbank Mem. Fund Quart. 47, Part 2, 143 (1969).

KATZ, L. N., STAMLER, J.: Experimental Atherosclerosis. Springfield: C.C.Thomas 1953.

KAWAMURA, A., Jr.: Fluorescent antibody techniques and their application, p. 11 - 64. Baltimore, Maryland (USA), and Manchester (England): University Park Press 1969.

KAY, A. B., PEPPER, D. S., EWART, M. R.: Generation of chemotactic activity for leukocytes by the action of thrombin on human fibrinogen. Nature New Biology 243, 56 - 57 (1973).

KEITZER, W. F., FRY, W. J., KRAFT, R. O., DeWEESE, M. S.: Hemodynamic mechanism for pulse changes seen in occlusive vascular disease. Surgery 57, 163 (1965).

KEMP, N. E., QUINN, B. L.: Morphogenesis and metabolism of amphibian larvae after excision of heart. Anat. Rec. 118, 773 (1954).

KENNEDY, L. J., BIEBER, C. P., MITCHINSON, M. J.: Aortic histopathology in human cardiac allografts. J. Thoracic Cardiovascular Surgery 62, 42 (1971).

KERSHBAUM, A., BELLET, S., DICKSTEIN, E. R., FEINBERG, L. J.: Effect of cigarette smoking and nicotine on serum free fatty acids. Based on a study in the human subject and the experimental animal. Circulat. Res. 9, 631 (1961).

KESSLER, G., LEDERER, H.: Fluorimetic measurement of triglycerides: automation in analytical chemistry. In: Technicon Symposia 1965, p. 341 (SKEGGS, L. T., Jr., Ed.). New York: Medial Inc. 1966.

KEYS, A.: Coronary heart disease in seven countries. Circulation 41 - 42, Suppl. I (1970).

KEYS, A., ARAVANIS, C., BLACKBURN, H. W., VAN BUCHEM, F. S. P., BUZINA, R., DJORDJEVIC, B. S., DONTAS, A. S., FIDANZA, F., KARVONEN, M. J., KIMURA, N., LEKOS, D., MONTI, M., PUDDU, V., TAYLOR, H. L.: Epidemiological studies related to coronary heart disease: Characteristics of men aged 40 - 55 in seven countries. Acta med. scand., Suppl. 460, 1 (1966).

KEYS, A., AVRANIS, C., BLACKBURN, H., VAN BUCHEM, F. S. P., BUZINA, R., DJORDJEVIC, B. S., FIDANZA, F., KARVONEN, M. J., MENOTTI, A., PUDDU, V., TAYLOR, H. L.: Probability of middle-aged men developing coronary heart disease in five years. Circulation 45, 815 (1972).

KHOO, J. C., AQUINO, A. A., STEINBERG, D.: The mechanism of activation of hormone-sensitive lipase in human adipose tissue. J.Clin.Invest. 53, 1124 (1974).

KHOO, J. C., STEINBERG, D., THOMPSON, B., MAYER, S. E.: Hormonal regulation of adipocyte enzymes. The effects of epinephrine and insulin on the control of lipase, phosphorylase kinase, phosphorylase and glycogen synthase. J. Biol. Chem. 248, 3823 (1973).

KIRBY, R. R., KEMMERER, W. T., MORGAN, J. C.: Transcutaneous doppler measurement of blood pressure. Anesthesiology 31, 86 (1969).

KIRK, J. E.: The 5'-nucleotidase activity of human arterial tissue in individuals of various ages. J. Geront. 14, 288 (1959).

KIRK, J. E.: Intermediary metabolism of human arterial tissue and its changes with age and atherosclerosis. In: Atherosclerosis and its Origin, p. 67 (SCANDLER, M., and BOURNE, G. H., Eds.). New York: Academic Press 1963.

KIRK, J. E.: Enzyme of the arterial wall, p. 494. New York: Academic Press 1969.

KIRKLAND, R. T., KIRKLAND, J. L.: Systolic blood pressuremeasurement in the newborn infant with the transcutaneous doppler method. J. of Ped. 80, 52 (1972).

KJEKSHUS, J. K., MJÖS, O. D.: Effect of inhibition of lipolysis on infarct size after experimental coronary artery occlusion. J. Clin. Invest. 52, 1770 (1973).

KJELDSEN, K., ASTRUP, P., WANSTRUP, J.: Reversal of rabbit atheromatosis by hyperoxia. J. Atheroscl. Res. 10, 173 (1969).

KJELDSEN, K., ASTRUP, P., WANSTRUP, J.: Ultrastructural intimal changes in the rabbit aorta after a moderate carbon monoxide exposure. Atherosclerosis 16, 67 – 82 (1972).

KJELDSEN, K., WANSTRUP, J., ASTRUP, P.: Enhancing influence of arterial hypoxia on the development of atheromatosis in cholesterol-fed rabbits. J. Atherosclerosis 8, 835 (1968).

KLEIN, W.: Über die enzymatische Hydrolyse der Cholesterinester des menschlichen Serums. Z. Physiol. Chem. 254, 1 (1938).

KLEIN, W.: Über die enzymatische Hydrolyse der Cholesterinester II. Z. Physiol. Chem. 259, 268 (1939).

KLEMENS, U. H., LÖWIS OF MENAR, P. V., BREMER, A., WNUCK, E., V., SCHRÖDER, R. Hyperlipoproteinamien und Koronarerkrankungen. Häufigkeit, Typenverteilung Abhängigkeit von Alter und Geschlecht. Klin. Wschr. 50, 139 (1972).

KLIMOV, A. N., LOVIAGINA, T. N., BAN'KOVSKAYA, E. B.: Preparation of lipoproteins with double radioactive label and study of their penetration into vessel wall. Vopr. med. Chim. 17, 434 (1972). (In Russian).

KLOTZ, O., MANNING, M. F.: Fatty streaks in the intima of arteries. J. Pathol. Bacteriol. 16, 211 – 220 (1911).

KNICK, B., LANGE, H.-J., SKOLUDA, D., KREMER, G.: Frühdiabetische Lipoidstoffwechselanomalien bei Myokardinfarkt und arterieller Verschlußkrankheit. Dtsch. med. Wschr. 93, 1954 (1968).

KNIKER, W. T., COCHRANE, C. G.: The localization of circulating immune complexes in experimental serum sickness. The role of vasoactive amines and hydrodynamic forces. J. Exp. Med. 127, 119 – 136 (1968).

KNÜCHEL, F.: Statistische Vergleichsuntersuchungen über den Einfluß von Lipostabil auf Serumlipoide und -lipoproteine. Med. Klinik 36, 1652 (1959).

KOBAYASHI, J.: On geographical relationship between the chemical nature of river water. Ber. Ohara Inst. 11, 12 – 21 (1957).

KOCSIS, J. J., HERNANDOVICH, J., SILVER, M. J., SMITH, J. B., INGERMAN, C.: Duration of inhibition of platelet prostaglandin formation and aggregation by ingested aspirin or indomethacin. Prostaglandins 3, 141 – 144 (1973).

KOEHLER, D. F., DEMPSEY, M. E.: Development of a specific assay for squalene and sterol carrier protein in lipoprotein fractions of human serum. Circulation 48, IV – 246 (1973).

KOGA, S., BOLIS, L., SCANU, A. M.: Isolation and characterization of subunit polypeptides from apoproteins of rat serum lipoproteins. Biochim. Biophys. Acta 236, 416 (1971).

KOLETSKY, C. R., RIVERA-VELEZ, J. M.: Rapid acceleration of atherosclerosis in hypertensive rats on high fat diet. Exp. Mol. Path. 9, 322 – 338 (1968).

KOPPERS, L. E., PALUMBO, P. J.: Lipid disturbances in endocrine disorders. Med. Clin. N. A. **56**, 1013 - 1020 (1972).

KORN, E. D.: Clearing factor, a heparin-activated lipoprotein lipase. I. Isolation and characterization of the enzyme from normal rat heart. J. Biol. Chem. **215**, 1 (1955).

KORN, E. D.: Clearing factor, a heparin activated lipoprotein lipase. II. Substrate specificity and activation of coconut oil. J. Biol. Chem. **215**, 15 (1955).

KORN, E. D.: The assay of lipoprotein lipase *in vivo* and *in vitro*. Meth. Biochem. Anal. **VII**, 145 - 192 (1959).

KOSEK, J., BIEBER, C.: Atheroma in a transplanted heart. Lancet **1970 I**, 563.

KOSEK, J. C., BIEBER, C., LOWER, R. R.: Severe atheroma in human transplants. Heart graft arteriosclerosis. Transplantation Proc. **3**, 512 - 514 (1971).

KOSTNER, G., ALAUPOVIC, P.: Studies of the composition and structure of plasma lipoproteins. Separation and quantification of the lipoprotein families occurring in the high density lipoproteins of human plasma. Biochemistry **11**, 3419 (1972).

KOTHARI, H. V., BONNER, M. J., MILLER, B. F.: Cholesterol ester hydrolase in homogenates and lysosomal fractions of human aorta. Biochim. Biophys. Acta **202**, 325 (1970).

KOTHARI, H. V., MILLER, B. F., KRITCHEVSKY, D.: Aortic cholesterol esterase: Characteristics of normal rat and rabbit enzyme. Biochem. Biophys. Acta **296**, 446 - 454 (1973).

KOTTKE, B. A.: Differences in bile acid excretion. Primary hypercholesterolaemia compared to combined hypercholesterolemia and hypertriglyceridaemia. Circ. **40**, 13 (1969).

KRAMSCH, D. M., FRANZBLAU, C., HOLLANDER, W.: The protein and lipid composition of arterial elastin and its relationship to lipid accumulation in the atherosclerotic plaque. J. Clin. Invest. **50**, 1666 - 1677 (1971).

KRAMSCH, D. M., HOLLANDER, W.: Occlusive atherosclerotic disease of the coronary arteries in monkey (Macaca irus) induced by diet. Exp. Mol. Pathol. **9**, 1 - 22 (1968).

KRAMSCH, D. M., HOLLANDER, W.: The interaction of serum and arterial lipoproteins with elastin of the arterial intima and its role in the lipid accumulation in atherosclerotic plaques. J. Clin. Invest. **52**, 236 - 247 (1973).

KRAMSCH, D. M., HUVOS, A., HOLLANDER, W.: A primate model for the study of coronary (atherosclerotic) heart disease. Circ. **42**, Suppl. III, 9 (1970).

KRASNO, L. R., KIDERA, G. J.: Clofibrate in coronary heart disease. Effect on morbidity and mortality. JAMA **219**, 845 (1972).

KRAUSS, R. M., ASSMANN, G., WINDMUELLER, H. G., FREDRICKSON, D. S., LEVY, R. I.: Substrate and positional specificities of heparin-released lipolytic activities. Circ. **48**, Suppl. IV, 112 (Abstr.) (1973).

KRAUSS, R. M., WINDMUELLER, H. G., LEVY, R. I., FREDRICKSON, D. S.: Selective measurement of two different triglyceride lipase activities in rat post-heparin plasma. J. Lipid Res. **14**, 286 (1973).

KREMER, G. J., NIEMCZYK, H., POEPLAU, W., NICOLESCU, R. F.: Hyperlipoproteinämien bei peripheren arteriellen Verschlußkrankheiten. Münch. med. Wschr. **115**, 662 (1973).

KRISTA, L. M., WAIBEL, P. E., SAUTTER, J. H., SHOFFNER, R. N.: Aortic rupture, body weight, and blood pressure in the turkey as influenced by strain, dietary fat, beta-aminopropionitrile fumarate, and diethylstilbestrol. Poult. Sci. **48**, 1954 - 1960 (1969).

KRITCHEVSKY, D.: Current concepts in the genesis of the atherosclerotic plaque in atherosclerotic vascular disease, p. 1 (BREST, A. N., and MAYER, J. H., Eds.). New York: Appleton-Century-Crofts 1967.

KRITCHEVSKY, D.: Role of cholesterol vehicle in experimental atherosclerosis. Am. J. Clin. Nutr. **23**, 1105 - 1110 (1970).

KRITCHEVSKY, D., KOTHARI, H.V.: Metabolism of the arterial wall. This volume p. 39.

KRITCHEVSKY, D., CASEY, R. P., TEPPER, S. A.: Isocaloric, isogravic diets in rats. II. Effect on cholesterol absorption and excretion. Nutr. Reports Intl. 7, 61 (1973).

KRITCHEVSKY, D., GENZANO, J. C., KOTHARI, H. V.: Influence of age on aortic cholesterol esterase in rats. Mech. Aging Development (1974 a, In press).

KRITCHEVSKY, D., SALLATA, P., TEPPER, S. A.: Experimental atherosclerosis in rabbits fed cholesterol-free diets. Part 2. Influence of various carbohydrates. J. Atheroscler. Res. 8, 697 (1968).

KRITCHEVSKY, D., TEPPER, S. A.: Experimental atherosclerosis in rabbits fed cholesterol-free diets: influence of chow components. J. Atheroscler. Res. 8, 357 (1968).

KRITCHEVSKY, D., TEPPER, S. A.: Influence of pyridinolcarbamate on oxidation of cholesterol by rat liver mitochondria, Arzneimittel-Forschung 21, 146 (1971).

KRITCHEVSKY, D., TEPPER, S. A., GENZANO, J. C., KOTHARI, H. V.: Aortic cholesterol esterase in rabbits: effect of duration of cholesterol fedding. Atherosclerosis (1974 b, In press).

KRITCHEVSKY, D., TEPPER, S. A., VESSELINOVITCH, D., WISSLER, R. W.: Cholesterol vehicle in experimental atherosclerosis. Part 11: Peanut oil. Atherosclerosis 14, 53 - 64 (1971).

KRITCHEVSKY, D., TEPPER, S. A., VESSELINOVITCH, D., WISSLER, R. W.: Cholesterol vehicle in experimental atherosclerosis, Part 13. Randomized peanut oil. Atherosclerosis 17, 225 - 243 (1973).

KRZYWANEK, H. J., BREDDIN, K.: Der Plättchenaggregationstest (PAT) Med. Laboratorium 15, 103 (1972).

KUDCHOKAR, B. J., SODHI, H. S., HORLICK, L.: Absorption of dietary-cholesterol in man. Metabolism 22, 155 (1973).

KUMAR, V., BERENSON, G. S., RUIZ, H., DALFERES, E. R., Jr., STRONG, J. P.: Acid mucopolysaccharides of human aorta, Variations with maturation, Part 1, Atheroscler. Res. 7, 573 - 581 (1967 a).

KUMAR, V., BERENSON, G. S., RUIZ, H., DALFERES, E. R., Jr., STRONG, J. P.: Acid mucopolysaccharides of human aorta. Variations with Atherosclerotic involvement, Part 2. J. Atheroscler. Res. 7, 583 - 590 (1967 b).

KUO, P. T.: Plasma lipids and atherosclerosis. In: Atherosclerosis and coronary heart diseases, p. 8. (LIKOFF, W., BERNARD, L. S., and INSULL, W., Jr., Eds.). New York: Grune and Stratton 1972.

KURAI, A.: Study on thrombosis (1). New experimental method of inducing thrombosis in vivo, Ochanomizu Medical Journal 13, 189, 368 (1965).

KWAAN, H. C., Mc FADZEAN, A. J. S.: Inhibition of fibronolysis in vivo by feeding cholesterol. Nature 179, 260 (1957).

KWITEROVICH, P. O., Jr., LEVY, R. I., FREDRICKSON, D. S.: Neonatal diagnosis of familial type-II hyperlipoproteinaemia. Lancet 1973 I , 118.

KYD, P. A., BOUCHIER, I. A. D.: Cholesterol metabolism in rabbits with oleic acid-induced cholelithiasis. Proc. Soc. Exp. Biol. Med. 141, 846 (1972).

KYUSOV, V. A., BELOUSOV, Y. B., MARTYNOV, A. I., KOROLEVA, S. A., ZIMIN, V. S., DUDAEV, V. A.: Treatment by Anginin (pyridinolcarbamate) of the coronary and obliterating atherosclerosis of the lower extremities. Cardiology 11, 39 (1972).

LACY, P. E., HOWELL, S. L., YOUNG, D. A., FINK, C. J.: New hypothesis of insulin secretion. Nature 219, 1177 - 1179 (1968).

LADEN, A. M. K.: Experimental atherosclerosis in rat and rabbit cardiac allografts. Arch. Path. 93, 240 (1972).

LAMB, R. G., FALLON, H. J.: Inhibition of monoacylglycerophosphate formation by chlorophenoxyisobutyrate and betabenzalbutyrate. J. Biol. Chem. 247, 1281 (1972).

LAMB, R. G., HILL, P. M., FALLON, H. J.: Inhibition of palmitoyl CoA deacylase by chlorophenoxyisobutyrate and betabenzalbutyrate. J. Lipid Res. 14, 459 - 467 (1973).

LAMBERT, G. F., MILLER, J. P., OLSEN, R. T., FROST, D. V.: Hypercholesteremia and atherosclerosis induced in rabbits by purified high rat rations devoid of cholesterol. Proc. Soc. Exp. Biol. Med. 97, 544 (1958).

LANDIS, E. M., PAPPENHEIMER, J. R.: Exchange of substances through the capillary Walls. In: Handbook of physiology, section 2: Circulation, Vol 2, p. 961 -

1034 (HAMMILTON, W. F., and DOW, P., Eds.). Baltimore: Williams & Wilkins 1963.

LANE, J. M., BORA, F. W., PROCKOP, D. J., HEPPERSTALL, R. B., BLACK, J.: Inhibition of scar formation by the proline analog cis-hydroxyproline. J. Surg. Res. 3, 135 - 137 (1972).

LANG, P. D., INSULL, W., Jr.: Lipid droplets in arteriosclerotic fatty streaks of human aorta. J. Clin. Invest. 49, 1479 (1970).

LANGER, T., LEVY, R. I.: Acute muscular syndrome associated with administration of clofibrate. N. Engl. J. Med. 279, 856 (1968).

LANGER, T., STROBER, W., LEVY, R. I.: The metabolism of low density lipoprotein in familial type II hyperlipoproteinaemia. J. Clin. Invest. 51, 1528 (1972).

LANGMAN, M. J. S., ELWOOD, P. C., FOOTE, J., RYRIE, D. R.: ABO and Lewis blood-groups and serum-cholesterol. Lancet 1969 II, 607.

LARAGH, J. H.: Biochemical profiling and the natural history of hypertensive diseases: Low-renin essential hypertension, a benign condition, Circulation 44, 971 (1971).

LaROSA, J. C., LEVY, R. I., HERBERT, P., LUX, S. E., FREDRICKSON, D. S.: Specific apoprotein activator for lipoprotein lipase. Biochem. Biophys. Res. Commun. 41, 57 (1970).

LaROSA, J. C., LEVY, R. I., WINDMUELLER, H. G., FREDRICKSON, D. S.: Comparison of the triglyceride lipase of liver, adipose tissue, and postheparin plasma. J. Lipid Res. 13, 356 (1972).

LARRUE, J., BERJON, J. J., DESGRANGES, C., MEUNIER, J. M., BRICAUD, H.:
a) Caractères histologiques et histoenzymologiques d'homogreffes de fragments de paroi aortique chez le rat. C R Acad. Sci. (Paris) 277, 321 - 324 (1973).
b) Modifications histométaboliques de fragments de paroi aortique en homo-greffes et cultures organotypiques. Proceedings of the symposium on the vessel wall, London 1973 (In press).

LAURELL, C. B.: Electroimmuno assay. Scand. J. Clin. Lab. Invest. 29, Suppl. 124, 21 (1972).

LAUTSCH, E. V., COOPER, D. R., BASSETT, J. G., MATTHIS, Le R.: Morphologic aspects of alcohol preserved vascular homografts in dogs. Lab. Invest. 8, 848 (1959).

LAZZARINI-ROBERTSON, A., Jr.: Blood vessel bank - its possibilities. Angiology 4, 516 (1953).

LAZZARINI-ROBERTSON, A., Jr.: Studies on the effects of lipid emulsions on arterial intimal cells in tissue culture in relation to atherosclerosis. Thesis, Cornell Grad. Med. School, Cornell University, 1959.

LAZZARINI-ROBERTSON, A., Jr.: The role of local cholesterol re-utilization in atherogenesis. Arch. Sur. 85, 41 (1962).

LAZZARINI-ROBERTSON, A., Jr., BUTKUS, A., EHRHART, L. A., LEWIS, L. A.: Experimental arteriosclerosis in dogs. Evaluation of anatomopathological findings. Atherosclerosis 15, 307 - 325 (1972).

LECHNER, K., NIESSNER, H.: Protokoll über das Symposion des Arbeitskreises Plättchenfunktion und Thrombose in Wien am 12.6.1971. I. Med. Universitäts-klinik, A-1090 Wien.

LEE, D. M., ALAUPOVIC, P.: Studies of the composition and structure of plasma lipoproteins. Isolation, composition, and immunochemical characterization of low density lipoprotein subfractions of human plasma. Biochemistry 9, 2244 (1970).

LEE, D. M., ALAUPOVIC, P.: Characterization of associated and free forms of LP-B in low density lipoproteins of normal human plasma. This volume p. 914.

LEE, K. T., JARMOLYCH, Y., KIM, D. N., GRANT, C., KRASNEY, J. H., THOMAS, W. A., BRUNO, A. M.: Production of advanced coronary atherosclerosis, myocardial infarction and "sudden death" in swine. Exp. Molec. Pathol. 15, 170 - 190 (1971).

LEES, R. S.: Immunoassay of plasma low-density lipoproteins. Science 169, 493 (1970).

LEHNER, N. D. M., CLARKSON, T. C., BELL, F. B., ST. CLAIR, R. W., LOFLAND, H. B.: Effect of insulin deficiency hypothroidism and hypertension on cholesterol metabolism in the squirrel monkey. Exp. Mol. Path. 16, 109 (1972).

LEHNER, N. D. M., CLARKSON, T. B., BULLOCK, B. C., LOFLAND, H. B., ST. CLAIR, R. W., PRICHARD, R. W.: Studies on atherosclerosis of some non-human primates. In: Medical Primatology 1970 (Selected papers from 2nd Conf. on Experimental Medicine and Surgery in Primates, New York 1968), p. 873 – 885 (GOLDSMITH, E. I., and MOOR-JANKOWSKI, J. K., Eds.). Basel: Karger 1971.

LEHNER, N. D. M., CLARKSON, T. B., LOFLAND, H. B.: The effects of insulin deficiency, hypothyroidism, and hypertension on atherosclerosis in the squirrel monkey. Exp. Mol. Pathol. 15, 230 (1971).

LEMPERT, H.: Plasma fibrinogen determination. In: Practical clinical biochemistry, 3rd Ed.. p. 191 (VARLEY, H., Ed.). London: Heinemann 1962.

LENDRUM, A. C.: In: Vascular histochemistry in relation to the chemical and structural pathology of cardiovascular disease, p. 195 (ADAMS, C. W. M., Ed.). London: Lloyd-Luke 1967.

LENEGRE, J., DE BRUX, J., HIMBERT, J., BEAUMONT, J. L.: Avant-project d'un rapport sur l'athérosclérose. Revue d'Atherosclerose 1, 3 (1959).

LEREN, P., HAARBREKKE, O.: Blood lipids in patients with atherosclerosis obliterans of the lower limbs. Acta med. scand. 189, 511 (1971).

LEVENE, C. I., POOLE, J. C. F.: The collagen content of the normal and atherosclerotic human aortic intima. Brit. J. Exp. Pathol. 43, 469 – 471 (1962).

LEVENTHAL, H.: Changing attitudes and habits to reduce risk factors in chronic disease. Amér. J. Card. 31, 571 (1973).

LEVIN, W. C., ABOUMRAD, M. H., RITZMANN, S. E., BRANTLY, C.: γ-Type I myeloma and xanthomatosis. Arch. Int. Med. 114, 688 (1964).

LEVINE, P. H.: An acute effect of cigarette smoking on platelet function. A possible link between smoking and arterial thrombosis. Circulation 48, 619 – 623 (1973).

LEVINE, S. B., ZAK, B.: Automated determination of serum total cholesterol. Clin. Chim. Acta 10, 381 (1964).

LEVINE, Y. K., BIRDSALL, N. J. M., LEE, A. G., METCALFE, J. C.: ^{13}C Nuclear magnetic resonance relaxations measurements of synthetic lecithins and the effect of spin-labeled lipids. Biochemistry 11, 1416 (1972).

LEVY, L.: A form of immunological atherosclerosis. In: The retuculoendothelial system and atherosclerosis, p. 426 (Di LUZZIO, G., and PAOLETTI, R., Eds.). New York: Plenum Press 1967.

LEVY, R. I., BILHEIMER, D. W., EISENBERG, S.: The structure and metabolim of chylomicrons and very low density lipoproteins (VLDL). In: Plasma lipoproteins, p. 3 (SMELLIE, R. M. S., Ed.). London: Academic Press 1971.

LEVY, R. I., FREDRICKSON, D. S.: Type II and type III hyperlipoproteinemia. I. Chemical differentiation. In: The metabolic basis of inherited disease, p. 545 (STANBURY, J. B., WYNGAARDEN, J. B., and FREDRICKSON, D. S., Eds.). New York: Mc Graw-Hill 1971.

LEVY, R. I., QUARFORDT, S. H., BROWN, W. V., SLOAN, H. R., FREDRICKSON, D. S.: Efficacy of clofibrate (CPIB) in familial hyperlipoproteinemias. In: Drugs affecting lipid metabolism, Vol 4 (HOLMES, W. L., CARLSON, L. A., and PAOLETTI, R., Eds.). New York: Plenum Press 1969.

LEVY, R. I., RIFKIND, B. M.: Diagnosis and management of hyperlipoproteinemia in infants and children. Amer. J. Card. 31, 547 (1973).

LEVY, R. S., LYNCH, A. C., Mc GEE, E. D., MEHL, J. W.: Amino acid composition of the proteins from chylomicrons and human serum lipoproteins. J. Lipid Res. 8, 463 (1967).

LEVY, S. W., SWANK, R. L.: The effects of in vivo heparin on plasma esterase activity and lipaemia clearing. J. Physiol. 123, 301 – 314 (1954).

LEWIS, L. A., GREEN, A. A., PAGE, I. H.: Ultracentrifuge lipoprotein pattern of serum of normal, hypertensive and hypothyroid animals. Am. J. Physiol. 171, 391 (1972).

LEWIS, L. A., LAZZARINI-ROBERTSON, A., Jr.: Hyperimmunoglobulinemia-lipoproteinemias and atherogenesis. This volume p. 595.

LEWIS, L. A., PAGE, I. H.: Serum proteins and lipoproteins in multiple myelomatosis. Am. J. Med. 17, 670 (1954).

LEWIS, L. A., PAGE, I. H.: An unusual serum lipoprotein-globulin complex in a patient with hyperlipemia. Am J. Med. 38, 286 (1965).

LEWIS, L. A., PAGE, I. H., BATTLE, J. D., DE WOLFE, V. G.: How should hyperli-poproteinemia-hyperimmunoglobulinemia manifestations of an antilipoprotein autoantibody be treated? Internat. Res. Communic. System 1, 40 (1973).

LEWIS, L. A., VAN OMMEN, R. A., PAGE, I. H.: Association of cold-precipitability with beta-lipoprotein and cryoglobulin. Amer. J. of medicine 40, 785 (1960).

LILJEFORS, I.: Coronary heart disease in male twins: Hereditary and environ-mental factors in concordant and discordant pairs. Acta med. scand., Suppl. 511, 1 (1970).

LILJEFORS, I., RAHE, R. H.: An identical twin study of psychosocial factors in coronary heart disease in Sweden. Psychosom. Med. 32, 523 (1970).

LILLEHEI, R. C., SIMMONS, R. L., NAJARIAN, J. S., WEIL, R., UCHIDA, H., RUIZ, J. O., KJELLSTRAND, C. M., GOETZ, F. C.: Pancreatico-duodenal allotrans-plantation: Experimental and clinical experience. Annals of Surgery 172, 405 (1970).

LINDGREN, F. T., JENSEN, L. C., HATCH, F. T.: The isolation and quantitative analysis of serum lipoproteins. In: Blood lipids and lipoproteins: quanti-tation, composition, and metabolism, p. 181 (NELSON, G. S., Ed.). New York: John Wiley & Sons, Inc. 1972.

LINDSTEDT, S.: Turnover of cholic acid in man. Acta Physiol. Scand. 40, 1 (1957).

LINK, R. P., PEDERSOLI, W. M., SAFANIE, A. H.: Effect of exercise on development of atherosclerosis in swine. Atherosclerosis 15, 107 - 122 (1972).

LLOYD, J. K., WOLFF, O. H.: A pediatric approach to the prevention of athero-sclerosis. J. Atheroscler. Res. 10, 135 (1969).

LO, C. H., MARSH, J. B.: Biosynthesis of plasma lipoproteins. Incorporation of ^{14}C-glucosamine by cells and subcellular fractions of rat liver. J. Biol. Chem. 245, 5001 (1970).

LOFLAND, H. B., Jr., CLARKSON, T. B.: A biochemical study of spontaneous athero-sclerosis in pigeons. Circulation Res. 7, 234 (1959).

LOFLAND, H. B., Jr., CLARKSON, T. B.: The bi-directional transfer of cholesterol in normal aorta, fatty streaks, and atheromatous plaques. Proc. Soc. Exp. Biol. Med. 133, 1 - 8 (1970).

LOFLAND, H. B., Jr., CLARKSON, T. B., BULLOCK, B. C.: Whole body sterol metabo-lism in squirrel monkeys (Saimiri sciureus). Exp. Molec. Path. 13, 1 (1970).

LONDON, J. W., ROSENBERG, S. E., DRAPER, J. W., ALMY, T. P.: The effect of estrogens on atherosclerosis. Am. J. of Int. Med. 55, 63 (1961).

LOPEZ, S. A., SRIVASAN, S. R., DUGAN, F. A., RADHAKRISHNAMURTHY, B., BERENSON, G. S.: Detection of subtle abnormalities of serum beta-and pre-beta-lipo-proteins in "normal" individuals by turbidimetric and electrophoretic me-thods. Clin. Chim. Acta 31, 123 (1971).

LOUGH, J., MOORE, S.: Platelet embolic injury; the healing process. Exp. Mol. Path. 17, 132 - 144 (1972).

LOWRY, O. H., ROBERTS, N. R., LEINER, K. Y., WU, M., FARR, A. L.: The quantita-tive histochemistry of brain. J. Biol. Chem. 207, 1 (1954).

LOWRY, O. H., ROSEBROUGH, J., FARR, A. L., RANDALL, R. J.: Protein measurement with the folin phenol reagent. J. Biol. Chem. 193, 265 (1951).

LUEKER, R. D., VOGEL, J. H. K., BLOUNT, S. G., Jr.: Regression of valvular pul-monary stenosis. Brit. Heart J. 32, 779 - 782 (1970).

LUGINBÜHL, H., JONES, J. E. T.: The morphology of spontaneous atherosclerotic lesions in aged swine. In: Comparative Atherosclerosis, p. 3 (ROBERTS, J. C., Jr., and STRAUS, R., Eds.). New York: Harper & Row 1965.

LUGINBÜHL, H., RATCLIFFE, H. L., DETWEIBER, D. K.: Failure of egg-yolk feeding to accelerate progress of atherosclerosis in older female swine. Virchow Arch. Abt. A. Path. Anat. 348, 281 (1969).

LUND, A.: Fluorimetric determination of adrenaline in blood. Acta Pharmacol. Toxicol. 6, 137 (1950).

LUX, S. E., HIRZ, R., SHRAGER, R. I., GOTTO, A. M., Jr.: The influence of lipid on the conformation of human plasma high-density apolipoproteins. J. Biol. Chem. 247, 2598 (1972).

LUX, S. E., LEVY, R. I., GOTTO, A. M., FREDRICKSON, D. S.: Studies on the pro-tein defect in Tangier disease. Isolation and characterization of an abnor-mal high density lipoprotein. J. Clin. Invest. 51, 2505 (1972).

MACA, R. D., CONNOR, W. E.: The accumulation of serum lipoprotein cholesterol by tissue culture cells. Proc. Soc. Exp. Biol. Med. 138, 913 (1971).

MAGNANI, B., COCCHERI, S.: On the pathogenesis of dietetic atheromasia in the rabbit: significance of phenomena of changed vascular permeability. G. Clin. Med. 41, 1103 - 1119 (1960).

MAGNANI, H. N., ALAUPOVIC, P.: A method for quantitative determination of the abnormal lipoprotein (LP-X) of obstructive jaundice. Clin. Chim. Acta 38, 405 (1972).

MAHLER, F. R.: Insulin action on arterial tissue in relation to diabetes and atheroma. In: Diabetes Mellitus (DUNCAN, L. P. J., Ed.). Edinburgh: Edinburgh University Press 1966.

MAHLER, R.: The effect of diabetes and insulin on biochemical reactions of the arterial wall. In: Blood vessel disease in diabetes mellitus, V Capri Conference 1971. Acta diab. lat. 8, Suppl. 1, 68 (1971).

MAHLER, R., PARKES, A. B.: Fat synthesis in cultures of cells of arterial intima. Europ. J. Clin. Invest. 1, 137 (1970).

MAHLEY, R. W., BENNETT, B. D., MORRE, D. J., GRAY, M. E.: Lipoproteins associated with the Golgi apparatus isolated from epithelial cells of rat small intestine. Lab. Invest. 25, 435 (1971).

MAHLEY, R. W., HAMILTON, R. L., LEQUIRE, V. S.: Characterization of lipoprotein particles isolated from the Golgi apparatus of rat liver. J. Lipid Res. 10, 433 - 439 (1969).

MAIER, N., HAIMOVICI, H.: Metabolism of arterial tissue with special reference to esterase and lipase. Proc. Soc. Exp. Biol. 118, 258 (1965).

MAJNO, G., SHEA, S. M., LEVENTHAL, M.: Endothelial contraction induced by histamine-type mediators. An electron microscopic study, J. Cell Biol. 42, 647 (1969).

MALAISSE-LAGAE, F., GREIDER, M. H., MALAISSE, W. J., LACY, P. E.: The stimulus-secretion coupling of glucose-induced insulin release. IV. The effect of Vincristine and Deuterium oxide on the microtubular system of the pancreatic beta cell. J. Cell Biol. 49, 530 - 535 (1971).

MALHERBE, C., DE GASPARO, M., BERTHET, P., DE HERTOGH, R., HOET, J. J.: The patterns of plasma insulin response to glucose in patients with a previous myocardial infarction, - the respective effects of age and disease. Europ. J. Clin. Invest. 1, 265 (1971).

MALINOW, M. R., Mc LAUGHLIN, P., PERLEY, A.: Effect of muscular contraction on cholesterol oxidation. J. Applied Physiol. 25, 733 - 735 (1968).

MALINOW, M. R., Mc LAUGHLIN, P., PIEROVICH, I.: Muscular activity and the degradation of cholesterol by the liver. Atherosclerosis 15, 153 - 162 (1972).

MALINOW, M. R., PERLEY, A., Mc LAUGHLIN, P.: Muscular exercise and cholesterol degradation: mechanisms involved. J. Applied Physiol. 27, 662 - 665 (1969).

MALMROS, H., STERNBY, N. H.: Induction of atherosclerosis in dogs by a thiouracil-free semisynthetic diet containing cholesterol and hydrogenated coconut oil. In: Progress in biochem. pharmacol. 4, 482. (MIRAS, C. J., HOWARD, A. N., PAOLETTI, R., Eds.). Basel: Karger 1968.

MALMROS, H., WIGAND, G.: Atherosclerosis and deficiency of essential fatty acids. Lancet 1959 II, 749.

MANGANIELLO, V. C., MURAD, F., VAUGHAN, M.: Effects of lipolytic and antilipolytic agents on cyclic 3', 5'-adenosine monophosphate in fat cells. J. Biol. Chem. 246, 2195 (1971).

MANN, G. V., ANDRUS, S. B., Mc NALLY, A., STARE, F. J.: Xanthomatosis and atherosclerosis produced by diet in an adult rhesus monkey. J. Lab. Clin. Med. 48, 533 - 550 (1956).

MANNING, P. J., CLARKSON, T. B.: Development, distribution and lipid content of diet-induced atherosclerotic lesions of rhesus monkeys. Exp. Mol. Pathol. 17, 35 - 54 (1972).

MANNING, P. J., CLARKSON, T. B.: Diet induced atherosclerosis in the cat. Arch. Path. 89, 271 (1973).

MANZ, H. J., ROBERTSON, D. M.: Vascular permeability to horse radish peroxidase in brainstem lesions of thiamine-deficient rats. Amer. J. Pathol. 66, 565 (1972).

MARCHESI, V. T., JACKSON, R. L., SEGREST, J.P., KAHANE, I.: Molecular features of the major glycoprotein of the human erythrocyte membrane. Fed. Proc. 32, 1833 (1973).

MARGARETTEN, W., Mc KAY, D. G.: The requirement for platelets in the active Arthus reaction. Amer. J. Path. 64, 257 - 263 (1971).

MARGOLIS, J.: Activation of Hageman factor by saturated fatty acids. Aust. J. Exp. Biol. Med. Sci. 40, 505 - 513 (1962).

MARMO, E., CAPUTI, A. P., CATELDI, S., AMELIO, A.: Attivitá ipolipidemizzante ed ipocolesterolemizzante di un copolimero della tetraetilenepentamine e dell' epicloroidrine (U-26, 597A). Giornale dell' arteriosclerosi 8, 229 (1970).

MAROKO, P. R., KJEKSHUS, J. K., SOBEL, B. E., WATANABE, T., COWELL, J. W., ROSS, J., Jr., BRAUNWALD, E.: Factors influencing infarct size following experimental coronary artery occlusions. Circulation 43, 67 (1971).

MARSHALL, M., HESS, H., MALLASCH, M.: On the content of biogenous amines in several arteries of the miniature pig. Res. Exp. Med. 161, 210 - 223 (1973).

MARSHALL, W. E., KUMMEROW, F. A.: The carbohydrate constituents of human serum beta-lipoprotein: galactose, mannose, glucosamine and sialic acid. Arch. Biochem. Biophys. 98, 271 - 273 (1962).

MARTIN, J. S., HARTROFT, W. S.: Atherogenicity of dietary fats in diabetic rats. In: On the nature and treatment of diabetes, p. 410 (LEIBEL, B. S., and WRENSHALL, C. A., Eds.). Amsterdam: Excerpta Medica Foundation 1965.

MARUFFO, C. A., PROTMAN, O. W.: Nutritional control of coronary artery atherosclerosis in the Squirrel monkey. J. Atheroscl. Res. 8, 237 (1968).

MASIRONI, R.: Tracé elements and cardiovascular diseases. Bull. Wld. Hlth. Org. 40, 305 - 312 (1969).

MASIRONI, R.: Cardiovascular mortality in relation to radioactivity and hardness of local water supplies in the United States. Bull. Wld. Hlth. Org. 43, 687 - 697 (1970).

MASTER, A. M., LASSER, R. P.: Single and multiple attacks of transmural myocardial infarction. JAMA 209 (V), 672 (1969).

MASUYA, T., NOBENAGA, T., KATO, K.: Clinical aspects of beta-glucuronidase. Saishin Igaku 16, 70 (1961).

MATEU, L., TARDIEU, A., LAZZATI, V., AGGERBECK, L., SCANU, A. M.: On the structure of human serum low-density lipoprotein. J. Molec. Biol. 70, 105 (1972).

MATHUES, J. K., WOLFF, C. E., CEVALLOS, W. H., HOLMES, W. L.: Platelet adhesiveness and thrombosis in rabbits on an atherogenic diet. Med. Exp. 18, 121 - 128 (1968).

MATTHEWS, L. M. E.: The theory of tracer experiments with ^{131}1-labelled plasma proteins. Phys. Med. Biol. 2, 36 (1957).

MAYO, O., FRASER, G. R., STAMATOYANNOPOULOS, G.: Genetic influences on serum cholesterol in two Greek villages. Hum. Hered. 19, 86 (1969).

Mc BRIDE, J. A., JACOBS, H. S.: Abnormal kinetics of red cell membrane cholesterol in acanthocytes: Studies in genetic and experimental abetalipoproteinemia and in spur cell anaemia. Br. J. Haematol. 18, 383 (1970).

Mc CANDLESS, E. L., LEHOCZKY, J. M., RODBARD, S.: Aortic cartilage produced by intramural carrageenan. Arch. Pathol. 75, 507 - 516 (1963).

Mc CANDLESS, E. L., ZILVERSMIT, D. B.: The effect of cholesterol on the turnover of lecithin, cephalin and sphingomyelin in the rabbit. Arch. Biochem. Biophys. 62, 402 (1956).

Mc COMBS, H. L., ZOOK, B. C., Mc GANDY, R. B.: Fine structure of atherosclerosis of the aorta in the squirrel monkey. Am. J. Path. 55, 235 (1969).

Mc CONATHY, W. J., ALAUPOVIC, P.: Isolation and partial characterization of apolipoprotein D. A new protein moiety of the human plasma lipoprotein system. FEBS Lett. 37, 178 (1973).

Mc COY, K. E., KOEHLER, D. F., CARLSON, J. P.: Purification, lipid binding and tissue distribution of squalene and sterol carrier protein (SCP). Fed. Proc. 32, 519 (1973).

Mc CULLAGH, K. G., EHRHART, L. A.: Increased arterial collagen synthesis in experimental canine atherosclerosis. Atherosclerosis 19, 13 (1974).

Mc DONALD, D.: In: Blood flow in arteries, p. 195. Baltimore, Maryland: Williams and Wilkins 1960.

Mc DONALD, L., EDGILL, M.: Dietary restriction and coagulability of the blood in ischaemic heart-disease. Lancet 1958 I, 996 - 998.

Mc DONALD, T. P., WOODARD, D., COTTRELL, M.: Effect of nicotine on clot retraction of rat blood platelets. Pharmacology 9, 357 - 366 (1973).

Mc DONOUGH, J. R., HAMES, C. G., GREENBERG, B. G., GRIFFIN, L. H., EDWARDS, A. J.: Observations on serum cholesterol levels in the twin population of Evans County, Georgia. Circ. 25, 962 (1962).

Mc GANDY, R. B.: Adolescence and the onset of atherosclerosis, Bull. N. Y., Acad. Med. 47, 590 (1971).

Mc GILL, H. C., Jr., Ed.: The geographic pathology of atherosclerosis. Lab. Invest. 18, 465 (1968).

Mc GILL, H. C., Jr.: Fatty streaks in the coronary arteries and aorta. Lab. Invest. 18, 560 - 564 (1968).

Mc GILL, H. C., Jr., FRANK, M. H., GEER, J. C.: Aortic lesions in hypertensive monkeys. Arch. Path. 71, 96 - 102 (1961).

Mc GILL, H. C., Jr., GEER, J. C., HOLMAN, R. L.: Sites of vascular vulnerability in dogs demonstrated by Evans blue. Arch. Path. 64, 303 (1957).

Mc GILL, H. C., Jr., GEER, J. C., STRONG, J. P.: The natural history of human atherosclerosis. In: Atherosclerosis and its origin, ch. 2, p. (SANDLER, M., and BOURNE, G. H., Eds.). New York: Academic Press 1963.

Mc GILL, H. C., Jr., HOLMAN, R. J.: Influence of alloxan diabetes on cholesterol atheromatosis in the rabbit. Proc. Soc. Exp. Biol. Med. 72, 72 - 80 (1949).

Mc GILL, H. C., Jr., STRONG, J. P., HOLMAN, R. L., WERTHESSEN, N. T.: Arterial lesions in the Kenya baboon. Circ. Res. 8, 670 - 679 (1960).

Mc KUSICK, V. A.: Natural selection and contemporary cardiovascular disease. Circ. 27, 161 - 163 (1963).

Mc KUSICK, V. A.: Mendelian inheritance in man, 3rd ed. Baltimore: Johns Hopkins Press 1971.

Mc KUSICK, V. A.: Homocystinuria. In: Heritable disorders of connective tissue, 4th ed., p. 224 (Mc KUSICK, V. A., Ed.). St. Louis: C. V. Mosby 1972.

Mc LELLAN, G. H.: Automated colorimetric method for estimating serum triglycerides. Clin. Chem. 17, 535 (1971).

Mc MENAMY, R. H., LUND, C. C., VAN MARCKE, J., ONCLEY, J. L.: The binding of L-tryptophan in human plasma at 37° C. Arch. Biochem. Biophys. 93, 135 (1961).

Mc MENAMY, R. H., ONCLEY, J. L.: The specific binding of L-tryptophan to serum albumin. J. Biol. Chem. 233, 1436 (1958).

Mc MILLAN, G. C.: Development of arteriosclerosis. Am. J. Cardiol. 31, 542 - 546 (1973).

Mc MILLAN, G. C., DUFF, G. L.: Mitotic activity in the aortic lesions of experimental cholesterol atherosclerosis of rabbits. Arch. Pathol. 46, 179 - 182 (1948).

Mc MILLAN, G. C., STARY, H. C.: Radioautographic observations on DNA synthesis in the cells of arteriosclerotic lesions of cholesterol-fed rabbits. Prog. Biochem. Pharmacol. (MIRAS, C. J., HOWARD, A. N., and PAOLETTI, R., Eds.). 4, 280 - 281. Basel, New York: S. Karger 1968.

Mc MILLAN, G. C., STARY, H. C.: Preliminary experience with mitotic activity of cellular elements in the atherosclerotic plaques of cholesterol-fed rabbits studied by labeling with tritiated thymidine. Ann. N. Y. Acad. Sci. 149, 699 -709 (1968).

MEEKER, D. R., KESTEN, H. D.: Effect of high protein diets on experimental atherosclerosis in rabbits. Arch. Pathol. 31, 147 - 162 (1941).

MEHNERT, H., HASLBECK, M., FÖRSTER, H.: Zur Prüfung der oralen Glukosetoleranz. Dtsch. med. Wschr. 97, 1763 (1972).

MEITES, S., FAULKNER, W. R.: Manual of practical micro and general procedures in clinical chemistry, p. 98 - 103. Springfield, Illinois: Chas. C. Thomas 1961.

MELCHIOR, G. W., CLARKSON, T. B., BULLOCK, B. C., LOFLAND, H. B.: Cholelithiasis in nonhuman primates-effect of species and type of dietary fat. Circ. 46, II - 19 (1972).

MENDELSOHN, D., MENDELSOHN, L.: The biosynthesis of cholesterol in human skin: a comparison between normal and hyperlipoproteinaemic subjects. S. Afr. Med. J. 46, 229 (1972).

MERIMEE, TH. J.: Comparative clinical and metabolic studies in diabetes mellitus and sexual ateliotic dwarfism. Israel J. med. Sci. 8, 420 (1972).

METZGER, A. L., HEYMSFIELD, S., GRUNDY, S. M.: The lithogenic index - a numerical expression for the relative lithogenicity of bile. Gastroenterology
62, 499 (1972).

MEYER, K.: Biochemistry and biology of mucopolysaccharides. Amer. J. of Med.
47, 664 - 672 (1969).

MEYERS, D. K., SCOTTE, A., MENDEL, B.: Studies on ali-esterases and other lipid-
hydrolyzing enzymes. Biochem. J. 60, 481 (1955).

MIALL, W. E., HENEAGE, P., KHOSLA, T., LOVELL, H. G., MOORE, F.: Factors influencing the degree of resemblance in arterial pressure of close relatives.
Clin. Sci. 33, 271 (1967).

MIDDLETON, C. C., CLARKSON, T. B., LOFLAND, H. B., PRICHARD, R. W.: Atherosclerosis in the squirrel monkey. Naturally occurring lesion in the aorta and
coronary arteries. A. M. A. Arch. Path. 76, 16 (1964).

MIDDLETON, C. C., ROSAL, J., CLARKSON, T. B., NEWMAN, W. P., III, Mc GILL, H.
C., Jr.: Arterial lesions in squirrel monkeys. Arch. Pathol. 83, 352 - 358
(1967).

MIETTINEN, M., TURPEINEN, O., KARVONEN, M. J., ELOSUO, R., PAAVILAINEN, E.:
Effect of cholesterol-lowering diet on mortality from coronary heart-
disease and other causes. Lancet 1972 II, 835 - 838.

MIETTINEN, T. A.: Detection of changes in human cholesterol metabolism. Ann.
Clin. Res. 2, 300 (1970).

MIETTINEN, T. A.: Cholesterol production in obesity. Circ. 44, 842 (1971).

MIETTINEN, T. A.: Clinical implications of bile acid metabolism in man: In: The
bile acids, vol. 2, p. 191 (NAIR, P. P., and KRITCHEVSKY, D., Eds.). New
York, London: Plenum Press 1973.

MIETTINEN, T. A., PELKONEN, R., NIKKILÄ, E. A., HEINONEN, O.: Low excretion of
fecal bile acids in a family with hypercholesterolemia. Acta med. scand.
182, 645 (1967).

MIETTINEN, T. A., PENTTILÄ, I. M., LAMPAINEN, E.: Familial occurrence of mild
hyperlipoproteinaemias. Clin. Genet. 3, 271 (1972).

MILLER, H. H., CALLOW, A. D., WELCH, C. S., Mc MAHON, H. E.: The fate of arterial grafts in small arteries. Surg. Gynaec. Obst. 92, 581 (1951).

MILLER, N. E., CLIFTON-BLIGH, P., NESTEL, P. J.: Effects of colestipol, a new
bile-acid-sequestering resin, on cholesterol metabolism in man. J. Lab.
Clin. Med. 82, 876 (1973).

MILLS, D. C. B.: Drugs that effect platelet behaviour. In: Platelet disorders,
p. 295 - 305 (O'BRIEN, J. R., Ed.). Clinics in Haematology. Vol. 1 (1972).

MILLS, D. C. B., ROBERTS, C. C. K.: Effects of adrenaline on human blood platelets. J. Physiol. 193, 443 - 453 (1967).

MILLS, G. L., CHAPMAN, M. J., Mc TAGGART, F.: Some effects of diet on guinea
pig serum lipoproteins. Biochim. Biophys. acta 260, 401 (1972).

MILLS, G. L., TAYLAUR, C. E.: The distribution and composition of serum lipoproteins in eighteen animals. Comp. Biochem. Physiol. 40 B, 489 - 501
(1971).

MINDELL, E. R., RODBARD, S., KWASMAN, B. C.: Chondrogenesis in bone repair: a
study of the healing fracture callus in the rat. Clin. Orthop. Rel. Res.
79, 187 - 196 (1971).

MINICK, C. R.: The induction of athero-atherosclerosis in rabbits by repeated
injection of foreign serum and diets rich in lipid. Bull. N. Y. Acad. Med.
42, 159 (1966).

MINICK, C. R., MURPHY, G. E.: Experimental induction of athero-atheriosclero-
sis by the synergy of allergic injury to arteries and lipid-rich diet.
II. Effect of repeatedly injected foreign protein in rabbits fed a lipid-
rich, cholesterol-poor diet. Amer. J. Pathol. 73, 265 (1973).

MINICK, C. B., MURPHY, G. E., CAMPBELL, W. C.: Experimental induction of atherosclerosis by the synergy of allergic injury to arteries and lipid-rich diet.
I. Effect of repeated injections of horse serum in rabbits fed dietary cholesterol supplement. J. of Exper. Med. 124, 635 (1966).

MITCHELL, J. R. A., SCHWARTZ, C. J.: Arterial disease. Oxford: Blackwell Scientific Publications 1965.

MITCHELL, S. C.: Symposium on prevention of atherosclerosis at the pediatric level. Amer. J. Card. 31, 539 (1973).

MITTAL, K. K., TERASAKI, P.I.: Cross reactions in the HL-A system. Tissue Antigens 2, 94 (1972).

MJÖS, O. D.: Effect of free fatty acids on myocardial function and oxygen consumption in intact dogs. J. Clin. Invest. 50, 1386 (1971 a).

MJÖS, O. D.: Effect of inhibition of lipolysis on myocardial oxygen consumption in the presence of isoproterenol. J. Clin. Invest. 50, 1869 (1971 b).

MJÖS, O. D., ILEBEKK, A.: Effects of nicotine on myocardial metabolism and performance in dogs. Scand. J. Clin. Lab. Invest. 32, 75 (1973).

MOCZAR, M., ROBERT, L.: Extraction and fractionation of the media of the thoracic aorta: isolation and characterzation of structural glycoproteins. Atherosclerosis 11, 7 - 25 (1970).

MOLNAR, J., SY, D.: Attachment of glucosamine to protein at the ribosomal site of rat liver. Biochemistry 6, 1941 - 1947 (1967).

MONTENEGRO, M. R., EGGEN, D. A.: Topography of atherosclerosis in the coronary arteries. Lab. Invest. 18, 126 (1968).

MOON, H. D.: Coronary arteries in fetuses, infants, and juveniles. Circulation 16, 263 - 267 (1957).

MOORE, J. H., WILLIAMS, D. L.: The effect of diet on the level of plasma cholesterol and the degree of atheromatous degeneration in the rabbit. Brit. J. Nutr. 18, 253 - 273 (1964).

MOORE, S.: The relation of superficial cortical scars of the kidney to aortic atherosclerosis. J. Path. Bact. 88, 471 - 478 (1964).

MOORE, S.: Hypertension and renal ischemia. Geriatrics 24, 81 - 90 (1969).

MOORE, S.: Thromboatherosclerosis in normolipemic rabbits: a result of continued endothelial damage. Lab. Invest. 29, 478 - 487 (1973).

MOORE, S., GENT, M.: Plasma renin activity in experimental nephrosclerosis and hypertension. Circulation 46, Suppl. II, 70 (1972).

MOORE, S., LOUGH, J.: Lipid accumulation in renal arterioles due to platelet aggregate embolism. Amer. J. Pathol. 58, 283 - 293 (1970).

MOORE, S., MERSEREAU, W. A.: Micro-embolic renal ischemia, hypertension and nephrosclerosis. Arch. Path. 85, 623 - 630 (1968).

MOOSSY, J.: Development of cerebral atherosclerosis in various age groups. Neurology 9, 569 - 574 (1959).

MOOSSY, J.: Morphology, sites, and epidemiology of cerebral atherosclerosis. In: Cerebrovascular Disease, ARNMD vol. 41, p. 1 - 22 (MILLIKAN, C. H., Ed.). Baltimore: The Williams & Wilkins Co., 1966.

MORE, R. H., HAUST, M. D.: The role of thrombosis in occlusive disease of coronary arteries. In: Anticoagulants and fibrinolysins, p. 143 - 153 (Mc MILLAN, R. L., and MUSTARD, J. F., Eds.). Philadelphia: Lea and Febiger 1961.

MORGAN, A. D.: The Pathogenesis of coronary occlusion. Oxford: Blackwell Scientific Publications 1956.

MORITA, T., BING, R. J.: Lipid metabolism in perfused human coronary arteries. Proc. Soc. Exp. Biol. Med. 140, 617 (1972)

MORLEY, N., KUSKIS, A.: Positional specificity of lipoprotein lipase. J. Biol. Chem. 247, 6389 (1972).

MORRIS, J. N., CRAWFORD, M. D., HEADY, J. A.: Hardness of local water-supplies and mortality from cardiovascular disease. Lancet 1961 I, 860 - 862.

MORRIS, M. D., FITCH, C. D.: Spontaneous hyperbetalipoproteinemia in the rhesus monkey. Biochem. Med. 2, 209 (1968).

MORRIS, M. D., GREER, W. E.: In: Atherosclerosis: Proceedings of the Second International Symposium, p. 192 (JONES, R. J., Ed.). New York: Springer-Verlag 1970.

MORRISETT, J. D., DAVID, J. S. K., POWNALL, H. J., GOTTO, A. M., Jr.: Interaction of an apolipoprotein (apoLP-alanine) with phosphatidylcholine. Biochemistry 12, 1290 (1973).

MORRISON, A. D., CLEMENTS, R. S., Jr., WINEGRAD, A. I.: Effects of elevated glucose concentrations on the metabolism of the aortic wall. J. Clin. Invest. 51, 3114 (1972).

MORRISON, L. M., BAJWA, G. S.: Absence of naturally occurring coronary atherosclerosis in squirrel monkeys (Saimiri sciurea) treated with chondroitin sulfate A. Experientia 28, 1410 - 1411 (1972).

MORRISON, L. M., BAJWA, G. S., ALFIN-SLATER, R. B., ERSHOFF, B. H.: Pervention of vascular lesions by chondroitin sulfate A in the coronary artery and aorta of rats induced by a hypervitaminosis D., cholesterol-containing diet. Atherosclerosis 16, 105 - 118 (1972).

MORRISON, L. M., BRANWOOD, A. W., ERSHOFF, B. H., MURATA, K., QUILLIGAN, J. J., Jr., SCHJEIDE, O. A., PATEK, P., BERNICK, S., FREEMAN, L., DUNN, O. J., RUCKER, P.: The prevention of coronary arteriosclerotic heart disease with chondroitin sulfate A: Preliminary Report. Exp. Med. Surg. 27, 278 - 289 (1969).

MORRISON, L. M., MURATA, K., QUILLIGAN, J. J., Jr., SCHJEIDE, O. A., FREEMAN, L.: Prevention of atherosclerosis in sub-human primates by chondroitin sulfate A. Circ. Res. 19, 358 - 363 (1966).

MORRISON, L. M., SCHJEIDE, O. A.: In: Coronary heart disease and the mucopoly-saccharides (glycosaminoglycans). Publisher Charles C. Thomas, Publisher, Inc. 1974.

MORRISON, L. M., SCHJEIDE, O. A., QUILLIGAN, J. J., Jr., FREEMAN, L., MURATA, K.: Metabolic parameters of the growth-stimulating effect of chondroitin sulfate A in tissue cultures. Proc. Soc. Exp. Biol. & Med. 119, 618 - 622 (1965).

MOSCHOS, C. B., LAHIRI, K., LYONS, M., WEISSE, A. B., OLDEWURTEL, H. A., REGAN, T. J.: Relation of microcirculatory thrombosis to thrombus in the proximal coronary artery: effect of aspirin, dipyridamole and thrombolysis. Amer. Heart J. 86, 61 - 86 (1973).

MOSKOWITZ, M. S., MOSKOWITZ, A. A., BRADFORD, W. L., WISSLER, R. W.: Changes in serum lipids and coronary arteries of the rat in response to estrogens. A. M. A. Arch. Pathol. 61, 245 (1956).

MOTULSKY, A. G.: Frequency of sickling disorders in US blacks. New Engl. J. Med. 288, 31 (1973).

MOURANT, A. E., KOPEC, A. C., DOMANIESKA-SOBCZAK, K.: Blood-groups and blood-clotting. Lancet 1971 I, 223.

MOVAT, H. Z., HAUST, M. D., MORE, R. H.: The morphologic elements in the early lesions of arteriosclerosis. Am. J. Path. 35, 93 - 101 (1959).

MOZERSKY, D. J., HOKANSON, D. E., SUMNER, D. S., STRANDNESS, D. E., Jr.: Ultra-sonic visualization of the arterial lumen. Surgery 72, 253 (1972).

MOZERSKY, D. J., SUMNER, D. S., STRANDNESS, D. E., Jr.: Long-term results of re-constructive aortoiliac surgery. Amer. J. Surg. 123, 503 (1972 a).

MOZERSKY, D. J., SUMNER, D. S., STRANDNESS, D. E., Jr.: Disease progression after femoropopliteal procedures. Surg. Gynecol. Obstet. 135, 700 (1972 b).

MUNDALL, J., QUINTERO, P., VON KAULLA, K. N., HARMON, R., AUSTIN, J.: Transient monocular blindness and increased platelet aggregability treated with aspirin. Neurology 22, 280 - 285 (1972).

MURPHY, E. A.: Thrombozyten, Thrombose und Gerinnung. In: Nikotin, Pharmakologie und Toxikologie des Tabakrauches, p. 178 - 192. (SCHIEVELBEIN, H., Ed.). Stuttgart: Georg Thieme 1968.

MURPHY, E. A., MUSTARD, J. F.: Coagulation tests and platelet economy in athero-sclerotic and control subjects. Circulation 25, 114 - 125 (1962).

MURPHY, J. R.: Erythrocyte metabolism. III. Relationship of energy metabolism and serum factors to the osmotic fragility following incubation. J. Lab. Clin. Med. 60, 86 (1962).

MURPHY, J. R.: Erythrocyte metabolism. VI. Cell shape and the location of chol-esterol in the erythrocyte membrane. J. Lab. Clin. Med. 65, 756 (1965).

MUSS, D. L.: Relationship between water qualitiy and deaths from cardiovascular disease. J. Amer. Wat. Wks. Ass. 54, 1371 - 1378 (1962).

MUSTARD, J. F.: The effect of clofibrate on platelets. Amer. Heart J. 76, 436 (1968).

MUSTARD, J. F., JØRGENSEN, L., PACKHAM, M. A.: Blood flow and platelet inter-action with surfaces. Thromb. Diath. Haemorrh. Suppl. 51, 151 - 160 (1972).

MUSTARD, J. F., KINLOUGH-RATHBONE, R. L., JENKINS, C. S. P., PACKHAM, M. A.: Modification of platelet function. Annals New York Acad. of Sciences 201, 343 - 359 (1972).

MUSTARD, J. F., MURPHY, E. A.: Effect of different dietary fats on blood coagula-tion, platelet economy, and blood lipids. Brit. Med. J. 1, 1651 - 1655 (1962).

MUSTARD, J. F., MURPHY, E. A.: Effect of smoking on blood coagulation and platelet survival in man. Brit. Med. J. 1, 846 - 849 (1963).

MUSTARD, J. F., PACKHAM, M. A.: Factors influencing platelet function: adhesion,
release and aggregation Pharmacol. Rev. 22, 97 (1970).

MUSTARD, J. F., ROWSELL, H. C., LOTZ, F, HEGARDT, B., MURPHY, E. A.: The effect
of adenine nucleotides on thrombus formation, platelet count and blood coagulation. Exp. Mol. Path. 5, 43 - 60 (1966).

MUSTARD, J. F., ROWSELL, H. C., MURPHY, E. A., DOWNIE, H. G.: Diet and thrombus
formation: quantitative studies using an extracorporeal circulation in pigs.
J. Clin. Invest. 42, 1783 - 1789 (1963).

MYASNIKOV, A.L., BLOCK, Y. E.: Influence of some factors on lipoidosis and cell
proliferation in aorta tissue cultures of adult rabbits. J. Atheroscler. Res.
5, 33 - 42 (1965).

NACHBAUR, J., COLBEAU, A., VIGNAIS, P. M.: Distribution of membrane-confined
phospholipases A in the rat hepatocyte. Biochim. Biophys. Acta 274, 426 -
446 (1972).

NACHMAN, R. L.: Platelet Proteins. Seminars Haematol. 5, 18 - 31 (1968).

NAM, S. C., LEW, W. M., JAMOLYCH, T., LEE, K. T., THOMAS, W. A.: Rapid production
of advanced atherosclerosis in swine by a combination of endothelial injury
and cholesterol feeding. Exp. Mol. Path. 18, 369 (1973).

NAMEROFF, M., HOLTZER, H.: The loss of phenotypic traits by differentiated cells.
IV. Changes in polysaccharides produced by living chondrocytes. Dev. Biol.
16, 250 (1967).

NELSON, G. J.: Quantitative analysis of plasma lipids, p. 25-74. In: Blood lipids
and lipoproteins: quantitation, composition, and metabolism (NELSON, G. J.,
Ed.). New York: Wiley-Interscience 1972.

NELSON, W. R., WERTHESSEN, N. T., HOLMAN, R. L., HADAWAY, H., JAMES, A. T.:
Changes in fatty acid composition of human aorta associated with fatty
streaking. Lancet 1961 I, 86.

NEMERSON, Y., PITLICK, F. A.: The tissue factor pathway of blood coagulation. In:
Progress in hemostasis and thrombosis, vol. 1, p. 1 - 37 (SPAET, T. H., Ed.).
New York: Grune and Stratton 1972.

NESTEL, P. J.: Relationship between plasma triglycerides and removal of chylomicrons. J. Clin. Invest. 43, 943 (1964).

NESTEL, P. J.: Relationship between FFA flux and TGFA influx in plasma before
and during the infusion of insulin. Metabolism 16, 1123 (1967).

NESTEL, P. J.: Turnover of plasma esterified cholesterol: Influence of dietary
fat and carbohydrate and relation to plasma lipids and body weight. Clin.
Sci. 38, 593 (1970).

NESTEL, P. J., CARROLL, K. F., HAVENSTEIN, N.: Plasma triglyceride response to
carbohydrates, fats and caloric intake. Metabolism 19, 1 (1970).

NESTEL, P. J., HAVENSTEIN, N., WHYTE, H. M., SCOTT, T. J., COOK, L. J.: Lowering
of plasma cholesterol and enhanced sterol excretion with the consumption of
polyunsaturated ruminant fats. New Engl. J. Med. 288, 379 (1973).

NESTEL, P. J., HIRSCH, E. Z.: Mechanism of alcohol-induced hypertriglyceridemia.
J. Lab. Clin. Med. 66, 357 (1965).

NESTEL, P. J., MONGER, E. A.: Turnover of plasma esterified cholesterol in normocholesterolemic and hypercholesterolemic subjects and its relation to body
build. J. Clin. Invest. 46, 967 - 974 (1967).

NESTEL, P. J., SCHREIBMAN, P. H., AHRENS, E. H., Jr.: Cholesterol metabolism in
human obesity. J. Clin. Invest. 52, 2389 (1973).

NESTEL, P. J., WHYTE, H. M., GOODMAN, De W. S.: Distribution and turnover of cholesterol in humans. J. Clin. Invest. 48, 982 (1969).

NEUFELD, H. N., WAGENVOORT, C. A., EDWARDS, J. E.: Coronary arteries in fetuses,
infants, juveniles, and young adults. Lab.Invest. 11, 837 - 844 (1962).

NEUMANN, R. E., LOGAN, M. A.: The determination of collagen and elastin in tissues.
J. Biol. Chem. 186, 549 (1950).

NEVIN, N. C., SLACK, J.: Hyperlipidaemic xanthomatosis. Ill. Mode of inheritance
in 55 families with essential hyperlipidaemia and xanthomatosis. J. Med.
Genet. 5, 9 (1968).

NEWKIRK, J. D., WAITE, M.: Identification of a phospholipase A in plasma membranes
of rat liver. Biochim. Biophys. Acta 225, 224 (1971).

NEWKIRK, J. D., WAITE, M.: Phospholipid hydrolysis by phospholipases A_1 and A_2 in plasma membranes and microsomes of rat liver. Biochim.Biophys.Acta 298, 562 (1973).

NEWMAN, H. A. I., DAY, A. J., ZILVERSMIT, D. B.: In vitro phospholipid synthesis in normal and atheromatous rabbit aortas. Circulat. Res. 19, 132 (1966).

NEWMAN, H. A. I., Mc CANDLESS, E. L., ZILVERSMIT, D. B.: The synthesis of ^{14}C-lipids in rabbit atheromatous lesions. J. Biol. Chem. 236, 1264 (1961).

NEWMAN, H. A. I., ZILVERSMIT, D. B.: Quantitative aspects of cholesterol flux in rabbit atheromatous lesions. J. Biol. Chem. 237, 2078 (1962).

NEWMAN, H. A. I., ZILVERSMIT, D. B.: Accumulation of lipid an nonlipid constituents in rabbit atheroma. J. Atheroscler. Res. 4, 261 (1964).

NICHOLS, C. W., Jr., GAN, J. C., MURTHY, P. V. N., CHAIKOFF, I. L.: Mucosubstances in the chicken aorta. Part 2. Changes induced by diethylstilbestrol implants or cholesterol feeding. Atherosclerosis 14, 39 - 51 (1971).

NICHOLS, C. W., Jr., LINDSAY, S., CHAIKOFF, I. L.: Histochemical study of the heart and thoracic aorta of the chick from hatch to 39 days of age. J. Atheroscler. Res. 1, 133 - 139 (1961).

NICOLOSI, R. J., SANTERRE, R. F., SMITH, S. C.: Lipid accumulation in muscular foci in White Carneau and Show Racer pigeon aortas. Exp. Mol. Pathol. 17, 29 (1972).

NIEWIAROWSKI, S., REGOECZI, E., STEWART, G. J., SENYI, A., MUSTARD, J. F.: Platelet interaction with polymerizing fibrin. J. Clin. Invest. 51, 685 (1972).

NIEWIAROWSKI, S., STUART, R. K., THOMAS, D. P.: Activation of intravascular coagulation by collagen. Proc. Soc. Exp. Biol. Med. 123, 196 - 200 (1966).

NIKKARI, T., HEIKKINEN, E.: The lipids of collagen preparations. Acta Chem. Scand. 22, 3047 - 3049 (1968).

NIKKILÄ, E. A.: Control of plasma and liver triglyceride kinetics by carbohydrate metabolism and insulin. Adv. Lipid Res. 7, 63 (1969).

NIKKILÄ, E. A., ARO, A.: Family study of serum lipids and lipoproteins in coronary heart-disease. Lancet 1973 I, 954.

NIKKILÄ, E. A., KEKKI, M.: Polymorphism of plasma triglyceride kinetics in normal human adult subjects. Acta Med. Scand. 190, 49 (1971).

NIKKILÄ, E. A., KEKKI, M.: Plasma triglyceride metabolism in thyroid disease. J. Clin. Invest. 51, 2103 (1972).

NIKKILÄ, E. A., KEKKI, M.: Plasma triglyceride transport kinetics in diabetes mellitus. Metabolism 22, 1 (1973).

NIKKILÄ, E. A., MIETTINEN, T. A., VESENNE, M. R., PELKONEN, R.: Plasma insulin in coronary heart-disease. Lancet 1965 II, 508 (1965).

NIKKILÄ, E. A., PYKALISTÖ, O.: Regulation of adipose tissue lopoprotein lipase synthesis by intracellular free fatty acid. Life Sci. 7, 1303 (1968).

NILSSON, I. M., PANDOLFI, M.: Fibrinolytic response of the vascular wall. Thromb. Diath. Haemorrh. Suppl. 40, 231 - 242 (1970).

NILSSON-EHLE, P., EGELRUD, T., BELFRAGE, P., OLIVECRONA, T., BORGSTRÖM, B.: Positional specificity of purified milk lipoprotein lipase. J. Biol. Chem. 248, 6734 (1973).

NITZBERG, S. I., PEYMAN, A. M., GOLDSTEIN, R., PROGER, S.: Studies of blood coagulation and fibrinolysis in patients with idiopathic hyperlipemia and primary hypercholesterolemia before and after a fatty meal. Circulation 19, 676 (1959).

NOBLE, R. P.: Electrophoretic separation of plasma lipoproteins in agarose gel. J. Lipid Res. 9, 693 - 700 (1968).

NOMA, A., BORGSTRÖM, B.: The exocellular lipase from Rhizopus arrhizus. Scand. J. Gastroent. 6, 217 - 223 (1971).

NORDÖY, A., HAMLIN, J. T., CHANDLER, A. B., NEWLAND, H.: The influence of dietary fats on plasma and platelet lipids and ADP-induced platelet thrombosis in the rat. Scand. J. Haematol. 5, 458 - 473 (1968).

NORUM, K. R., GJONE, E.: Familial plasma lecithin, cholesterol acid transferase deficiency. Biochemical study of a new inborn error of metabolism. Scand. J. Clin. Lab. Invest. 20, 231 - 243 (1967).

NORUM, K. R., GLOMSET, J. A., GJONE, E.: Familial lecithin: cholesterol acyl transferase deficiency. In: The metabolic basis of inherited disease, 3rd edition, p. 531 (STANBURY, J. R., WYNGAARDEN, J. H., and FREDRICKSON, D. S., Eds.). New York: Mc Graw-Hill Book Company 1972.

NORUM, K. R., GLOMSET, J. A., NICHOLS, A. V., FORTE, T., KING, W. C., APPLEGATE, K. R., MITCHELL, C. D., ALBERS, J.: To be submitted.

NOSEDA, G., BÜTLER, R., SCHLUPF, E., RIESEN, W.: Bindung von Beta-Lipoprotein durch ein IgA-Paraprotein: eine Antigen-Antikörper Reaktion? Schweiz. Med. Wochenschrift 101, 893 (1971).

NOVAK, M.: Colorimetric ultramicro method for the determination of free fatty acids. J. Lip. Res. 6, 431 (1965).

NOVIKOFF, A. B., ROHEIM, P. S., QUINTANA, N.: Changes in rat liver cells induced by orotic acid feeding. Lab. Invest. 15, 27 - 49 (1966).

NUMANO, F., KATSU, K., TAKENOBU, M., SAGARA, A., SHIMAMOTO, T.: Comparative studies on the preventive effect of pyridinolcarbamate and estrogen against aortic and coronary atherosclerosis of cholesterol-fed rabbits. Part II: Histoenzymatic studies, Acta Path. Jap. 21, 193 (1971).

NYE, E. R., JACKSON, D., HUNTER, J. D.: Treatment of hypercholesterolaemia with colestipol: a bile acid sequestering agent. New Zealand med. J. 76, 12 (1972).

O'BRIEN, J. R.: Some possible enzyme systems involved in platelet aggregation. J. Atheroscler. Res. 3, 262 (1961).

OCKNER, R. K., HUGHES, F. B., ISSELBACHER, K. J.: Very low density lipoproteins in intestinal lymph: Origin, composition, and role in lipid transport in the fasting state. J. Clin. Invest. 48, 2079 - 2088 (1969).

OGSTON, C. M., OGSTON, D.: Plasma fibrinogen and plasminogen levels in health and in ischaemic heart disease. J. Clin. Path. 19, 352 (1966).

OGSTON, D., OGSTON, C. M., RATNOFF, O. D., FORBES, C. D.: Studies on a complex mechanism for the activation of plasminogen by kaolin and by chloroform: the participation of Hageman factor and additional cofactors. J. Clin. Invest. 48, 1786 - 1801 (1969).

OGURA, M., SHIGA, J., YAMASAKI, K.: Studies on the cholesterol pool as the precursor of bile acids in the rat. J. Biochem. 70, 967 (1971).

OKOSHIO, T., NAIR, P. P.: Studies on bile acids. Some observations on the intracellular localization of major bile acids in rat liver. Biochem. 5, 3662 (1966).

OLIVECRONA, T., EGELRUD, T., IVERIUS, P. H., LINDAHL, U.: Evidence for an ionic binding of lipoprotein lipase to heparin. Biochem. Biophys. Res. Commun. 43, 524 - 529 (1971).

OLIVER, M. F.: Modern Trends in Cardiology II, p. 46. London: Butterworths 1969.

OLIVER, M. F.: Ischaemic heart disease: a secondary prevention trial using clofibrate. Report by a research committee of the Scottish Society of Physicians. Brit. Med. J. 4, 775 - 784 (1971).

OLIVER, M. F., GEIZEROVA, H., CUMMING, R. A., HEADY, J. A.: Serum-cholesterol and ABO and Rhesus blood-groups. Lancet 1969 II, 605.

O'NEAL, R. M., THOMAS, W. A., HARTROFT, W. S.: Dietary production of myocardial infarction in rats. Anatomical features of the disease. Am. J. Cardiol. 3, 94 (1959).

ORNSTEIN, L.: Disc electrophoresis. Ann. N. Y. Acad. Sci. 121, 321 (1964).

OSBORNE, R. H., ADLERSBERG, D., DeGEORGE, F. V., WANG, C.: Serum lipids, heredity and environment: A study of adult twins. Amer. J. Med. 26, 54 (1959).

OST, C. R., STENSON, S.: Regression of peripheral atherosclerosis during therapy with high doses of nicotinic acid. Scand. J. Clin. & Lab. Invest. Suppl. 99, 241 - 245 (1967).

OSUGA, T., PORTMAN, O. W.: Experimental formation of gallstones in the squirrel monkey. Proc. Soc. Exp. Biol. Med. 136, 722 (1971).

OSUGA, T., PORTMAN, O. W.: Relationship between bile composition and gallstone formation in squirrel monkeys. Gastroenterology 63, 122 (1972).

OSUGA, T., PORTMAN, O. W., MITAMURA, K., ALEXANDER, M.: A morphological study of gallstone development in the squirrel monkey. Lab. Invest. (1974, In press).

OTT, H., LOHSS, F., GERGELY, J.: Der Nachweis von Serumlipoproteiden in der Aortenintima. Klin. Wschr. 36, 383 (1958).

PACKHAM, M. A., MUSTARD, J. F.: Drug-induced alteration of platelet function. In: Platelets: production, function, transfusion and storage (BALDINI, M., EBBE, S., Eds.). New York: Grune and Stratton 1974 (In press).

PACKHAM, M. A., NISHIZAWA, E. E., MUSTARD, J. F.: Response of platelets to tissue injury. Biochem. Pharmacol. (Suppl.), 171 - 184 (1968).

PACKHAM, M. A., ROWSELL, H. C., JØRGENSEN, L., MUSTARD, J. F.: Localized protein accumulation in the wall of the aorta. Exp. Mol. Pathol. 7, 214 - 232 (1967).

PADYKULA, H. A., HERMAN, E.: Factors affecting the activity of ATPase and other
   phosphatases as measured by histochemical techniques. J. Histochem. Cytochem. 3, 161 - 169 (1955).
PAGE, I. H.: The Lewis A. Conner Memorial Lecture: Atherosclerosis. An introduction. Circulation 10, 1 - 27 (1954).
PAGNAN, A., FELLIN, R., CREPALDI, G.: Studio elettroforetico delle lipoproteine
   plasmatiche su agarosio nei soggetti normali e in diverse condizioni morbose.
   Acta Med. Patav. 31, 71 (1971).
PALMER, A. J., BLACKET, R.: Regression of xanthomata of the eyelids with modi-
   fied fat diet. Lancet 1972 I, 66 - 68.
PAPAHADJOPOULOS, D., HANAHAN, D. J.: Observations on the interaction of phospho-
   lipids and certain clotting factors in prothrombin activator formation.
   Biochim. Biophys. Acta 90, 436 - 439 (1964).
PARKER, F., ORMSBY, J. W., PETERSON, N. F., ODLAND, G. F.,WILLIAMS, R. H.: In
   vitro studies of phospholipid synthesis in experimental atherosclerosis.
   Possible role of myo-intimal cells. Circulat. Res. 19, 700 (1966).
PARKER, F., SCHIMMELBUSCH, W., WILLIAMS, R. H.: The enzymic nature of phospho-
   lipid synthesis in normal rabbit and human aorta. Results of in vitro stud-
   ies. Diabetes 13, 182 (1964).
PARKINSON, T. M., GUNDERSEN, K., NELSON, N. A.: Effects of U-26, 597 A, a new
   bile acid sequestrant, on serum lipids of experimental animals and man.
   Atherosclerosis 11, 531 (1970).
PARKINSON, T. M., SCHNEIDER, J. C., Jr., PHILLIPS, W. A.: Effects of colestipol
   hydrochloride (U-26, 597 A) on serum and fecal lipids in dogs. Atherosclerosis 17, 167 (1973).
PARRA, A., SCHULZ, R. B., GERAXSTONE, J. E., CHEEK, D. D.: Correlative studies
   in obese children and adolescents concerning body composition and plasma insulin and growth hormone levels, Ped. Res. 5, 605 (1971).
PARSONS, W. B.: Long-term therapy with nicotinic acid and aluminum nicotinate
   in hypercholesteremic individuals: Results in ninety-nine patients treated
   for one to nine years. Circulation 31, II, 26 (1965).
PARTRIDGE, S. M.: Isolation and characterization of elastin. In: Chemistry and
   molecular biology of the intercellular matrix E. A. (BALAZS, E. A., Ed.).
   Academic Press 1, 593 - 616 (1970).
PARVING, H.-H.: The effect of hypoxia and CO exposure on plasma volume and
   capillary permeability to albumin. Scand. J. Clin. Lab. Invest. 30, 49
   (1972).
PARVING, H.-H., OHLSSON, K., BUCHARDT-HANSEN, H. J., RORTH, M.: Effect of CO ex-
   posure on capillary permeability to albumin α_2 macroglobulin. Scand. J. Clin.
   Lab. Invest. 29, 381 (1972).
PATELSKI, J.: Cholesterol esterase of the aorta. Panstwowy Zaklad Wydawnicta
   Lekaeskich Warszawa (1964).
PATELSKI, J., BOWYER, D. E., HOWARD, A. N., GRESHAM, G. A.: Changes in phospho-
   lipase A, lipase and cholesterol esterase activity in the aorta in experimen-
   tal atherosclerosis in the rabbit and rat. J. Atheroscler. Res. 8, 221 (1968a).
PATELSKI, J., BOWYER, D. E., HOWARD, A. N., JENNINGS, I. W., THORNE, C. J. R.,
   GRESHAM, G. A.: Modification of enzyme activities in experimental atheroscle-
   rosis in the rabbit. Atherosclerosis 12, 41 (1970).
PATELSKI, J., HOWARD, A. N.: Effect of polyunsaturated phosphatidyl choline on
   regression of atherosclerosis in baboons. This volume p. 893.
PATELSKI, J., TIPTON, K. F.: The subcellular localisation of lipolytic enzymes in
   pig aorta. Atherosclerosis 13, 288 (1971).
PATELSKI, J., WALIGORA, Z., SZULC, S.: Demonstration and some properties of the
   phospholipase A, lipase and cholesterol esterase from the aortic wall. J.
   Atheroscler. Res. 7, 453 (1967).
PATELSKI, J., WALIGORA, Z., SZULC, S., BOWYER, D. E., HOWARD, A. N.: Lipolytic
   enzymes of the aortic wall. Prog. Biochem. Pharmacol. 4, 287 (1968 b).
PATTEN, R. L.: The reciprocal regulation of lipoprotein lipase activity and hormone-sensitive lipase activity in rat adipocytes. J. Biol. Chem. 245, 5577
   (1970).
PATTERSON, D., SLACK, J.: Lipid abnormalities in male and female survivors of myocardial infarction and their first-degree relatives. Lancet 1972 I, 393.

PAULIK, F., PAULIK, J., ERDEY, L.: Der Derivatograph. Z. anal. Chem. 160, 241 (1958).

PEARLSTEIN, E., ALADJEM, F.: Subpopulations of human serum very low density lipoproteins. Biochemistry 11, 2553 (1972).

PEETERS, H.: The apoprotein and lipid moieties of the lipoproteins. In: Protides of the biological fluids, vol. 18, p. 3 (PEETERS, H., Ed.). Oxford: Pergamon Press 1971.

PEETERS, H., BLATON, V.: Comparative lipid values of human and nonhuman primates. In: Medical Primatology, part III, p. 336 - 342 (GOLDSMITH, E.I., and MOOR-JANKOWSKI, J., Eds.). Basel: Karger 1972.

PEETERS, H., BLATON, V., DECLERCQ, B., VANDAMME, D.: The effect of essential phospholipids on the lipid and fatty acid patterns of lipoproteins in type II patients. 4th Int. Symposium on drugs affecting lipid metabolism, Philadelphia USA, p. 93 (1971).

PEETERS, H., BLATON, V., SOETEWEY, F., DECLERCQ, B., VANDAMME, D.: Die Wirkung der "essentiellen" Phospholipide auf Plasmalipide und Fettsäuren beim Typ II der Hyperlipoproteinämie. Münch. Med. Wochenschrift 115, 1358 (1973).

PEETERS, H., ROSSENEU-MOTREFF, M. Y., SOETEWEY, F.: In: Protides of the biological fluids, vol. 20, p. 471 (PEETERS, H., Ed.). Oxford: Pergamon Press 1972.

PELLETIER, G., BORNSTEIN, M. B.: Effect of colchicine on rat anterior pituitary gland in tissue culture. Exp. Cell Res. 70, 221 (1972).

PEPINE, C. J., VIENER, L.: Relationship of anginal symptoms to lung mechanics during myocardial ischemia. Circulation 46, 863 - 869 (1972).

PERL, W., SAMUEL, P.: Input-output analysis for total input rate and total traced mass of body cholesterol in man. Circ. Res. 25, 191 (1969).

PERSSON, B.: Lipoprotein lipase activity of human adipose tissue in health and in some diseases with hyperlipidemia as a common feature. Acta Med. Scand. 193, 457 (1973).

PERSSON, B.: Lipoprotein lipase activity of human adipose tissue in different types of hyperlipidemia. Acta med. Scand. 193, 447 (1973).

PERSSON, B., SCHRODER, G., HOOD, B.: Lipoprotein lipase activity in human adipose tissue: assay methods. Atherosclerosis 16, 37 (1972).

PETERS, N., HALES, C. N.: Plasma insulin concentrations after myocardial infarction. Lancet 1965 I, 1144.

PETERS, T. J., TAKANO, T., De DUVE, C.: Subcellular fractionation studies on the cells isolated from normal and atherosclerotic aorta. In: Ciba Foundation Symposium on Mechanisms in the Development of Early Atheroma, London, 1972. Atherogenesis: Initiating factors, pp. 197 - 222. (Ciba Foundation Symposium 12). Amsterdam: Associated Scientific Publishers 1973.

PETERSON, M., DAY, A. J., TUME, R. K., EISENBERG, E.: Ultrastructure, fatty acid content, and metabolic activity of foam cells and other fractions separated from rabbit atherosclerotic lesions. Exp. Mol. Pathol. 15, 157 - 169 (1971).

PFEIFFER, E. F.: In: On the nature and treatment of diabetes. Excerpta Media Found., Amsterdam, 1965, S. 368.

PHILLIPS, W. A., STAFFORD, W. W., STUUT, J., Jr.: Jugular vein technique for serial blood sampling and intravenous injection in the rat. Proc. Soc. exp. Biol. Med. (N. Y.) 143, 733 (1973).

PHILP, R. B., LEMIEUX, V.: Comparison of some effects of dipyridamole and adenosine on thrombus formation, platelet adhesiveness and blood pressure in rabbits and rats. Nature 218, 1072 (1968).

PICARD, J., BRETON, M., HERMELIN, B., LEVY, P., DEUDON, E., GROLEAS, A.: Glysosaminoglycanes des membranes plasmiques rugueuses et lisses de l'Intima et du Compartiment extracellulaire de la paroi artérielle. Arterial Wall 1, 1973 (In press).

PICARD, J., GARDAIS, A.: Les mucopolysaccharides arteriels et leur variations dans l'athérosclérose. Arch. Mal. Coeur (Revue de l'Atherosclérose) 3, 2 - 62 (1962).

PICARD, J., LEVY, P.: Incorporation de glucuronate et d'Acetylhexosamine dans les glucosaminoglycanes de la paroi artérielle C. R. Acad. Sc. 277, 373 - 376 (1973).

PICK, R., GLICK, G.: The influence of hypertension on diet-induced aortic, coronary and cerebral atherosclerosis in the stumptail macaque. Circulation 46, (Suppl. II), 248 (1972).

PICK, R., STAMLER, J., RODBARD, S., KATZ, L. N.: The inhibition of coronary atherosclerosis by estrogens in cholesterol-fed chickens.Circulation 6,276 (1952).

PICKERING, G.: The inheritance of arterial pressure. I.: Epidemiology of hypertension, p. 18 (STAMLER, J., STAMLER, R., and PULLMAN,T. N., Eds.). New York: Grune and Stratton 1967.

PIKKARAINEN, J., TAKKUNEN, J., KULONEN, E.: Serum cholesterol in Finnish twins. Amer. J. hum. Genet. 18, 115 (1966).

PISANO, J. J., CROUT, J. R., ABRAHAM, D.: Determination of 3-methoxy-4-hydroxy-mandelic acid in urine. Clin. Chim. Acta 7, 285 (1962).

PLATT, R.: Heredity in Hypertension, Quarterly J. Med. 16, 111 (1947).

PLATT, R.: The influence of heredity. In: The Epidemiology of Hypertension, p. 9 (STAMLER, J., STAMLER, R., and PULLMAN, T. N., Eds.). New York: Grune and Stratton 1967.

POCOCK, D. M.-E., RAFAL, S., VOST, A.: Separation of mammalian neutral lipids by chromatography on glass fiber paper impregnated with silica gel. J. Chromatograph. Science 10, 72 - 76 (1972).

POHJANPECTO, P., RAINA, A.: Identification of a growth factor produced by human fibroblasts in vitro as putrescine. Nature (New Biol.) 235, 247 (1972).

POLLARD, H. B., DEVI, S. K.: Construction of a three-dimensional isodensity map of the low-density liporotein particle from human serum. Biochem. Biophys. Res. Commun. 44, 593 (1971).

POLLARD, H. B., SCANU, A. M., TAYLOR, E. W.: On the geometrical arrangment of the protein subunits of human serum low-density lipoprotein: evidence for a dodecahedral model. Proc. Nat. Acad. Sci. U. S. 64, 304 (1969).

POLLER, L., THOMSON, J. M., TABIOWO, A., PRIEST, C. M.: Progesterone, oral contraception and blood coagulation. Brit. Med. J. 1, 554 - 556 (1969).

POOL, W. R., NEWMARK, H. L., DALTON, C., BANZIGER, R. F., HOWARD, A. N.: Effect of biotin and ascorbic acid on the development of atherosclerosis in rabbits. Atherosclerosis 14, 131 - 135 (1971).

POOLE, J. C. F., CROMWELL, S. B., BENDITT, E. P.: Behaviour of smooth muscle cells and formation of extracellular structures in the reaction of arterial walls to injury. Amer. J. Pathol. 62, 391 - 414 (1971).

POPOV, A. V., GERCHIKOVA, E. A.: The perfusion of rabbit isolated aorta for study of lipoprotein entry into the vessel wall. Pathol. physiol. (In Russian, in press).

PORTE, D., Jr., O'HARA, D. D., WILLIAMS, R. H.: The relation between post-heparin lipolytic activity and plasma triglyceride in myxedema. Metabolism 15, 107 - 113 (1966).

PORTMAN, O.: Arterial composition and metabolism: esterified fatty acids and cholesterol. In: Advances in lipid research, Vol. 8, p. 41 (PAOLETTI, R., and KRITCHEVSKY, D., Eds.). New York: Academic Press 1970.

PORTMAN, O. W., ALEXANDER, M., MARUFFO, C. A.: Nutritional control of arterial lipid composition in the squirrel monkey: Major ester classes and types of phospholipids. J. Nutr. 91, 31 (1967).

PORTMAN, O. W., ANDRUS, S. B.: Comparative evaluation of three species of new world monkeys for studies of dietary factors, tissue lipids, and atherogenesis. J. Nutr. 87, 429 (1965).

POSNER, I.: Abnormal fat absorption and utilization in rats bearing Walker carcinoma. Cancer Research 20, 551 (1960).

POTTENGER, L. A., GETZ, G. S.: Serum lipoprotein accumulation in the livers of orotic acid-fed rats. J. Lipid Res. 12, 450 - 459 (1971).

PRADER, A., ZACHMANN, M., POLEY, J. R., ILLIG, R., SZEKY, J.: Long-term treatment with human growth hormone (Raben) in small doses. Evaluation of 18 hypopituitary patients. Helv. paediat. Acta 22, 423 (1967).

PRAGA, C., VALENTINI, L., MAIORANO, M., CORTELLARO, M.: A new automatic device for the standardized Ivy bleeding time. In: Platelet function and thrombosis, p. 271 - 279 (MANNUCI, P. M., GORINI, S., Eds.). Adv. Expt. Med. Biol. 34 (1972).

PRATHAP, K.: Spontaneous and experimental atherosclerosis in the Malaysian long-tailed monkey (Macaca irus). Dissertation for an M. D. degree, University of Malaya, 1972.

PRATHAP, K.: Spontaneous aortic lesions in wild adult Malaysian long-tailed monkeys (Macaca irus). J. Path. 110, 135 - 143 (1973).

PRATHAP, K.: The morphology of two-year-old healed platelet-rich thrombi in femoral arteries of normocholesterolaemic monkeys: light- and electron-microscope observations. J. Path. 110, 145 - 151 (1973 a).

PRATHAP, K.: The natural history of platelet rich thrombi in systemic arteries in hypercholesterolaemic monkeys. J. Pathol. 110, 203 - 212 (1973 b).

PRICHARD, R. W.: Spontaneous atherosclerosis in pigeons, In: Comparative atherosclerosis, p. 45 - 49 (ROBERTS, J. C., Jr., and STRAUS, R., Eds.). New York: Harper and Row 1965.

PRICHARD, R. W., CLARKSON, T. B., LOFLAND, H. B.: Estrogen in pigeon atherosclerosis estradiol valerate effects at several dose levels on cholesterol-fed male white carneau pigeons. Arch. Path. 82, 15 (1966).

PRIOR, J. T., HARTMANN, W. H.: The effect of hypercholesterolemia on intimal repair of the aorta of the rabbit following experimental trauma. Amer. J. Path. 32, 417 - 431 (1966).

PROUDLOCK, J. W., DAY, A. J.: Cholesterol esterifying enzymes of atherosclerotic rabbit intima. Biochim. Biophys. Acta 260, 716 (1972).

PROUDLOCK, J. W., DAY, A. J., NAUGHTON, J. M.: Lipid composition and metabolic activity of subcellular fractions isolated from rabbit atherosclerotic lesions. Exp. Molec. Pathol. (1973, In press).

PUCAK, G. J., LEHNER, N. C. M., CLARKSON, T. B., BULLOCK, B. C., LOFLAND, H. B.: Spider monkeys (Ateles sp.) as animal modela for atherosclerosis research. Exp. molec. Path. 18, 32 - 49 (1973).

PUGATCH, E. M. J., SAUNDERS, A. M.: A new technique for making häutchen preparations of unfixed aortic endothelium. J. Atheroscler. Res. 8, 735 - 738 (1968).

PUNSAR, S., KARVONEN, M. J.: Angina pectoris and ECG abnormalities in relation to prognosis of coronary heart disease in population studies in Finland. Adv. Cardiol. 8, 148 - 161 (1973).

QUARFORDT, S. H., FRANK, A., SHAMES, D. M., BERMAN, M., STEINBERG, D.: Very low density lipoprotein triglyceride transport in type IV hyperlipoproteinemia and the effects of carbohydrate-rich diets. J. Clin. Invest. 49, 2281 (1970).

QUARFORDT, S., LEVY, R. I., FREDRICKSON, D. S.: On the lipoprotein abnormality in Type III hyperlipoproteinemia. J. Clin. Invest. 50, 754 (1971).

QUINTAO, E., GRUNDY, S. M., AHRENS, E. H., Jr.: Effects of dietary cholesterol on the regulation of total body cholesterol in man. J. Lipid Res. 12, 233 (1971).

RABINOWITZ, D., KLASSEN, G. A., ZIEGLER, K. L.: Effect of human growth hormone on muscle and adipose tissue metabolism in the forearm of man. J. Clin. Invest. 44, 51 (1965).

RACHMILEWITZ, D., EISENBERG, S., STEIN, Y., STEIN, O.: Phospholipases in arterial tissue. I. Sphingomyelin cholinephosphohydrolase activity in human, dog, guinea pig, rat and rabbit arteries. Biochim. Biophys. Acta 144, 624 (1967).

RACHMILEWITZ, D., STEIN, O., ROBEIM, P. S., STEIN, Y.: Metabolism of Iodinated high density lipoproteins in the rat. II. Autoradiographic localization in the liver. Biochem. Biophys. Acta 270, 414 (1972).

RALL, T. W., SUTHERLAND, E. W., WOSILAIT, W. D.: The relationship of epinephrine and glucagon to liver phosphorylase. J. Biol. Chem. 218, 483 (1956).

RAPP, W., KAHLKE, W.: Lipoprotein-Elektrophorese in Agarosegel. Clin. chim. Acta 19, 493 (1968).

RATCLIFFE, H. L., LUGINBÜHL, H.: The domestic pig: A model for experimental atherosclerosis. Atherosclerosis 13, 133 - 136 (1971).

REAGAN, T. J.: Relation of microcirculatory thrombosis to thrombus in the proximal coronary artery: Effect of aspirin, dipyridamole and thrombolysis. Amer. Heart J. 86, 61 - 86 (1973).

REAVEN, G. M., HILL, D. B., GROSS, R. C., FARQUHAR, J. W.: Kinetics of triglyceride turnover of very low density lipoproteins of human plasma. J. Clin. Invest. 44, 1826 (1965).

REAVEN, G. M., OLEFSKY, J., FARQUHAR, J. W.: Does hyperglycaemia or hyperinsulin-
aemia characterise the patient with chemical diabetes? Lancet 1972 II, 1247.
REDGRAVE, T. G.: Formation of cholesteryl ester-rich particulate lipid during
metabolism of chylomicrons. J. Clin. Invest. 49, 465 (1970).
REDGRAVE, T. G.: Cholesterol feeding alters the metabolism of thoracic-duct lym-
phy lipoprotein cholesterol in rabbits but not in rats. Biochem. J. 136, 109
(1973).
REDMAN, C. M.: The synthesis of serum proteins on attached rather than free ribosomes of rat liver. Biochem. Biophys. Res. Commun. 31, 845 - 850 (1968).
REDMAN, C. M., CHERIAN, M. G.: The secretory pathways of rat serum glycoproteins
and albumin. J. Cell Biol. 52, 231 (1972).
RENAIS, J., HADJIISKY, P., SCEBAT, L.: Immunological properties of connective
tissue and smooth muscle cells. Workshop on arterial mesenchyme and arterio-
sclerosis, New Orleans, April 2 - 3, 1973 (To be published).
RENAUD, S.: Diet, drugs and thrombosis, Can. Med. Ass. J. 108, 458 - 459 (1973).
RENAUD, S., ALLARD, C.: Hypertension, thrombosis and atherosclerosis in the rat.
Canad. Med. A. J. 88, 1275 - 1279 (1963).
RENAUD, S., ALLARD, C.: Effect of dietary protein on cholesterolemia, thrombosis,
atherosclerosis and hypertension in the rat. J. Nutr. 83, 149 - 157 (1964).
RENAUD, S., ALLARD, C., LATOUR, J. G.: Influence on the type of dietary saturated
fatty acid on lipemis, coagulation and the production of thrombosis in the
rat. J. Nutr. 90, 433 - 440 (1966).
RENAUD, S., KINLOUGH, R. L., MUSTARD, J. F.: Relationship between platelet aggre-
gation and the thrombotic tendency in rats fed hyperlipemic diets. Lab. Invest. 22, 339 - 343 (1970).
RENAUD, S., LECOMPTE, F.: Hypercoagulability induced by hyperlipemia in rat,
rabbit and man. Role of platelet factor 3. Circ. Res. 27, 1003 - 1011 (1970).
RESCH, J. A., OKABE, N., LOEWENSON, R., KIMOTO, K., KATSUKI, S., BAKER, A. B.:
A comparative study of cerebral atherosclerosis in a Japanese and Minnesota
population, J. Atheroscler. Res. 7, 687 (1967).
RIESEN, W., NOSEDA, G., BUTLER, R.: Anti-beta-lipoprotein activity of human mono-
clonal immunoglobulins. Vox Sanguinis 22, 420 (1972).
RIGHETTI, A., SCHERRER, J. R., MICHELI, H., POMETTA, D.: Etude clinique des rè-
lations entre le diabète, les hyperlipoprotéinémies et l'atheromatose.
Schweiz. med. Wschr. 103, 668 (1973).
RITTER, M. C., DEMPSEY, M. E.: Purification and characterization of a naturally
occurring activator of cholesterol biosynthesis from $\Delta^{5,7}$-cholestadienal and
other precursors. Biochem. Biophys. Res. Commun. 38, 1921 - 1929 (1970).
RITTER, M. C., DEMPSEY, M. E.: Specificity and role in cholesterol biosynthesis
of a squalene and sterol carrier protein. J. Biol. Chem. 246, 1536 - 1539
(1971).
RITTER, M. C., DEMPSEY, M. E.: Squalene and sterol carrier protein: Structural
properties, lipid binding, and function in cholesterol biosynthesis. Proc.
Nat. Acad. Sci. USA 70, 265 (1973).
RITTER, M. C., DEMPSEY, M. E., FRANTZ, I. D., Jr.: Control of pathways of cholesterol biosynthesis by a squalene and sterol carrier protein (SCP). Fed. Proc.
31, 430 (1972).
RIVIN, A. U., DIMITROFF, S. P.: The incidence and severity of atherosclerosis in
estrogen-treated males, and in females with a hypoestrogenic or a hyperestro-
genic state. Circulation 9, 533 (1954).
ROBERT, A. M., GROSGOGEAT, Y., REVERDY, V., ROBERT, B., ROBERT, L.: Lésions ar-
térielles produites chez le lapin par immunisation avec l'élastine et les
glycoprotéines de structure de l'aorte. Etudes biochimiques et morphologiques.
Atherosclerosis 13, 427 (1971).
ROBERT, A. M., ROBERT, B., ROBERT, L.: Composition et biosynthèse de l'élastine.
Son rôle dans l'athérosclérose. Arch. Mal. du Coeur 62, Suppl. 3, 25 - 43
(1969).
ROBERT, B., ROBERT, L.: Studies on the structure of elastin and the mechanism
of action of elastolytic enzymes. In: Chemistry and molecular biology of the
intercellular matrix (BALAZS, E.A., Ed.). (Academic Press) 1,665-670 (1970).
ROBERT, B., ROBERT, L., LEGRAND, Y., PIGNAUD, G., CAEN, J.: Elastolytic protease
in blood platelets. Ser. Haemat. 4, 175 - 185 (1971).

ROBERT, L.: The macromolecular matrix of the arterial wall: Collagen, elastin, mucopolysaccharides, In: Atherosclerosis: Proceedings of the second international symposium, P. 59 - 74 (JONES, R. J., Ed.). New York: Springer-Verlag 1970.

ROBERT, L.: Immunology and aging. Lecture delivered at the Gottlieb Dettwieler Symposium on Aging, Ruschliken, September 1971.

ROBERT, L., ROBERT, M., MOCZAR, M., MOCZAR, E.: Constituants macromoleculaires de la paroi artérielle: antigénicité et role dans l'athérosclerose. In: Le role de la paroi artérielle dans l'athérogénése, p. 395. Paris: C.N.R.S. 1968.

ROBERT, L., ROBERT, B., MOCZAR, E., MOCZAR, M.: Les glycoprotéines de structure du tissu conjonctif. Pathol. Biol. 20, 1001 - 1012 (1972).

ROBERT, L., ROBERT, B., ROBERT, A. M.: Interactions entre lipids, lipoproteines et macromolécules fibreuses du tissu conjonctif. Exp. Ann. Biochim. Méd. 31, 111 - 144 (1972).

ROBERTS, J. C.: The effects of serum sickness on cholesterol atherosclerosis in the rabbit. Circulation 22, 657 (1960).

ROBERTS, J. C., Jr., STRAUS, R. (Eds.): Comparative Atherosclerosis, New York: Harper & Row 1965.

ROBERTS, W. C., BUJA, L. M.: The frequency and significance of coronary arterial thrombi and other observations in fatal acute myocardial infarctions: a study of 107 necropsy patients. Amer. J. Med. 52, 425 - 443 (1972).

ROBERTS, W. C., FERRANS, V. J., LEVY, R. I., FREDRICKSON, D. S.: Cardiovascular pathology in hyperlipoproteinemia. Amer. J. Card. 31, 557 (1973).

ROBERTSON, A. L., Jr.: Some aspects of the metabolism and ultrastructure of human and animal lining. In Fundamentals of vascular grafting, p. 79 - 105 (WESOLOWSKI, S. A., DENNIS, C., Eds.). New York: Mc Graw-Hill Book Co. 1963.

ROBERTSON, A. L., Jr.: Intracellular incorporation of plasma lipoproteins by arterial intima in relation to early stages of intravascular thrombosis. In: Biophysical mechanisms in vascular homeostasis and intravascular thrombosis, p. 267 - 274 (SAWYER, P. N., Ed.).   Appleton-Century-Crofts 1965.

ROBERTSON, A. L., Jr.: Transport of plasma lipoproteins and ultrastructure of human arterial intimacytes in culture. In: Lipid metabolism in tissue culture cells. The Wistar Inst. Press, (ROTHBLAT, G. H., and KRITCHEVSKY, D., Eds.). Wistar Inst. Symp. Monogr. 6, 115 - 128.

ROBERTSON, A. L., Jr.: The artery and process of arteriosclerosis. Pathogenesis. In: Advances in experimental medicine and biology, Vol. 16A, pp. 24 - 25, 104 - 107, and 229 - 239 (WOLF, S., Ed.). New York - London: Plenum Press 1971.

ROBERTSON, A. L., KHAIRALLAH, P. A.: Effects of angiotensin II and some analogues on vascular permeability in the rabbit, Circ. Res. 31, 923 (1972).

ROBERTSON, A. L., Jr., KHAIRALLAH, P. A.: Arterial endothelial permeability and vascular disease. The "trap door" effect. Exp. Mol. Pathol. 18, 241 (1973).

ROBERTSON, A. L., Jr., KHAIRALLAH, P. A.: Effects of angiotensin II on the permeability of the vascular wall. In: Handbook of experimental pharmacology. Vol. 37. Angiotensin, (PAGE, I. H., and BUMPUS, F. M., Eds.). Heidelberg: Springer-Verlag 1973, In press.

ROBERTSON, J. H.: The significance of intimal thickening in the arteries of the newborn. Arch. Dis. Child. 35, 588 - 590 (1960).

ROBERTSON, R. P., GAVARESKI, D. J., HENDERSON, J. D., PORTE, D., Jr., BIERMAN, E. L.: Accelerated triglyceride secretion. A metabolic consequence of obesity J. Clin. Invest. 52, 1620 - 1626 (1973).

ROBERTSON, W. B., GEER, J. C., STRONG, J. P., Mc GILL, H. C., Jr.: The fate of the fatty streak. Exp. Mol. Pathol. Suppl. 1, 1, 28 - 39 (1963).

ROBERTSON, W. B., STRONG, J. P.: Atherosclerosis in persons with hypertension and diabetes mellitus. In: Geographic pathology of atherosclerosis, p. 78 (Mc GILL, H. C., Jr. Ed.). Baltimore: Williams and Wilkins Company 1968.

ROBERTSON, W. B., STRONG, J. P.: Atherosclerosis in persons with hypertension and diabetes mellitus. Lab. Invest. 18, 538 - 551 (1968).

ROBINSON, D. S.: In: Comprehensive Biochemistry, vol. 18, p. 51 - 116, Amsterdam: Elsevier 1970.

ROBINSON, D. S., HARRIS, P. M.: The production of lipolytic activity in the circulation of the hind limb in response to heparin. Quart. J. Exp. Physiol. 44, 80 (1959).

ROBINSON, D. S., HARRIS, P. M.: Ethionine administration in the rat. 2. Effects on the incorporation of (^{32}P) orthophosphate and d(1-^{14}C) leucine into the phosphatides and proteins of liver and plasma. Biochem. J. 80, 361 (1961).

ROBINSON, D. S., SEAKINS, A.: The development in the rat of fatty livers associated with reduced plasma-lipoprotein synthesis. Biochim. Biophys. Acta 62, 163 - 165 (1962).

ROBINSON, D. S., WING, D. R.: Regulation of adipose tissue clearing factor lipase activity. In: Adipose Tissue, p. 41 (JEANRENAND, B., and HEPP, D., Eds.). New York: Academic Press 1970.

RODBARD, S.: Distribution of flow through a pulmonary manifold. American Heart J. 51, 106 - 126 (1956).

RODBARD, S.: Vascular modifications induced by flow. Amer. Heart J. 51, 926 - 942 (1956).

RODBARD, S.: Chondrogenesis induced in arteries by reduction in vascular extensibility. Fed. Proc. 17, 134 (1958).

RODBARD, S.: Negative feedback mechanisms in the architecture and function of the connective and cardiovascular tissues. Perspect. Biol. Med. 13, 507 - 527 (1970).

RODBARD, S.: Physical factors in arterial sclerosis and stenosis. Angiology 22, 267 - 284 (1971).

RODBARD, S., EPSTEIN, S.: The role of friction in the induction of cutaneous papilliferous growths. Amer. J. Med. Sci. 249, 685 - 690 (1965).

RODBARD, S., IKEDA, K., MONTES, M.: An analysis of mechanisms of post stenotic dilatation. Angiology 18, 349 - 369 (1967).

RODBARD, S., JOHNSON, A. C.: Deposition of flowborne materials on vessel walls. Circ. Res. 11, 664 - 668 (1962).

RODBARD, S., KINOSHITA, Y., MONTES, M.: Induction of papillary growths in the heart. Science 143, 1341 - 1342 (1964).

RODBARD, S., LEHOCZKY, J. M., TERNER, J. Y., Mc CANDLESS, E. L.: Mechanical factors effecting conversion of arterial smooth muscle into fibroblasts or cartilage. In: Metabolisms Parietis Vasorum, p. 696 - 698 (PRUSIK, B., REINIS, Z., and RIEDL, O., Eds.) (1962).

RODBELL, M.: The localisation of lipoprotein lipase in fat cells of rat adipose tissue. J. Biol. Chem. 239, 753 (1964).

ROE, J. H., KUETHER, C. A.: The determination of ascorbic acid in whole blood and urine through the 2,4-dinitrophenylhydrazine derivative of dehydroascorbic acid. J. Biol. Chem. 17, 399 (1943).

ROHEIM, P. S., BIEMPICA, L., EDELSTEIN, D., KOSOWER, N. S.: Mechanism of fatty liver development and hyperlipemia in rats treated with allylisopropylacetamide. J. Lipid Res. 12, 76 - 83 (1971).

ROHEIM, P. S., GIDEZ, L. I., EDER, H. A.: Extrahepatic synthesis of lipoproteins of plasma and chyle: role of the intestine. J. Clin. Invest. 45, 297 - 300 (1966 a).

ROHEIM, P. S., RACHMILEWITZ, D., STEIN, O., STEIN, Y.: Metabolism of iodinated high denisty lipoproteins in the rat. 1. Half-life in the circulation and uptake by organs. Biochim. Biophys. Acta 248, 315 (1971).

ROHEIM, P. S., SWITZER, S., GIRARD, A., EDER, H. A.: Alterations of lipoprotein metabolism in orotic acid-induced fatty liver. Lab. Invest. 15, 21 - 26 (1966 b).

ROSE, G.: Familial patterns in ischaemic heart disease. Brit. J. prev. soc. Med. 18, 75 (1964).

ROSE, G.: Predicting coronary heart disease from minor symptoms and electrocardiographic findings. Brit. J. prev. soc. Med. 25, 94 - 96 (1971).

ROSE, G. A., BLACKBURN, H.: Cardiovascular Study Methods. Geneva: WHO 1968.

ROSE, H. G.: Influence of plasma lipoprotein levels on lipoprotein cholesterol esterification in normal and hyperlipemic subjects. Circ. 46, II - 274 (1972).

ROSE, H. G., KRANZ, P., WEINSTOCK, M., JULIANO, J., HAFT, J. I.: Inheritance of combined hyperlipoproteinemia: evidence for a new lipoprotein phenotype. Am. J. Med. 54, 148 (1972).

ROSENBLOOM, J., PROCKOP, D. J.: Incorporation of cis-hydroxyproline into protocollagen and collagen. J. Biol. Chem. 246, 1549 (1971).

ROSENMAN, R. H., FRIEDMAN, M., STRAUS, R., WURM, M., KOSITCHEK, R., HAHN, W.,
WERTHESSEN, N. T.: A predictive study of coronary heart disease: The Western
Collaborative Group Study. J. Amer. med. Ass. 189, 15 (1964).

ROSNER, P., BOUVIER, C. A., BERTHOUD, S.: Mesure de l'adhésivité plaquettaire au
verre (modification de la méthode de Hellem). Nouv. Rev. Franc. Hemat. 7,
184 (1967).

ROSS, R.: The smooth muscle cell II. Growth of smooth muscle in culture and formation of elastic fibers. J. Cell Biol. 50, 172 (1971).

ROSS, R., GLOMSET, J. A.: Atherosclerosis and the arterial smooth muscle cell.
Science 180, 1332 (1973).

ROSS, R., GLOMSET, J. A.: Studies of primate arterial smooth muscle cells in relation to atherosclerosis. In: Workshop on Arterial Mesenchyme, New Orleans,
May 1, Plenum Press (1973 b, In press).

ROSS, R., GLOMSET, J., KARIYA, B., HARKER, L.: A platelet-dependent serum factor
that stimulates the proliferation of arterial smooth muscle cells in vitro.
Proc. Nat. Acad. Sci. USA 71, 1207 - 1210 (1974).

ROSS, R., KLEBANOFF, S. J.: The smooth muscle cell. I. In vivo synthesis of
connective tissue proteins. J. Cell. Biol. 50, 159 (1971).

ROSSENEU-MOTREFF, M. Y., BLATON, 'V., LIEVENS-TAVEIRNE, J., PEETERS, H.: Binding
of lysolecithin to apo-HDL. Microcalorimetric study. Programme Conference on
Serum Lipoproteins, Graz, p. 48 (1973).

ROTHBLAT, G. H., BUCHKO, M. K., KRITCHEVSKY, D.: Cholesterol uptake by L5178Y
tissue culture cells: studies with delipidized serum. Biochem. Biophys. Acta
164, 327 (1968).

ROTHBLAT, G. H., KRITCHEVSKY, D.: Cholesterol metabolism in tissue culture cells.
In: Lipid metabolism in tissue culture cells, (ROTHBLAT, G. H., and KRITCHEVS-
KY, D., Eds.). Philadelphia: Wistar Press 1967.

ROTHBLAT, G. H., KRITCHEVSKY, D.: The metabolism of free and esterified cholesterol in tissue culture cells: a review. Exp. Molec. Pathol. 8, 314 (1968).

ROUILLER, C., JEZEQUEL, A. M.: Electron microscopy of the liver. In: The liver,
Vol. I, p. 195 - 264 (ROUILLER, C., Ed.). New York: Academic Press 1963.

ROWBLATT, U. F., RIMOLDI, H. J. A., LEV, M.: The quantitative anatomy of the
normal childs heart. Pediat. Clin. N. Amer. 10, 499 - 588 (1963).

RUBULIS, A., LIM, E. C., FALOON, W. W.: Effect of a bile acid sequestrant, colestipol, on serum cholesterol, fecal bile acids and neutral sterols in human
subjects. Fed. Proc. 31, (Abs) 727 (1972).

RUCKDESCHEL, J. C., PETERS, T., Jr., LEE, K. T.: Fibrinogen catabolism in rats
fed thrombogenic diets. Atherosclerosis 16, 277 - 285 (1972).

RUDERMAN, N. B., RICHARDS, K. C., VALLES DE BOURGES, V., JONES, A. L.: Regulation
of production and release of lipoprotein by the perfused rat liver. J. Lipid
Res. 9, 613 - 619 (1968).

RUDMAN, D., DI GIROLAMO, M.: Comparative studies on the physiology of adipose
tissue, Vol. 5, p. 35 In: Advances in lipid research (FAOLETTI, R. and
KRITCHEVSKY, D., Eds.). New York: Academic Press 1967.

RUDNICK, P. A., ANDERSON, P. S., Jr.: Diabetes mellitus in Hiroshima, Japan: A
detection program and clinical survey. Diabetes 11, 533 (1962).

RUMBALL, A., ACHESON, E.: Electrocardiograms of healthy men after strenous exercise. Brit. Heart H. 22, 415 - 425 (1960).

RUSH, R. L., LEON, L., TURRELL, J.: Automated simultaneous cholesterol and triglyceride determinations on the Auto-analyzer II instrument. Advances in
automated analysis. VI, 503 - 507 (1970).

RUSSEK, H. I., ZOHMAN, B. L.: Relative significance of heredity, diet and occupational stress in coronary heart disease of young adults. Am. J. med. Sci.
235, 266 (1958).

RUSSELL, R. W. R.: Observations on the retinal blood-vessels in monocular blindness. Lancet 1961 II, 1422 - 1428.

RUTENBERG, H. L., SOLOFF, L. A.: Possible mechanisms of egress of free cholesterol from the arterial wall. Nature 230, 123 (1971).

RYAN, J. R., JAIN, A.: The effect of colestipol or cholestyramine on serum cholesterol and triglycerides in a long-term controlled study. J. clin. Pharmacol. 12, 268 (1972).

RYGAARD, J., OLSEN, W.: Determination of characteristics of interference filters. Ann. New York Acad. Sci. 177, 430 - 433 (1971).

SAILER, S., SANDHOFER, F., BRAUNSTEINER, H.: Umsatzraten für freie Fettsäuren und Triglyzeride im Plasma bei essentieller Hyperlipämie. Klin. Wochenschr. 44, 1032 (1966).

SAITO, H., YAMAGATA, T., SUZUKI, S.: Enzymatic methods for the determination of small quantities of isomeric chondroitin sulfates. J. Biol. Chem. 243, 1536 (1968).

SAMUEL, P., LIEBERMAN, S.: Improved estimation of body masses and turnover of cholesterol by computerized input-output analysis. J. Lipid Res. 14, 189 (1973).

SANDBERG, L. B., WEISSMAN, N., SMITH, D. W.: The purification and partial characterization of a soluble elastin-like protein from copper-deficient porcine aorta. Biochemistry 8, 2940 (1969).

SANDERSON, J. H., DELAMORE, I. W.: Changes in platelet thrombotic tendency during oral contraception. J. Obst. Gyn. 80, 639 - 643 (1973).

SANDHOFER, F., BOLZANO, K., SAILER, S., BRAUNSTEINER, H.: Studies on cholesterol turnover in normo-cholesterolaemic subjects. Europ. J. Clin. Invest. 2, 426 (1972).

SANO, T., YAMAZAKI, H., SHIMAMOTO, T.: Enhancement of ADP-induced platelet aggregation by cholesterol and its prevention by pyridinolcarbamate, Thromb. Diath. haemorrh. 29, 684 (1973).

SANTERRE, R. F.: Pre-atherosclerotic differences in respiratory control between susceptible White Carneau and resistant Show Racer pigeons. Ph. D. Thesis, Univ. of New Hampshire, 1971.

SANTERRE, R. F., WIGHT, T. N., SMITH, S. C., BRANNINGAN, D.: Spontaneous atherosclerosis in pigeons. A model system for studying metabolic parameters associated with atherogenesis. Am. J. Pathol. 67, 1 (1972).

SAPHIR, O., STRYZAK, D., OHRINGER, L.: Hypersensitivity changes in coronary arteries of rabbits and their relationship to atherosclerosis. J. of Lab. Investigation 7, 434 (1958).

SARDA, L., DESNUELLE, P.: Action de la lipase pancreatique sur les esters en emulsion. Biochim. Biophys. Acta 30, 513 (1958).

SARDET, C., HANSMA, H., OSTWALD, R.: Effects of plasma lipoproteins from control and cholesterol-fed guinea pigs on red cell morphology and cholesterol content in vitro study. J. Lipid Res. 13, 705 (1972).

SARMA, J. S. M., TILLMANNS, H. H., IKEDA, S., BING, R. J.: The effect of carbon monoxide on lipid metabolism of human coronary arteries. Atherosclerosis (To be published).

SAUVAGE, L. R., HARKINS, H. N.: Experimental vascular grafts: an evaluation relating to types, means of preservation and methods of suture in the growing pig. Surgery 33, 587 (1953).

SCALLEN, T. J., SCHUSTER, M. W., DHAR, A. K.: Evidence for a noncatalytic carrier protein in cholesterol biosynthesis. J. Biol. Chem. 246, 224 (1971).

SCANU, A.: Binding of human serum high density lipoprotein apoproteins with aqueous dispersions of phospholipids. J. Biol. Chem. 242, 711 (1967).

SCANU, A. M.: Human plasma high-density lipoproteins. In: Plasma lipoproteins (SMELLIE, R. M. S., Ed.). London : Academic Press 1973.

SCANU, A., CUMP, E., TOTH, J., KOGA, S., STILLER, E., ALBERS, L.: Degradation and reassembly of a human serum high-density lipoprotein. Evidence for differences in lipid affinity among three classes of polypeptide chains. Biochem. 9, 1327 (1970).

SCANU, A. M., EDELSTEIN, C., AGGERBECK, L.: Application of the technique of isoelectric focusing to the study of human-serum lipoproteins and their apoproteins. Ann. N. Y. Acad. Sci. 209, 311 (1973).

SCANU, A. M., TOTH, J., EDELSTEIN, C., KOGA, S., STILLER, E.: Fractionation of human serum high density lipoprotein in urea solutions. Evidence for polypeptide heterogeneity. Biochemistry 8, 3309 (1969).

SCEBAT, L., RENAIS, J., GROULT, N., LENEGRE, J.: Experimental arteriopathy induced in the rabbit through rat aorta homogenate injections: a study of the aortic tissue specificity. In: The reticuloendothelial system and atherosclerosis, p. 451 (DI LUZZIO and PAOLETTI, R. Eds.). New York: Plenum Press 1967.

SCEBAT, L., RENAIS, J., IRIS, L., GROULT, N., LENEGRE, J.: Athérosclérose expérimentale du rat. III. Rôle de lésions préalables de la paroi artérielle par
un processus immunologique. Revue d'atherosclerose 9, 242 (1967 b).

SCHAEFER, L. E., ADLERSBERG, D., STEINBERG, A. G.: Heredity, environment, and
serum cholesterol: A study of 201 healthy families. Circulation 17, 537
(1958).

SCHAFFNER, F., SCHARNBECK, H. H., HUTTERER, F., DENK, H., GREIM, H. A., POPPER,
H.: Mechanism of cholestasis. 7. α-naphthylisothiocyanate induced jaundice.
Lab. Invest. 28, 321 - 331 (1973).

SCHAPER, W.: The collateral circulation of the heart. New York: American
Elsevier Publishing Company, 1971.

SCHARRER, J. C., SCHEPPING, M., BREDDIN, K.: Thromboseprophylaxe mit Aspirin?
Klin. Wschr. 47, 1318 (1969).

SCHETTLER, G.: Atherosclerosis. Berlin, Heidelberg: Springer-Verlag 1970.

SCHETTLER, G., KAHLKE, W., SCHLIERF, G.: Essential hypercholesterolemia. In:
Lipids and lipidoses, p. 412 (SCHETTLER, G., Ed.). Berlin, Heidelberg:
Springer-Verlag 1967.

SCHIMKE, R. N.: Genetics of hormone-secreting tumours. Clin. Gastroenterol. 2,
661 (1973).

SCHLIERF, G., DOROW, E.: Diurnal patterns of triglycerides, free fatty acids,
blood sugar, and insulin during carbohydrate-induction in man and their
modification by nocturnal suppression of lipolysis. J. Clin. Invest. 52, 732
(1973).

SCHLIERF, G., KAHLKE, W.: The effect of chlorophenoxyisobutyrate (CPIB) in va-
rious types of primary hyperlipidemia. In: Drugs affecting lipid metabolism,
Vol. 4. (HOLMES, W. L., CARLSON, L.A., and PAOLETTI, R., Eds.). New York:
Plenum Press 1969.

SCHLIERF, G., REINHEIMER, W., STOSSBERG, V.: Diurnal patterns of plasma triglycerides and free fatty acids in normal subjects and in patients with endogeneous (Type IV) hyperlipoproteinemia. Nutr. Metabol. 13, 80 - 91 (1971).

SCHLIERF, G., WEINANS, G., WEINANS, T., REINHEIMER, W., KAHLKE, W.: Häufigkeit
und Typenverteilung von Hyperlipoproteinämien bei stationären Patienten
einer Medizinischen Klinik. Dtsch. med. Wschr. 97, 1371 - 1375 (1972).

SCHLOSSER, V., BERTRAM, E., GOERTTLER, U., MITTERMAYER, C., SPILLNER, G.: Zwei
Typen der chronischen arteriellen Verschlußkrankheit. Dtsch. med. Wschr.
98, 593 (1973).

SCHLUNK, F. F., LONGNECKER, D. S., LOMBARDI, B.: On the ethionine-induced inhibition of protein synthesis in male and female rats - lack of intestinal mucosa. Biochim. Biophys. Acta 158, 425 - 434 (1968).

SCHMITT, A.: Virchows Arch. Path. Anat. 296, 603 (1936) cited by Moensfaber,
The human aorta. Arch. Pathology 48, 342 (1942).

SCHOEFL, G. I., FRENCH, J. E.: Vascular permeability to particulate fat: morphological observations on vessels of lactating mammary gland and of lung. Proc.
Roy. Soc. (Biol.) 169, 153 (1968).

SCHOENFIELD, G., PFLEGER, B., LEES, R. S.: Plasma beta-protein in the classification of the hyperlipidemias. Circulation 46, Suppl. II, 17 (1972).

SCHONHOFER, P. S., SKIDMORE, I. F., FORN, J., FLEICH, J. H.: Adenyl cyclase activity of rabbit aorta. J. Pharm. Pharmacol. 23, 28 (1971).

SCHREIBMAN, P. H., ARONS, D. L., SAUDEK, C. D., ARKY, R. A.: Abnormal lipoprotein lipase in familial exogenous hypertriglyceridemia. J. Clin. Invest. 52,
2075 (1973).

SCHRETZENMAYR, A.: Über kreislaufregulatorische Vorgänge an den großen Arterien
bei der Muskelarbeit. Pflüg. Arch. ges. Physiol. 236, 930 (1935).

SCHRIRE, V.: Heart disease in Southern Africa with special reference to ischaemic
heart disease; South African Medical Journal 45, 634 - 644 (1971).

SCHROEDER, H. A.: Relation between mortality from cardiovascular disease and
treated water supplies. J. Amer. Med. Assoc. 172, 1902 - 1908 (1960).

SCHROEDER, H. A.: Municipal drinking water and cardiovascular death rates. J.
Amer. Med. Assoc. 195, 125 - 129 (1966).

SCHROEDER, H. A.: Cadmium, chromium and cardiovascular disease. Circulation 35,
570 - 582 (1967).

SCHROTT, H. G., GOLDSTEIN, J. L., HAZZARD, W. R., Mc GOODWIN, M. M., MOTULSKY, A. G.: Familial hypercholesterolemia in a large kindred. Evidence for a monogenic mechanism. Ann. intern. Med. 76, 711 (1972).

SCHUBERT, W. K.: Fat nutrition and diet in childhood. Amer. J. Card. 31, 581 (1973).

SCHULTZ, R. D., HOKANSON, D. E., STRANDNESS, D. E., Jr.: Pressure-flow and stress-strain measurements of normal and diseased aortoiliac segments. Surg. Gynecol. Obstet. 124, 1267 (1967).

SCHUMAKER, V. N., ADAMS, G. H.: Very low density lipoproteins: surface-volume changes during metabolism. J. Theor. Biol. 26, 89 (1970).

SCHWARTZ, S. M., BENDITT, E. P.: Studies on aortic intima. I. Structure and permeability of rat thoracic aortic intima. Amer. J. Pathol. 66, 241 - 256 (1972).

SCHWARTZ, S. M., BENDITT, E. P.: Cell replication in the aortic endothelium; a new method for study of the problem. Lab. Invest. 28, 699 - 707 (1973).

SCOTT, P. J., HURLEY, P. J.: Incorporation of radioiodinated serum albumin and low-density lipoprotein into human thrombi in vivo. J.Pathol.97,603-609 (1969).

SCOTT, P. J., HURLEY, P. J.: The distribution of radio-iodinated serum albumin and low-density lipoprotein in tissues and the arterial wall. Atherosclerosis 11, 77 (1970).

SCOTT, R. F., DAOUD, A. S., FLORENTIN, R. A.: Animal models in atherosclerosis. In: The pathogenesis of atherosclerosis. (WISSLER, R. W., GEER, J. C., Eds.), Baltimore: Williams and Wilkins 1972.

SCOTT, R. F., FLORENTIN, R. A., DAOUD, A. S., MORRISON, E. S., JONES, R. M., HUTT, M. S. R.: Coronary arteries of children and young adults. A comparison of lipids and anatomic features in New Yorkers and East Africans. Exp. Molec. Pathol. 5, 12 (1966).

SCOTT, R. F., JONES, R., DAOUD, A. S., ZUMBO, O., COULSTON, F., THOMAS, W. A.: Experimental atherosclerosis in rhesus monkeys. II. Cellular elements of proliferative lesions and possible role of cytoplasmic degeneration in pathogenesis as studied by electron microscopy. Exp. Mol. Pathol. 7, 34 - 57 (1967 b).

SCOTT, R. F., MORRISON, E. S., JARMOLYCH, J., NAM, S. C., KROMS, M., COULSTON, F.: Experimental atherosclerosis in rhesus monkeys. I. Gross and light microscopy features and lipid values in serum and aorta. Exp. Mol. Pathol. 7, 11 - 33 (1967 a).

SCOW, R. O., HAMOSH, M., BLANCHETTE-MACHLE, E. J., EVANS, A. J.: Uptake of blood triglyceride by various tissues. Lipids 7, 497 - 505 (1972).

SEIDEL, D.: A new immunological technique for a rapid, semi-quantitative determination of the abnormal lipoprotein (LB-X) characterizing cholestasis. Clin. Chim. Acta 31, 225 (1971).

SEIDEL, D., AGOSTINI, B., MÜLLER, P.: Structure of an abnormal plasma lipoprotein (LP-X) characterizing obstructive jaundice. Biochim. Biophys. Acta 260, 146 (1972 a).

SEIDEL, D., ALAUPOVIC, P., FURMAN, R. H.: A lipoprotein characterizing obstructive jaundice. I. Method for quantitative separation and identification of lipoproteins in jaundiced subjects. J. Clin. Invest. 48, 1211 (1969).

SEIDEL, D., ALAUPOVIC, P., FURMAN, R. H., Mc CONATHY, W. J.: A lipoprotein characterizing obstructive jaundice. II. Isolation and partial characterization of the protein moieties of low density lipoproteins. J. Clin. Invest. 49, 2396 (1970).

SEIDEL, D., GJONE, E., BLOMHOFF, J. P., GEISEN, H. P.: Plasma lipoproteins in patients with familial plasma lecithin: cholesterol acyltransferase (LCAT) deficiency - studies on the apolipoprotein composition of isolated fractions with identification of LP-X. In: Hormone and metabolic research.(GRETEN, H., LEVINE, R., PFEIFFER, E. F., RENOLD, R. E., Eds.) p.6. Stuttgart: Thieme 1974.

SEIDEL, D., GRETEN, H., GEISEN, H. P., WENGELER, H., WIELAND, H.: Further aspects on the characterization of high and very low density lipoproteins in patients with liver disease. Europ. J. Clin. Invest. 2, 359 (1972).

SEIDEL, D., WIELAND, H., RUPPERT, C.: Improved techniques for assessment of plasma lipoprotein patterns. I. Precipitation in gels after electrophoresis with polyanionic compounds. Clin. Chem. 19, 737 (1973).

SEGALL, M. M., FOSBROOKE, A. S., LLOYD, J. K., WOLFF, O. H.: Treatment of familial hypercholesterolaemia in children. Lancet 1970 I, 641.

SELIGMAN, A. M., TSOU, K. L., RUTENBURG, S. H., COHEN, B. B.: Histochemical demonstration of beta-glucuronidase with a synthetic substrate. J. Histochem.
Cytochem. 2, 209 - 229 (1954).

SHAFRIR, E., SUSSMAN, K. E., STEINBERG, D.: The nature of epinephrine-induced
hyperlipidemia in dogs and its modification by glucose. J. Lipid Res. 1, 109
(1959).

SHAFRIR, E., SUSSMAN, K. E., STEINBERG, D.: Role of the pituitary and adrenal in
the mobilization of free fatty acids and lipoproteins. J. Lipid Res. 1, 459 -
465 (1960).

SHAMES, D., FRANK, H., STEINBERG, D., BERMAN, M.: Transport of plasma free fatty
acids and triglycerides in man: a theoretical analysis. J. Clin. Invest. 49,
2298 (1970).

SHANBERGE, J. N., TANAKA, K., GRUHL, M. C., IKEMORI, R., INOSHITA, K.: The effect
of oral contraceptives on fibrin-clot stabilization. Annals New York Acad.
Sciences 202, 220 - 229 (1972).

SHANOFF, H. M., LITTLE, A., MURPHY, E. A., RYKERT, H. E.: Studies of male survivors of myocardial infarction due to "essential" atherosclerosis. I. Characteristics of the patients. J. Canad. med. Ass. 84, 519 (1961).

SHARP, C. L. E. H.: In: Presymptomatic detection and early diagnosis. A critical
appraisal, p. 3 - 24 (SHARP, C. L. E. H., and KEEN, H., Eds.). Baltimore:
Williams and Wilkins 1968.

SHELBURNE, F. A., QUARFORDT, S. H.: A new apoprotein of human plasma very low
density lipoprotein. Fed. Proc. 32, 547 (Abs) 1973.

SHIFF, T. S., ROHEIM, P. S., EDER, H. A.: Effects of high sucrose diets and 4-
aminopyrazolopyrimidine on serum lipids and lipoprotein in the rat. J. Lipid
Res. 12, 596 - 603 (1971).

SHIMAMOTO, T.: The relationship of edematous reaction in arteries to atherosclerosis and thrombosis, J. Atheroscler. Res. 3, 87 (1963).

SHIMAMOTO, T.: Experimental study on atherosclerosis. An attempt at its prevention and treatment, Acta Path. Jap. 19, 15 (1969).

SHIMAMOTO, T., New concept on atherogenesis and treatment of atherosclerotic
diseases. Japan Heart J. 13, 537 - 562 (1972).

SHIMAMOTO, T.: Contracting and swallowing activity of arterial endothelial cells
induced by cholesterol or epinephrine or angiotensin II or bradykinin. An
electron microscopic study. J. Japan Atheroscler. Soc. 1, 29 - 56 (1973).

SHIMAMOTO, T., ATSUMI, T., YAMASHITA, S., MOTOMIYA, T., ISOKANE, N., ISHIOKA, T.,
SAKUMA, A.: Clinical pharmacologic evaluation of the anti-atherosclerotic
agent, pyridinolcarbamate. A double-blind crossover trial in the treatment
of atherosclerosis obliterans, Am. Heart J. 79, 5 (1970).

SHIMAMOTO, T., KOBAYASHI, M., NUMANO, F.: Infiltration of γ-globulin, fibrinogen
and β-lipoprotein into blood vessel wall by atherogenic stress visualized by
immunofluorescence, Proc. Jap. Acad. 48, 336 (1972).

SHIMAMOTO, T., NUMANO, F.: Preventive effect of estrogen against cholesterol-induced contraction of arterial endothelial cells. An electron microscopic observation. Proc. Japan Acad. 48, 742 - 746 (1972).

SHIMAMOTO, T., NUMANO, F.: Contraction and relaxation of endothelial cells covering atheroma and their significance. Proc. Jap. Acad. 49, 77 (1973).

SHIMAMOTO, T., NUMANO, F., FUJITA, T.: Atherosclerosis-inhibiting effect of an
antibradykinin agent, pyridinolcarbamate, Am. Heart J. 71, 216 (1966).

SHIMAMOTO, T., SUNAGA, T.: Contraction of endothelial cells as a key mechanism
in atherogenesis. Proc. Japan Academy 48, 633 - 699 (1972).

SHIMAMOTO, T., SUNAGA, T.: The contraction and blebbing of endothelial cells
accompanied by acute infiltration of plasma substances into the vessel wall
and their prevention. In: Atherogenesis II, Excerpta Medica, p. 3 (SHIMAMOTO,
T., NUMANO, F., and ADDISON, G. M., Eds.). Amsterdam 1973.

SHIMAMOTO, T., YAMAZAKI, H.: Bradykinin-antagonistic antiinflammatory substance
B23 in treatment of angina pectoris. Proc. 3rd Asian-Pacific Congr. Cardiology, Kyoto, p. 748 (1964).

SHIPLEY, G. G., ATKINSON, D., SCANU, A. M.: Small-angle X-ray scattering of human
serum high-density lipoproteins. J. Supramol. Struct. 1, 98 (1972).

SHKHVATSABAYA, I. K.: Anginin in the treatment of patients with chronic coronary
insufficiency. In: Atherogenesis II, p. 347. Excerpta Medica 1973.

SHORE, B., NICHOLS, A. V., FREEMAN, N. K.: Evidence for lipolytic action by
human plasma obtained after intravenous administration of heparin. Proc. Soc.
Exp. Biol. Med. 83, 216 - 220 (1953).

SHORE, B., SHORE, V.: Heparin-released lipolytic and esterolytic activities of
human and rabbit plasmas. Amer. J. Physiol. 201, 915 - 922 (1961).

SHORE, B., SHORE, V.: Heterogeneity in protein subunits of human serum high-density lipoproteins. Biochemistry 7, 2773 (1968).

SHORE, B., SALEL, A., SHORE, V., ZELIS, R., MASON, D.: Apolipoprotein and
lipoprotein heterogeneity. This volume p. 88o.

SHORE, P. A., ALPERS, H. S.: Platelet damage induced in plasma by certain fatty
acids. Nature 200, 1331 (1963).

SHORE, V. G., SHORE, B.: Isolation and characterization of polypeptides of human
serum lipoproteins. Biochemistry 8, 4510 (1969).

SHORE, V. G., SHORE, B.: Heterogeneity of human plasma very low density lipoproteins. Separation of species differing in protein components. Biochemistry
12, 502 (1973).

SHORT, R. H. D.: Orientation of structure and of thrombi in the deep veins of
the leg in man. J. Path. Bact. 68, 41 - 54 (1954).

SHULMAN, R., HERBERT, P., WEHRLY, K., CHESEBRO, B., LEVY, R. I., FREDRICKSON,
D. S.: The complete amino acid sequence of ApoLP-Ser.: An apolipoprotein obtained from human very low density lipoprotein. (Abs.) Circulation 46, II -
246 (1972).

SIGGAARD-ANDERSEN, J., PETERSEN, F. B., HENSEN, T. I., MELLEMGAARD, K.: Plasma
volume and vascular permeability during hypoxia and carbon monoxide exposure.
Scand. J. Clin. Lab. Invest. Suppl. 103, 39 (1968).

SIGMA CHEMICAL CO., ST. LOUIS, Mo.: The colorimetric determination of phosphatase.
Tech. Bull. 104 (1961).

SIMPSON, C. F., NEILSON, J. T. M.: Aortic atherosclerosis of turkeys induced by
single treatment with diethylstilbestrol. Atherosclerosis 17, 245-255 (1973).

SIMS, E. A. H., GOLDMAN, R. F., GLUCK, C. M., HORTON, E. S., KELLEHER, P. C.,
ROWE, D. W.: Experimental obesity in man. Trans. Ass. Amer. Phys. 81, 153
(1968).

SIMS, E. A. H., HORTON, E. S., SALANS, L. B.: Inducible metabolic abnormalities
during development of obesity. Ann. Rev. Med. 22, 235 (1971).

SINAPIUS, D.: Häufigkeit und Morphologie der Coronarthrombose und ihre Beziehungen zur antithrombotischen und fibrinolytischen Behandlung. Klin. Wschr. 43,
37 - 43 (1965).

SINGER, S. J.: In: Structure and Function of Biological Membranes, p. 145.
(ROTHFIELD, L. I., Ed.). New York: Academic Press 1971.

SIPERSTEIN, M. D.: Regulation of cholesterol biosynthesis in normal and malignant tissues, In: Current Topics in Cellular Regulation (STADTMAN, E., and
HORECKER, B., Eds.). New York: Academic Press 2, 65 - 100 (1970).

SIPERSTEIN, M. D., UNGER, R. H., MADISON, L. L.: Studies of muscle capillary
basement membranes in normal subjects, diabetic and prediabetic patients.
J. Clin. Invest. 47, 1973 - 1999 (1968).

SLACK, J.: Risks of ischaemic heart disease in familial hypercholesterolemic
states. Lancet 1969 II, 1380.

SLACK, J., EVANS, K. A.: The increased risk of death from ischaemic heart disease
in first degree relatives of 121 men and 96 women with ischaemic heart disease. J. med. Genet. 3, 239 (1966).

SLACK, J., MILLS, G. L.: Anomalous low density lipoproteins in familial hyperlipoproteinaemia. Proceedings of the Second International Symposium on Atherosclerosis, p. 189 (JONES, R., Ed.). New York: Springer-Verlag 1970.

SLACK, J., MILLS, G. L.: Anomalous low density lipoproteins in familial hyperbetalipoproteinemia. Clin. Chim. Acta 29, 15 (1970).

SLOAN, H. R., FREDRICKSON, D. S.: Enzyme deficiency in cholesteryl ester storage
disease. J. Clin. Invest. 51, 1923 (1972).

SMITH, E. B.: Intimal and medial lipids in human aortas. Lancet I, 799.

SMITH, E. B.: The influence of age and atherosclerosis on the chemistry of aortic intima. Part 1. The lipids. J. Atheroscler. Res. 5, 224 (1965).

SMITH, E. B.: The influence of age and atherosclerosis on the chemistry of aortic intima. Part 2. Collagen and mucopolysaccharides. J. Atheroscler. Res. 5, 241 - 248 (1965).

SMITH, E. B.: Acid glycosaminoglycan, collagen, and elastin content of normal artery, fatty streaks, and plaques. Workshop on Arterial Mesenchyme, New Orleans, 1973. Plenum Press (In press).

SMITH, E. B., EVANS, P. H., DOWNHAM, M. D.: Lipid in the aortic intima. The correlation of morphological and chemical characteristics. J. Atheroscler. Res. 7, 171 (1967).

SMITH, E. B., SLATER, R. S.: The lipoproteins of the lesions. In: Atherosclerosis: Proceedings of the Second International Symposium, pp. 42 - 49 (JONES, R. J., Ed.). Berlin: Springer-Verlag 1970.

SMITH, E. B., SLATER, R. S.: The chemical and immunological assay of low density lipoproteins extracted from human aortic intima. Atherosclerosis 11, 417 - 438 (1970).

SMITH, E. B., SLATER, R. S.: An immuno-electrophoretic assay of beta-lipoprotein and albumin in human aortic intima by direct electrophoresis from the tissue sample into an antibody-containing gel. Biochem. J. 123, 39 (Abs.) 1971.

SMITH, E. B., SLATER, R.S.: The microdissection of large atherosclerotic plaques to give morphologically and topographically defined fractions for analysis: Part 1. The lipids in the isolated fractions. Atherosclerosis 15,37 (1972).

SMITH, E. B., SLATER, R. S.: Relationship between low-density lipoprotein in aortic intima and serum-lipid levels. Lancet 1972 I, 463 - 469.

SMITH, E. B., SLATER, R. S.: Lipids and low-density lipoproteins in intima in relation to its morphological characteristics. In: Atherogenesis: Initiating Factors. Ciba Foundation Symposium 12 (New Series), p. 39 - 62. Amsterdam: Associated Scientific Publishers 1973.

SMITH, E. B., SLATER, R. S.: Relationship between plasma lipids and arterial tissue lipids. Nutr. Metabol. 15, 17 (1973 b).

SMITH, E. B., SLATER, R. S., CHU, P. K.: The lipids in raised fatty and fibrous lesions in human aorta. A comparison of the changes at different stages of development. J. Atheroscler. Res. 8, 399 - 419 (1968).

SMITH, E. B., SLATER, R. S., HUNTER, J. A.: Quantitative studies on fibrinogen and low-density lipoprotein in human aortic intima. Atherosclerosis 18, 479 - 487 (1973).

SMITH, H. G., LAKATOS, C.: Effects of acetylsalicyclic acid on serum protein binding and metabolism of tryptophan in man. J. Pharm. Pharmacol. 23, 180 - 189 (1971).

SMITH, J. B.., WILLIS, A. L.: Aspirin selectively inhibits prostaglandin production in human platelets. Nature New Biology 231, 235 (1971).

SMITH, R., DAWSON, J. R., TANFORD, C.: The size and number of polypeptide chains in human serum low density lipoprotein. J. Biol. Chem. 247, 3376 (1972).

SMITH, R. L., HILKER, D. M.: Experimental dietary production of aortic atherosclerosis in Japanese quail. Atherosclerosis 17, 63 - 70 (1973).

SMITH, S. C., STROUT, R. G., DUNLOP, W. R., SMITH, E. C.: Fatty acid composition of cultured aortic cells from White Carneau and Show Racer pigeons. J. Atheroscler. Res. 5, 379 (1965).

SMITH, S. C., STROUT, R. G., DUNLOP, W. R., SMITH, E. C.: Mitochondrial involvement in lipid vacuole formation in cultured aortic cells from White Carneau pigeons. J. Atheroscler. Res. 6, 489 (1966).

SMIT SIBINGA, C.: Prevention of vessel wall damage in experimental irradiation. Dissertation. Groningen: Drukkerij Jan Haan N. V. 1972.

SMYTHE, H. A., OGRYZLO, M. A., MURPHY, E. A., MUSTARD, J. F.: The effect of sulfinpyrazone (anturan) on platelet economy and blood coagulation in man. Can. Med. Ass. J. 92, 818 - 821 (1965).

SNEDECOV, G. W.: Statistical Methods. 5th Ed. Ames: Iowa State Coll. Press 1956.

SNIDERMAN, A. D., CAREW, T. E., CHANDLER, J. G., HAYES, S., STEINBERG, D.: J. Clin. Invest. 52, 79 a (1973). The role of the liver in metabolism of low density lipoproteins (LDL).

SNIDERMAN, A. D., CAREW, T. E., CHANDLER, J. G., STEINBERG, D.: Paradoxical increase in rate of catabolism of low density lipoproteins after hepatectomy.
Science 183, 526 (1974).

SNIDERMAN, A. D., CAREW, T. E., STEINBERG, D.: Metabolism of low density lipoprotein apoprotein in the pig. Circ. 46, II - 249 (1972).

SNYDER, D., BREST, A. N., NOVAK, P.: Systolic hypertension: A presenting finding
in the hyperkinetic heart syndrome (P), Circ. 32, Suppl. II - 199 (Abs.)
(1965).

SOBRA, J.: Inborn errors of lipid metabolism. XIII. Familial hypercholesterolemic xanthomatosis. A review of the genealogical tree of 142 patients. Acta
Univ. Carol. Med. Praha 13, 295 - 318 (1967).

SOBRA, J.: Familiárni hypercholesterolémická xanthomatosa. Thomayerova sb. c,
456, Praha: Avicenum (1970).

SOBRA, J., HEYROVSKY, A.: Inborn errors of lipid metabolism XXV. Familial hyperlipoproteinaemia type III - Detection of heterozygotes. Rev. Czech. Med. 18,
34 - 39 (1972).

SOBRA, J., HEYROVSKY, A., HORAKOVA, D., KOPECKA, J.: Vrozené vady lipidového metabolism. XVIII. Diferenciálni diagnosa familiérnich hyperlipoproteinémii.
Cas. Lék. Ces. 109, 69 - 72 (1970).

SOBRA, J. HEYROVSKY, A., KVASILOVA, M.: Inborn errors of lipid metabolism. XXVI.
Two sub-fraction of pre-beta-lipoproteins. Rev. Czech. Med. 18, 167 -
171 (1972).

SOBRA, J., Jîlek, M.: Inborn errors of lipid metabolism. XXIII. Coincidence of
hyperlipoproteinaemia type III and albinism. Rev. Czech. Med. 17, 214 - 218
(1971).

SODHI, H. S., KUDCHODKAR, B. J.: Synthesis of cholesterol in hypercholesterolemia
and its relationship to plasma triglycerides. Metabolism 22, 895 (1973).

SODHI, H. S., KUDCHODKAR, B. J.: Correlating metabolism of plasma and tissue-
cholesterol with that of plasma-lipoproteins. Lancet 1973 I, 513 - 519.

SODHI, H. S., SUNDARAM, G. S., McKENZIE, S. L.: Isoelectric fractionation of
plasma high density lipoproteins. This volume p. 881.

SOEDERLING, T. R., CORBIN, J. D., PARK, C. R.: Regulation of adenosine 3', 5'-
monophosphate-dependent protein kinase. II. Hormonal regulation of the adipose tissue enzyme. J. Biol. Chem. 248, 1822 (1973).

SOLBERG, L. A., EGGEN, D. A.: Localization and sequence of development of atherosclerotic lesions in the carotid and vertebral arteries. Circulation 43,
711 - 724 (1971).

SOLBERG, L. A., Mc GARRY, P. A.: Cerebral atherosclerosis in Negroes and Cau-
casians. Atherosclerosis 16, 141 - 154 (1972).

SOLBERG, L. A., Mc GARRY, P. A., MOOSSY, J., TEJADA, C., LØKEN, A. C., ROBERT-
SON, W. B., DONOSO, S.: Distribution of cerebral atherosclerosis by geographic location, race, and sex. Lab. Invest. 18, 604 - 612 (1968).

SOLOMON, H. M., SCHROGIE, J. J.: The effect of various drugs on the binding of
warfarin - 14C to human albumin. Biochem. Pharm. 16, 1219 - 1225 (1967).

SOMER, J. B., EVANS, G., SCHWARTZ, C. J.: Influence of experimental aortic
coarctation on the pattern of aortic Evans Blue uptake in vivo. Atherosclerosis 16, 127 - 133 (1972 b).

SOMER, J. B., SCHWARTZ, C. J.: Focal 3H-cholesterol uptake in the pig aorta.
Atherosclerosis 13, 293 - 304 (1971).

SOMER, J. B., SCHWARTZ, C. J.: Focal (3H)cholesterol uptake in the pig aorta.
Part 2. Distribution of (3H)cholesterol across the aortic wall in areas of
high and low uptake in vivo. Atherosclerosis 16, 377 - 388 (1972).

SPAIN, D. M., BRADESS, V. A.: Relationship of coronary thrombosis to coronary
atherosclerosis and ischemic heart disease. Amer. J. Med. Sc. 240, 701 - 707
(1960).

SPANO, P. F., SZYSZKA, K., GALLI, C. L., RICCI, A.: Effect of clofibrate on free
and total tryptophan in serum and brain tryptophan metabolism. Pharm. Res.
Comm. 6, 163 - 173 (1974).

SPELLACY, W. N., BUTTI, W. C., BIRK, S. A., CABAL, R.: The effects of estrogens,
progesteron, oral contraceptives and intrauterine devices on fasting triglyceride and insulin levels, Fertil. Steril. 24, 178 (1973).

SPELLACY, W. N., FACOG, W., BUTTI, W. C., BRADLEY, B., HOLSINGER, K. U.: Maternal fetal and amniotic fluid levels of glucose, insulin and growth hormone, Obstet. & Gynec. 41, 323 (1973).

SPELLACY, W. N., GALL, S. A., CARLSON, K. L.: Carbohydrate Metabolism of the Normal Term Newborn: Plasma, insulin and blood glucose levels during an intravenous tolerance test, Obstet. & Gynec. 30, 580 (1967).

SPERRY, W. M., WEBB, M. A.: Revision of Schoenheimer-Sperry method for cholesterol determination. J. Biol. Chem. 187, 97 (1950).

SPITZER, J. A., SPITZER, J. J.: Effect of liver on lipolysis by normal and post-heparin sera in the rat. Amer. J. Physiol. 185, 18 - 22 (1956).

SPÖTTL, F., HOLZKNECHT, F., BRAUNSTEINER, H.: Essentielle Hyperlipaemie und verminderte Fibrinolyse-Aktivität. Acta Haematol. 38, 178 (1967).

SRINIVASAN, S. R., DALFERES, E. R., PARGAONKAR, P. S., RADHAKRISHNAMURTHY, B., BERENSON, G. S.: Rapid serum lipoprotein changes in spider monkeys on short term feeding of cholesterol-high saturated fat diet. Proc. Soc. Exp. Biol. Med. 141, 154 (1972).

SRINIVASAN, S. R., DOLAN, P., RADHAKRISHNAMURTHY, B., BERENSON, G. S.: Isolation of lipoprotein-acid mucopolysaccharide complexes from fatty streaks of human aortas, Atherosclerosis 16, 95 - 104 (1972).

SRINIVASAN, S. R., LOPEZ-S., A., RADHAKRISHNAMURTHY, B., BERENSON, G. S.: Complexing of serum pre-beta- and beta-lipoproteins and acid mucopolysaccharides, Atherosclerosis 12, 321 - 334 (1970).

SRINIVASAN, S. R., RADHAKRISHNAMURTHY, B., PARGAONKAR, P. S., BERENSON, G. S.: Glycoproteins from connective tissue of twins, Nature 229, 58 (1971).

STAMLER, J.: Epidemiology of coronary heart disease. Med. Clin. N. Amer. 57, 5 (1973).

STAMLER, J., BERKSON, D. M., LINDBERG, H. A.: Risk factors: Their role in the etiology and pathogenesis of the atherosclerotic diseases. In: The Pathogenesis of atherosclerosis, p. 41 - 119 (WISSLER, R. W., and GEER, J. C., Eds.). Baltimore: Williams and Wilkins 1972.

STAMLER, J., PICK, R., KATZ, L. N.: Insulin and cholesterol-oil diet atherosclerosis in cockerels. Circ. Res. 8, 572 (1960).

STARR, J. J., JUHN, D. J., MAKO, M. E., GUERIN, M., SCANU, A. M., RUBENSTEIN, A. H.: Circulating high density lipoprotein (HDL): Measurement of an apoprotein component by radioimmuno-assay. J. Clin. Invest. 52, 81a (1973).

STARY, H. C.: Cell proliferation in the experimental atheroma as revealed by radioautography after injection of thymidine-^{3}H. Circulation 36 (Suppl. II) 39 (1967).

STARY, H. C.: Radioautographic observations on DNA synthesis of aortic cells in Rhesus monkeys. Circulation 40 (Suppl. III), 25 (1969).

STARY, H. C.: Electron microscopic observations on the progression of aortic atherosclerosis in rhesus monkeys. Circulation 42 (Suppl. III), 9 (1970).

STARY, H. C.: Progression and regression of experimental atherosclerosis in rhesus monkeys. In: Medical primatology 1972. Proc. IIIrd Conf. Exp. Med. Surg. Primates, Lyon 1972, part III, p. 356. Basel: Karger 1972.

STARY, H. C.: Proliferation of arterial cells in atherosclerosis. In: Arterial mesenchyme and arteriosclerosis. Proc. Int. Workshop on Arterial Mesenchyme and Arteriosclerosis, New Orleans, 1973 a. Adv. Exp. Med. Biol. New York: Plenum Press (In press).

STARY, H. C.: The fine structure of coronary atherosclerosis in rhesus monkeys. Prim. Med., Basel: Karger 1974 (In press).

STARY, H. C., Mc MILLAN, G. C.: Kinetics of cellular proliferation in experimental atherosclerosis. Radioautography with grain counts in cholesterol-fed rabbits. Arch. Pathol. 89, 173 - 183 (1970).

STARY, H. C., STRONG, J. P.: The fine structure of coronary arteries in rhesus monkeys. Symp. Comparative Pathology of the Heart, Boston 1973. Adv. Cardiol. Basel: Karger 1973 (In press).

ST. CLAIR, R. W., CLARKSON, T. B., LOFLAND, H. B.: Effects of regression of atherosclerotic lesions on the content and esterification of cholesterol by cell-free preparations of pigeon aorta. Circ. Res. 31, 664 (1972).

ST. CLAIR, R. W., LOFLAND, H. B., Jr., CLARKSON, T. B.: Composition and synthesis of fatty acids in atherosclerotic aortas of the pigeon. J. Lipid Res. 9, 739 - 747 (1968).

ST. CLAIR, R. W., LOFLAND, H. B., Jr., CLARKSON, T. B.: Influence of atherosclerosis on the composition, synthesis, and esterification of lipids in aortas
of squirrel monkeys (Saimiri sciureus). J. Atheroscler. Res. 10, 193 - 206
(1969).
ST. CLAIR, R. W., LOFLAND, H. B., Jr., CLARKSON, T. B.: Influence of duration of
cholesterol feeding on esterification of fatty acids by cell-free preparation of pigeon aorta. Circ. Res. 27, 213 (1970).
STEELE, P. P., WEILY, H. S., GENTON, E.: Platelet survival and adhesiveness in
recurrent venous thrombosis. New Engl. J. Med. 288, 1148 - 1152 (1973).
STEGALL, H. F., KARDON, M. B., KEMMERER, W. T.: Indirect measurement of arterial
blood pressure by doppler ultrasonic sphygmomanometry. J. of Appl. Phys. 25,
793 (1968).
STEIN, F., PEZESS, M. P., ROBERT, L., POULLAIN, N.: Anti-elastin antibodies in
normal and pathological human sera. Nature, 207, 312 (1965).
STEIN, O., SELINGER, Z., STEIN, Y.: Incorporation of (1-^{14}C)-linoleic acid into
lipids of human umbilical arteries. J. Atheroscler. Res. 3, 189 (1963 a).
STEIN, O., STEIN, Y.: Visualization of intravenously injected 9, 10-^{3}H$_2$-palmitic
acid in rat liver by electronmicroscopic autoradiography. Israel J. Med. Sci.
2, 239 - 242 (1966).
STEIN, O., STEIN, Y.: Lipid synthesis, intracellular transport storage and secretion. I. Electron microscopic radioautographic study of liver after injection of tritiated palmitate or glycerol in fasted and ethanol treated rats.
J. Cell Biol. 33, 319 (1967).
STEIN, O., STEIN, Y.: The role of the liver in the metabolism of chylomicrons,
studied by electron microscopic autoradiography. Lab. Invest. 17, 436 (1967b).
STEIN, O., STEIN, Y.: An electron microscopic study of the transport of peroxida-
ses in endothelium of mouse aorta. Z. Zellforsch. 133, 211 - 222 (1972).
STEIN, O., STEIN, Y.: Colchine induced inhibition of very low density lipopro-
tein released by rat liver in vivo. Biochim. Biophys. Acta 306, 142 (1973).
STEIN, O., STEIN, Y., GOODMAN, D. S., FIDGE, A.: The metabolism of phylomicron
cholesteryl ester in rat liver. A combined radioautographic-electron micro-
scopic and biochemical study. J. Cell Biol. 43, 410 (1969).
STEIN, Y., SHAPIRO, B.: The synthesis of neutral glycerides by fractions of rat
liver homogenates. Biochim. Biophys. Acta 24, 197 - 198 (1957).
STEIN, Y., SHAPIRO, B.: Glyceride synthesis by mocrosome fractions of rat liver.
Biochim. Biophys. Acta 30, 271 - 277 (1958).
STEIN, Y., SHAPIRO, B.: Assimilation and dissimilation of fatty acids by the
rat liver. Amer. J. Physiol. 196, 1238 - 1241 (1959).
STEIN, Y., STEIN, O.: Incorporation of fatty acids into lipids of aortic slices
of rabbits, dogs, rats and baboons. J. Atheroscler. Res. 2, 400 (1962).
STEIN, Y., STEIN, O.: Transport of lipids in the arterial wall. A biochemical
and radioautographic study. Exposé Ann. Biochem. Med. 31, 97 (1972).
STEIN, Y., STEIN, O.: Lipid synthesis and degradation and lipoprotein transport
in mammalian aorta. In: Ciba Foundation Symposium on Mechanisms in the
Development of Early Atheroma, London, 1972. Atherogenesis: Initiating factors, p.. 165 - 183. (Ciba Foundation Symposium 12). Amsterdam: Associated
Scientific Publishers 1973.
STEIN, Y., STEIN, O., SHAPIRO, B.: Enzymic pathways of glyceride and phospholipid synthesis in aortic homogenates. Biochim. Biophys. Acta 70, 33 (1963 b).
STEINBERG, D., CAREW, T. E., CHANDLER, J. G., SNIDERMAN, A. D.: The role of the
liver in metabolism of plasma lipoproteins. Alfred Benzon symposium VI, Regulation of hepatic metabolism, Munksgaard, Copenhagen 1974, In press.
STEMERMAN, M. B.: Thrombogenesis of the rabbit arterial plaque. Amer. J. Path.
73, 7 - 26 (1973).
STEMERMAN, M. B., BAUMGARTNER, H. R., SPAET, T. H.: The subendothelial micro-
fibril and platelet adhesion. Lab. Invest. 24, 179 - 186 (1971).
STEMERMAN, M. B., ROSS, R.: Experimental arteriosclerosis. I. Fibrous plaque formation in primates, an electron microscopic study. J. Exp. Med. 136, 769 -
789 (1972).
STERN, M. P., KOLTERMAN, O. G., Mc DEVITT, H., REAVEN, G. M.: Acquired type III
hyperlipoproteinemia. Arch. Intern. Med. 130, 817 - 821 (1972).
STILL, W. J.: Hyperlipaemia and the arterial Arch. Path. 89, 392 (1970).

STILL, W. J. S.: An electron microscopic study of the organization of experimen-
tal thromboemboli in the rabbit. Lab. Invest. 15, 1492 - 1507 (1966).
STILL, W. J. S.: The early effect of hypertension on the aortic intima of the rat.
Amer. J. Path. 51, 721 - 734 (1967).
STILL, W. J. S.: The pathogenesis of the intimal thickenings produced by hyper-
tension in large arteries in the rat. Lab. Invest. 19, 84 - 91 (1968).
STILL. W. J. S.: Hyperlipemia and the arterial intima of the hypertensive rat.
Arch. Path. 89, 392 - 404 (1970).
STILL, W. J. S., MARTIN, J. M., GREGOR, W. H.: Effect of alloxan diabetes on ex-
perimental atherosclerosis in the rat. Exp. Mol. Path. 3, 141 - 147 (1964).
STIPPES, M., WEMPNER, G., STERN, M., BECKETT, R.: In: An introduction to the
mechanics of deformable bodies, chap. 4.
Columbus (Ohio): Charles E. Merrill Books, Inc. 1961.
STITT, F. W., CLAYTON, D. G., CRAWFORD, M. D., MORRIS, J. N.: Clinical and bio-
chemical indicators of cardiovascular disease among men living in hard and
soft water areas. Lancet 1973 I, 122 - 126.
STOCKS, P.: A biometric investigation of twins and their brothers and sisters.
Ann. Eugen. 4, 49 (236) (1930).
STOFFEL, W., ZIERENBERG, O., TUNGGAL, B. D.: ^{13}C-Nuclear magnetic resonance
spectroscopic studies on saturated-, mono-, di- and polyunsaturated fatty
acids, phospho- and sphingolipids. Hoppe-Seyler's Z. Physiol. Chem. 353,
1962 (1972).
STOKKE, K. T., NORUM, K. R.: Determination of lecithin: cholesterol acyltrans-
ferase in human blood plasma. Scand. J. Clin. Lab. Invest. 27, 21 (1971).
STONE, N. J., LEVY, R. I., FREDRICKSON, D. S., VERTER, J.: Coronary artery disease in 166 kindred with familial type II hyperlipoproteinemia. Circulation
(In press).
STOUT, C.: Atherosclerosis in exotic carnivora and pinnepedia. Amer. J. Path.
57, 673 - 687 (1969).
STOUT, C., BOHORQUEZ, F.: Aortic atherosclerosis in hoofed hammels. J. Athero-
scler. Res. 9, 73 (1969).
STOUT, C., BOHORQUEZ, F.: Arteriosclerosis and other vascular diseases in zoo
and laboratory animals. In: Research animals in medicine, (HARMISON, L. T.,
Ed.). National Heart and Lung Institute Publication (In press).
STOUT, C., LEMMON, W. B.: Predominant coronary and cerebral atherosclerosis in
captive non-human primates. Exp. Mol. Pathol. 10, 312 - 322 (1969).
STOUT, R. W.: Insulin-stimulation of cholesterol synthesis by arterial tissue.
Lancet 1969 II, 467.
STOUT, R. W.: Development of vascular lesions in insulin-treated animals fed a
normal diet. Brit. Med. J. 3, 685 (1970).
STOUT, R. W., BIERMAN, E. L., ROSS, R.: The arterial smooth muscle cell: insulin
stimulation of cell proliferation, This volume p. 935.
STOUT, R. W., BUCHANAN, K. D., VALLANCE-OWEN, J.: The relationship of arterial
disease and glucagon metabolism in insulin-treated chickens. Atherosclerosis
18, 153 - 162 (1973).
STOUT, R. W., VALLANCE-OWEN, J.: Insulin and atheroma. Lancet 1969 I, 1078.
STRANDNESS, D. E., JR.: Exercise testing in the evaluation of patients under-
going direct arterial surgery. J. Cardiovasc. Surg. 11, 192 (1970).
STRANDNESS, D. E., Jr.: Techniques in the evaluation of vascular disease. In:
Surgery Annual, p. 181 (COOPER, P., and NYHUS, L. M., Eds.). New York:
Appelton-Century Crofts 1971.
STRANDNESS, D. E., Jr., BELL, J. W.: Peripheral vascular disease: diagnosis and
objective evaluation using a mercury strain gauge. Ann. Surg. 161 (Suppl),
1 - 35 (1965).
STRANDNESS, D. E., Jr., STAHLER, C. A.: Arteriosclerosis obliterans: manner and
rate of progression. J. A. M. A. 196, 121 (1966).
STRASSER, T.: Atherosclerosis and coronary heart disease: the contribution of
epidemiology. WHO Chronic. 26, 7 (1972).
STRAUSS, E. W.:   In: Handbook of Physiology Alimentary Canal. Vol. III,
p. 1377. Washington D. C.: Amer. Physiol. Soc. 1968.
STRISOWER, E. H., ADAMSON, G., STRISOWER, B.: Treatment of hyperlipidemias.
Amer. J. Medicine 45, 488 (1968).

STRISOWER, E. H., STRISOWER, B.: The separate hypolipoproteinemic effects of dextrotyroxine and ethyl chlorophenoxyisobutyrate. J. Clin. Endocr. 24, 139 - 144 (1964).

STRIVASTAVA, S. C., SMITH, M. J., Mc NICOL, G. P.: The effect of Atromid on fibrinolytic activity of patients with ischemic heart disease and hypercholesterolemia. J. Atheroscler. Res. 3, 640 (1963).

STRONG, J. P., EGGEN, D. A.: Risk factors and atherosclerotic lesions. Atherosclerosis: Proceedings of the Second International Symposium, p. 355 - 364. (JONES, R. J., ed.). New York: Springer-Verlag 1970.

STRONG, J. P., EGGEN, D. A., OALMANN, M. C.: The natural history, geographic pathology, and epidemiology of atherosclerosis. In: The pathogenesis of atherosclerosis, p. 20 - 40 (WISSLER, R. W., and GEER, J. C., Eds.). Baltimore: Williams and Wilkins 1972.

STRONG, J. P., Mc GILL, H. C., Jr.: The natural history of coronary atherosclerosis. Amer. J. Pathol. 40, 37 (1962).

STRONG, J. P., Mc GILL, H. C., Jr.: The natural history of aortic atherosclerosis: Relationship to race, sex, and coronary lesions in New Orleans. Exp. Molec. Pathol. 2, No. 1, 15 (1963).

STRONG, J. P., Mc GILL, H. C., Jr.: The pediatric aspects of atherosclerosis, J. Atheroscler. Res. 9, 251 (1969).

STRONG, J. P., RICHARDS, M. L., Mc GILL, H. C., Jr., EGGEN, D. A., Mc MURRY, M. T.: On the association of cigarette smoking with coronary and aortic atherosclerosis. J. Atheroscler. Res. 10, 303 - 317 (1969).

STRONG, J. P., SOLBERG, L. A., RESTREPO, C.: Atherosclerosis in persons with coronary heart disease. Lab. Invest. 18, 527 - 537 (1968).

STURDEVANT, R. A. L., PEARCE, M. L., DAYTON, S.: Increased prevalence of cholelithiasis in men ingesting a serum-cholesterol-lowering diet. New Engl. J. Med. 288, 24 (1973).

SULLIVAN, J. M., HARKEN, D. E., GORLIN, R.: Pharmacologic control of thromboembolic complications of cardiac-valve replacement. New Engl. J. Med. 284, 1391 - 1394 (1971).

SUMIYOSHI, A., MORE, R. H., WEIGENSBERG, B. I.: Aortic fibrofatty type atherosclerosis from thrombus in normolipidemic rabbits. Atherosclerosis 18, 43 - 57 (1973).

SUMNER, D. S., STRANDNESS, D. E., Jr.: The relationship between calf blood flow and ankle blood pressure in patients with intermittent claudication. Surgery 65, 763 (1969).

SURI, V. P., SINGH, D., TANDON, O. P.: Familial patterns in coronary artery disease. Indian J. med. Sci. 20, 321 (1966).

SUZUKI, M., FUKUUCHI, Y., SHIMAZU, K., KIM, H. S., MEYER, J. S.: Cerebral atherosclerosis in the dog. Arch. Path. 96, 14 (1973).

SUZUKI, M., O'NEAL, R. M.: Accumulation of lipids in the leukocytes of rats fed atherogenic diets. J. Lipid Res. 5, 624 (1964).

SVENNERHOLM, L.: Distribution and fatty acid composition of phosphoglycerides in normal human brain. J. Lipid Res. 9, 570 (1968).

SWELL, L., TREADWELL, C. R.: Cholesterol esterase VI. Relative specificity and activity of pancreatic cholesterol esterase. J. Biol. Chem. 212, 141 (1955).

SZIGETI, M., MONNIER, G., JACOTOT, B., ROBERT, L.: Distribution of ingested 14C-cholesterol in the macromolecular fractions of rat connective tissues. Conn. Tissue Res. 1, 145 - 152 (1972).

SZIGETI, I., PIKO, K., DOMAN, J.: The immunopathological importance of different structural protein antigens of human arterial vessel-wall in heterologous immunisation of rabbits compared with immunological data of human coronary heart patients. In: le role de la paroi artérielle dans l'athérogénese, p. 493 (Ed. C. N. R. S.). Paris: 1968.

TAGLIAMONTE, A., BIGGIO, G., VARGIU, L., GESSA, G. L.: Increase of brain tryptophan and stimulation of serotonin synthesis by salicylate. J. Neurochem. 20, 909 - 912 (1972).

TAGLIAMONTE, A., TAGLIAMONTE, P., PEREZ-CRUET, J., GESSA, G. L.: Increase of brain tryptophan caused by drugs which stimulate serotonin synthesis. Nature (New Biology) 229, 125 - 126 (1971).

TANNER, J. M., WHITEHOUSE, R. H.: Growth response of 26 children with short
   stature given human growth hormone. Brit. med. J. II, 69 (1967).
TANNER, J. M., WHITEHOUSE, R. H.: The effect of human growth hormone on subcutaneous fat thickness in hyposomatotropic and panhypopituitary dwarfs.
   J. Endocr. 39, 263 (1967).
TARIZZO, R. A., ALEXANDER, R. W., BEATTIE, E. J., ECONOMOU, S. G.: Atherosclerosis in synthetic vascular grafts. Arch. Surg. 82, 826 (1961).
TAYLOR, C. B., BALDWIN, D., HASS, G. M.: Localised arteriosclerotic lesions induced in the aorta of the juvenile rabbit by freezing. Arch. Path. 49, 623
   (1950).
TAYLOR, C. B., COX, G. E., COUNTS, M., YOGI, N.: Fatal myocardial infarction in
   the rhesus monkey with diet induced hypercholesterolaemia. Am. J. Path. 35,
   674 (1959).
TAYLOR, C. B., COX, G. E., MANALO-ESTRELLA, P., SOUTHWORTH, J.: Atherosclerosis
   in rhesus monkeys. II. Arterial lesions associated with hypercholesteremia
   induced by dietary fat and cholesterol. Arch. Path. 74, 16 (1962).
TAYLOR, C. B., PATTON, D. E., COX, G. E.: Atherosclerosis in rhesus monkeys. V.
   Marked diet-induced hypercholesteremia with xanthomatosis and severe athero-
   sclerosis. Arch. Path. 76, 239 (1963).
TAYLOR, C. B., PATTON, D. E., COX, G. E.: Atherosclerosis in rhesus monkeys.
   VI. Fatal myocardial infarction in a monkey fed fat and cholesterol. Arch.
   Path. 76, 66 (1963).
TECHNICON AUTOANALYZER METHODOLOGY: Bulletin 34 a (1962). Total cholesterol.
   Chauncy, New York, Technicon Instruments Corporation.
TEJADA, C., STRONG, J. P., MONTENEGRO, M. R., RESTREPO, C., SOLBERG, L. A.: Di-
   stribution of coronary and aortic atherosclerosis by gergraphic location,
   race, and sex. Lab. Invest. 18, 509 - 526 (1968).
TEPPERMAN, J., PEARLMAN, D.: Effects of exercise and anemia on coronary arteries
   of small animals as revealed by the corrosion-cast technique. Circ. Res. 9,
   576 - 584 (1961).
THOMAS, C. B., COHEN, B. H.: The familial occurrence of hypertension and coronary artery disease, with observations concerning obesity and diabetes. Ann.
   intern. Med. 42, 90 (1955).
THOMAS, D. P.: The role of platelet catecholamines in the aggregation of platelets by collagen and thrombin. In: Platelets in Haemostasis. Exp. Biol. Med.
   3, 129 - 134 (1968).
THOMAS, W. A., FLORENTIN, R. A., NAM, S. C., KIM, D. N., JONES, R. M., LEE, K.
   T.: Preproliferative phase of atherosclerosis in swine fed cholesterol. Arch.
   Pathol. 86, 621 - 643 (1968).
THOMAS, W. A., FLORENTIN, R. A., NAM, S. C., REINER, J. M., LEE, K. T.: Alterations in population dynamics of arterial smooth muscle cells during atherogenesis. I. Activation of interphase cells in cholesterol-fed swine prior
   to gross atherosclerosis demonstrated by postpulse salvage labeling. Exp.
   Mol. Pathol. 15, 245 - 267 (1971).
THOMAS, W. A., HARTROFT, W. S.: Myocardial infarction in rats fed diets con-
   taining high fat, cholesterol, thiouracil and sodium cholate. Circulation
   19, 65 (1959).
THOMAS, W. A., O'NEAL, R. M., LEE, K. T.: Thromboembolism, pulmonary arterio-
   sclerosis, and fatty meals. Arch. Pathol. 61, 380 - 389 (1956).
THOMSEN, H. K.: Ultrastructural changes in the coronary arteries of primates
   after a prolonged, mild carbon monoxide exposure. This volume p. 333.
THOMSON, J. G.: Production of severe atheroma in a transplanted human heart.
   Lancet 1969 II, 1088.
THORP, J. M.: An experimental approach to the problem of disordered lipid me-
   tabolism. J. Atheroscl. Res. 3, 351 - 360 (1963).
TOMUS, L., CORDOS, D., BANU, V., RUSU, M., DANIELLO, R., IANCU, P., TALOS, D.:
   Influence of cerebral ischemia on the development of experimental athero-
   sclerosis in the rabbit. Atherosclerosis 13, 267 - 281 (1971).
TOOLE, B. P., GROSS, J.: The extracellular matrix of the regenerating newt limb:
   synthesis and removal of hyaluronate prior to differentiation. Dev. Biol.
   25, 57 (1971).
TOOR, M., KATCHALSKY, A., AGMON, J., ALLALOUF, D.: Serum-lipids and athero-sclerosis among Yemenite immigrants in Israel. Lancet 1957 I, 1270.

TORQUEBIAU-COLARD, O., PAYSANT, M., WALD, R., POLONOVSKI, J.: Phospholipase des membranes plasmiques isolées de fois de rat. Action sur les phospholipides exogènes. Bull. Soc. Chim. Biol. 52, 1061 – 1071 (1970).

TORSVIK, H., BERG, K., MAGNANI, H. N., Mc CONATHY, W. J., ALAUPOVIC, P., GJONE, E.: Identification of the abnormal cholestatic lipoprotein (LP-X) in familial lecithin: cholesterol acyltransferase deficiency. FEBS Letters 24, 165 (1972).

TORVIK, A., JØRGENSEN, L.: Thrombotic and embolic occlusions of the arteries in an autopsy series. Part 2. Cerebral lesions and clinical course. J. Neurol. Sci. 3, 410 – 432 (1966).

TRACY, R. E., MERCHANT, E. B., KAO, V. C. Y.: On the antigenic identity of human serum beta and alpha-2 lipoproteins and their identification in the aortic intima. Circ. Res. 9, 472 (1961).

TRANZER, J. P., BAUMGARTNER, H. R.: Filling gaps in the vascular endothelium with blood platelets. Nature 216, 1126 – 1128 (1967).

TRILLO, A., RENAUD, S., HAUST, M. D.: Ultrastructure of aortic lesions in normotensive and hypertensive hyperlipemic rats. Fed. Proc. 29 (ABS.), 487 (1970).

TRILLO, A., RENAUD, S., HAUST, M. D.: The morphogenesis of aortic lesions in hypertensive and hypertensive-hyperlipemic rats. Lab. Invest. 24 (Abs.), 451 (1971).

TROWELL, H.: Crude fibre, dietary fibre and atherosclerosis. Atherosclerosis 16, 138 – 140 (1972).

TRUETT, J., CORNFIELD, J., KANNEL, W.: A multivariate analysis of the risk of coronary heart disease in Framingham. J. Chronic Dis. 20, 511 (1967).

TRULSON. M. F., CLANCY, R. E., JESSOP, W. J. E., CHILDERS, R. W., STARE, F. J.: Comparisons of siblings in Boston and Ireland. J. Amer. diet. Ass. 45, 225 (1964).

TSAI, C.-C., TAICHMAN, N. S., PULVER, W. H., SCHONBAUM, E.: Heterophile antibodies and tissue injury. III. A role for platelets in the development of lethal vascular injury during Forssman shock in guinea pigs. Amer. J. Path. 72, 179 – 200 (1973).

TUCKER, C. F., CATSULIS, C., STRONG, J. P., EGGEN, D. A.: Regression of early cholesterol-induced aortic lesions in rhesus monkeys. Amer. J. Pathol. 65, 493 – 514 (1971).

TURPEINEN, O., MIETTINEN, M., KARVONEN, M. J., ROINE, P., PEKKARINEN, M., LEHTO-SUO, E. J., ALIVIRTA, P.: Dietary prevention of coronary heart disease: long-term experiment. I. Observations on male subjects. Amer. J. Clin. Nutr. 21, 255 – 276 (1968).

TYTGAT, G. N., RUBIN, C. E., SAUNDERS, D. R.: Synthesis and transport of lipoprotein particles by intestinal absorptive cells in man. J. Clin. Invest. 50, 2065 – 2078 (1971).

UITTO, J., DEHM, P., PROCKOP, D. J.: Incorporation of cishydroxyproline into collagen by tendon cells. Failure of the intracellular collagen to assume triple-helical conformation. Biochim. Biophys. Acta 278, 601 – 605 (1972).

UNIVERSITY GROUP DIABETES PROGRAM: A study of the effects of hypoglycemic agents on vascular complications in patients with adult onset diabetes. Diabetes 19 (Suppl. 2), 78 (1970).

UTERMANN, G., SCHOENBORN, W., LANGER, K. H., DIEKER, P.: Lipoproteins in LCAT-deficiency. Humangenetik 16, 295 (1972).

VAHOUNY, G. V., KOTHARI, H. V., TREADWELL, C. R.: Specificity of bile salt protection of cholesterol ester hydrolase from proteolytic inactivation. Arch. Biochem. Biophys. 121, 242 (1967).

VANDAMME, D., BLATON, V., PEETERS, H.: Symposium V. Chromatographie Electrophorèse, p. 268, Presses Académiques Européennes 1968.

VAN DER WATT, J. J., KOTZE, J. P., KEMPFF, P. G., PLESSIS, J. P., DU, LAUBSCHER, N. F.: Aortic intimal lesions and serum lipids in wild baboons. J. Med. Prim. 2, 25 – 38 (1973).

VAN HANDEL, E., ZILVERSMIT, D. B.: Micromethod for the direct determination of serum triglycerides. J. Lab. and Clin. Med. 50, 152 (1957).

VARTIAINEN, T., KANERVA, K.: Arteriosclerosis and wartime (Siege 1941 – 1942). Am. Rev. Soviet. Med. 4, 70 (1946).

VASQUEZ-COLON, L., ZIEGLER, F. R., ELLIOT, W. B.: On the mechanism of fatty acid inhibition of mitochondrial metabolism. Biochem. 5, 1134 (1966).

VASTESAEGER, M. M., VERCRUYSSE, J., MARTIN, J. J.: Pitfalls of experimental atherosclerosis in the chimpanzee. In: Medical primatology, part III, p. 376 - 381 (GOLDSMITH and MOOR-JANKOWSKI, Eds.). Basel: Karger 1972.

VAUGHAN, M., STEINBERG, D.: Effect of hormones on lipolysis and esterification of free fatty acids during incubation of adipose tissue in vitro.J. Lipid Res. 4, 193 (1963).

VEDIN, A., WILHELMSSON, C.-E., WILHELMSEN, L., BJURE, J., EKSTRÖM-JODAL, B.: Relation of resting and exercise-induced ectopic beats to other ischemic manifestations and to coronary risk factors. Amer. J. Cardiol. 30, 25 - 31 (1972).

VESSELINOVITCH, D., DZOGA, K., HUGHES, R.: Oxygen, cholestyramine and estrogen effects on experimental atherosclerosis in rabbits. Fed. Proc. 29, 488 (1970).

VESSELINOVITCH, D., GETZ, G. S., HUGHES, R. H., WISSLER, R. W.: Atherosclerosis in the Rhesus monkey fed three food fats. Submitted for publication.

VESSELINOVITCH, D., HUGHES, R., FRAZIER, L., WISSLER, R. W.: Studies of the reversal of advanced atherosclerosis in the Rhesus monkey. Am. J. Path. 70, (2) 75 (ABS.) (1973).

VESSELINOVITCH, D., WISSLER, R. W.: Experimental atherosclerosis in rabbits: the effects of oxygen on its production and reversibility. Eighteenth World Veterinary Congress, Paris (1967).

VESSELINOVITCH, D., WISSLER, R. W.: Experimental atherosclerosis in rabbits: the effect of oxygen and/or cholestyramine on its reversibility. Circulation 38, VI - 198 (1968).

VESSELINOVITCH, D., WISSLER, R. W., DZOGA, K., HUGHES, R.: Oxygen and estrogen effects on coronary artery atherosclerosis in rabbits. Circulation 44, II - 27 (1971).

VESSELINOVITCH, D., WISSLER, R. W., DZOGA, K., HUGHES, R. H., DUBIEN, L.: Repression of atherosclerosis in rabbits. Part 1, Treatment with low-fat diet, hyperoxia and hypolipidemic agents. Atherosclerosis 19, 259 (1974).

VESSEY, M. P., DOLL, R.: Investigation of relation between use of oral contraceptives and thromboembolic disease. A further report. Brit. Med. J. 2, 651 - 657 (1969).

VETERANS ADMINISTRATION COOPERATIVE UROLOGICAL RESEARCH GROUP: Treatment and survival of patients with cancer of the prostate. Surg. Gynec. Obstet. 124, 1011 - 1017 (1967).

VICTORIA, E. J., VAN GOLDE, L. M. G., HOSTETLER, K. Y., SCHERPHOF, G. L., VAN DEENEN, L. L. M.: Some studies on the metabolism of phospholipids in plasma membranes from rat liver. Biochim. Biophys. Acta 239, 443 (1971).

VIJAYAGOPAL, P., SARASWATHI DEVI, K., KURUP, P. A.: Fibre content of different dietary starches and their effect on lipid levels in high fat - high cholesterol diet fed rats. Atherosclerosis 17, 156 - 160 (1973).

VLAHCEVIC, Z. R., BELL, C. C., Jr., GREGORY, G. H., BUKER, G., JUTTIJUDATA, P., SWELL, L.: Relationship of bile acid pool size to the formation of lithogenic bile in female Indians of the Southwest. Gastroenterology 62, 73 - 83 (1972).

VLODAVER, Z., KAHN, H. A., NEUFELD, H. N.: The coronary arteries in early life in three different ethnic groups. Circulation 39, 541 - 550 (1969).

VOGEL, F., KRÜGER, J.: Statistische Beziehungen zwischen den ABO-Blutgruppen und Krankheiten mit Ausnahme der Infektionskrankheiten. Blut 16, 351 (1968).

VOGEL, W. C., BIERMAN, E. L.: Post-heparin serum lecithinase in man and its positional specificity. J. Lipid Res. 8, 46 - 53 (1967).

VOGEL, W. C., BIERMAN, E. L.: Evidence for in vivo activity of post-heparin plasma lecithinase in man. Proc. Soc. Exp. Biol. and Med. 127, 77 (1968).

VOGEL, W. C., BIERMAN, E. L.: Correlation between post-heparin lipase and phospholipase activities in human plasma. Lipids 5, 385 - 391 (1970).

VOGEL, W. C., BRUNZELL, J. D., BIERMAN, E. L.: A comparison of triglyceride, monoglyceride, and phospholipid substrates for post-heparin lipolytic activities from normal and hypertriglyceridemic subjects. Lipids 6, 805 - 814 (1971).

VOGEL, W. C., ZIEVE, L.: Post-heparin phospholipase. J. Lipid Res. 5, 177 (1964).
VOGELBERG, K. H., UTERMANN, G., GRIES, F. A.: Zur Differenzierung des Lp(a)-Li-
    poproteins mit Hilfe der Agarosegel-Elektrophorese. Z. Klin. Chem. Klin.
    Biochem. 11, 291 (1973).
VOLLRATH, L.: Über Bau und Funktion von Basalmembranen. Dtsch. med. Wschr. 93,
    360 - 365 (1968).
VON DECASTELLO, A.: Über Experimentelle Nierentransplantation. Wiener Klin.
    Wochenschr. 15, 317 (1902).
VOST, A.: Uptake and metabolism of circulating chylomicron triglyceride by rab-
    bit aorta. J. Lipid Res. 13, 695 (1972).
VOST, A., HOLLENBERG, C. H.: Insulin and atherosclerosis. Lancet 1969 II, 218.
VOST, A., POCOCK, D.: Aortic uptake of chylomicron triglyceride in vivo and
    aortic lipoprotein triglyceride lipase in rat. This volume p. 150.
WAGNER, H., HÖLZL, J., LISSAU, Ä., HÖRHAMMER, L.: Papierchromatographie von
    Phosphatiden. III. Quantitative papierchromatographische Bestimmung von
    Phosphatiden und Phosphatidsäuren in Rattenorganen. Biochem. Z. 339, 34
    (1963).
WAGNER, R. R., CYNKIN, M. A.,: Glycoprotein biosynthesis. Incorporation of glyco-
    syl groups into endogenous acceptors in a golgi apparatus-rich fraction of
    liver. J. Biol. Chem. 246, 143 (1971).
WAGNER, W. D., CLARKSON, R. B.: Slowly miscible cholesterol pools in progressing
    and regressing atherosclerotic aortas. Proc. Soc. Exp. Biol. Med. 143, 804
    (1973).
WAHLBERG, F.: Intravenous glucose tolerance in myocardial infarction, angina
    pectoris and intermittent claudication. Acta med. scand. 180 (Suppl. 453),
    (1966).
WAHLQVIST, M. L., DAY, A. J., TUME, R. K.: Incorporation of oleic acid into
    lipid by foam cells in human atherosclerotic lesions. Circ. Res. 24, 123 -
    130 (1969).
WAKLEY, E. J., LANGMAN, M. J. S., ELWOOD, P. C.: Blood group A sub-groups and
    serum cholesterol. Cardiovasc. Res. 7, 679 (1973).
WALKER, A. R. P.: Coronary heart disease: Limitations to the application to
    white populations of lessons learned from the underprivileged. Circulation
    29, 1 (1964).
WALLDIUS, G., OLSSON, A. G., CARLSON, L. A.: Metabolic defects in adipose tissue
    in hypertriglyceridemia (HTG). New aspects on pathogenesis of HTG. In: Re-
    gulation of the adipose tissue mass. Excerpta Medica. Amsterdam: 1973.
WALSH, D. A., PERKINS, J. P., KREBS, E. G.: An adenosine 3', 5'-monophosphate-
    dependent protein kinase from rabbit skeletal muscle. J. Biol. Chem. 243,
    3763 (1968).
WALSH, P. N., BIGGS, R.: The role of platelets in intrinsic factor-Xa formation.
    Brit. J. Haemat. 22, 743 - 760 (1972).
WALTON, K. W.: The biological properties of a new anticoagulant possessing he-
    parin-like properties. Brit. J. Pharmacol. 7, 370 (1952).
WALTON, K. W.: The biology of atherosclerosis. In: The biological basis of me-
    dicine, Vol. 6, p. 193 - 223 (BITTAR, E. E., and BITTAR, N., Eds.). New
    York: Academic Press 1969.
WALTON, K. W.: Atherosclerosis of heart valves and the formation of the corneal
    arcus as models for the study of atherosclerosis. Nutr. Metabol. 15, 37 -
    41 (1973).
WALTON, K. W.: Atherosclerosis and aging. In: Textbook of geriatric medicine and
    gerontology, p. 77 - 112 (BROCKLEHURST, J. C., Ed.). Edinburgh: Churchill-
    Livingstone 1973 a.
WALTON, K. W.: The role of serum lipoproteins in very early and late atheroscle-
    rotic lesions. In: Connective tissue and ageing (VOGEL, H. G., Ed.), p. 34.
    Amsterdam: Excerpta Medica 1973 b.
WALTON, K. W., DARKE, S. J.: Immunological characteristics of human low-density
    lipoproteins. Immunochemistry 1, 267 - 277 (1964).
WALTON, K. W., HITCHENS, J., MAGNANI, H. N.: Significance of the Lp(a) lipopro-
    tein in health and hyperlipidaemia. Proceedings of Conference on serum lipo-
    proteins, October 22 - 23, Graz, Austria (1973 a).

WALTON, K. W., SCOTT, P. J.: Estimation of the low-density (β) lipoproteins of
serum in health and disease using large molecular weight dextran sulphate.
J. Clin. Path. 17, 627 (1964).
WALTON, K. W., SCOTT, P. J., JONES, J. V., FLETCHER, R. F., WHITEHEAD, T.:
Studies on low-density lipoprotein turn over in relation to Atromid therapy.
J. Atheroscler. Res. 3, 296 (1963).
WALTON, K. W., THOMAS, C., DUNKERLEY, D. J.: The pathogenesis of xanthomata, J.
Path. 109, 271 - 289 (1973 b).
WALTON, K. W., WILLIAMSON, N.: Histological and immunofluorescent studies on
the evolution of the human atheromatous plaque. J. Atheroscler. Res. 8, 599
(1968).
WALTON, K. W., WILLIAMSON, N., JOHNSON, A. G.: The pathogenesis of atherosclero-
sis of the mitral and aortic valves. J. Path. 101, 205 - 220 (1970).
WANSTRUP, J., KJELDSEN, K., ASTRUP, P.: Acceleration of spontaneous intimal-
subintimal changes in rabbit aorta by a prolonged moderate carbon monoxide
exposure. Acta Path. Microbiol. Scandinav. 75, 353 (1969).
WARTMAN, A., LAMPE, T. L., McCANN, D. S., BOYLE, A.J.: Plaque reversal with
MgEDTA in experimental atherosclerosis: Elastin and collagen metabolism.
J. Atheroscler. Res. 7, 331 (1967).
WARTMAN, W. B., JENNINGS, R. B., HUDSON, B.: Experimental arterial disease. I.
The reaction of the pulmonary artery to minute emboli of blood clot. Circ.
4, 747 - 763 (1951).
WASSERMAN, F. W., Mc DONALD, T. F.: The electron microscopic study of adipose
tissue (fat organs) with special reference to the transport of lipid be-
tween blood and fat cells. Z. Für Zellforschung 59, 326 (1963).
WATTS, H. F.: Histochemical studies of the pathogenesis of human coronary ar-
tery atherosclerosis. Amer. J. Path. 35, 719 (1959).
WATTS, H. F.: The mechanism of arterial lipid accumulation in human coronary
artery atherosclerosis. In: Coronary heart disease, p. 98 - 113 (LIKOFF,
and MOYER, Eds.). New York, London: Grune and Stratton 1963.
WEATHERALL, D., CLEGG, J. B.: The thalassaemia syndromes, 2nd ed. Philadelphia:
F. A. Davis 1972.
WEBER, K., OSBORN, M.: The reliability of molecular weight determinations by
dodecyl sulfate-polyacrylamide gel electrophoresis. J. Biol. Chem. 244,
4406 (1969).
WEBSTER, M. E., RATNOFF, O. D.: Role of Hageman factor in the activation of va-
sodilator activity in human plasma. Nature 192, 180 (1961).
WEBSTER, W. S., CLARKSON, T. B., LOFLAND, H. B.: Carbon monoxide-aggravated athe-
rosclerosis in the squirrel monkey. Exp. Mol. Pathol. 13, 36 - 50 (1970).
WEILY, H. S., STEELE, P. P., GENTON, E.: Platelet survival in patients with a
Beall valve. Relation to low incidence of thromboembolism. Amer. J. Cardiol.
30, 229 - 231 (1972).
WEISS, H. J.: The pharmacology of platelet inhibition. In: Progress in hemosta-
sis and thrombosis, Vol. 1, p. 199 - 231 (SPAET, T. H., Ed.). New York:
Grune and Stratton 1972.
WEISS, S. B., KENNEDY, E. P., KIYASU, J. Y.: The enzymatic synthesis of trigly-
ceride. J. Biol. Chem. 235, 40 (1960).
WEKSLER, B. B., COUPAL, C. E.: Platelet-dependent generation of chemotactic activity in serum. J. Exp. Med. 137, 1419 - 1430 (1973).
WELLER, R. O., CLARK, R. A., OSWALD, W. B.: Stages in the formation and metabolism of intracellular lipid droplets in atherosclerosis. An electron microscopical and biochemical study. J. Atheroscler. Res. 8, 249 - 263 (1968).
WERB, Z., COHN, Z. A.: Cholesterol metabolism in the macrophage. III. Ingestion
and intracellular fate of cholesterol and cholesterol esters. J. Exp. Med.
135, 21 (1972).
WERLE, E., SCHIEVELBEIN, H.: Activity of nicotine and inactivity of kallikrein
and kallidin in aggregation of blood platelets. Nature 207, 871 - 872 (1965).
WEST, R. J., LLOYD, J. K.: Use of cholestyramine in treatment of children with
familial hypercholesterolaemia. Arch. Dis. Childh. 48, 370 (1973).
WESTPHAL, U.: Steroid-Protein Interactions, p. 115. New York: Springer-Verlag
1971.

WESTPHAL, U., HARDING, G. B.: Steroid-protein interactions. XXVII. Progesterone
    binding to polymers of human serum albumin. Biochim. Biophys. Acta 310, 518–
    527 (1973).
WEXLER, B. C.: Pathophysiologic responses to severe chronic alloxan diabetes in
    arteriosclerotic and non-arteriosclerotic rats. Atherosclerosis 14, 289 –
    307 (1971).
WEXLER, B. C.: Protective effects of propranolol on isoproterenol-induced myo-
    cardial infarction in arteriosclerotic and non-arteriosclerotic rats. Athe-
    rosclerosis 18, 11 – 42 (1973).
WEXLER, B. C., LUTMER, R. F.: Myocardial and plasma lactate changes in arterio-
    sclerotic and non-arteriosclerotic rats during isoproterenol-induced infarc-
    tion. Angiology 23, 36 – 46 (1972).
WHAYNE, T. F., FELTS, J. M.: Activation of lipoprotein lipase; comparative study
    of man and other mammals. Circ. Res. 26, 545 – 551 (1970).
WHEREAT, A. F.: Lipid biosynthesis in aortic intima from normal and cholesterol-
    fed rabbits. J. Atheroscler. Res. 4, 272 (1964).
WHEREAT, A. F., HULL, F. E., ORISHIMO, M. W.: The role of succinate in the re-
    gulation of fatty acid synthesis by heart mitochondria. J. Biol. Chem. 242,
    4013 (1967).
WHEREAT, A. F., STAPLE, E.: The preparation of serum lipoproteins labelled with
    radioactive cholesterol. Arch. Biochem. 90, 224 (1960).
WHO BULLETIN: Classification of hyperlipidaemias and hyperlipoproteinemias.
    43, 891 (1970).
WHUR, P., HERSCOVICS, A., LEBLOND, C. P.: Radioautographic visualization of the
    incorporation of galactose-^{3}H by rat thyroids in vitro in relation to the
    stages of thyroglobulin synthesis. J. Cell Biol. 43, 289 (1969).
WIELAND, H., SEIDEL, D.: Plasmalipoproteine bei Patienten mit Hyperthyreose: Iso-
    lierung und Charakterisierung eines abnormen High-Density-Lipoproteins. Z.
    Klin. Chem. Biochem. 10, 311 (1972).
WIELAND, H., SEIDEL, D.: Improved techniques for assessment of plasma lipoprotein
    patterns. II. Rapid method for diagnosis of type III hyperlipoproteinemia
    without ultracentrifugation. Clin. Chem. 19, 1139 (1973).
WIGGERS, K. D., JACOBSON, N. L., GETTY, R., RICHARD, M.: Mode of cholesterol
    ingestion and atherosclerosis in the young bovine. Atherosclerosis 17, 281 –
    295 (1973).
WIGHT, T. N.: Vascular smooth muscle cell development and degeneration in vitro:
    An ultrastructural and histochemical study. Ph. D. Thesis. Univ. of New
    Hampshire (1972).
WIKSTRAND, J., WALLENTIN, I., BERGLUND, G., WILHELMSEN, L.: Non-invasive methods,
    cardiac methods in hypertension and after myocardial infarction compared
    with random sample from the general population. Swedish Medical Association
    Meeting 1973.
WILCOX, H. G., DAVIS, D. C., HEIMBERG, M.: The isolation of lipoproteins from
    human plasma by ultracentrifuation in the Ti-14 and Ti-15 zonal rotors.
    Biochim. Biophys. Acta 187, 147 (1969).
WILCOXON, F.: Individual comparisons by ranking methods. Biometrics Bull. 1,
    80 (1945).
WILENS, S. L.: The resorption of arterial atheromatous deposits in wasting di-
    sease. Am. J. Path. 23, 793 (1947).
WILENS, S. L., Mc CLUSKEY, R. T.: The permeability of excised arteries and other
    tissues to serum lipid. Circ. Res. 2, 175 (1954).
WILHELMSEN, L., BJURE, J., EKSTRÖM-JODAL, B., GRIMBY, G., AURELL, M., TIBBLIN,
    G.: Prognostic significance of a standardized exercise test in a random
    population sample of men aged 50 years. To be published.
WILHELMSEN, L., WEDEL, H., TIBBLIN, G.: Multivariate analysis of risk factors
    for coronary heart disease. Circulation 48, 950 – 958 (1973).
WILKINSON, P. A., MILLS, G. L.: Analysis of serum-lipoproteins by crossed elec-
    trophoresis. Biochem. J. 126, 28 P (1972).
WILLIAMS, C. D., AVIGAN, J.: In vitro effects of serum proteins and lipids on
    lipid synthesis in human skin fibroblasts and leukocytes grown in culture.
    Biochem. Biophys. Acta 260, 413 (1972).

WILLIAMS, G.: Experimental studies in arterial ligation. J. Path. Bact. 72, 659 - 674 (1956).

WILLIAMS, J. A., WOLFF, J.: Possible role of microtubules in thyroid secretion. Proc. Nat. Acad. Sci. 67, 1901 (1970).

WILLIAMSON, J. R., VOGLER, W. J., KILO, C.: Estimation of vascular basement membrane thickness. Theoretical and practical considerations. Diabetes 18, 567 - 578 (1969).

WILLIS, A. L.: Platelet synthesis of pro-aggregating material from arachidonate and its blockage by aspirin. Circulation 48, Suppl. IV-55 (1973).

WILLIS, G. C.: The reversibility of atherosclerosis. Canad. Med. Ass. J. 77, 106 (1957).

WILSON, D. E., LEES, R. S.: Metabolic relationships among the plasma lipoproteins. Reciprocal changes in the concentrations of very low and low density lipoproteins in man. J. Clin. Invest. 51, 1051 (1972).

WILSON, R. B., HARTROFT, W. S.: Pathogenesis of myocardial infarcts in rats fed a thrombogenic diet. Arch. Path. 89, 457 - 469 (1970).

WINDAUS, A.: Über den Gehalt normaler und atheromatöser Aorten an Cholesterin und Cholesterinestern. Z. Physiol. Chem. 67, 174 (1910).

WINDMUELLER, H. G., HERBERT, P. N., LEVÝ, R. I.: Biosynthesis of lymph and plasma lipoprotein apoproteins by isolated perfused rat liver and intestine. J. Lipid Res. 14, 215 - 223 (1973).

WINDMUELLER, H. G., LEVY, R. I.: Total inhibition of hepatic beta-lipoprotein production in the rat by orotic acid. J. Biol. Chem. 242, 2246 (1967).

WINDMUELLER, H. G., LINDGREN, F. T., LOSSOW, W. J., LEVY, R. I.: On the nature of circulating lipoproteins of intestinal origin in the rat. Biochim. Biophys. Acta 202, 507 (1970).

WINDMUELLER, H. G., SPAETH, A. E.: De novo synthesis of fatty acid in perfused rat liver as a determinant of plasma lipoprotein production. Arch. Biochem. Biophys. 122, 362 (1967).

WINDMUELLER, H. G., SPAETH, A. E.: Fat transport and lymph and plasma lipoprotein biosynthesis by isolated intestine. J. Lipid Res. 13, 92 - 105 (1972).

WINEGRAD, A. I., YALCIN, S., MULCAHY, P. D.: Alterations in aortic metabolism in diabetes. In: On the nature and treatment of diabetes, p. 452 - 462 (LEIBEL, B. S., and WRENSHALL, G. A., Eds.).Amsterdam: Excerpta Medica Foundation 1965.

WING, D. R., FIELDING, C. J., ROBINSON, D. S.: The effect of cyclohemimide on tissue clearing factor lipase activity. Biochem. J. 104, 45C - 46C (1967).

WINKELSTEIN, W., Jr., KANTOR, S., IBRAHIM, M., SACUETT, D. L.: Familial aggregation of blood pressure: Preliminary report, Jama 195, 848 (1965).

WISSLER, R. W.: The arterial medial cell, smooth muscle or multifunctional mesenchyme? J. Atheroscler. Res. 8, 201 (1968).

WISSLER, R. W.: Recent progress in studies of experimental primate atherosclerosis. In: Prog. in Biochem. Pharmacol. 4 (MIRAS, C. J., HOWARD, A. N., PAOLETTI, R., Eds.). 378 - 392. Basel: Karger 1968.

WISSLER, R. W.: Development of the atherosclerotic plaque. Hospital Practice 8, 61 (1973).

WISSLER, R. W., EILERT, M. L., SCHROEDER, M. A., COHEN, L.: Production of lipomatous and atheromatous arterial lesions in the albino rat. A.M.A. Arch. Path. 57, 333 (1954).

WISSLER, R. W., FRAZIER, L. E., HUGHES, R. H., RASMUSSEN, R. A.: Atherogenesis in the Cebus monkey. I. A comparison of three food fats under controlled dietary conditions. A.M.A. Arch. Pathol. 74, 312 (1962).

WISSLER, R. W., GEER, J. C., Eds.: The Pathogenesis of Atherosclerosis, Baltimore: Williams and Wilkins 1972.

WISSLER, R. W., HUGHES, R. H., FRAZIER, L. E., GETZ, G. S., TURNER, D.: Aortic lesions and blood lipids in Rhesus monkeys fed "table prepared" human diets. Circulation 32, II - 220 (1965).

WISSLER, R. W., VESSELINOVITCH, D.: Comparative pathogenic patterns in atherosclerosis. Adv. Lipid Res. 6, 181 (1968).

WISSLER, R. W., VESSELINOVITCH, D.: Experimental models of human atherosclerosis. Ann. N. Y. Acad. Sci. 149, 907 (1968).

WISSLER, R. W., VESSELINOVITCH, D., GETZ, G. S., HUGHES, R. H.: Aortic lesions and blood lipids in rhesus monkeys fed three food fats. Fed. Proc. 26, 2 (1967).

WISSLER, R. W., VESSELINOVITCH, D., HUGHES, R. H.: A comparison of the aortic atherosclerotic response in the rhesus and stump-tailed monkeys using rations rich in vegetable fat with or without added cholesterol. Am. J. Path. 66, 156 (1972).

WISSLER, R. W., VESSELINOVITCH, D., HUGHES, R. H., ROTH, T.: Atherosclerosis and blood lipid in rhesus monkeys confined in widely varying space. Fed. Proc. 28, 447 (1969).

WISSLER, R. W., VESSELINOVITCH, D., HUGHES, R., TURNER, D., FRAZIER, L. E.: Atherosclerosis and blood lipids in rhesus monkeys fed human "table prepared" diets. Circulation 44, II - 57 (1971).

WITTENBERG, J. B.: Myoglobin-facilitated diffusion of oxygen. In: Oxygen. Proceedings of a symposium sponsored by the New York Heart Association, p. 57. Boston: Little Brown and Co. 1965.

WOLFE, B. M., AHUJA, S. P.: Mechanism of carbohydrate induction of hyperlipaemia. Clin. Res. 20, 947 (1972).

WOLFE, B. M., HAVEL, R. J., MARLISS, E. B., KANE, J. P., SEYMOUR, J.: Effects of ethanol on splanchnic metabolism in healthy men. (1973, In press).

WOLLENWEBER, J., DOENECKE, P., GRETEN, H., HILD, R., NOBBE, F., SCHMIDT, F. H., WAGNER, E.: Zur Häufigkeit von Hyperlipidämie, Hyperurikämie, Diabetes mellitus, Hypertonie und Übergewicht bei arterieller Verschlußkrankheit. Dtsch, med. Wschr. 96, 103 (1971).

WOLLENWEBER, J., STIEHL, A.: Größe des Pools und Turnover der primären Gallensäuren bei Hyperlipoproteinämien: Unterschiedliche Befunde bei Typ II und Typ IV Hyperlipoproteinämie. Klin. Wschr. 50, 33 (1972).

WONG, H. Y. C., MENDEZ, H. C., WALTERS, C. S., ORVIS, H. H.: A revised method for determination of total cholesterol in blood. Life Sci. 4, 431 (1965).

WOOD, P. D. S., STERN, M. P., SILVERS, A., REAVEN, G. M., VON DER GROEBEN, J.: Prevalence of plasma lipoprotein abnormalities in a free-living population of the Central Valley, California. Circ. 45, 114 (1972).

WOOLF, N., BRADLEY, J. W. P., CRAWFORD, T., CARSTAIRS, K. C.: Experimental mural thrombi in the pig aorta. The early natural history. Brit. J. Exp. Path. 49, 257 - 264 (1968).

WOOLF, N., CRAWFORD, T.: Fatty streaks in the aortic intima studied by an immunohistochemical technique. J. Pathol. Bacteriol. 80, 405 - 408 (1960).

WOOLF, N., PILKINGTON, T. R. E.: The immunohistochemical demonstration of lipoproteins in vessel walls. J. Pathol. Bacteriol. 90, 459 - 463 (1965).

WORLD HEALTH ORGANISATION: Classification of Hyperlipidaemias and Hyperlipoproteinaemias. Bull. W. H. O. 43, 891 (1970).

WRIGHT, A. D., HILL, D. M., LOWY, C., FRASER, T. R.: Mortality in acromegaly. Q. J. Med. 3, 1 (1970).

WRIGHT, H. P.: The adhesiveness of blood platelets in normal subjects with varying concentrations of anti-coagulants. J. Pathol. Bacteriol. 53, 255 - 262 (1941).

WRIGHT, H. P.: Endothelial mitosis around aortic branches in normal guinea-pigs. Nature 220, 78 (1968).

WRIGHT, H. P.: Endothelial turnover. Thrombosis et diathesis haemorrhagica Suppl. 40, 79 - 84 (1970).

WRIGHT, R. D.: The blood supply of abnormal tissues in the lungs. J. Path. Bact. 47, 489 - 499 (1938).

WU, C. C., HUANG, T. S., HSU, C. J.: Prevention of experimental atherosclerosis with pyridinolcarbamate. Amer. Heart J. 77, 657 (1969).

WYLLIE, J. C., MORE, R. H., HAUST, M. D.: Demonstration of fibrin in yellow aortic streaks by the fluorescent antibody technique. J. Path. Bact. 88, 335 - 338 (1964).

WYNN, V., DOAR, J. W. J., MILLS, G. L.: Some effects of oral contraceptives on serum-lipid and lipoprotein levels, Lancet 1966 II, 720.

YAMAMURA, T.: Inhibitory effects of pyridinolcarbamate in angiolathyrism and osteolathyrism, In: Atherogenesis, p. 29 (SHIMAMOTO, T., and NUMANO, F., Eds.). Excerpta Medica (1969).

YAMANOUCHI, H.: Über die zirkulären Gefäßnähte und Arterienvenen - Anastamosen, sowie über die Gefäßtransplantation. Dent. Ziet. Chir. 112, 1 (1911).

YAMAZAKI, H., TAKAHASHI, T., SHIMAMOTO, T.: Inhibitory of acetylsalicylic acid, pyridinolcarbamate and its derivative on human platelet aggregation. Blood & Vessel 3, 1377 (1972).

YAMAZAWA, S., SHIMAMOTO, T., HIDAKA, H., MOHRI, K.: The search for anti-atherosclerotic agents. Histological and chemical analysis of the preventive effect of estrogen, progresterone and pyridinolcarbamate on experimentally induced atherosclerosis. In: Atherogenesis II, p. 98. Excerpta Medica (1973).

YASUOKA, S., FUJII, S.: Esterase and lipase activities released into the blood by intravenous injection of heparin. J. Biochem. Tokyo 70, 937 - 944 (1971).

YOSHIKAWA, H.: Estimation methods of serum total cholesterol with ferric chloride. Igaku no Ayumi 33, 375 (1960).

YOUNGER, R. K., SCOTT, W. H., Jr., BUTTS, W. H., STEPHENSON, S. E., Jr.: Rapid production of experimental hypercholesterolemia and atherosclerosis in the rhesus monkey. Comparison of five dietary regimens. J. Surg. Res. 9, 263 - 271 (1969).

ZAHAVI, J., DREYFUSS, F., KALEF, M., SOFERMAN, N.: Adenosine diphosphate-induced platelet aggregation in healthy women with and without a combined and sequential contraceptive pill. Am. J. Obstet. Gynecol. 117, 107 - 113 (1973).

ZAK, B., DICKENMAN, R. C., WHITE, E. G., BUMETT, H., CHEMEY, P. J.: Rapid estimation of free and total cholesterol. Amer. J. Clin. Pathol. 24, 1307 (1954).

ZARET, B. L., STRAUSS, H. W., MARTIN, N. D., WELLS, H. P., Jr., FLAMM, M. D., Jr.: Noninvasive regional myocardial perfusion with radioactive potassium. New Engl. J. Med. 288, 809 - 812 (1973).

ZEBE, H., PFLEIDERER, TH.: Beeinflussung der Thrombozytenadhäsivität durch Aspirin während der akuten Phase eines Myocardinfarktes. Verh. Dtsch. Ges. inn. Med. 76, 649 (1970).

ZELIS, R., MASON, D. T., BRAUNWALD, E., LEVY, R. I.: Effects of hyperlipoproteinemias and their treatment on peripheral circulation. J. Clin. Invest. 49, 1007 - 1015 (1970).

ZEMPLENYI, T. Z.: Enzyme biochemistry of the arterial wall, p. 214 - 225. London: Lloyd-Duke Ltd. 1968.

ZEMPLENYI, T., GRAFNETTER, D.: The lipolytic activity of the aorta: its relation to aging and to atherosclerosis . Gerontologia 3, 55 (1959).

ZEMPLENYI, T., LOJDA, Z., MRHOVA, O.: Enzymes of the vascular wall in experimental atherosclerosis in the rabbit. In: Atherosclerosis and its origins, p. 459 (SANDLER, M., and BOURNE, G. H., Eds.). New York: Academic Press 1963.

ZIEVE, F. J., ZIEVE, L.: Post-heparin phospholipase and post-heparin lipase have different tissue origins. Biochem. Biophys. Res. Commun. 47, 1480 - 1485 (1972).

ZILVERSMIT, D. B., HUGHES, L. B.: Incorporation in vivo of labeled plasma cholesterol into aortas of young and old rabbits. Atherosclerosis 18, 141 - 152 (1973).

ZILVERSMIT, D. B., Mc CANDLESS, E. L.: Independence of arterial phospholipid synthesis from alterations in blood lipids. J. Lipid Res. 1, 118 (1959).

ZILVERSMIT, D. B., Mc CANDLESS, E. L., JORDAN, P. H., HENLY, W. S., ACKERMAN, R. F.: The synthesis of phospholipids in human atheromatous lesions. Circ. 23, 370 (1961).

ZILVERSMIT, D. B., NEWMAN, H. A. I.: Does a metabolic barrier to circulating cholesterol protect the arterial wall? Circ. 33, 7 (1966).

ZILVERSMIT, D. B., SHORE, M. L., ACKERMAN, R. F.: The origin of aortic phospholipid in rabbit atheromatosis. Circ. 9, 581 (1954).

ZINNER, S. H., LEVY, P. S., KASS, E. H.: Familial aggregation of blood pressure in childhood, New Engl. J. Med. 284, 401 (1971).

ZINSERLING, W. D.: Untersuchungen über Atherosklerose. I. Über die Aortaverfettung bei Kindern. Virchows Arch. Pathol. Anat. Physiol. Lin. Med. 255, 677-705 (1925).

ZLATKIS, A., ZAK, B., BOYLE, A. J.: A new method for the direct determination of serum cholesterol. J. Clin. Lab. Med. 41, 486 (1953).

ZÖLLNER, N., GUDENZI, M.: Behandlung der Hypercholesterinämie mit Beta-Pyridylcarbinol. Med. Klinik 61, 1996 (1966).
ZÖLLNER, N., SCHMIDT-GARVE, H. J., WOLFRAM, G.: Behandlung der Hypercholesterinämie mit Beta-Pyridylcarbinol III. Erfolge einer fünfjährigen Dauerbehand-
lung. Med. Klinik 66, 474 (1971).
ZORILLA, E., HULSE, M., HERNANDEZ, A., GERSHBERG, H.: Severe endogenous hyper-
triglyceridemia during treatment with estrogen and oral contraceptives.
J. Clin. Endocrin Metab. 28, 1793 (1968).
ZUCK, T. F., BERGIN, J. J.: Thrombotic predisposition associated with oral con-
traceptives. Obst. and Gyn. 41, 427 - 435 (1973).
ZUCKER, M. B., PETERSON, J.: Effect of acetylsalicylic acid, other nonsteroidal
anti-inflammatory agents, and dipyridamole on human blood platelets. J. Lab.
Clin. Med. 76, 66 - 75 (1970).
ZUKEL, W. J., COHEN, B. M., MATTINGLY, T. W., HRUBEC, Z.: Survival following
first diagnosis of coronary heart disease. Amer. Heart J. 78, 159 (1969).

Atherosclerosis

Proceedings of the Second International Symposium. Held in
Chicago, Illinois, November 2-5, 1969. Editor: R.J. Jones
150 figures. XXXII, 706 pages. 1970
ISBN 3-540-05049-3 Cloth DM 72,—
ISBN 0-387-05049-3 (North America) Cloth US $22.70
Necessary pathogenetic, prophylactic, and therapeutic considerations for the control of atherosclerosis, the major cause of
death in the advanced countries of the world, discussed by author-
ities of international reknown from sixteen countries.

Hypertension — 1972

Symposium organized by the Clinical Research Institute
of Montreal. Editors: J. Genest, E. Koiw
304 figures. XVI, 617 pages. 1972
ISBN 3-540-05755-2 DM 98,—
ISBN 0-387-05755-2 (North America) Cloth US $33.90
The essential features of this book are the important and new
contributions concerning the basic disturbances of aldosterone
regulation in benign essential hypertension, the discovery of isoenzymes of renin in brain and arterial tissue, independent of the
renal renin system, the discovery of a new ß-converting enzyme
in submaxillary glands, a discussion-in-depth of the mechanisms
controlling renin release and of the disturbances of mineralo-
corticoid hormones other than aldosterone in benign essential
hypertension.

Spontaneous Hypertension

Its Pathogenesis and Complications. Editor: K. Okamoto
128 figures. XIV, 266 pages. 1972
ISBN 3-540-05942-3 Cloth DM 78,—
ISBN 0-387-05942-3 (North America) Cloth US $27.20
Published by Igaku Shoin Ltd., Tokyo
Sole distribution rights for the USA, Canada, and Europe
(including the United Kingdom): Springer-Verlag

Contents: Development and Heredity. Catecholamine Metabolism.
Neural Factor and Behavior. Cardiovascular Dynamics. Cardiovascular Pathology. Endocrine Factors. Renal Factors and Electrolytes. Essential Hypertension and Spontaneous Hypertension.

Prices are subject to change without notice

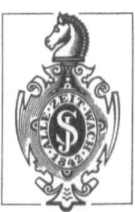

Springer-Verlag Berlin Heidelberg New York

München Johannesburg London Madrid New Delhi Paris
Rio de Janeiro Sydney Tokyo Utrecht Wien

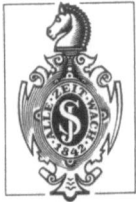